VOLUME
2

Pediatric Orthopedics

MIHRAN O. TACHDJIAN, M.S., M.D.

Head, Division of Orthopedics, Children's Memorial Hospital, Chicago, Illinois; Professor of Orthopedic Surgery, Northwestern University Medical School, Chicago, Illinois

W. B. SAUNDERS COMPANY
Philadelphia — London — Toronto

W. B. Saunders Company: West Washington Square
Philadelphia, Pa. 19105

12 Dyott Street
London, WC1A   1DB

833 Oxford Street
Toronto, Ontario M82 5T9, Canada

Pediatric Orthopedics Volume 2   ISBN-0-7216-8731-8

Print No.:   9   8   7   6   5   4

Contents

4

VOLUME 2

5

6

5. The Neuromuscular System

Levels of Affection

The neuromuscular system may be affected at various levels, each of which is characterized by changes in motor function peculiar to the site and extent of involvement.

At the *spinomuscular level* motor activity is simple; the impulses arising in the anterior horn cells of the spinal cord are transmitted through the peripheral nerves to the myoneural junctions and then to the individual muscles. In disorders at the spinomuscular level, the loss of motor power is focal and segmental, with complete paralysis of the muscles or muscle groups that are supplied by a peripheral nerve or by the anterior horn cells in the spinal cord. Muscular paralysis is flaccid or hypotonic, with reaction of degeneration, atrophy, fibrillations, and fasciculations. The deep tendon and superficial reflexes are diminished or absent. Pyramidal tract signs, abnormal involuntary movements, and ataxia are absent. There may be trophic changes in the skin, nails, and bone.

Pathologic processes at the spinomuscular level may be further classified into various sublevels. When the disease originates in the anterior horn cells, as in poliomyelitis, the *spinal level* of the motor system is affected. Other examples of diseases at the spinal level are: progressive spinal muscular atrophy of the Werdnig-Hoffmann type, progressive bulbar palsy, syringomyelia, and intramedullary neoplasm. The loss of function of the anterior horn cells and the motor nuclei of the brain stem results in clinical findings of flaccid paralysis, atrophy, areflexia, reaction of degeneration, and fasciculations.

At the *neural level* of the motor system, the peripheral nerves and nerve roots are affected, common examples of which are obstetrical brachial plexus palsy and progressive neural muscular atrophy (Charcot-Marie-Tooth disease). In affections of nerves sensory fibers are usually involved, with resultant sensory changes such as anesthesia or hyperesthesia. Otherwise, the clinical findings are similar to those of spinal level affections, i.e., there is flaccid paralysis, atrophy, reaction of degeneration, and areflexia as a result of loss of conduction of motor impulses. In the absence of sensory changes it is difficult to distinguish between diseases of the peripheral nerves, anterior roots and anterior horn cells.

When the pathologic process arises at the myoneural junction, as in myasthenia gravis and familial periodic paralysis, then it is a disease at the *myoneural level*. In diseases of primarily muscular origin, the motor system is involved at the *muscular level*. The muscular dystrophies are familiar examples of disturbance of the muscular level in disease at the spinomuscular level. Paralysis is flaccid, but reflexes persist until the late stages, when marked atrophy has occurred. There is loss of contractibility without loss of excitability, i.e., the muscle fibers have degenerated and have been replaced by fibroadipose tissue, but the peripheral nerves and anterior horn cells are normal.

In disorders of the motor system at the *extrapyramidal level* there is generalized involvement of the muscles of the limbs and trunk. The muscle tone is hypertonic. Atrophy, fasciculations, and reaction of degeneration are absent. Motion of the limbs is hyperkinetic, with loss of associated or automatic movements. The deep tendon and superficial reflexes are normal. There are no pyramidal tract responses and no sensory deficit. Athetoid cerebral palsy is a common example of a disease at the extrapyramidal level.

At the *pyramidal* or *corticospinal level* of involvement, motor deficit arises from affection of motor nuclei of the cerebral cortex. Paresis is usually generalized and associated with hypertonicity of spasticity of muscles. Pyramidal tract signs and pathologic reflexes are usually present. There is usually some atrophy that is not focal; it is caused by chronic paralysis and disuse. Fasciculations, trophic disturbances, reaction of degeneration, and abnormal movements are absent. The deep tendon reflexes are hyperactive and the superficial reflexes are diminished or absent. Spastic cerebral palsy illustrates the pyramidal level of motor involvement.

Cerebellar level lesions are characterized by loss of coordination and control, or ataxia. There is no real loss of motor power. Fasciculations, reaction of degeneration, atrophy, or trophic disturbances are absent. The deep tendon reflexes may be diminished or pendular, but the superficial reflexes are normal. Pyramidal tract responses cannot be elicited.

The *psychomotor level* of motor performance is the highest level of neuromuscular activity—at which volitional movements are initiated and affected by integration, memory, and symbolization. Paralysis caused by hysteria is an example of psychomotor disturbance. Loss of motor power is bizarre, with no actual paralysis. There is no real neurologic deficit. There are no fasciculations, no atrophy, and no true ataxia.

Differential features of various levels of motor function are illustrated in Table 5–1.

Neuromuscular System as a Functional Unit

Muscles are the expressive unit of the neuromuscular system and the moving force of the body. Muscles whose contraction directly produces a specific action are classified as *agonists* or *prime movers* (protagonists). An example is the biceps brachii in flexion of the elbow. Those muscles that oppose the agonists must be relaxed for contraction of the agonists (these are called *antagonists* or *moderators*) as, for example, the triceps brachii is in flexion of the elbow.

A motor action, even in an apparently simple motion, is quite complex. It involves the *muscles of fixation*, which stabilize the adjacent joints and afford a firm base for muscle action. The action of *synergists* is to assist the agonists and to reduce to a minimum all unnecessary motions. The execution of a motor movement requires the coordinated action of all four physiologic muscle groups—the contraction of agonists and the relaxation of antagonists as well as the associated function of the synergists and the muscles of fixation. Loss of function of any of these muscle groups will result in disturbance of motor performance.

Responses of Muscles

The responses of muscles to injury and disease are predictable. Muscles that are not used atrophy. The rapidity of development of such disuse atrophy is well illustrated by the atrophy of the quadriceps femoris that follows a painful lesion of the knee or immobilization of the knee in a long leg cast. With progressive resistive exercises, muscles hypertrophy. Painful stimuli will cause protective spasm of a muscle, which, when maintained in its shortened position for a period of time, will tend to develop myostatic contracture. The antagonist muscles to those in spasm are weakened by being maintained in their longer, stretched position and by inhibition of their function and recovery.

Muscular action affects bone growth. In the growing skeleton, muscle imbalance will cause deformity in the direction of action of the stronger muscle. Muscles are very sensitive to ischemia, as illustrated by Volkmann's ischemic contracture. Chronic systemic disease causes generalized muscle weakness and increased fatigability.

Affections of the Brain and Spinal Cord

CEREBRAL PALSY

Definition

Cerebral palsy is difficult to define, as it is not a single disease entity but, rather, a convenient category denoting conditions having certain common characteristics. The generally accepted criteria of the symptom complex of cerebral palsy are as follows:

1. It must be due to a fixed, nonprogressive brain lesion or lesions. There should not exist any active disease at the time of diagnosis. Thus, transient disorders or those that are the result of a progressive disease of the brain or spinal cord are excluded.

2. The original lesion must occur prenatally, at birth, or early in the postnatal period. The exact limits of this early period are not agreed upon, and it is best to avoid arbitrary age limits. The interference with the developing central nervous system by the early fixed lesion is the significant pathologic feature.

3. In certain children, the primary disorder involves the musculoskeletal system

Table 5–1. *Differentiation of Motor Disorders at Various Levels of Neuromuscular Function**

	Spinomuscular			Extrapyramidal	Pyramidal	Cerebellar	Psychomotor
	Muscular	*Neural*	*Spinal*				
Loss of motor power	Focal-segmental Usually proximal and axial muscle groups	Focal-segmental Usually distal limb musculature	Focal-segmental Usually distal limb musculature	Generalized Entire limb and movements	Generalized Entire limb and movements	None Ataxia may simulate loss of power	No true loss Bizarre, may simulate any type
	Complete	Complete	Complete	Incomplete	Incomplete		
Tone	Flaccid	Flaccid	Flaccid	Rigid	Spastic	Hypotonic (ataxia)	Normal or variable, may be increased
Atrophy	Present	Present	Present	Absent	Minimal (due to disuse and chronic paresis)	Absent	Absent
Fasciculations	May be present	Absent	May be present	Absent	Absent	Absent	Absent
Reaction of degeneration	Present	Present	Present	Absent	Absent	Absent	Absent
EMG							
Interference pattern	Normal until late in disease	Reduced	Reduced				
Fibrillation potential	Not usually present	Present	Usually present				
Action potential	Short duration	Prolonged with normal or polyphasic potentials	Prolonged with occasional giant potentials				
Evoked sensory and mixed nerve potentials	Normal	Absent, diminished amplitude, or prolonged conduction time	Normal				

Reflexes							
Deep	Normal or increased range	Diminished or pendular	Hyperactive	Normal or variable	Absent early	Absent early	Diminished and preserved until late
Superficial	Normal or increased	Normal	Diminished or absent	Normal or increased	Absent	Absent	Diminished
Pyramidal tract response	No	No	Yes	No	No	No	No
Sensory deficit	Absent	Absent	May be present (stereognosis or other cortical)	Absent	Absent	Usually present	Absent
Trophic disturbance	Absent	Absent	Usually absent	Absent	Present	Present	Present
Ataxia	Absent (may simulate ataxia)	Present	Absent	Absent	Absent	Absent	Absent
Abnormal movements	May be present	May be present (intention tremor and ataxia)	None	Present	Absent	Absent	Absent
Associated movements	Normal	Normal	Presence of pathologic associated movements	Absence of normal associated movements	Normal	Normal	Normal

*Adapted from DeJong, R. N.: The Neurological Examination. 3rd edition. New York, Hoeber Medical Division, Harper & Row, 1967, p. 382; and Farmer, T. W.: Pediatric Neurology. New York, Hoeber Medical Division, Harper & Row, 1964, p. 612.

and lack of motor control is the greater handicap, whereas in others mental retardation, convulsions, sensory disturbance, speech impediments, or defects of hearing, language, or eyesight may be the more important difficulty.

The term *cerebral palsy* has certain administrative usefulness. The foregoing criteria of this category of disease should, however, be carefully examined, as conditions such as Friedreich's ataxia, progressive hereditary paraplegia, or amaurotic familial idiocy should not be included under the heading of "cerebral palsy."

Classification

The differing approaches of clinicians and therapists concerned with the diagnosis and treatment of cerebral palsy are reflected in the various classifications they have used.[2, 5, 75, 83, 186] During the past 25 years, the ones must commonly employed are essentially modifications of Phelps's description of the clinical manifestations of cerebral palsy, which consists primarily of helpful suggestions to therapists and others concerned with the practical management of these patients.[142–144] Phelps based his classification primarily on the state of muscle tone, the presence or absence of involuntary movement, and the topographical distribution of motor deficits, taking into account etiologic factors, the presumed site of neuropathologic changes, and associated sensory defects (Table 5–2).

The defect of a classification that defines categories primarily in terms of changes in muscle tone is that the muscle tone of individual patients varies greatly with maturation and may alter considerably from day to day—and even from hour to hour—according to position, posture, state of alertness of fatigue, environmental temperature, and emotional state.

Perlstein and Minear have attempted to produce more comprehensive descriptive classifications by considering the site of pathologic change, clinical manifestations, topographical description, severity of motor involvement, muscle tone and etiology. (Tables 5–3 and 5–4).[127, 138, 139]

Crothers and Paine, stressing that the characteristic signs in cerebral palsy manifest themselves only gradually, have offered

Table 5–2. *Recent American Classification of Cases of Cerebral Palsy**

Spastic	
Aspastic	
Spastic	
Monoplegia	
Hemiplegia	
Paraplegia	
Triplegia	
Quadriplegia	
Basilar	
Athetosis	
Tension	Rotary
Nontension	Emotional release
Dystonic	Tremor
Flail	Unclassified
Arm neck	Paraplegia
Deaf	Quadriplegia
Shudder	Monoplegia
Hemiathetoid	Recovered
Cerebellar release	
Rigidity	
Intermittent	
Continuous	
Miscellaneous	
Hemiplegia	
Paraplegia	
Triplegia	
Quadriplegia	
Tremor	
Intention	
Constant	
Ataxia	
Cerebellar	
Eighth nerve	

*Based on that of Phelps by Hellebrandt, F. A.: Trends in the management of cerebral palsy. Lectures in Medical College of Virginia (unpublished manuscript). 1950–1951.

a more explicit neurologic classification (Table 5–5).[49]

Ingram and Balf and Ingram have suggested a classification by neurologic syndromes based on that of Freud, with modifications made necessary by advances in knowledge since his time (Table 5–6).[12, 89]

Classification of cerebral palsy is difficult but very important. There is no general agreement. In the care of the child with cerebral palsy, the orthopedist is part of a multidisciplinary team. The neurologist or pediatrician may be using any one of the foregoing classifications, and the orthopedic surgeon should be familiar with their vocabulary.

The distribution of paralysis is described as follows, according to the number of

Table 5–3.   *Classification of Perlstein, 1952**

By Clinical Symptoms	Topographical Involvement of Extremities	By Muscle Tone	Severity	Etiology
Spastic conditions	Paraplegia	Isotonic	Mild	Prenatal
				Hereditary
Dyskinesias	Diplegia	Hypertonic	Moderate	Static
Choreas	Quadriplegia or	Hypotonic	Severe	Progressive
	tetraplegia	–	–	Acquired in utero
Athetoids	Hemiplegia	–	–	Infection
Dystonia	Triplegia	–	–	Anoxia
Tremors	Monoplegia	–	–	Cerebral hemorrhage
Rigidity	Double hemiplegia	–	–	Rh factor
Ataxia	Limited to both	–	–	Metabolic disturbance
	upper extremities			Gonadal irradiation
				Natal factors
				Anoxia
				Cerebral hemorrhage
				Trauma
				Pressure change, etc.
				Postnatal factors
				Trauma
				Infections
				Toxic causes
				Vascular accident
				Anoxia
				Neoplasms and developmental
				defects

*From Perlstein, M. A., and Barnett, H. E.: Nature and recognition of cerebral palsy in infancy. J.A.M.A., *148*:1389, 1952.

limbs involved. If a patient has one limb involved, the condition is termed *monoplegia;* if two limbs on the same side are affected, *hemiplegia;* if two legs, *paraplegia;* if three limbs, *triplegia;* or four limbs, *quadriplegia* or *tetraplegia.* There is little agreement about the use of the words *diplegia* or *double hemiplegia.* The term "cerebral diplegia" or "diplegia" is employed by some authors to describe the condition of patients with more or less symmetrical paralysis, dating from birth or shortly afterward, which is more severe in the lower than in the upper limbs.[48, 64, 88] *Double* or *bilateral hemiplegia* is used when the arms are more severely affected than the legs or when there is asymmetry of involvement.

Etiology and Pathology

The nonprogressive brain lesion in cerebral palsy may be due to birth injury, developmental malformations, or damage acquired postnatally. Etiologic diagnosis is circumstantial in the majority of patients.

Pathologic findings are available in only a few patients, and even then, one has difficulty in determining the primary underlying cause. Ingram and Crothers and Paine have given a critical etiologic analysis of their own cases, as well as a comprehensive review of the literature.[49, 89]

BIRTH INJURY

Little first described three types of paralysis that could occur as a result of abnormal birth, denoting them as "hemiplegic rigidity," "paraplegia," or "generalized rigidity," as well as a condition characterized by "disordered movement."[115–117] These would now be considered forms of cerebral palsy.

Birth injury is direct or indirect damage of pregnancy or during labor and the process of delivery. It must be differentiated from abnormalities of the brain that are due to genetically determined developmental malformations dating from early pregnancy or others caused by a variety of teratogenic insults. Cerebral palsy due to birth injury should also be distinguished from postnatal

Table 5–4. *Classification of Cerebral Palsy (Minear, 1956)**

Physiologic (motor)
  Spastic
  Athetotic

Tension	Ataxic
Nontension	Tremor
Dystonic	Atonic (rare)
Tremor	Mixed
Rigidity	Unclassified

Topographical

Monoplegia	Quadriplegia
Paraplegia	Diplegia
Hemiplegia	Double hemiplegia
Triplegia	

Etiologic
  Prenatal
    Hereditary
    Acquired in utero
  Natal
    Anoxia
  Postnatal
    Trauma (subdural hematoma, skull fractures, wounds, contusions of the brain)
    Infections (meningitis, encephalitis, brain abscess)
    Toxic causes (lead, arsenic, coal tar derivatives, streptomycin, etc.)
    Vascular accidents
    Anoxia (carbon monoxide poisoning, strangulation, high altitudes, deep pressure anoxia, hypoglycemia)
    Neoplastic or late development defects (brain tumors, hydrocephalus, brain cysts, internal hydrocephalus)

Supplemental
  Psychological evaluation
    Degree of mental deficiency, if any

Physical status
  Physical growth evaluation (Wetzel Grid or other)
  Developmental level (Gesell)
  Bone age
  Contracture
Convulsive seizures
Posture and locomotive behavior patterns
Eye-hand behavior patterns
Visual status
  Sensory
    Amblyopia
    Field defects
  Motor
Auditory status
  Pitch range loss
  Decibel loss
Speech disturbances

Functional capacity (degree of severity)
  Class   I.   Patients with cerebral palsy with no practical limitation of activity
  Class II.   Patients with cerebral palsy with slight to moderate limitation of activity
  Class III.   Patients with cerebral palsy with moderate to great limitation of activity
  Class IV.   Patients with cerebral palsy unable to carry on any useful physical activity

Therapeutic
  Class A.   Patients with cerebral palsy not requiring treatment
  Class B.   Patients with cerebral palsy who need minimal bracing and minimal therapy
  Class C.   Patients with cerebral palsy who need bracing and apparatus, and the services of a cerebral palsy treatment team
  Class D.   Patients with cerebral palsy limited to such a degree that they require long-term institutionalization and treatment

*Adapted from Minear, W. L.: A classification of cerebral palsy. Pediatrics, *18*:841, 1956.

Table 5–5. *Classification of Cerebral Palsy Patients by Types (Crothers and Paine, 1959)**

Spastic monoplegia		
Spastic hemiplegia		
Prenatal or natal	right	left
Postnatal	right	left
Spastic tetraplegia		
Symmetric		
Asymmetric		
Spastic triplegia		
Spastic paraplegia		
Extrapyramidal cerebral palsies, not mixed		
Kernicterus		
Mixed types		
Cerebral palsy plus cord injury		

*Adapted from Crothers, B., and Paine, R. S. The Natural History of Cerebral Palsy. Cambridge, Mass., Harvard University Press, 1959.

or acquired cerebral palsy, the consequence of insults sustained by the infant following birth.

Abnormalities of pregnancy, labor, and delivery may cause "hypoxic," "traumatic," or "toxic" damage to the brain.

Hypoxia. In the last trimester of pregnancy, probable causes of fetal hypoxia are: (1) antepartum hemorrhage due to placenta previa or other causes, with the attendant disturbance in placental nutrition; (2) pre-eclamptic toxemia—infarction of placentae of toxemic mothers tends to be more extensive than in mothers without toxemia; and there is greater decline of the oxygen saturation of the umbilical vein in pregnancy complicated by pre-eclampsia,

Table 5–6. *Classification of Cerebral Palsy in Childhood (Ingram, 1955; Balf and Ingram, 1956)**

Neurological Diagnosis	Extent	Severity
Hemiplegia	Right Left	Mild Moderately severe Severe
Bilateral hemiplegia		Mild Moderately severe Severe

Diplegia
  Hypotonic
  Dystonic
  Rigid or spastic
	Paraplegic
	Triplegic
	Tetraplegic
		Mild
		Moderately severe
		Severe

Ataxia	Unilateral Bilateral	Mild Moderately severe Severe

Dyskinesia
  Dystonic
  Choreoid
  Athetoid
  Tension
  Tremor
Other
	Monoplegic
	Hemiplegic
	Triplegic
	Tetraplegic
		Mild
		Moderately severe
		Severe

*Adapted from Ingram, T. T. S.: A study of cerebral palsy in the childhood population of Edinburgh. Arch. Dis. Child., 30·87, 1955, and Balf, C. L., and Ingram, T. T. S.: Problems in the classification of cerebral palsy in childhood. Brit. Med. J., 2:163, 1955.

as compared with normal pregnancies;[182] (3) postmaturity; and (4) maternal causes of anoxemia such as cardiopulmonary disease.

Hypoxic damage to the fetus during labor and delivery may be caused by umbilical cord prolapse or torsion, or both, resulting in obstruction of circulation to the cord.

Neonatal apnea is not only the end result of many different forms of fetal injury, but is also a cause of further hypoxic damage in the newborn infant. The common causes of a failure to breathe after birth are prematurity and hypoxia during pregnancy or delivery. There may be poisoning or structural damage to the respiratory center, or the air passages may be obstructed as a result of the infant's premature efforts to breathe before delivery. Other neonatal complications that may cause hypoxia in the period immediately following birth are: persistent atelectasis due to immaturity, bronchial obstruction, or the baby's failure to expand the lungs; or hindrance of pulmonary respiratory exchange by hyaline membrane formation, pulmonary edema, intrauterine pneumonia, and aspiration of gastrointestinal contents.

Traumatic Birth. In recent years, the tendency has been to attribute less importance to trauma as an etiologic factor in birth injury and to emphasize the dangers of hypoxia. However, there is quite adequate evidence to suggest that subdural hemorrhage is predominantly the result of birth trauma. The forms of abnormal labor and delivery that are especially prone to cause subdural hemorrhage are: prolonged labor because of disproportion or malpresentation, precipitate delivery, forceps delivery, breech extraction, and version and extraction. Subdural hemorrhage most often results from tears of the dural ligaments that involve either the tributaries of the sagittal sinus or the great cerebral vein itself. Tears are especially liable to occur when undue or oblique stresses are placed on the tentorium cerebelli or the falx.[86]

Toxic Injury. Fetal damage may be caused by toxic agents that operate during late pregnancy, labor, and delivery. These include: (1) conditions that act by causing toxic accumulations of naturally occurring substances (e.g., rhesus incompatibility producing an excess of bilirubin and ammonia in the fetus; maternal uremia, causing an excess of nitrogenous waste products to accumulate; or diabetes, in which an excess of a variety of hormonal substances that are damaging to the fetus are produced) or (2) the presence of abnormal toxins that cause fetal injury (as in syphilis and toxoplasmosis, in which secondary infection of the fetus is relatively common; or in some other maternal infection, e.g., pyelitis, diphtheria, or meningococcemia, in which there is no invasion of the fetus by microorganisms).

DEVELOPMENTAL MALFORMATIONS

Findings that suggest developmental malformations as a possible cause of cerebral palsy are: (1) known family history of cerebral palsy, congenital malformations, or neurologic disease (excluding mental retardation) in siblings, parents, uncles, aunts, or cousins; (2) births of patients after apparently uncomplicated pregnancy, labor, and delivery that were not thought to have been likely to cause gross hypoxia or trauma; (2) associated congenital malformations of patients, excluding those possibly secondary to cerebral palsy; (4) patients' having extremely small heads with an occipitofrontal circumference of less than one percentile for age.

The problem of etiologic diagnosis of developmental malformations as a cause of cerebral palsy is complex, and positive diagnostic criteria are difficult to establish. Clinically, developmental malformations might be responsible, in a significant proportion of patients, for bilateral hemiplegia and ataxic diplegia.

Experimental work and clinical observations have shown that a number of agents are likely to provoke developmental abnormalities in the unborn child, usually in the first three months of pregnancy. The connection between roentgen irradiation and congenital fetal defects is well established.[4, 130, 188] The most frequent neurologic manifestations are diplegia and ataxia, often complicated by epilepsy.[63] Rubella in the early months of pregnancy tends to produce offspring with congenital cataracts and abnormalities of other systems, with the brain being affected in a significantly high proportion of cases. Spastic paraplegia and athetosis may be the presenting clinical picture.

CAUSES OF ACQUIRED CEREBRAL PALSY

Well-recognized causes occurring in postnatal life include intracranial trauma, cerebral embolism, arterial thrombosis, intracranial abscess, venous thrombosis of the lateral sinus, meningitis, and viral encephalitides.

Perlstein and Barnett state that there is a statistically significant correlation between certain etiologic causes and specific clinical syndromes. In general, brain damage caused by anoxia is usually followed by extrapyramidal syndromes, whereas that caused by primary trauma and hemorrhage results in pyramidal affections. The following list shows some of the more common neurologic sequelae of various etiologic factors:[139]

Prematurity	spastic paraplegia
Breech delivery	athetoid or spastic paraplegia
Toxemia of pregnancy	spastic hemiplegia or quadriplegia
Birth trauma	spastic hemiplegia or quadriplegia
Anoxia	athetosis
Rh factor and kernicterus	athetosis with deafness and paralysis of supravergence
Maternal rubella	spasticity, with deafness or auditory aphasia, cataract, and congenital heart disease
Precipitate or cesarean delivery	spastic quadriplegia, ataxia, or rigidity
Placenta previa and abruptio	athetosis

Blumel, Eggers, and Evans, in a study of 100 cerebral palsy patients, reported the chief causes to be trauma at birth (13 per cent), anoxia (24 per cent), prematurity (32 per cent), congenital defects (11 per cent), and postnatal causes (7 per cent).[24] More than one agent may be operative in producing cerebral palsy, and for the most part, the possible causes cannot be definitely identified.

In the past, the teaching has been dogmatic, it being said that spasticity is the result of damage to the motor cortex or pyramidal tracts, that athetosis is caused by lesions of the basal ganglia, that ataxia is due to damage or disease of the cerebellum or its connections, and that tremor and rigidity are the sequelae of more widespread lesions of the central nervous system. Recently, the gradual accumulation of more reliable and accurate information has failed to show a definite correlation between the pathologic findings and clinical features.[48] Generally, destructive, infectious, or vascular lesions will produce unilateral or asymmetrical paralysis, whereas developmental malformations will result in symmetrical involvement, although two or more destructive injuries could produce symmetrical paralysis.

Neurophysiologic Considerations

For a basic understanding of the musculoskeletal manifestations of brain damage in children, it is imperative to have a clear knowledge of the following fundamentals of the pathophysiology of the central nervous system.

SPASTICITY

Spasticity may be defined as a state of increase in tension of a muscle when it is passively lengthened, which is caused by an exaggeration of the muscle stretch reflex. It occurs in association with lesions of the cerebrum and descending pathways of the so-called pyramidal level of function. In the past, spasticity has been ascribed to the loss of, or release from the normal inhibiting action of, the pyramidal cortex on the anterior horn cells. Recent work indicates that spasticity results from an imbalance of the inhibitory and fasciculatory centers in the midbrain and brain stem reticular formations with consequent alteration of the alpha and gamma motor neuron balance.

Increased tension of a spastic muscle may be demonstrated on rapid or forceful passive movement; there is "blocking" and limitation of further movement. If passive movement of the limb is performed slowly, it is comparatively free. If the part is moved abruptly or suddenly, this "blocking" may be felt from the beginning of the passive movement, following which the muscle resists to a certain point and then relaxes. This "clasp knife" type of waxing and waning resistance of spasticity is distinguished from rigidity.

Objective means for accurate measurement of the degree of spasticity are not available. Thus far, clinical evaluation remains the most reliable method. The degree of hypertonicity and the range of motion of spastic limbs may vary between examinations and among different examiners. On palpation a spastic muscle may be hard, or it may be soft and flabby, depending not so much on the actual amount of spasticity as on the degree of contraction or relaxation at the time of palpation. The degree of electrical neuromuscular activity of a spastic muscle depends on whether the muscle is relaxed or stimulated.

In spasticity, the deep tendon reflexes are exaggerated and pathologic reflexes such as the Babinski and Hoffmann signs are present. On sudden dorsiflexion of the ankle or rapid distal movement of the patella, one may elicit *clonus*—alternate spasm and relaxation of the agonist and antagonist muscles.

Testing of motor power is difficult in spasticity, but it is important and an attempt should be made. In charting the muscle examination, both the motor power and the physiologic status should be designated. Motor power is graded by the standard accepted by the National Foundation for Infantile Paralysis, and the same abbreviations are used: zero, *0*; trace, *T*; poor, *P*; fair, *F*; good, *G*; and normal, *N*. For physiologic status, the author uses the following notations and abbreviations: *S* for spastic (stretch reflex); *H* for hypotonic; *0C* for cerebral zero (i.e., the patient has no voluntary control over the muscle); and *IN* for innervation normal. Table 5–7 shows various possible physiologic status and motor strength combinations of muscles in cerebral palsy patients.[174]

In the motor evaluation of a child with spasticity, the following pitfalls should be

Table 5–7. *Physiological Status Variations in Motor Strength of Muscles in Cerebral Palsy*

Physiological Status	Motor Strength
Innervation normal (*IN*)	P to N
Spastic (*S*)	P to N
Hypotonic (*H*)	O to G
Cerebral zero (*OC*)	O to G

borne in mind. Tension athetosis should be distinguished from spasticity. Tension athetosis is produced by the intentional effort of the athetoid patient to prevent any undesired motion of the athetoid limb. By shaking the limb, this voluntary tension can be released. The spastic extremity cannot be shaken loose because the exaggerated stretch reflex of a spastic muscle is involuntary and will occur whenever it is stretched by sudden passive elongation. It is also essential to differentiate between voluntary resistance of a normal muscle and exaggerated stretch reflex of a spastic muscle.

Spastic paralysis has a certain predilection for specific groups of muscles, with any variations depending upon the disease syndrome. In congenital spastic paralysis, for example, the spasticity is more marked in the flexor muscles of the upper limb. The shoulder is adducted, flexed, and internally rotated; the elbow is flexed; the wrist and fingers are flexed; and the thumb is adducted in the palm. In the lower limb, the hip is adducted, flexed, and internally rotated; the knee is flexed; and the ankle is held in plantar flexion. In acquired spastic cerebral palsy, the deltoid muscle may be spastic and hold the shoulder in abduction; and in the foot and ankle, the anterior tibial muscle may be spastic.

ABNORMAL MOVEMENTS OR HYPERKINESIA

These may be defined as involuntary contractions of the voluntary muscle caused by lesions in various parts of the motor system—the motor cortex and its descending pathways, basal ganglia, midbrain and brain stem centers, cerebellum and its connections, spinal cord, peripheral nerves, or the muscles themselves. Hyperkinesia is frequently present in the extrapyramidal type of cerebral palsy and must be regarded as a sign of disease and not as a disease entity. The character of the disordered movement depends both on the site of the lesion and on the type of pathologic change.

In the clinical study of hyperkinesia, one should observe the part and extent of the body involved, analyze the pattern and rhythmicity of the movement, and describe its various components.

Motion picture picture records are of great help in evaluating effects of treatment. Other devices used to record the frequency, rhythmicity, and amplitude of the various hyperkinesias are electromyography and myography (in which the oscillations are transmitted directly to a moving drum or kymograph).

The more common forms of hyperkinesia seen in cerebral palsy are described next.

ATHETOSIS

Athetosis may be defined as a fluctuation of posture superimposed upon a persistent attitude; there are "swings" of movement from one posture to another, such as from hyperextension of the fingers and wrist and pronation of the forearm to full flexion of the fingers and wrist and supination of the forearm, caused by release of two opposing actions.[51]

Clinically, athetosis is characterized by involuntary writhing or squirming movements that are irregular, coarse, relatively continuous, and somewhat rhythmic. They are intensified by voluntary motion or tension and disappear during sleep. Coordination is very poor. There is marked impairment of voluntary movements. In the limbs, the distal portions (i.e., the hands, fingers, and toes) are more markedly affected. The face, neck, and trunk may be involved. Facial grimacing is slower and more sustained than in chorea. There may be associated hypertonicity of the musculature or some muscle weakness.

Tension may develop to control involuntary motions. The state of tension is not constant, and can be released by repeated rapid passive flexion and extension of the joints of the involved extremity. As was emphasized earlier, tension in athetosis must be distinguished from spasticity, in which the exaggerated stretch reflex is constantly present, and also from rigidity, in which a lead-pipe-like resistance of the muscle is found.

Undulating and writhing movements of the limbs may also be present when there is loss of position sense in conditions such as peripheral nerve disease or posterolateral sclerosis. These become more marked when the eyes are closed. Muscle tone is usually not increased. This is called *pseudoathetosis* and is not a true hyperkinesia.

In athetosis, the predominant pathologic changes are in the basal ganglia, especially the caudate nucleus and putamen, although there may also be cortical involvement. It may be associated with status marmoratus or with brain changes resulting from erythroblastosis fetalis, kernicterus, or infantile encephalitis. Acquired athetosis may occur later in life as a result of disease or trauma.

Various clinical types of athetosis have been described by Phelps, such as rotatory, shudder, flair, tension, nontension, hemiathetosis, neck and arm, deaf athetosis, balance release, and emotional release.[144]

In dystonic movements usually seen in dystonia musculorum deformans, there is excessive muscular tone in certain muscle groups. It involves larger portions of the body with distorted postures of the limbs and trunk. There may be dysarthria, facial grimacing, and torticollis.

Tremor may be defined as a series of involuntary, rhythmic, purposeless, oscillatory movements that result from alternate contraction of agonist and antagonist groups of muscles that have reciprocal innervation. Muscles of fixation and synergists also play a part in the movement of tremor. One may distinguish tremors according to their rate, amplitude, rhythmicity, relationship to rest and movement, etiology, and underlying pathologic change.

Tremors may be elicited by asking the patient to hold his fingers extended and separated with his arms outstretched, to draw circles, or to make up slow movements. Tremors should be observed at rest and on activity.

The type of tremor seen frequently with lesions of the basal ganglia and extrapyramidal structures is *resting, static,* or *nonintention tremor,* which is slow, coarse, and compound in type. It is present with inactivity when the limb is in an attitude of repose or static posture and becomes less marked with activity. It is independent of voluntary movement and may disappear temporarily while the part is engaged in some voluntary effort. The tremor may involve the hands, feet, lip, mandible, or head.

If there is involvement of the cerebellar efferent pathways and their connections with the thalamus, the tremor encountered may be of the *intention, motor,* or *kinetic type.* It is absent while the patient is resting, but reappears with activity.

Toxic tremors such as those seen in hyperthyroidism are fine and are usually rapid. *Psychogenic tremors* are of medium amplitude and rate. There is also a *physiologic normal tremor,* which may be brought out by placing the limb in a position of tension or by performing voluntary movements at the slowest possible rate.

ATAXIA

Lesions of the cerebellum produce loss of coordination and control, or ataxia, in which all kinesthetic sense is destroyed. The various disturbances of equilibrium, muscle function, and movement seen in cerebellar disease are as follows:

1. There is loss of posture and balance both with the eyes open and with the eyes closed. With midline lesions, there is a wide-based, staggering, and unsteady gait that resembles that seen in alcoholic intoxication. The patient is unable to walk tandem or follow a straight line on the floor. He may sway backward, forward, or to either side. In unilateral cerebellar disease, there is persistent swaying or deviation toward the affected side. In standing the patient tends to fall toward the side of the lesion. On attempting to walk a straight line, he turns toward the involved side.

The cerebellar ataxic gait should be distinguished from the gait of sensory ataxia. The latter is also referred to as the gait of spinal ataxia, as it results most frequently from interruption of the proprioceptive pathways in the spinal cord. It is seen in conditions such as peripheral neuritis, brain stem lesions, tabes dorsalis, and posterolateral and multiple sclerosis. There is loss of position sense. The patient does not appreciate motion of the parts of the body, particularly of the joints and muscles of the lower limbs. Spatial orientation is disturbed, with loss of awareness of position of his feet and legs in space. If the patient walks with his eyes open, keeps his eyes on the floor watching his feet, and thus correlates visual impulses with proprioceptive ones, the gait may not be too abnormal. When the eyes are closed, the patient staggers, is unsteady, his feet seem to shoot out, and he may be unable to walk. With severe involvement, the patient walks with a broad base and the gait is irregular and jerky, even when his eyes are open. He stamps his feet in two phases, first on the heel and then on the toes, with a slapping sound or "double tap." An experienced person may diagnose the condition by hearing the patient walk.

2. *Asynergy* and *dysynergy*—in which there is loss or disturbance of coordinated action between various groups of muscles or several movements that normally act synchronously—are present. There may be decomposition of movement.

3. There is *dysdiadochokinesia* or *adiadochokinesia*—in which alternate movements, such as successive pronation and supination of the forearms or opening and closing of the hands are carried out slowly, irregularly, and clumsily. The patient is unable to terminate one movement and follow it immediately by its diagrammatic opposite because of a disturbance of reciprocal innervation of agonists and antagonists.

4. There is *dysmetria*—loss of ability to gauge the distance, speed, or power of movement. The patient may overshoot the desired point or stop before it is reached.

5. The muscles are *hypotonic* and tire easily.

6. *Intention type tremor* is commonly seen.

7. The muscles of phonation are synergic, with the result that speech is slurred, jerky, or explosive in type.

8. *Nystagmus* is usually present.

9. *Hyporeflexia* is common, probably caused by hypotonicity of the flexor and extensor muscles and loss of the restraining effect that they normally exert upon each other.

Rigidity is caused by diffuse damage to the brain. It is a state of fairly steady increased muscular tension equal in degree in agonist-antagonist groups such as flexor and extensor muscles in a limb, with resis-tance to passive movement in all directions and present throughout the entire range of motion. Resistance to passive motion is present on either slow or rapid movement of the limb. The muscles are firm, prominent, and tense. If the resistance to passive movement is continuous, it is referred to as waxy resistance, lead-pipe resistance, or flexibilitas cerea; whereas, if the resistance to passive motion is discontinuous, interrupted at regular intervals in a jerky fashion, the muscles giving way in a series of steps as if the manipulator were moving a limb attached to a heavy cogwheel or pulling it over a ratchet, the rigidity is referred to as *cogwheel rigidity*.

Incidence

There are seven children with cerebral palsy born in every 100,000 of the population. Out of seven, one is likely to die in the first year of life. There are currently about 25,000 new cases in the United States each year, a population of 180,000,000. In Britain, Ingram reports 2.5 per 1,000.[88]

In a cerebral palsy clinic, there is some variation of the incidence of each type. One may expect 50 to 60 per cent to be spastic; 20 to 25 per cent, athetoid; 1 to 5 per cent, ataxic; 5 to 7 per cent, rigid; the remainder will be of mixed type. With maturation of the child, changes in diagnosis of the type of cerebral palsy will be made.

Clinical Features

There are certain differences in the clinical findings between congenital and acquired cerebral palsy, but they are not so important that they should be considered separately. The common types of cerebral palsy are here described briefly to facilitate understanding of the total problem involved in the management of the child with cerebral palsy. The reader is referred to the works of Crothers and Paine, Ingram, Illingworth, Denhoff and Robinault, and Woods for a more detailed description.[49,50,83,89,185]

SPASTIC HEMIPLEGIA

Certain authors distinguish between "hemiplegia" and "hemiparesis" on the basis that hemiplegia is more severe than hemiparesis and is of sudden onset, whereas others use the two terms interchangeably, as the late picture of the two conditions is quite similar.

Side of Involvement. Hemiplegia is slightly more frequent on the right side (56 per cent, Hood and Perlstein, 1956; 59 per cent, Ingram, 1964).[82,89] The majority of people have a natural right-handed preference; thus right hemiplegia constitutes a great disadvantage. Clinically, when the dominant side is affected, reading and writing difficulties, aphasia, and behavioral disturbances occur more frequently.

Musculoskeletal Manifestations. The evolution of physical findings in hemiplegia has been studied experimentally in monkeys by studying the reorganization of motor functions in a cerebral cortex deprived of motor and premotor areas in infancy.[106,107,179] The sequence of events is as follows: The initial acute findings are flaccid paralysis and absence of movement of the affected side. Soon, within hours or days, automatic movements recover if they ever appear. (Those that monkeys normally

acquire relatively late in development are the last.) Spasticity will take weeks or even months to develop.

Byers and Tizard observed a similar sequence of clinical findings in human infants with hemiplegia.[36,177] Initially, the affected limb is relatively flaccid, motionless, and hyporeflexic (often a diagnosis of a lesion of the brachial plexus is made). Soon it passes through a period of reflex activity, but this stage is seldom observed clinically. Then it progresses to the period of hypertonus and hyperreflexia with the typical spastic hemiplegia posture and the tendency to contractural deformities in that position.

In congenital hemiplegia, the arm is adducted and internally rotated at the shoulder, the elbow is flexed, the forearm pronated, the wrist and fingers flexed, and the thumb adducted in the palm. In the lower limb the hip is adducted, slightly flexed, and internally rotated. The knee is flexed because of spasticity of the hamstrings. The spastic child tends to stand on his toes (Fig. 5–1). When he touches the heel on the floor, the heel is everted and the knee may be hyperextended because of

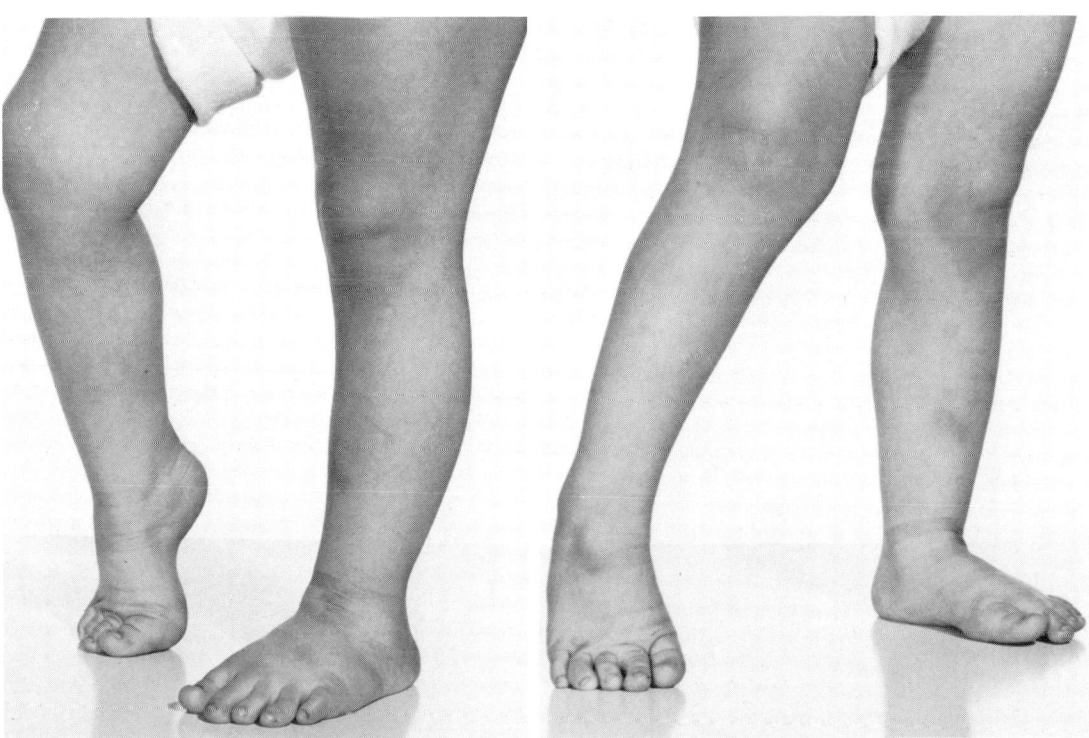

FIGURE 5–1. Right spastic hemiplegia showing equinus deformity.

the spasticity of the gastrocnemius muscle. The gait may be toe-toe, toe-heel, or plantigrade on the affected side, depending on the severity of involvement. On weight-bearing on the hemiplegic leg, there is an abductor lurch with a contralateral drop of the pelvis. The Trendelenburg test is positive.

Congenital hemiplegia is seldom diagnosed at birth. The usual history obtained is that the mother observed the baby to be dominantly right- or left-handed. In fact, a strong hand dominance under 12 months of age should make one very suspicious of contralateral hemiplegia or some other abnormality. In other patients the clenched fist or lack of use of the hemiplegic arm, or the equinus posture of the foot and ankle may be the first abnormal finding noted by the parents. Occasionally, these abnormalities may escape attention and hemiplegia is diagnosed when the child begins to walk and is seen to have a toe-toe or toe-heel gait on the affected side.

Motor development, in general, is slightly delayed. About one third of hemiplegics are walking by 18 months of age, two thirds by two years, and 90 per cent by three years.

All children with spastic hemiplegia show a varying degree of underdevelopment and atrophy of the involved upper and lower limbs. The severely involved and functionally poor limbs have the greatest amount of shortening and atrophy.

Reflex Examination. In congenital hemiplegic children, the asymmetrical tonic neck reflex, the grasp reflex, and the sucking reflex tend to persist on the affected side after they have already disappeared on the contralateral normal side. The plantar response tends to remain extensor in the hemiplegic foot as it becomes flexor in the opposite normal foot.

Sensory Disturbances. Sensory defects are quite common in cerebral palsy. Tizard, Paine, and Crothers, in a detailed study of the sensory function of 106 cerebral palsied children with congenital or postnatally acquired hemiplegia, found 57 patients (53.8 per cent) with sensory disorders.[178] Tachdjian and Minear reported an incidence of 41.7 per cent in 96 children with different types of cerebral palsy.[175] The most common sensory defects are astereognosis, impaired two-point discrimination,

and impaired position sense. These are perceptual functions that are affected by lesions of the somatosensory cortices. Hemianopsia, usually homonymous on the hemiplegic side, is present in about 25 per cent of the cases.

A *modality* is a distinct subjective response to stimulation. *Perception* is an elaboration of sensation involving the synthesis of information of several modalities or a temporal pattern of single modality. Stereognosis, for example, is a perception based mainly upon the fusion of the modalities of touch and proprioception. The parietal lobes are the primary somatosensory cortices, with the thalamus being their sensory gateway. The postcentral gyrus area is primarily a sensory center, whereas the precentral gyrus is primarily motor. Both are closely united by connecting neurons to form a *sensorimotor functional unit*. Stimulation of the postcentral gyrus produces most sensory responses, but stimulation of the precentral gyrus will also produce some sensory responses. The reverse is true for motor responses.

Permanent sensory defects produced by cortical lesions are only discriminative and have a strong spatial element—for example, defects in stereognosis, two-point discrimination, topognosis, and identification of numbers traced lightly on the skin. Perceptions of temporal pattern (vibratory sensibility) are affected less frequently by cortical lesions unless they extend into the white matter. Any permanent damage of crude or simple sensations such as touch, pain, and temperature implies subcortical damage.

In the pathogenesis of sensory defects in the hands of children with cerebral palsy, there are two factors to consider: (1) organic brain lesions in the parietal cortices, the thalamus, or both, and (2) inexperience in using the hand. It is hard to determine which of these two plays the greater role in a specific case.

Epilepsy. Seizures are frequent in spastic hemiplegia (Perlstein and Hood, 43 per cent; Illingworth, 35 per cent).[83,140] They are more frequent in children with acquired hemiplegia than with congenital hemiplegia. In the series of Crothers and Paine, 29 per cent of the patients with congenital hemiplegia and 55 per cent of those with postnatally acquired hemiplegia were epileptic at the time of examination. The types of seizure seen are the generalized grand mal, the focal or jacksonian, and less commonly, myoclonic jerks and petit mal. The presence of seizures seems to correlate unfavorably with the intellectual status and general prognosis.

Intelligence and Speech Development. The degree of intellectual impairment varies greatly in spastic hemiplegia from the apparently normal to the grossly subnormal and untestable. In general, the greater the severity of hemiplegia, the greater is the degree of mental impairment, but this is by no means constant. Ingram reports 41 per cent (28 of the 68 tested patients) had I.Q.'s below 70 and only 23 (33 per cent) above 85. Specific impairments found in hemiplegic patients are the inability to deal with written symbols, difficulty of organization and retention of memory, and perceptual problems, such as the failure to correctly visualize masses in space and to delineate horizontal and vertical directions and the third dimension.

Severe dysarthria is rare in spastic hemiplegia, but minor articulatory abnormalities are common. Hood and Perlstein found the mean age of verbalizing single words to be 22.4 months in patients with hemiplegia on the right side as compared with 20.5 in those with hemiplegia on the left, and the mean age of saying sentences to be 32.8 and 28.8 months respectively.[82]

Prognosis. All hemiplegics are able to walk independently in time. All of them have one normal hand, and they are able to participate in some type of occupation, although they cannot perform work requiring skilled use of both upper limbs. Abnormalities of behavior, mental retardation, and epilepsy are the principal obstacles to competitive performance in adult life.

SPASTIC QUADRIPLEGIA

In almost all the patients, spastic quadriplegia originates prenatally or at the time of birth, but there is usually a delay of some months before the classic picture is apparent. Ingram has proposed three stages in the evolution and gradual development of the final picture—the hypotonic stage, the dystonic stage, and a third stage in which rigidity and spasticity are present together in varying degrees in different patients.[88,89]

The Hypotonic Stage. Paucity of movement is the striking clinical feature. Unless seizures or other marked neurological findings are present, these children are thought to be normal and the condition is rarely diagnosed. The duration of the hypotonic stage usually varies between six weeks and six months, although it may be much longer. In general, the longer its duration, the greater the severity of involvement.

The Dystonic Stage. On examination, there is constant muscular rigidity that is more severe in the lower limbs. Sudden extension of the neck and head will produce a typical dystonic posture—the shoulders are adducted and internally rotated, the elbows extended, the forearms pronated, wrists and fingers flexed, and the thumbs adducted in the palm; in the lower limbs, the hips are extended, adducted, and internally rotated, the legs scissored, the knees extended, the ankles in equinus position, and the toes flexed. When the child is held in vertical position, rigidity is markedly increased in the limbs. The generalized dystonic attacks are present between 2 and 12 months.

The Rigid-Spastic Stage. The phase of predominant rigidity evolves gradually from the stage of dystonia.

Within a period of several weeks or months the spastic state insidiously appears. The posture and physical findings are similar to those in hemiplegia except that they are bilateral and usually the legs are more severely affected than the arms. The face is expressionless. There is a tendency to drool, and defects in speech are common. Visual disturbances and strabismus are present in some patients. Seizures are a frequent manifestation. Disturbance of hand sensation, so common in spastic hemiplegia, is relatively less so in spastic quadriplegia. Mental impairment is great in these children. It is rare that they have nearly normal intelligence.

About one third of patients with spastic quadriplegia fail to achieve standing balance for independent walking. Contractural deformities of the lower limbs provide a poor base upon which balance can be developed (Fig. 5–2). The musculoskeletal abnormalities are discussed later under

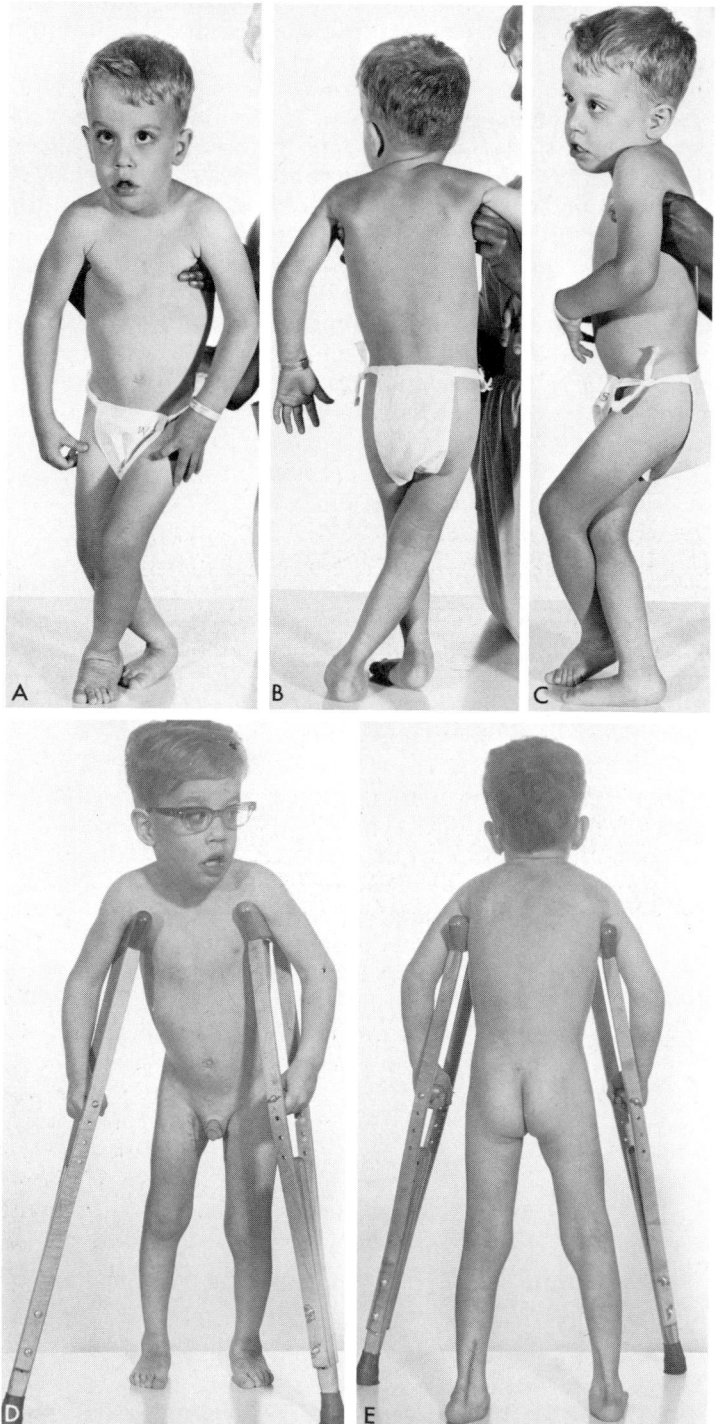

FIGURE 5–2.   Spastic quadriplegia.

A to **C**. At four years of age. The marked scissoring of the hips and equinus deformity of the ankles provide a poor base upon which balance can develop. Note the pes valgus.

D and **E**. Following correction of contractural deformities by adductor myotomy and heel cord lengthening the patient is able to stand and walk with the assistance of crutches.

treatment for the sake of convenience and brevity.

Pure spastic paraplegia without involvement of the upper extremities is rare. One should be cautious in entertaining such a diagnosis at a young age, for the majority of these patients have arm involvement at a later age.

Triplegia is almost always a variant of asymmetrical quadriplegia.

EXTRAPYRAMIDAL CEREBRAL PALSY

This disorder constitutes the second largest classification of cerebral palsy. The presenting clinical picture is one of marked retardation of motor development. Most of the children are seen between 6 and 12 months of age because of a delay in achieving head and neck balance or sitting balance.

At this stage of the disease, the infant will be found to be hypotonic, with an expressionless facies and an open, drooling mouth. The deep tendon reflexes are normal, but immature reflexes such as the asymmetrical tonic neck reflex persist. Between 12 and 18 months of age, the hypotonia is gradually replaced with varying degrees of tension. Soon involuntary movements develop. When the infant is placed prone in the mother's lap, an emotionally and posturally secure position, the tension and involuntary motions decrease or disappear, but when placed supine on the examination table, an insecure posture, tension athetosis becomes marked (Fig. 5-3). The reciprocal action of the agonist and antagonist muscles is lost in the slow, purposeless, involuntary movements, interfering with functional activities. In pure extrapyramidal cerebral palsy, there is no evidence of spasticity and contractural deformities do not usually develop.

The rate of development of balance and postural reflexes is very variable. Uncontrolled involuntary movements may hinder function to the extent that sitting, walking, or effective use of the hands may be impossible during their entire life. As handwriting is impossible, these patients are taught to use an electric typewriter. Substitution for hand function by the mouth may enable the child to perform such activities as turning the pages of a book or holding a pencil steady. Often these children ambulate by creeping, or pivoting on the abdomen or buttocks.

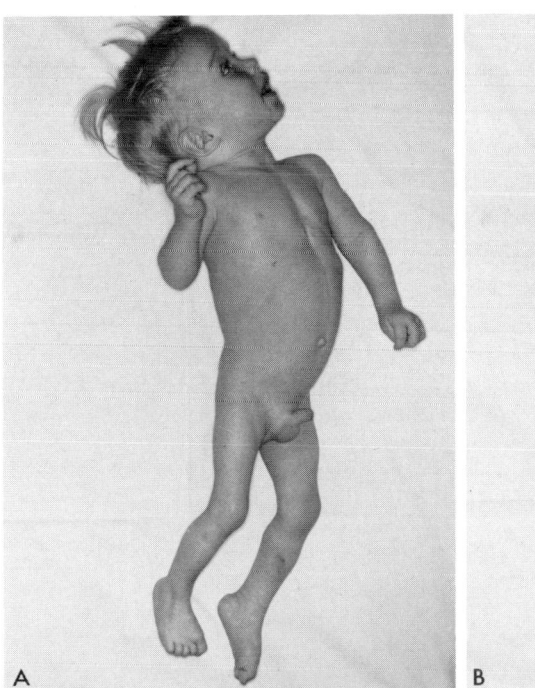 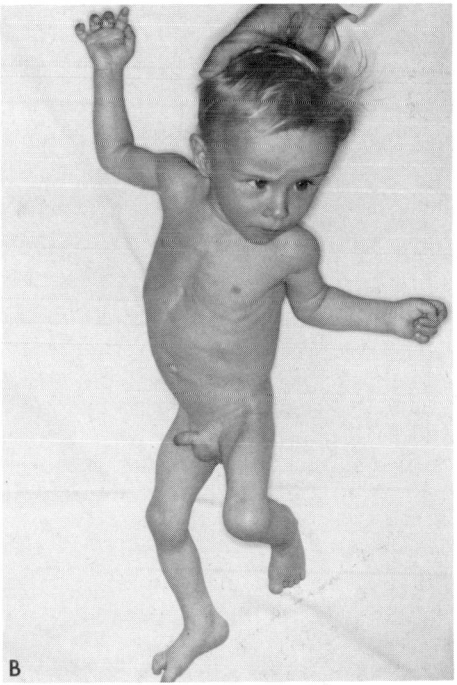

A   B

FIGURE 5-3. Extrapyramidal type of cerebral palsy.

A two-year-old infant with tension athetosis. Note the persistence of asymmetrical tonic neck reflex in **A**.

Patients with extrapyramidal involvement are the most intelligent group of those with cerebral palsy. Hearing loss is common in these children, though other sensory defects such as astereognosis are quite rare.

Kernicterus as a cause of extrapyramidal cerebral palsy is getting less and less frequent because of effective prophylaxis. In the Crothers and Paine series, it constituted 4.3 per cent of all cases of cerebral palsy and 19 per cent of those of the extrapyramidal type.

In the differential diagnosis one should consider Werdnig-Hoffmann disease, amyotonia congenita, and birth injury to the spinal cord. The generalized flabbiness of the muscles, the labored abdominal respirations with intercostal retraction, and the absence of deep tendon reflexes may suggest amyotonia congenita. In neonatal spinal cord injury, there is a level of anesthesia distal to a certain segment, crossed extension reflex, and a respiratory pattern similar to that in amyotonia congenita.

Mixed cerebral palsy with involvement of both extrapyramidal and pyramidal systems is not uncommon. In some of these children, a diagnosis of spastic tetraplegia will be made in the first year of life, and then, later on, signs of extrapyramidal tract involvement will develop. Others will begin as pure athetoids and will develop spasticity later.

General Principles of Treatment

Generalizations concerning treatment of cerebral palsy that are applicable to all affected children cannot be made. Many disciplines are involved, including pediatrics, neurology, orthopedic surgery, physical therapy, psychology, speech therapy, audiology, sociology, and vocational counseling. The care of children with cerebral palsy extends over a period of many years. In the course of this multidisciplinary treatment, the patient must be evaluated as an individual, as a member of the family, and as a future member of the community.

The problem is a dynamic one, changing with the growth, development, and maturation of the central nervous system. As the child grows, he acquires higher levels of performance and greater skills.

As was stated before a great variety of conditions are included under the term "cerebral palsy." Each child should be carefully and thoroughly assessed to determine his individual difficulties. Vagaries must be avoided. An attempt should be made to find out why a child cannot do a certain task and what the implications of this failure are for his present disability and future performance. It is important to think in terms of doing something *for* the patient and not *to* the patient.

The orthopedic surgeon's primary concern is the care of the musculoskeletal system, helping to achieve the maximum potential of locomotion as well as functional use of the upper limbs, with the ultimate aim of normalizing performance of daily activities to the greatest possible degree. Frequently, because he sees the patient more often than others, the orthopedic surgeon may be undertaking most of the patient's care. It is important that he be aware of his limitations and seek the help of other disciplines, as other problems involving speech, sight, hearing, mentality, and the like most certainly affect orthopedic management. This concept of *total care* must constantly be borne in mind.

Surgery has a definite role in the management of cerebral palsy. It can prevent and correct deformity and improve function. In the past, conservative management of cerebral palsy has been overemphasized, and the role and value of operative treatment overlooked. In 1942, Green and McDermott evaluated their experience with surgical treatment of cerebral palsy and pointed out the principles to be followed.[70] The importance of the role of surgery has also been delineated by Baker, Banks and Green, Bost, Chandler, Eggers, Keats, McCarroll, Phelps, Silver, and others.*

The following factors determine the result of surgery and should be carefully assessed preoperatively:

TYPE OF CEREBRAL PALSY

It is in the spastic type of cerebral palsy that operative measures are most useful.

---

*See References 6–11, 41, 42, 56–59, 95–104, 118, 145–147, 161, 162.

In the other forms of cerebral palsy, such as athetoid, rigid, ataxic, or tremor, soft-tissue operations on the limbs are seldom indicated.

The active movements of athetoid children are distorted because of a lack of voluntary control of the involved muscle or muscle groups. If a deforming athetoid muscle is transferred or lengthened, the athetosis may shift to other muscles of similar function, resulting in the same deformity. For example, in a patient with flexor athetosis of the wrist flexors (but not of the finger flexors), the flexor carpi ulnaris muscle is transferred to the dorsum of the wrist; persistent flexor athetosis may then develop due to shifting of the athetosis to the flexor digitorum profundus and sublimis muscles. Less frequently, the athetosis may not be transferred, and severe extension deformity of the wrist may develop. Neurectomy and tendon lengthening or transfer operations are likely to be followed by a recurrence of the original deformity or, at times, the development of an opposite deformity. In pure athetosis there is no constant spasm of the muscles and myostatic contractures do not usually develop.

In the cerebral palsied child with extrapyramidal involvement, surgery is indicated mainly in certain fixed deformities, and the operation should be primarily limited to bony procedures such as fusion of joints. Surgery, however, should only be performed after carefully assessing its anticipated results by using plaster splints or orthoses over a period of time. Because plaster of Paris cast fixation is usually not tolerated by athetoid patients, it is wise to test preoperatively to determine whether such a problem exists and whether it can be overcome by using tranquilizing relaxant drugs such as diazepam (Valium) or chlordiazepoxide (Librium).

REFLEX MATURATION AND MOTOR LEVEL DEVELOPMENT

There is a great variation in severity, extent of involvement, and prognosis in cerebral palsy. The asymmetrical tonic neck reflex and the Moro and grasp reflexes normally disappear between four and six months of age. One should note if they are still present at the age of two years. Does the child have good sitting and standing balance? Does he crawl? Is there reciprocal motion between his upper and lower limbs? What degree of control and function does he have in his upper extremities? Will he be able to hold the rails of parallel bars or the handles of crutches for assisted gait training?

In retarded children, one should note the rate of maturation of his neurophysiologic and motor system. What is his potential for further improvement with growth and development? Are his deformities interfering with his already precarious balance and hindering his stance and locomotion? It must be remembered that the nursing and perineal care of a retarded child may be greatly simplified by a simple adductor myotomy of the hips. Surgical procedures are also performed prior to attainment of the desired level of motor and neurophysiologic maturation to prevent deformities, primarily that of hip dislocation; prevention of hip dislocation is, in fact, the principal indication for surgery before evidence of sitting balance has developed. Even though these children will never be able to walk, they will be much more comfortable and have much less difficulty with nursing care than if their hips were dislocated.

ADEQUACY OF POSTOPERATIVE CARE

The feasibility of *adequate* and *meticulous postoperative care* should be determined. Several factors influence this, namely:

Age of Patient. He should be old enough to cooperate in the postoperative period to obtain the maximum benefit from the surgery. Usually this age range is from four to six years.

Level of Intelligence. In order to be able to cooperate with his physical therapist during the postoperative training period, the child should possess a reasonable mentality. Will he be trainable after his operation? What is his span of attention? The motivational factor often determines the difference between success and failure.

Home and Family Situation. Is it adequate and conducive to good follow-up care? Are the parents sufficiently intelligent? How interested are they in the child? How faithfully have they kept their appointments? What has been their past performance with conservative management? In the preoperative period it is imperative to indoctrinate the patient and his family concerning exercises and night support. They should be well prepared for an aggressive postoperative training program.

TYPE AND TIMING OF SURGICAL PROCEDURES

In the past, it has been emphasized that soft-tissue procedures should not be performed during the growth period because the deformities will recur. The results of Green and Banks have shown, however, that if the patients receive adequate postoperative care with a well-supervised program of exercises and night supports, the recurrence of deformities can be prevented. Unless a surgeon is willing to supervise minute details of postoperative care, he should never operate on these children.

The parents should realize that the motor handicap of cerebral palsied children can be substantially improved by surgery, but that, unless their involvement is minimal, they will never be completely normal.

The specific deformities and their treatment are discussed next.

The Foot and Ankle

The triceps surae muscle comprises the gastrocnemius, a three-joint muscle (knee, ankle, and subtalar), and the soleus, a two-joint muscle (ankle and subtalar). The coordinated, harmonious action of the triceps surae with its principal antagonist, the anterior tibial, is necessary to have a normal heel-toe gait with adequate push-off. In the majority of children with spastic cerebral palsy, this normal gait pattern is lost because of equinus deformity of the ankle and foot, which may be *functional*— a result of spasticity and exaggerated stretch reflex of the triceps surae without myostatic shortening—or may be *fixed*— because of permanent shortening of the triceps surae muscle.

Equinus deformity may be caused by contractural involvement of both the soleus and gastrocnemius muscles or due to contracture of the gastrocnemius alone. These two types of involvement may be differentiated by passive dorsiflexion of the ankle joint, first with the knee flexed and then with it extended. The gastrocnemius portion of the triceps surae originates from the femoral condyles and is, therefore, relaxed when the knee is passively flexed. If the equinus deformity is chiefly due to contracture of the gastrocnemius, it disappears. With the knee extended, the part played by the gastrocnemius is tested (Fig. 5–4). Care should be taken to apply the dorsiflexion force to the hindfoot and not to the forefoot, as the latter brings the peroneal, tibialis posterior, and toe flexor muscles into play (Fig. 5–5). Contracture of the gastrocnemius is the primary cause of equinus deformity in spastic cerebral palsy.

The gait pattern may be *toe-toe* if the body weight of the child is unable to overcome the exaggerated stretch reflex of the calf muscles (Fig. 5–6); or, depending upon the degree of involvement, the gait may be *toe-heel* or *plantigrade* (planting the foot as a unit). A taut triceps surae muscle may prevent dorsiflexion of the ankle, and the tibia, acting as a lever, thrusts the knee into recurvatum when the heel touches the floor. More frequently, however, the knee is held in flexion by the spastic hamstrings and a stretched-out, poorly functioning quadriceps muscle. The spastic gastrocnemius muscle plays a lesser role in producing flexion deformity of the knee. On plantar flexion of the foot, the gastrocnemius is relaxed, any persistence of deformity most probably being caused by the hamstrings.

In equinus deformity, the hindfoot is often forced into valgus position when the heel touches the floor, resulting from the bowstring effect of the triceps surae on the ankle and subtalar joints. With rigid resistance to dorsiflexion of the foot, the calcaneus rotates underneath the talus and is displaced posterolaterally (see Fig. 5–2). With loss of support of the sustentaculum tali beneath the head of the talus, the talus drops into a vertical position. Dorsiflexion occurs in the midfoot, and a rocker-bottom deformity results; the calcaneus is still in equinovalgus position. The stress of weight-bearing is on the head of the talus (the midfoot) and not on the heel. This valgus deformity is increased when the peroneal muscles are spastic.

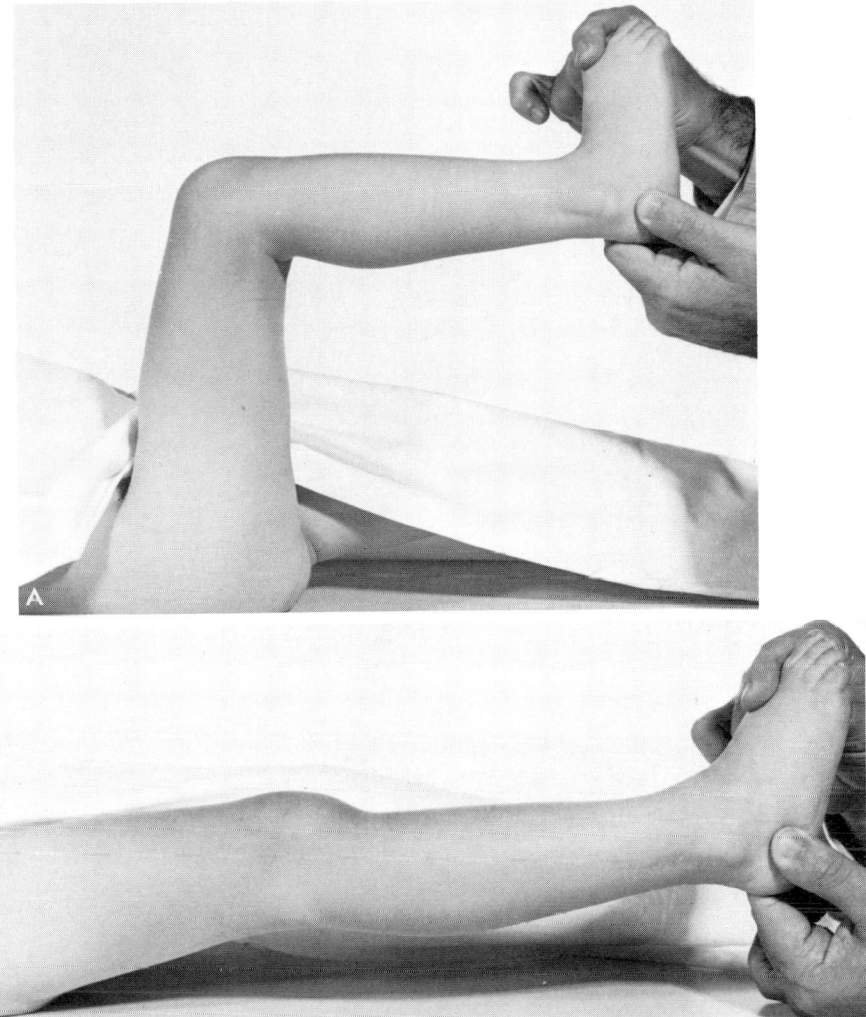

FIGURE 5–4. *Testing spasticity and contracture of triceps surae muscle by passive dorsiflexion of the ankle.*

A. With the knee in flexion, the gastrocnemius muscle is relaxed and equinus deformity is caused by contracture of the soleus muscle. **B**. With the knee in extension the part played by the gastrocnemius is tested.

Less often, the foot position is equino-varus, owing to spastic posterior tibial and toe flexor muscles (Fig. 5–7). On weight-bearing or passive dorsiflexion of the ankle, the posterior tibial stands out as a tight band in its groove behind the medial malleolus and the toes may be curled. In stance, the varus deformity is usually more marked in the forefoot, and on walking, these children toe in. Functional or fixed internal rotation deformity of the hip or tibia vara, or both, will aggravate the toeing-in.

In acquired cerebral palsy, the anterior tibial muscle may be spastic; these children usually have varying degrees of varus deformity of both the hindfoot and forefoot, and a plantigrade gait.

It is essential to perform a muscle test prior to determination of the type and extent of surgery in order to evaluate the motor strength of the overactive muscle and its antagonist. Often voluntary active con-traction of the anterior tibial muscle cannot be elicited with the knee in extension (Fig. 5–8). The child is asked to dorsiflex the ankle with the knee in extension and flexion. The gastrocnemius portion of the triceps surae is relaxed when the knee is flexed. If the anterior tibial does not contract with the knee flexed, the child is asked to flex the hip and knee against resistance. This maneuver (called synkinesia, "confu-sion" or automatic reflex, or Strümpell test) will cause the anterior tibial muscle to contract, bringing the ankle and foot into dorsiflexion. In order to prevent recurrence of equinus deformity, it is essential to de-velop active voluntary function of the anterior tibial in gait in the postoperative period.

The effect of hip and knee flexion con-tracture on equinus deformity of the foot should be assessed, for if they are not cor-rected, the equinus deformity is likely to recur (Fig. 5–9).

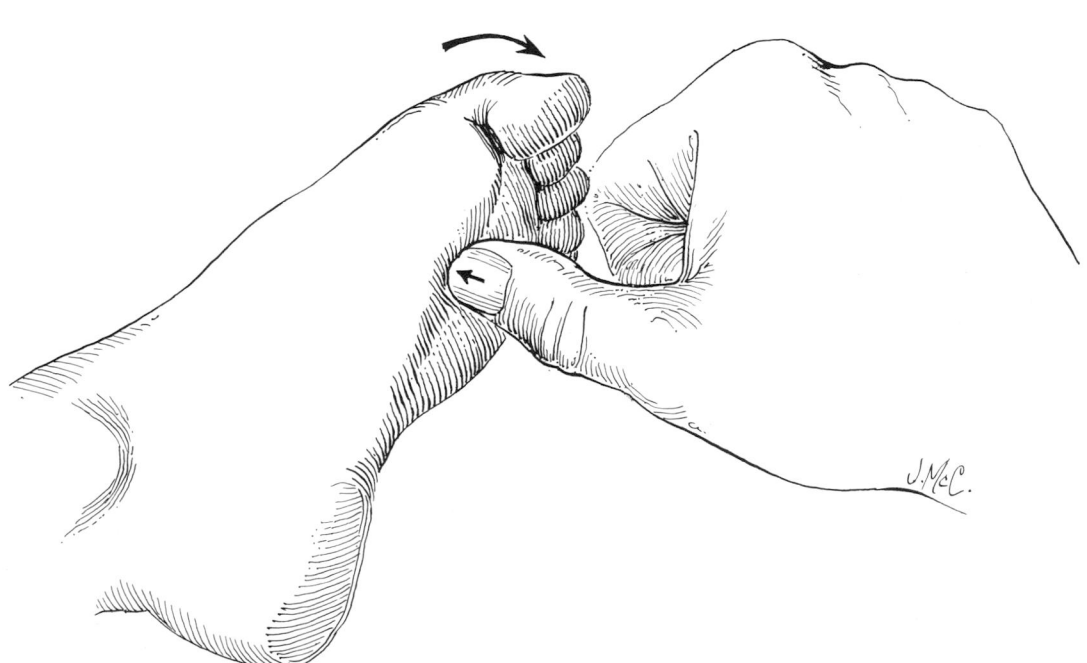

FIGURE 5–5. *Spasticity of toe flexors shown by dorsiflexion of the foot by pressure over the metatarsal head.*

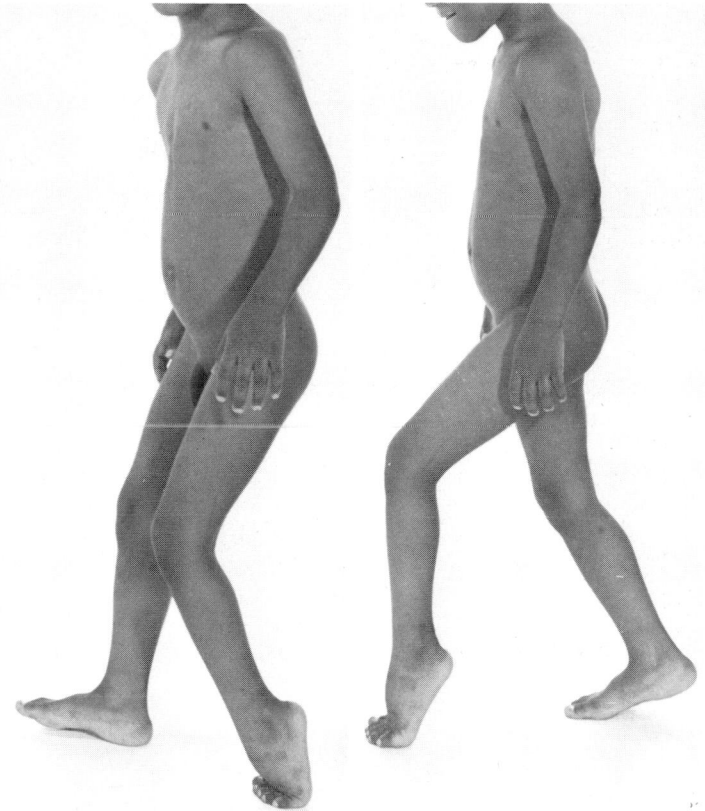

FIGURE 5-6. *Toe-toe gait in spastic hemiplegia.*

CONSERVATIVE MANAGEMENT

Initially, all children should have a trial period of nonoperative treatment. The surgeon should condition the patient and his family for future care and indoctrinate them concerning exercises and night support.

Conservative measures consist of passive manual stretching of the gastrocnemius-soleus muscles with the knee in extension, active exercises to develop function of the anterior tibial muscle, wearing of a bivalved cast at night to hold the foot and ankle in dorsiflexed neutral position, gait training, and use of dorsiflexion assist below-knee orthoses during the day.

A bivalved removable long leg cast is an effective means of night support that prevents the foot from resting in equinus and maintains it in neutral position. It is more comfortable than a night brace and should fit the limb snugly. Its purpose is support, not correction. A common pitfall is to make the cast in maximal dorsiflexion at the ankle; this will not be tolerated and will cause a pressure sore on the heel. Initially, it is advisable to place the knee in 5 to 15 degrees of flexion, the ankle being in neutral or 5 to 10 degrees of plantar flexion. As equinus deformity lessens, each subsequent bivalved cast is made with the ankle in more dorsiflexion, as tolerated.

Most surgeons use a short leg night orthosis with a single caliper (rod), a right-angled stop, and a T-strap; the rod is progressively bent into increasing dorsiflexion as the triceps surae stretches out. The toe portion of the shoe may be cut out, and a large woolen sock may be worn every night until growth of the tibia is completed.

To control the contracture of the gastrocnemius muscle, the night orthosis should be above-knee, holding the knee in extension. A below-knee orthosis does not control the commonly associated contracture of the hamstring muscles.

Dynamic day orthoses are the dorsiflexion

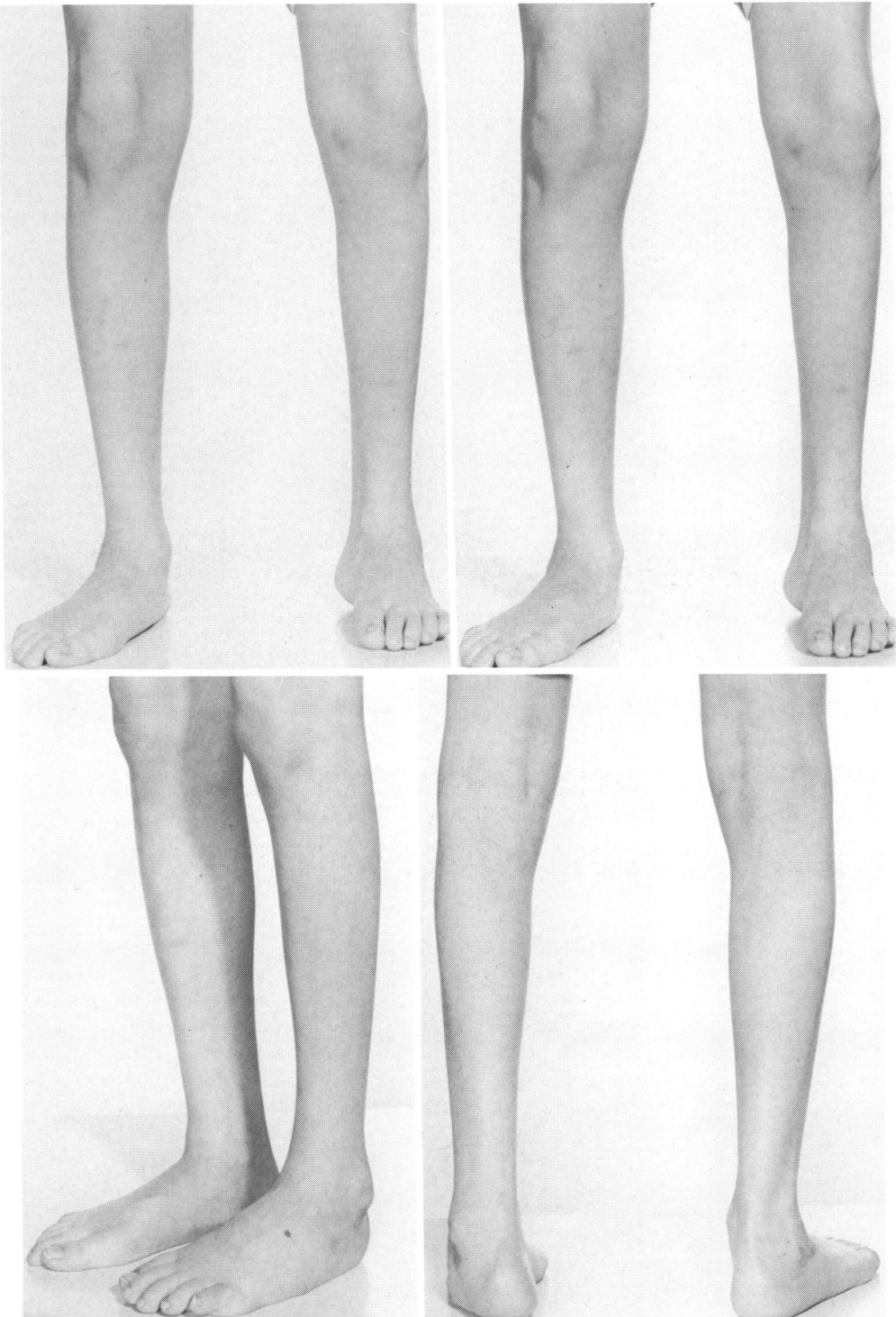

FIGURE 5-7. *Left spastic hemiplegia with equinovarus deformity of the foot.*

Note the taut posterior tibial tendon behind the medial malleolus.

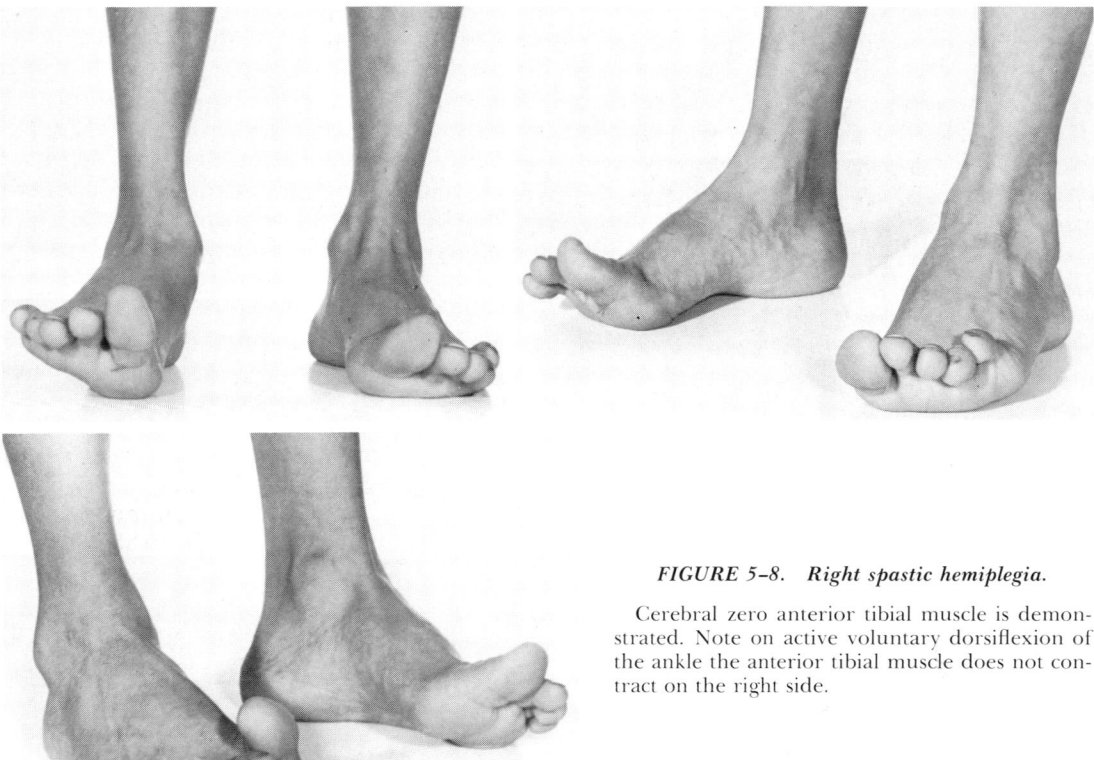

FIGURE 5–8.   *Right spastic hemiplegia.*

Cerebral zero anterior tibial muscle is demonstrated. Note on active voluntary dorsiflexion of the ankle the anterior tibial muscle does not contract on the right side.

spring type, used in the young child, and the dorsiflexion Klenzak orthosis, used in the older patient. The orthosis should be short to allow synergistic flexion of the knee, hip, and ankle, and to develop voluntary control and motor strength of the anterior tibial muscle. Spring dorsiflexion dynamic orthoses have not been used by some surgeons, as it is believed the spring action provides constant stimulation of the triceps surae muscle, thus aggravating the equinus deformity rather than correcting it. This has not been the experience of the author. The amount of tension found in the dorsiflexion spring orthosis or in the Klenzak ankle joint is not strong enough to cause constant stretch stimulation of the triceps surae muscle.

The dorsiflexion Klenzak ankle orthosis has also been criticized because the tension within the spring is not adequate to correct the myostatic contracture of the triceps surae. One should understand, however, that the primary purpose of the dorsiflex-

ion spring or Klenzak ankle joint brace is to develop dynamic action of the anterior tibial muscle in gait and to hold the part in corrected position; it is not designed to correct fixed equinus deformity.

In order to obtain effective use of day orthoses, the shoe should be high-topped and should fit snugly. Often, because of the smaller size of the foot, it may be necessary to obtain mismated shoes. To secure the forefoot in the shoe, an extra strap may be used over the dorsum of the foot or one may have to lace the shoes in the reverse direction with the bow at the base of the tongue. A sole plate is inserted between the inner and outer soles, extending to the end of the shoe and beyond the metatarsophalangeal joints in order to prevent breaking of the shank. A T strap may be used to hold the foot out of varus or valgus position.

Wedging plaster casts to correct fixed equinus deformity are not tolerated well by cerebral palsied children; they should only be used in selected cases, if at all.

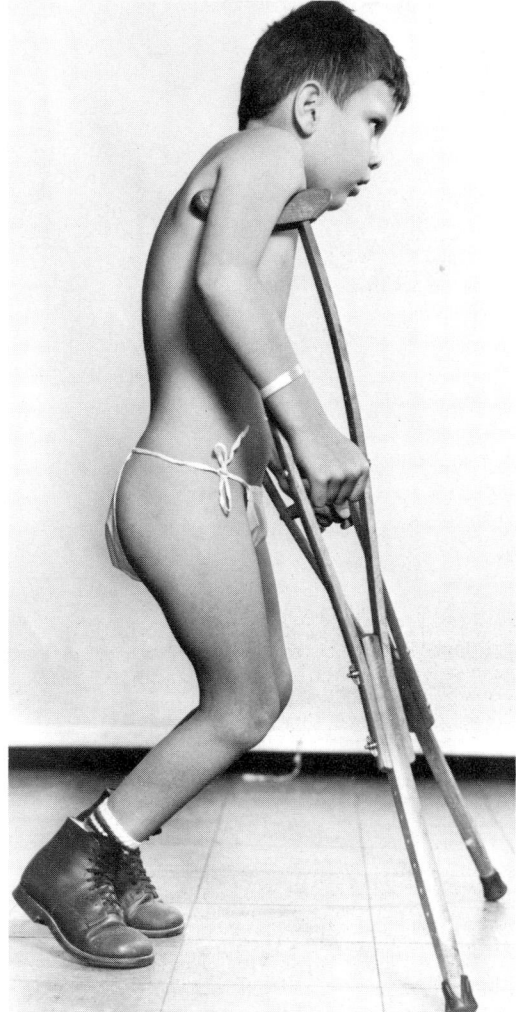

FIGURE 5–9. *Equinus posture of the ankles and feet secondary to flexion contracture of the knee and hip.*

SURGICAL TREATMENT

Equinus Deformity. Operative correction of equinus deformity is indicated if a toe-toe or toe-heel gait persists following an adequate period of conservative management. In stance, if the heel goes into marked valgus position and the talus into plantar flexion because of shortening of the spastic gastrocnemius muscle, heel cord lengthening should be considered to prevent development of fixed valgus deformity of the foot. Correction of functional equinus deformity may also be indicated. If overactivity and exaggerated stretch reflex of the gastrocnemius and soleus cause equinus

deformity of the foot when walking, heel cord lengthening is indicated, despite the fact that the foot can be passively dorsiflexed to neutral position. Before surgical procedures on the foot can be considered, the child must have good sitting and standing balance and potentiality of walking, as determined by a period of gait training on parallel bars and later with crutches.

The key to success in surgical treatment of equinus deformity is adequate postoperative care. It is imperative that the parents realize that surgery is only the initial stage of treatment. The type of technique used is not so important. The author prefers sliding lengthening of the heel cord — the White procedure, as advocated by Banks and Green.[13, 184] Because anatomic continuity of the heel cord is not disturbed, one can control the amount of lengthening, allowing relatively early mobilization. The operative procedure of sliding heel cord lengthening is described and illustrated in Plate 28.

Vulpius and Stöffel, in 1913, described an operation to correct spastic equinus deformity, in which the aponeurotic tendon of the gastrocnemius and soleus was divided transversely just below the middle of the leg, leaving the underlying muscle fibers intact. By forceful dorsiflexion of the ankle, the segments of the aponeurotic tendon were separated, but continuity of the soleus muscle fibers was not disturbed.[181] Later, one or two V-shaped incisions were made instead of transverse incisions (Fig. 5–10). Compere and Schnute popularized the Vulpius procedure in the United States, and Baker further modified this procedure by tongue-in-groove lengthening.[6] In both the Vulpius and Baker operations, aponeurotic lengthening of the soleus is often performed also.

In 1913, Stöffel described neurectomy of the motor branches of peripheral nerves for the correction of spastic contractures. Since then, division of motor nerves to one or both heads of the gastrocnemius to correct equinus deformity has been advocated by numerous authors. The author recommends it only when there is severe ankle clonus on weight-bearing, which hinders walking. It is imperative that one distinguish the clonus caused by the gastrocnemius from that caused by the soleus. When it diminishes or disappears on flexion of the knee, the clonus is primarily caused by the gastrocnemius; when the clonus is unaltered by changes in the position of the knee, the soleus is its chief cause. Motor branches of the tibial nerve to the spastic muscle causing the clonus are the ones to be resected. The tendo Achillis is usually not lengthened at the same time, although, on occasion, it may have to be done later. Operative technique of neurectomy of motor branches of the tibial nerve is described and illustrated in Plate 29.

When equinus deformity is primarily caused by contracture of the gastrocnemius muscle, Silfverskiöld recommends lowering or recession of the gastrocnemius muscle heads below the level of the knee joint and partial neurectomy of the tibial motor nerves to the gastrocnemius muscle to further decrease its motor power. This procedure does not disturb the soleus muscle, which retains its function for effective push-off in gait.[163]

In 1950, Strayer described recession of the gastrocnemius muscle in its distal portion. The gastrocnemius tendon is divided transversely at its junction with the conjoined gastrocnemius-soleus tendon. The foot is dorsiflexed to neutral portion, and the retracted proximal part of the gastrocnemius tendon resutured to the underlying soleus.[168] In 1958, Strayer reported on distal gastrocnemius recession in 23 patients, with good or excellent results in 16.[169]

Silver and Simon, in 1959, reported their experience with the proximal gastrocnemius recession of Silfverskiöld in 66 children on whom 110 operations were performed. In addition, they performed neurectomy of one head of the gastrocnemius. The equinus deformity recurred in five cases; on their evaluation, the failures were caused by muscle imbalance and weakness of the dorsiflexor muscles of the foot.[161]

The advantage of the Strayer and Silfverskiöld procedures is that they preserve soleus function for push-off in gait; however, there are definite disadvantages to each. The Silfverskiöld operation removes the posterior dynamic support to the knee provided by the gastrocnemius with the result that genu recurvatum is a potential complication. It should not be performed when the hamstrings need to be lengthened at a later date or when, in gait, the knee goes into hyperextension when the heel touches the floor. Following the Strayer procedure, in which the gastrocnemius is completely freed from the soleus, the gastrocnemius muscle may retract proximally as a small functionless knot in the upper calf. For these reasons, the Strayer procedure is not advocated. Percutaneous tenotomy and Z-plasty should not be performed to correct equinus deformity in cerebral palsy.

Varus Deformity. Associated valgus or varus deformity of the equinus foot is usually caused by an imbalance of the muscles of inversion and eversion—the tibialis posterior and the peroneal muscles. The toe flexors may contribute to varus deformity of the foot, particularly after tendo Achillis lengthening. Bleck has pointed out that spasticity of the abductor hallucis may cause varus deformity of the forefoot. This may well be a deforming force in an occasional case. Treatment of these deforming spastic muscles may be carried out at the same time as correction of equinus deformity.

When the spastic posterior tibial muscle is causing pes varus, it may be lengthened at the same time as the heel cord. It is not necessary to make a separate incision. Through the posteromedial incision for heel cord lengthening, the posterior tibial muscle and tendon can be exposed above the medial malleolus in the distal third of the leg immediately posterior to the tibia. At two levels, 5 cm. apart, and well above the site where muscle fibers terminate on the tendon, two incisions are made over the tendinous portion of the posterior tibial muscle but not into the muscle fibers themselves. The proximal incision is transverse, and the distal one long and oblique. The sliding lengthening of the tendon is obtained by forcing the foot into valgus position and by gentle stretching between two moist sponges (Fig. 5–11). Total section and release of the posterior tibial tendon should be avoided, as it will cause marked valgus deformity in the growing foot. Baker recommends freeing of the sheath of the posterior tibial tendon behind the medial malleolus and allowing it to be displaced anterior to it. The author does

(*Text continued on page 799.*)

Sliding Lengthening of the Heel Cord

A. With the patient preferably in prone position, a posteromedial incision about 7.5 cm. long is made just medial to the tendo Achillis. The subcutaneous tissue and tendon sheath are divided in one plane so that the latter remains attached to subcutaneous tissue and can be reconstructed effectively later on. It is not necessary to disturb the deep surface of the tendon or to dissect around the sheath.

B. The rotation of fibers of the tendo Achillis is studied next, as it varies greatly. The tendon usually rotates about 90 degrees on its longitudinal axis between its origin and insertion, so that the fibers that occupy a medial position proximally twist laterally as they approach their insertion on the calcaneus and are posterior to those fibers that proximally occupied a lateral position. Straight Keith needles may be used to mark rotation of fibers.

The Achilles tendon is then transversely sectioned at two levels. The site of division must be chosen according to the degree of rotation of fibers. Usually the anteromedial half to two thirds of the tendon is divided distally near its insertion and then the posteromedial half of its fibers is divided in the proximal end of the wound.

C. The foot is then passively dorsiflexed with the knee in extension. The medial portion of the tendon will slide on the lateral portion, lengthening the tendon in continuity. (A third incision, midway between the others, is indicated at times if stretching does not occur easily; its site can be readily determined by palpation.) There is no fraying of the tendon as in the Z-plasty type of tendon lengthening. The actual amount of lengthening depends upon the degree of equinus deformity. At the end of the procedure the foot should rest comfortably in neutral position or 5 degrees of dorsiflexion. Correction beyond this point should be avoided, as it may cause calcaneus deformity. The pneumatic tourniquet is released and all bleeding vessels are clamped and coagulated.

D. The sheath, including a small portion of the subcutaneous tissues, is meticulously closed over the lengthened Achilles tendon.

E. The lower extremity is immobilized in a well-padded long leg cast with the knee in full extension or 5 degrees' flexion (but no hyperextension) and the foot-ankle in neutral position or 5 to 10 degrees of dorsiflexion. It is essential to mold the plaster cast well, particularly at the ankle, heel and the knee.

Postoperative care is discussed in the text.

Plate 28.   Sliding Lengthening of the Heel Cord

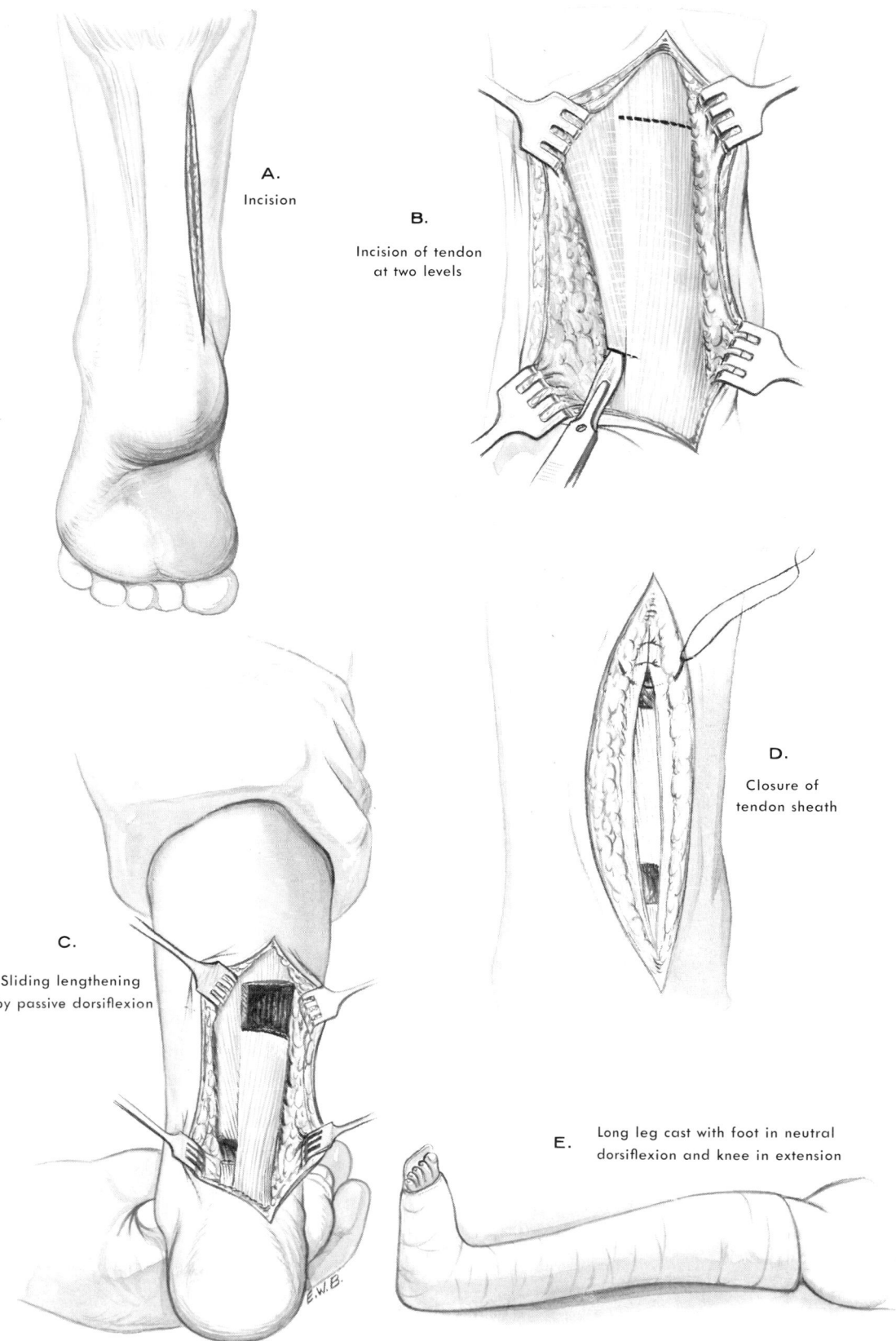

A.
Incision

B.
Incision of tendon
at two levels

D.
Closure of
tendon sheath

C.
Sliding lengthening
by passive dorsiflexion

E.   Long leg cast with foot in neutral
dorsiflexion and knee in extension

E.W.B.

797

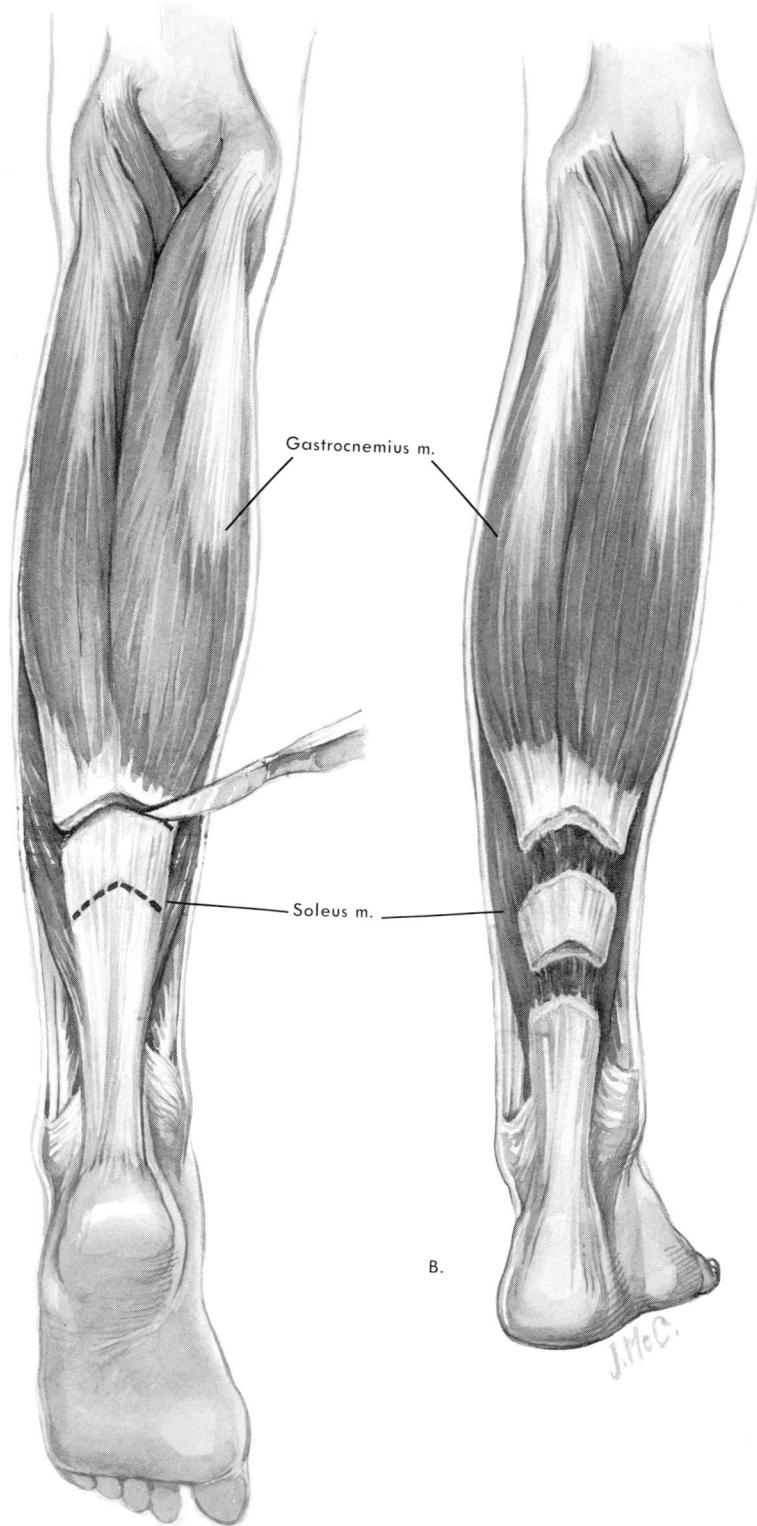

Gastrocnemius m.

Soleus m.

A.

B.

J.McC.

FIGURE 5–10.   *Lengthening of the gastrocnemius by the Vulpius technique.*

not advise this procedure because in its new transposed position, the posterior tibial muscle still acts as an invertor of the foot, causing varus deformity.

In spastic paralysis, tendon transfers in the lower extremity for the correction of varus or valgus deformities of the foot should not be performed. The results are unpredictable, and not infrequently, a reverse deformity may develop. In acquired spastic paralysis, when the anterior tibial muscle is spastic and the foot is in varus but not in equinus position, one may transfer the anterior tibial tendon laterally to the base of the second or third metatarsal — never more laterally.

On occasion, the patient is unable to develop cerebral control over the anterior tibial muscle, in which case, the author transfers the extensor hallucis longus to the base of the first metatarsal, rerouting it through the anterior tibial muscle. This procedure is a modification of that of Alfonso Tohen.[179] If any equinus deformity is present, it should be corrected by serial wedging casts. The ankle joint should passively dorsiflex to at least 20 degrees beyond neutral prior to surgery. The details of operative technique are as follows:

A longitudinal incision about 7 cm. long is made over the dorsum of the foot. It starts at the base of the proximal phalanx of the big toe and extends proximally to the first cuneiform bone. The extensor hallucis longus tendon is detached from its insertion as far distally as possible. The stump of the longus is sutured to the tendon of the extensor hallucis brevis as described in Plate 58. The tendon of the extensor hallucis longus is dissected free of its sheath as high as possible. Then a second incision is made over the course of the anterior tibial tendon in the distal third of the leg. The tendons of the extensor hallucis longus and the anterior tibial are identified. The extensor hallucis longus is pulled into the proximal wound by gentle traction. With a scalpel, three slits of appropriate size are made in the anterior tibial tendon. The extensor hallucis longus tendon is rewound by passing through these slits and then delivered into the distal wound with an Ober tendon passer. The extensor hallucis longus tendon is sutured to the insertion of the anterior tibial muscle with the ankle in neutral position or 10 degrees of dorsiflexion. Any excess of extensor hallucis longus tendon is excised. The wound is closed in layers. The limb is immobilized in a long leg cast for a period of three weeks. Then active assisted and passive exercises are begun.

The author has not found it necessary to detach the anterior tibial and reattach it to the base of the second metatarsal.

Valgus Deformity. Valgus deformity of the foot may be caused by contracture of the triceps surae muscle because the height of the foot is shortened when the hindfoot is everted, or by spasticity of the peroneal muscles in the presence of cerebral zero or weak anterior and posterior tibial muscles.

In early childhood, management of valgus foot follows a conservative approach. A Thomas heel is given with a $\frac{1}{8}$ inch inner heel wedge and a $\frac{3}{8}$ inch longitudinal arch support. If an orthosis is worn, a valgus strap is added to it. Surgical correction of equinus deformity, however, should not be long delayed, as fixed pes valgus may develop. A sliding heel cord lengthening is performed at the appropriate time. This is combined with fractional lengthening of the peroneal muscles if they are spastic and are a deforming force. In the postoperative period, the foot is supported with a longitudinal arch support and inner heel wedges as already described. The motor strength of the anterior tibial is developed by appropriate exercises.

By six or seven years of age, if the pes valgus persists, a subtalar extra-articular arthrodesis is performed. This will control the alignment of the foot and will help to avoid a triple arthrodesis later, on completion of growth. The operative technique of extra-articular subtalar arthrodesis (Grice procedure) is described in Plate 30.

The Hip

Adduction, flexion, and internal rotation deformities of the hip are common in spastic paralysis. With growth the biologically plastic skeleton of the child will respond to the forces of muscle imbalance, and coxa valga, increased anteversion of the femoral neck, acetabular dysplasia, subluxation, and eventually dislocation of the hip may develop.

Adduction deformity of the hip is caused

Neurectomy of Motor Branches of Tibial Nerve to Gastrocnemius

A. The patient is placed in prone position with a pneumatic tourniquet on the proximal thigh. A transverse incision 5 to 7 cm. long is made immediately proximal to the popliteal crease in line with the flexion creases of the skin.

B. The deep fascia is divided and the tibial nerve, lying superficial to the vessels, is exposed. The first branch is cutaneous; it is not disturbed. The next two branches are the motor nerves to the gastrocnemius. One branch emerges from the medial side and enters the medial head close to its origin; just prior to disappearing into the muscle, it divides into three branches. The other branch emerges from the lateral side and similarly enters the lateral head close to its origin, but it divides into only two branches. The motor branch to the soleus muscle emerges distal to that of the gastrocnemius. It is best to stimulate each branch to determine which is the principal cause of clonus.

C. The appropriate motor branches are resected by dividing them proximally at their origin and distally at their entrance into the muscle. The wound is closed in layers in the usual manner. The limb is immobilized in a long leg cast with the foot at 5 to 10 degrees of dorsiflexion at the ankle and with the knee in full extension. The cast is removed in three weeks; the postoperative care is similar to that after heel cord lengthening. (Some surgeons apply only a pressure dressing and allow the patient to walk when he is comfortable and when the wound is healed.)

Plate 29.   Neurectomy of Motor Branches of
Tibial Nerve to Gastrocnemius

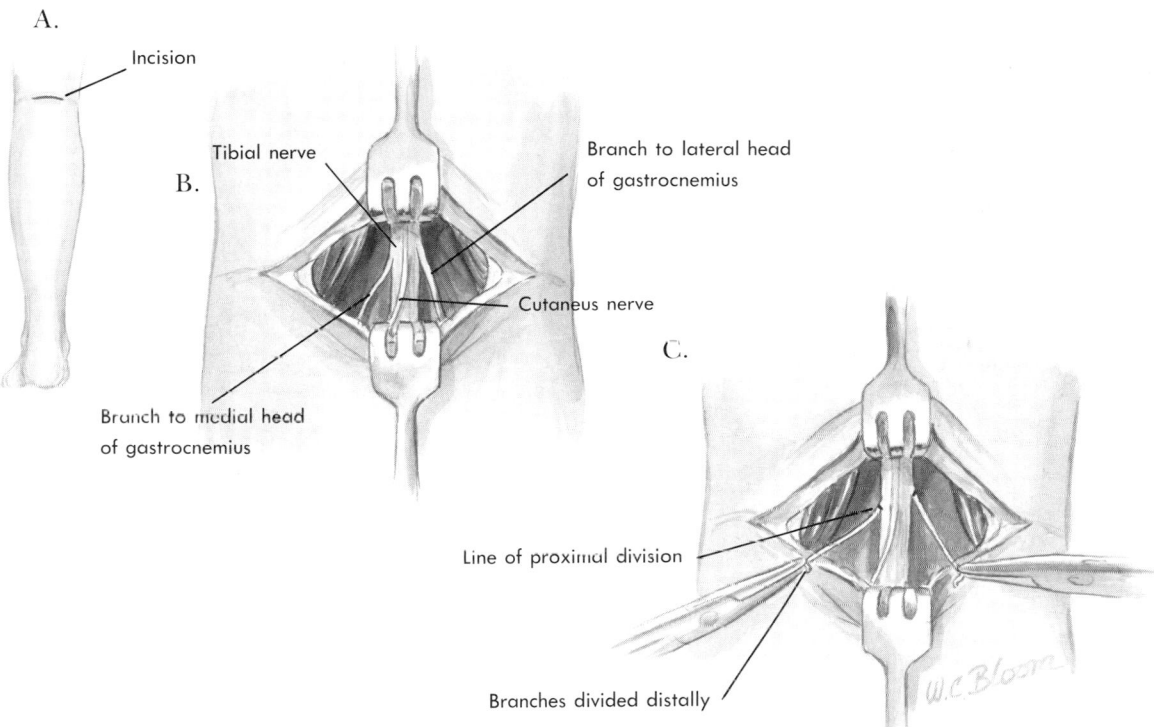

A.

Incision

Tibial nerve

B.

Branch to lateral head
of gastrocnemius

Cutaneus nerve

C.

Branch to medial head
of gastrocnemius

Line of proximal division

W.C.Bloom

Branches divided distally

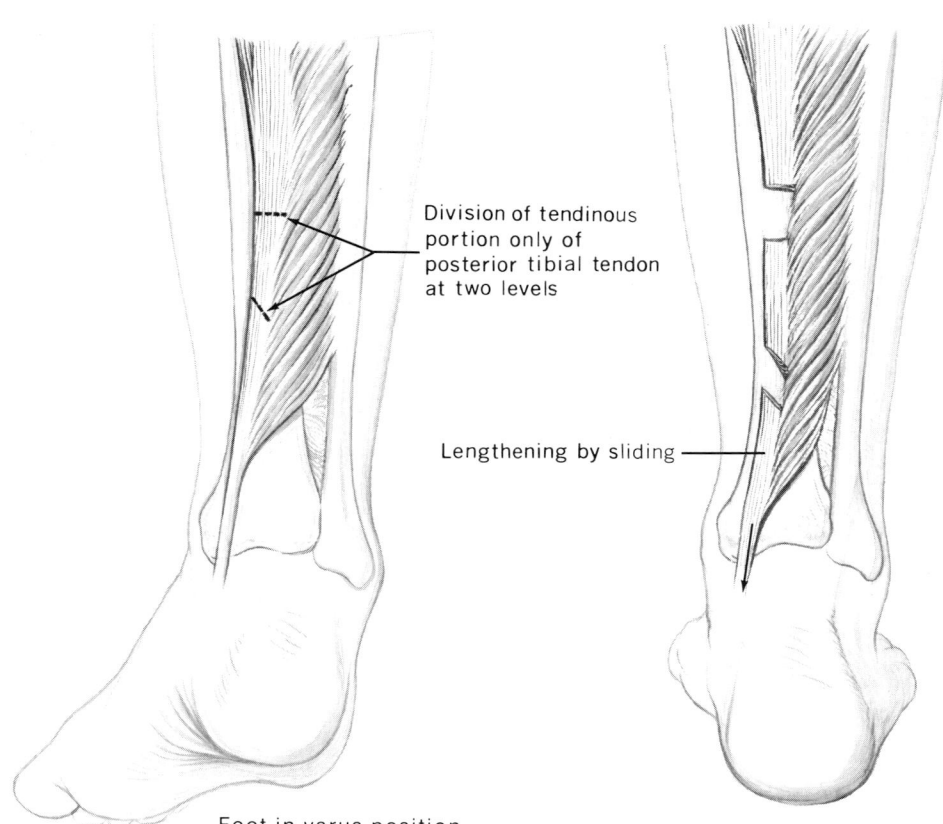

Division of tendinous
portion only of
posterior tibial tendon
at two levels

Lengthening by sliding

Foot in varus position

FIGURE 5-11.   *Sliding lengthening of the posterior tibial tendon.*

by spasticity and contracture of the hip adductors (adductor longus, adductor brevis, adductor magnus, and pectineus), the gracilis, and the medial hamstrings (semitendinosus and semimembranosus muscles). It is important to distinguish between limitation of hip abduction caused by overaction and pull of the hip adductors and that caused by the gracilis and medial hamstrings. The two deforming components are differentiated by performing passive hip abduction with the knees in extension and then with the knees in 90 degrees of flexion, which relaxes the gracilis and medial hamstring muscles (Fig. 5–12). Any asymmetry of involvement between the right and left sides should be carefully noted at this time.

To determine further the degree of contracture of the gracilis muscle (one of the major forces in the production of hip adduction deformity), Phelps has suggested the following maneuver: The patient is placed in prone position with the hips in maximum abduction and the knees in 90 degrees of flexion; if the gracilis muscle is shortened upon passive full extension of the knee, the hip will automatically adduct. The degree of hip adduction is noted.

Scissoring is a term commonly used to describe the adduction posture of the hips when the patient is upright. True scissoring must be distinguished from approximation of the knees for stability and balance.

Flexion deformity of the hip is primarily caused by spasticity and contracture of the iliopsoas and rectus femoris muscles. To distinguish between the two forces, the Thomas test is performed with the knee in extension and then in flexion (Fig. 5–13). When the rectus femoris is the cause, hip flexion deformity is increased with the knee in flexion and decreased with the knee in extension; whereas, when it is due to the iliopsoas muscle, the position of the knee has no effect on the degree of hip flexion contracture. Palpation for tautness of the muscle fibers of the iliopsoas and pelvic origin of the rectus femoris muscles is also of some assistance (Fig. 5–14). Often it is the iliopsoas muscle that is the principal deforming force in the causation of hip flexion deformity.

Other spastic muscles that may contribute to flexion deformity of the hip, particularly in stance, include the following: (1) tensor fasciae latae, (2) sartorius (flexing the hip to 90 degrees of flexion), (3) pectineus, (4) adductors longus and brevis (flexing the hip from hyperextension to 50 degrees of flexion), (5) adductor (flexing the hip from hyperextension to 20 degrees of flexion), and (6) gracilis (flexing to 30 degrees of flexion).

In stance and gait a flexed attitude of the hip may be secondary to flexion deformity of the knee or equinus deformity of the ankle; also, when balance is poor, the spastic child will flex his knees and hips to lower his center of gravity. "Jump position" is a term referring to the posture of a spastic child who stands with his knees and hips flexed and the ankles in equinus position (Fig. 5–15).

One of two roentgenographic methods may be used for accurate determination of the degree of hip flexion deformity in stance. In the Milch method, a line is drawn from the ischial tuberosity to the anterior superior iliac spine and a second line is drawn parallel along the axis of the femoral shaft. The angle formed by the intersection of these two lines is the *pelvic-femoral angle*, which normally measures 55 degrees. In the Fick method the *sacro-femoral angle* is the angle formed between the lines drawn across the superior surface of the first sacral vertebra and the axis of the femoral shaft. Normally, the sacro-femoral angle diminishes. These roentgenographic methods of mensuration of hip flexion deformity are ordinarily impractical for routine use, as the spastic child has poor balance and often requires the support of crutches or parallel bars for standing and walking. Inspection of the standing posture of the patient and the Thomas test are of more clinical value.

Internal rotation deformity of the hips often accompanies hip adduction contracture. Several factors should be considered in its pathogenesis. It is primarily caused by spasticity and myostatic contracture of the muscles that internally rotate the hip; these are the tensor fasciae latae, gluteus minimus, and the anterior portion of the gluteus medius. When the hip is in flexion, the hip adductors are also internal rotators; Banks and Green have demonstrated this by stimulation of the various branches of

Extra-Articular Arthrodesis of the Subtalar Joint
(Grice Procedure)

THE PROCEDURE

A. A 2½-inch long and slightly curved incision is made over the subtalar joint, centering over the sinus tarsi.

B. The incision is carried down to the sinus tarsi. The capsules of the posterior and anterior subtalar articulations are identified and left intact. The operation is extra-articular. If the capsule is opened inadvertently, it should be closed by interrupted sutures.

The periosteum on the talus corresponding to the lateral margin of the roof of the sinus tarsi is divided and reflected proximally. The fibrofatty tissue in the sinus tarsi with the periosteum of the calcaneus corresponding to the floor of the sinus tarsi and the tendinous origin of the short toe extensors from the calcaneus is elevated and reflected distally in one mass.

C. The remaining fatty and ligamentous tissue from the sinus tarsi is thoroughly removed with a sharp scalpel and curet.

Plate 30.   Extra-Articular Arthrodesis of the Subtalar Joint (Grice Procedure)

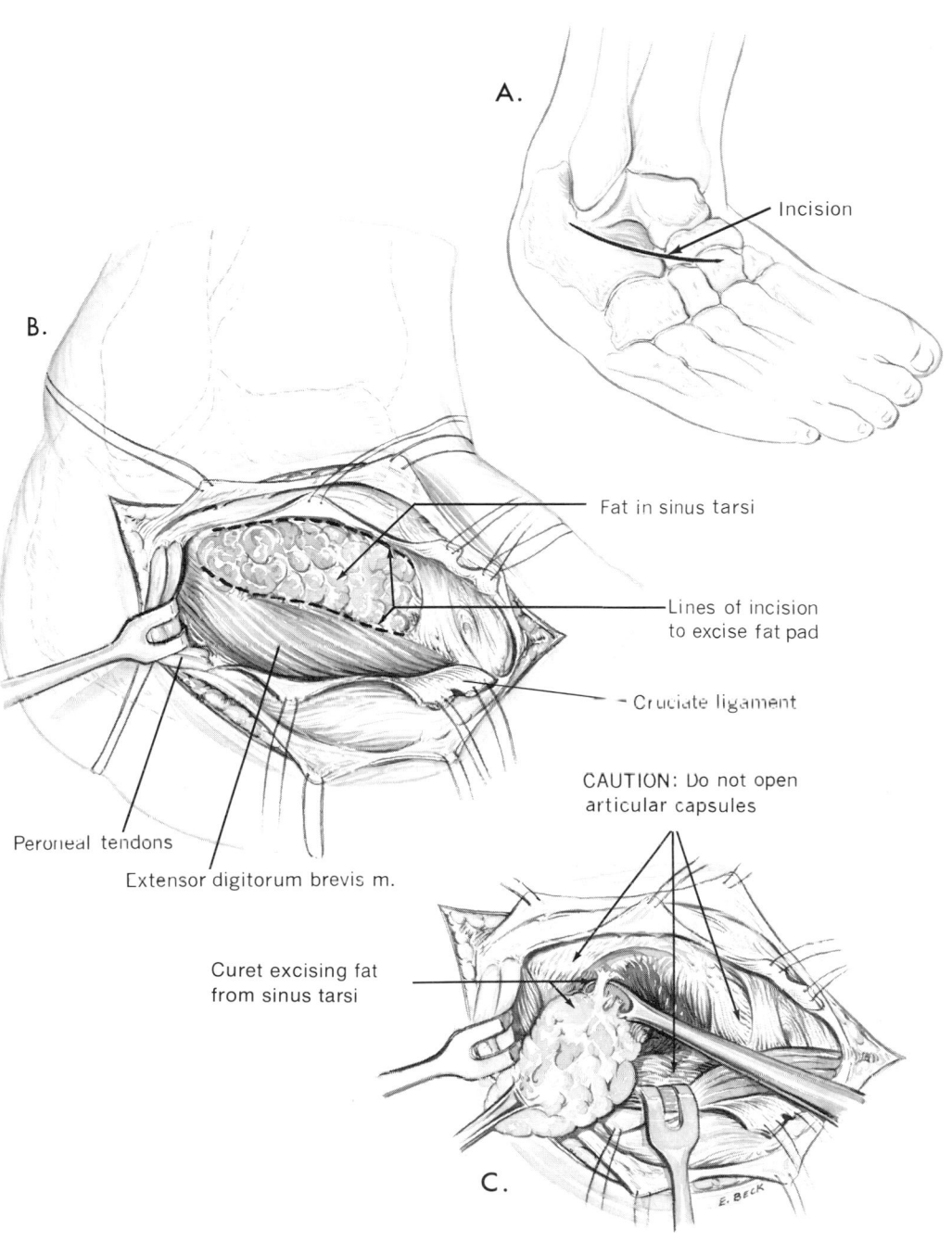

A.

Incision

B.

Fat in sinus tarsi

Lines of incision
to excise fat pad

Cruciate ligament

Peroneal tendons

Extensor digitorum brevis m.

CAUTION: Do not open
articular capsules

Curet excising fat
from sinus tarsi

C.

E. BECK

Extra-Articular Arthrodesis of the Subtalar Joint *(Grice Procedure)* *(Continued)*

D. Next the foot is manipulated into equinus position and inversion, rotating the calcaneus into its normal position beneath the talus and correcting the valgus deformity. Broad straight osteotomes of various sizes ($\frac{3}{4}$ to $1\frac{1}{4}$ inches or more) are inserted into the sinus tarsi, blocking the subtalar joint and determining the length and optimum position of the bone graft and the stability that it will provide. The long axis of the graft should be parallel with that of the leg when the ankle is dorsiflexed into neutral position, and the hindfoot should be 5 degrees valgus or neutral, but never varus. Even a slight degree of varus deformity of the heel seems to increase with growth.

E. The optimum site of the bone graft bed is marked with the broad osteotome. A thin layer of cortical bone ($\frac{1}{8}$ to $\frac{3}{16}$ inch) is removed with a dental osteotome from the inferior surface of the talus (the roof of the sinus tarsi) and the superior surface of the calcaneus (the floor of the sinus tarsi) at the marked site for the bone graft. It is best to preserve the most lateral cortical margin of the graft bed to support the bone block and to prevent it from sinking into soft cancellous bone.

F. A bone graft of appropriate size can be taken from the anteromedial surface of the proximal tibial metaphysis as a single cortical graft, which is then cut into two trapezoidal bone grafts with their cancellous surfaces facing each other. Lately the author prefers to use fibular bone grafts with the cortices intact. The corners of the base of the graft are removed with a rongeur so that it is trapezoidal in shape and can be countersunk into cancellous bone, preventing lateral displacement after operation.

The bone graft is placed in the prepared graft bed in the sinus tarsi by holding the foot in varus position. An impacter may be used to fix the cortices of the graft in place. The longitudinal axis of the graft should be parallel with the shaft of the tibia with the ankle in neutral position.

With the foot held in the desired position, the distal soft-tissue pedicle of fibrofatty tissue of the sinus tarsi, the calcaneal periosteum, and the tendinous origin of the short toe extensors are sutured to the reflected periosteum from the talus. The subcutaneous tissue and skin are closed with interrupted sutures, and a long leg cast is applied.

POSTOPERATIVE CARE

The cast is removed eight to ten weeks after operation. Roentgenograms are taken; if there is solid healing of the graft, gradual weight-bearing is allowed with the protection of crutches. Active and passive exercises are performed to strengthen the muscles and to increase the range of motion of the ankle and of the knee.

Plate 30. Extra-Articular Arthrodesis of the Subtalar Joint (Grice Procedure)

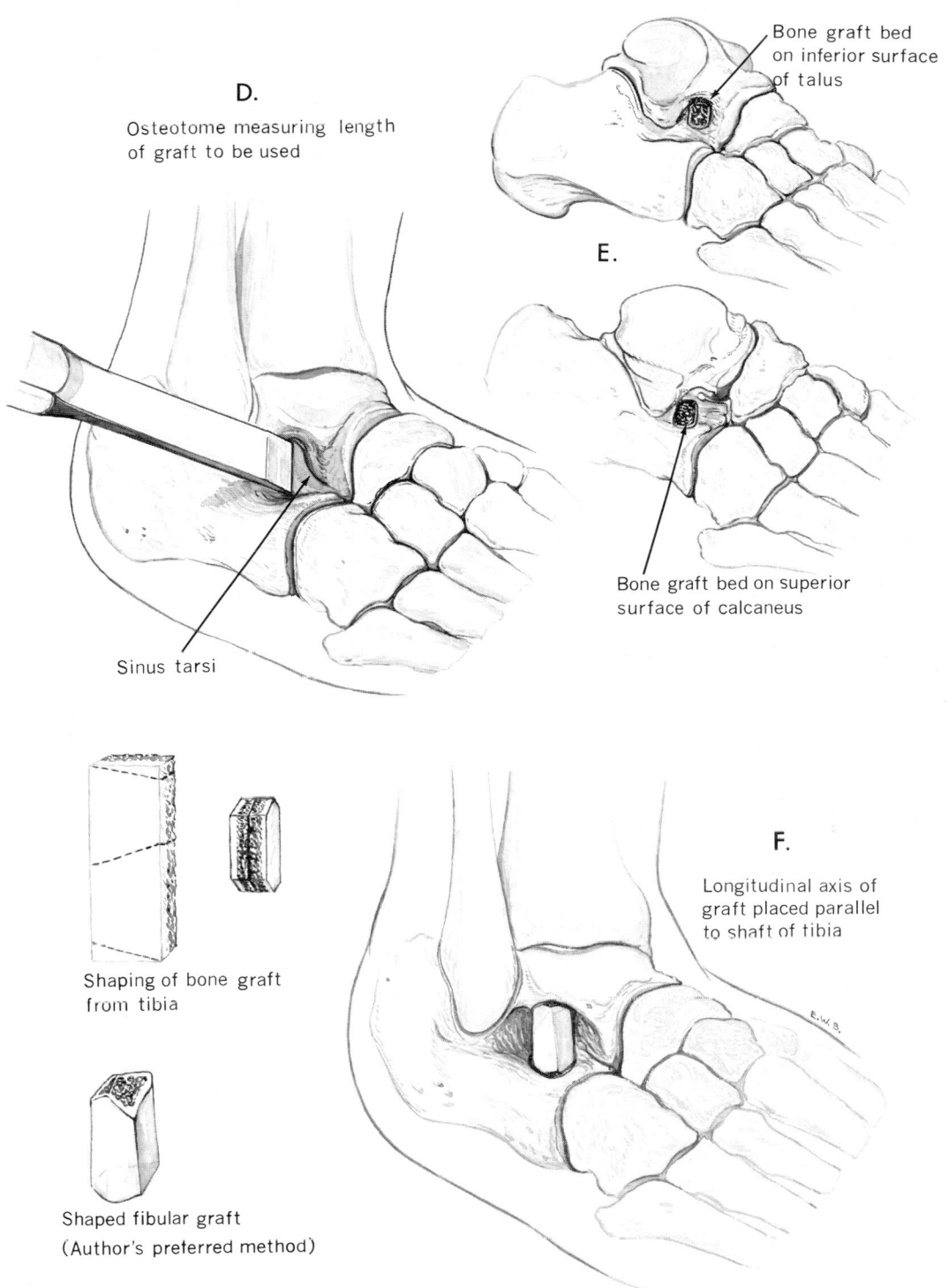

D.

Osteotome measuring length of graft to be used

Sinus tarsi

Bone graft bed on inferior surface of talus

E.

Bone graft bed on superior surface of calcaneus

Shaping of bone graft from tibia

Shaped fibular graft (Author's preferred method)

F.

Longitudinal axis of graft placed parallel to shaft of tibia

E.W.B.

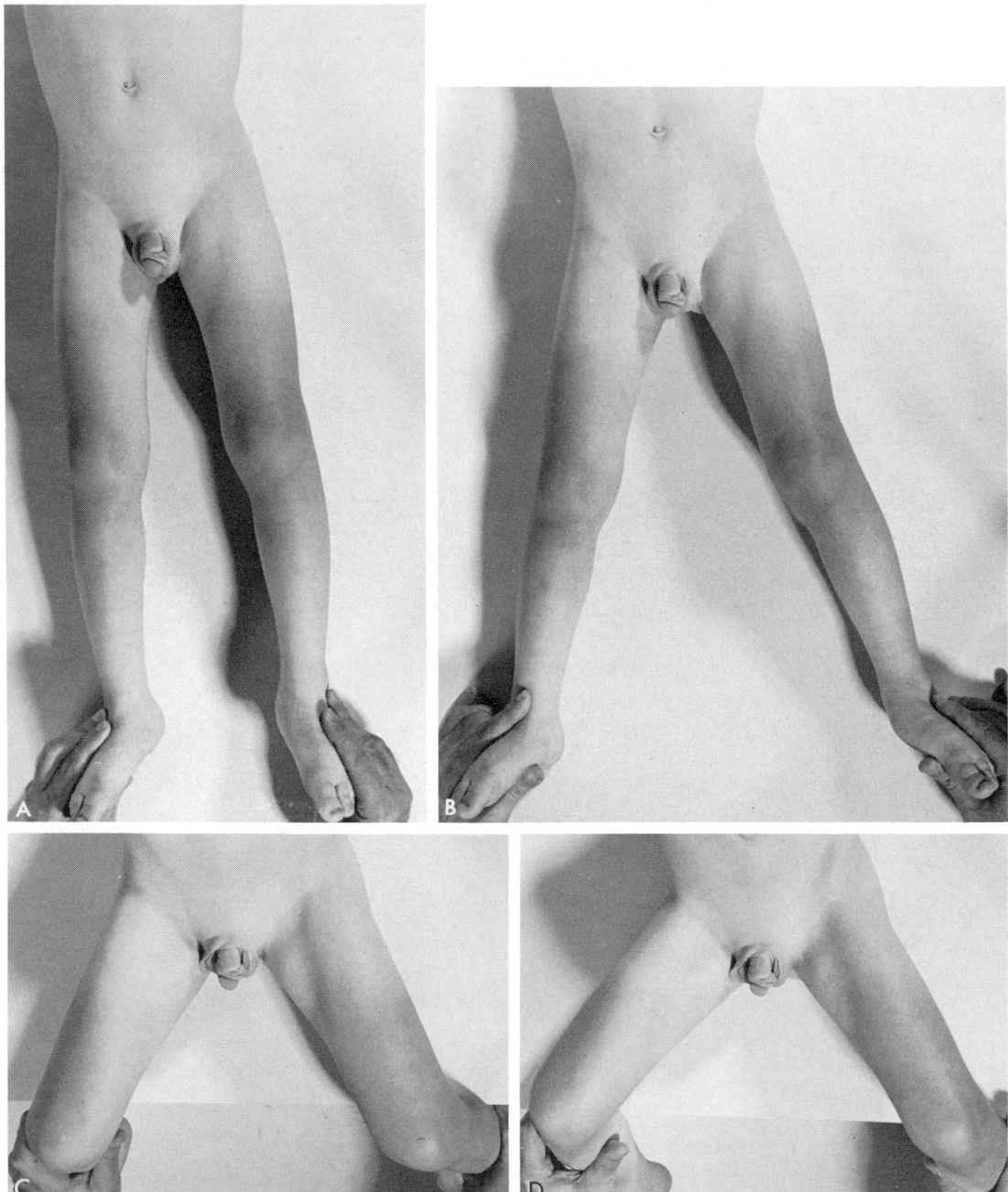

FIGURE 5-12. *Passive abduction of the hips with the knees in extension and in 90 degrees of flexion.*

Flexion of the knee will relax the gracilis and medial hamstring muscles, enabling differentiation between limitation of hip abduction caused by spasticity and contracture of the hip adductors and that due to the gracilis and medial hamstrings. **A** and **C** show the range of motion when the spastic muscles grab; **B** and **D** demonstrate the maximum range of passive hip abduction.

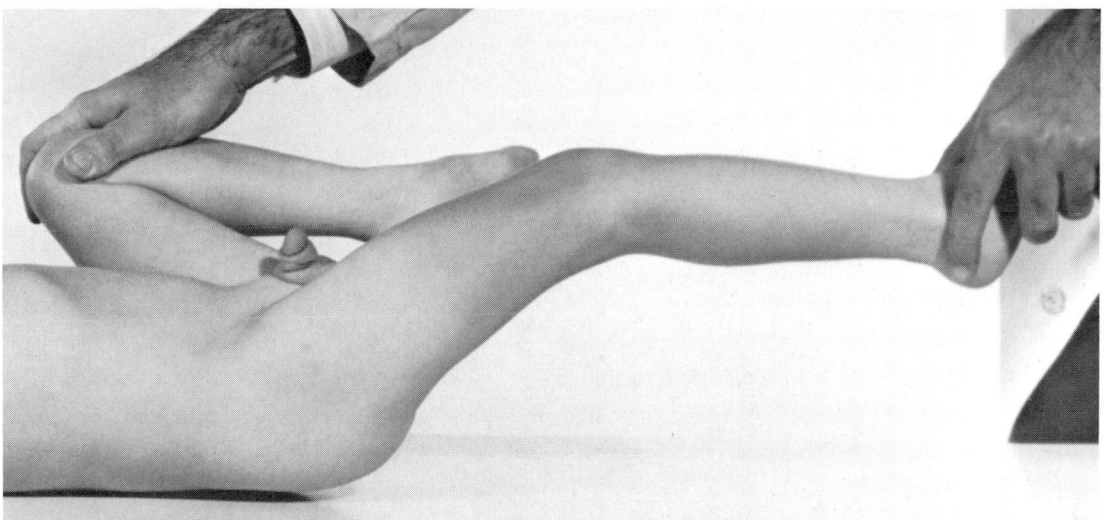

FIGURE 5–13. *Thomas test demonstrating flexion deformity of the hip in spastic cerebral palsy.*

It is primarily caused by spasticity and contracture of the iliopsoas and rectus femoris muscles. To distinguish between the two components, the Thomas test is performed with the knee in extension and then in flexion. If flexion contracture of the hip is due to spasticity of the iliopsoas muscle, the degree of hip flexion deformity is not altered by a change in position of the knee.

the obturator nerve during surgery.[15] The cerebral palsied child sleeps, sits, and stands with his hips in internal rotation; this prolonged continuous positioning of the hips may be an additional static force. Permanent contractures of the ligaments and capsule of the hip joint soon develop; with growth, increased antetorsion of the femoral neck takes place, resulting in fixed structural internal rotation deformity of the hips.

During clinical examination, the various etiologic forces are studied by passive external rotation of the hip in various positions; first, with the patient in prone position with the hip in extension and in neutral abduction, 30 degrees of adduction, and 25 degrees of abduction; and then with the patient in supine position with the hip in 90 degrees of flexion. Passive external rotation of the hip is performed first suddenly to determine the degree of rotation at which the spastic muscles grab, and then gradually and steadily to note the presence or absence of fixed deformity. The spastic child with internal rotation-adduction-flexion deformity of his hips walks with a "stepover" gait.[60]

Bony deformities of the hip are usually acquired. Coxa valga and increased ante-

version of the femoral neck develop first, followed by dysplasia of the acetabulum and gradual progressive leveling of the femoral head out of the acetabular socket (Fig. 5–16). The dynamic imbalance between the spastic hip adductors and weakened hip abductors combined with spastic hip flexors is the prime deforming force in the causation of coxa valga. With loss of hip abductor power, growth from the greater trochanteric apophysis is not normally stimulated, and valgus deformity of the femoral neck results from disparity of relative growth between the capital femoral epiphysis and the greater trochanteric apophysis. Absence of normal weight-bearing forces is another factor in the pathogenesis of coxa valga.

Brooks and Wardle studied the effect of muscle action on the shape of the femur by performing experiments on ten decalcified femora. The effect of iliopsoas action alone on femoral shape was that of valgus deformity, a posterior deflection of the neck, an untwisting of the upper diaphysis, and an increased anterior curvature of the shaft. The tendency to femoral deformity produced by an iliopsoas force was abolished by a gluteal force acting at the greater

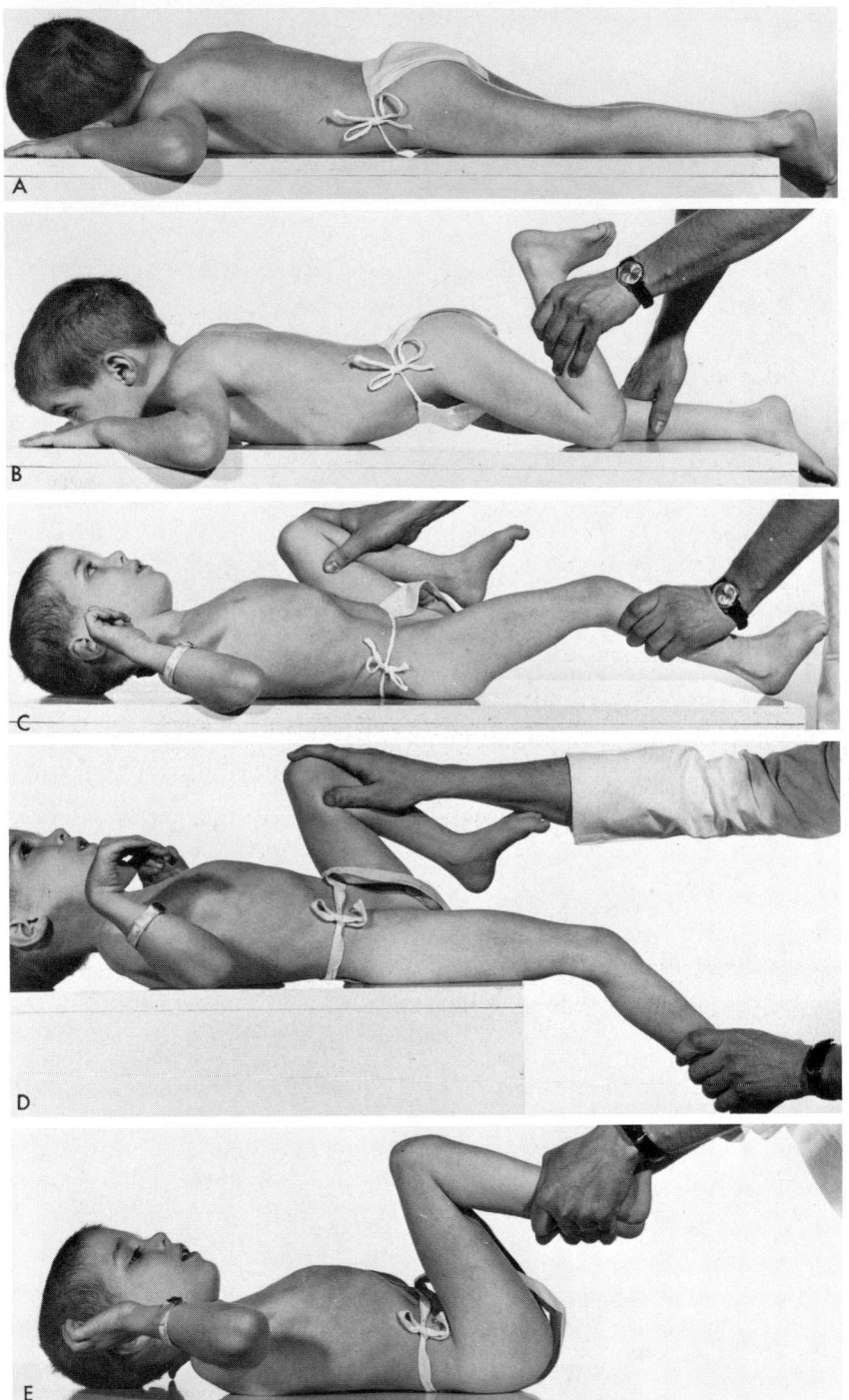

FIGURE 5–14.   Spasticity and contracture of the pelvic origin of the rectus femoris muscle.

A and **B**. Positive Ely test. The child is placed in prone position with the hip and knee in extension. On passive flexion of the knee the pelvis will elevate from the table. **C**. On the Thomas test 35 degrees of flexion of the hip is demonstrated. To distinguish between the iliopsoas and rectus femoris as causes of flexion contracture of the hip, the Thomas test is performed with the knee in extension and then in flexion. If flexion contracture of the hip is due to spasticity of the iliopsoas muscle, the degree of hip flexion deformity is not altered by a change in position of the knee. **D**. Spasticity and contracture of the rectus femoris is demonstrated by sudden passive flexion of the knee with the hip in extension. Note the lumbar lordosis to compensate for fixed flexion contracture of the hip. **E**. The degree of passive knee flexion is near normal when the hip is flexed, relaxing the pelvic origin of the rectus femoris muscle.

810

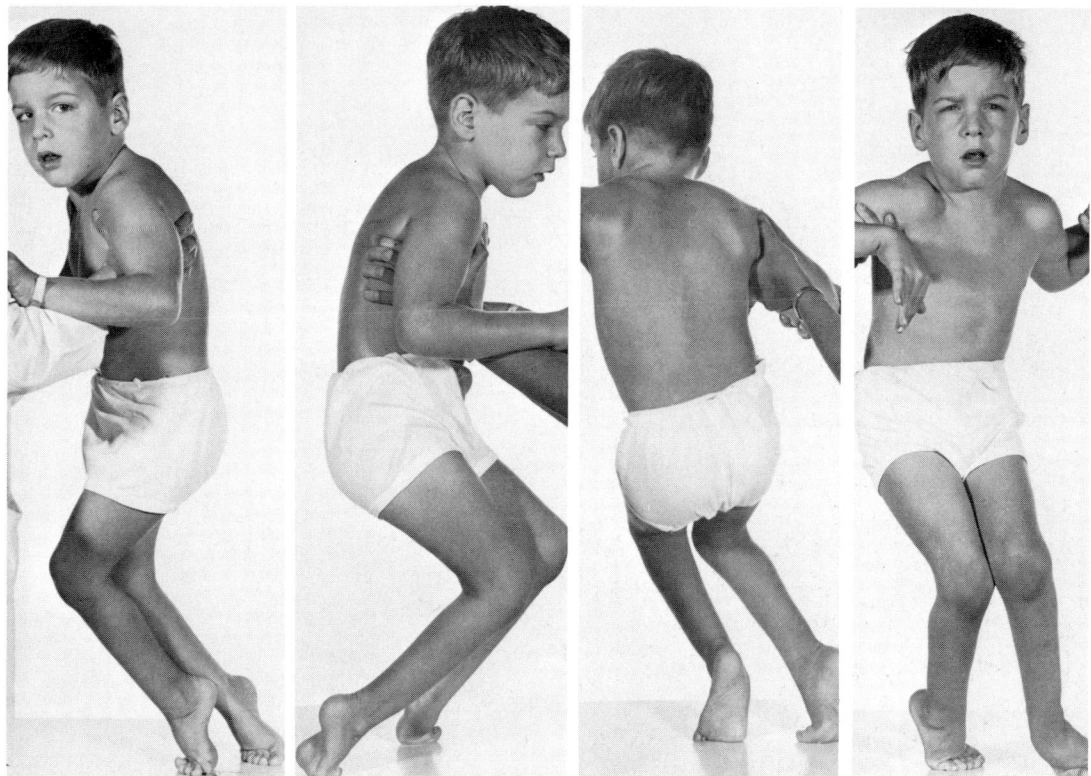

FIGURE 5–15. *A five-year-old boy with cerebral palsy—spastic paraplegia.*

Note the severe flexion, internal rotation, and adduction contracture of the hips, flexion deformity of the knees, and equinus deformity of the ankles and feet. It is obvious that the severity of the deformities prevents the child from walking and interferes with his already precarious balance. He was treated by bilateral adductor myotomy, obturator neurectomy (anterior branch), and heel cord lengthening; this was followed six months later by fractional lengthening of the hamstrings. The patient is able to ambulate now with minimal support of crutches.

trochanter when these forces were in the ratio of 5:3.[32]

Dislocation of the hip in cerebral palsy should be suspected when there is marked limitation of hip abduction, a positive Galeazzi sign, prominence of the greater trochanter, and asymmetry of the skin folds on the thigh. It usually occurs in the spastic type of cerebral palsy. Periodic roentgenograms of the hips should be routinely taken for early diagnosis. Widening of the joint space is the earliest sign of lateral displacement. In such an instance, early surgical intervention is indicated in the form of adductor myotomy, iliopsoas lengthening, and neurectomy of the anterior branch of the obturator nerve. Hip dislocation in cerebral palsy is preventable.

Congenital dislocation in cerebral palsy can occur and should be distinguished from acquired dislocation; the latter is characterized by the greater ease of its reduction and the absence of significant acetabular dysplasia.

TREATMENT

Conservative measures consist of passive stretching and range of motion exercises to prevent the development of contractural deformity. The hip adductors, flexors, and internal rotators are stretched several times a day. Night splints that hold the hips in abduction, external rotation, and extension are used in selected cases. In the preoperative period, routine use of the bivalved night cast is not recommended, as it is usually not well tolerated by the severely spastic child. The need for orthoses to support the lower limbs for ambulation has

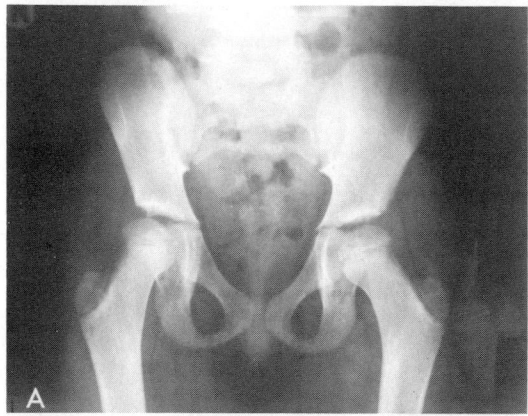

FIGURE 5–16. *Acquired dislocation of the right hip in spastic cerebral palsy.*

A. Roentgenogram of the hips at four years of age. Note the severe bilateral coxa valga and subluxation of the right hip. **B** and **C.** At nine years of age the right hip is completely dislocated. Bilateral adductor myotomy of the hip and neurectomy of the anterior branch of the obturator nerve was performed, followed by closed reduction of the right hip and subtrochanteric varization osteotomy. **D** and **E.** Postoperative roentgenograms.

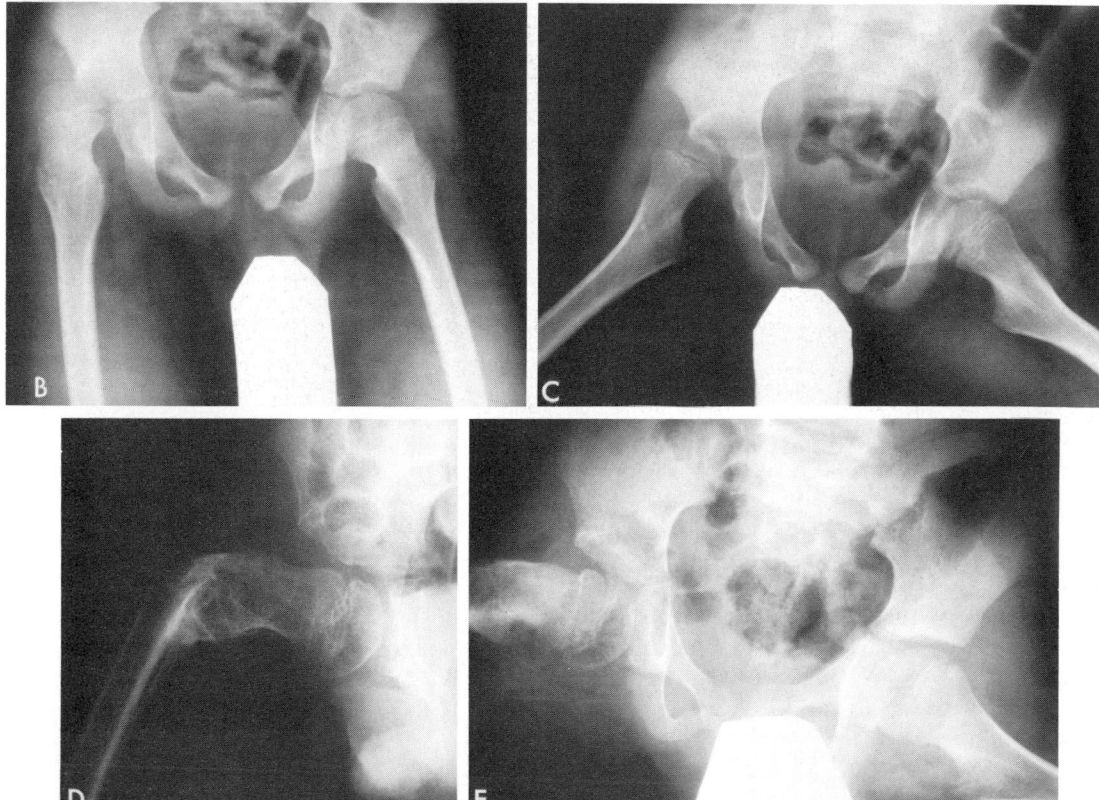

been greatly decreased by early surgery. As soon as the child has good sitting balance, reciprocal motion between the upper and lower limbs, and adequate hand function to hold parallel bars or crutches, the deformities of the lower limbs are assessed to determine whether surgical intervention is indicated. It is preferable that these children develop weight-bearing and demonstrate the potential of locomotion in parallel bars before consideration of surgery. The child may need his hip adductors for stability. Often the scissor-like deformity and the equinus position of the feet prevent the child from walking. If the hips begin to develop subluxation, surgical intervention is indicated, even prior to the development of sitting balance; it is paramount to prevent dislocation of the hip, as these patients will have much less difficulty with hygienic care, will have a wider and more secure base for assisted sitting, and will be much more comfortable than if their hips were dislocated.

Adductor myotomy and neurectomy of the anterior branch of the obturator nerve are often performed in combination with sliding lengthening of the Achilles tendon. Also, when adductor myotomy is performed simultaneously, there is greater surgical accessibility to the lesser trochanter and iliopsoas tendon. When flexion contracture of 25 to 30 degrees is present in the hip, the author recommends fractional lengthening of the iliopsoas tendon at the same time as adductor myotomy. The operative technique and postoperative care of adductor myotomy and neurectomy of the anterior branch of the obturator nerve and fractional lengthening of the iliopsoas tendon are described and illustrated in Plate 31.

If the pelvic origin of the rectus femoris is very spastic and is a major force in the causation of hip flexion deformity, it may be sectioned through a separate longitudinal incision. In such an instance, hip flexion contracture will be accompanied by extension contracture of the knee.

Internal rotation deformity of the hip is managed more conservatively. Following adductor myotomy, the night bivalved cast holds the hips in extension and 15 to 20 degrees of external rotation. If, after intensive physical therapy and gait training, the patient still walks with the hip in marked internal rotation, external rotation torsion

cables with a pelvic band or external rotation elastic twisters with an abdominal corset are given. The latter is prescribed if there is hyperextension of the knee.

In the adolescent patient surgical measures may be indicated if severe internal rotation of the hips persists despite the preceding conservative measures.

The Durham procedure should not be performed, as division of the gluteus medius and minimus fibers will further weaken the abductor power and lateral stability of the hip joint.[55]

In 1923, Legg transferred the origin of the tensor fasciae latae from the anterior portion of the ilium to the posterior third to improve the power of hip abduction in patients with anterior poliomyelitis.[111] Barr, in 1943, advocated the Legg procedure for treatment of flexion–internal rotation deformity of the hip in spastic paralysis.[17] Green added the sartorius muscle to the tensor fasciae latae to increase the motor strength of the abductors and external rotators.[15, 70] In his experience, the author has found the Green modification of the Legg-Barr procedure to be very satisfactory in correction of internal rotation contracture of the hip; in addition, it gives some power of hip abduction.

Baker has described transfer of the semitendinosus tendon to the anterolateral aspect of the distal shaft of the femur through a subcutaneous tunnel to act as an external rotator. He termed the procedure "barber pole" or "stripe transfer."[11] This procedure is ineffective in correcting internal rotation deformity of the hip, and is not recommended by the author.

When internal rotation deformity of the hip is fixed because of structural bony deformity and marked anteversion of the femoral neck, or when the patient is over ten years of age, rotational osteotomy of the femur is indicated. There is often associated marked coxa valga; in such an instance, the rotational osteotomy at the subtrochanteric level is performed in combination with varization osteotomy. Occasionally genu recurvatum is the accompanying deformity and it is indicated to carry out the rotational osteotomy at the supracondylar level so that the distal femoral segment can be tilted posteriorly. Overcorrection should be avoided. A safe rule to follow is that postoperatively the

(*Text continued on page 818.*)

Adductor Myotomy of Hip and Neurectomy of Anterior Branch of Obturator Nerve (Banks and Green)

THE PROCEDURE

A. With the patient in supine position, both lower limbs and hips are prepared and carefully draped to allow full manipulation of the hips. Meticulous attention should be paid to avoiding contamination from the perineal area. In the groin, the prepared area should be proximal enough to include the origin of the adductor longus muscle. With both hips in flexion, abduction, and external rotation, a longitudinal incision is made over the posterior border of the adductor longus, beginning about ½ inch below the pubis and extending distally for about 3 inches.

B. The subcutaneous tissue and deep fascia are incised in line with the skin incision. Any bleeding vessels are clamped and coagulated.

C. With a blunt instrument or finger, the interval between the adductor longus (anteriorly) and the adductor brevis (posteriorly) is developed.

D. Next, the adductor longus is retracted forward and the anterior branch of the obturator nerve is identified. The motor branches to the adductor longus, adductor brevis, and gracilis muscles are isolated. It is best to identify these nerves positively by gently pinching with a smooth forceps or by using a nerve stimulator and observing the contraction of the corresponding muscles.

E. These motor branches are individually clamped distally with hemostats and dissected proximally to their origin, where they are sectioned, an approximately 2 cm. segment of the nerve being excised. The posterior branch of the obturator nerve should not be damaged.

F. The adductor longus is then sectioned transversely in its tendinous portion over a blunt instrument close to its origin from the pubis. The adductor brevis is divided obliquely at a lower level to minimize the extent of dead space (the author uses a coagulation knife, sectioning the muscle over a nonconductive object such as plastic tubing). Next, the gracilis muscle is isolated in the posteromedial portion of the wound. With the knees in extension, it is sectioned obliquely in an opposite direction to that of the adductor brevis and at a lower level.

Plate 31. *Adductor Myotomy of Hip and Neurectomy of Anterior Branch of Obturator Nerve (Banks and Green)*

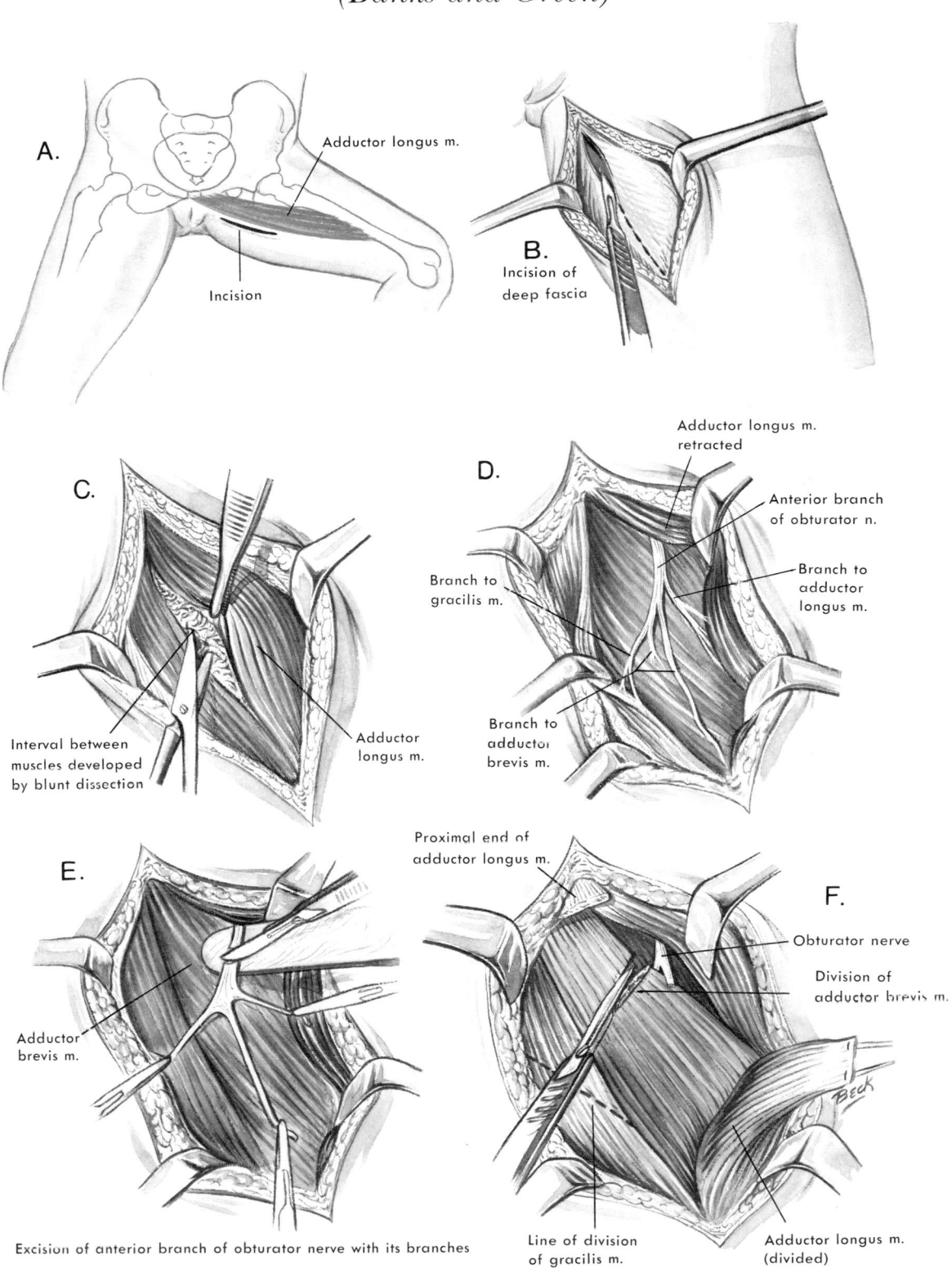

A.

Adductor longus m.

Incision

B.

Incision of deep fascia

C.

Interval between muscles developed by blunt dissection

Adductor longus m.

D.

Adductor longus m. retracted

Anterior branch of obturator n.

Branch to adductor longus m.

Branch to gracilis m.

Branch to adductor brevis m.

E.

Adductor brevis m.

Excision of anterior branch of obturator nerve with its branches

F.

Proximal end of adductor longus m.

Obturator nerve

Division of adductor brevis m.

Line of division of gracilis m.

Adductor longus m. (divided)

Beck

815

Adductor Myotomy of Hip and Neurectomy of Anterior Branch of Obturator Nerve (Banks and Green) (Continued)

G. At this time, the degree of correction obtained is checked by abducting both hips in extension. If there is still some limitation to complete hip abduction, the most anterior fibers of the adductor magnus may be divided.

H. If iliopsoas lengthening is indicated, the hips are again flexed, externally rotated, and abducted. This position of the hip rotates the proximal femur, bringing the lesser trochanter anteriorly and making it more accessible. The interval between the pectineus and adductor brevis is developed and widened by blunt dissection to expose the lesser trochanter and the iliopsoas tendon. If the pectineus muscle is hypertrophic and covers the iliopsoas tendon, it may be released or retracted medially with the adductor brevis.

I. A small periosteal or staphylorrhaphy elevator is inserted deep to the iliopsoas tendon, bringing it into view. With a curved hemostat the iliopsoas tendon is dissected free of its adjacent tissues. Care should be taken not to injure the sciatic nerve. Next, with the elevator under the iliopsoas tendon, two transverse incisions are made 1.5 to 2 cm. apart, dividing only its tendinous fibers, not its muscle fibers. The hip is hyperextended and the tendon is lengthened 2 to 4 cm.

J. All bleeding vessels should be clamped and coagulated, establishing complete hemostasis. The author routinely uses suction tubes, which are connected to a Hemovac. The deep fascia is not sutured. Only subcutaneous tissue and skin are closed.

K. A plaster of Paris hip spica cast is applied with the hips in full abduction and extension and in 10 to 15 degrees of external rotation. If there is flexion contracture of the knees, the patellae should be well padded. Toe-to-groin casts joined by an abduction bar should not be used, as pelvic obliquity may result.

POSTOPERATIVE CARE

One or two days after operation, the suction catheters are removed. The period of immobilization in solid casts varies. Ordinarily in three to four weeks, the solid casts are removed and bilateral long leg bivalved casts are made in which the hips are kept in the desired amount of abduction with an adjustable abduction bar. In the presence of subluxation or dislocation of the hip, immobilization in a solid cast is continued for three months. When the patient is cooperative and has a good motor picture the casts may be bivalved and exercises instituted as early as the fifth to seventh postoperative day.

Active hip abduction, adduction, and extension exercises are performed first in the supine position. The range of motion of joints is maintained by gentle passive stretching exercises. As muscle strength increases, exercises are performed first against gravity and then against resistance. As soon as functional range of motion in the weight-bearing joints is developed, standing and walking are allowed under supervision, first in parallel bars and then with crutches. Gait training with crutches is continued until as normal a gait pattern as is possible is obtained. The crutches are discontinued when good balance is present. Some patients, especially severe quadriplegics, have to use crutches for support indefinitely.

The length of time that bivalved casts should be worn at night is variable. As a rule, they are used for at least six months to a year. They are not discontinued until the patient has effective full active abduction of the hips against gravity. If there is any tendency to recurrence of contracture, bivalved night casts are reapplied.

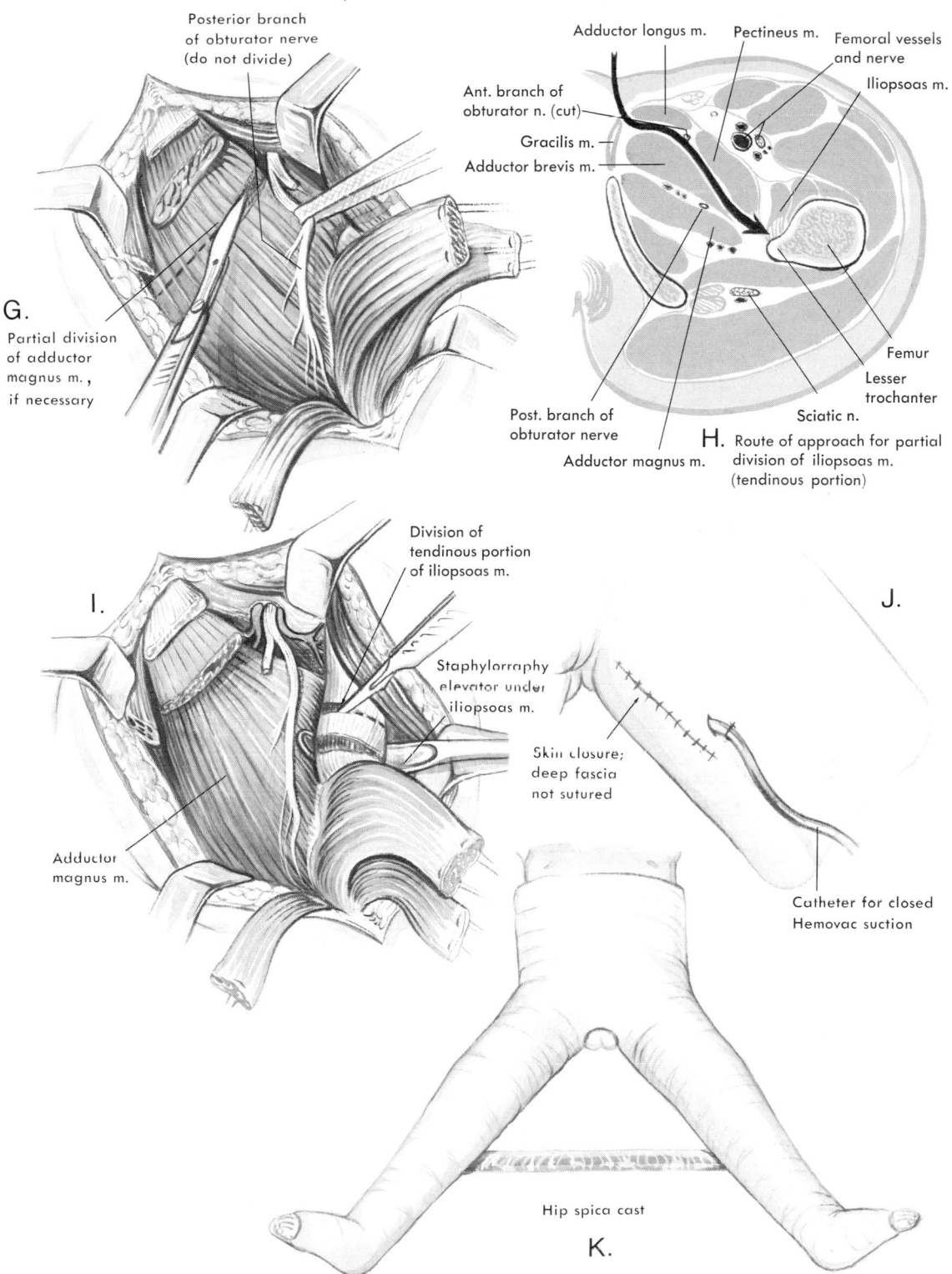

G. Partial division of adductor magnus m., if necessary

Posterior branch of obturator nerve (do not divide)

Adductor longus m.

Pectineus m.

Femoral vessels and nerve

Iliopsoas m.

Ant. branch of obturator n. (cut)

Gracilis m.

Adductor brevis m.

Post. branch of obturator nerve

Adductor magnus m.

Sciatic n.

Lesser trochanter

Femur

H. Route of approach for partial division of iliopsoas m. (tendinous portion)

I.

Division of tendinous portion of iliopsoas m.

Staphylorraphy elevator under iliopsoas m.

Adductor magnus m.

J.

Skin closure; deep fascia not sutured

Catheter for closed Hemovac suction

Hip spica cast

K.

817

range of external rotation of the hip in extension should equal that of internal rotation. The type of osteotomy varies according to the deformity to be corrected. Simple rotational osteotomy is transverse, whereas when it is combined with varization there should be a lateral buttress on the proximal fragment. When it is done with correction of genu recurvatum, an anterior buttress is provided. The method of internal fixation used is a matter of individual preference. In the younger patient, the author uses large threaded Steinmann pins and Roger Anderson apparatus; in the older patient, a modified Jouett or Coventry nail with an angle of 125 degrees. Other surgeons may use two staples inserted at right angles to each other or a bone plate; in both instances, the proximal fragment should be held in maximal internal rotation with a large threaded Steinmann pin while the osteotomy is performed. A double hip spica cast is always applied.

In lateral rotation of the distal fragment of the hip in patients over 15 years of age with severe fixed flexion–internal rotation deformity, the hip should be tilted into extension to correct the fixed flexion deformity.

Following varization osteotomy, the already weakened hip abductors can be further relaxed. In such as instance, the gluteus medius and minimus muscles are tightened by transplanting their insertion on the greater trochanter down the femoral shaft. The author has not found it necessary to transfer the iliopsoas muscle from the lesser trochanter to the greater trochanter to increase the power of hip abduction. In general, caution should be exercised in performing the Mustard iliopsoas transfer in spastic cerebral palsy because of the inherent danger of weakening functional active hip flexion, which is so important in gait.

Intrapelvic obturator neurectomy in spastic cerebral palsy is rarely indicated. The procedure was advocated by Chandler because, after neurectomy of the obturator nerve, some adductor power remains, as the pectineus is innervated by the femoral nerve and the ischial origin of the adductor magnus by the sciatic nerve. The operative technique is as follows:

A transverse incision is made in the abdomen just above the symphysis pubis, parallel with one of the distal transverse skin creases.

The subcutaneous tissue and fascia are divided in line with the skin incision. The wound flaps are retracted proximally and inferiorly, exposing the two rectus abdominis muscles. The sheath of one of the rectus muscles is split longitudinally in its lateral third, reflected, and the margin of the muscle is identified.

The rectus abdominis muscle is retracted medially and, with the index finger used as a blunt dissector, the peritoneum and bladder are pushed posteriorly and held so with a retractor. Again, with the index finger, the obturator nerve is palpated and its course identified within the pelvic wall as it enters the neural foramen of the obturator fascia. The obturator nerve is dissected free of its accompanying vessels with a nerve hook and is delivered out into the wound. One should be cautious not to tear accompanying vessels. The nerve is stimulated for positive identification.

Silk sutures (0000) are placed around the nerve, 1 cm. apart, and the nerve in between is excised. The deep retractors are removed, allowing the bladder and peritoneum to fall into place. The rectus sheath is closed. The opposite obturator nerve is resected following the same technique and the wound is closed in the usual manner. A bilateral long leg hip spica cast is applied immobilizing the lower limbs with the hips in 110 to 120 degrees abduction, neutral extension, and 10 to 15 degrees external rotation.

In three to four weeks, the hip spica cast is removed and active and passive exercises are begun. The same general principles of care are followed as outlined in adductor myotomy of the hips.

Abduction deformity of the hip with loss of active hip adduction is a very disabling complication. Pollock, in such an instance, recommends transfer of the origin of the hamstrings to the inferior ramus of the pubis and their insertion to the medial femoral condyle to "make" it a hip abductor.[148]

Pelvic obliquity in the postoperative period is a difficult problem that, if not prevented, will cause lumbar scoliosis and subluxation of the adducted hip. Several measures can be taken to deter this complication. Bilateral long leg casts should not be used following adductor myotomy, as they permit the pelvis to tilt. It is important to immobilize the hips in a bilateral long leg hip spica cast. Failure to recognize asymmetry of involvement is another cause; on the less affected side, adductor myotomy should be performed to a lesser extent. Even if all the preceding precautions are taken, pelvic obliquity may still result because of differences in recovery of hip abductor power following adductor myotomy. In the postoperative muscle re-education period this can usually be detected.

The Knee

The knee joint should not be regarded as an isolated problem in cerebral palsy since it is affected by deformities of the hip or ankle. The mechanism of the knee joint is complex because of the pressure of "two-joint" muscles, i.e., the hamstrings, which extend the hip and flex the knee; the gastrocnemius, which plantarflexes the ankle and flexes the knee; and the quadriceps (direct head of rectus femoris), which extends the knee and flexes the hip.

Disabilities of the knee encountered in spastic paralysis are: (1) flexion deformity, which may be fixed or functional; (2) extensor contracture due to spasticity of the quadriceps; (3) genu recurvatum; and (4) loss of complete active extension of the knee due to elongation of the patellar tendon.

FLEXION DEFORMITY

Flexion deformity is frequently present. It is imperative that one determine whether flexion deformity of the knee is *primary*, caused by spasticity and contracture of the hamstrings, *secondary*, to compensate for equinus deformity of the ankle and flexion deformity of the hip, or *functional*, to lower the center of gravity to achieve balance. One should carefully study the active and passive range of motion of the hip, knee, ankle, and foot, determining at which point the spastic muscles grab. The location of the patella should be determined; is it riding high owing to elongation of the patellar tendon? Are the patellar retinacula contracted? One should perform a complete muscle test in order to assess any imbalance between flexors and extensors of the knee. Stance and gait must be analyzed. Roentgenograms of the knee are taken to detect the presence of any structural bony changes in the proximal end of the tibia and the distal end of the femur.

Conservative measures in the treatment of flexion contracture of the knee consist of passive stretching of the hamstrings to prevent permanent shortening, active exercises to increase the motor strength of the quadriceps, and the use of a bivalved night cast, which holds the knee in extension and the ankle at neutral position.

Surgical procedures about the knee should be performed conservatively and with great caution. It is always safe to correct talipes equinus and hip deformities first. While performing adductor myotomy, the gracilis muscle is routinely lengthened. Postoperatively, hamstring stretching and the already described conservative measures are carried out. If, at 6 to 12 months following a thorough trial period of conservative treatment, the child still walks with the knees flexed and the hamstrings grab at 30 to 40 degrees on straight leg raising, or a flexion deformity of the knee persists, fractional lengthening of the hamstrings is performed, as advocated by Green.[70] The biceps femoris, the semimembranosus, and the semitendinosus are all lengthened. The operative procedure is presented in Plate 32.

It is recommended that the hamstrings not be lengthened at the same time that hip adductor myotomy and heel cord lengthening are performed. This is discouraged because only one third of the patients will require fractional lengthening of the hamstrings at a later date, and furthermore, postoperative training is made very difficult.

The author does not perform transfer of hamstring tendons to the femoral condyles as described and advocated by Eggers (Fig. 5–17).[57] In a certain percentage of cases, the Eggers hamstring transfer will cause varying degrees of genu recurvatum, decreased posterior pelvic support, increase in lumbar lordosis, and loss of knee flexion

(Text continued on page 824.)

Fractional Lengthening of Hamstrings

THE PROCEDURE

A. The patient is placed in prone position with a pneumatic tourniquet high on the proximal thigh. A 3 to 4 inch-long midline incision is made, starting just proximal to the popliteal crease. The subcutaneous tissue is divided and the incision carried to the deep fascia. The posterior femoral cutaneous nerve will be in the proximal aspect of the wound and should not be damaged.

B. The deep fascia is incised and the hamstring tendons are identified by blunt dissection. It is imperative to divide the tendon sheath of each hamstring tendon separately and mark it with 000 silk sutures for meticulous closure later.

C. In the lateral compartment of the wound, the biceps femoris tendon is exposed. It should be gently dissected away from the common peroneal nerve, which lies on its posteromedial surface. A blunt instrument, such as a staphylorrhaphy probe or a joker, is passed deep to the biceps tendon.

D. With a sharp knife, the tendinous portion of the biceps femoris is incised transversely at two levels, 3 cm. apart, leaving the muscle fibers intact. The tendon is lengthened in continuity by straight leg raising with the knee in extension.

Plate 32. Fractional Lengthening of Hamstrings

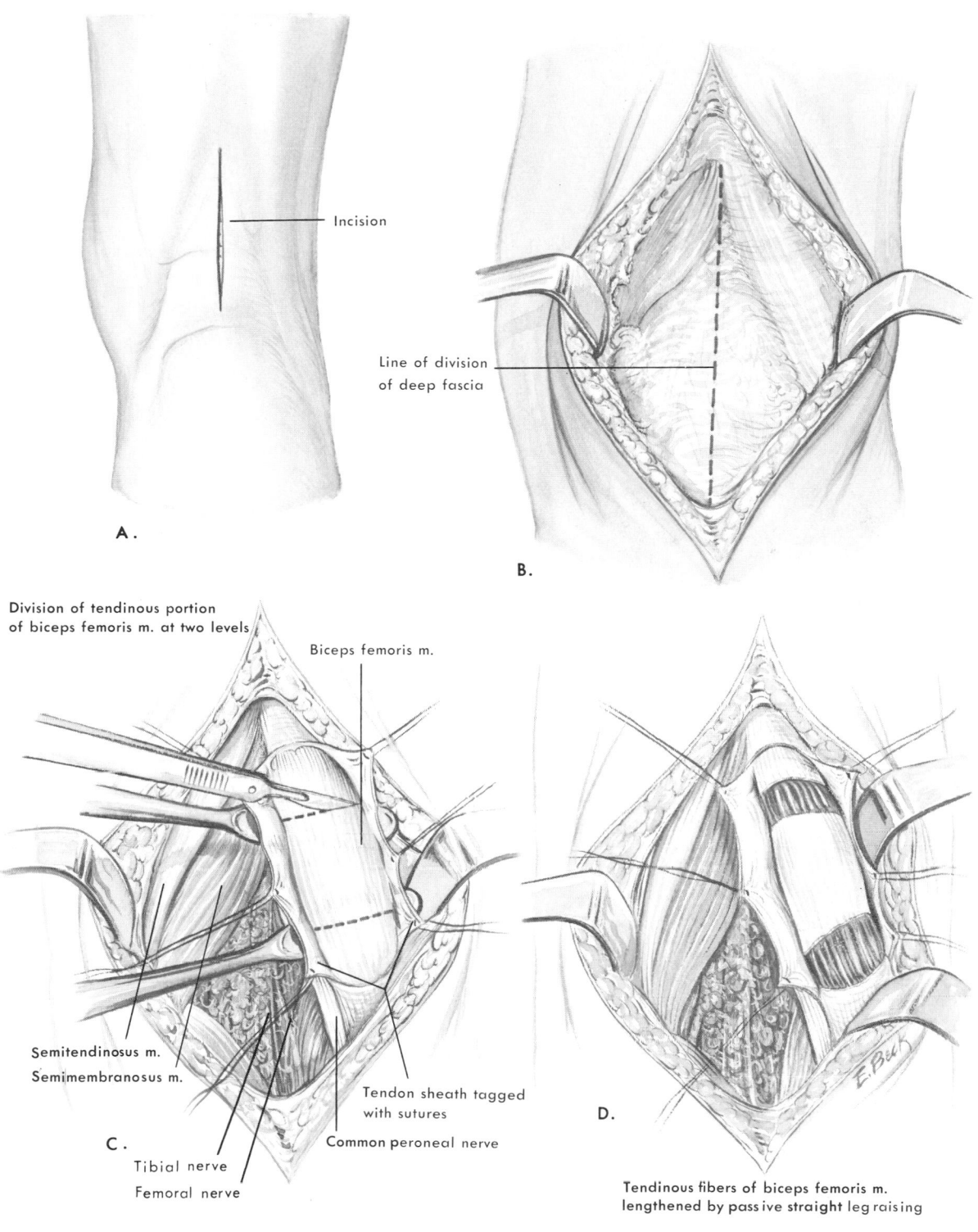

Incision

A.

Line of division
of deep fascia

B.

Division of tendinous portion
of biceps femoris m. at two levels

Biceps femoris m.

Semitendinosus m.
Semimembranosus m.

Tendon sheath tagged
with sutures

Common peroneal nerve

Tibial nerve
Femoral nerve

C.

D.

Tendinous fibers of biceps femoris m.
lengthened by passive straight leg raising

Fractional Lengthening of Hamstrings *(Continued)*

E. The semimembranosus tendon is then isolated in the medial compartment of the wound. The tendinous portion lies on its deep surface; to expose it the muscle is everted. The tendinous fibers are divided at two levels (similar to the biceps tendon), leaving the muscle fibers in continuity. Again, by extending the knee and flexing the hip, a sliding lengthening of the semimembranosus is performed.

F. Next, the semitendinosus is exposed. The tendinous portion is divided proximal to the musculotendinous junction.

G. If inadvertently the semitendinosus tendon ruptures, a Z-plasty is performed.

H. The tendon sheath of each tendon is meticulously closed. The deep fascia is not sutured. The subcutaneous tissue and skin are closed in routine manner and bilateral long leg casts are applied with the knees in full extension.

POSTOPERATIVE CARE

While the patient is in the solid cast, straight leg raising exercises are performed 15 times once a day for further stretching of the hamstrings. At the end of three to four weeks the casts are removed and new long leg bivalved casts are made. Active and passive exercises are performed to develop knee flexion, first side-lying with gravity eliminated and then against gravity. The motor strength of the quadriceps is developed. Whenever functional range of motion of the knees is present, the patient is allowed to be ambulatory with crutches.

Plate 32.   Fractional Lengthening of Hamstrings

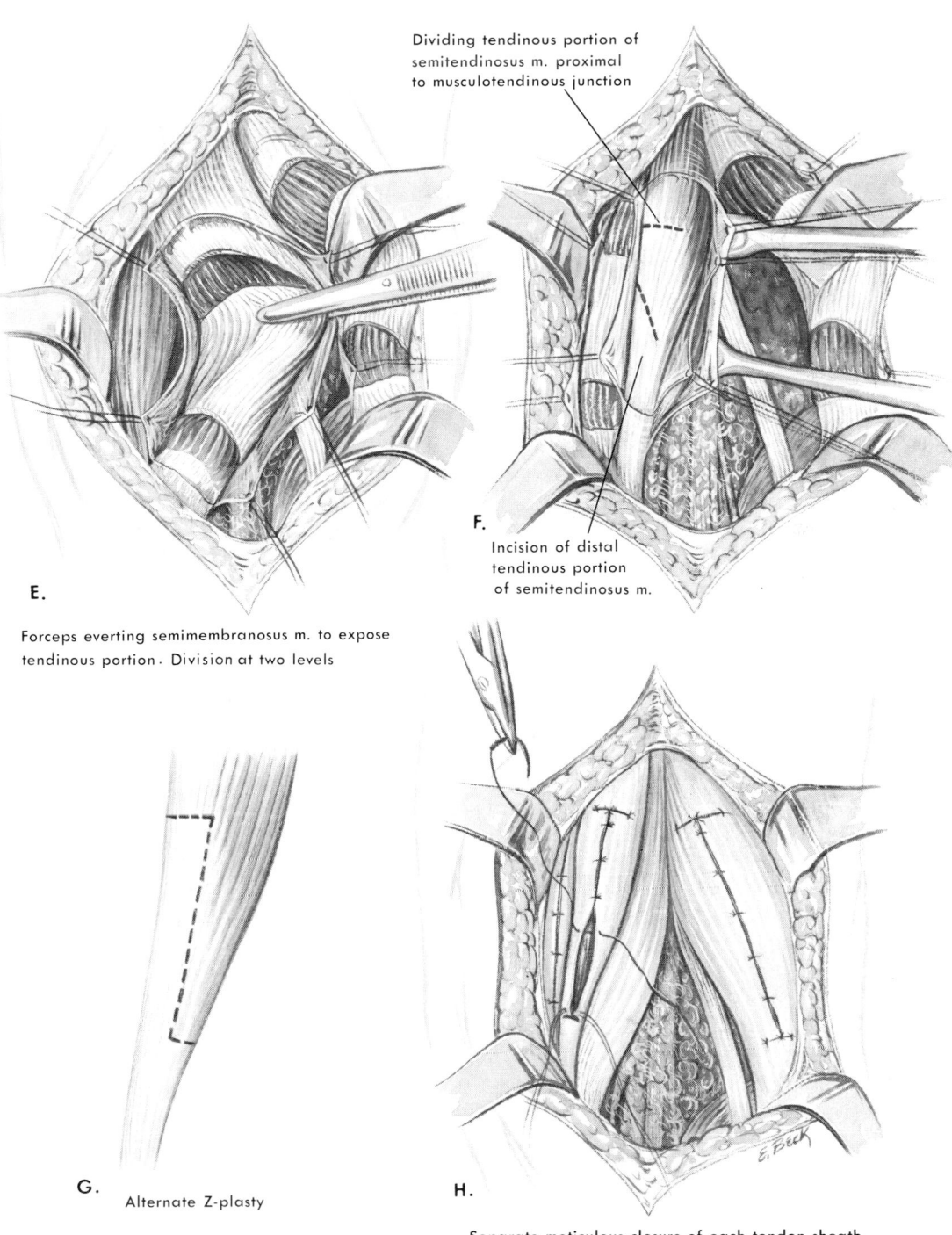

Dividing tendinous portion of
semitendinosus m. proximal
to musculotendinous junction

F.

Incision of distal
tendinous portion
of semitendinosus m.

E.

Forceps everting semimembranosus m. to expose
tendinous portion. Division at two levels

G.

Alternate Z-plasty

H.

Separate meticulous closure of each tendon sheath
Deep fascia is not sutured

power. Because of these complications, various authors have modified the original Eggers procedure. Pollock, for example, will preserve at least one hamstring, either the semitendinosus or semimembranosus.[149, 151]

Keats and Kambin perform a Z-lengthening of the biceps femoris.[102] Evans tenotomizes the gracilis, lengthens the biceps femoris and semimembranosus in their aponeurotic portion, and transfers only the semitendinosus to the ipsilateral femoral condyle.[60] Mortens performs the same modification as Evans.[128]

The hamstrings should have enough motor strength to balance the quadriceps. It is essential to maintain knee flexion

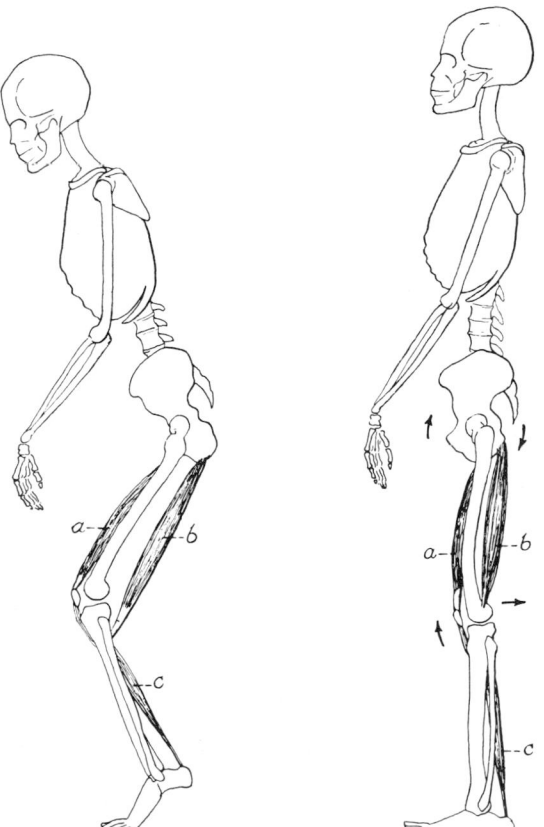

FIGURE 5–17. Egger's transfer of hamstrings to femoral condyles.

a. Quadriceps femoris muscle; *b.* hamstring muscles; *c.* soleus muscle. (*From* Eggers, G. N. M.: Transplantation of hamstring tendons to femoral condyles in order to improve hip extension and to decrease knee flexion in cerebral spastic paralysis. J. Bone Joint Surg., *34-A*:827, 1952.)

against gravity. Reciprocal hip and knee flexion and dorsiflexion of the ankle are essential for a normal gait pattern.

EXTENSION CONTRACTURE OF THE KNEE

This is caused by spasticity of the quadriceps femoris muscle. The child walks with a stiff extended knee with loss of normal reciprocal hip and knee flexion. In prone position with the hips in extension, the quadriceps muscle grabs on passive flexion of the knee. Upon further passive flexion of the knee, the pelvis will be elevated off the table because of the pelvic origin of the direct head of the rectus femoris (positive Ely test) (Fig. 5–18).

Treatment consists of passive stretching exercises of the spastic rectus femoris and active exercises to develop simultaneous knee and hip flexion in gait with dorsiflexion of the ankle. On occasion, the direct portion of the rectus femoris has to be released. The operative technique is as follows:

A 3 to 5 cm. longitudinal incision is made directly over the origin of the rectus femoris. Subcutaneous tissue and deep fascia are divided. The medial and lateral borders of the rectus femoris are identified and, with a blunt instrument, dissected free of adjacent tissues. A curved Kocher hemostat is inserted under the origin of the rectus femoris and the muscle is sharply divided. The wound is closed in the usual manner.

Postoperatively, the lower limbs are immobilized with the knees in 60 to 90 degrees of flexion for a period of two or three weeks. Active and passive exercises are performed to develop balance of motor strength between the extensors and flexors of the knee and reciprocal knee-hip flexion in gait. To maintain the lengthened position of the rectus femoris, the patient sleeps in a night cast for several months.

GENU RECURVATUM

In cerebral palsy, this is usually caused by spasticity of the quadriceps muscle or equinus deformity due to contracture of the triceps surae. It may be produced by Eggers transfer of the hamstrings to the femoral condyles or recession of the heads of the gastrocnemius, or by arresting the

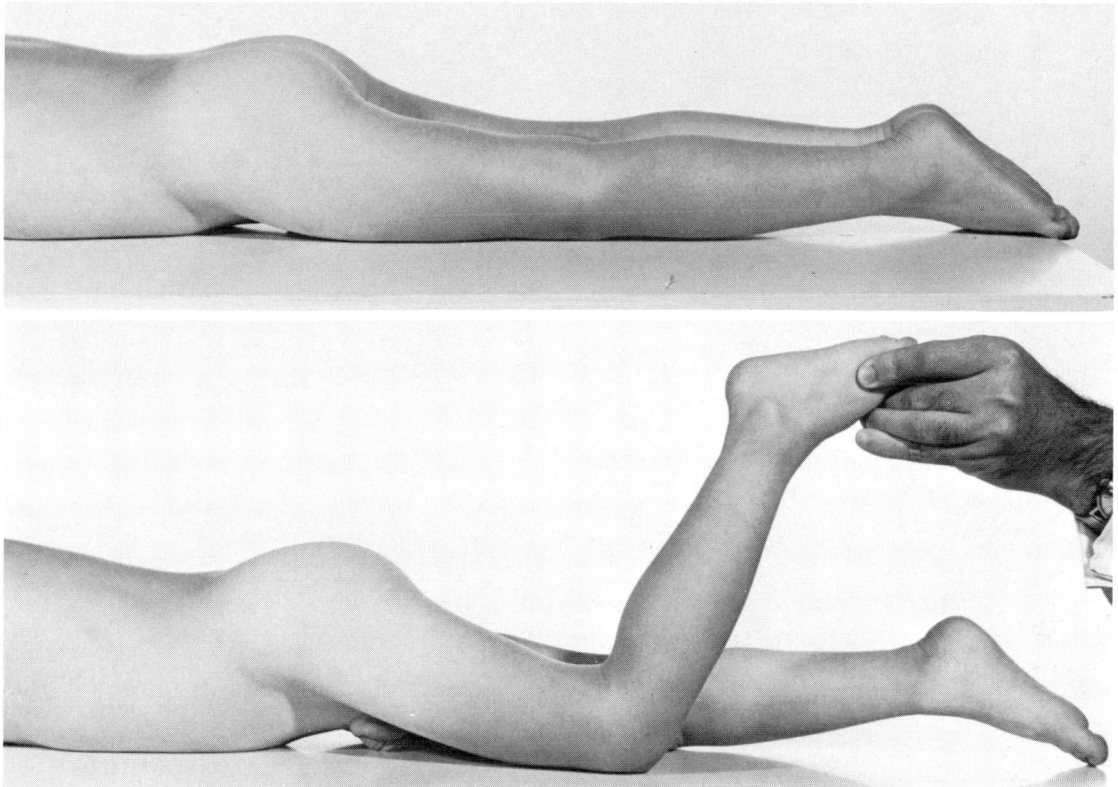

FIGURE 5-18. *Positive Ely test.*

In prone position, the quadriceps muscle will grab on passive flexion of the knee with the hips in extension. Upon further passive flexion of the knee, the pelvis will be elevated off the table because of the pelvic origin of the direct head of the rectus femoris muscle.

growth of the anterior part of the proximal tibial epiphyseal plate by performing distal transplantation of the proximal tibial tubercle. Genu recurvatum is a very difficult problem to treat. Equinus deformity, if present, should be corrected by heel cord lengthening, followed by an aggressive regimen of physical therapy to develop simultaneous knee flexion with dorsiflexion of the ankle. If the patient is uncooperative, use of an above-knee orthosis may be indicated to prevent hyperextension of the knee. In the adolescent with marked genu recurvatum, osteotomy of the proximal tibia and fibula or of the distal femur may be indicated.

ELONGATED PATELLAR TENDON AND QUADRICEPS FEMORIS INSUFFICIENCY

When the patellar tendon is elongated and the patella is high-riding, there will be loss of full active extension of the knee joint. In such a case, the patellar tendon may be plicated or transferred distally to correct the deformity. However, it is imperative that knee flexion deformity and contracture of the hamstrings be corrected prior to advancing the patella distally. If, following fractional lengthening of the hamstrings, the patient is still unable to completely extend the knee and there is still quadriceps insufficiency that causes the patient to stumble or fall, a Chandler patellar advancement operation is indicated. This operative technique is described in Plate 33.

The Upper Limb

In spastic paralysis, the upper limb is usually characterized by the following deformities: thumb-in-palm, flexion of the fingers and wrist, pronation of the forearm,

Patellar Advancement by Plication of Patellar Tendon and Division of Patellar Retinacula

THE PROCEDURE

A. A transverse skin incision is made, centering over the knee joint and extending from the medial to the lateral condyle of the femur. Subcutaneous tissue and fascia are divided in line with the skin incision.

B. The wound flaps are retracted proximally and distally, exposing the high-riding patella, elongated patellar tendon, and patellar retinacula.

C. The wound flaps are approximated, and through separate stab wounds in the skin, a large threaded Steinmann pin is inserted transversely through the center of the patella and a similar pin is placed in the proximal tibia. The distal pin should be drilled from the lateral side and should be directed somewhat anteroposteriorly to prevent pressure irritation of the common peroneal nerve.

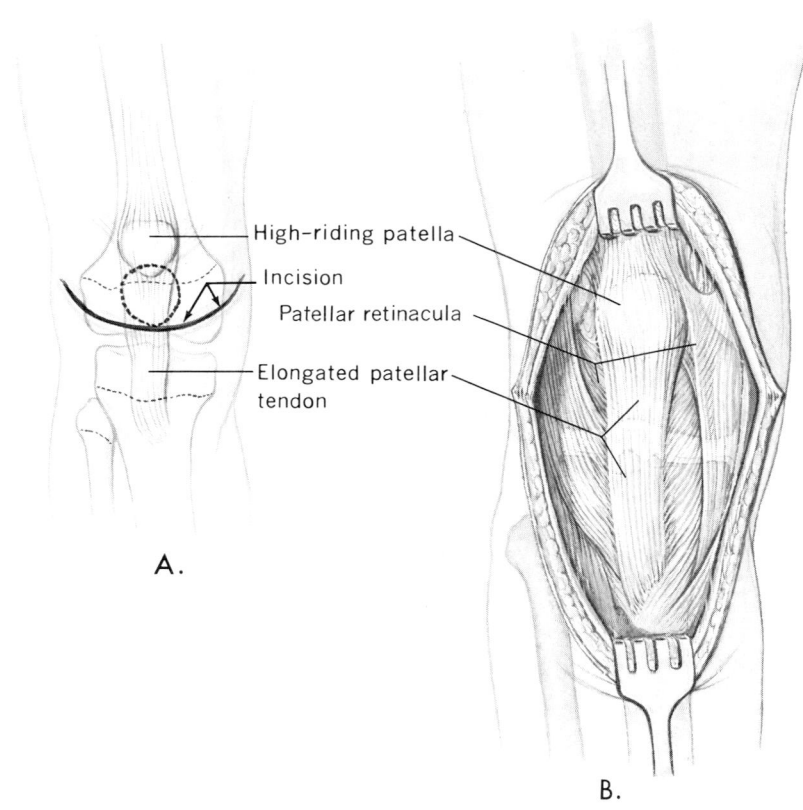

A.

High-riding patella

Incision

Patellar retinacula

Elongated patellar tendon

B.

C.

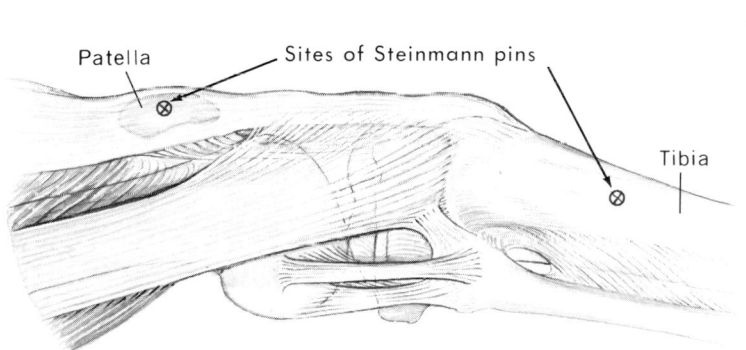

Patella

Sites of Steinmann pins

Tibia

Patellar Advancement by Plication of Patellar Tendon and Division of Patellar Retinacula *(Continued)*

D. The medial and lateral margins of the patellar tendon are identified. Longitudinal incisions are made on each side of the tendon, which is isolated and mobilized from subjacent and surrounding structures. Care should be taken not to open the capsule of the knee joint. Next, the patellar retinacula are divided medially and laterally.

E. The patella is pulled distally to its normal position in the intercondylar notch by traction on the proximal pin and manual pressure. The two pins are securely held together by a plate or Roger Anderson apparatus. The patellar tendon is thoroughly freed from the underlying fat pad.

F. The patellar tendon is plicated, shortening it to the desired length. Its plicated ends are sutured together with 00 silk. Any bulky segment of the tendon is excised, if necessary. The wound is closed in layers and a long leg cast is applied, which holds the knee in 5 to 10 degrees of hyperextension. The pins are covered with petrolatum gauze to prevent skin slough from being incorporated in the cast. Adequate padding should be applied to prevent pressure sores.

POSTOPERATIVE CARE

About four to six weeks after surgery, the cast and pins are removed. Active and passive exercises are performed to regain muscle strength and range of motion. Weight-bearing is gradual and is protected with crutches. Full weight-bearing is allowed when the quadriceps is fair in motor strength.

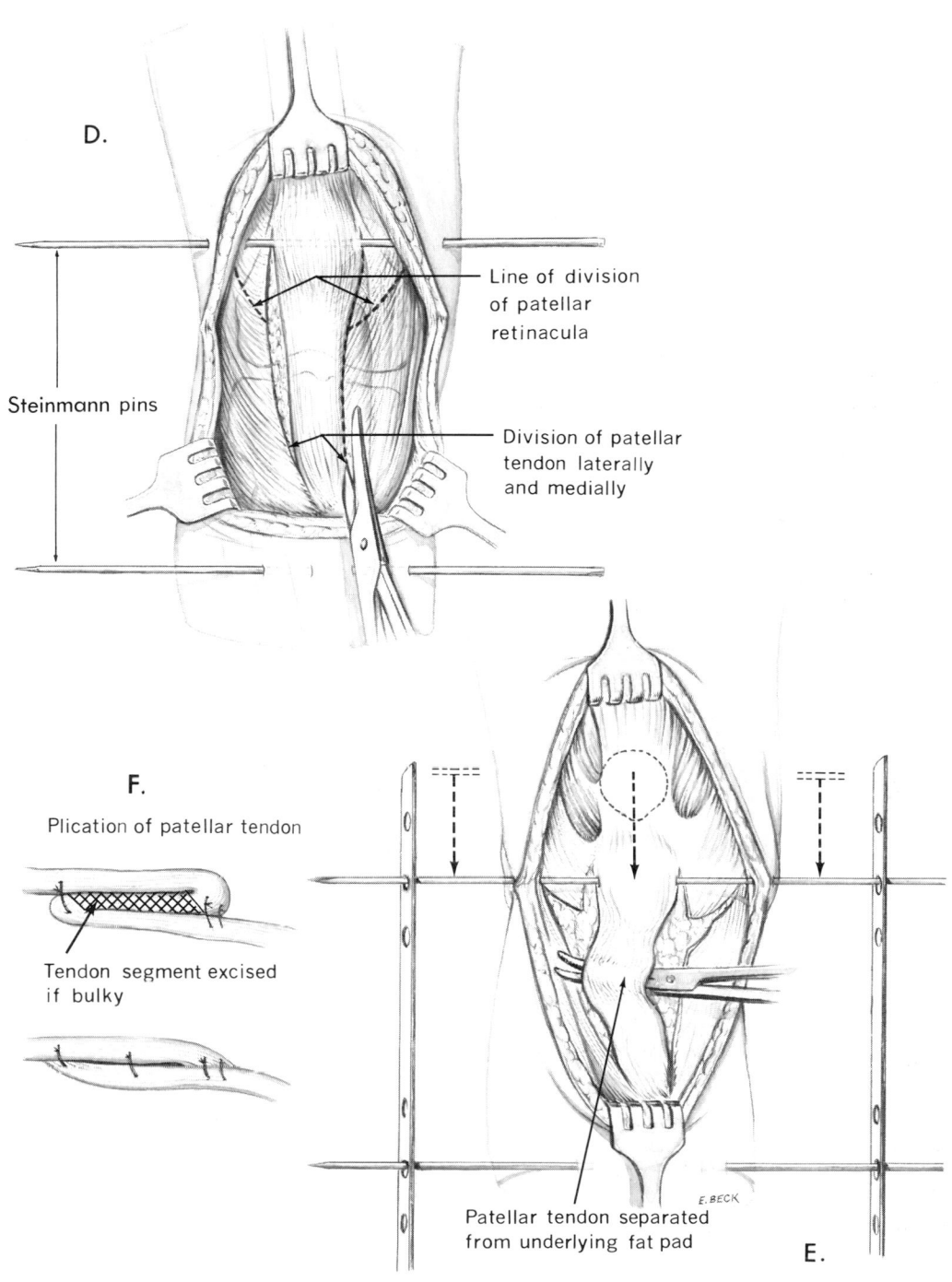

D.

Steinmann pins

Line of division
of patellar
retinacula

Division of patellar
tendon laterally
and medially

F.

Plication of patellar tendon

Tendon segment excised
if bulky

Patellar tendon separated
from underlying fat pad

E. BECK

E.

flexion of the elbow, and adduction and internal rotation of the shoulder.

The primary purpose of treatment of the upper limb in cerebral palsy is to improve function, i.e., reach, grasp, and release with the hand. Function in the upper limb is more complicated than that of the lower limb, demanding finely coordinated motions and good muscular control. As a rule, surgical measures in the upper limb should be delayed until maturation of the central nervous system permits adequate functional training in the postoperative period. Astereognosis may hinder functional use of the hand. Coordination and cerebral control are not provided by surgical measures. In the hemiplegic child, the presence of a contralateral normal hand is not a contraindication for surgery on the involved hand.

Occasionally cosmetic appearance becomes a consideration for surgical intervention. In an adolescent female, the acutely flexed wrist and clenched fingers in the palm may be very disturbing psychologically. Cosmetic improvement effected by placing the hand in a nearly normal position may be indicated despite poor functional potential.

These deformities are discussed individually.

THUMB-IN-PALM DEFORMITY

Thumb-in-palm deformity results from spasticity and contracture of the adductor pollicis or spasticity of the flexors of the thumb, or both. It is very disabling, as the thumb is in a poor position for effective function. Pulp-to-pulp action and lateral pinch are lost. Grasp is hindered and entry of objects into the palm is blocked. In some patients, particularly those with tension athetosis, the thumb-in-palm position stimulates the so-called "gripping reflex," in which the fingers are clenched in the palm over the thumb (Fig. 5–19 A). On hyperflexion of the wrist, the fingers and thumb extend out of the palm (Fig. 5–19 B).

Stretching of the capsule may cause instability of the metacarpophalangeal joint of the thumb, resulting in hypermobility and subluxation, which interfere with complete extension of the thumb. Soft-tissue contracture in the web between the thumb and index metacarpals may develop in

severe deformities; if left untreated, it will eventually cause subluxation of the carpometacarpal joint.

Treatment of thumb-in-palm deformity is by passive stretching exercises to place the thumb metacarpal into abduction and the whole thumb into extension. A persistent regimen of such therapy will prevent development of myostatic contracture and fixed deformity.

As soon as the child is old enough, normally by two or three years of age, a well-fitted opponens splint is used, which holds the thumb metacarpal in maximal abduction and the thumb phalanges in extension (Fig. 5–20). This opponens splint is worn in the night bivalved cast, which holds the wrist in dorsiflexion and the forearm in full supination. Attempts to hold the thumb in corrected position in the bivalved long arm cast are usually unsuccessful and often result in deformity, as the thumb slips proximally through the cast and causes subluxation of the metacarpophalangeal joint (Fig. 5–21).

Adductor release of the thumb is indicated when the child is five years of age and thumb-in-palm deformity persists despite adequate conservative management. The author prefers tenotomy of the adductor pollicis at its insertion by the technique shown in Plate 34. The procedure is usually performed at the same time as flexor carpi ulnaris transfer. Some surgeons prefer to release the adductor pollicis and intrinsic muscles of the thumb at their origin.[172] The operative technique is as follows:

A curvilinear incision is made in the palm along the thenar crease. Injury to the muscular branch of the ulnar nerve in the hand should be avoided; it is a short stout nerve that branches out from the radial side of the median and supplies the abductor pollicis brevis, opponens pollicis, and the superficial head of the flexor pollicis brevis. By appropriate retraction, the origins of the transverse and oblique heads of the adductor pollicis are identified and released by blunt dissection with a periosteal elevator. The transverse head of the adductor pollicis takes its origin from a broad base on the distal two thirds of the volar surface of the third metacarpal, whereas the oblique head of the adductor pollicis arises from the bases of the second and third meta-

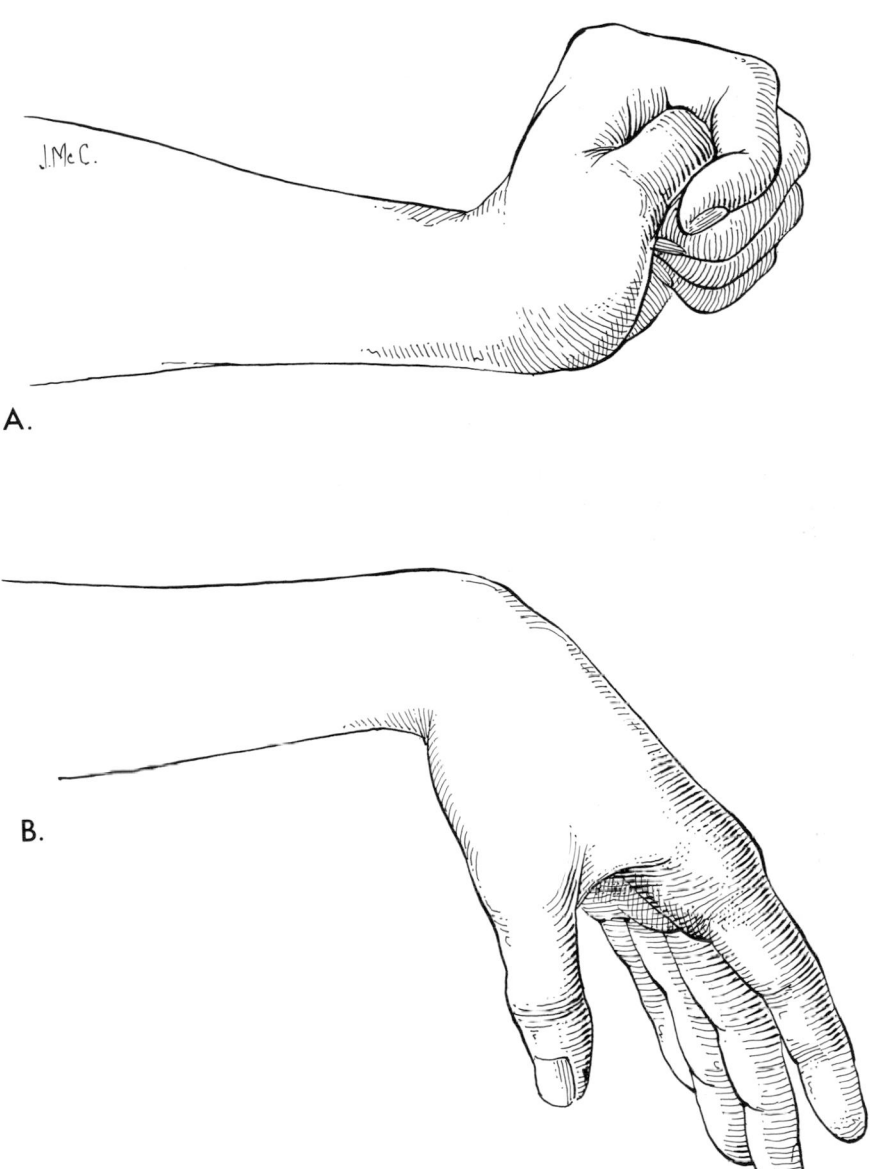

FIGURE 5-19. *Thumb-in-palm deformity in the spastic hand.*

A. Note the fingers are clenched in the palm over the thumb. **B.** On hyperflexion of the wrist, the fingers and thumb extend out of the palm.

carpal bones, from the capitate bone, and from the sheath of the tendon of the flexor carpi radialis. The deep palmar branch of the ulnar nerve is the motor nerve of the adductor pollicis; it should be protected from inadvertent injury. Perforating branches of the radial artery should be avoided. Next, if necessary, the flexor pollicis brevis, opponens pollicis, and abductor pollicis brevis muscles are recessed distally by division and elevation of their origin from the volar carpal ligament. The

tourniquet is released and, after complete hemostasis is obtained, the wound is closed in the usual manner. A long arm cast is applied with the *thumb metacarpal* (not the phalanges) in maximal abduction and the thumb in a posture of functional opposition.

Those who advocate release of the spastic adductor pollicis at its origin claim that it maintains power of thumb adduction, which is very important functionally. With myotomy of the thumb adductor at its insertion, however, loss of active thumb adduction

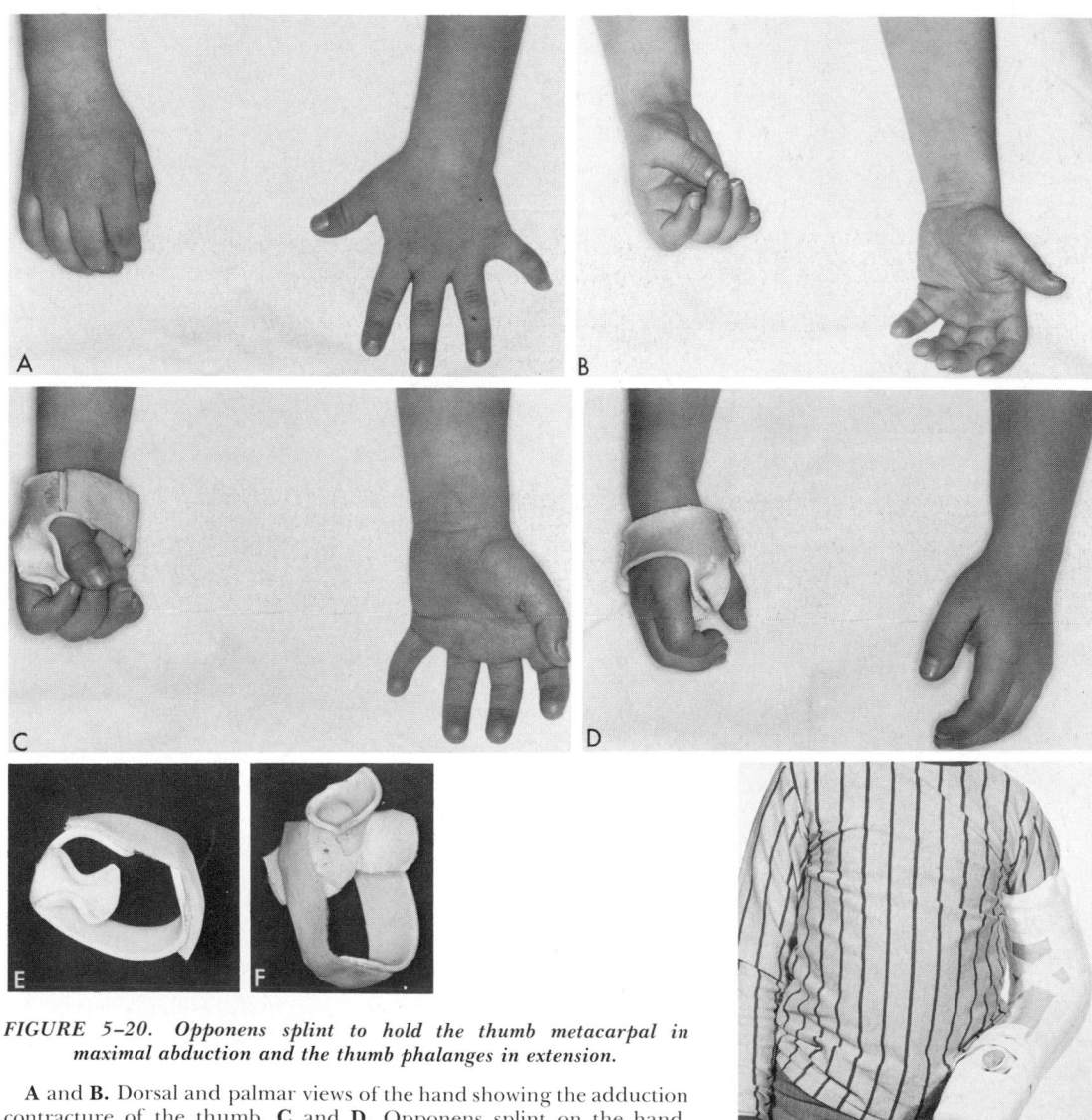

FIGURE 5–20. *Opponens splint to hold the thumb metacarpal in maximal abduction and the thumb phalanges in extension.*

A and **B.** Dorsal and palmar views of the hand showing the adduction contracture of the thumb. **C** and **D.** Opponens splint on the hand. **E** and **F.** Views of the opponens splint. **G.** The opponens splint is worn at night in a bivalved cast, which holds the wrist in dorsiflexion and the forearm in full supination.

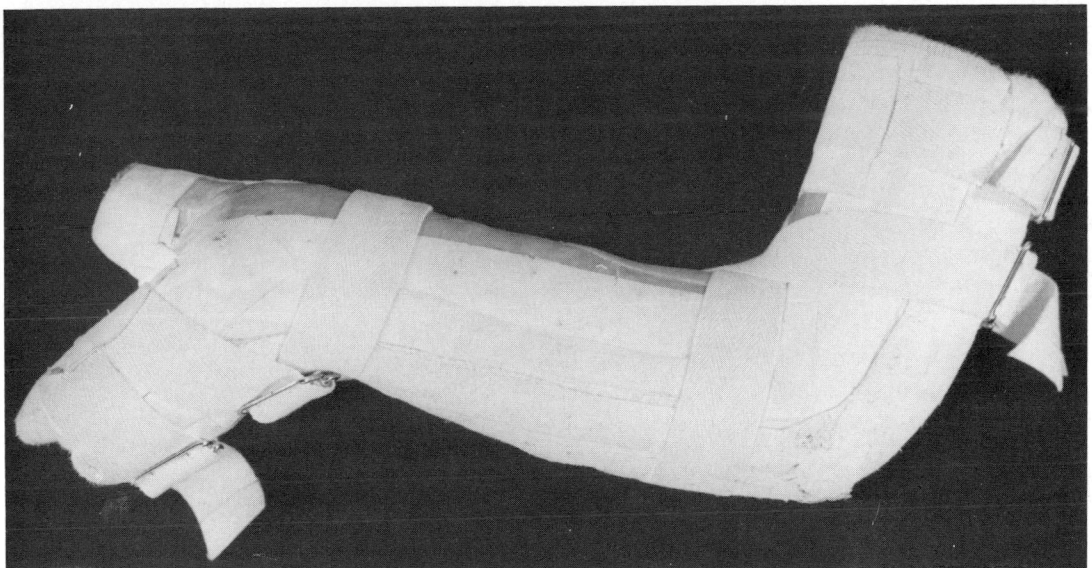

FIGURE 5-21. *Bivalved long arm cast without opponens splint.*

Often the thumb will slip proximally through the cast and cause subluxation of the metacarpophalangeal joint.

has not become a complication, and technically the procedure is much easier.

Neurectomy of the motor branches of the ulnar and median nerves to the adductor pollicis and intrinsic muscles of the thumb should not be performed.

After 6 to 12 months of aggressive therapy, if the thumb abductors and extensors continue to be cerebral zero in function and active voluntary motion does not develop, a tendon transfer to enhance their function should be considered. This should not be done simultaneously with adductor myotomy of the thumb, as release of the spastic adductor pollicis and proper postoperative training may be adequate to gain thumb abduction.

Prior to tendon transfers to the abductor and extensor pollicis, there should be full passive abduction of the first metacarpal and full passive extension of the thumb. The metacarpophalangeal joint of the thumb should be stable. If the flexor pollicis longus is very spastic and contracted, it is passively stretched in a corrective cast; on occasion, especially in recalcitrant cases, fractional lengthening of the flexor pollicis longus in the forearm is indicated.

In children, subluxation of the metacarpophalangeal joint of the thumb is treated by capsulorrhaphy. Growth of the physis of the first phalanx of the thumb is proximal; this should not be disturbed. The deformity is usually one of hyperextension of the metacarpophalangeal joint. The whole width of the capsule on the volar surface is dissected free from the head of the first metacarpal (its growth plate is proximal) and, with the metacarpophalangeal joint in hyperflexion, is reattached proximally to the metacarpal bone with 0 silk suture through two drill holes. One or two smooth Kirschner wires may be inserted across the metacarpophalangeal joint to maintain its hyperflexed position securely. The thumb is immobilized in a below-elbow or above-elbow cast (length of the cast depending upon the associated deformities) for a period of six weeks. Then the cast and Kirschner wires are removed and active exercises are started. A splint is worn at night to maintain the flexed position of the metacarpophalangeal joint of the thumb and to prevent recurrence of deformity. The interphalangeal joint of the thumb should be in only 5 degrees of flexion.

In those of an older age group in whom growth is completed, arthrodesis of the metacarpophalangeal joint of the thumb is performed when there is marked hypermobility and gross subluxation. Fusion is

Adductor Myotomy of the Thumb

THE PROCEDURE

A and **B.** A 2 to 3 cm. long oblique incision is made over the dorsum of the hand. It begins at the ulnar border of the first metacarpal head, extends proximally to the middle third of the metacarpal, and then swings ulnarward toward the base of the second metacarpal. One should avoid the distal margin of the thumb web, as the cicatrix may cause contracture of the web. This surgical approach permits stripping of the first dorsal interosseous muscle if necessary. When only an adductor tenotomy is to be done, an alternate approach is a 1.5 to 2 cm. long transverse incision immediately proximal to the flexor crease of the thumb. Again, the ulnar border of the incision should stop short of the distal margin of the thumb web. (When a Z-plasty of the contracted thumb web is indicated, a transverse skin incision is made at the distal border of the web, extending between the ulnar border of the proximal flexion crease of the thumb and the radial border of the proximal transverse crease of the palm, and two oblique cuts at a 45- to 60-degree angle are made for Z-lengthening.)

C. The subcutaneous tissue is divided. The first dorsal interosseous muscle is retracted proximally, and the tendon of the adductor pollicis is identified near its insertion.

D. With a staphylorrhaphy elevator, the adductor pollicis longus tendon is lifted dorsally and 1 cm. of the adductor tendon is excised near its insertion. Care should be exercised not to disturb the tendon mechanism of the extensors and the abductors of the thumb.

If the first dorsal interosseous muscle is contracted, it is stripped from the metacarpal with a periosteal elevator through the same incision.

The wound is closed in routine manner. A well-molded cast is applied to hold the thumb metacarpal in maximal abduction, the metacarpophalangeal joint in neutral extension, and the interphalangeal joint in 10 degrees of flexion.

POSTOPERATIVE CARE

Three weeks after surgery the cast is bivalved and an opponens splint is made to hold the thumb in a position of maximal abduction and functional opposition. Active exercises are begun to develop active motion of the thumb in all directions— adduction, abduction, opposition, flexion, and extension. Passive exercises are also performed to maintain maximal range of motion. In the beginning two weeks, the opponens splint is worn continuously, except during the exercise periods; later the use of the splint is gradually decreased and an aggressive regimen of occupational therapy is instituted to develop function.

Plate 34. Adductor Myotomy of the Thumb

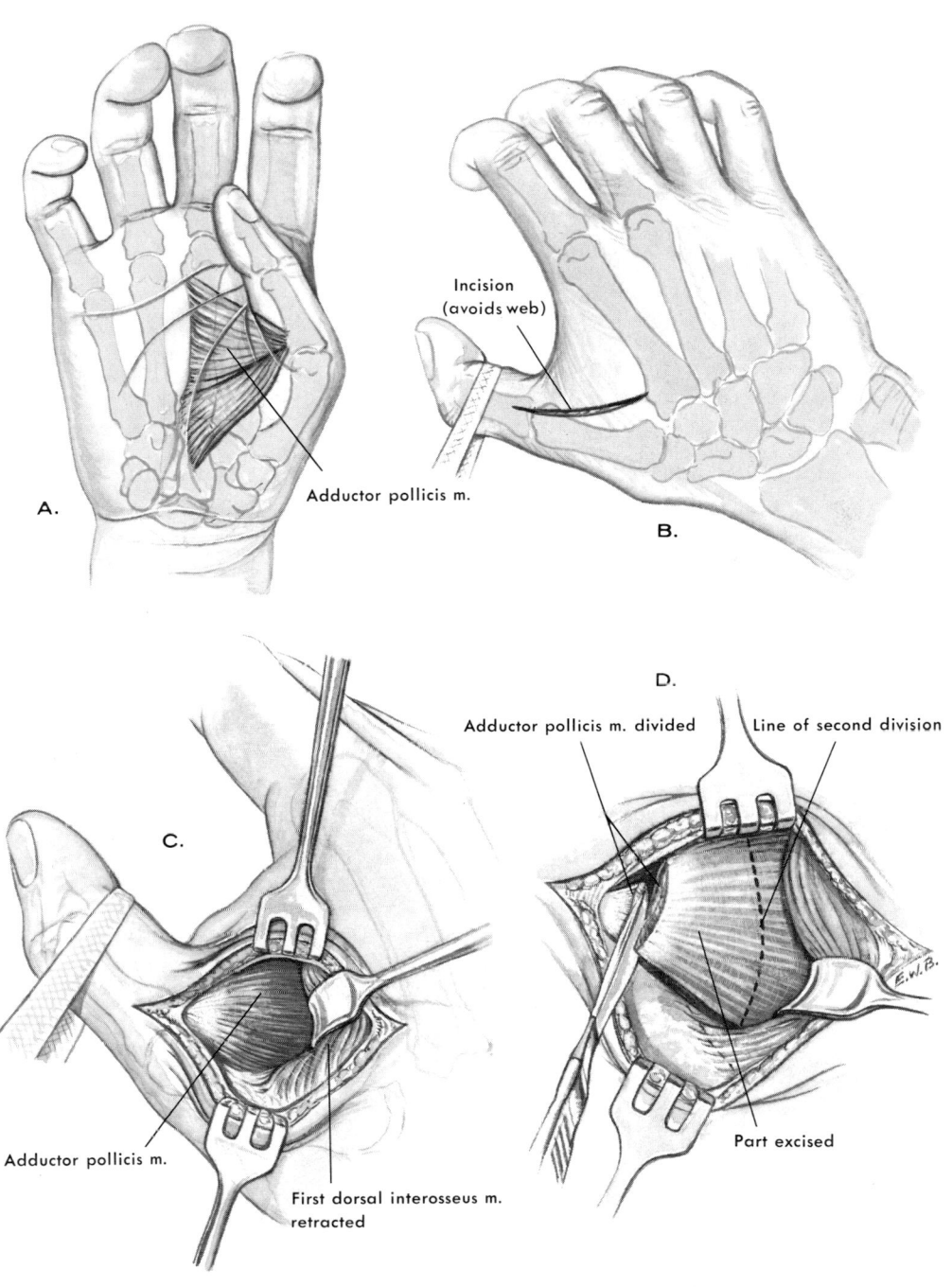

A.

Adductor pollicis m.

Incision
(avoids web)

B.

C.

Adductor pollicis m.

First dorsal interosseus m.
retracted

D.

Adductor pollicis m. divided

Line of second division

Part excised

E.W.B.

achieved by excising the articular cartilage and utilizing the "peg" technique. Criss-cross Kirschner wires are inserted for secure fixation.

TENDON TRANSFERS FOR THUMB ABDUCTION AND EXTENSION

The motor muscles usually available for transfer are the brachioradialis, the flexor digitorum sublimis of the ring or long finger, and the flexor carpi radialis.

In spastic paralysis, the brachioradialis muscle is usually strong and under voluntary control. The amplitude of excursion of the divided tendon of the brachioradialis is approximately 1.5 cm. After thorough mobilization of the muscle from its surrounding fascia, its amplitude can be increased to 3 cm. The nerve and blood supply enter the brachioradialis muscle above the lateral epicondyle of the humerus; this allows thorough mobilization of the brachioradialis muscle without endangering its neurovascular supply. The surgical technique of brachioradialis transfer is illustrated in Plate No. 35.

If the flexor digitorum sublimis of the ring or long finger is used for a motor, the tendon is sectioned at the wrist and the distal end of the proximal segment sutured to the extensor pollicis longus and abductor pollicis brevis tendons in the same manner.

The flexor carpi radialis ordinarily should not be used as a motor if the flexor carpi ulnaris is transferred to the extensor carpi radialis or if there is the possibility of such a transfer in the future. Such a transfer will increase ulnar deviation of the wrist, which often is an already existing deformity of the spastic hand; also, it is best to maintain the action of a wrist flexor.

An intermetacarpal bone block between the first and second metacarpals or between the first and third metacarpals to place the thumb metacarpal rigidly in maximal abduction and opposition is not recommended in the spastic hand, as it often hinders its functional use.

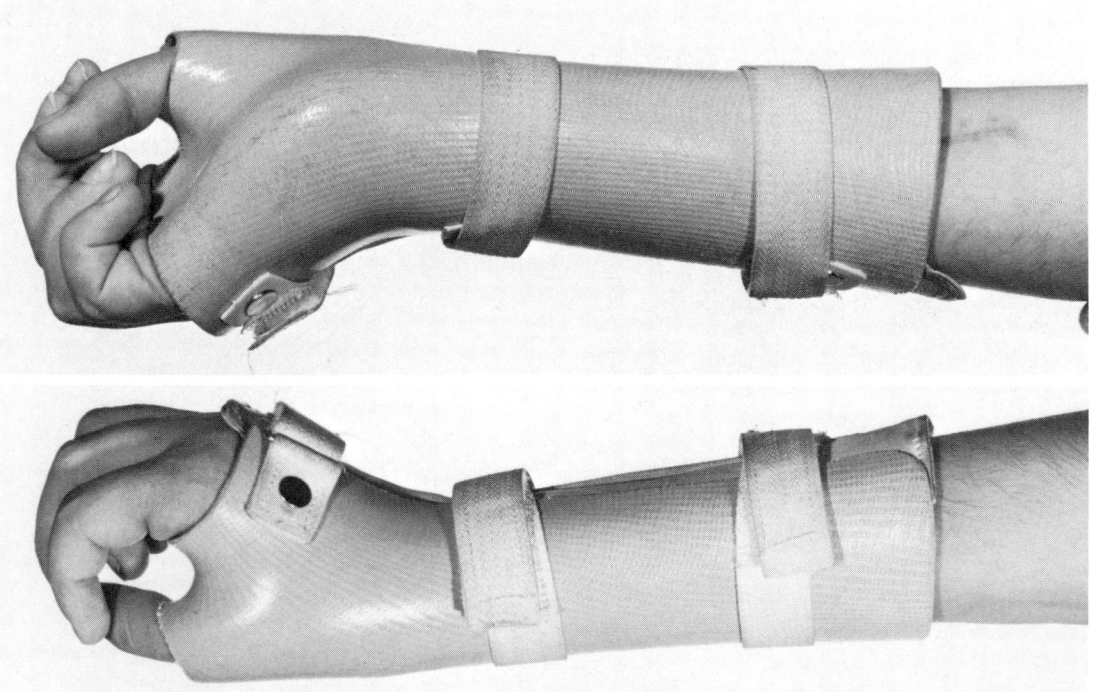

FIGURE 5–22.   Below-elbow plastic splint worn following flexor carpi ulnaris transfer.

In the postoperative period the splint holds the wrist in 45 degrees dorsiflexion and the thumb in maximal abduction and opposition.

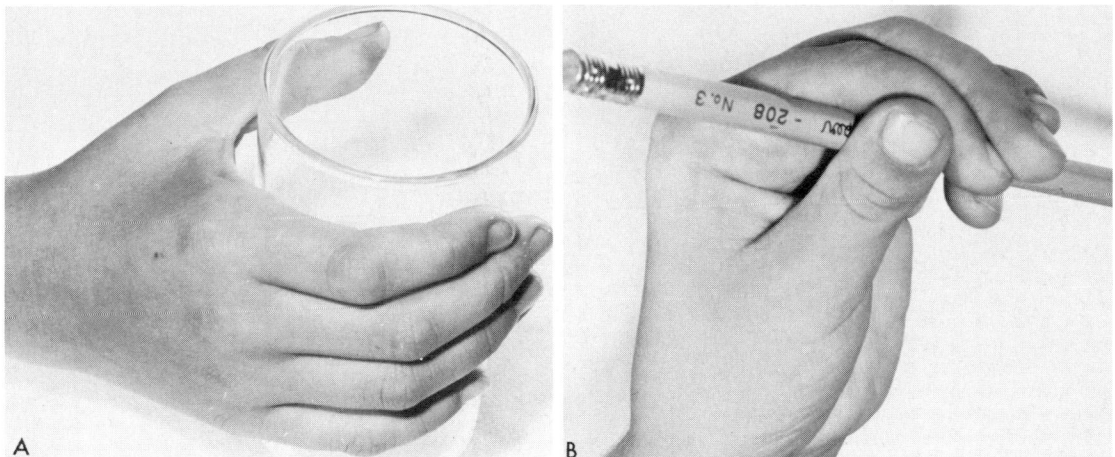

FIGURE 5-23. *Functional therapy for thumb abduction (A) and adduction (B).*

This is important following brachioradialis transfer to extensor pollicis longus and abductor pollicis brevis tendon.

FINGER DEFORMITIES

Flexion Deformity. Flexion at the metacarpophalangeal and interphalangeal joints is the common deformity in the spastic hand. It is caused by spasticity and myostatic contracture of the flexor digitorum profundus and sublimis muscles. This is usually associated with flexion deformity of the wrist due to spasticity of the wrist flexors and pronation contracture of the forearm. Flexion deformity of the digits is increased by extension of the wrist, and it is diminished on hyperflexion of the wrist. With the wrist in maximal flexion, there will be a varying degree of active extension of the fingers out of the palm. Fixed joint contractures are usually not present.

Conservative methods of treatment should always be attempted prior to consideration of surgery.

If flexion deformity is severe, it is best to apply a corrective long arm solid cast to stretch the flexion contracture of the digits and wrist and pronation contracture of the forearm. The thumb is placed in abduction and extension. The metacarpophalangeal and interphalangeal joints of the fingers are held in some flexion to prevent the disabling hyperextension deformity. Stretching of the finger flexors is accomplished by *progressive extension of the wrist* and by changing the cast weekly or biweekly. The

deformity is corrected gradually and the cast is well padded to prevent pressure sores. In about four to six weeks, a fair degree of correction can be obtained. Then a bivalved cast is made for night use and passive stretching exercises are performed several times a day to maintain the correction. Active exercises are performed to develop voluntary finger control.

Surgical measures are indicated if preceding conservative measures fail. The author prefers fractional lengthening of the finger and wrist flexors in the forearm. The operative technique is described and illustrated in Plate 36.

Release of the flexor-pronator origin for flexion deformities of the hand and wrist was originally described by Page.[133] Later, Inglis and Cooper evaluated their experience with 18 cases.[85] The procedure requires extensive soft-tissue and nerve dissection, creates antecubital and forearm dead space, and may cause supination contracture of the forearm due to loss of pronator power. Because of these possible complications, flexor-pronator origin release should not be routinely performed. Fractional lengthening of the flexors in the forearm is a much simpler procedure. The surgical technique as described by Inglis and Cooper is as follows:

The incision begins 5 cm. proximal to the medial epicondyle, curving radially at

(Text continued on page 846.)

Brachioradialis Transfer to Restore Thumb Abduction and Extension

THE PROCEDURE

A. A long dorsoradial incision is made, beginning at the radial styloid process and extending proximally to a point 2 cm. distal to the lateral epicondyle of the humerus. The subcutaneous tissue is divided and the wound edges are undermined and retracted.

B and **C.** The flat tendon of the brachioradialis is sectioned at its insertion into the base of the styloid process of the radius. The tendons of the abductor pollicis longus and extensor pollicis brevis are divided at their musculotendinous junction and marked with 00 silk whip sutures as they traverse from the dorsal to the volar aspect on the brachioradialis tendon. Injury to neurovascular structures should be avoided. The radial artery lies on the volar margin of the brachioradialis tendon, and on the ulnar side of the radial vessels is the flexor carpi radialis tendon. The radial nerve runs along the lateral aspect of the forearm deep to the brachioradialis muscle. In the upper third of the forearm, the nerve is radial to the radial artery; in the middle of the forearm it is immediately lateral to the artery, whereas in the lower third of the forearm the superficial branch of the nerve curves dorsally underneath the brachioradialis tendon to divide into the medial or lateral branches after penetrating the deep fascia on the dorsum of the wrist.

Plate 35. *Brachioradialis Transfer to Restore Thumb Abduction and Extension*

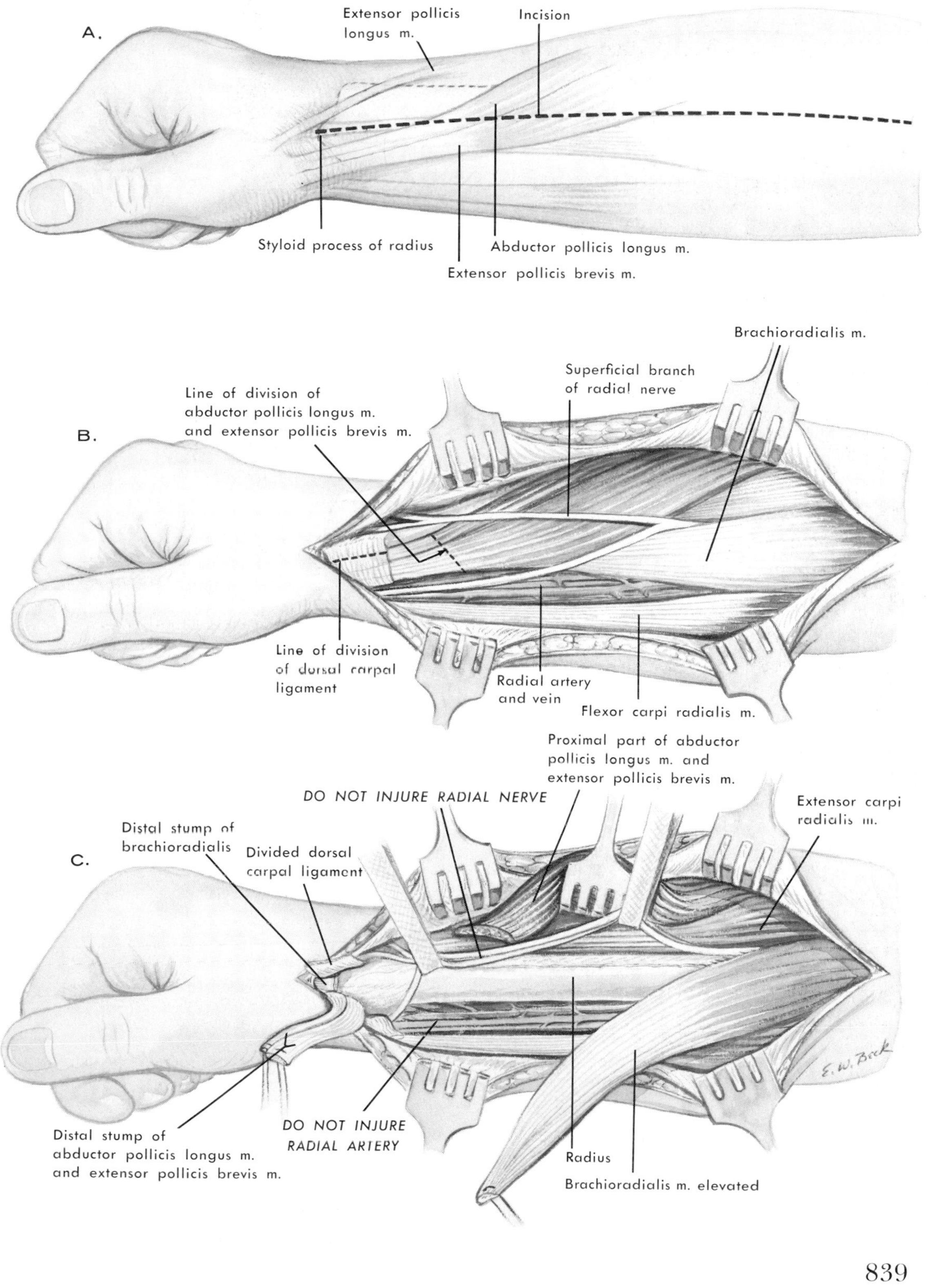

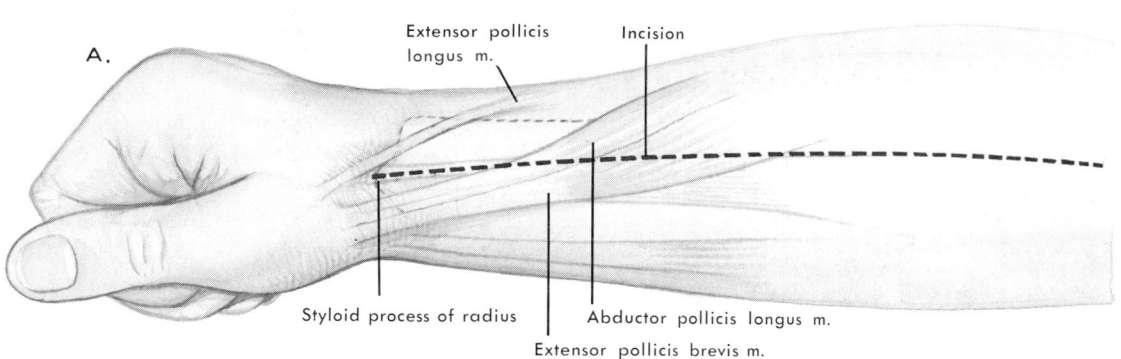

A.

Extensor pollicis longus m.

Incision

Styloid process of radius

Abductor pollicis longus m.

Extensor pollicis brevis m.

B.

Line of division of abductor pollicis longus m. and extensor pollicis brevis m.

Superficial branch of radial nerve

Brachioradialis m.

Line of division of dorsal carpal ligament

Radial artery and vein

Flexor carpi radialis m.

C.

Distal stump of brachioradialis

Divided dorsal carpal ligament

Proximal part of abductor pollicis longus m. and extensor pollicis brevis m.

DO NOT INJURE RADIAL NERVE

Extensor carpi radialis m.

Distal stump of abductor pollicis longus m. and extensor pollicis brevis m.

DO NOT INJURE RADIAL ARTERY

Radius

Brachioradialis m. elevated

E. W. Beck

Brachiorahialis Transfer to Restore Thumb Abduction and Extension (Continued)

D. By sharp and dull dissection, the brachioradialis muscle is freed from the antebrachial fascia and the adjacent muscles (extensor carpi radialis dorsally and flexor carpi ulnaris anteriorly). It is imperative to mobilize the brachioradialis as proximally as possible (preferably immediately distal to the elbow joint) to gain maximal excursion of the muscle action and to have a straight line of muscle pull.

E. The extensor pollicis longus and abductor pollicis brevis tendons are sutured to the brachioradialis tendon by interrupted 00 silk sutures, and the tendon ends interwoven. The tension on the transferred tendon should be moderate, so that the first metacarpal can be passively adducted 1.5 cm. from the palm with the wrist in neutral position and passive pulp pinch is possible between the thumb and index finger. The wound is closed in layers and a long arm cast is applied with the elbow in 90 degrees of flexion, the wrist in neutral position, the first metacarpal in maximal abduction, and the thumb in neutral extension.

POSTOPERATIVE CARE

Three to four weeks following surgery, the cast is removed and active exercises are performed to develop function of the transferred brachioradialis muscle as an abductor and extensor of the thumb. Passive exercises are performed to maintain full range of motion of the joint. In the beginning a short arm splint is worn to maintain the thumb metacarpal in maximum abduction (see Fig. 5–22). Functional therapy is very important, such as holding water glasses of various sizes for thumb abduction and holding a pencil for thumb adduction (see Fig. 5–23).

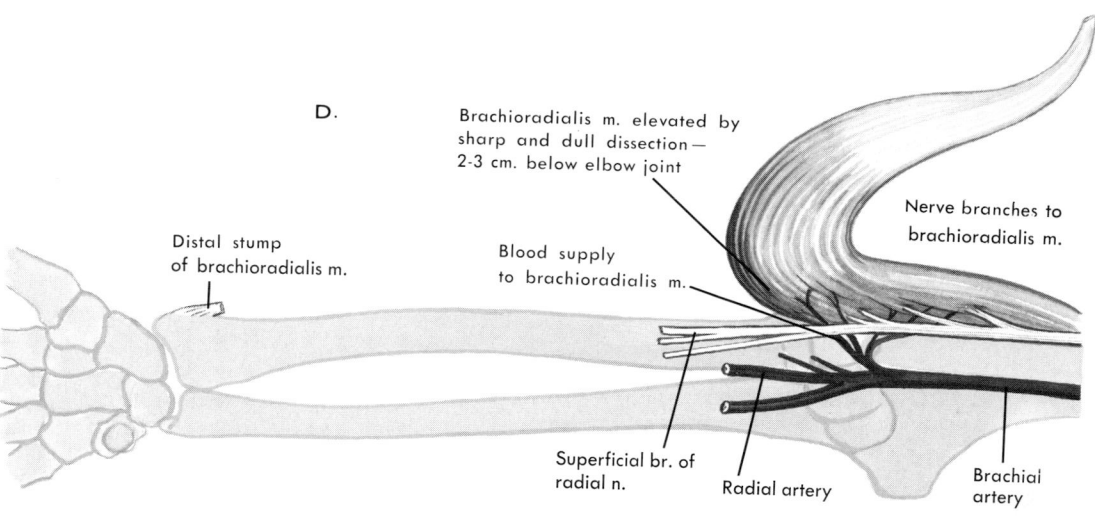

D.

Brachioradialis m. elevated by sharp and dull dissection— 2-3 cm. below elbow joint

Nerve branches to brachioradialis m.

Distal stump of brachioradialis m.

Blood supply to brachioradialis m.

Superficial br. of radial n.

Radial artery

Brachial artery

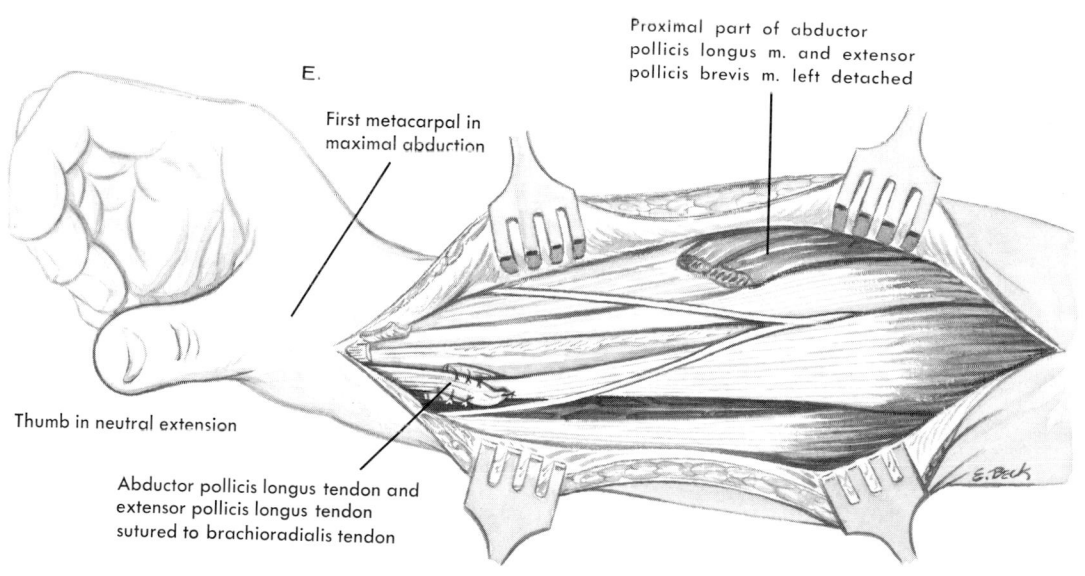

E.

Proximal part of abductor pollicis longus m. and extensor pollicis brevis m. left detached

First metacarpal in maximal abduction

Thumb in neutral extension

Abductor pollicis longus tendon and extensor pollicis longus tendon sutured to brachioradialis tendon

841

Fractional Lengthening of Finger and Wrist Flexors in Forearm

THE PROCEDURE

A. A midline longitudinal incision is made in the middle three fourths of the volar surface of the forearm. The subcutaneous tissue and deep fascia are divided in line with the skin incision. The wound flaps are undermined, elevated, and retracted with four-prong rake retractors to expose the superficial groups of muscles. On the radial side of the flexor carpi ulnaris tendon, the ulnar vessels and nerves are identified and protected from injury; similarly, on the radial side of the flexor carpi radialis tendon, the radial vessels and nerve are isolated to protect them from inadvertent damage. Sliding lengthening of the flexor carpi radialis and flexor carpi ulnaris muscles is performed at the musculotendinous junction by making two incisions of their tendinous fibers, about 1.5 cm. apart, without disturbing underlying muscle tissue. The proximal incision is transverse and the distal one is oblique. The palmaris longus and flexor digitorum muscles are lengthened by only one transverse incision in each.

B. The wrist and the fingers are passively hyperextended. The tendinous parts will separate while the intact underlying muscle fibers will maintain continuity of the muscles.

Plate 36. Fractional Lengthening of Finger and Wrist Flexors in Forearm

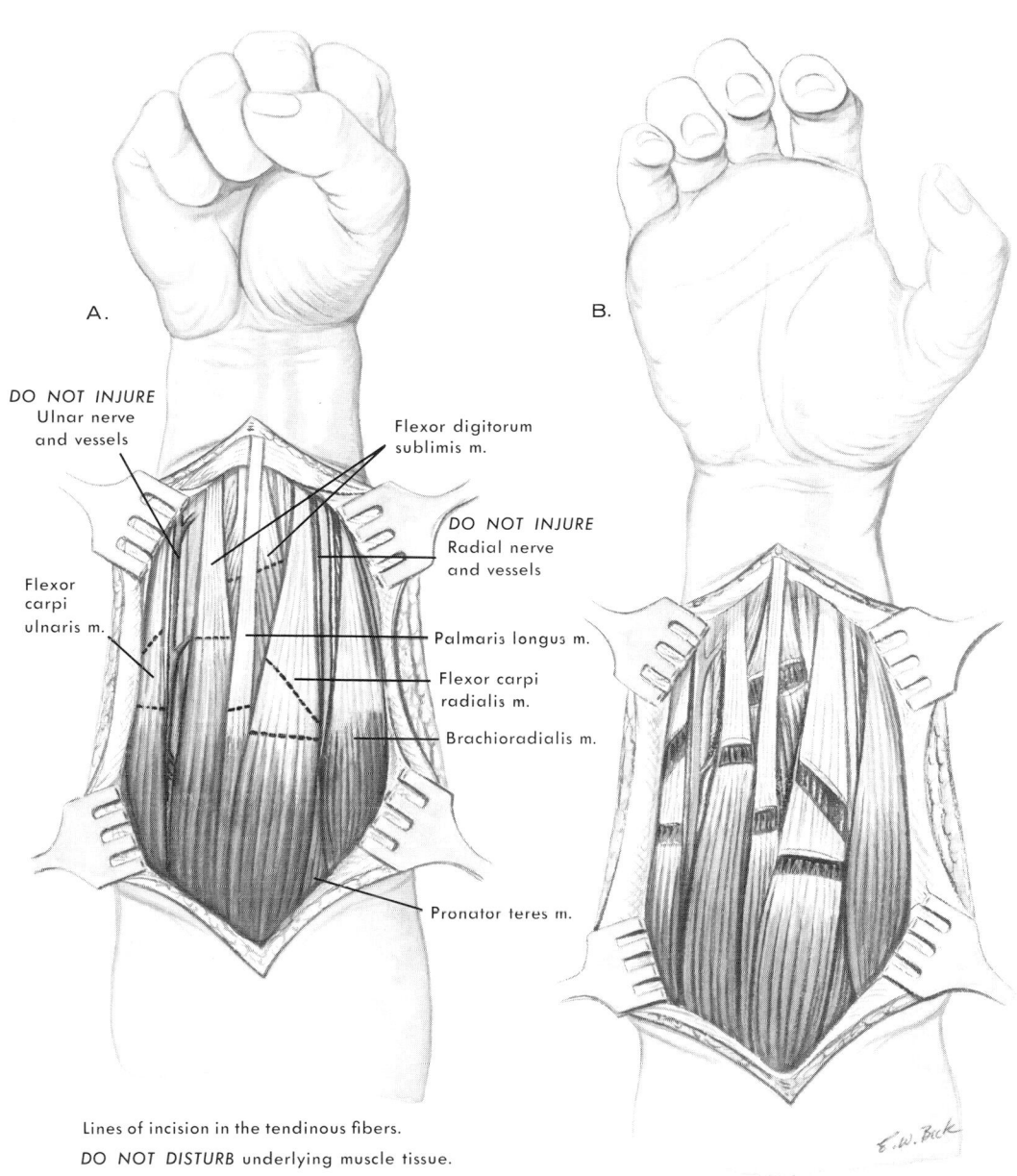

A.

DO NOT INJURE
Ulnar nerve
and vessels

Flexor digitorum
sublimis m.

DO NOT INJURE
Radial nerve
and vessels

Flexor
carpi
ulnaris m.

Palmaris longus m.

Flexor carpi
radialis m.

Brachioradialis m.

Pronator teres m.

Lines of incision in the tendinous fibers.
DO NOT DISTURB underlying muscle tissue.

B.

E. W. Beck

Separation of tendinous parts on extension
of wrist and digits

Fractional Lengthening of Finger and Wrist Flexors in Forearm
(Continued)

C and **D.** The deep volar muscles are exposed by retracting the brachioradialis muscle and radial vessels radially, and the flexor carpi radialis and flexor digitorum sublimis muscles ulnarward. The median nerve is identified and protected from injury by retracting it medially with the flexor carpi radialis muscle. The flexor pollicis longus and flexor digitorum profundus muscles are lengthened by making two incisions in their tendinous parts and sliding them in the same manner as that described for the superficial volar forearm muscles. Continuity of muscles is maintained by gentle handling of tissues and by taking care that there is adequate muscle substance underlying the divided tendinous parts. Sliding lengthening is achieved by separating the tendinous fibers by slow but firm extension of the thumb and four ulnar digits.

Next, the range of passive supination of the forearm is tested. If there is pronation contracture, the pronator teres muscle is lengthened by two oblique incisions, 1.5 cm. apart, of its tendinous fibers. Again, underlying muscle tissue should not be disturbed. The forearm is forcibly supinated; the tendinous segments will slide and separate, elongating the muscle.

The tourniquet is released and complete hemostasis is obtained. The deep fascia is not closed. The subcutaneous tissue and skin are approximated by interrupted sutures. An above-elbow long arm cast that includes all the fingers and the thumb is applied to immobilize the forearm in full supination, the elbow in 90 degrees of flexion, the wrist in 50 degrees of extension, and the fingers and thumb in neutral extension.

POSTOPERATIVE CARE

Four weeks following surgery, the cast is removed and active exercises are started to develop motor power in the elongated muscle. Squeezing soft balls of varying sizes and other functional exercises are carried out several times a day. An aggressive occupational therapy program is essential. The corrected position is maintained in a bivalved cast. As motor function develops in the elongated muscles and its antagonists, the periods out of the cast are gradually increased.

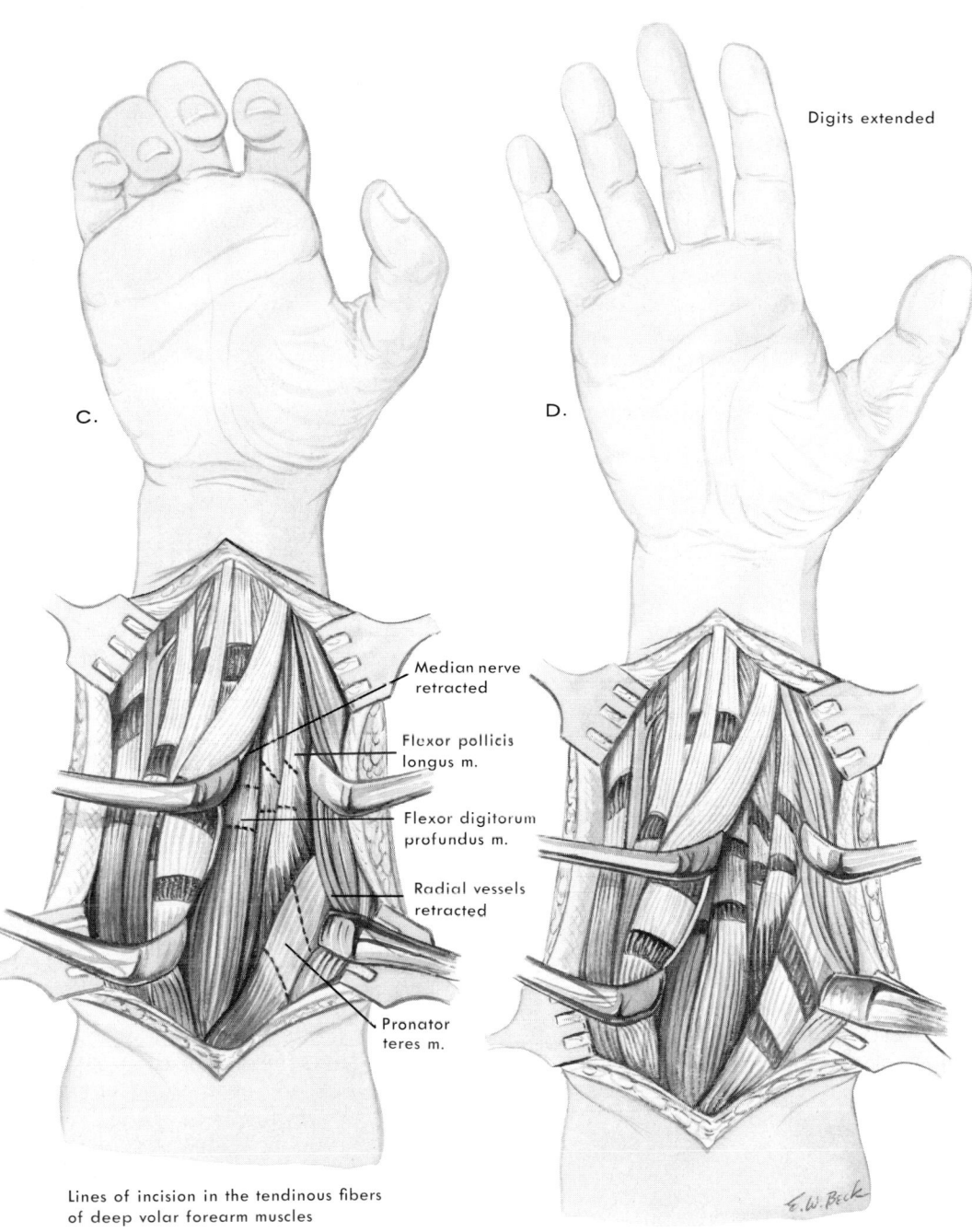

Digits extended

C.

D.

Median nerve
retracted

Flexor pollicis
longus m.

Flexor digitorum
profundus m.

Radial vessels
retracted

Pronator
teres m.

E.W.Beck

Lines of incision in the tendinous fibers
of deep volar forearm muscles

Note the sliding lengthening by separation
of tendinous fibers

the elbow joint across the antecubital space and is extended distally on the volar surface of the ulna to end at the midpoint of the forearm. The subcutaneous tissue is divided and the wound edges are retracted. Caution should be exercised not to injure the medial brachial cutaneous nerve (located posterior to the medial epicondyle) and the medial antebrachial cutaneous nerve in the forearm. The ulnar nerve is identified, carefully dissected free, and elevated from its groove behind the medial epicondyle. The motor branches of the ulnar nerve to the flexor carpi ulnaris and to the two medial heads of the flexor digitorum profundus are exposed and gently dissected free to prevent traction injury to the nerve after release of the muscles.

Starting at the midpoint of the ulna, with a periosteal elevator, the flexor carpi ulnaris and flexor digitorum profundus are bluntly dissected free of their origins from the ulna and interosseous membrane. The release is continued proximally to the medial epicondyle. The ulnar nerve is retracted posteriorly and the entire flexor-pronator muscle mass is sectioned at its origin from the medial epicondyle of the humerus. The median nerve is identified in the antecubital space as it passes through the pronator teres and is retracted forward. Next, the lacertus fibrosus is divided and the remaining portions of the flexor muscle origin are elevated and released distally. The fascia of the brachialis is incised if there is any persistence of flexion deformity of the elbow. The ulnar nerve is then transplanted anteriorly from its groove. At this point, the fingers and wrist are passively extended and the flexor muscle mass origin is displaced 3 to 4 cm. distally from its original location. The distal displacement should not exceed 4 cm., as marked loss of pronation will occur and result in fixed supination contracture of the forearm. This retains some pronation power and helps to avoid such a postoperative supination contracture. The wound is drained with closed suction catheters to prevent formation of a hematoma in the dead space, which can cause marked flexion contracture of the elbow with accompanying neuritis of the median and ulnar nerves. The wound is closed and the limb immobilized in a long arm cast with the forearm in neutral rotation and the wrist and fingers in neutral position. Three weeks after surgery, the solid cast is removed and bivalved casts are made to maintain the correction. Passive and active exercises are performed.

Swan-Neck Deformity.   Swan-neck deformity of the fingers is caused by chronic overpull on the middle extensor band by the spastic intrinsic muscles and by the tenodesis effect of the extensor digitorum longus when the wrist is in flexion. The middle extensor band, as compared to the lateral extensor bands, is relatively short. Thus, the proximal interphalangeal joint hyperextends and the distal interphalangeal joint goes into flexion. The volar capsule and retinacular ligaments become stretched and elongated. The lateral bands eventually are displaced dorsally, increasing the force hyperextending the proximal interphalangeal joint.

The sublimis tenodesis of the proximal interphalangeal joint, as described by Swanson, will restrict extension of the proximal interphalangeal joint and will correct the swan-neck deformity. Prior to performing the Swanson procedure, the flexor carpi ulnaris should be transferred to the extensor carpi radialis longus to reinforce the power of the wrist dorsiflexors. By doing this at an early age in the pure spastic hand, the swan-neck deformity can be prevented or can be kept from being severe enough to warrant sublimis tenodesis. The swan-neck deformity in the mixed type of cerebral palsy, i.e., spastic and athetoid, or in pure tension athetosis presents a difficult and different problem; in these patients Swanson's sublimis tenodesis should be performed with caution and only after thorough assessment of the pathomechanics and motor picture, because the results have not been satisfactory in the author's experience.

The surgical technique of sublimis tenodesis of the proximal interphalangeal joint, as described by Swanson, is as follows:[171, 172]

A midlateral incision is made immediately dorsal to the flexion crease and extending from the distal end of the middle phalanx to the base of the proximal phalanx. The flexor sheath is incised, exposing the flexor tendons, which are retracted dorsally. The distal half of the volar surface of the proximal phalanx is subperiosteally exposed by resection of the periosteum, the palmar capsule, and the volar plate. Two small drill holes approximately 1 cm. apart are made through the neck of the proximal phalanx in the palmar to dorsal direction. With a curet, the two drill holes are connected on the palmar aspect and the bone is roughened to give a raw surface of bone for attachment of the tendon. With a scalpel the sublimis tendon is scarified. Silk sutures are passed through these drill holes and through the sublimis tendon, firmly anchoring it to bone with the interphalangeal joint in 20 to 30 degrees of flexion. The flexed position of the proximal interphalangeal joint is further secured by placing across it a small Kirschner wire, which is cut off subcutaneously. The retinacular ligament and flexor sheath are closed with 0000 or 00000 plain catgut sutures and the skin with 0000 nylon. A long arm cast is applied; it should extend to the tip of the fingers with the wrist in neutral dorsiflexion, the forearm in full supination, and the elbow in 90 degrees of flexion.

The cast and Kirschner wire are removed in six weeks. Passive and active exercises are performed under supervision of the therapist and the parents to develop functional range of motion. Extension of the proximal interphalangeal joints should be avoided. Aluminum finger splints that hold the proximal interphalangeal joints in flexion are taped to the digits. These splints are worn during the day except for exercise periods for four to six weeks. At night a bivalved cast is used for a long period to maintain the fingers in flexion.

FLEXION DEFORMITY OF WRIST AND PRONATION CONTRACTURE OF FOREARM

This is the common deformity of spastic paralysis. Ability to extend the wrist and to supinate and pronate the forearm is fundamental to the effective use of the hand and fingers. The transfer of the flexor carpi ulnaris to the extensor carpi radialis longus or brevis was first described by Green in 1942. Thirty years' experience with 39 patients was reviewed by Green and Banks in 1962. This transfer removes the deforming force at the wrist, which pulls the hand into flexion and ulnar deviation; also, the rerouting of the tendon around the medial side of the ulna provides an active force that promotes supination and dorsiflexion (Fig. 5–24).

Prior to performing Green's flexor carpi ulnaris transfer, the following essential prerequisites should be met. There should be full range of passive supination of the forearm, dorsiflexion of the wrist, and extension of the fingers. If any fixed deformity is present, it should be corrected by successive stretching casts and an aggressive regimen of passive exercises. In severe and resistant cases, the pronator teres may have to be lengthened or reinserted to a wrist dorsiflexor, and occasionally stripping of the interosseous membrane is indicated. Such procedures are usually indicated in neglected cases in which the patient has had no conservative therapy prior to surgery.

Motor control of the fingers is an equally important prerequisite for success of the operation. With the wrist in 30 to 45 degrees of dorsiflexion, the patient should be able to extend the fingers actively (Fig. 5–24C). If active finger action is not present, a passive stretching cast is applied, or fractional lengthening of the flexor digitorum profundus and sublimis is initially performed. Adequate sensory function in the hand is desirable; astereognosis is a great handicap to postoperative training, but is not a contraindication to the procedure.

The operative technique and postoperative care of Green's flexor carpi ulnaris transfer are depicted in Plate 37.

Transfer of the flexor carpi ulnaris through the interosseous route is not indicated in spastic cerebral palsy.

Arthrodesis of the wrist in functional position is rarely performed in spastic paralysis. Wrist and forearm motion are important complements to effective use of the hand. In the experience of Green and Banks since the development of the flexor carpi ulnaris transfer, it has not been necessary to do a wrist fusion. The author performs wrist fusion only in the athetoid patient in whom stabilization of the wrist in functional position enables active grasp and release and improves finger control.

Pronation contracture of the forearm may exist without flexion deformity of the wrist. The patient is able to extend the

(*Text continued on page 854.*)

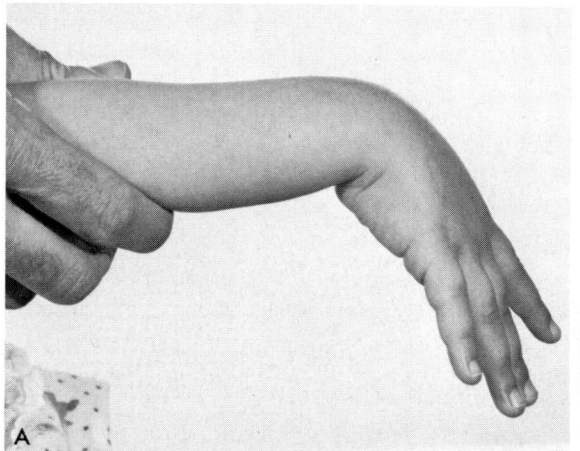

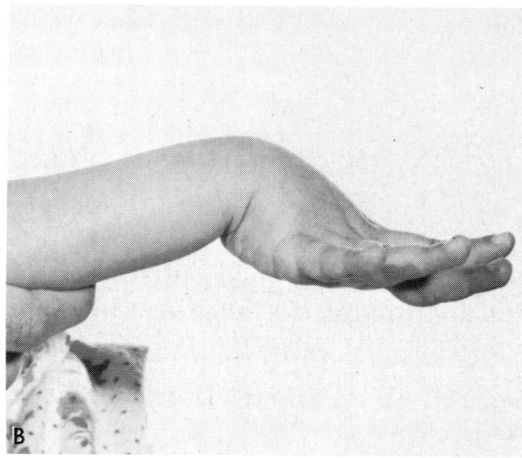

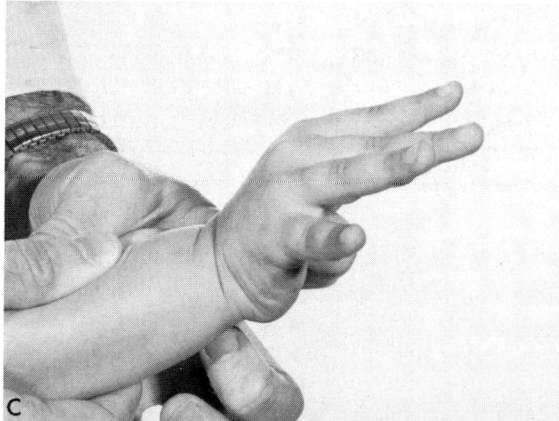

FIGURE 5–24. *Flexor carpi ulnaris transfer to extensor carpi radialis longus (Green procedure).*

A to **C.** Preoperative photographs.

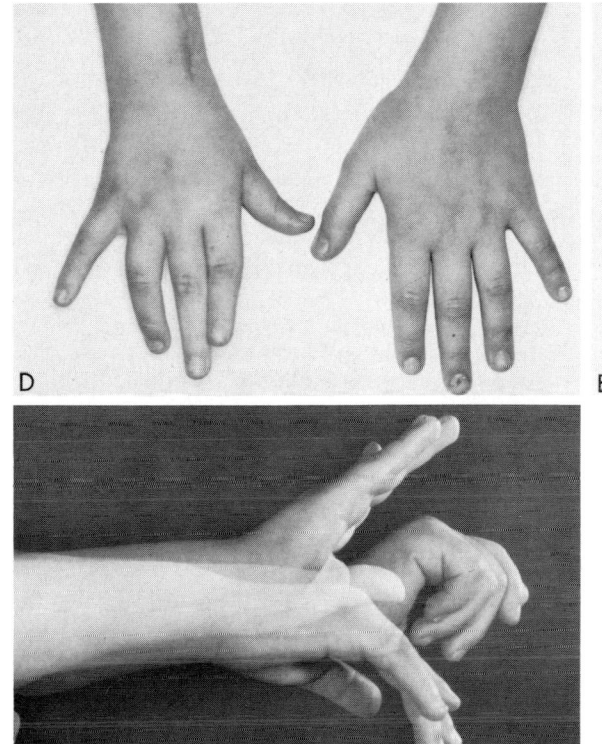

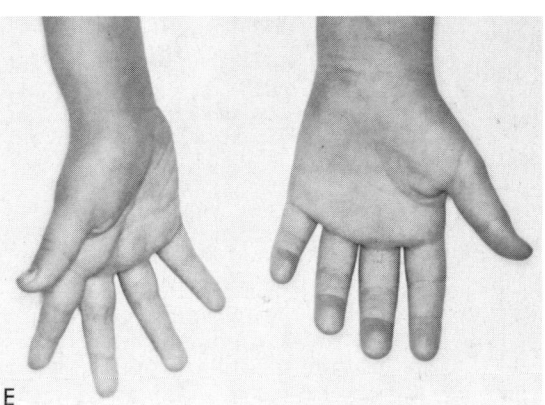

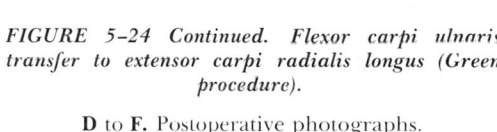

FIGURE 5-24 Continued. *Flexor carpi ulnaris transfer to extensor carpi radialis longus (Green procedure).*

D to **F.** Postoperative photographs.

Flexor Carpi Ulnaris Transfer (Green Procedure)

THE PROCEDURE

The operation is usually performed with the patient in supine position; some surgeons, however, prefer the patient to be in prone position, as it facilitates manipulating the forearm and holding the wrist in dorsiflexed position. The author uses the prone position when there is pronation deformity of the forearm and internal rotation contracture of the shoulder.

A. An anteromedial incision is made over the flexor carpi ulnaris tendon. It starts at the flexor crease of the wrist and extends proximally and somewhat ulnarward over the belly of the muscle to the junction of the middle and upper thirds of the forearm (Green and Banks make two incisions, one distal and the other proximal).

B and **C.** The subcutaneous tissue is divided and the tendon of the flexor carpi ulnaris is exposed. The ulnar nerve, lying immediately posterior to the tendon, is visualized and protected from injury. The tendon is detached at its insertion to the pisiform bone and mobilized proximally. The muscle fibers of the flexor carpi ulnaris take their origin from the ulna quite distally; they are stripped extraperiosteally from the underlying bone by sharp and dull dissection. The muscle is freed proximally as far as possible without disturbing its nerve supply from the ulnar nerve (which is the limiting factor of proximal dissection). The mobilization of the flexor carpi ulnaris should be high enough to allow its passage in a straight line from its origin to the dorsum of the wrist. The extensor compartment of the forearm is entered by excising a segment of the intermuscular septum at the medial margin of the ulna.

Plate 37. *Flexor Carpi Ulnaris Transfer (Green Procedure)*

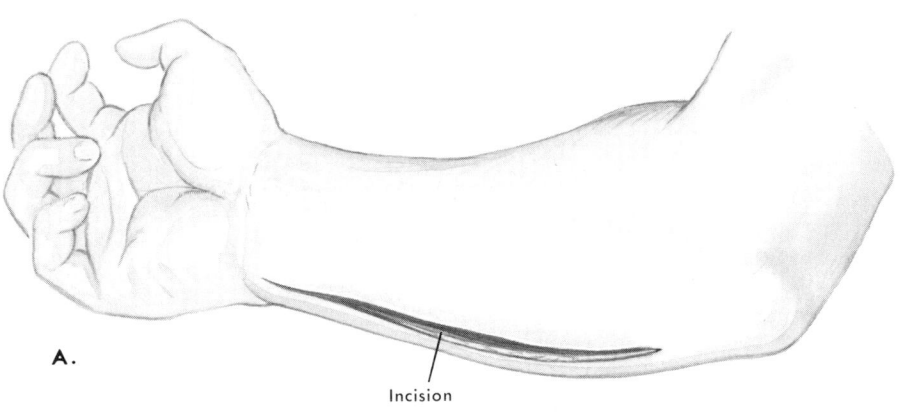

A.

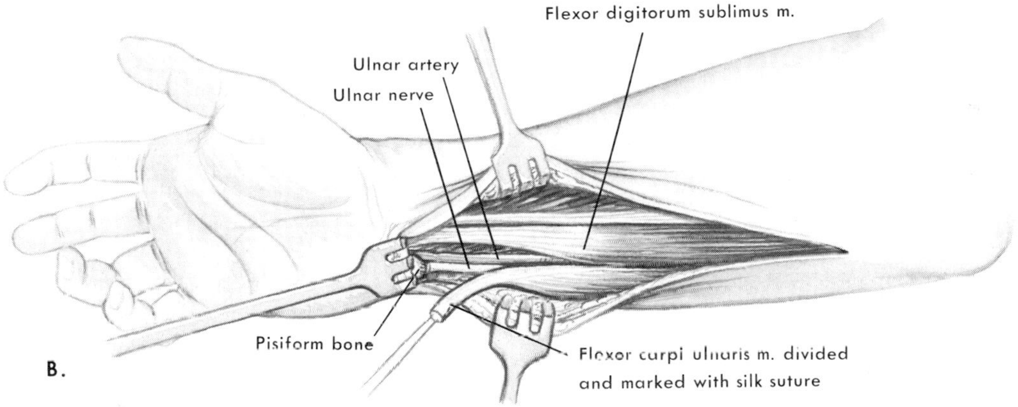

Incision

B.

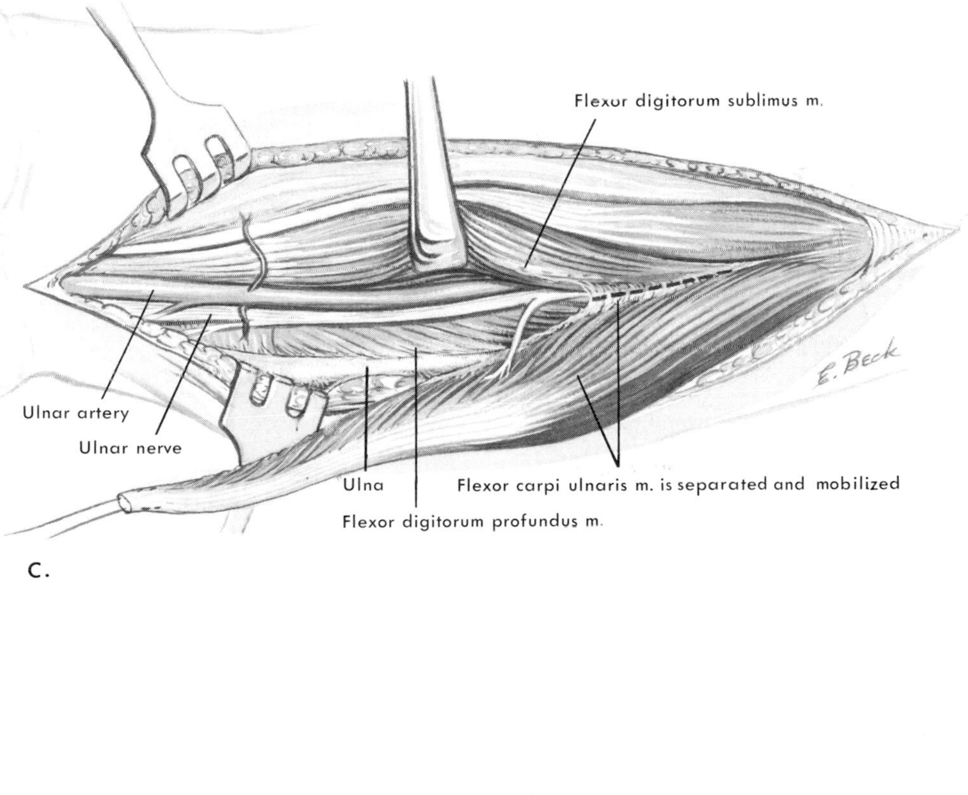

Flexor digitorum sublimus m.

Ulnar artery

Ulnar nerve

Pisiform bone

Flexor curpi ulnaris m. divided
and marked with silk suture

C.

Flexor digitorum sublimus m.

Ulnar artery

Ulnar nerve

Ulna

Flexor carpi ulnaris m. is separated and mobilized

Flexor digitorum profundus m.

E. Beck

851

Flexor Carpi Ulnaris Transfer (Green Procedure) (Continued)

D. Next, a longitudinal incision is made on the dorsum of the wrist over the extensor carpi radialis longus and brevis tendons. It starts at the distal end of the radius immediately above the transverse crease and extends proximally for a distance of 3 cm.

E and **F.** The incision is carried through subcutaneous tissue and fascia. The extensor carpi radialis longus (in line with the second metacarpal) and the extensor carpi radialis brevis (in line with the third metacarpal) tendons are identified and isolated.

An Ober tendon transfer is passed from the proximal portion of the ulnar incision to the wound on the dorsum of the wrist. The flexor carpi ulnaris tendon is passed around the ulna through the channel created by the Ober tendon transfer. The line of pull of the tendon should be as straight as possible. On the dorsum of the wrist and forearm the ulnaris tendon should be along the extensor communis tendons.

G and **H.** With a No. 11 blade knife a buttonhole is made in the extensor carpi radialis longus or brevis tendons. When there is ulnar deviation of the wrist, the ulnaris tendon is attached to the longus; when the wrist is in neutral posture, it is inserted into the brevis tendon. Not infrequently, the author attaches it to both tendons.

With the forearm in full supination and the wrist in 45 degrees of dorsiflexion, the ulnaris tendon is sutured to the extensor tendon. The tension on the ulnaris tendon should be such that the wrist can be passively palmar-flexed 15 degrees, but when the tension is released, it should resume a position of 35 to 45 degrees of dorsiflexion. The method of suturing is not important. The author prefers that the ulnaris tendon pass through the buttonhole and be sutured to itself. In addition, three interrupted sutures are used to transfix the ulnaris and radialis tendons securely.

I. The wound is closed in layers as an assistant holds the forearm in full supination and the wrist in marked dorsiflexion. A long arm cast is applied with the forearm in full supination, the wrist in 60 degrees of dorsiflexion, the thumb in abduction, the metacarpophalangeal joint in 15 degrees of flexion, and the interphalangeal joint in neutral extension.

POSTOPERATIVE CARE

About three to four weeks after operation, the cast is bivalved and physical therapy is started to develop function in the transferred muscle. In the beginning, it consists of guided active exercises, attempting ulnar deviation and dorsiflexion of the wrist and supination of the forearm. Exercises are performed three to four times a day under supervision of the therapist and later of the parents (after thorough instruction by the therapist). The limb is maintained in the bivalved cast in the desired position except for the exercise periods for the following three weeks. The time out of the cast is then gradually increased. When out of the cast and not exercising, the patient wears a light short arm orthosis or plastic splint, which holds the wrist in 45 degrees of dorsiflexion and the thumb in maximal abduction and opposition (see Fig. 5–22). The support is discontinued when the flexor carpi ulnaris muscle is fair in motor strength and the wrist can be maintained in dorsiflexed functional position. If there is a tendency for the wrist to drop into flexion, the support with the dorsiflexion orthosis is continued part-time during the day. The use of a night cast is continued until good function is developed and until there is no tendency for recurrence of the original deformity. This may take many months or even several years. During the growth period, exercises are continued, with emphasis on active exercises to improve function of the hand and passive stretching exercises to maintain range of motion and to prevent recurrence of contractural deformity.

Plate 37. Flexor Carpi Ulnaris Transfer
(Green Procedure)

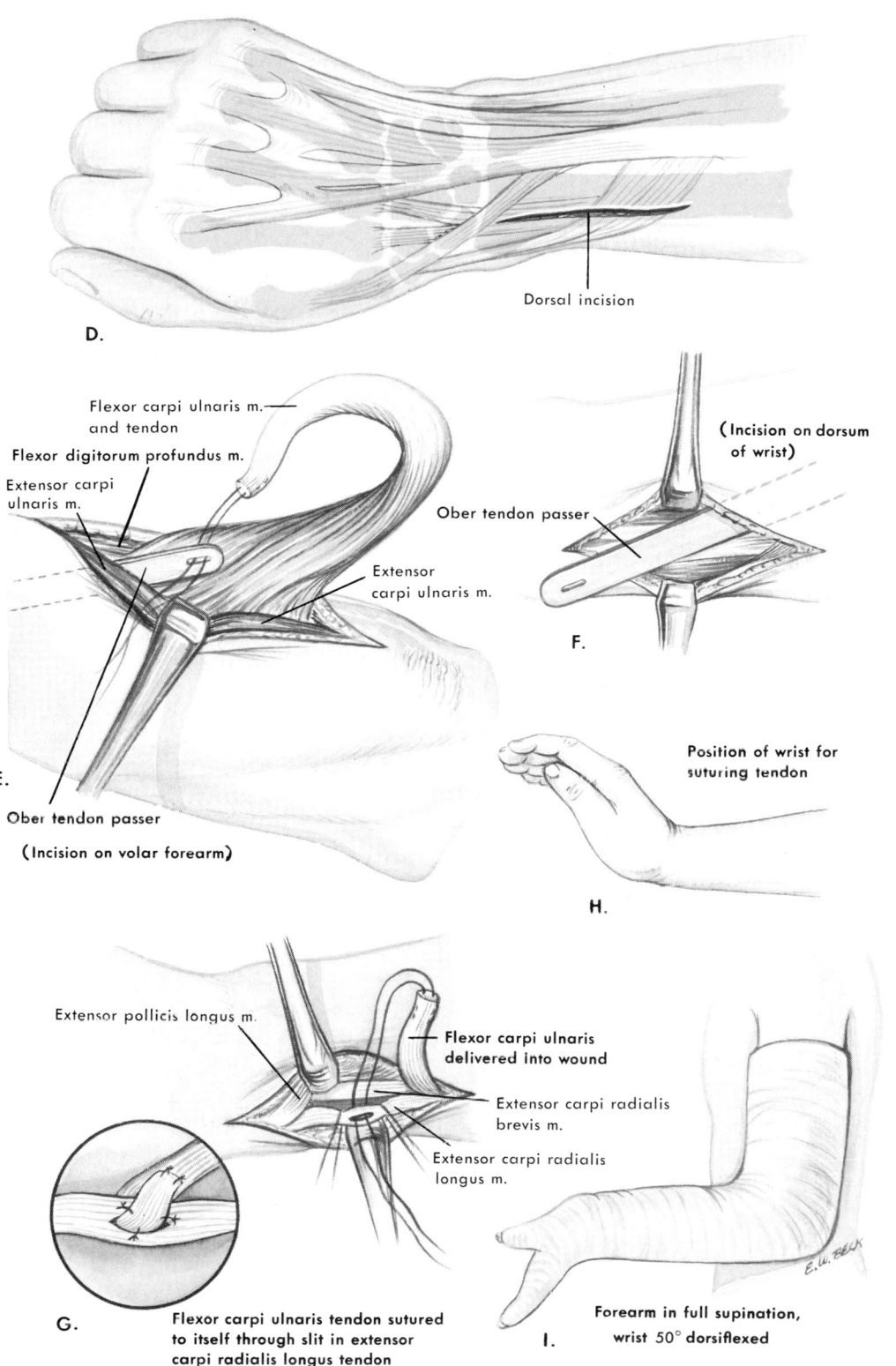

Dorsal incision

D.

Flexor carpi ulnaris m. and tendon

Flexor digitorum profundus m.

Extensor carpi ulnaris m.

Extensor carpi ulnaris m.

Ober tendon passer

E.

Ober tendon passer

(Incision on volar forearm)

(Incision on dorsum of wrist)

Ober tendon passer

F.

Position of wrist for suturing tendon

H.

Extensor pollicis longus m.

Flexor carpi ulnaris delivered into wound

Extensor carpi radialis brevis m.

Extensor carpi radialis longus m.

G. Flexor carpi ulnaris tendon sutured to itself through slit in extensor carpi radialis longus tendon

I. Forearm in full supination, wrist 50° dorsiflexed

wrist, with normal muscle balance between the wrist flexors and extensors. In such an instance, lengthening of the pronator teres is performed and later, reinforcement of active force of supination may be indicated by transfer of the flexor carpi ulnaris to the radius at the insertion of the brachioradialis tendon.

FLEXION DEFORMITY OF THE ELBOW

This is commonly present in cerebral palsy. The deformity is usually minimal or moderate and is effectively controlled by passive stretching exercises. Occasionally, especially in the tension athetoid or mixed spastic and athetoid patient, it is very severe and presents a significant functional handicap. In such an instance, the biceps and brachialis muscles are lengthened in their tendinous portion.

SHOULDER DEFORMITY

The shoulder deformity is one of internal rotation and adduction. Ordinarily this is effectively managed by passive stretching exercises. Rarely, in neglected cases, lengthening of the pectoralis major and subscapularis muscles may be indicated.

Abduction contracture of the shoulder may develop in *acquired* cerebral palsy because of spasticity of the deltoid muscle. In the severe case it may be so disturbing cosmetically that a deltoid release at its insertion may be indicated (Fig. 5–25). This is performed through a longitudinal incision. The tendinous fibers of the anterior two thirds of the deltoid muscle are detached from their insertion to the tuberosity of the humerus and the deltoid muscle is recessed (Fig. 5–26). The shoulder is immobilized for four weeks in a Velpeau bandage reinforced by a plaster of Paris cast.

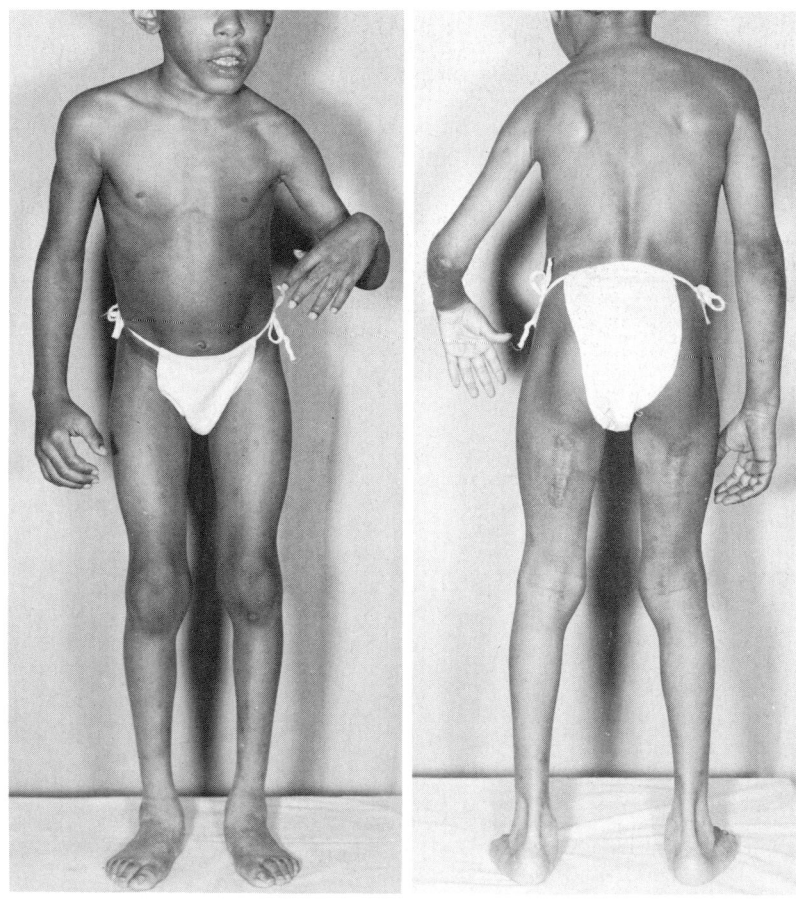

FIGURE 5–25. *Abduction contracture of the shoulder in acquired cerebral palsy.*

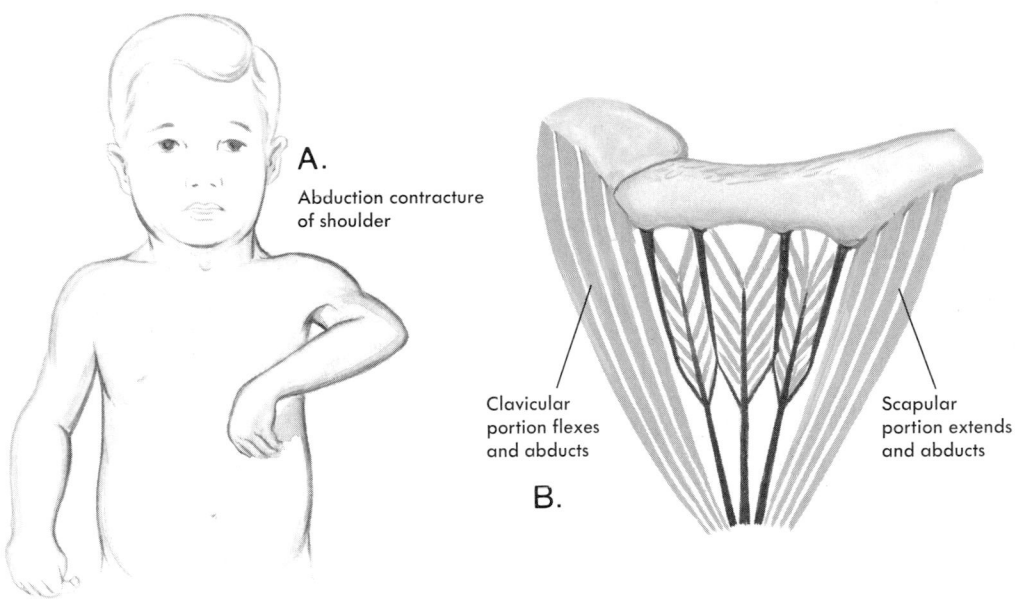

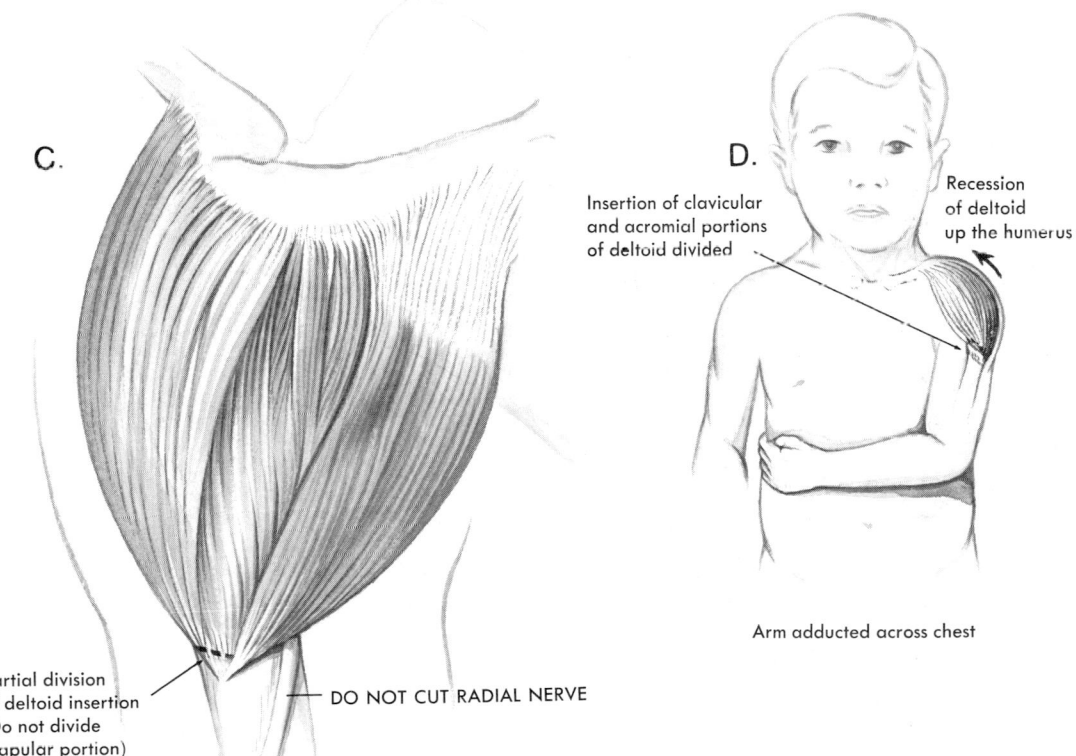

FIGURE 5-26. *Recession of deltoid muscle at its insertion.*

Scoliosis

The incidence of structural scoliosis in adolescents and young adults with cerebral palsy is reported to be 15.2 per cent by Robson, and 21 per cent by Balmer and MacEwen. In 4 per cent of the cases of Robson, the scoliosis was considered to be moderately severe; and in 6 per cent of the series of cases of Balmer and MacEwen the curvature was over 30 degrees.[13, 154]

Scoliosis may result from: (1) *pelvic obliquity*, that may be caused by asymmetrical involvement and contracture of the hip

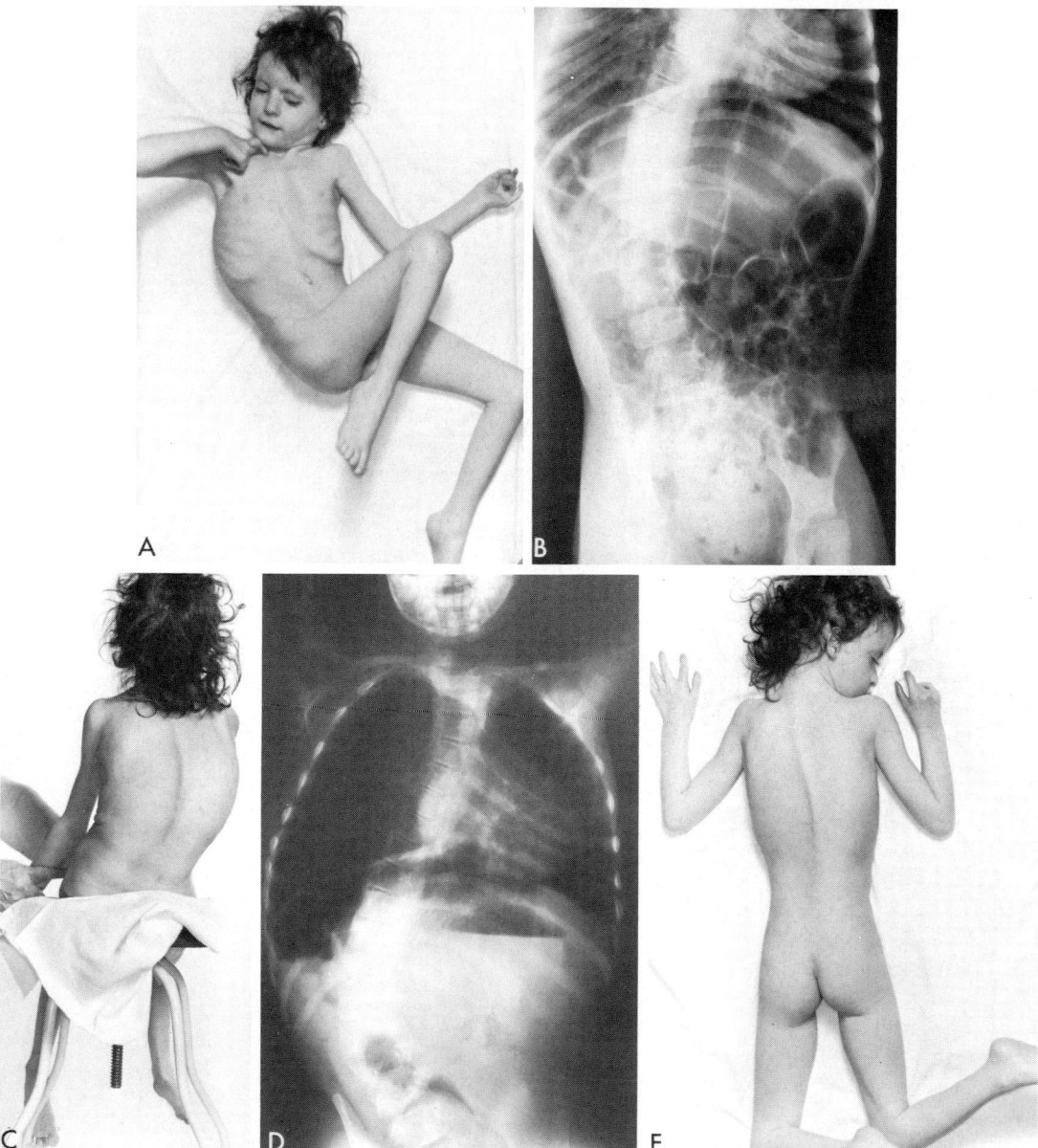

FIGURE 5–27. *Scoliosis in a child with mixed type of cerebral palsy — spastic and tension athetoid.*

A and **b.** Anteroposterior photograph and roentgenogram of patient. **C** and **D.** Posteroanterior photograph and roentgenogram with the patient sitting. **E.** When lying face down, the position is secure and tension athetosis is diminished. Note the decrease in the degree of curvature.

adductors or abductors, or by unilateral dislocation of the hip, (2) *unilateral or asymmetrical spasticity or tension athetosis of the trunk musculature* (Fig. 5–27); (3) *congenital deformities of the vertebrae* such as hemivertebrae or unilateral bar; (4) or it may be *idiopathic.*

Ordinarily, the Milwaukee brace is not tolerated by the child with cerebral palsy. Cooperation by the patient in wearing the brace and performing the back exercises (so important for success of treatment with the brace) is poor. Immobilization in a corrective Risser cast is not very well tolerated. For these reasons, Balmer and MacEwen recommend Harrington instrumentation combined with spinal fusion as the only feasible effective form of treatment.[13]

MINIMAL BRAIN DYSFUNCTION

by J. Gordon Millichap, M.D.*

The term "minimal brain dysfunction" has been coined for certain learning and behavioral disorders in children that are associated with a short attention span, impulsiveness, and impairment of control of motor function. Of several combinations of symptoms recognized, the hyperkinetic syndrome is the most common, and the clumsy child syndrome the one of greatest interest to the orthopedist. An organic cause is frequently apparent, but a theory of delayed maturation of the brain is supported by the natural history of the syndrome and the tendency to improvement with increasing age.

Etiology

The causes of minimal brain dysfunction as manifested by incoordination and hyperactivity are diverse and uncertain. Evidence is frequently retrospective and presumptive, being generally based on a history of ab-

*Dr. Millichap is Professor of Neurology and Pediatrics, Northwestern University Medical School; and Neurologist, Children's Memorial Hospital and Passavant Memorial Hospital, Chicago, Illinois.

normalities or illnesses that occurred during pregnancy, on delivery at birth, or in early childhood.

Organic causes include genetic cerebral defects, cerebral dysgenesis, bleeding during pregnancy, toxemia, and delayed maturation. Cerebral anoxia, hemorrhage, trauma, prematurity, and jaundice with kernicterus are birth complications of related importance in some cases. Postnatal factors less commonly associated are trauma, encephalitis, meningitis, hypernatremic dehydration, lead encephalopathy, degenerative disorders, and cerebral tumors.

Psychogenic factors are sometimes contributory, but in patients with abnormal neurologic signs, emotional disorders are secondary complications. The influence of the environment on the brain-damaged, hyperactive, and uncoordinated child is particularly evident in family relations, as often parental attitudes tend to be undermined by loss of patience and frustration, and this, in turn, exacerbates anxiety reactions in the child.

Pathophysiology

The frontal areas of the brain, hypothalamus, and the reticular activating system all seem to be implicated in the hyperkinetic syndrome. However, the specific areas involved and the mechanism of the increased motor activity are undetermined. It has been postulated that destruction or damage to certain cortical and subcortical areas of the brain removes the normal inhibitory mechanisms and results in hyperactivity.

Abnormal neurologic signs are minimal and subtle in type, diffuse in localization, and rarely point to a discrete cerebral lesion. Motor incoordination and ataxia may be explained by dysfunction or damage to the cerebellum or its connections with the frontal cerebral cortex, the vestibular system, or the spinocerebellar pathways. Mirror or synkinetic movements, tightness of heel cords, and Babinski responses are manifestations of dysfunction of the corticospinal or pyramidal system. Choreiform movements, tremors, athetosis, and dystonic postures are extrapyramidal in origin. Apraxia, an inability to perform purposeful movements in spite of normal muscle power and coordination, is caused by a lesion in the corresponding or major precentral gyrus. Gerstmann's syndrome of acalculia, confusion of laterality, finger agnosia, and agraphia results from a lesion at the border of the major angular gyrus on the occipital lobe.

The opportunity to examine the brain at autopsy is rare, since the pathologic change is always minimal and generally nonprogressive in nature. Indirect evidence of scar tissue and cerebral structural changes may be obtained by electroencephalography and are revealed by the persistent occurrence of focal spike or slow wave activity. The electroencephalogram shows abnormalities of varying degrees in 30 to 50 per cent of patients. Biochemical rather than anatomic lesions have been postulated in view of the general tendency for neurologic abnormalities to become less remarkable in later childhood and adult life. The marked difference in incidence between the sexes with a preponderance in boys is indicative of genetic influences.

Clinical Manifestations

Hyperkinesis, the symptom most commonly encountered, is associated with one or more additional disorders of motor function, behavioral abnormality, and perceptual handicap.

The symptoms of motor dysfunction include the following: clumsy or apraxic gait and general awkwardness; impairment of hopping ability; a tendency to walk on the toes; dysgraphia; mild choreiform movements, tremors, and tics; and disorders of speech and communication. The most frequent abnormal neurologic signs are mirror or synkinetic movements, dysdiadochokinesia, Babinski responses, finger-to-nose incoordination, apraxia of tandem gait, contracture of triceps surae muscle, graphanesthesia, and left and mixed laterality.

Additional symptoms and signs are categorized as follows: disorders of attention and concentration, motor impersistence, failure to organize and complete work assignments, impulsiveness, low frustration tolerance, and lack of inhibition with no fear of heights or other hazards.

Neuropsychologic tests reveal visual motor and auditory perception deficits, distortions of body image, poor spatial orientation, difficulties in concept formation, disorganized thinking, and poor short-term and long-term memory. Despite average to above average intelligence, the child fails to achieve up to the level of his potential at school.

Differential Diagnosis

The diagnosis of minimal brain dysfunction is usually established by the history of a hyperkinetic child with a short attention span, who distracts the class, has a learning disability despite a normal intelligence quotient, and is awkward and uncoordinated in his movements. The neurologic examination reveals mild and subtle, so-called "soft," abnormal signs; the electroencephalogram may show dysrhythmia indicative of seizure discharges or other nonspecific irregularities. Neuropsychologic test scores are often low in the areas of visual and auditory perception.

Hyperkinesis and a tendency to walk on the toes may be manifestations of a primary emotional disorder such as autistic behavior, juvenile schizophrenia, or anxiety and depressive reactions. Periods of inattention and memory deficits may be caused by petit mal or psychomotor seizures. The lesion responsible for abnormalities of gait and incoordination associated with Babinski responses and sensory deficits may be localized in the spinal cord; diastematomyelia, spinal cord tumor, and Friedreich's ataxia must be considered in diagnosis. Impairments of hearing and sight must be excluded in children who appear to be inattentive and who lack eye-hand coordination.

Management

The clinical management of the child with hyperactivity and minimal brain dysfunction is complex, requiring a multifaceted approach and the skills of experts from many disciplines, including pharmacotherapy, orthopedic and physical therapy, remedial education, parental counseling, and psychotherapy.

PHARMACOTHERAPY

Drugs are usually essential for the control of hyperactivity and impulsive behavior. Central nervous system stimulants, methylphenidate (Ritalin) being the drug of choice, have a paradoxical quieting effect in 75 per cent of hyperkinetic children with signs of minimal brain damage. The control of hyperactivity is usually accompanied by improvement in attention, memory, visual perception, and coordination. Short-term trials of methylphenidate are advised, beginning with a dose of 5 mg. at breakfast and at lunch, given on school days as an adjunct to remedial education. The response to treatment should be monitored carefully by a pediatric neurologist, using reports from teachers and parents and periodic neuropsychologic tests. Tranquilizing agents are indicated in those patients with hyperkinetic behavior who exhibit no other signs of organic brain damage and whose symptoms may be attributed to primary emotional disorders. Phenobarbital often exacerbates the hyperkinesis and should be avoided.

ORTHOPEDIC CARE

The orthopedist is usually consulted for the presenting complaints of clumsiness in gait and toe-walking. Passive stretching exercises of the triceps surae muscles are performed several times a day. When the myostatic contracture is of such severity that the feet cannot be dorsiflexed to neutral position, a below-knee stretching cast with a walking heel placed anteriorly is applied. The child is allowed to walk, stretching the Achilles tendon with each footstep. The cast is changed at weekly or biweekly intervals, each time immobilizing the ankle in further dorsiflexion. Following removal of the solid cast, a bivalved cast is worn at night to maintain correction. In severe cases, a below-knee dynamic dorsiflexion assist orthosis may be used during the day to establish a heel-toe gait pattern, and occasionally, in persistent recurrent contracture of the triceps surae muscle, sliding lengthening of the heel cord is indicated.

Motor coordination and postural exercises, including the use of a balancing beam, are performed at school. Certain eye exercises and motor development programs that are popular with some physicians and optometrists are of doubtful and unproved value.

REMEDIAL EDUCATION

The complex educational needs of the child require discussions among teachers, psychologist, parents, and physician. Class size should be small, with lessons interrupted by frequent periods of supervised physical exercise, and discipline firm but related to the child's disability. Motor, sensory, and perceptual handicaps should be explained to the teacher; this will usually lead to the provision of the optimal remedial education available.

PSYCHOTHERAPY AND PARENTAL COUNSELING

The hyperactive and clumsy child must receive love and understanding, but tolerance should be tempered by appropriate discipline.

The child's image of himself has a major influence on his behavior. In order to attract attention, these children often clown and become garrulous and brash. Inability to control their hyperactive and aggressive behavior leads to a sense of guilt and fear of the consequences of the outburst.

The parents' confidence must be earned; the physician must listen to them while avoiding criticism. The nature and cause of the disorder should be explained and the prognosis discussed. It may be pointed out that amelioration will occur as the child reaches puberty, but that effective control and management of hyperactivity and incoordination in childhood are essential for satisfactory achievement in school.

Prognosis

Improvement is generally to be expected with age. Hyperkinetic behavior is less prevalent in children after 10 or 12 years of age, and abnormal neurologic signs become more subtle and difficult to recognize in adolescence and young adult life. Achievement in school is dependent on the quality of remedial education, the success of pharmacotherapy and exercise programs, and the correction of secondary emotional disorders.

INTRACRANIAL TUMORS

Intracranial tumors in childhood are common, being third in frequency to leukemia and neoplasms arising in the renal and suprarenal area. The highest incidence is in the age period from five to eight years. There is no significant sex predilection.

The orthopedic surgeon should keep in mind the possibility of an intracranial neoplasm when examining the child with an abnormality in gait, spasticity in the limbs, or torticollis. Also, since rehabilitation of the musculoskeletal system in the postoperative period is the concern of the orthopedist, he should be knowledgeable about the biology and prognosis of intracranial tumors.

Pathologic Considerations

Gliomas constitute a large proportion (about 75 per cent) of intracranial neoplasms found in children. Cerebellar astrocytomas, fourth ventricle medulloblastomas and ependymomas, and pontine gliomas are the common tumors, whereas the malignant glioblastoma multiforme (a common neoplasm in the cerebral hemisphere of adults) is relatively infrequent in children. Also, the benign lesions—meningiomas, acoustic neurinomas, and pituitary adenomas—which are the commoner types of adult tumors, are almost unknown in childhood. Other specific tumors encountered in childhood are craniopharyngioma, papilloma of the choroid plexus, glioma of the optic chiasm, and teratoma.

The anatomic location of intracranial neoplasms in children differs from that in the adult. About two thirds of the tumors in children arise within the cerebellum, fourth ventricle, lower brain stem, cisterna magna, and cerebellopontine angle, whereas in the adult only one fourth of the tumors occur in these areas. In children, there is also a preponderance of tumors along the central neural axis. These account for the initial clinical manifestations being the result of increased intracranial pressure rather than a focal neurologic abnormality.

The common malignant intracranial tumors of childhood are medulloblastoma, pontine glioma, and third and fourth ventricular ependymomas, the prognoses for all of which are very poor. In the experience of Matson, 45 per cent of intracranial tumors should be considered benign; that is, they can be surgically excised with an 80 to 90 per cent cure rate. Figure 5–28 shows the incidence of various pathologic types of intracranial tumors in children under 12 years of age seen at the Children's Hospital Medical Center in Boston. They are arbitrarily divided into benign and malignant, being so designated because of their histologic features and their anatomic accessibility for surgical excision.

Clinical Features

Often the initial manifestation of an intracranial tumor is increased intracranial pressure, the clinical features of which are headache, irritability, vomiting, somnolence, lethargy, papilledema, strabismus, diplopia, and increased head size. The pediatrician is ordinarily consulted for evaluation of these symptoms, and thus it is important that he keep in mind the possibility of an intracranial neoplasm when confronted with this complex of symptoms.

Neurologic manifestations depend upon the location of the tumor. When the lesion is located in the *posterior fossa*, neurologic symptoms and signs include ataxia (the child walks in a wide-based gait, develops a lurch, and falls frequently); dysmetria and adiadochokinesia; torticollis (the head is held tilted to one side with resistance to attempts to move it; there is also palpable spasm of the cervical muscle); generalized muscular weakness, especially of the lower limbs, with hypotonia and hyporeflexia; nystagmus; cranial nerve paralysis (particularly the sixth); and tonic seizures. Tumors of the *cerebral hemispheres* cause disturbances of behavior, speech, or visual perception; motor, sensory, or reflex changes; and convulsive seizures. *Suprasellar tumors* (craniopharyngioma, optic pathway and hypothalamic gliomas, and epidermoid

	BENIGN		MALIGNANT
ASTROCYTOMA	87	MEDULLOBLASTOMA	63
Cerebellar	68	EPENDYMOMA	35
Cerebral	19	Sub-tentorial	20
EPENDYMOMA	7	Supra-tentorial	15
Sub-tentorial	2	GLIOMA of BRAIN STEM	39
Supra-tentorial	5	MIXED GLIOMA	15
GLIOMA of OPTIC PATHWAY	16	Cerebral	7
CRANIOPHARYNGIOMA	23	Cerebellar	8
DERMOID and EPIDERMOID CYST	12	GLIOBLASTOMA MULTIFORME	13
PAPILLOMA of CHOROID PLEXUS	12	GANGLIOGLIOMA	5
CAVERNOUS HEMANGIOMA	4	SARCOMA of MENINGES	4
MENINGIOMA	2	HAMARTOMA, III VENTRICLE	3
PARAPHYSIAL CYST	1	RETINOBLASTOMA	3
TUBERCULOMA	1	TERATOMA, MALIGNANT	2
CHORDOMA	1	METASTATIC WILMS TUMOR	1
NEUROFIBROMA	1	SPONGIOBLASTOMA	1
		MICROGLIOMA	1
		EMBRYONAL CELL CARCINOMA	1
		PINEALOMA	1
TOTAL	167(47%)	TOTAL	187(53%)

FIGURE 5–28.   Incidence of intracranial tumors in children.

Three hundred and fifty-four consecutive intracranial tumors in children under 12 years of age were seen by the neurosurgical service, Children's Hospital Medical Center, Boston, between 1948 and 1961. Note that 47 per cent are considered benign. (From Matson, D. D., Intracranial tumors. *In*, Farmer, T. W., ed.: Pediatric Neurology. New York, Hoeber Medical Division, Harper and Row, Publishers, 1964, p. 475.)

and teratoid tumors) produce visual disorders and disturbances of carbohydrate and water metabolism and of autonomic and pituitary function. Neoplasms in the *brain stem* are associated with pyramidal tract signs (spastic paralysis and hyporeflexia) and bilateral cranial nerve involvement.

Diagnostic Considerations

Roentgenograms of the skull will show changes in about 86 per cent of children with intracranial tumors. The increase in intracranial pressure causes the cranial sutures to separate—initially and most prominently, the coronal suture, followed by the sagittal and lambdoid, and rarely, the squamosal. The head of the infant generally enlarges from increased intracranial

tension. Other abnormalities may include increased convolutional markings, localized thinning of one or more of the skull bones by erosion from the adjacent mass, and intracranial calcification (commonly seen on ependymomas and craniopharyngiomas).

Electroencephalography is invaluable in diagnosis of brain lesions. When the neoplasm is located in the cerebral hemisphere the electroencephalogram is almost always abnormal, whereas with tumors of the brain stem, ventricular system, and suprasellar area, the electroencephalogram may be normal. Pneumoencephalography, contrast (Pantopaque) ventriculography, and arteriography are extremely important in the diagnosis and determination of the exact anatomic site of intracranial tumors.[191–198]

Caution should be exercised in performing lumbar puncture for cerebrospinal fluid examination in brain tumors in children, as a high percentage of these neoplasms are located in the posterior fossa and a sudden reduction in pressure by lumbar puncture is very dangerous.

Treatment

Treatment is by surgical excision. When total excision of the tumor is impossible, however, and spinal fluid circulation is still disturbed, operative procedures are carried out to short-circuit the spinal fluid circulation around an area of obstruction. Radiation therapy and chemotherapy are indicated in malignant tumors.

In the postoperative period, meticulous care should be given to the musculoskeletal system to prevent development of limb deformities and for functional rehabilitation. Often such care has been neglected because of the common misconception that all intracranial tumors in childhood have a poor prognosis for useful survival. In the modern era of neurosurgery and progress in anesthesia, temperature control, hemostasis, blood replacement, and endocrine and metabolic supportive treatment, the results of intracranial surgery of benign brain tumors are good. Details of orthopedic care depend upon the degree and distribution of neurologic deficit and paralysis. Active and passive exercises are performed and bivalved night casts are worn to prevent the development of deformities. Orthotic devices are used as indicated. In the residual stage, operative procedures are carried out, provided the lesion is stabilized and there is no change in the pattern of paralysis.

INTRASPINAL TUMORS

Intraspinal tumors in children are rare, occurring about one fifth as frequently as intracranial tumors in the same age group. Intraspinal gliomata (astrocytoma, ependymoma, and medulloblastoma) are the commonest; next in decreasing order of frequency are neuroblastoma, extradural sarcomata arising in paraspinal lymphoid tissue, dermoid cyst, teratoma, lipoma, and intramedullary cysts. Neurofibroma and meningiomata, which are so common in adults, are rarely encountered in children.

Intraspinal tumors are twice as common in males as in females, and are frequently found during the first four years of life (about half of the tumors).

Clinical Picture

The initial symptoms of intraspinal tumors are usually manifested in the musculoskeletal system, and diagnosis is often not readily made. The presenting complaints and physical findings in 115 children with intraspinal tumors treated at the Children's Hospital Medical Center in Boston are shown in Figures 5–29 and 5–30.

Persistent or intermittent pain in the back, neck, trunk, or limbs not readily explained by local injury or some other disease process should suggest the possibility of an intraspinal tumor. The pain is usually ill-defined and poorly described; it is accentuated by physical activity, sneezing, coughing, straining, flexing the neck or back, or straight leg-raising.

The commonest physical sign is motor weakness, which may be either flaccid or spastic, depending upon the level of the lesion. The parents may note that the child is unable to run or climb stairs as well as usual, or a limp may be the initial manifestation of motor weakness. An infant may tend to use one hand to the exclusion of the other when playing with toys. Muscle atrophy usually accompanies motor weakness.

Muscle spasm is a common finding, particularly in the paravertebral muscles. When the lesion is located in the cervical spine, it causes torticollis (Fig. 5–31). Scoliosis may be the initial deformity (Fig. 5–32). The presence of pathologic reflexes is an important neurologic sign; an unequivocal upturning of the toe elicited by plantar stimulation at any time after infancy suggests the presence of a cervical or thoracic spinal cord lesion. Diminution or absence of deep tendon reflexes in the upper or lower limbs is another valuable sign.

A change in bladder or bowel habits, such as incontinence, enuresis, urgency, dribbling, or increasingly severe constipation, may be the presenting complaint. A lax anal sphincter may be noted on rectal examination. Deformities of the foot, cavus,

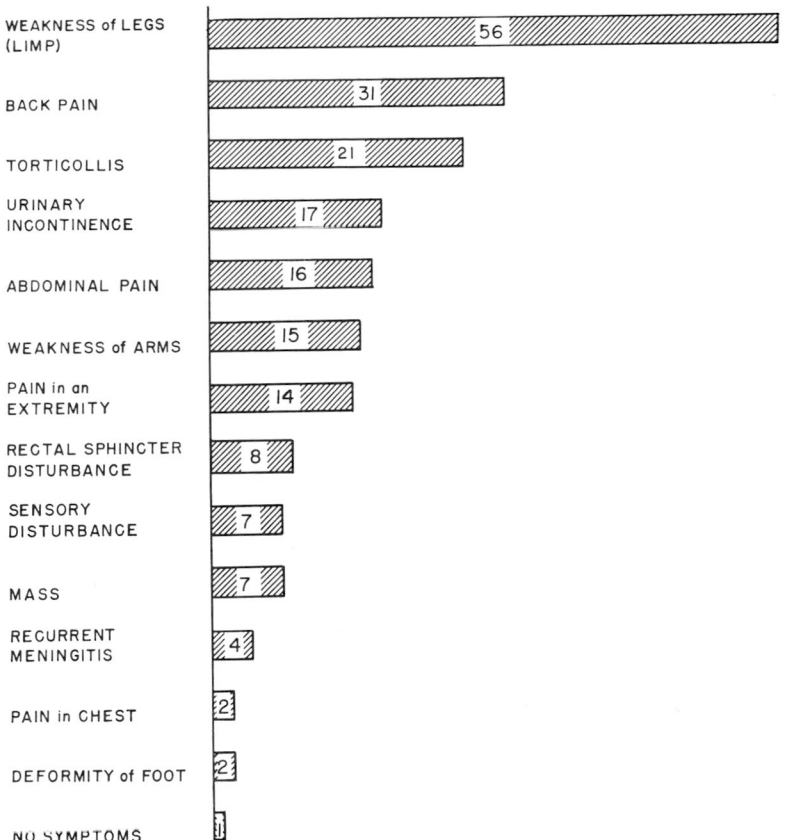

WEAKNESS of LEGS (LIMP) 56

BACK PAIN 31

TORTICOLLIS 21

URINARY INCONTINENCE 17

ABDOMINAL PAIN 16

WEAKNESS of ARMS 15

PAIN in an EXTREMITY 14

RECTAL SPHINCTER DISTURBANCE 8

SENSORY DISTURBANCE 7

MASS 7

RECURRENT MENINGITIS 4

PAIN in CHEST 2

DEFORMITY of FOOT 2

NO SYMPTOMS 1

FIGURE 5–29. Initial complaints of intraspinal tumors of childhood of 115 patients treated at the Children's Medical Center in Boston.

(From Tachdjian, M. O., and Matson, D. D.: Orthopaedic aspects of intraspinal tumors in infants and children. J. Bone Joint Surg., *47-A*:230, 1965.)

varus, or equinus, may be seen. A definite sensory level may be elicited in about one third of the patients. This usually consists of diminished awareness of pinprick or anesthesia caudal to a given dermatome. Other occasional physical findings of intraspinal tumors are visible or palpable paraspinal soft-tissue mass, local tenderness over the affected area of the spine, and vasomotor changes.

Roentgenographic Findings

On the initial plain roentgenograms, pathologic changes are often visible to make one suspicious of an intracranial neoplasm.

Widening of the spinal canal is a frequent finding. With the slowly growing intraspinal tumors of childhood, vertebral growth be-comes altered in such a way that, for long periods, an expanding intraspinal mass is accommodated without visible evidence of bone erosion. With diligent measurements of the interpediculate spaces and sagittal diameter of the spinal canal, a local lesion may often be diagnosed early. The upper and lower limits of normal interpediculate measurements in infants and children were published by Simril and Thurston.[203] A simple, rapid, and accurate method of using drawings on transparencies to compare the interpediculate spaces in infants, children, and adults in a group of average normal persons of similar age and height was described by Haworth and Keillor.[200] Normal values for the sagittal diameter of the cervical spinal canal in children and young adults between the ages of 3 and 18 years of age have been published by Hinck

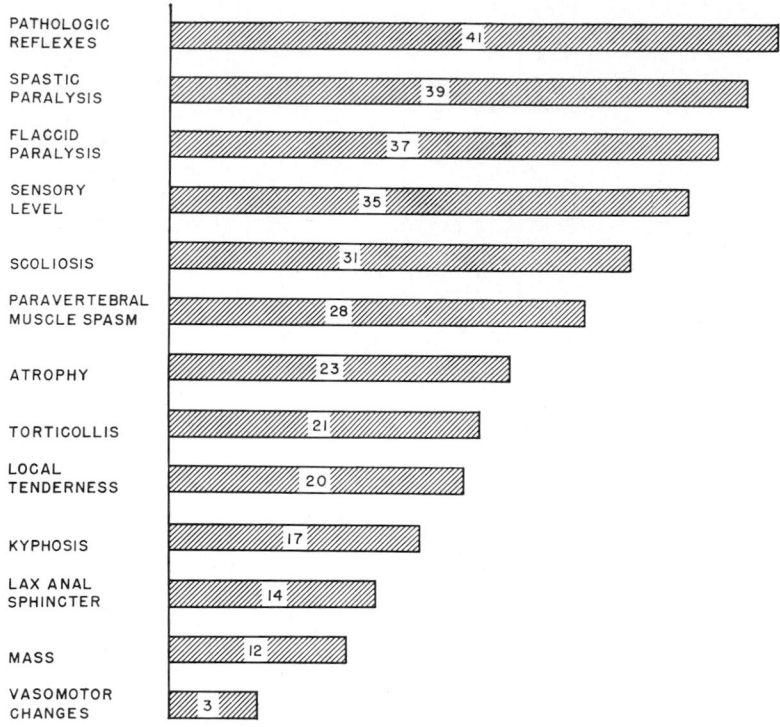

FIGURE 5-30. *Physical findings of intraspinal tumors of childhood of 115 patients treated at the Children's Medical Center in Boston.*

(From Tachdjian, M. O., and Matson, D. D.: Orthopaedic aspects of intraspinal tumors in infants and children. J. Bone Joint Surg., *47-A*:231, 1965.)

and associates.[201] The sagittal diameter is measured from the middle of the posterior surface of the vertebral body to the nearest point on the ventral line of the cortex at the junction of the spinous process and laminae. Meticulous measurements made of both the interpediculate spaces on anteroposterior roentgenograms and the sagittal diameters on lateral projections may disclose minute localized increases that may be of diagnostic value.

Other roentgenographic changes that may be seen in intraspinal tumors are: thinning or erosion of the pedicles, erosion of the vertebral bodies or laminae, erosion of rib ends, paravertebral soft-tissue masses, calcification in the tumor, kyphoscoliosis, loss of cervical or lumbar lordosis, and often, in the case of intraspinal dermoid cysts, spina bifida, or other congenital vertebral abnormality.

The roentgenographic examination should include the *entire* spine whenever a tumor is suspected. A common error is failure to make roentgenograms at sufficiently high levels; in other words, roentgenograms may be obtained of only the lumbosacral spine because the presenting complaint is related to the feet or to sphincter disturbance, although intraspinal lesions at the cervical or thoracic level may cause symptoms and signs limited to the lower lumbar and sacral segments for a considerable time. It is also easy, particularly in a young child, to overlook minor sensory and motor disturbances involving the trunk. Obviously, the presence of hyperactive deep tendon reflexes in the lower limbs, toes upturned on plantar stimulation, ankle clonus, or spasm indicates an upper motor neuron deficit and, therefore, a lesion cephalad to the first lumbar skeletal level.

Myelography with Pantopaque has particular value in a child in accurate determination of the level of the intraspinal tumor. The level of sensory and motor loss demonstrated by neurologic examinations

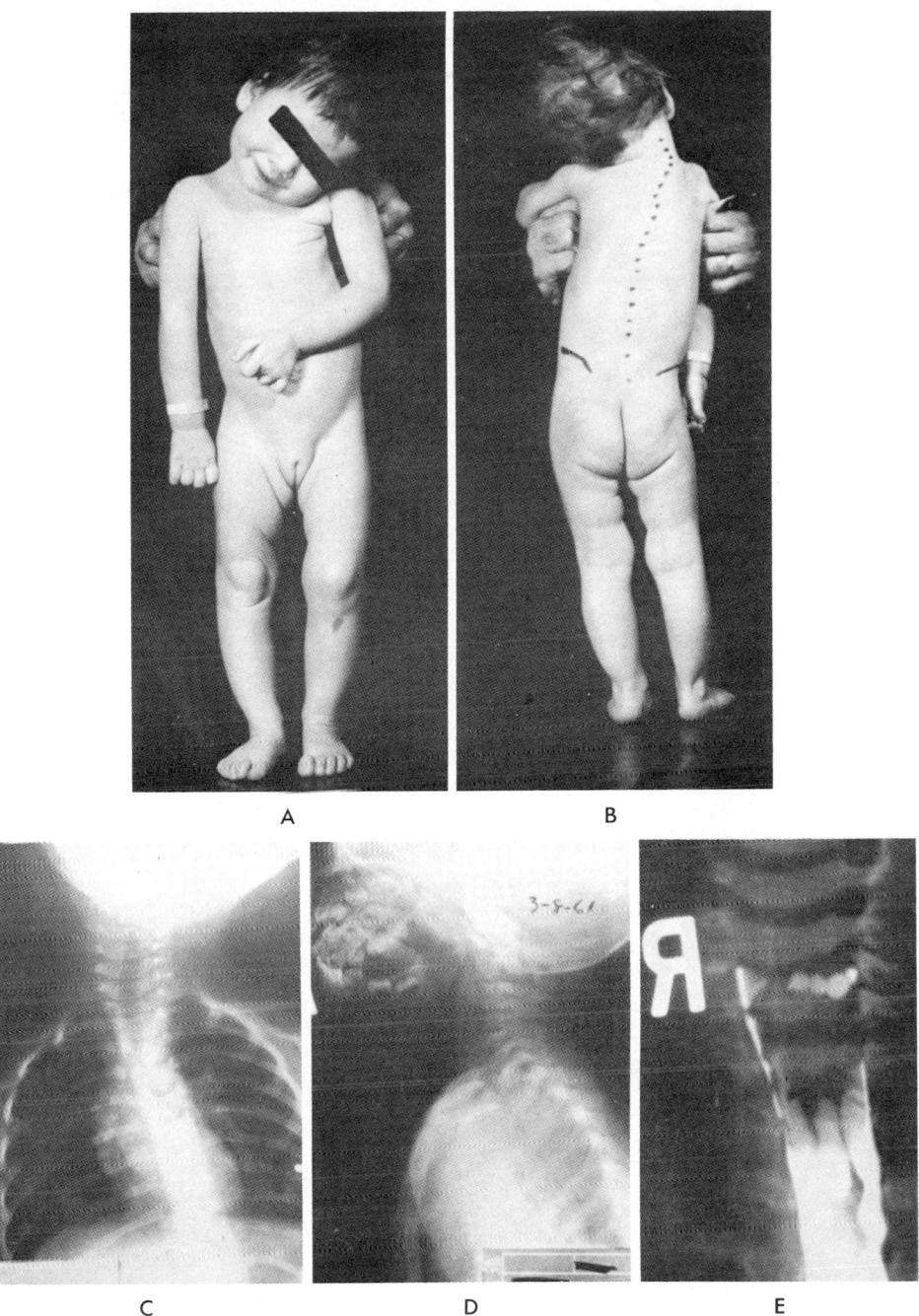

A   B

C   D   E

FIGURE 5-31. *Grade III–IV astrocytoma of the cervical spinal cord in a one-and-one-half-year-old girl.*

A and **B.** The initial symptom was left torticollis, as shown in these photographs of the patient. During the six months prior to admission she had been treated for left congenital torticollis by passive stretching exercises. **C** and **D.** Anteroposterior and lateral roentgenograms of the spine. Note the widening of the spinal canal without evidence of bone destruction. **E.** Myelogram shows the complete block at the second thoracic level. (From Tachdjian, M. O., and Matson, D. D.: Orthopaedic aspects of intraspinal tumors in infants and children. J. Bone Joint Surg., *47-A*: 227, 1965.)

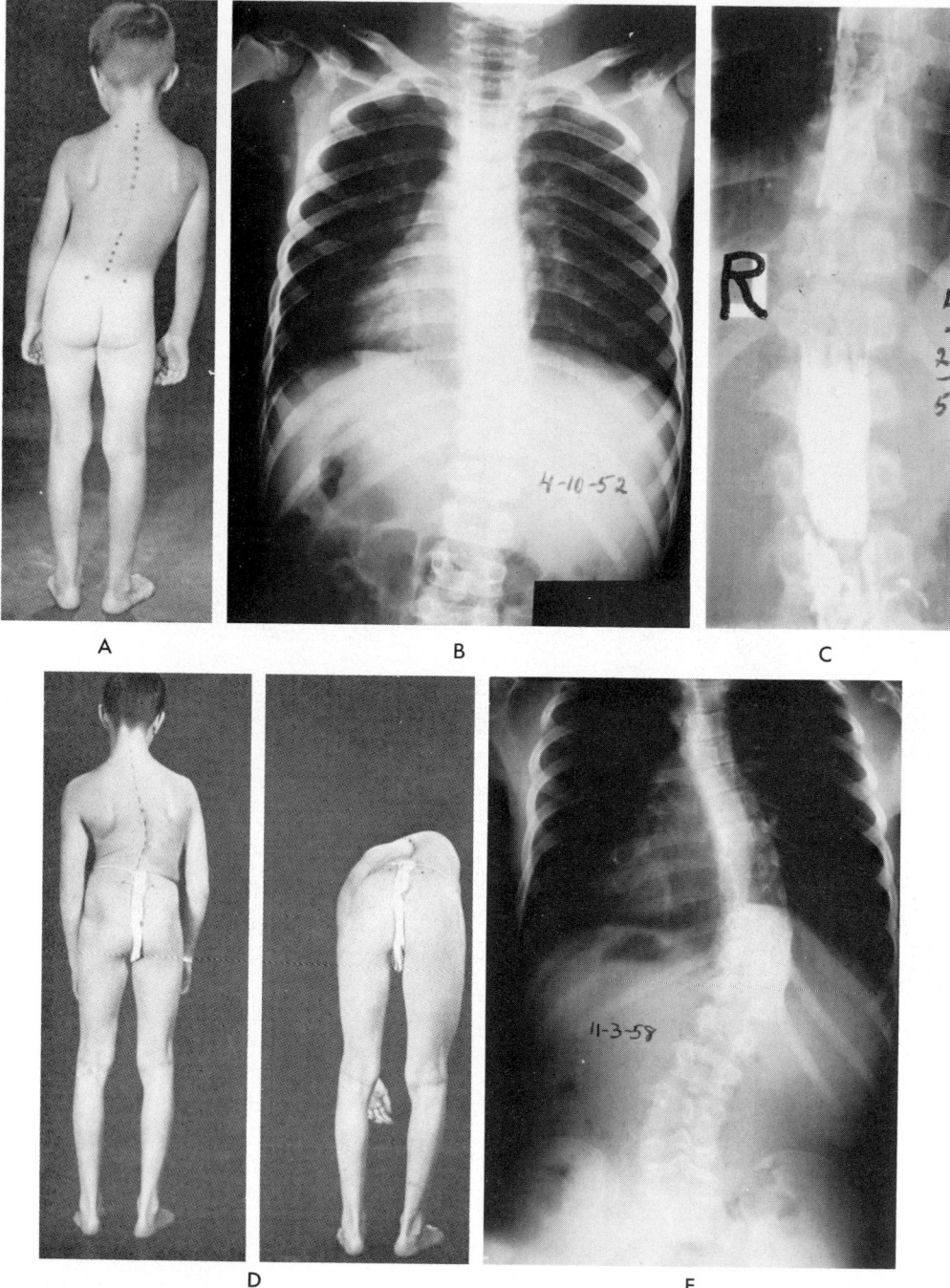

FIGURE 5–32. *Scoliosis as the initial manifestation of a cystic astrocytoma of the spinal cord in a five-and-one-half-year-old boy.*

A and **B.** Photograph and roentgenogram of the spine showing the right thoracolumbar scoliosis. Paravertebral muscle spasm and hyperactive deep tendon reflexes were found on careful neurologic examination. The total cerebrospinal fluid protein on lumbar puncture was 159 mg. per 100 ml. **C.** Myelogram showing block at the interspace between the twelfth thoracic and first lumbar vertebrae with fusiform expansion of the cord from this level to the tenth thoracic level. **D** and **E.** Photographs and anteroposterior roentgenograms of the spine four years after laminectomy and aspiration of the intraspinal cyst. The scoliosis has markedly increased. (From Tachdjian, M. O., and Matson, D. D.: Orthopaedic aspects of intraspinal tumors in infants and children. J. Bone Joint Surg., *47-A*:241, 1965.)

alone may be inaccurate and mislead the surgeon in placing the laminectomy incision. The caudal extent of the intraspinal mass may be determined accurately by myelography, and the cephalad pole may be located if necessary by noting the descent of a small amount of opaque medium instilled into the cisterna magna.

Cerebrospinal Fluid Findings

It is imperative to perform lumbar puncture and analysis of cerebrospinal fluid, though it should be done cautiously when a spinal cord tumor is suspected, and only after critical examination of plain roentgenograms of the entire spine. Whenever the presence of a block is suggested by the finding of xanthocromia and the results of the Queckenstedt test, Pantopaque myelography is performed at the same time, eliminating the need for an additional lumbar puncture. If neurologic signs suggest the presence of a tumor, myelography should be performed, regardless of the manometric studies. Cell count and direct smear are performed to detect the presence of tumor cells; this is of particular importance in the presence of medulloblastoma and epidemoid and dermoid cysts.

The total protein content will be elevated whenever an intraspinal lesion encroaches upon the cerebrospinal fluid pathways below the level of the foramen magnum. The normal level in cerebrospinal fluid is 20 to 35 mg. per 100 ml.; when an intraspinal tumor is present, it may be elevated from 50 to 4,000 mg. per 100 ml.

Differential Diagnosis

The possibility of an intraspinal tumor should always be considered when evaluating an abnormality of the musculoskeletal system. One cannot overemphasize this. Often an erroneous diagnosis is entertained initially and needless treatment is carried out for prolonged periods before the lesion is identified. Such a delay in diagnosis will result in permanent damage to the cord (Fig. 5–33). Torticollis, idiopathic scoliosis, spastic cerebral palsy, traumatic subluxation of the cervical spine, acute back strain, spondylitis, poliomyelitis, muscular dystrophy, and infectious polyneuritis are some of the common orthopedic conditions for which intraspinal neoplasms are mistaken. Figure 5–34 illustrates a case of cystic astrocytoma of the cervical spinal cord that was erroneously diagnosed and treated as traumatic subluxation of the cervical spine.

Appendicitis is another diagnosis mistakenly made when the tumors involve the lower thoracic spinal cord and nerve roots. In the work-up of a child with otherwise unexplored persistent abdominal pain, a thorough neurologic examination should be made and roentgenograms of the spine taken. A lumbar puncture should not be neglected.

Treatment

The treatment of intraspinal tumors is by surgical removal of the lesion. Benign lesions may be completely excised by a competent neurosurgeon. Infiltrating intramedullary lesions are ordinarily removed in two stages to prevent surgical damage to the cord. Surgery is supplemented by irradiation for malignant infiltrating gliomata and for extradural extensions of such tumors of paraspinal origin as neuroblastoma, reticulum cell sarcoma, and lymphoma. Urologic care in the form of constant bladder drainage is indicated in the immediate postoperative period. When cystometrograms indicate that urination is voluntary, the catheter is removed to facilitate skin care and to minimize the possibilities of urinary infection.

Postoperative care of the musculoskeletal system is very important. It is preferable, whenever possible, for the orthopedic surgeon to examine the patient preoperatively to assess the musculoskeletal deformities that may have been present for some time. Complete and thorough muscle examination should be carried out to record the degree of preoperative motor weakness. This measurement will serve as a base line during the postoperative period. At operation, every effort should be made to preserve the integrity of the pedicles and the posterior joints, meticulous attention being paid to all anatomical structures that give stability to the spine. In childhood,

(*Text continued on page 876.*)

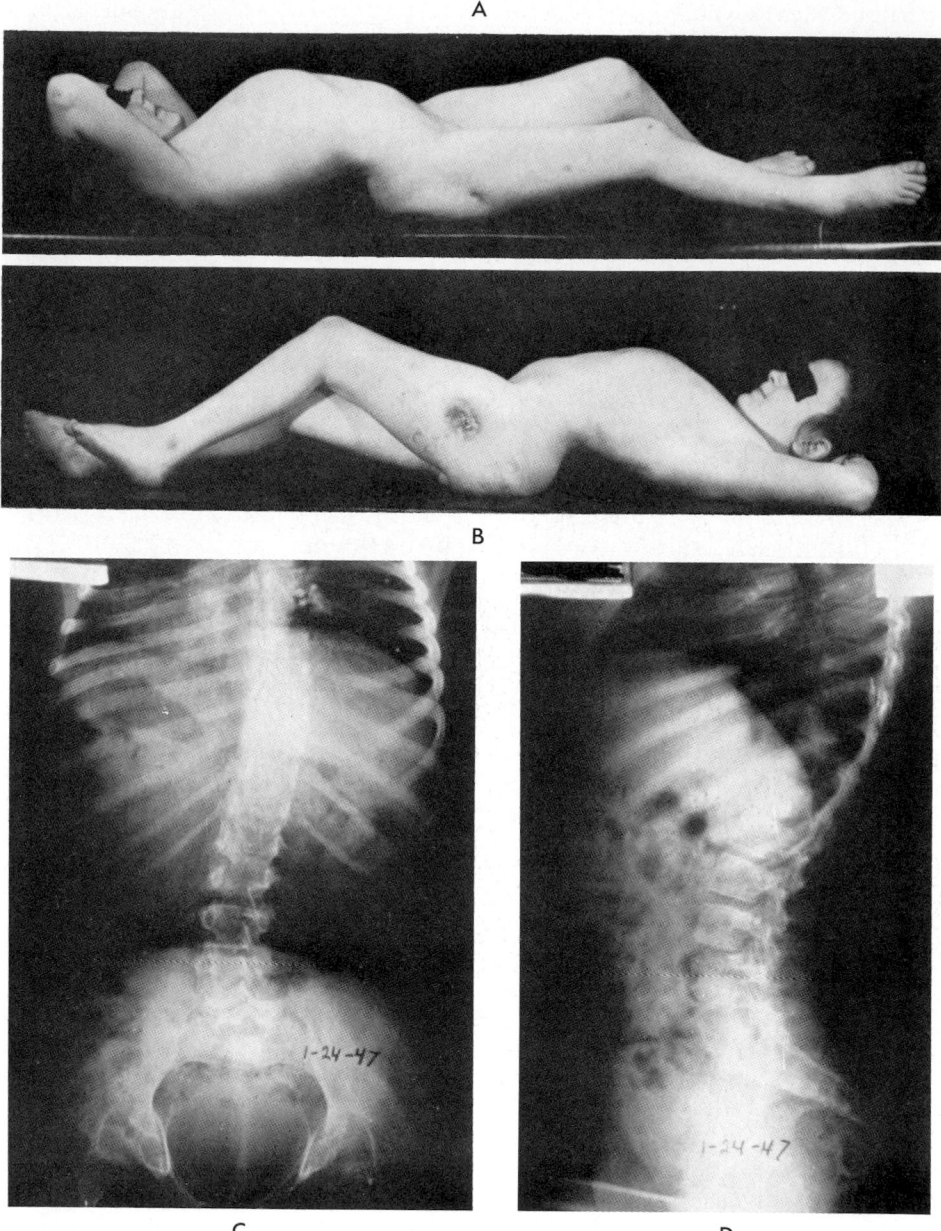

FIGURE 5–33. *A girl, 11 years old, with cystic teratoma of the spinal cord.*

Teratoma extends from the fifth thoracic to the second lumbar level. The lesion is a benign, slowly growing neoplasm. With early diagnosis and immediate surgical treatment, persistent injury to the spinal cord could have been prevented. **A** and **B.** Photographs of patient showing the flexion deformities of the hips and knees, the severe lumbar lordosis, and the deep ulcers over both greater trochanters. A diagnosis of chronic poliomyelitis had been made because of motor weakness in the lower limbs. This erroneous diagnosis could have been prevented by neurologic examination, which disclosed spasticity, hyperactive reflexes, and sensory disturbances. **C** and **D.** Anteroposterior and lateral roentgenograms of the spine. Note the marked widening of the spinal cord extending from the fifth thoracic to the second lumbar level, with thinning of the pedicles and erosion of the posterior aspect of the vertebral bodies, indicating an extensive, intraspinal mass of very long duration. The total spinal fluid protein was 3,900 mg. per 100 ml. (From Tachdjian, M. O., and Matson, D. D.: Orthopaedic aspects of intraspinal tumors in infants and children. J. Bone Joint Surg., *47-A*:224, 1965.)

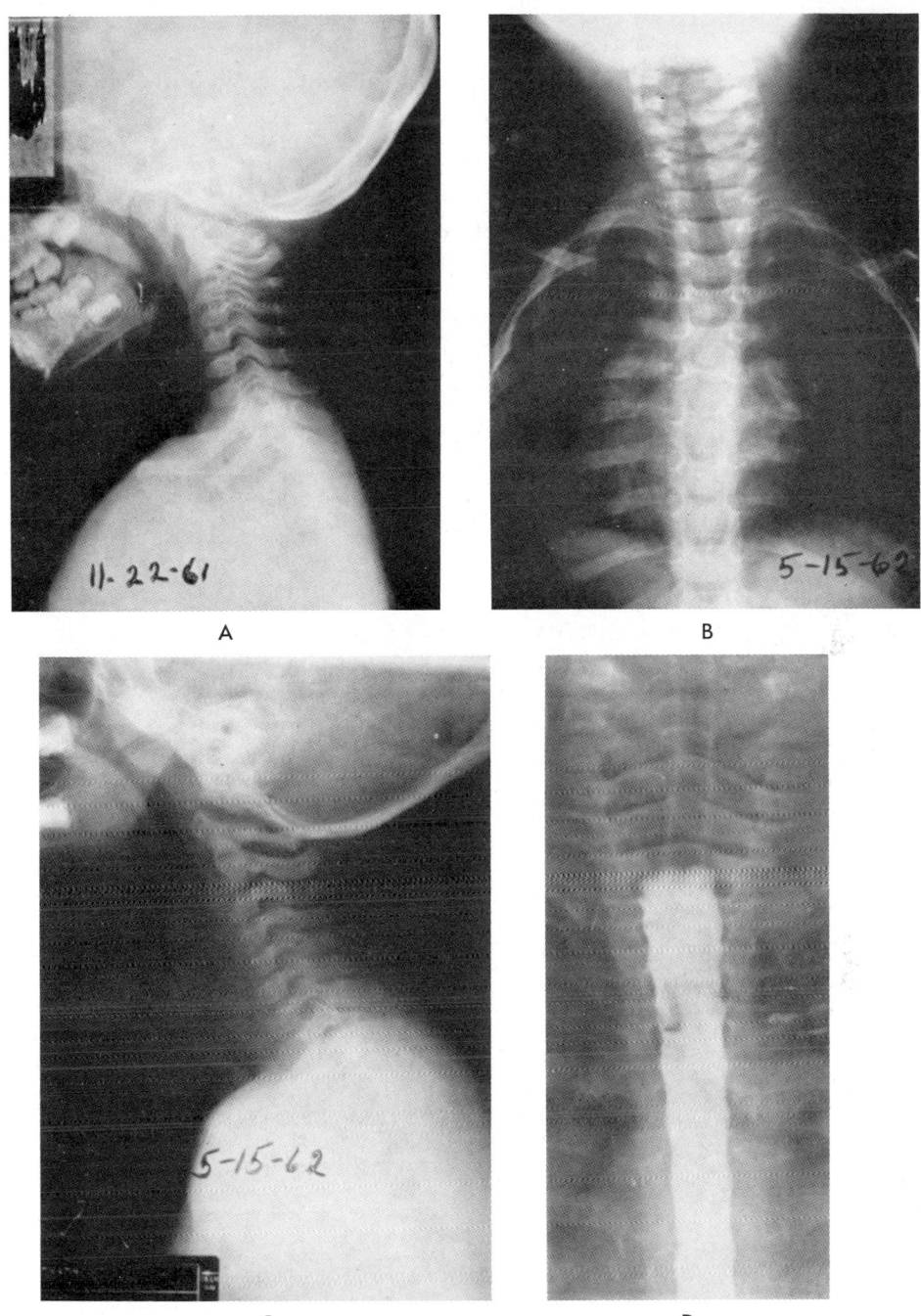

FIGURE 5–34. *Cystic astrocytoma of the cervical spinal cord in a three-and-one-half-year-old girl.*

The initial manifestations were torticollis on the right and paralysis of the right upper limb, precipitated by a fall from a kitchen stool. For six months after diagnosis of traumatic subluxation of the second or the third cervical vertebra she was treated by traction, first with head halter and then with Crutchfield tongs. **A.** Lateral roentgenogram of the cervical spine made at the time of injury. This was erroneously interpreted as showing subluxation of the second or the third cervical vertebra. The widening of the sagittal diameter of the spinal canal was missed. **B** and **C.** Anteroposterior and lateral roentgenograms of the cervical spine made six months later. Note the absence of bone erosion or destruction. There is no true subluxation or dislocation. The marked widening of both anteroposterior and sagittal diameters of the cervical spinal canal is evident. **D.** Myelogram shows almost complete block with greatly widened spinal canal above it. (From Matson, D. D., and Tachdjian, M. O.: Intraspinal tumors in infants and children. Postgrad. Med., *34*:282, 1963.)

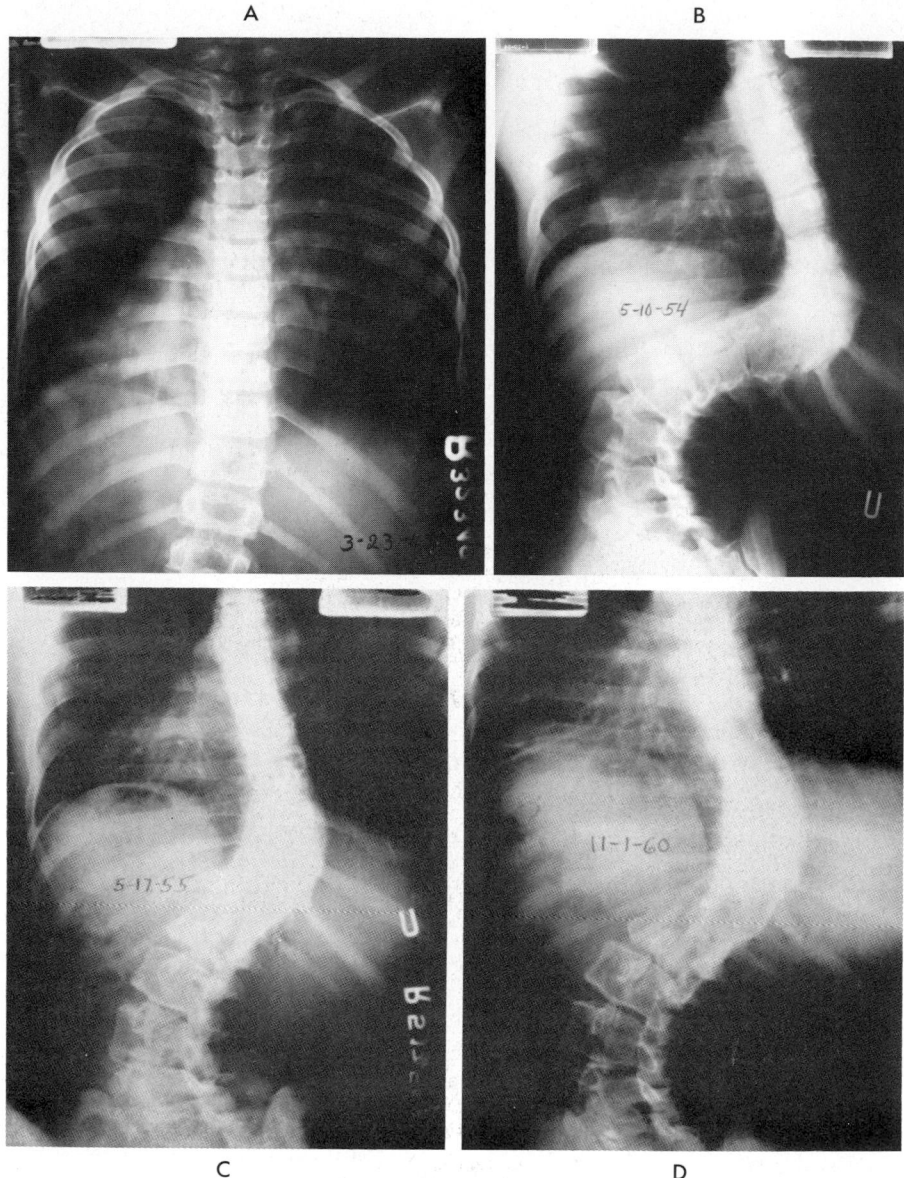

FIGURE 5–35. *Cystic intramedullary astrocytoma of the spinal cord in an 11-year-old boy.*

A. Initial roentgenogram of the spine. Note the minimal right thoracic curve and the widened interpediculate spaces of the tenth and eleventh thoracic vertebrae. **B.** Anteroposterior roentgenogram of the spine six years after operation, showing marked progression of the scoliosis. **C.** Anteroposterior roentgenogram of the spine made one year after spinal fusion from the fifth thoracic to the first lumbar vertebra. **D.** Anteroposterior roentgenogram of the spine made six years after fusion. The patient had increasing paraplegia in both lower limbs with complete block at the twelfth thoracic level, as shown by the myelogram. The area was surgically explored and the cyst aspirated through a burr hole. (From Tachdjian, M. O., and Matson, D. D.: Orthopaedic aspects of intraspinal tumors in infants and children. J. Bone Joint Surg., *47-A*:239, 1965.)

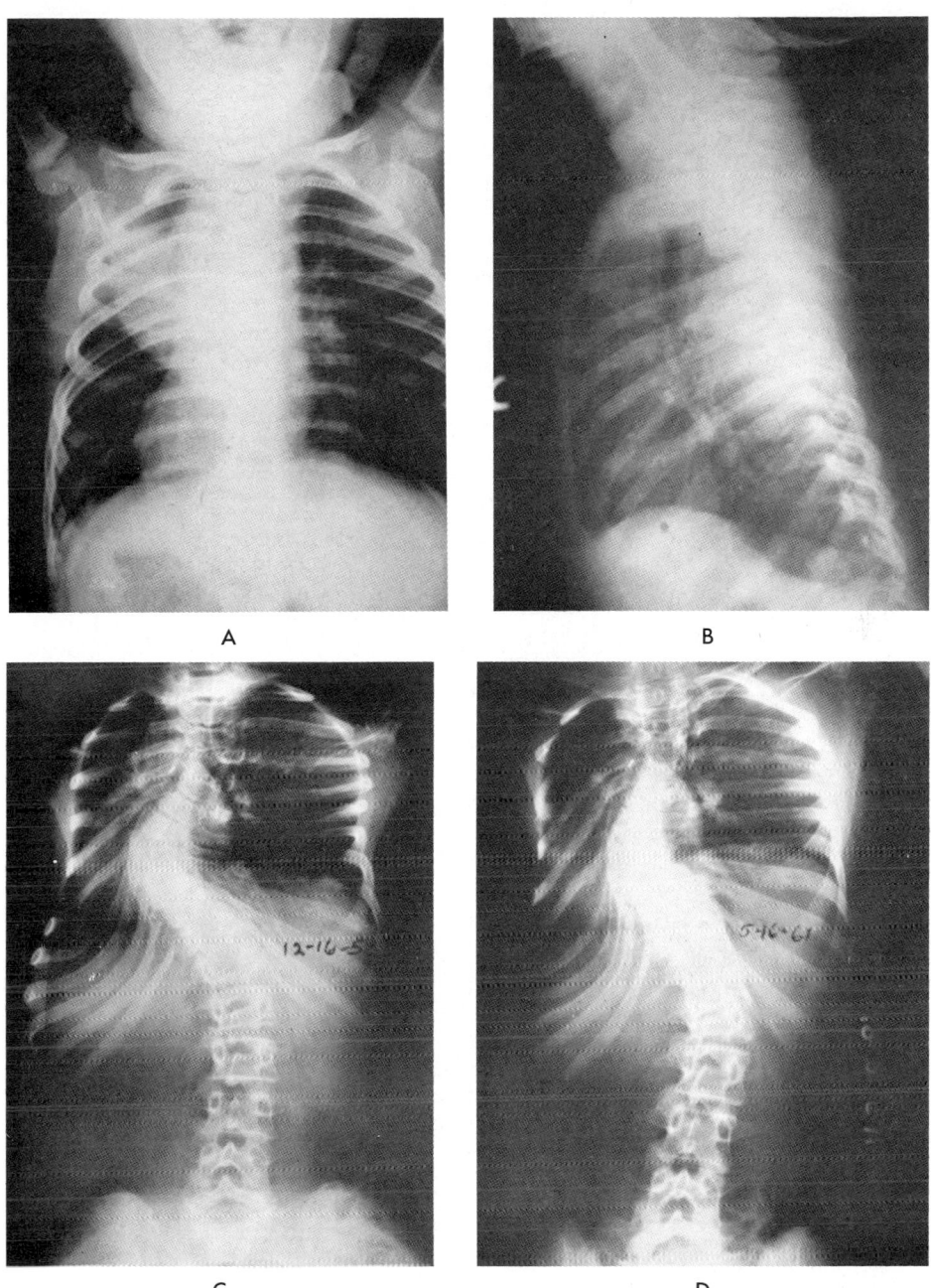

A   B

C   D

FIGURE 5–36. Extradural neuroblastoma in an infant.

A and **B.** Anteroposterior and lateral roentgenograms of the chest. Note the soft-tissue mass in the left paravertebral region with erosion of the ribs and thinning of the pedicles at the fourth and fifth thoracic vertebrae. On laminectomy an extradural neuroblastoma was found and was completely removed. The large retropleural tumor was excised two weeks later. Postoperatively she received 4,300 r of irradiation. **C.** Anteroposterior roentgenogram of the spine made nine years after laminectomy and irradiation. Note the severe left thoracic scoliosis. Spinal fusion was performed from the fourth to the eleventh thoracic vertebra. **D.** Anteroposterior roentgenogram of the spine made two years following fusion. (From Tachdjian, M. O., and Matson, D. D.: Orthopaedic aspects of intraspinal tumors in infants and children. J. Bone Joint Surg., 47-A:242, 1965.)

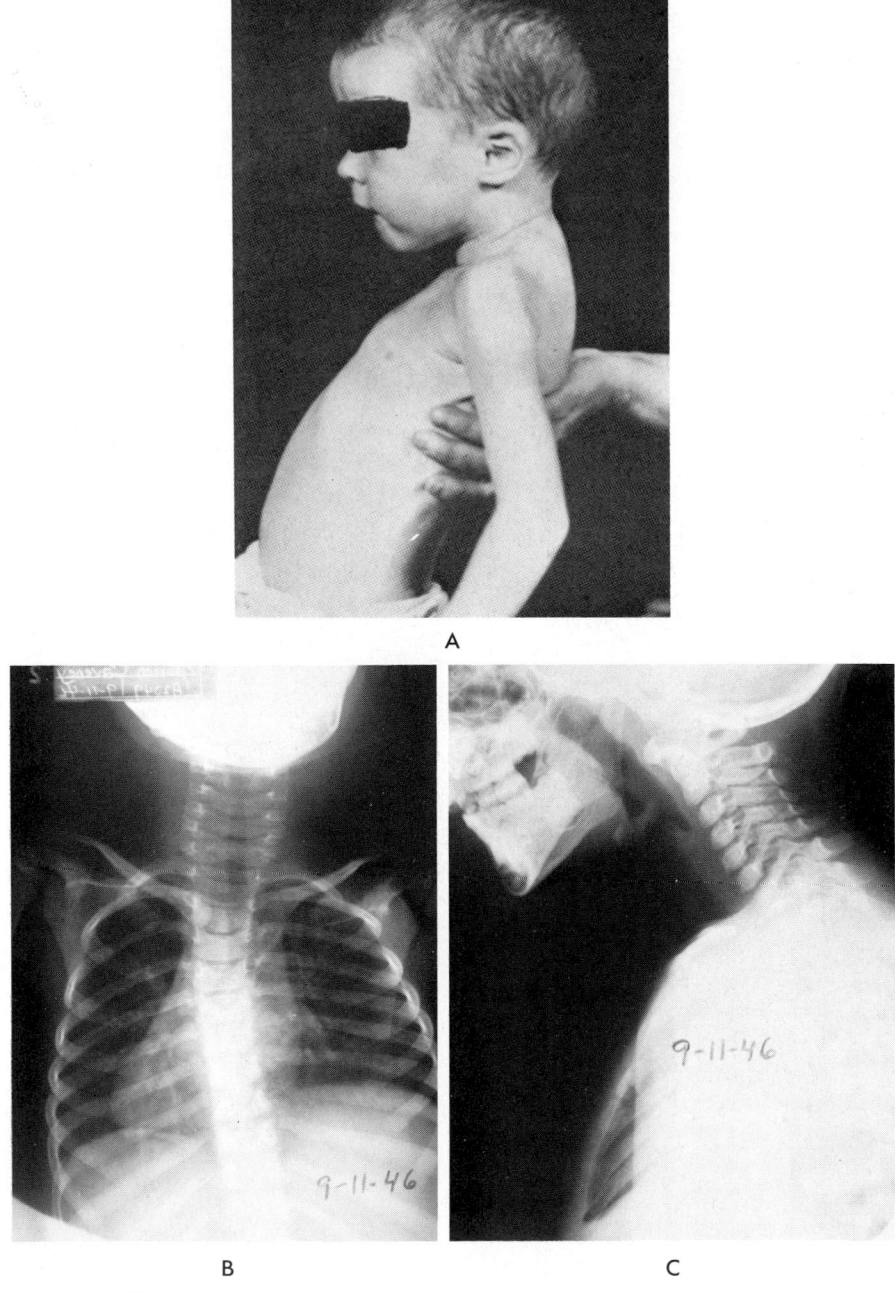

A

B   C

FIGURE 5–37.   Glioma of the cervical spinal cord in a four-year-old girl.

A to **C.** Preoperative photographs and roentgenograms. Note the kyphosis and widening of the spinal canal in both anteroposterior and sagittal diameters with no evidence of bone erosion or destruction. (From Tachdjian, M. O., and Matson, D. D.: Orthopaedic aspects of intraspinal tumors in infants and children. J. Bone Joint Surg., *47-A*:243, 1965.)

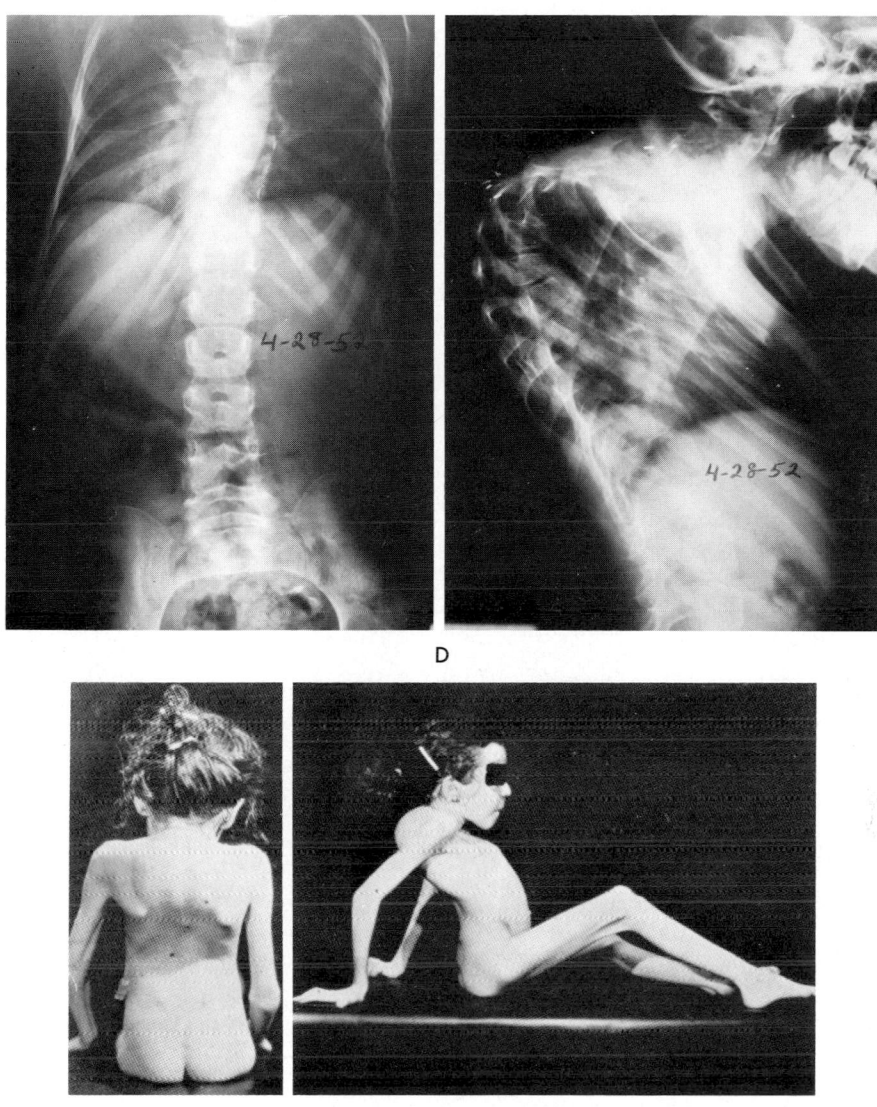

D

E

FIGURE 5–37 Continued.   Glioma of the cervical spinal cord in a four-year-old girl.

D and **E.** Roentgenograms and photographs of patient six years after operation. Note the severe kyphosis. (From Tachdjian, M. O., and Matson, D. D.: Orthopaedic aspects of intraspinal tumors in infants and children. J. Bone Joint Surg., *47-A*:243, 1965. Lateral views in **D** and **E** from Matson, D. D., and Tachdjian, M. O.: Intraspinal tumors in infants and children. Postgrad. Med. *34*:283, 1963.)

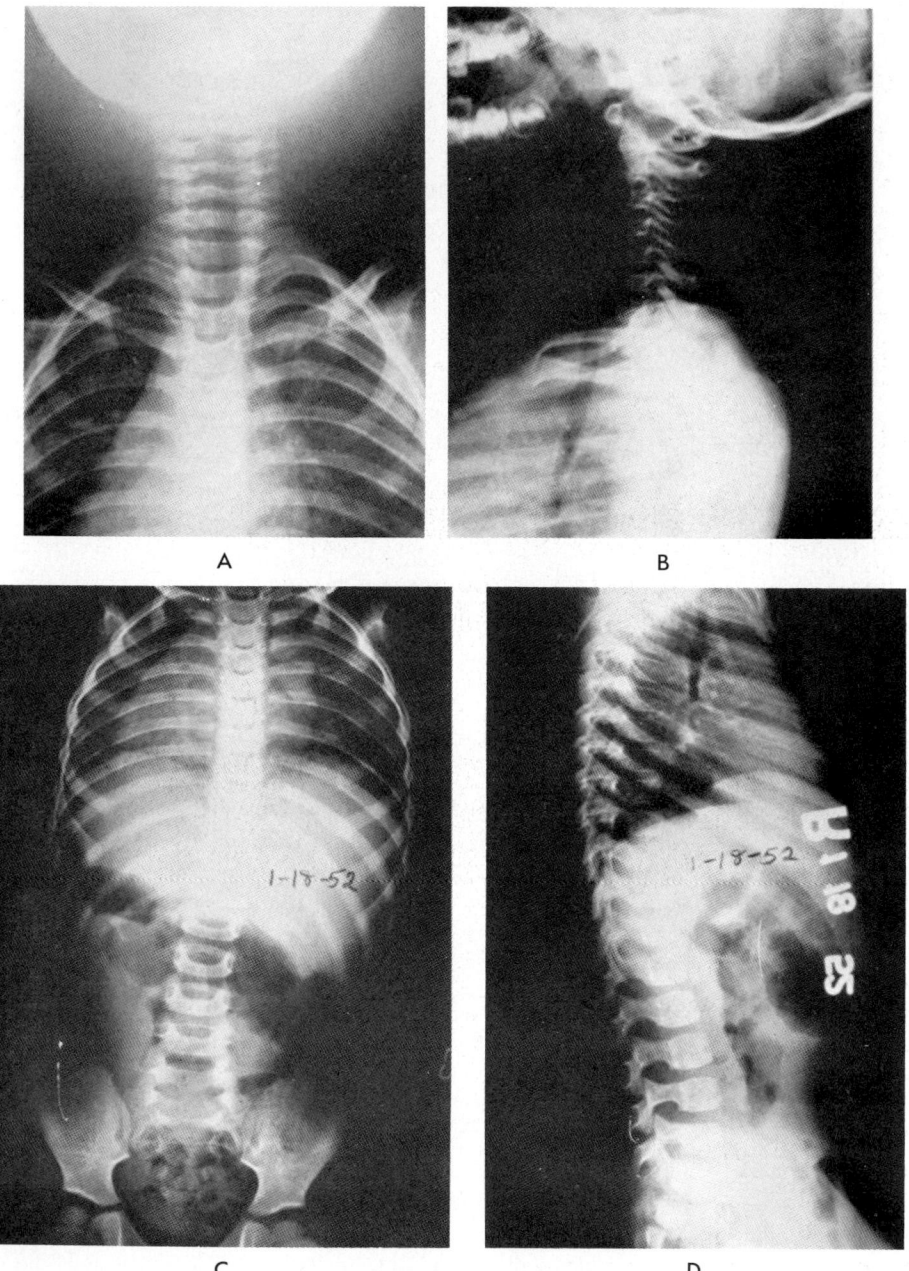

A

B

C

D

FIGURE 5–38.   *Intramedullary Grade II astrocytoma of the lower cervical and upper thoracic spinal cord in a one-year-and-eight month-old girl.*

A to **D.** Preoperative roentgenograms of the spine showing the widening of the spinal canal in the cervicothoracic region.

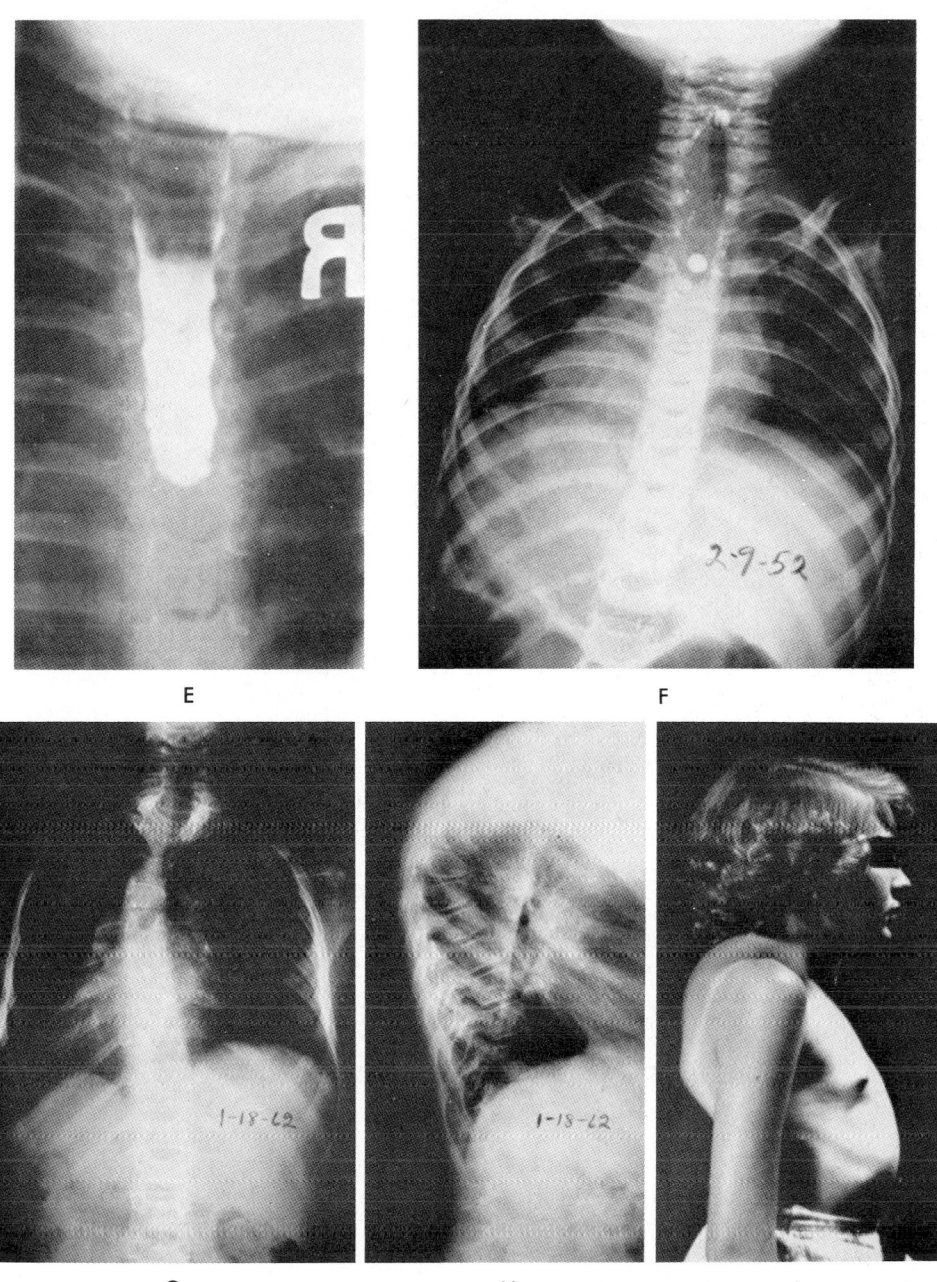

FIGURE 5–38 Continued. Intramedullary Grade II astrocytoma of the lower cervical and upper thoracic spinal cord in a one-year-and-eight-month-old girl.

E. Myelogram. Note the block with fusiform dilation of the spinal canal above the block. **F.** Immediate postoperative roentgenogram of the spine showing the extent of laminectomy. **G** to **I.** Roentgenograms and photograph of the patient ten years after the original operation. Note the severe kyphosis. (From Tachdjian, M. O., and Matson, D. D.: Orthopaedic aspects of intraspinal tumors in infants and children. J. Bone Joint Surg., *47-A*:245, 1965.)

when laminectomy extends over three or four vertebral segments, as is frequently the case, the spine should always be supported postoperatively by a Thomas cervical collar, a cervical orthosis, a plaster of Paris body jacket, or a spinal orthosis, depending upon the level of the laminectomy. Such support is particularly important when there is already associated muscle weakness, when there is existing deformity of the spine, or when the spine has been irradiated. All appliances should be carefully fitted and well padded to prevent pressure sores in anesthetic areas.

Postoperatively, if there is weakness of motor function in the lower limbs, its extent and any improvement or worsening should be assessed and recorded by periodic muscle examinations. Fundamental measures of orthopedic care include active exercises directed toward improving voluntary function in weak muscles, passive exercises to preserve the maximum range of motion in joints with emphasis on correcting existing deformity, and the use of such supports as bivalved casts to prevent the development of additional deformity. When motor recovery takes place, the patient is permitted to walk under supervision with the aid of any necessary crutches and orthotic devices.

Orthopedic operative procedures are indicated in some patients to correct severe musculoskeletal deformities. Before performing any such surgery, it is imperative that one be sure that the disease process is stable and that the pattern of paralysis or deformity is not changing. The neurologic status of each patient should be thoroughly evaluated; when progressive neurologic deficit exists, examination of the spinal fluid and myelography should be performed. If there is any doubt, it is best to wait and observe the patient and re-evaluate the neurologic picture at intervals, especially when the intraspinal tumor is an astrocytoma, teratoma, intramedullary cyst, or ependymoma.

Progressive scoliosis and kyphosis are deformities that should be closely observed following surgery (Fig. 5–35 to Fig. 5–38). They occur in about one third of the patients as a result of postoperative irradiation, associated muscle weakness, or instability of the spine after extensive laminectomy. Other factors involved are the level of the lesion, the age of the patient, recurrence of the tumor with progressive increase of the intraspinal mass, and lack of postoperative support for the spine. A Milwaukee brace is used to prevent or improve an increasing kyphoscoliosis. When it is felt that a checkrein on progression is necessary, spinal fusion is indicated — but only when the tumor or neurologic disease process is reasonably stable and not obviously progressing. If in doubt, it is preferable to fuse only one side to facilitate subsequent laminectomy.

FRIEDREICH'S ATAXIA
(Hereditary Spinocerebellar Ataxia)

In Friedreich's ataxia, the most common of the hereditary cerebellar ataxias, both the cerebellar and spinal cord pathways are involved.[205-223] In the spinal cord, there are degenerative changes of the dorsal and ventral spinocerebellar tracts, the corticospinal tracts, and the posterior column. The anterior horn cells are usually normal. In the cerebellum there is atrophy of the Purkinje's cells and the dentate nuclei Changes in the brain stem may occur. Degeneration of the corticospinal tract may occasionally extend above the level of the medulla to involve the cerebral cortex.

The etiology of the disease is unknown. Males and females are affected equally. It is definitely hereditary and is usually transmitted by an autosomal recessive gene. Often it can be traced through a number of generations. In some members of a family, it may occur only in the mild and incomplete form.

Clinical Features

The onset of symptoms is usually in childhood between the ages of seven and ten years, but often is so insidious that it is difficult to determine when the condition was first present.

An unsteady gait is almost always the first symptom to attract attention. The child has a tendency to stagger and fall, has difficulty in making sudden turns, and is unable to keep pace with his playmates in motor activities. Over a period of years, these symptoms progress and ataxia of the upper limbs develops. Parents notice that the child cannot handle a fork or spoon without spilling the food. He has difficulty in learning to write.

On examination certain characteristic musculoskeletal deformities are observed. A slowly progressive scoliosis, usually in the thoracic region, is most common and is present in approximately 80 to 90 per cent of cases. The feet, as a rule, show symmetrical cavus deformity with marked elevation of the longitudinal arch, equinus deformity of the forefoot, and claw toes. The plantar fascia is contracted in about half the cases. Varus deformity is present with the pes cavus and increases the disability. In the early phases the cavus deformity is flexible and can be passively corrected by elevation of the metatarsal heads. Later, however, the deformity increases with growth and becomes fixed.

Muscle imbalance is an important factor in the pathogenesis of pes cavus. On muscle examination of 43 patients with Friedreich's ataxia, Makin found definite muscle weakness in 27 cases. Ten patients had normal musculature, and in six the muscle picture was unrecorded. Peroneal muscle weakness was the most common finding, either in isolated form or in combination with paresis of the anterior tibial.[212] According to Duchenne, clawfoot results from weakness of the intrinsic musculature of the foot whose action is to flex the metatarsophalangeal joint. The overactive long toe extensors, which are taut like a bowstring, hold the toes in hammer toe position. It is a combination of intrinsic and extrinsic muscle imbalance that causes pes cavus.[206, 218]

The gait is unsteady and has a wide base. Heel-to-toe walking is usually impossible. The patient sways and reels and places the feet irregularly. Stance is unsteady and Romberg's sign may be present. The ataxia is both spinal and cerebellar in type. There is always a greater degree of ataxia in the legs than in the upper limbs. Heel-to-shin ataxia and later finger-to-nose ataxia may be demonstrated. There is slowness of the alternating movements of the hands.

Speech is often explosive, slurred, and staccato. Head tremor may be seen. Cranial nerves are normal; eventually, however, a horizontal or rotatory nystagmus develops.

The deep tendon reflexes—the knee and ankle jerks—in the lower limbs are usually absent very early in the course of the disease. Subsequently, the biceps and triceps jerks in the arms disappear. The plantar response is extensor, but this sign may be delayed for a few years.

On sensory examination, position and vibration sense and two-point discrimination are lost, initially in the feet, and later in the hands. Touch, pain, and temperature modalities of sensation are preserved.

Later in the course of the disease, tachycardia and evidence of cardiac failure develop.

Diagnosis

The diagnosis is suggested when a child is presented with pes cavus, scoliosis, signs of involvement of the tracts in the posterior half of the spinal cord, and a positive family history of similar disorders.

Cardiac manifestations will further substantiate the likelihood of Friedreich's ataxia. In the electrocardiogram, conduction defects with bundle branch block or complete heart block may be seen as a result of myocardial fibrosis, and there may be changes consistent with acute or chronic occlusive coronary artery disease.

Roentgenograms of the spine will reveal the structural scoliosis. The cerebrospinal fluid findings are within normal limits.

Roussy-Lévy syndrome consists of familial pes cavus and absence of deep tendon reflexes and it may be considered an abortive form of Friedreich's ataxia.[217] The differential diagnosis of chronic progressive ataxia is presented in Table 5-8.

Prognosis

The course of classic Friedreich's ataxia is steadily progressive to complete disability. An early onset is a poor prognostic sign. The history of the course of the disease in other members of the family will aid in estimating the rate of progression.

Table 5–8. *Differential Diagnosis of Chronic Progressive Ataxia**

Clinical Disorder	Preceding History	Usual Year of Onset in Children	Examination	Usual Laboratory Examination	Usual Prognosis
Arnold-Chiari malformation	Headache, dysphagia		Palatal and tongue weakness, pyramidal signs, ataxia	May have hydrocephalus, spina bifida	Slowly progressive; stationary after surgery
Hereditary spinocerebellar ataxia	Stumbling, dizziness, familial incidence	7–10	Ataxia, loss of position sense, extensor plantar responses, kyphoscoliosis, pes cavus	Occasional associated EKG changes	Progressive with death usually by 30 years of age
Bassen-Kornzweig syndrome	Fatty diarrhea at 6 weeks to 2 years of age	2–17	Cerebellar ataxia, posterior column signs, retinitis pigmentosa, scoliosis, pes cavus	Acanthocytosis, lack of beta-lipoprotein in serum	Slowly progressive
Dentate cerebellar ataxia	Myoclonus, convulsions	7–17	Ataxia with severe intention tremor		Slowly progressive
Hereditary cerebellar ataxia	Familial incidence	3–17	Ataxia, optic atrophy, occasionally associated posterior column and pyramidal tract signs	Pneumoencephalogram: small cerebellar folia	Slowly progressive
Ataxia telangiectasia	Recurrent sinopulmonary infections in ⅔ of cases; familial incidence	1–3	Oculocutaneous telangiectasia at 4 to 6 years; ataxia, choreoathetosis, dysarthria	Chest X-ray may reveal bronchiectasis	Death before 25 years of age
Cerebellar tumors	Headache, vomiting		Papilledema, ataxia, nystagmus	Skull X-rays: separation of sutures	Progressive until operation
Multiple sclerosis	Preceding neurologic symptoms	14–17	Optic neuritis; brain stem, cerebellar, pyramidal or sensory signs	Spinal fluid may reveal increased cells, protein or gamma globulin	Exacerbations and remissions
Spinal cord tumor	May have numbness or bladder disorder		Ataxia with weakness or sensory loss	Defect on myelography	Progressive until operation

*From Farmer, T. W.: Pediatric Neurology. New York, Hoeber Medical Division, Harper & Row, 1964, p. 525.

Death usually results from myocardial failure due to interstitial myocarditis or from respiratory infection. The average duration of the disease from its onset until death is 16 years. Abortive cases are not uncommon; the disease may become arrested at almost any stage or may have such a slow course of progression that the patient will have a normal life span.

Treatment

There is no specific treatment for the fundamental disease process. Prevention and adequate correction of the foot deformity will aid in prolonging the period of ambulation and delay the day the patient will eventually become bedridden. Pes cavus is the most frequent deformity; its management is discussed in Chapter 7. Tendon transfers are occasionally performed on the hand to improve function. Spinal fusion for progressive scoliosis may be indicated, especially when the scoliosis hinders cardiopulmonary function.

Makin, in a review of the end results of operative procedures on 34 patients with Friedreich's ataxia with an average follow-up of 7.2 years, emphasized that structural foot deformities and instability often contribute to abnormalities of gait and stance, and that the correction of these deformities has a markedly beneficial effect on the ataxia.

INFANTILE MUSCULAR ATROPHY (Werdnig-Hoffmann Disease)

This is a rare degenerative disease of the anterior horn cells of the spinal cord and of the motor neurons of the cranial nerves (fifth to twelfth inclusive), characterized by progressive hypotonia and paralysis of voluntary muscles in infancy and usually terminating fatally at an early age. The condition was first described by Werdnig, in 1891, in two brothers.[243] A family of four affected children was reported by Hoffmann, in 1893.[232] Brandt, in 1950, and Byers and Banker, in 1961, studied the disease in great detail.[225, 227]

Its etiology is unknown. The condition is

transmitted by an autosomal recessive gene, affecting both sexes equally.

Pathology

The anterior horn cells of the spinal cord and the motor cells of the cranial nerves undergo degenerative changes, with diminution in their number, pyknosis, central chromatolysis, neuronophagia, and gliosis. The condition begins and is most marked at the caudal end of the spinal cord and extends proximally to affect the motor nuclei of the cranial nerves. Involvement is always symmetrical. Secondary wallerian degeneration takes place in the anterior roots and nerves, which become pale and thin; the medullated fibers disappear and are replaced by fibrous tissue. The skeletal muscles develop denervation atrophy characterized by smallness and narrowness of the muscle fibers, an increase in the sarcolemmal nuclei, and preservation of the longitudinal and transverse striations and of their internal architecture. The bundles of atrophic muscle fibers are separated by fat and fibrous tissue.

At autopsy, the diaphragm is normal in all cases and the involuntary musculature of the intestine, bladder, heart, and sphincters is not affected.

Clinical Features

As a rule, the age of onset can be correlated with the extent of the disease, and the length of the period of survival. Byers and Banker, in a review of their personal experience with 52 cases, separated the patients into three groups. The first group has the onset in utero or in the first months of life, the weakness is generalized, and death occurs early. The second category comprises those cases with onset somewhere between the second and twelfth postnatal months; the weakness is more localized and there is a longer survival period. In the third group symptoms begin in the second year of life or later, weakness is acutely localized, and there is a survival period of many years.[227]

The patients of the first group are the most severely involved. Some abnormality of the fetus is reported by most mothers, who usually state that in late pregnancy fetal movements were unusually diminished and then became totally absent. At birth or within the first few weeks of life, inactivity and "flopping" of the baby are noted. There is conspicuous generalized weakness of the voluntary muscles, the limb girdle and trunk muscles being most severely affected. The degree of paralysis is less severe distally, with persistence of function of the muscles controlling the fingers and toes until late in the disease. Extraocular movements are usually normal.

These infants lie in a characteristic posture with the hips flexed, abducted, and externally rotated, the shoulders abducted, externally rotated, the knees and elbows flexed, the forearms pronated, and the hands elevated above the head. The infant is so limp and flaccid that he can be manipulated into any posture. Respiratory movements are paradoxical because of the coexistence of intercostal paralysis and a well-functioning diaphragm. The chest is compressed anteroposteriorly and the lower ribs are often flared in a "bell shape."

The deep tendon reflexes are absent. Sensation, sphincter function, and intelligence are normal. Corticospinal tract signs are absent. Dysphagia is present in some. Paralysis of the facial muscles gives a "bland" facial expression. Fasciculations of the tongue are frequently seen. The sucking and gag reflexes are eventually lost.

Bulbar muscle weakness and respiratory insufficiency result in recurrent pneumonia and atelectasis. The course of the disease is rapidly progressive, and the infant usually dies of respiratory infection at the average age of ten months.

In the second group in which muscular weakness is first detected between 2 and 12 months, the lower limbs are more severely affected than the arms. The patellar tendon reflex is absent, but the biceps and triceps reflexes are retained for some time. On attempting active motions, the infant commonly exhibits a fine tremor in the arms and hands owing to inequality of weakness of the antagonistic muscles. Fasciculations may be noted in the tongue, the deltoid muscle, and the intrinsic muscles of the hand. About three fourths of these children develop sitting balance, and a few are able to crawl or stand up by holding onto furniture. The course of the disease is less rapidly progressive, the average age of death being 42 months (i.e., four times the longevity of Group I).

The third group constitutes a small percentage of cases of spinal muscular atrophy. In these children, symptoms begin from 12 months on. The gluteus maximus and thigh muscles are principally affected. Tremor and muscular fasciculations are usually present. The biceps and triceps tendon reflexes are normal. The ankle jerk may be depressed. These children are usually able to sit up at 6 months of age and to stand and walk between 12 and 24 months. The clinical course is quite benign. The average length of survival is seven years. Some patients live to the age of 20 to 30 years. These cases have been mistaken for the Duchenne type of muscular dystrophy. Kugelberg and Welander have described a form of "pseudomyopathic" spinal atrophy with onset even later in childhood.[233]

Laboratory Findings

The cerebrospinal fluid and serum electrolytes are normal. Electromyography will show fasciculations and muscle biopsy will show evidence of neural atrophy.

Differential Diagnosis

Infantile muscular atrophy must be distinguished from a number of conditions. Cerebral palsy, particularly the extrapyramidal type, is initially manifested by a stage of hypotonia and flaccid paralysis prior to the development of athetosis and rigidity. Hypotonia may also be a prominent symptom of glycogen storage disease with involvement of the anterior horn cells. Traumatic transverse myelitis may result from obstetrical injury and may produce flaccid paralysis of the limbs and trunk. Muscular dystrophy in infancy is rare, but can occur. Peripheral neuropathy, such as acute infectious polyneuritis and chronic hypertrophic neuritis, may have its onset in early infancy and cause flaccid paralysis. Benign congenital hypotonia is distinguished from Werdnig-Hoffmann disease by the preservation of tendon reflexes and lack of progression of paralysis. The differential diagnosis of hypotonia in infants and children is given in Table 5–9.

Treatment

There is no specific therapy. Each case should be individually assessed as to potential ability. In Group I, orthopedic measures are not indicated. In Groups II and III, orthoses and crutches are given for support and for assistance in locomotion (Fig. 5–39). Scoliosis, a common deformity, is treated by a plastic body jacket. Occasionally stabilization of the spine by spinal fusion and Harrington instrumentation is indicated.

DIASTEMATOMYELIA*

Diastematomyelia is a congenital malformation of the neural axis in which there is a sagittal division of the spinal cord or its intraspinal derivatives by a projection of an osseous or fibrocartilaginous mass that is attached anteriorly to one or more vertebral bodies and posteriorly to the dura. This entity should be distinguished from *diplomyelia,* a very rare anomaly in which the spinal cord is duplicated, that usually occurs in association with extensive spina bifida.

The pathogenesis of diastematomyelia is unknown. It appears that during the organization of the neural tube from the primitive neuroectoderm, aberrant mesodermal cells protrude into the neural tissue on its anterior surface instead of becoming arranged entirely around its periphery. They persist in this location, developing into a bony and dural septum. Associated multiple congenital anomalies of the vertebrae with some degree of incomplete spinal fusion are often present.

The bony spicule is usually located in the lumbar region, though it may be seen at a segmental level as high as the fifth thoracic

---

*See References 245 to 254.

Table 5–9. *Clinico-Anatomic Classification and Differential Diagnosis of the Hypotonic Child Syndrome**

	Cerebral Hypotonic Diplegia	Infantile Muscular Atrophy	Acute Infective Polyneuritis	Juvenile Myasthenia Gravis	Progressive Muscular Dystrophy	Polymyositis	Benign Congenital Hypotonia
Site of lesion	Cerebrum	Anterior horn cells	Peripheral nerves	Myoneural junction	Skeletal muscle	Skeletal muscle	Skeletal muscle
Inheritance	None	Recessive	None	Not defined	Sex-linked	None	None
Sex preponderance	None	None	None	Females	Males	Females	None
Limb musculature involved	Distal more than proximal	Generalized	Distal more than proximal	Generalized	Proximal	Proximal	Generalized
Cranial muscle pareses	Facial and pseudobulbar	Bulbar in late stages	Facial often, bulbar less often	Eyelids very often, ocular, facial, bulbar	None	Pharyngeal 50%	None
Respiratory paralysis	None	Common	Less common	Common 43%	Late	Occasional	Mild
Muscle fasciculations	None	Common	Less common	None	None	None	None
Muscle atrophy	Moderate	Severe	Moderate to severe	Mild	Severe	Mild (with tenderness)	Moderate
Pseudohypertrophy	None	None	None	None	Characteristic	Occasional	None
Deep tendon reflexes	Brisk or normal	Absent	Absent	Normal	Variable, usually depressed	Variable, usually depressed	Normal or depressed
Sensory defect	Cortical	None	Frequent	None	None	Usually none	None
Mental defect	Severe	None	None	None	Moderate	None	None or moderate
Muscle biopsy	Normal	Grouped atrophy	Atrophy	Lymphorrhages	Degeneration, variation in fiber size	Degeneration, and inflammatory cells	Small fibers
Electromyography	Normal	Fibrillations; sparse, giant action potentials	Fibrillations; sparse action potentials	Decline in amplitude of potentials	Short, low amplitude potentials	Fibrillations; short, low amplitude potentials	Normal or low amplitude potentials
Serum creatine kinase, SGOT, aldolase	Normal	Normal	Normal	Normal	Increased	Increased	Normal
Spinal fluid protein	Normal	Normal	Often high	Normal	Normal	Usually normal	Normal
Specific therapy	None	None	Steroids (?)	Rest and anticholinesterase drugs	None	Steroids	None
Course	Nonprogressive	Rapid	Acute or subacute	Prolonged, remittent	Chronic	Acute, subacute, or chronic	Nonprogressive
Prognosis	Severe chronic disability	Fatal, usually within 2 yr. (4 wk. to 20 yr.)	Recovery in 80%	Complete remission in 25% within 6 yr.; fatal in 5%	Fatal within 20 to 30 yr.	Remission in 80%	Gradual improvement

*From Millichap, J. G.: The hypotonic child. Reproduced by special permission from *Brennemann's Practice of Pediatrics*, Vol. IV, chapter 16. Hagerstown, Md. Medical Department Harper & Row, Publishers, Inc., 1966.

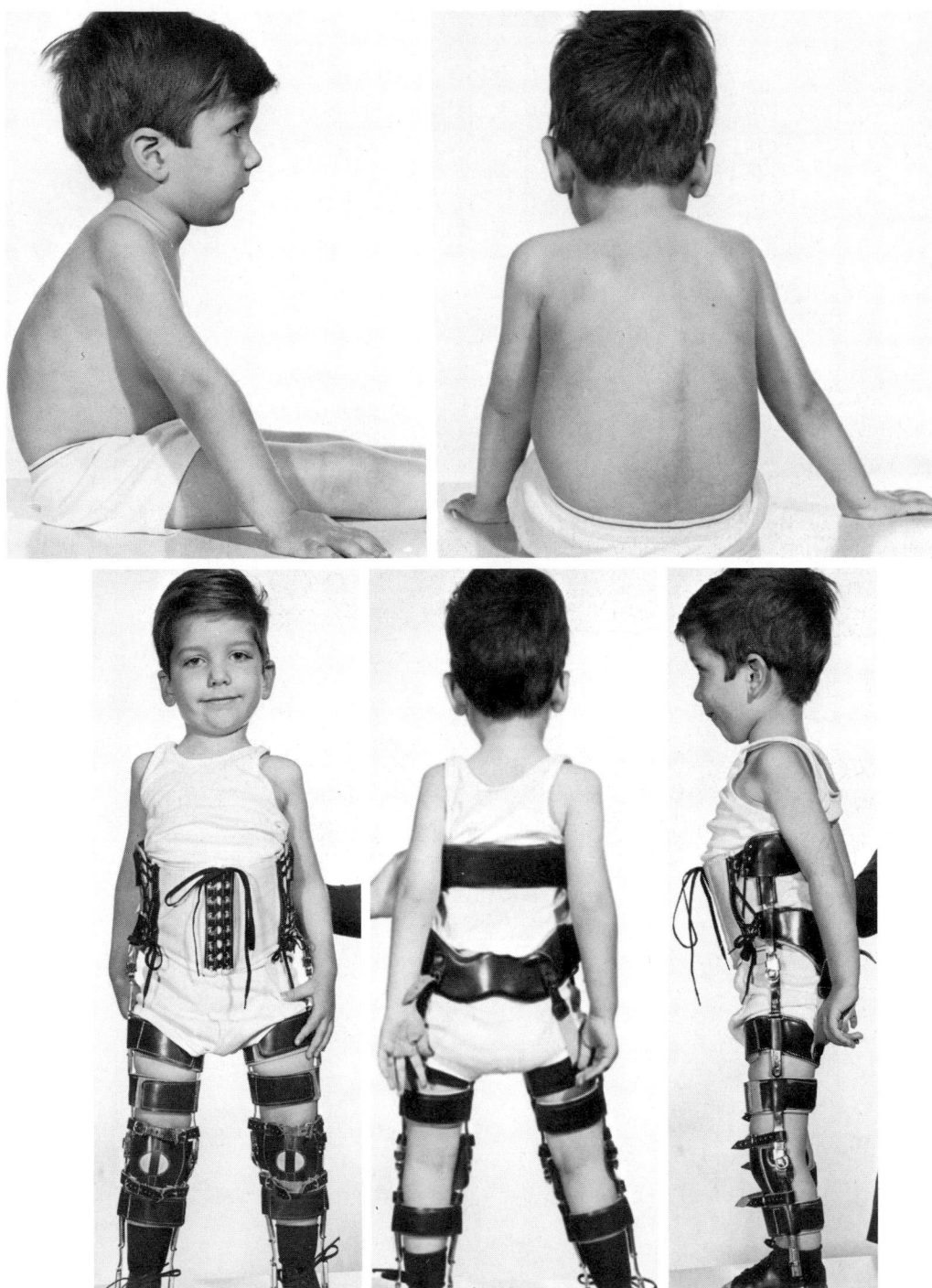

FIGURE 5–39.   Child with Werdnig-Hoffmann disease.

With orthotic support and crutches he is able to ambulate.

vertebra. The osseous septum transfixes the spinal cord or cauda equina at a low anatomic level, checkreining its normal ascent during growth of the vertebral column. Progressive neurologic deficit distal to the level of the lesion develops as a result of traction on the cord.

The condition is more common in the female, accounting for about 75 per cent of the cases.

Clinical Picture

Abnormalities of motor function in the lower limbs are not ordinarily detected at birth. Hallmarks of the condition are the various types of skin defects that are found near the midline at the level of the lesion. The cutaneous abnormalities include abnormal tufts of hair, dimpling of the skin, ill-defined subcutaneous fatty tumors, and cutaneous vascular malformations. Localized scoliosis due to congenital anomalies of the vertebrae is not uncommon.

During the first two years of life increasing disturbance of function of the lower limbs develops. The child may fail to walk at the expected normal time, or some abnormality of gait may develop after the child has learned to walk properly. Muscle paralysis is often present and it may be spastic or flaccid, depending upon the level of the lesion. The anterior tibial and peroneal muscles are often paralyzed. The type of limp depends upon the muscles involved. Atrophy of one or both lower limbs is a common finding. A varus, valgus, or cavus deformity of the foot is frequent. In thoracic lesions, the deep tendon reflexes are hyperactive with a positive ankle clonus and dorsiflexion response to the Babinski stimulus. In lumbar lesions the deep tendon reflexes may be diminished or absent. Poor rectal sphincter tone and urinary incontinence are frequent findings. Sensory examination may demonstrate a definite deficit, particularly in the saddle area.

Roentgenographic Findings

Roentgenograms of the spine will disclose widening of the spinal canal and interpedicular distance that is maximal at the level of the lesion, but that may extend over several adjacent segments (Fig. 5–40). The absence of thinning of the pedicles and lack of erosion of the posterior aspect of the vertebral bodies will suggest a congenital origin for widening of the spinal canal rather than an expanding intraspinal mass, which would cause pressure erosion.

The bony spicule is best visualized in the anteroposterior projection as an irregular fragment of increased density, lying in the midline of the spinal canal. It is approximately 1 cm. in length (Fig. 5–40). In the lateral projection, the bony spicule may be seen as a radiopaque septum arising from the posterior surface of the vertebral body.

Various other anomalies of the vertebrae are also present. These include decrease in the anteroposterior diameter of the vertebral bodies, hemivertebrae, failure of segmentation of vertebrae, and incomplete or lack of fusion of laminae resulting in spina bifida.

Pantopaque myelography will usually visualize the pathologic changes and help to determine the exact level and extent of diastematomyelia. A characteristic finding is the division of the opaque medium into two columns that flow readily around the midline bony spicule and dural septum. Myelography is of significant help in surgery, but is not always essential for diagnosis, as plain roentgenograms are often satisfactory.

Treatment

The purpose of surgery in diastematomyelia is the prevention of progressive neurologic deficit. It is prophylactic rather than curative. In diastematomyelia, the spinal cord and cauda equina are transfixed by the midline bony spicule and the normal migration of the cord is obstructed, producing progressive neurologic deficit. The aim of surgery is not so much to attempt to reverse changes that are already present, but to prevent further neurologic deficit by allowing the spinal cord to ascend and mature normally.

The operation is a neurosurgical procedure (Fig. 5–41). A local laminectomy is performed and most of the bony spicule is subperiosteally resected. Next the dura is

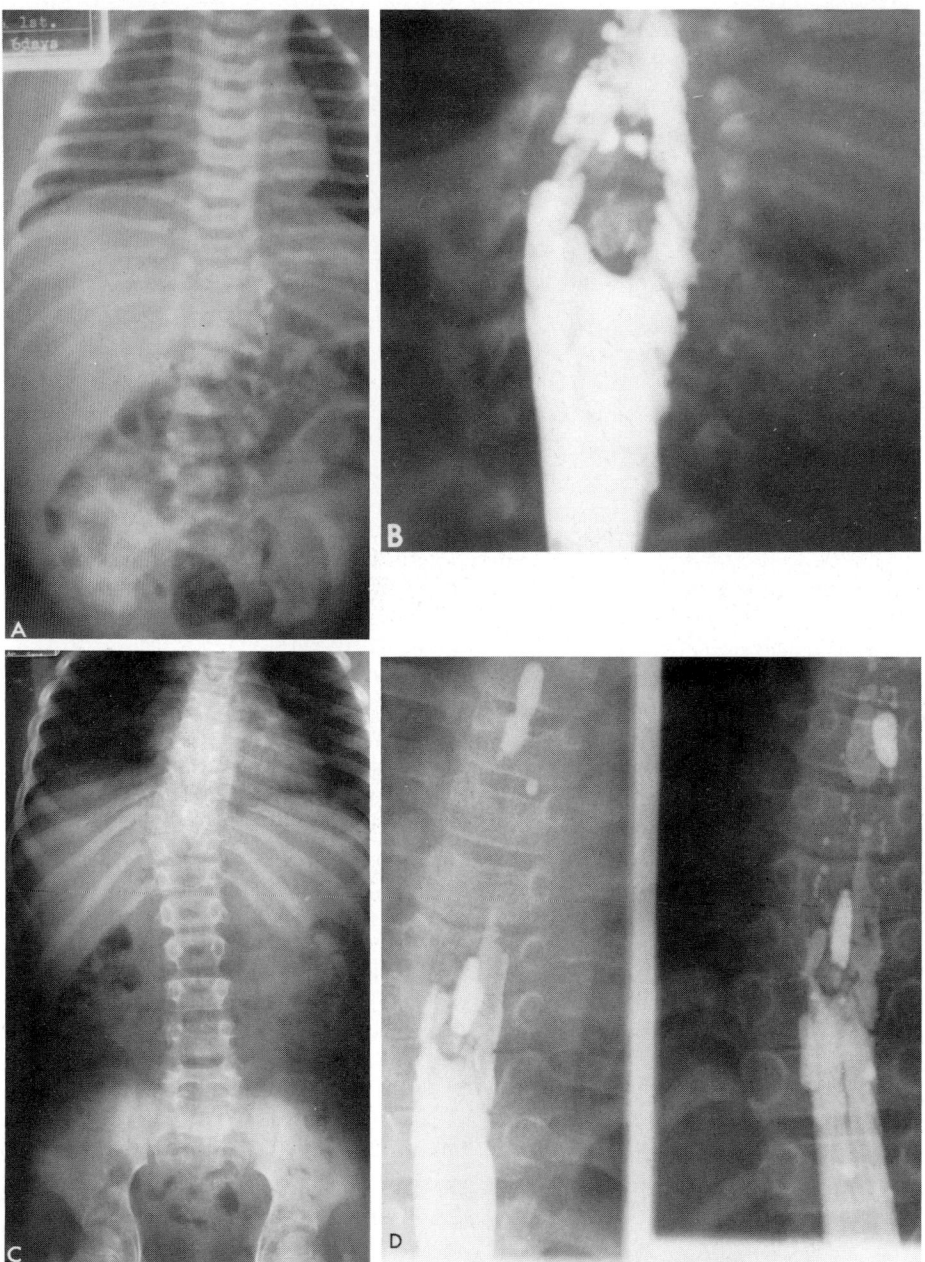

FIGURE 5–40. *Diastematomyelia.*

A and **B.** Diastematomyelia in a six-day-old infant. In the plain roentgenogram of the spine, note the widening of the interpediculate distance and hemivertebra, and in the myelogram, the midline bony spicule around which the opaque medium is divided into two columns. **C** and **D.** Diastematomyelia in an eight-year-old boy. Note the bony spicule and widening of the intraspinal canal.

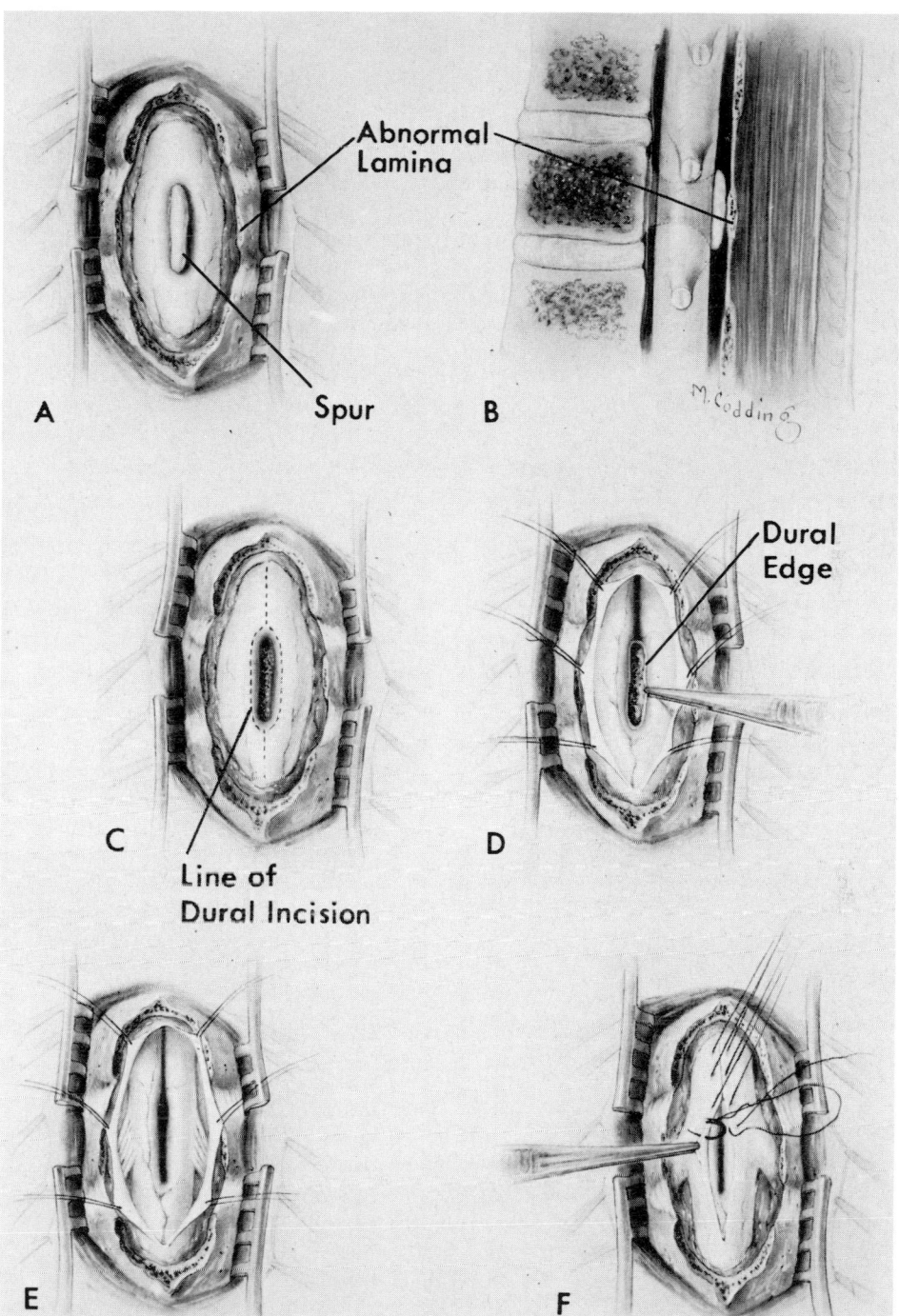

FIGURE 5-41. *Operative technique of excision of diastematomyelia.*

(From Matson, D. D., Woods, R., Campbell, J., and Ingraham, F. D.: Diastematomyelia (congenital clefts of the spinal cord): Diagnosis and surgical treatment. Pediatrics, *6*:98, 1950.)

incised, arachnoidal adhesions to medial dural reflections are divided, and the remaining portion of the bony spicule and dural septa are excised. Thus the separate halves of the cord are freely movable and approximate each other. The dura is not closed anteriorly; posteriorly, however, it is approximated in a linear manner. Hydrocephalus or other clinical evidence of the Arnold-Chiari malformation are not postoperative complications.

The role of the orthopedic surgeon is the care of muscle paralysis and deformities affecting the lower limbs. Treatment follows the same principles discussed in the section on poliomyelitis.

MYELOMENINGOCELE

Spina bifida is a developmental defect of the spinal column characterized by a failure of fusion between the vertebral arches, with or without protrusion and dysplasia of the spinal cord or its membranes.

The condition has been described as far back as 2000 B.C. The reader is referred to Doran and Guthkelch for a historical survey of the subject.[270]

Classification and Terminology

Spina bifida may be classified as follows:
Spina bifida occulta is characterized by incomplete closure of the laminae of one or more vertebrae without protrusion of intraspinal contents to the surface and by the absence of a discernible external cyst. There may or may not be overlying cutaneous defects, neurologic deficit, or dysplastic changes in the spinal cord.

Meningocele is an unfused condition of the vertebral arches with a visible meningeal sac along the spinal axis. The sac is filled with cerebrospinal fluid and composed of dura or dura and arachnoid, but no nerve tissue. There is no myelodysplasia of the spinal cord, nor is there any neurologic deficit, i.e., on neurologic examination there is no evidence of any sensory, motor, or reflex abnormality or sphincter disturbance.

Myelomeningocele is the unfused condition of the vertebral arches with cystic distention of the meninges and the presence of

nerve tissue within or adherent to the sac. There is myelodysplasia of the spinal cord with clinically demonstrable neurologic deficit caudal to the level of the lesion.

Obviously it is often difficult to be certain by direct inspection of the surface or by transillumination whether neural elements are present in the sac; and, not infrequently, a thorough neurologic assessment of the newborn infant is difficult or impossible; thus, one may be unable to detect minimal abnormalities of motor, sensory, reflex, or sphincter function. The designation of either meningocele or myelomeningocele may be quite arbitrary until operative or pathologic data are available.

The term *spina bifida cystica* is used by some, grouping together meningocele and myelomeningocele. It serves to designate the condition of unfused vertebral arches with an external cystic protrusion of the nervous tissue elements overlying the bony defect in the posterior arch of the vertebra. The prognoses of the two, however, are vastly different, and they should not be grouped together.

Rachischisis is a synonym for spina bifida. The word *rachis* is Greek for "spinal column." The term *rachischisis* is sometimes used by neurosurgeons to describe the condition in which there is complete absence of all the covering structures so that the neural tissues themselves present on the surface of the body. The terms *myelocele*, *myelocystocele*, *hydromyelia*, and *myeloschisis* describe pathologic variations of the spinal cord; these are discussed in the section on pathology.

SPINA BIFIDA OCCULTA

Failure of fusion of one or more of the vertebral arches is perhaps among the most common congenital anomalies. It is so frequent that it is often regarded as a normal variation.

Fusion of the vertebral arches does not take place until the first year of life and is not complete until adolescence. This fact accounts for the higher incidence of spina bifida occulta in the roentgenograms of the spine in children than in adults. Ingraham and Matson state that probably about 25 per cent of all infants and young children show some minor defect of the vertebral arches on roentgen examination.[308]

The commonest sites of spina bifida occulta are the fifth lumbar, first sacral, and cervical axis vertebrae. Much less frequently, the last two segments of the sacrum, the twelfth thoracic, and the first lumbar vertebra are affected.

Clinical Features

The majority of spina bifida occulta cases are of no clinical significance and show no evidence of neurologic deficit or musculoskeletal abnormality. Diagnosis is made incidentally on x-ray films of the spine made for some other purpose. There is, however, a small percentage in which the central neural axis is involved as well as the bone, and in whom surgical intervention may be indicated. Early recognition of these patients is desirable.

The skin over the lesion is usually normal but may show various types of abnormalities such as: (1) abnormal growth of a patch of hair, which may be coarse and several inches in length or may be silky and limited to a definite area; (2) a dimple that manifests itself as a depression in the skin in the midline with fixation of the epithelium to underlying layers. Such dimples may mark either the level of an underlying spina bifida or the outlet of a continuous fibrous or fistulous tract extending directly into the spinal canal. The dimples may be minute or they may present as open sinus tracts. (3) Subcutaneous lipomas that are soft, nontender, and poorly circumscribed and (4) hemangiomas in the midline along the spine, particularly in the lumbosacral level, may occur. In the suboccipital area, cutaneous "port-wine" stains are frequent, but are of no clinical significance.

Even though the diagnosis of spina bifida occulta is established on radiologic examination, there is still much controversy over whether it is the cause of neurologic deficit, deformities of lower limbs, or disturbances of bladder or bowel control. The vast majority of clinicians believe it has no etiologic bearing. Myelography is indicated whenever there is objective evidence of motor loss, sensory deficit, changes in reflexes, regression of bladder or bowel con-

trol, actual demonstration of urinary dribbling on pressure of the suprapubic region of the abdomen, palpable relaxation of the anal sphincter, or the presence of musculoskeletal deformity of the lower limb (such as atrophy or pes varus or pes cavus). Myelography is performed to assess the significance of the spina bifida and to rule out intraspinal tumors. It will detect and localize filling defects caused by lesions such as intraspinal lipomatous masses, fibrous defects, bony spicules, dermoid cysts, or intraspinal meningoceles.

Treatment

Most patients with spina bifida occulta do not require treatment. Surgery is performed in a very few selected patients for specific indications which are as follows: (1) objective evidence of neurologic deficit, especially if it is increasing; (2) filling defect (demonstrated by Pantopaque myelography) in the region of spina bifida in a patient with impaired neurologic function; or (3) aesthetic reasons—the presence of a large hairy patch or skin nevus that may be removed. During this purely cosmetic procedure for removal of large deforming cutaneous defects, one should observe if there are any connecting tracks from the skin to the spinal canal.

SPINAL MENINGOCELE AND MYELOMENINGOCELE (Spina Bifida Cystica)

Incidence

The incidence of myelomeningocele varies in different parts of the world. The regional and national differences are possibly due to the different genetic composition of the population.

Lorber reports that in Great Britain, where every year about one million babies are born, some 3,000 of these newborns will be afflicted with myelomeningocele, of whom 2,000 could be expected to survive if optimum total surgical and medical care were available.[330]

The incidence of myelomeningocele in the United States appears to be less. O'Hare, in a survey of nearly a million and a half births at teaching centers in the United States, reported an incidence of 1.22 per thousand births.[350] In community surveys Alter reports a rate of 1.05 per 1,000 live births in Charleston, South Carolina; a similar rate is given by Wallace et al. in New York.[255, 284] In Sweden, the incidence is 0.72 per 1,000 live births.[297]

The mortality rate is getting progressively lower with improvement of total care of these children, and an increasing number of them are surviving.

Myelomeningocele is slightly more common in females than in males. The sex ratio of male to female is reported as 1:1.15 by Doran and Guthkelch, and 1:1.17 by Record and McKeown.[270, 354]

Etiology

The exact cause of myelomeningocele is unknown. Several theories have been proposed, none of which is totally satisfactory. There is a significantly greater incidence of myelomeningocele in the siblings of affected children than in the general population.

Ingraham et al. reported that 6 per cent of the families of 546 patients with spina bifida and cranium bifidum had a family history of similar malformation and that the expectancy of a second child being born was about one chance in 30.[310] The familial incidence in Doran and Guthkelch's series was 8.14 per cent, and in that of Smith, 7.8 per cent.[270]

Lorber studied the family histories of 722 infants born with spina bifida cystica. Of the 1,256 siblings, 85 (6.8 per cent) had gross malformation of the central nervous system; spina bifida cystica was found in 54; anencephaly, in 22; and uncomplicated hydrocephalus, in 9. Eight per cent of the infants born after the index case were affected.[331] In a couple who already have an infant affected by myelomeningocele, the chance that any subsequent sibling will be affected by a major malformation of the central nervous system is approximately 1:14. Three fifths of any affected siblings are liveborn.

Lorber also reported a progressive increase in multiple cases in the family in accordance with increasing size. In sibships of five or more, multiple cases occurred in 24.1 per cent. A positive family history among uncles, aunts, and cousins was obtained in 118 of the 722 families studied, with up to six cases in a single family.[330]

That spina bifida cystica is possibly a recessively inherited condition was proposed by Lorber. Failure to obtain a ratio of 1:4 was explained by the early fetal loss associated with such a highly lethal gene.[331]

Lorber and Levick reported the incidence of spina bifida occulta in parents of children affected with spina bifida cystica to be 20.4 per cent among 367 parents (14.3 per cent among 188 mothers and 26.7 per cent among 171 fathers). The incidence of spina bifida occulta in a control group of 200 adults living in the same district was 5 per cent. They could not derive any help in genetic counseling from this highly significant difference, because spina bifida occulta was not common among parents with more than one affected child, and because in the majority of families, neither parent had spina bifida cystica.[333]

MacMahon et al. report 6.6 per cent incidence of major malfunctions of the central nervous system in siblings born after a child with spina bifida cystica.[334] Milham reported the incidence of malformation of the central nervous system in siblings of affected cases to be 16 times higher than in the general population.[341]

Yen and MacMahon, in a study of 1,095 cases of anencephaly and spina bifida, reported a 4.6 per cent risk of recurrence in siblings born after the first index case. After a thorough analysis of their cases, they concluded that the recurrence of these anomalies in sibships is as likely to be due to persistence or recurrence of environmental factors as it is likely to be due to a common genetic inheritance.[393] Maternal age and parity seem to have relatively little effect.

In 108 instances of affected twins, none of the co-twins were affected. Case reports of affected concordant twins have been published, but such instances are extremely rare.[271, 275, 281, 292, 318] Chromosomal abnormalities have not been demonstrated in myelomeningocele.

In summary, in families already having one child with myelomeningocele, the chance of another afflicted child being born rises to 80 per thousand; and after two affected children, the incidence is much greater (up to 400 per thousand). These figures stress the desirability of genetic counseling.

The neural plate appears first in the late presomite phase approximately 18 days following conception, and neural tube closure is complete just after cessation of somite formation at about the end of the fourth week. Any exogenous factor that influences the spine of the developing embryo must be present in the first few weeks of pregnancy.[351] Failure of fusion of the neural groove dorsally because of developmental arrest and hence the failure to form a neural tube was originally proposed by von Recklinghausen.[353] This concept has been supported by experimental production of spina bifida in animals. Gillman et al., in 1948, developed the trypan blue method of inducing spinal anomalies.[289] Gunberg produced the defect of spina bifida in 21 per cent of the offspring of Lang-Evans female rats by giving 1 cc. of 1 per cent aqueous solution of trypan blue subcutaneously from three days prior to pregnancy to the seventh day after onset of conception.[293] Warkany et al. have also produced myeloschisis in the progeny of trypan blue treated pregnant rats. On the basis of his experiments, Warkany proposed that the lesion of spina cystica starts as a myeloschisis, becoming transformed into myelomeningocele by the development of the pia mater and epidermis during the second half of pregnancy.[385] The notochord is proximal to the neural groove and antedates the neural plate in development. It has been suggested that failure of fusion of the neural groove is due to faulty induction of the neural plate by the notochord.

The theory of myeloschisis being a developmental error in closure of the neural tube fails to explain the presence of a central canal in many localized myelomeningoceles, such as is so commonly seen in the lumbosacral area.[370]

Patten was the first to demonstrate the presence of tremendous excessive growth of the neural plate tissue in the region of spina bifida and for a short distance above in early human embryos with spina bifida. The process may be related to hamartomatous growth. Patten proposed that a myelomeningocele arises because of abnormal proliferative activity of the neural plate zone, which prevents closure of the neural groove.[351]

That spinal bifida is caused by failure of fusion of the vertebral arches, leaving a defect posteriorly through which herniation of the meninges and spinal cord occurs, is refuted by the following facts: (1) Embryologically, the neural tube is well formed before the notochord begins to segment. (2) The pathologic changes in the cord, such as hydromyelia, cannot be explained by simple herniation. (3) Dura mater does not contribute to the sac wall when there is an ectodermal defect; if myelomeningocele were a simple herniation, it ought to retain an external dural sac.

The theory that obstructive hydrocephalus and hydromyelia are etiologic factors of spina bifida is also untenable.

Pathology

A masterful and thorough description of pathologic findings of spina bifida cystica was given, in 1888, by von Recklinghausen, who accurately dissected out both the cord and meninges in cases of myeloschisis and myelocystocele, and who first recognized every variety of spina bifida.[353] The following descriptions are based on the writings of Ingraham, Campell, Cameron, and Smith.[264-266, 310, 370]

The lesions may occur at any point along the spinal axis, but are seen predominantly in the lumbosacral region. They are next most frequently found in the cervical spine area, and a smaller number of lesions are scattered along the thoracic region. The higher the level of the lesion, the less likelihood there is of severe neurologic involvement. In cervical lesions, for example, neurologic deficit is minimal because the majority are simple meningoceles with narrow necks to the sac. The converse is true for lesions below the first lumbar vertebra.

The great majority of the lesions are posterior, but in a very rare instance one may encounter an anterior or lateral meningocele, which should be considered in the differential diagnosis of atypical masses in the chest, retroperitoneal tissues, and pelvis. In these cases, myelography will confirm the diagnosis. The anterior cysts protrude through the vertebral bodies, not through the vertebral arches. The pathologic features are described in anatomic order:

SKIN

The skin over a myelomeningocele sac is almost always incomplete. In the usual type of lesion, there is a raised mass on the back, covered laterally at its base by normal skin, but the apex of the mass is devoid of skin. It is covered by a tissue-paper-thin membrane (arachnoid) through which one may see nerve roots. Within a day or two, it presents the appearance of an ulcerated granulating surface. The lesion may heal over completely by epithelial growth from the periphery. Not infrequently, however, the mass will slough from secondary infection. If the infant does not die from meningitis, recurrent episodes of superficial infection and cellulitis will cause the mass to become puckered and crevassed. In the skin directly over the sac or surrounding it, one will often encounter pigmentary or hemangiomatous lesions.

MENINGES

The three layers of meninges are normal above and below the lesion. In the usual lumbosacral myelomeningocele with a skin defect, the dura mater fuses with the edges of the skin defect, and only an arachnoid membrane covers the roof of the sac. Granulation tissue may obscure the identity of the arachnoid membrane in ulcerated myelomeningocele; however, on careful inspection, the continuity of the arachnoid membrane is demonstrable at the edges of the ulceration. When the skin is intact at the site of the lesion, all three layers of meninges similarly remain intact.

The size and contents of the "sac" of the meninges vary. It may be seen as a gross myeloschisis that has a wide and unfused embryonic neural plate involving the entire length of the spinal canal with a narrow slit of arachnoid cavity containing a few strands of nerve tissue; at the other extreme there is a definite neck to the sac, as the meninges protrude from the spinal canal through a small vertebral defect to line the myelomeningocele mass. The gradations between these two extremes depend on the extent of the vertebral defect and the amount of dysplastic cord and nerve tissue that emerges through the neck. The dysplastic cord is usually closely adherent to the inner lining of the sac. At times, lipomatous or fibrolipomatous tissue may be found either outside or within the dura mater.

SPINAL CORD

Myelodysplasia is always present. These variations in the dysplastic spinal cord may be classified into three types:

Absent Cord. In extreme degrees of anencephaly with complete spina bifida, the cord may be totally absent.

Split Cord. This may arise as a result of failure of fusion of the embryological neural plates ("myeloschisis"), in which the cord is represented by only unformed strands of neural tissue with no central canal; or "schisis" of the cord may occur following its formation—a condition known as diastematomyelia. Diastematomyelia does occur without spina bifida as well. On surgery for myelomeningocele, or even in simple meningocele, a search must be made for a bony, cartilaginous, or fibrous spur that splits the cord. Its removal might prevent the possible subsequent increasing distortion of the cord and roots with later growth of the vertebral column.

Formed But Dysplastic Cord. Commonly the cord may be formed but dysplastic in several ways. It may be cystic or cavitated; it may be solid, but degenerated and disorganized; or it may be grossly proliferated. Frequently all these features are found together in varying degrees.

PERIPHERAL ROOTS

Peripheral nerve development is not affected in myelomeningocele. At surgery and on dissection of the postmortem specimen, normal peripheral roots have been found in every case. However, inside the dura mater the roots appear to have tenuous connections with the actual cord itself and on occasion are hard to identify.

VERTEBRAE

The principal defect is the arrest of development of the laminae. It varies from one extreme of failure of the laminae and vertebral spines to fuse posteriorly to the other extreme of total failure of formation of laminae, the pedicles alone being present. The intraspinal canal is widened as a result of lateral displacement of the pedicles on the vertebral bodies.

HYDROCEPHALUS

Some degree of hydrocephalus is present in almost every infant born with myelomeningocele, the most common cause of this being the Arnold-Chiari malformation. There is herniation of the hindbrain through the foramen magnum and into the cervical spinal canal. In the Arnold-Chiari malformation, hydrocephalus may develop from obstruction of the flow of cerebrospinal fluid at the roof of the fourth ventricle by dislocation of the ventricle, by occlusion of the subarachnoid space at the site of herniation, by occlusion of the same space at the tentorial level by adhesive arachnoiditis, or by an associated aqueduct stenosis. Other causes of hydrocephalus in myelomeningocele are: the Dandy Walker malformation, which consists of marked distention of the fourth ventricle due to occlusion of the foramina of Luschka and Magendie; the "forking" of the aqueduct of Sylvius, in which the aqueduct is represented by two narrow channels situated in a sagittal plane; and adequate stenosis. The reader is referred to E. Durham Smith for a critical discussion of the causes of the Arnold-Chiari malformation in myelomeningocele.[370]

Clinical Features

The external appearance of the local lesion has been described previously. The size, location, and covering of the myelomeningocele sac are determined (Fig. 5–42). Any areas of ulceration or leakage of cerebrospinal fluid should be noted. The amount of neural tissue within the sac is determined by transillumination in a darkened room. The meningocele surface should be scanned for the presence of any neural elements. The extent of the bony defect in the vertebrae is noted by gentle palpation and confirmed by anteroposterior and lateral roentgenograms of the entire spine.

The adequacy of cerebrospinal fluid circulation is evaluated. One should look

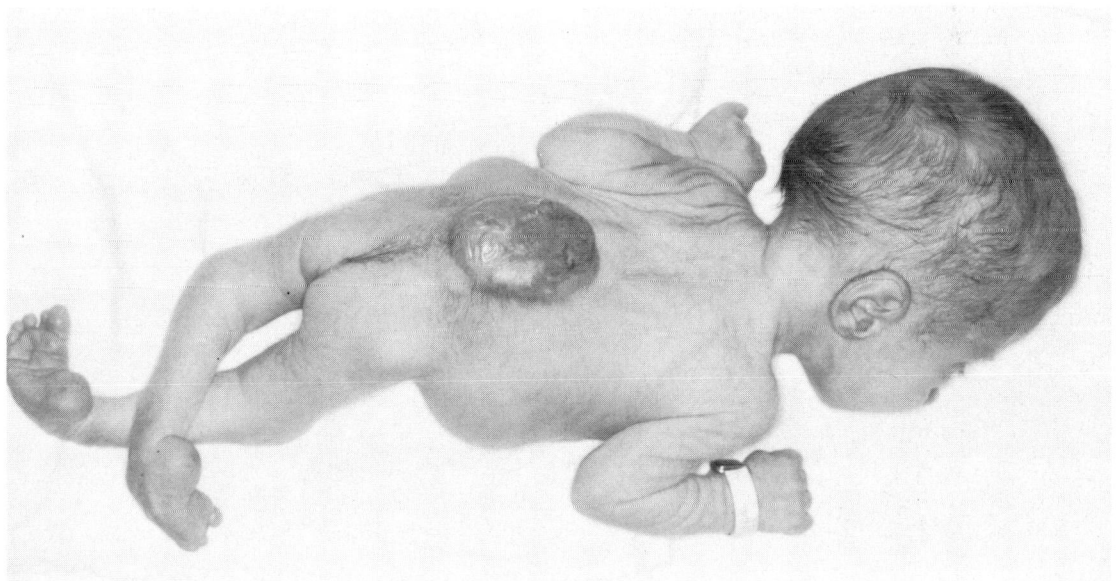

FIGURE 5–42. *Newborn infant with lumbosacral myelomeningocele.*

Note the severe equinovarus deformity of both feet.

for any signs of hydrocephalus, such as dilatation of scalp veins, tension of the fontanelles, separation of cranial sutures, downward displacement of the eyes, and hollowness of the cranial percussion note. The occipitobregmatic circumference of the head is measured and compared with standard growth charts. It is important to record the rate of growth of the head by measuring its circumference at regular intervals. Roentgenograms of the skull are obtained.

The anus is inspected for rectal prolapse and eversion of anal skin. With loss of innervation of the rectal sphincter, there is lack of resistance and absence of reflex contraction as the examining finger is introduced into the rectum. The anal skin reflex is lost. Bladder sphincter control is checked by watching the infant pass urine.

Intermittent dribbling of urine accentuated by suprapubic pressure indicates loss of vesical sphincter control. Suprapubic pressure has no effect on an infant with a normal bladder sphincter. Maceration of the perineal skin is another finding indicating lack of urinary control.

The degree and distribution of paralysis should be noted. A thorough neurologic evaluation of a newborn is difficult; however, by careful repeated examinations, a segmental level of neurologic deficit can be detected.

In lumbosacral lesions, paralysis of the lower limbs is flaccid, whereas in cervicothoracic lesions, it is of the spastic type because of partial cord involvement. Paralysis may be partial or complete below a certain neurosegmental level with normal function above it.

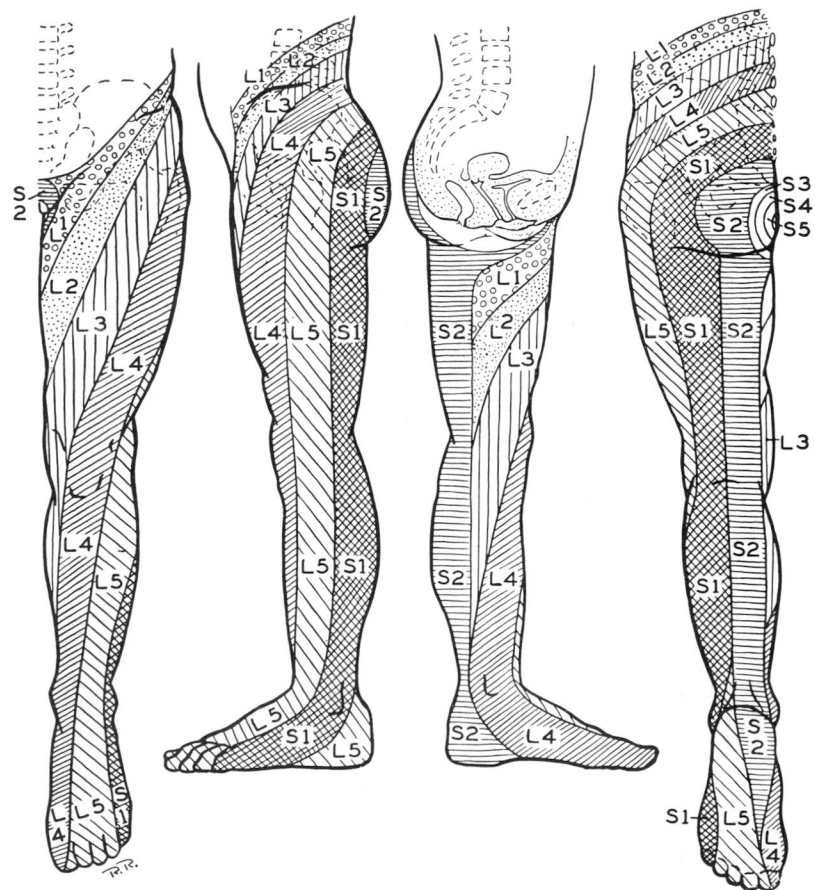

FIGURE 5–43. The segmental innervation of cutaneous sensation of the lower limb.

(From Keegan, J. J., and Garrett, F. D.: Segmental distribution of nerves in man. Anat. Rec., *102*:409, 1948.)

The presence or absence of deep tendon reflexes and superficial skin reflexes is determined. In flaccid paralysis, there is total areflexia, whereas in spastic paralysis there will be hyperactive deep tendon reflexes, ankle clonus, and extensor-plantar response. Sensory examination in a newborn is inadequate, but should be attempted. The segmental innervation of cutaneous sensation in the lower limb is shown in Figure 5–43.

Motor strength of muscles is evaluated, both by observing active motions of the limbs and by the use of reflex stimulation techniques. Faradic current may be applied over nerve trunks and at motor points of muscles to stimulate muscle groups. The neurosegmental level of innervation of muscle groups is given in Figure 5–44; correlation between segmental innervation of reflexes, joint movement, and consequent deformities is shown in Figure 5–45.

Deformities in myelomeningocele may be present at birth (congenital) or may develop postnatally (acquired). They may be teratologic in origin, or they may result from dynamic muscle imbalance or from static forces of faulty posture. The various deformities observed and their treatment are discussed individually later.

Associated Congenital Anomalies

These may occur in any form and are present in about one third of the patients with myelomeningocele. A list, based on a

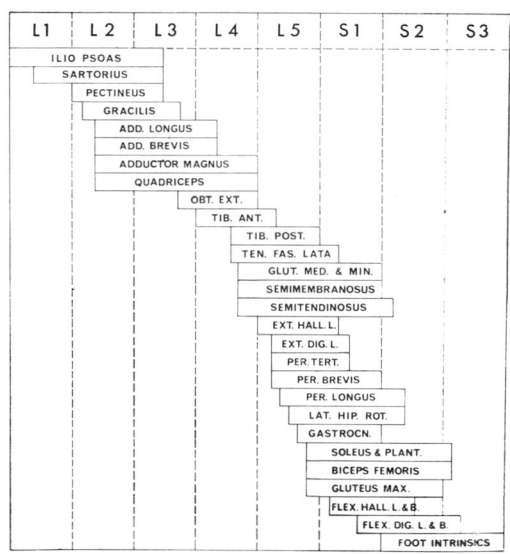

FIGURE 5–44. *Neurosegmental innervation of muscles of lower limb.*

(From Sharrard, W. J. W.: Posterior iliopsoas transplantation in the treatment of paralytic dislocation of the hip. J. Bone Joint Surg., *46-B*:427, 1964.)

study by Smith, of 170 anomalies in 101 children with spina bifida cystica is shown in Table 5–10. The high incidence of congenital dislocation of the hip, talipes equinovarus, hemivertebrae, other anomalies of the spine, and abnormalities of the genitourinary system should be noted. An intravenous pyelogram and a thorough urologic evaluation is imperative in these patients. The possibility of congenital heart disease, malformations of the gastrointestinal tract,

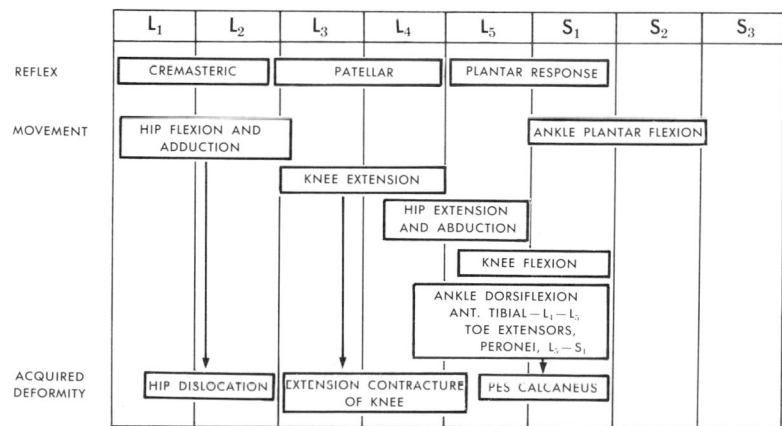

FIGURE 5–45. *Segmental innervation of reflexes, joint movements, and consequent deformities.*

Table 5–10. *Associated Anomalies in 101 Children With Spina Bifida Cystica**

System Involved		Number of Anomalies
Vertebral	Sacral agenesis and hemisacra	18
	Hemivertebrae, transitional vertebrae, fusion defects, fused ribs, etc. (including scoliosis and kyphosis)	18
Skeletal	Congenital talipes	37
	Congenital dislocation of hip	29
	Arthrogryposis	4
	Absent fibula	1
	Absent foot	1
	Extra rudimentary leg	1
	Syndactyly	2
Urinary	Megaureters and hydronephrosis	
	(a) with vesicoureteric reflux	22
	(b) without vesicoureteric reflux	4
	Vesicoureteric reflux in normal ureters	8
	Hypospadias	2
	Urethral diverticulum	1
	Posterior urethral valves	1
	Double ureters and kidneys	3
	Horseshoe kidney	1
	Exstrophy of bladder	1
Alimentary	Imperforate rectum	5
	Tracheo-oesophageal fistula	1
Cerebral	Encephalocele	1
	Congenital mental defect	5
Miscellaneous	Exomphalos	2
	Cleft palate	1
	Congenital cardiac lesions	3
	Sacral sinus	3
	Total	170

*From Smith, E. D.: Spina Bifida and the Total Care of Spinal Myelomeningocele. Springfield, Ill., Charles C Thomas, 1965, p. 49.

cleft palate, pilonidal sinus, or an imperforate rectum should be ruled out.

In the older child, the level of intelligence should be evaluated by a psychologist.[256]

General Principles of Treatment

When an infant is born with myelomeningocele, a serious ethical question should be resolved, i.e., whether or not the child is to be treated. In the past there have been two possible avenues of approach: the child was treated and given every opportunity to live, or he was encouraged to die by neglecting treatment. Intentional neglect of medical care is ethically wrong. The problem of myelomeningocele is, admittedly, a formidable one; however, the myelomeningocele child should be afforded every possible opportunity to live, and treatment should be aggressive to reduce his handicaps to a minimum.

The infant with myelomeningocele has multiple handicaps, each dysfunction and deformity requiring the frequent attention of many medical and surgical specialties. The cost of such care is prohibitive in terms of time as well as money for the average family that has to visit separate clinics. Also, the vision of a single physician can be myopic, his attention being directed upon only one phase of therapy. To administer adequate total care to the myelomeningocele child, it is imperative to have frequent interdisciplinary consultation. For these reasons, it is best to care for the myelomeningocele child in a special multidisciplinary clinic in a children's hospital, where the specialized services of the neurosurgeon, urologic surgeon, pediatric surgeon, orthopedic surgeon, neurologist, pediatrician, and physical and occupational therapists are available.

Social and psychologic factors also have a tremendous impact on the lives of these multiply handicapped children who are plagued by a pessimistic prognosis and inadequate motivation toward life and adjustment in the community. The roles of the special educator, vocational counselor, psychologist, and social worker are extremely important, as these workers enable the myelomeningocele child to compensate for his extreme physical disability by providing him with specialized education and vocational guidance. Finally, the total care of these children should be coordinated and supervised by an interested pediatrician who functions as director of the team (Fig. 5–46).

A positive approach beginning at birth is important. Immediate steps toward total care and habilitation will prevent or minimize deformity and improve the emotional attitude of the family. It should be emphasized to the parents that with proper medical care these children *can* become useful, independent, and self-supporting members of the community.

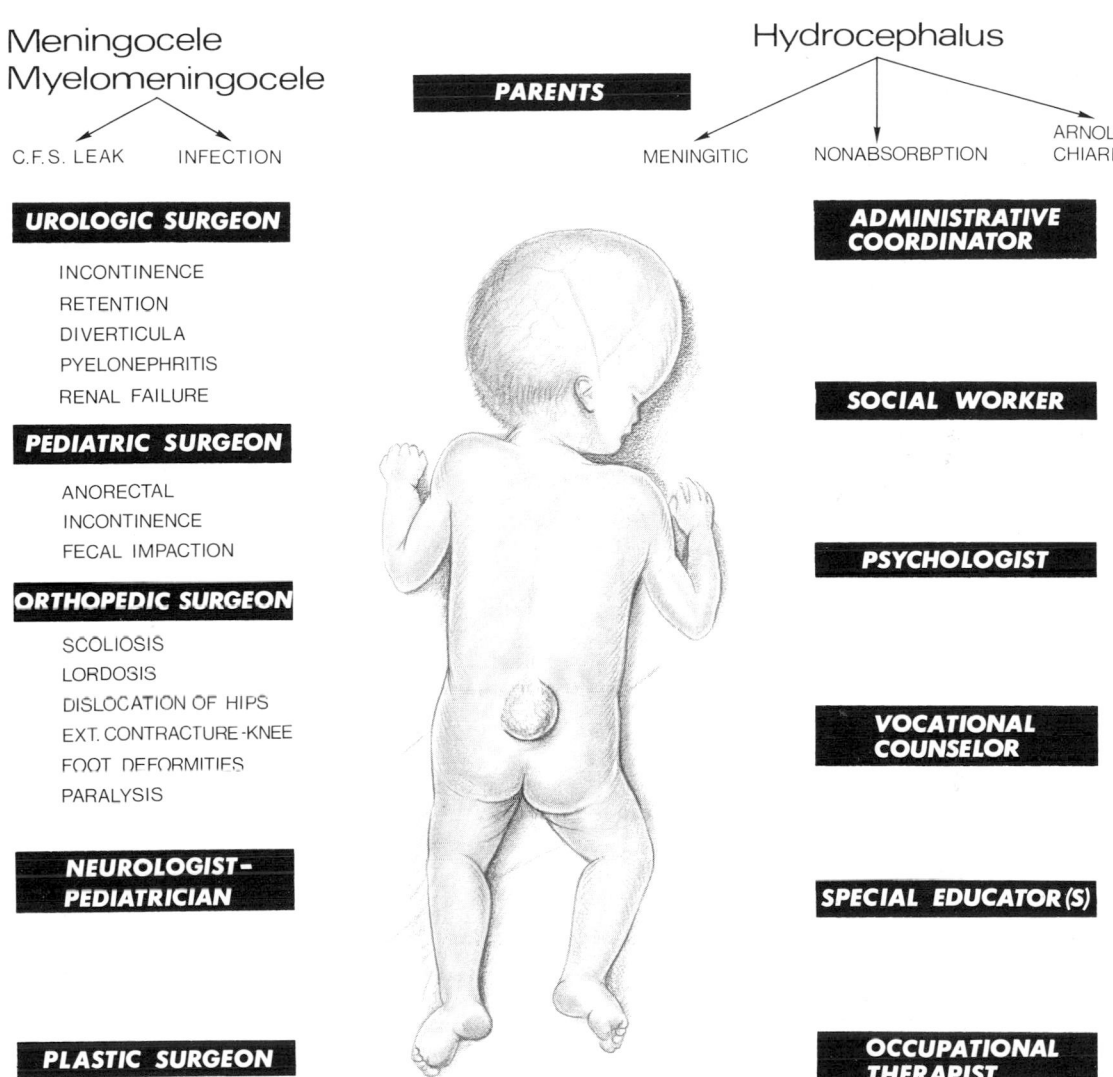

NEUROSURGEON

Meningocele
Myelomeningocele

C.F.S. LEAK   INFECTION

PARENTS

Hydrocephalus

MENINGITIC   NONABSORBPTION   ARNOLD-CHIARI

UROLOGIC SURGEON

INCONTINENCE
RETENTION
DIVERTICULA
PYELONEPHRITIS
RENAL FAILURE

PEDIATRIC SURGEON

ANORECTAL
INCONTINENCE
FECAL IMPACTION

ORTHOPEDIC SURGEON

SCOLIOSIS
LORDOSIS
DISLOCATION OF HIPS
EXT. CONTRACTURE-KNEE
FOOT DEFORMITIES
PARALYSIS

NEUROLOGIST-PEDIATRICIAN

PLASTIC SURGEON

ADMINISTRATIVE COORDINATOR

SOCIAL WORKER

PSYCHOLOGIST

VOCATIONAL COUNSELOR

SPECIAL EDUCATOR (S)

OCCUPATIONAL THERAPIST

Myelomeningocele

ORTHOTIST   **PHYSICAL THERAPIST**

FIGURE 5-46.   *Total care of the infant with myelomeningocele—the team approach.*

Spina bifida parents' associations are extremely valuable for educating the parents, giving them the continued moral support so necessary for the adequate and proper care of these children. A stable and cooperative family is the most important part of the team in the total care of the child with myelomeningocele.

It is beyond the scope of this book to present neurosurgical, urologic, and other aspects of medical treatment of the child with myelomeningocele. The reader is referred to the literature.* The general consensus of neurosurgeons is that the meningocele should be closed immediately as an emergency measure, as with such treatment there is a much more satisfactory preservation of innervation, and the eventual mortality rate is much lower than with delayed closure or conservative treatment. Immediate repair of the meningocele combined with successful control of hydrocephalus by shunting procedures has decreased the mortality rate of myelomeningocele from 90 to 20 per cent. The technique of meningocele excision is given in Figure 5–47 for general information to the orthopedist. The procedure is a neurosurgical one.

The care of the musculoskeletal system of the infant with myelomeningocele begins from the day of birth. The orthopedist should be called in consultation at the same time as the neurosurgeon, giving him an opportunity to evaluate the patient prior to closure of the lesion and to determine the neurosegmental level of the lesion and the presence or absence of deformities of the limbs and spine.

All children with myelomeningocele are potentially capable of locomotion, provided they have normal function of their upper limbs, adequate stability of the spine, and motor strength of the trunk and hip musculature to enable them to elevate the pelvis and flex the hips. The goal of orthopedic treatment is to have these children walk with appropriate orthotic support by the age of 18 months. Upright posture opens new vistas with promise of a useful and satisfying life (Fig. 5–48), whereas recumbency will result in emaciation and large pressure

sores that increase in size with malnutrition and infection; the bones become exposed, and death occurs within a few years (Fig. 5–49).

The care of each patient is individualized, depending upon his unique problems. Several factors may act as deterrents to the achievement of a satisfactory level of functional performance; these may include problems of balance and posture resulting from hydrocephalus and brain damage, a poor attention span, and a lack of the necessary motivation to walk owing to a low level of intelligence. Also, various behavioral aberrations and an unsatisfactory home environment may be detrimental to functional achievement.

The Foot and Ankle

A variety of deformities of the foot and ankle may be present in children with myelomeningocele, some of them congenital and others acquired in postnatal life. Intrauterine paralysis and malposture are the most common causative factors; however, some deformities may be of teratologic origin (Fig. 5–50).

In a consecutive series of 71 infants examined during the first 12 hours of life, Sharrard and Grosfield found deformities of the feet in 77 limbs (55 per cent) and no deformity in 65 feet.[366]

The type of paralytic foot deformity observed may be correlated with the neurosegmental level of the lesion. When it is at or above the third lumbar segment, there is flail foot and ankle; they may be in calcaneus, equinovarus, or valgus position as a result of static forces of intrauterine or postnatal malposture (Fig. 5–51). When these children are upright and begin to walk, pes valgus deformity will develop in response to static forces of body weight.

When the level of the lesion is at the fourth lumbar segment, the anterior tibial muscle will be active and strong, pulling the forefoot in dorsiflexion and inversion. The hindfoot is usually in calcaneovalgus, but occasionally may be in equinus position, with the talus plantarflexed with subluxation or dislocation of the talonavicular joint (paralytic vertical talus).

When involvement is at the fifth lumbar

---

*See references 262, 272, 291, 294, 306–310, 323, 335–337, 340, 342, 352, 367, 391, 392.

(*Text continued on page 902.*)

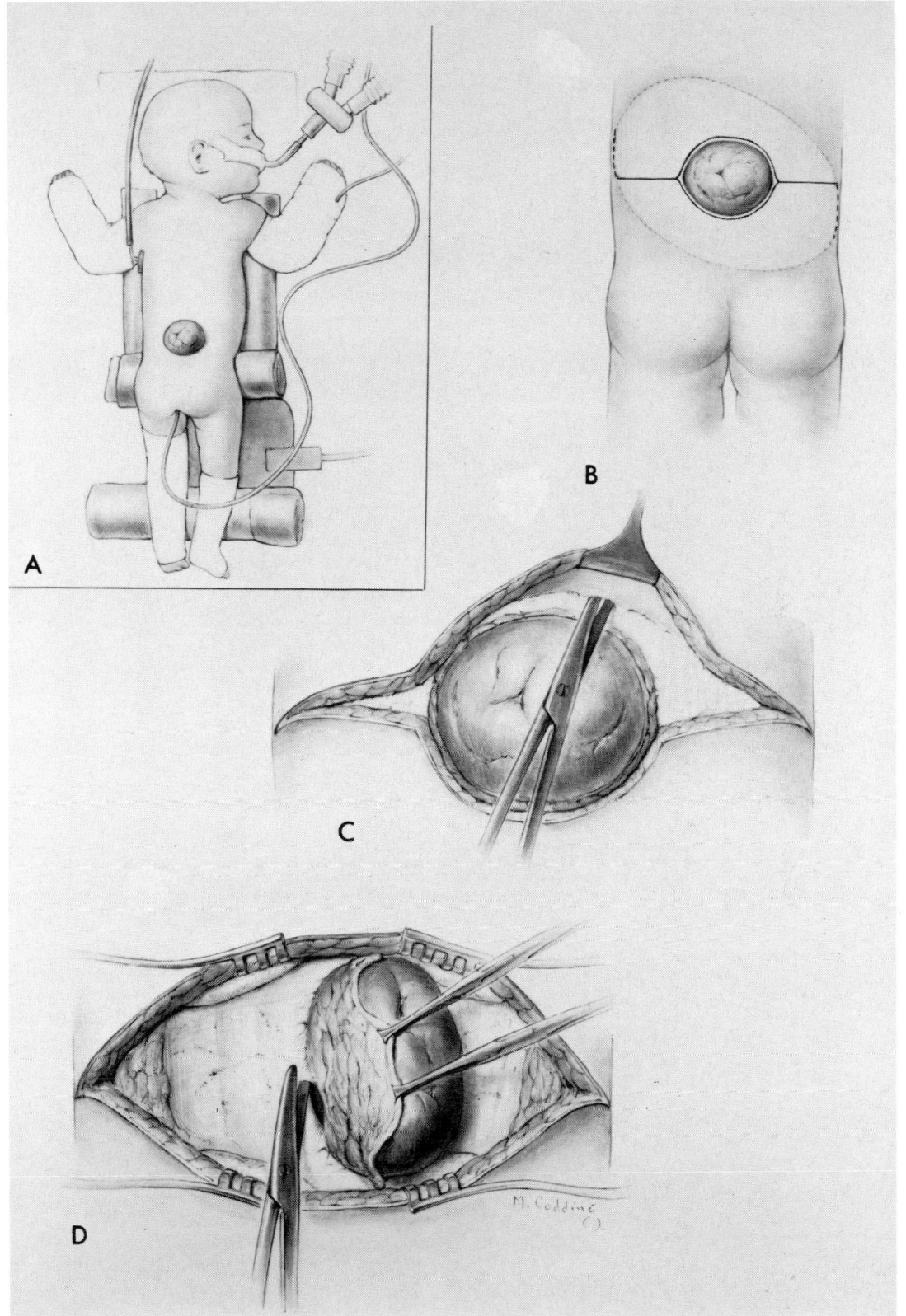

FIGURE 5–47. *Technique of meningocele excision.*

Surgical repair of myelomeningocele in the lumbar region. **A.** Operative position. **B.** Incision. **C.** Retraction of skin flap at the fascial level. **D.** Dissection at the fascial-level, revealing neck of meningocele. (From Matson, D. D.: Surgical repair of myelomeningocele. J. Neurosurg., 27:180, 1967.)

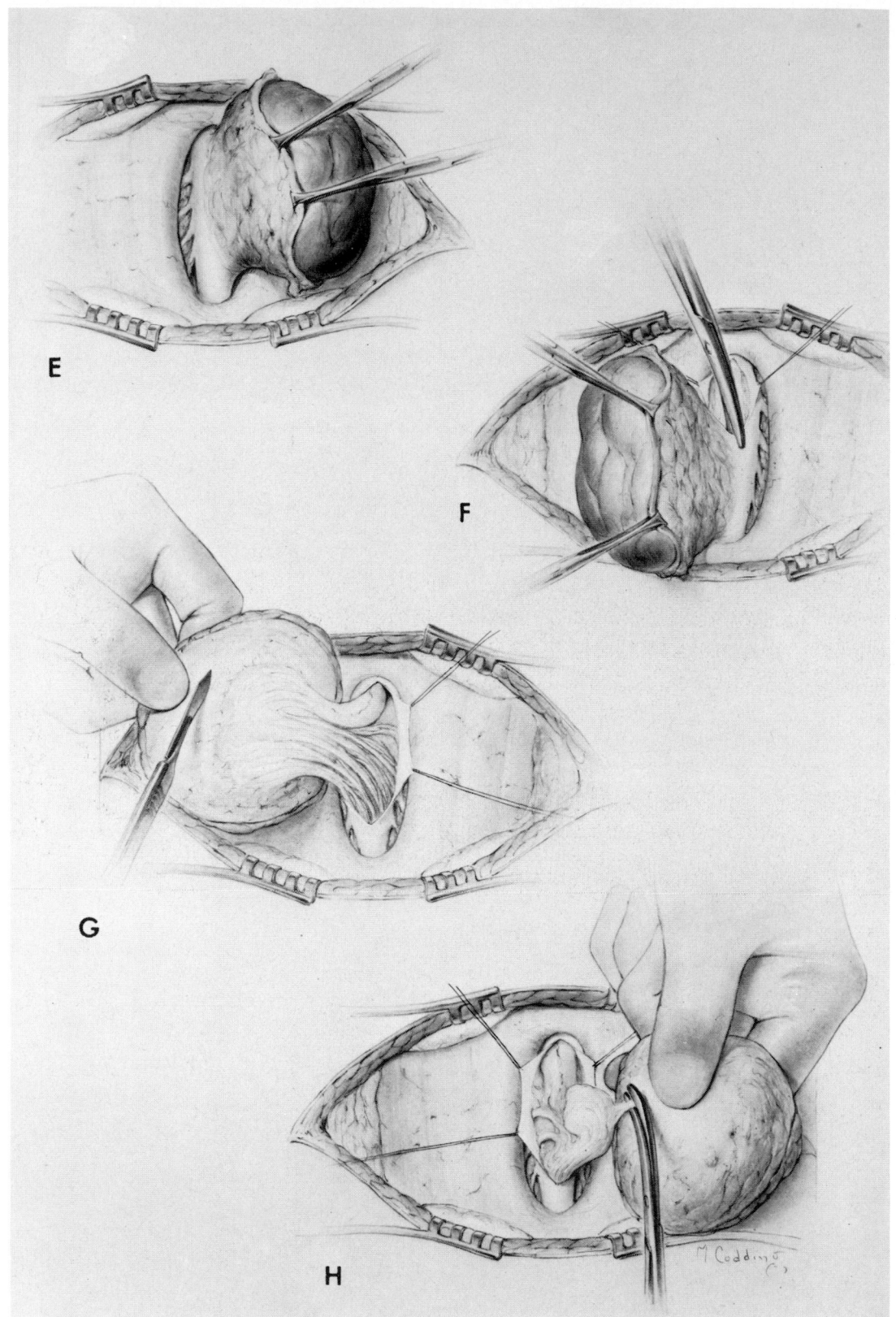

FIGURE 5–47 Continued. *Technique of meningocele excision.*

Dissection of the meningocele. **E.** Separation of the meningocele from its membranous attachments. **F.** Incision of the neck of the meningocele sac. **G.** Separation of neural elements from inner membrane of sac. **H.** Final adhesion divided and sac removed. (From Matson, D. D.: Surgical repair of myelomeningocele. J. Neurosurg., *27*:180, 1967.)

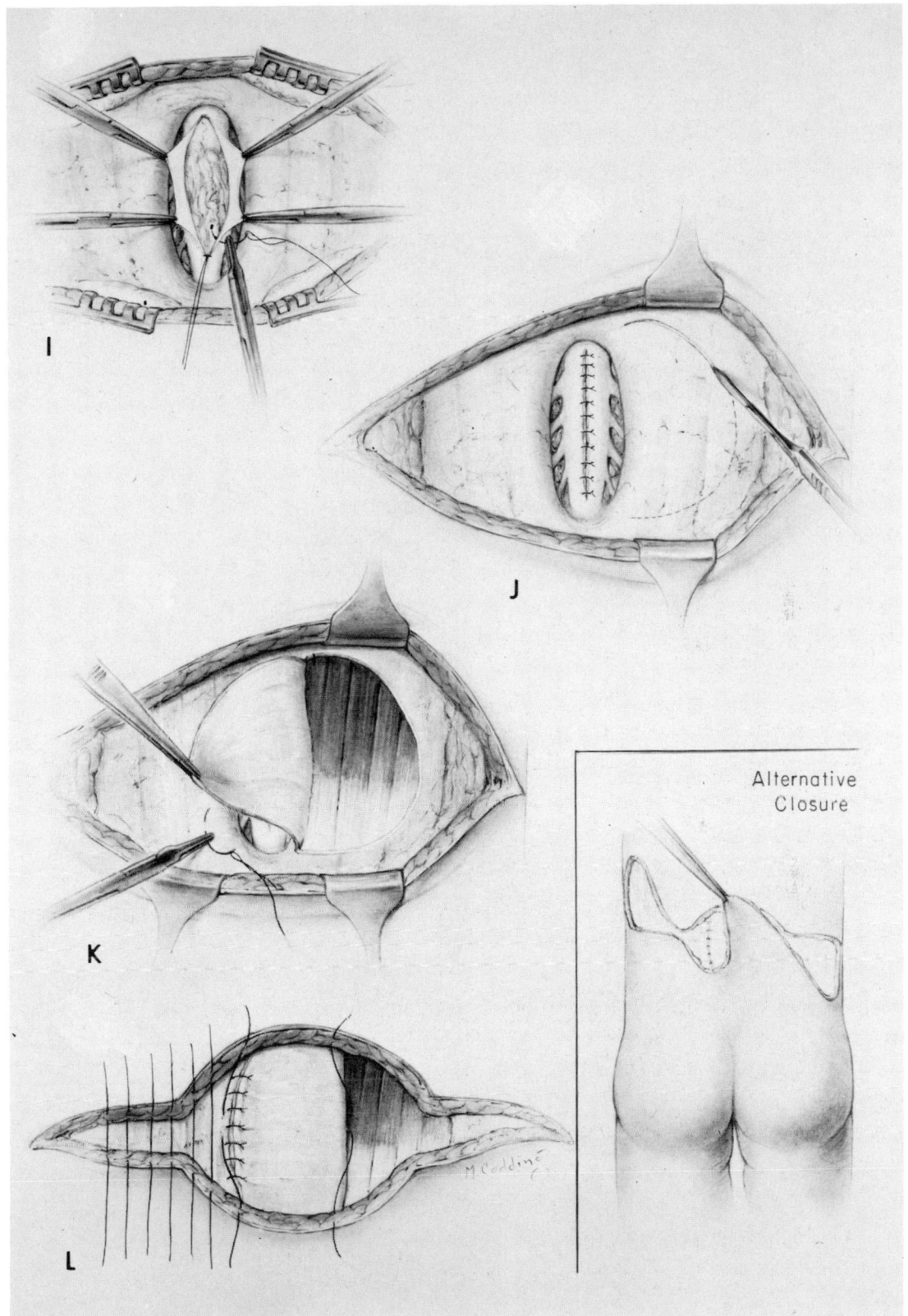

FIGURE 5–47 Continued. Technique of meningocele excision.

Closure. **I.** Dural closure. **J.** Creation of flap of fascia from the paraspinal muscles. **K.** Swinging of flaps to opposite side for suture to the paraspinal fascia. **L.** Closure of the skin. *Insert:* Alternative (plastic) closure of skin flaps. (From Matson, D. D.: Surgical repair of myelomeningocele. J. Neurosurg., 27:180, 1967.)

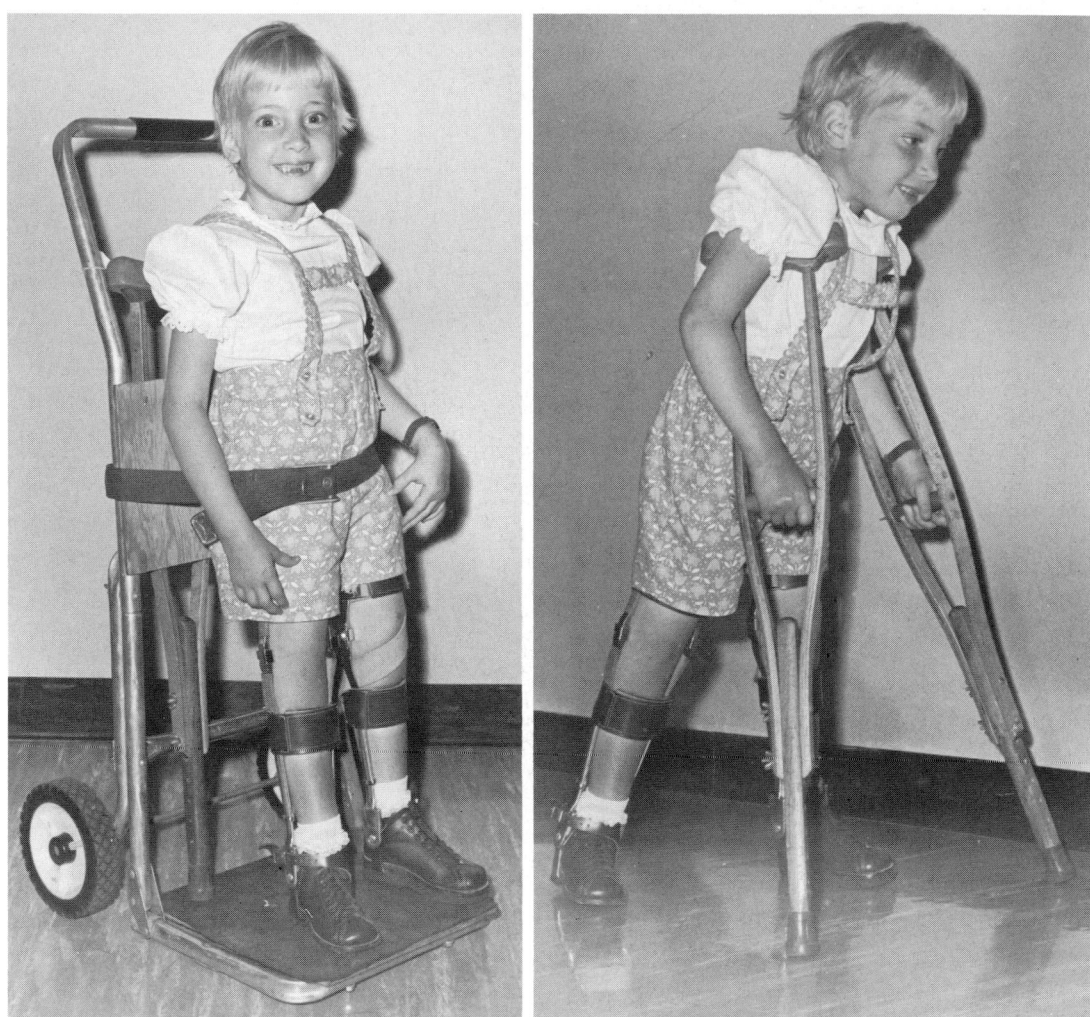

FIGURE 5–48.   A child with myelomeningocele is capable of locomotion.

This child has been standing and walking since one and one half years of age. Upright posture opens new vistas with hope of a useful and satisfying life.

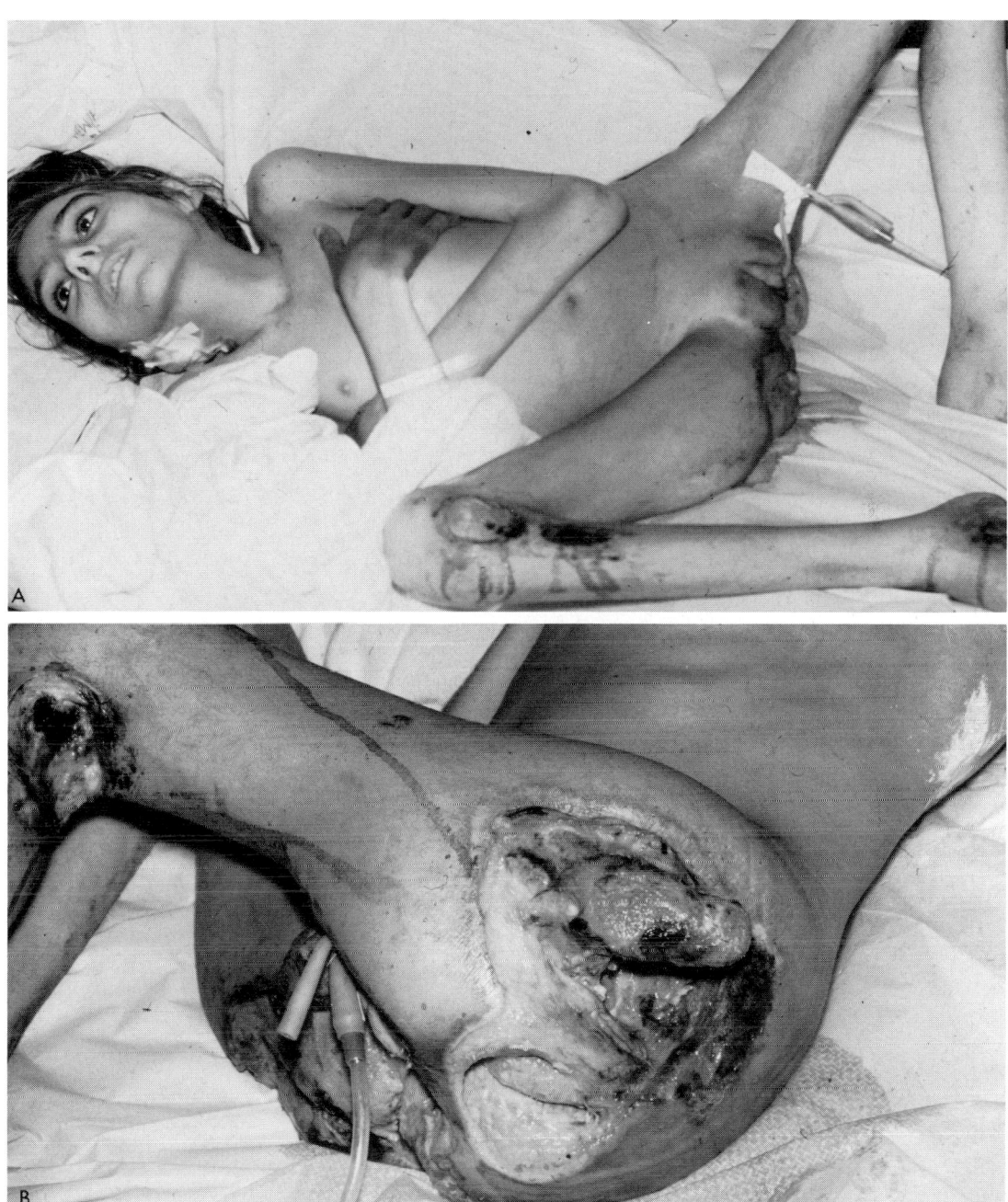

FIGURE 5–49. *An untreated patient with myelomeningocele.*

Recumbency will lead to rotting in bed with large pressure sores, resulting in death within a few years.

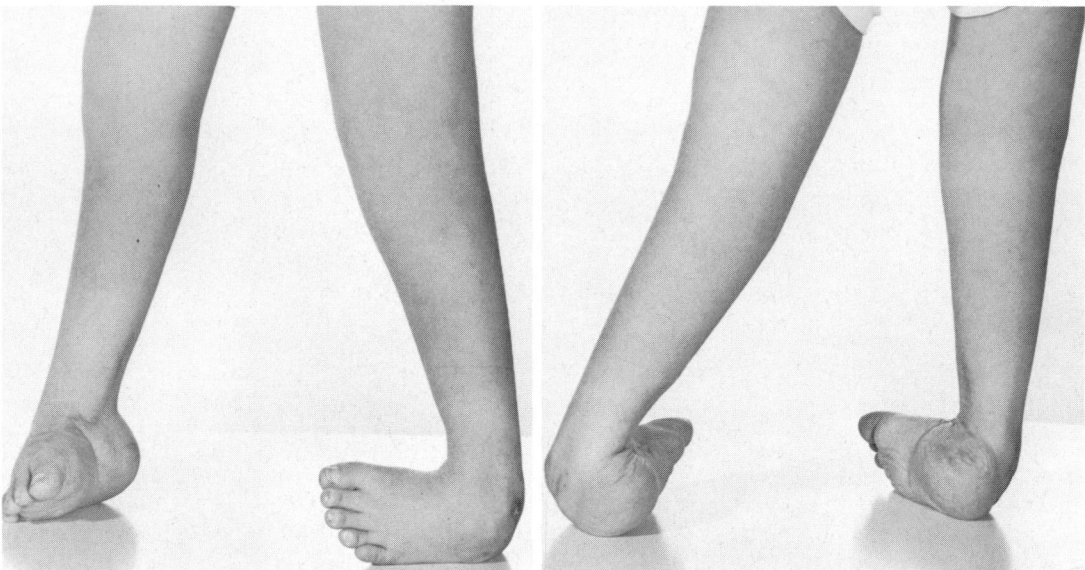

FIGURE 5–50.   A myelomeningocele child with severe bilateral talipes equinovarus.

This is an example of deformity of the foot that is of teratologic origin.

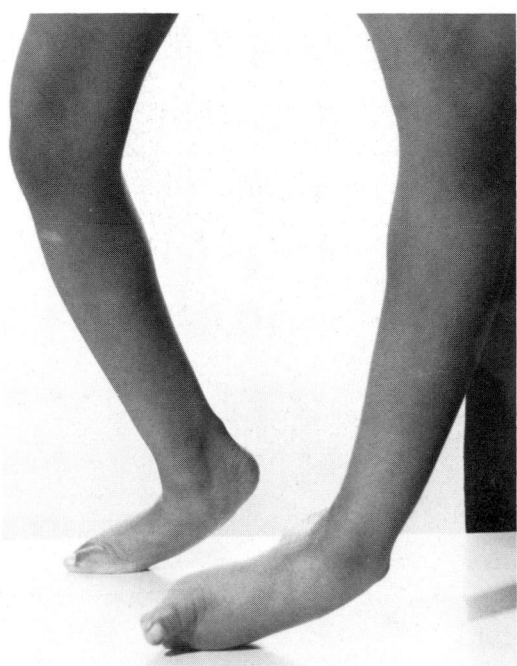

FIGURE 5–51.   A child with myelomeningocele with level of the lesion at the first lumbar neurosegment.

Both lower limbs are flail. Note the equinovalgus deformity of the right foot and the equinovarus deformity on the left as a result of static forces of intrauterine and postnatal malposture.

level, the long toe extensors and peroneal and anterior tibial muscles are strong, whereas the triceps surae and long toe flexor muscles are paralyzed. A progressive calcaneus deformity will result if dynamic imbalance is not corrected (Fig. 5–52).

When the level of the lesion is at the first two sacral neurosegments there is complete or partial paralysis of the long toe flexor and intrinsic muscles of the foot, with the long and short toe extensor muscles active; the resultant deformity is pes cavus with clawing of the toes. Equinovarus deformity of the feet may be present as a teratologic deformity at any level.

The treatment of specific deformities of the foot is discussed in Chapter 7. Management of the myelomeningocele foot, however, does present certain different and difficult problems because of associated motor paralysis and sensory loss. Every effort should be made to achieve a plantigrade normal foot that can bear weight safely. Deformed feet will develop pressure sores, cellulitis, and osteomyelitis, eventually necessitating amputation. One cannot overemphasize the importance of diligent and persistent care of the feet of these children.

Treatment should *begin at birth.* There is

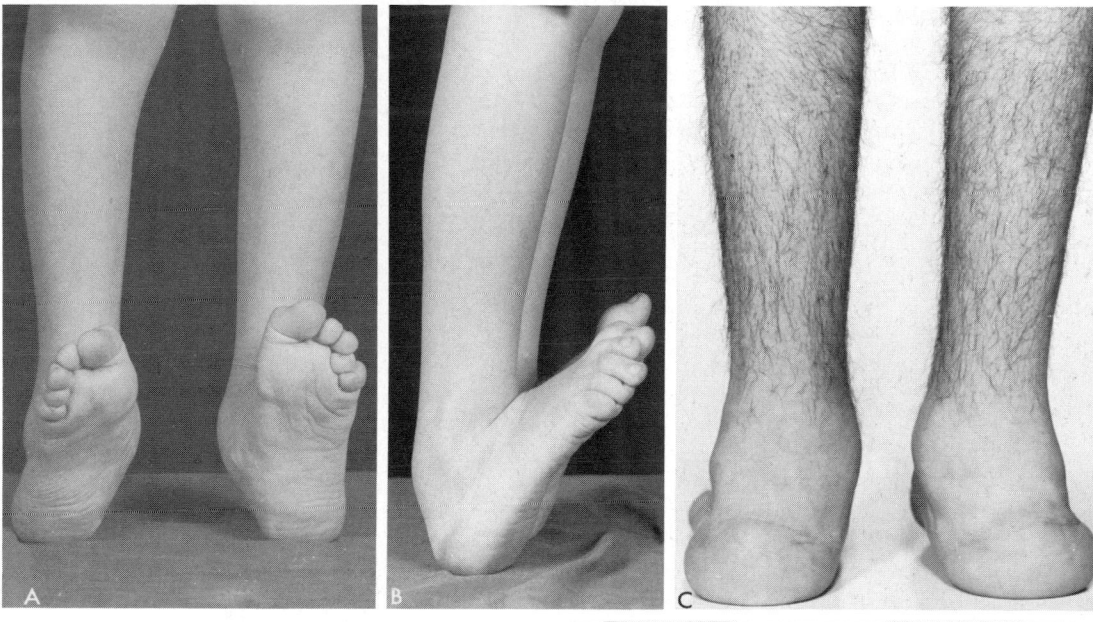

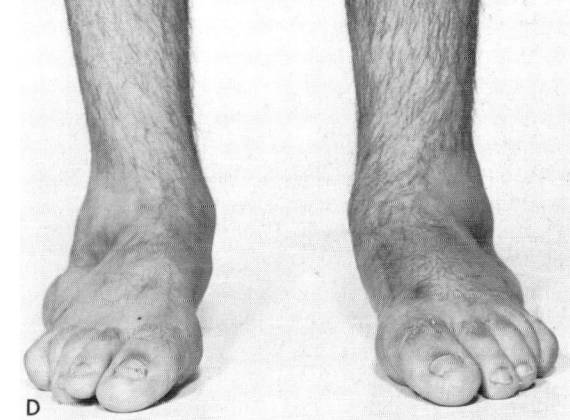

FIGURE 5–52. *A myelomeningocele child with involvement at the fifth lumbar level.*

The long toe extensor, peroneal, and anterior tibial muscles are normal in motor strength, whereas the triceps surae and long toe flexors are paralyzed. Severe calcaneus deformity of both feet has developed as a result of dynamic imbalance of muscles acting on the foot and ankle. A posterior transfer of the anterior tibial and peroneal muscles was performed to restore dynamic balance. **A** and **B.** Preoperative photographs at five years of age. **C** and **D.** Postoperative photographs when 14 years old.

no excuse for delay. The general tendency is to postpone the application of corrective casts to clubfoot because of the fear that it may interfere with the nursing and surgical management of the spinal defect and hydrocephalus. The neurosurgeon should be requested to place the needles for administration of intravenous fluids in the upper limb when there is deformity of the lower limb.

PES EQUINUS OR EQUINOVARUS

Gentle passive stretching exercises are performed to correct the deformity. The orthopedist often fails to take the necessary time to manipulate the feet prior to application of the cast. The skin should be painted with a nonirritating adhesive liquid before a well-padded molded plaster cast is applied. Plaster casts are changed successively at three- to four-day intervals, and the feet manipulated each time. Because of the difficulty of determining the extent of sensory loss in a newborn infant, it should be presumed that his foot is totally or partially anesthetic. To prevent skin ulceration the cast is applied to hold the degree of correction obtained by passive stretching exercises. Sharrard reports disastrous results of attempted conservative treatment of equinus and equinovarus deformity in children with myelomeningocele.[366] The same experience is *not* shared by the author. It is strongly advocated that they be corrected as much as possible by conservative methods.

Fibrotic contracture of a paralyzed muscle in myelomeningocele is often present. A resistant equinus deformity that fails to respond to treatment with a cast should be surgically corrected. In the foot with congenital equinovarus deformity the author attempts treatment with a corrective cast for three months prior to consideration of surgery, whereas in talipes equinovarus associated with myelomeningocele the period of conservative management is shortened to six to eight weeks. In recalcitrant equinus deformity, often an open sliding lengthening or section of the Achilles tendon and posterior capsulotomy of the ankle and subtalar joints are indicated. The posterior tibial and toe flexor muscles, if contracted, are lengthened at the same time. Sharrard recommends division of the toe flexors in the sole of the foot through a small incision; the author uses a plantar incision only when the forefoot is in equinus position. When the equinus deformity does not exceed 10 degrees, simple percutaneous tenotomy of the tendo calcaneus, performed under local anesthesia, may be adequate to correct the deformity. This should be double-checked by roentgenograms taken in the operating room. The normal range of dorsiflexion of the ankle in an infant is at least 30 degrees; the same range of dorsiflexion should be obtained following tendo Achillis section. The os calcis is always transfixed with a Kirschner wire, which is incorporated in the cast to hold the correction. The wire is removed in four to six weeks. Night splints are worn to prevent recurrence of deformity.

In the older child with fixed deformity, other surgical procedures may be indicated such as tarsometatarsal capsulotomies, cuboid decancellation, midtarsal osteotomy, metatarsal osteotomy, Dwyer osteotomy, excision of the talus, and triple arthrodesis. The indications for these operations and their surgical technique are discussed in Chapter 7. In general, in the infant and young child, surgical procedures are limited to the soft tissues; and operations on bones are performed only when skeletal maturation of the foot is completed, so that growth and development of the foot will not be disturbed. In myelomeningocele, however, certain exceptions to the preceding rule are made.

In *pes calcaneus and calcaneovarus deformities* a definite pattern of muscle imbalance is usually present. Muscle balance should be restored by appropriate tendon transfer at an early age to prevent recurrence and progression of deformity. In the neonatal period the feet are manipulated to passively stretch the contracted soft tissues. The severity of deformity may warrant the use of a corrective plaster cast. Upon correction of the deformity, night bivalved casts or splints are used and passive stretching exercises are performed to maintain normal alignment of the foot. If the anterior tibial muscle is the deforming force, it is transferred to the os calcis. This may be performed as early as two years of age if calcaneus deformity cannot be prevented from progressing. The operative technique of tendon transfer posteriorly to the os calcis is described and illustrated in Plate 38.

PES EQUINOVALGUS (PARALYTIC VERTICAL TALUS)

This is a rare deformity in which the talus is plantar-flexed with subluxation or dislocation of the talonavicular joint, the os calcis is everted in equinus position, and the forefoot is abducted and dorsiflexed (Fig. 5–54). Its pathogenesis is not clearly defined; it may be acquired or congenital in origin. The usual pattern of muscle imbalance found in association with paralytic vertical talus is normal strength of the anterior tibial, long toe extensor, and peroneal muscles, with paralysis of the triceps surae, the long and short toe flexors, and the intrinsic muscles of the foot.

The condition does not respond to conservative therapy, and early surgical correction is indicated. Dislocation of the talonavicular joint is reduced; meticulous capsular repair and retrograde internal fixation with a Kirschner wire are performed to maintain the reduction. The muscular forces acting on the foot are balanced by appropriate tendon transfers commonly consisting of posterior transfer of the anterior tibial and peroneal muscles to the os calcis. *Calcaneovalgus deformity* may be caused by malposture in utero or be due to fibrosis of the long toe extensors and peroneal muscles (Fig. 5–55). Treatment is by a passive stretching cast. Resistant and recurrent cases often require section of part of the deforming fibrosed muscles.

PES CAVUS AND CLAW TOES

These deformities are usually paralytic in origin, resulting from muscle imbalance between the long toe extensors and flexors and the intrinsic muscles of the foot. Most of these children have quite adequate motor function in their lower limbs and are very active on their feet. Meticulous care should be given to the toe and forefoot deformities to prevent development of pressure sores on the toes or on the plantar surface of the metatarsal heads. The type of treatment varies with the severity of deformity. In mild to moderate cases, treatment is by passive stretching exercises and a metatarsal pad. More severe deformity may require plantar fasciotomy and transfer of long toe extensors to the metatarsal heads. In the older child with fixed pes cavus, a dorsal wedge midtarsal osteotomy may be indicated.

FLAIL ANKLE

When the foot is plantigrade and free of deformity it may be stabilized by appropriate fusion, enabling the patient to discard orthotic support and use only crutches for walking. If the hip flexors and quadriceps femoris muscles are satisfactory, the author will consider the Chuinard type of ankle fusion at the age of eight or ten years. If the valgus deformity of the hindfoot is marked, the fusion is combined with a Green-Grice extra-articular subtalar arthrodesis. These procedures do not disturb the growth of the foot or the tibia.

The Hip

Deformities of the hip in myelomeningocele may be any one of the following types: dislocation or subluxation, coxa valga, flexion deformity, and external rotation abduction deformity. Involvement may be asymmetrical, depending upon the pattern of paralysis.

HIP DISLOCATION AND COXA VALGA

Hip dislocation, a common deformity in myelomeningocele, may be categorized as one of the following types:

Teratologic (developing in utero)

Congenital (occurring at birth)
   with a completely flail lower limb with muscle imbalance due to partial paralysis of the limb

Acquired (occurring postnatally with gradual dislocation of the femoral head) caused by muscle imbalance between hip flexor-adductors and hip extensor-abductors
   due to pelvic obliquity with the hip on the high side gradually becoming dislocated

Sharrard has classified the patterns of muscle paralysis into six groups, correlating them with resultant acquired paralytic deformity of the hip (Fig. 5–56). *Group I* is characterized by total flail lower limbs due to complete paralysis below the level of the twelfth thoracic root. Malpositional or static deformities of the limbs result from faulty posture in utero or in supine or prone position in postnatal life (Fig. 5–57). When these children begin to stand with support, coxa valga may develop with subsequent subluxation of the hips. Complete dislocation usually does not occur. In *Group II* there is flaccid paralysis of the muscles that are innervated distal to the first and second lumbar nerve roots. Thus, the hip flexors are good or fair in motor strength, and the hip adductors are fair or poor; all other muscles are paralyzed. Flexion deformity of the hip is found in all patients at birth. During the first year of life all patients develop progressively increasing flexion-adduction hip deformity with valgus deformity of the femoral neck. Moderate or marked subluxation of the hips will occur in four fifths of these children. If left untreated, some of the subluxated hips will become dislocated (about 10 per cent). In *Group III* the upper three of four lumbar nerve roots are intact, with paralysis distal to this level. Motor strength is as follows: normal hip flexors, good hip adductors, good quadriceps femoris, and fair sartorius and tensor fasciae latae; the hip abductors and extensors are completely paralyzed; the anterior tibial muscle is

(*Text continued on page 911.*)

Posterior Tendon Transfer to Os Calcis for Correction of Calcaneus Deformity (Green and Grice)

THE PROCEDURE

It is best to place the patient in the prone position to facilitate the surgical exposure of the heel. The posterior tibial, and peroneus longus and brevis tendons are divided distally at their insertion and delivered into the proximal wound following the technique and steps described in Plate 40, page 982. When the flexor hallucis longus tendon is to be transferred, its distal portion is sutured to the flexor hallucis brevis muscle. The anterior tibial tendon is delivered into the calf and heel through the interosseous route.

A. A 5 cm. long posterior transverse incision is made around the heel along one of the skin creases in the part that neither presses the shoe nor touches the ground.

B. The skin and subcutaneous flaps are undercut and reflected, exposing the os calcis and the insertion of the tendo calcaneus. An L-shaped cut is made in the lateral two thirds of the insertion of the tendo calcaneus. The divided portion is reflected proximally, exposing the apophysis of the os calcis.

C. Next, with a $9/64$-inch drill, a hole is made through the calcaneus, beginning in the center of the apophysis and coming out laterally at its plantar aspect. With a diamond head hand drill and curet, the hole is enlarged to receive all the transferred tendons.

Plate 38. Posterior Tendon Transfer to Os Calcis for Correction of Calcaneus Deformity
(Green and Grice)

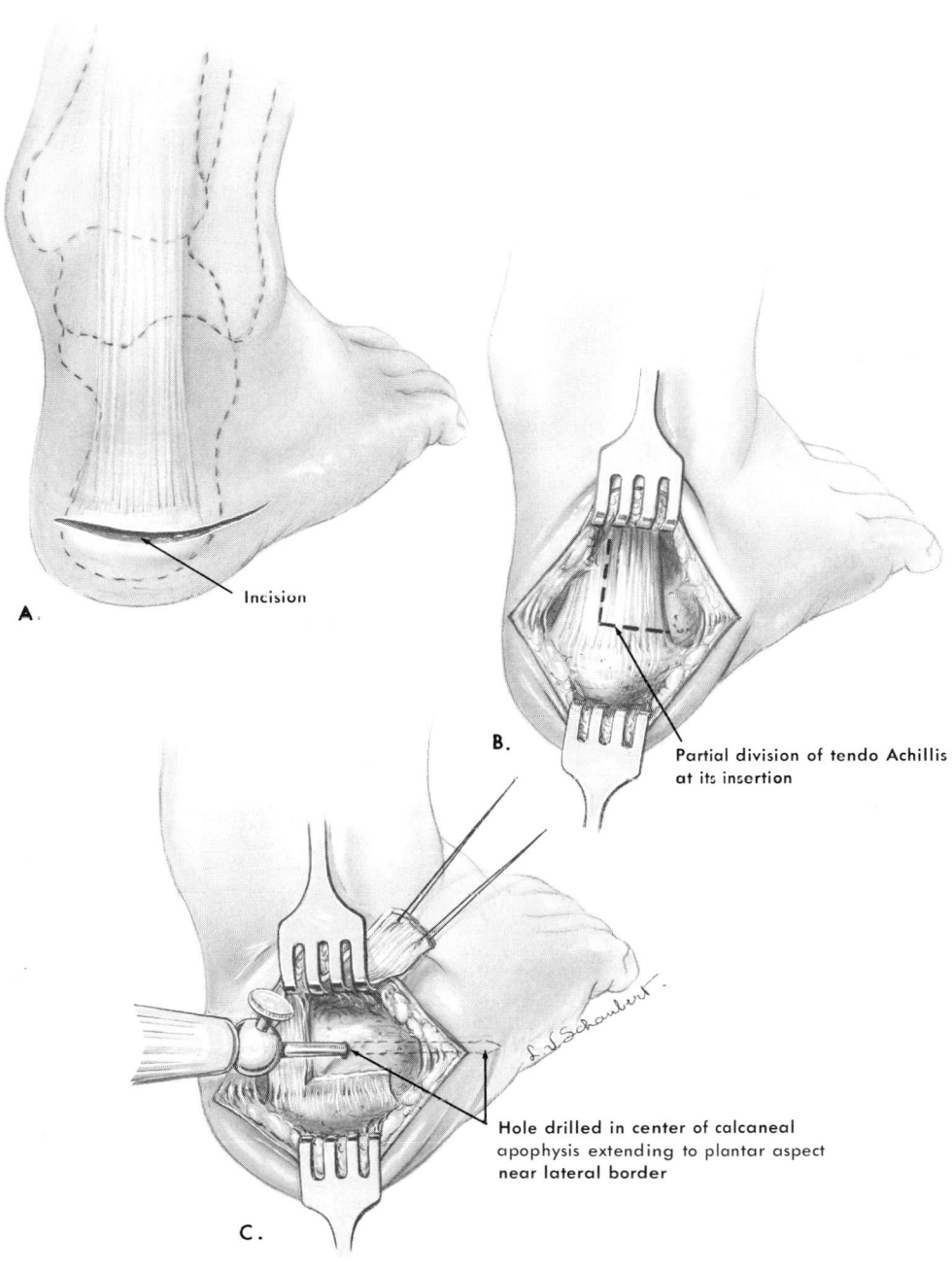

A.

Incision

B.

Partial division of tendo Achillis at its insertion

C.

Hole drilled in center of calcaneal apophysis extending to plantar aspect near lateral border

Posterior Tendon Transfer to Os Calcis for Correction of Calcaneus Deformity (Green and Grice) *(Continued)*

D. Through a lateral incision, the intermuscular septum is widely divided between the lateral and posterior compartments. An Ober tendon transfer is inserted through the wound and directed anterior to the tendo calcaneus into the transverse incision over the os calcis. The threads of the whip sutures at the ends of the peroneal tendons are passed through the hole in the tendon passer and the tendons are delivered at the heel. The posterior tibial tendon is delivered at the heel by a similar route, through an incision in the intermuscular septum between the medial and posterior compartments and anterior to the tendo calcaneus. Next, with a twisted wire probe, the tendons are inserted in the hole and pulled through the tunnel in the calcaneus.

E. At their point of exit on the lateral aspect of the calcaneus the tendons are sutured to the periosteum and ligamentous tissues. The tendons are sutured under enough tension to hold the foot 15 degrees equinus when the remaining ankle dorsiflexors are fair in motor strength, and 30 degrees equinus if they are good or normal. The tendons are sutured to each other and to the periosteum of the apophysis of the calcaneus at the posterior end of the tunnel.

F and **G.** The divided portion of the tendo calcaneus is resutured in its original position posterior to the transferred tendons.

The wounds are closed and a long leg cast is applied, the knee in 45 to 60 degrees of flexion, the hindfoot 15 to 30 degrees equinus, but the forefoot neutral. Cavus deformity of the forefoot should be avoided.

POSTOPERATIVE CARE

Three to four weeks following surgery the solid cast is removed and a new long leg bivalved cast is made to protect the limb at all times when exercises are not being performed. It is imperative to prevent forced dorsiflexion of the ankle and stretching of the transferred tendons.

Exercises are first performed side-lying and with gravity eliminated, and then in prone position against gravity (see Fig. 5–53 A and B). In order to teach the patient the new action of the transferred muscle, he is asked to move the foot in the direction of a component of the original action of the muscle and then to plantar-flex the foot. For example, when the peroneals are transferred, he is asked to evert and plantar-flex the foot; or when the anterior tibial is transferred, to invert and plantar-flex the foot. Soon, under supervision, guided dorsiflexion of the foot is performed along with plantar flexion. It is important to develop reciprocal motion and motor strength of agonists and antagonist muscles. Weight-bearing is not allowed. Ambulation is permitted in the long leg bivalved cast with crutches.

In about four to six weeks when the transferred tendons are fair in motor strength the patient is allowed to stand on both feet. The heel of the foot that was operated on rests on a 3 cm. thick block to prevent stretching of the transferred tendons. Bearing partial weight on his foot, the patient should rise up on his tiptoes while holding on to a table with his hands or using two crutches.

When the transplant functions effectively on tiptoe standing, walking with crutches is begun with three-point gait and partial weight-bearing on the affected limb (Fig. 5–53 D). The heel of the shoe is elevated with a 1 to 1.5 cm. lift that tapers in front (toward the toes). Walking periods are gradually increased. When the transplant works effectively in gait and take-off has been developed in walking, standing tiptoe rising exercises are started without the support of crutches (Fig. 5–53 E). The knee should not be flexed and the patient should not lean forward while rising up on his toes at least three times (Fig. 5–53 F). This may take a long time (as much as a year or more), but it is a very important phase of postoperative management.

A plantar-flexion spring brace or a brace with a posterior elastic is worn when the patient is uncooperative in the use of crutches or when muscular control of the knee and hip is poor because of extensive paralysis. A stop at the ankle prevents dorsiflexion of the ankle beyond neutral position.

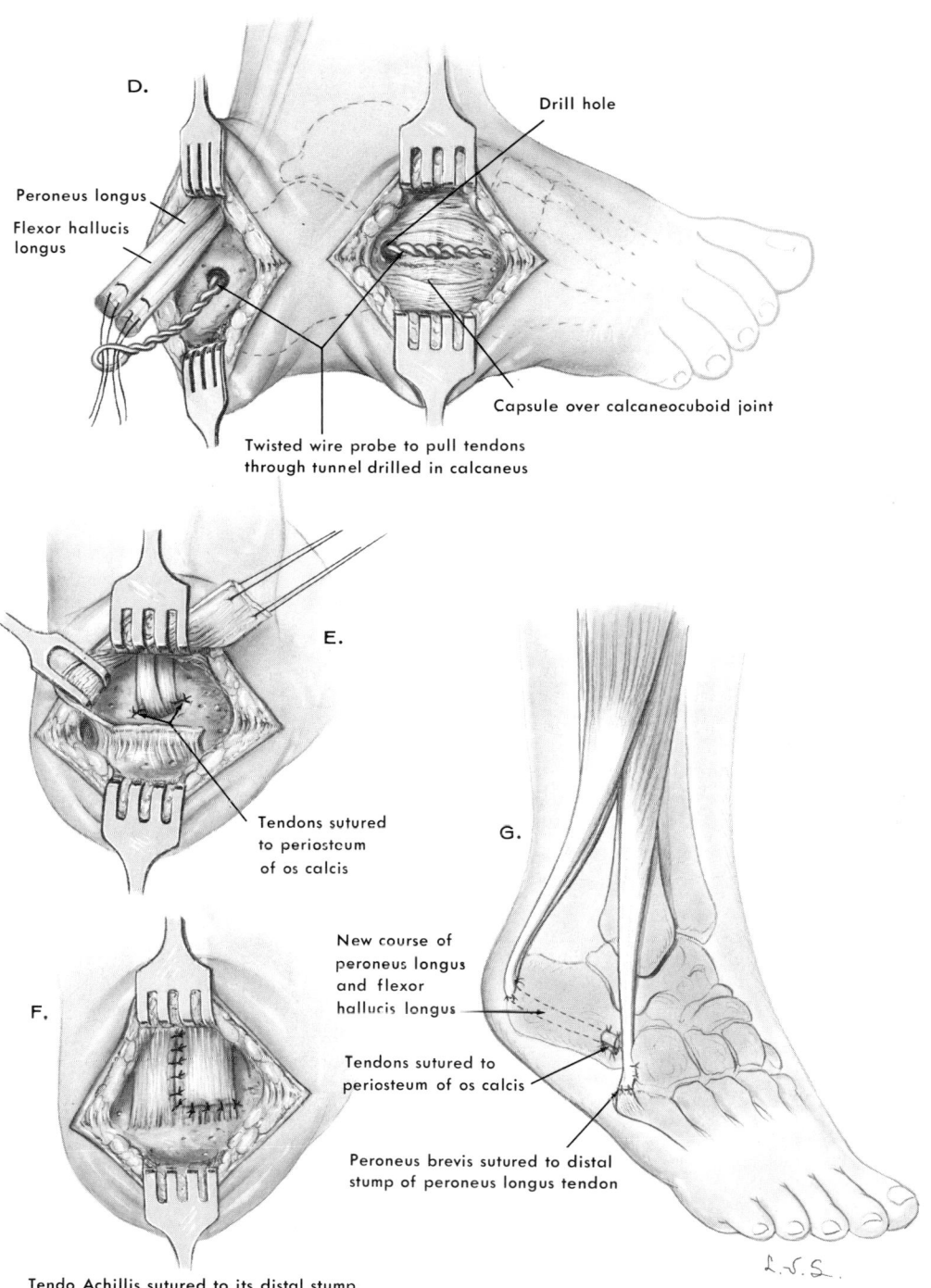

D.

Drill hole

Peroneus longus

Flexor hallucis
longus

Capsule over calcaneocuboid joint

Twisted wire probe to pull tendons
through tunnel drilled in calcaneus

E.

Tendons sutured
to periosteum
of os calcis

G.

New course of
peroneus longus
and flexor
hallucis longus

Tendons sutured to
periosteum of os calcis

F.

Peroneus brevis sutured to distal
stump of peroneus longus tendon

Tendo Achillis sutured to its distal stump

L.S.S.

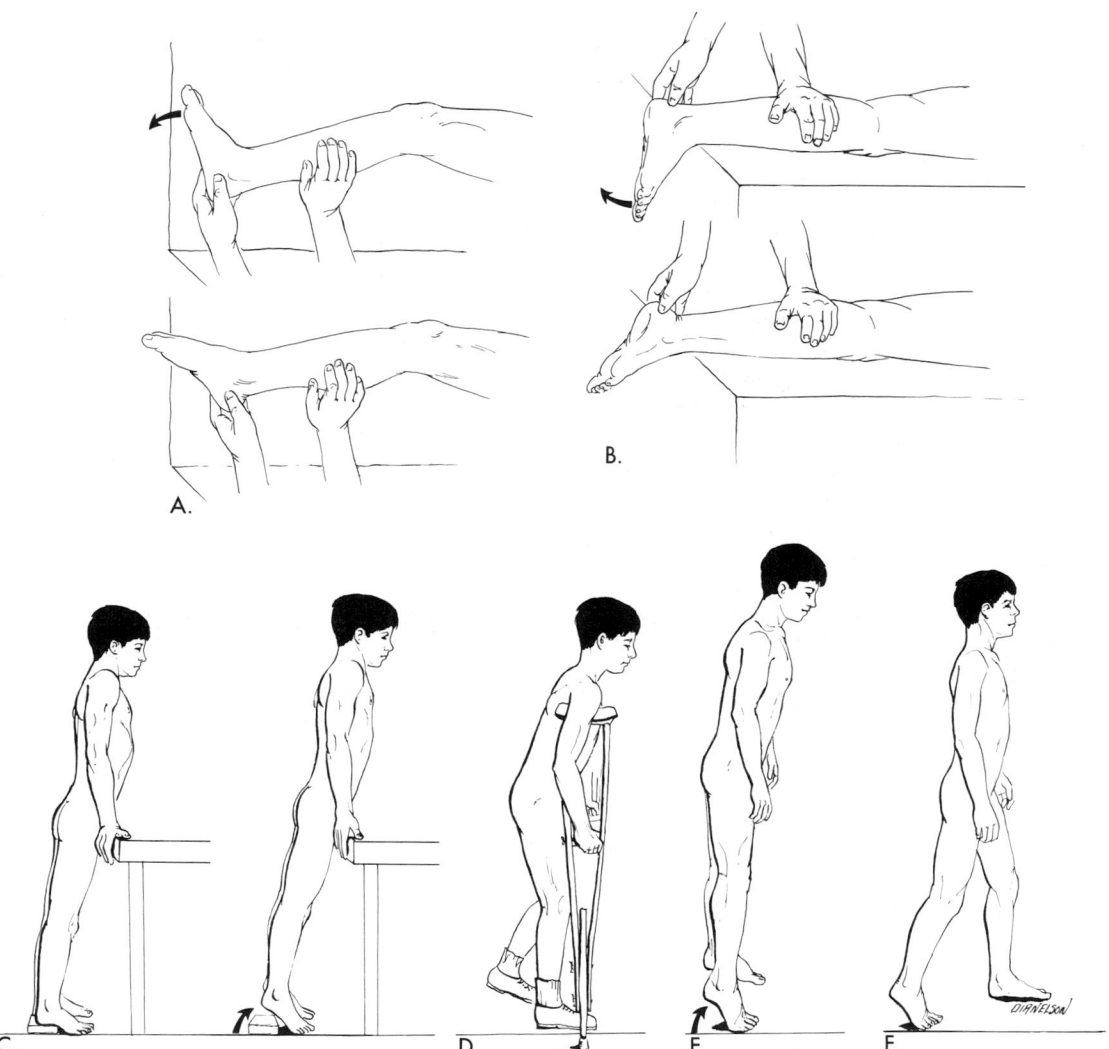

FIGURE 5-53.   Postoperative exercises following posterior tendon transfer to the os calcis.

fair or good. At birth all patients have marked flexion-adduction deformity of the hips. Extension contracture of the knee and pes varus are common associated deformities. During the first two years of life, frank dislocation of the hip will develop in 80 per cent of the patients; in the remaining 20 per cent of cases, the hips are subluxated, and if left untreated, they will become dislocated. Coxa valga is uniformly found in all patients. The acetabulum appears normal or will develop normally during the first year of postnatal life. In *Group IV* all the lumbar nerve roots are normal and the sacral segments are paralyzed. In these patients the hip abductors are poor or fair and the hamstrings are fair in motor strength, while the hip extensors are paralyzed. Progressively increasing flexion deformity of the hip occurs in all, and coxa valga develops in 30 per cent of the patients. In *Group V*, characterized by paralysis distal to the first sacral root, the gluteus maximus is the only hip muscle that is weak. Mild flexion is the only acquired deformity in these patients. Paralytic subluxation or dislocation does not take place. *Group VI* is characterized by normal musculature in the lower limbs with no acquired hip deformity.[362]

Diagnosis of hip dislocation in the newborn with myelomeningocele is not difficult. Often, however, the hips are examined inadequately because the infant is in prone position to protect the delicate posterior sac. It is difficult to perform the Barlow and Ortolani tests with the infant lying face down on the Bradford frame. He should be turned supine and gently supported by the nurse for thorough examination of the hips. Roentgenograms of the hips should always be obtained. The distinguishing features of teratologic and typical congenital dislocation of the hip are discussed in Chapter 2. Ordinarily a congenitally dislocated hip with associated complete or partial paralysis is much easier to reduce than if the limb had normal musculature.

Treatment varies according to the type of dislocation. In general, *teratologic* dislocation of the hip in myelomeningocele should not be treated. An attempt at closed reduction following an initial period of skin traction may be made. If the hips are irreducible by closed methods, open reduction should not be carried out, as the result

will often be a stiff, "frozen" hip, which will prove to be a greater handicap that will make sitting almost impossible.

In *congenital* dislocation with total or partial paralysis of the lower limbs, closed reduction in the neonatal period is a simple procedure. This is often postponed until closure of the posterior defect is complete. The performance of shunting procedures to control increasing hydrocephalus may be another cause of delay. During this period, however, the hips are maintained in wide abduction on the Bradford frame. In the presence of proximal displacement of the femoral heads or adduction contracture of the hips, skin traction may be applied on the lower limbs with the infant lying prone on the Bradford frame, which is securely elevated on blocks. The hips should be in a partially flexed position while in traction; forced extension of the hips should be avoided.

Following closed reduction, the exact position of immobilization of the hips in a plaster of Paris cast is an important consideration. Flexion–abduction–external rotation (the so-called frog-leg position) should be avoided; it will cause contracture of the iliotibial band. The hips should be placed in neutral or slight internal rotation and 60 to 70 degrees of abduction. In the presence of a strong iliopsoas muscle and moderate flexion contracture of the hips, the hips are maintained in 80 to 90 degrees of flexion, depending upon the stability of reduction; whereas, if the lower limbs are completely flail, the hips should be in only 70 to 80 degrees of flexion. The period of rigid immobilization in the cast is usually from six to eight weeks; then a bivalved hip spica cast worn during sleeping hours is utilized to maintain the reduction.

The course of treatment following this stage depends on the presence or absence of muscle imbalance. In involvement at the higher levels, i.e., the first lumbar level and above, with almost total paralysis of the lower limbs, the hips, once reduced, will remain so. Static deformities are prevented by proper splinting and by avoidance of faulty positions while lying or sitting. Coxa valga may develop when these children are upright and it may cause instability of the hip. In such an instance, varization osteotomy of the proximal femur is performed.

With lower neurosegmental levels of in-

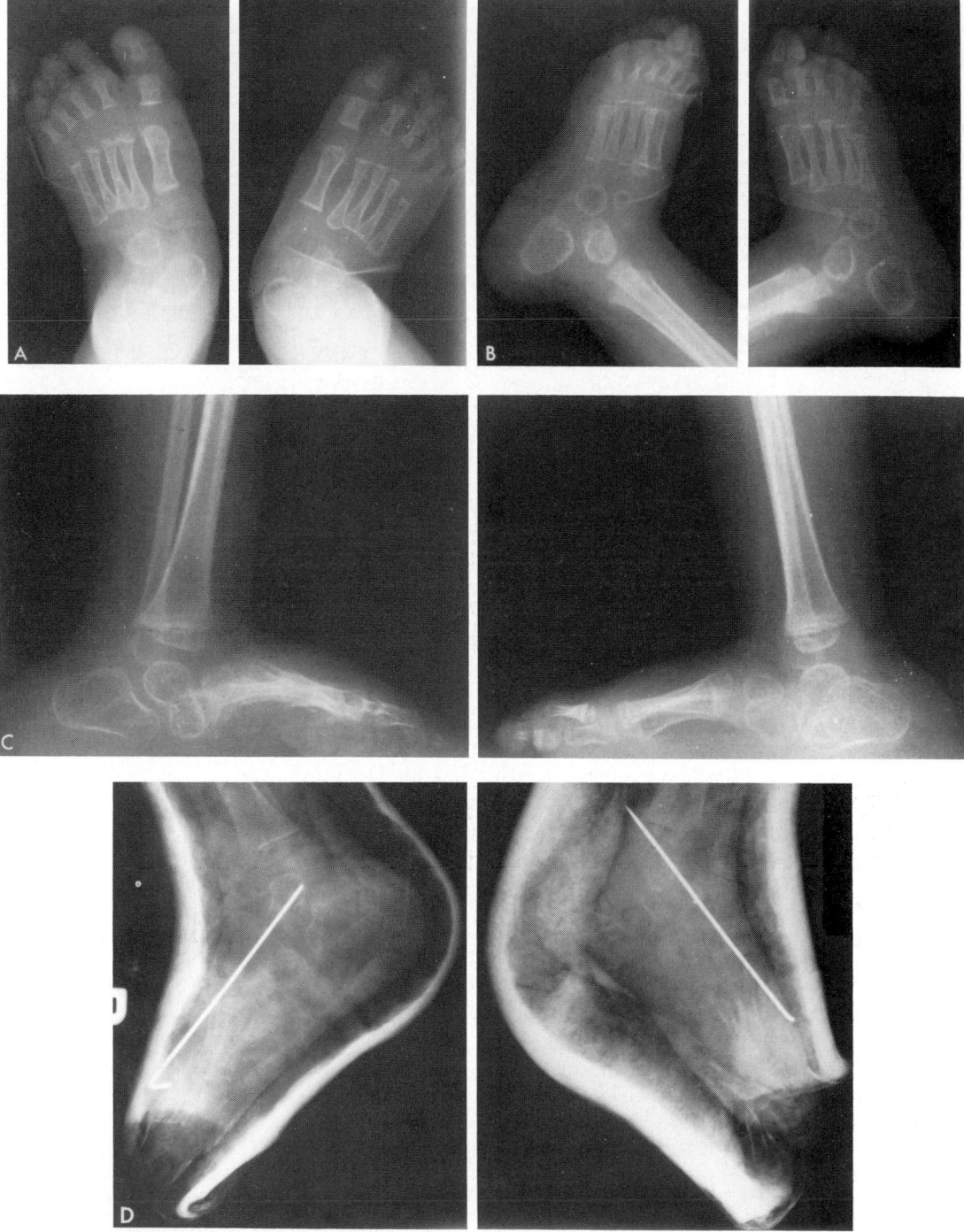

FIGURE 5-54. *Equinovalgus deformity (paralytic vertical talus) of both feet in a child with myelomeningocele.*

A and **B.** Roentgenograms of both feet when ten months old. **C.** Lateral roentgenograms of the feet at two and one half years of age. Note the plantarflexed talus with dislocation of the talonavicular joint. The os calcis is everted and somewhat equinus. The forefoot is abducted and slightly dorsiflexed. **D.** Postoperative lateral roentgenograms of both feet in cast. Open reduction of the talonavicular joint was performed. The Kirschner wire was introduced retrograde to maintain the reduction. The anterior tibial and peroneal muscles were transferred posteriorly to the os calcis.

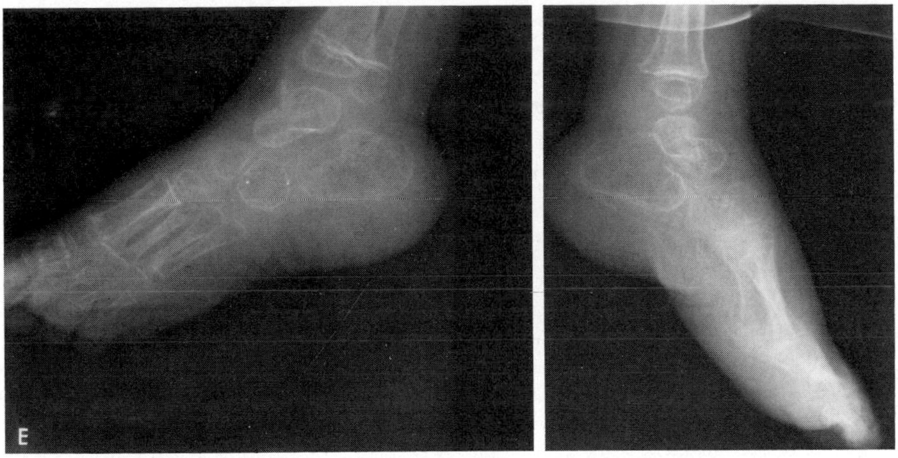

FIGURE 5–54 Continued. *Equinovalgus deformity (paralytic vertical talus) of both feet in a child with myelomeningocele.*

E. Six months after surgery. The roentgenograms of both feet show maintenance of reduction. The foot has normal alignment.

volvement, i.e., the third lumbar level and below, stability of the hip joint depends entirely on the distribution of paralysis. The hip flexors and adductors are innervated by the upper three lumbar neurosegments, whereas the hip abductor-extensor muscle groups are innervated by the fourth and fifth lumbar and first sacral neurosegments. In the presence of strong hip flexor-adductors and paralyzed hip extensor-abductors, subsequent dislocation of the hip is inevitable.

Following reduction of the congenitally dislocated hip with muscle imbalance, the hip is maintained in a stable position in a bivalved hip spica cast at night until the infant is of suitable age (usually 10 to 12 months) for iliopsoas transfer. With this method, open reduction and capsular plication of the hip are not necessary, and the possible complication of postoperative stiffness of the hip joint is avoided.

The performance of this major operative procedure at such an early age is justified because a strong iliopsoas muscle is a deforming force. The transferred iliopsoas muscle is seldom powerful enough to lift the limb against gravity; following the Sharrard procedure, however, stability of the hip is ensured and progressive flexion deformity of the hip with resultant excessive lumbar lordosis is prevented. The purpose of early iliopsoas transfer is to give stable hips that will not become deformed and to enable these children to walk as soon as possible after the age of 15 to 18 months.

Prior to transfer of the iliopsoas muscle, the passive range of hip abduction should be at least 60 degrees and it is imperative that the sartorius and tensor fasciae latae muscles be normal in motor strength, enabling active hip flexion against gravity. Posterior transfer of the iliopsoas muscle is combined with open reduction of the hip and Salter innominate osteotomy if there is frank congenital dislocation of the hip and an inadequate acetabulum (Fig. 5–58). In hip subluxation the lax capsule may be tightened superiorly and anteriorly by an extrasynovial purse-string capsular suture.

The operative technique of posterolateral transfer of the iliopsoas muscle through a hole in the ilium from the lesser to the greater trochanter is described and illustrated in Plate 39.

When the sartorius and tensor fasciae latae muscles are paralyzed, it is wise not to weaken active hip flexion by transfer of the iliopsoas muscle. Stability of the hip joint is given by early varization osteotomy of the proximal femur. Recurrence of coxa valga with growth is treated by repeating the varization osteotomy. The degree of anteversion of the proximal femur should be determined; if it is excessive and is a

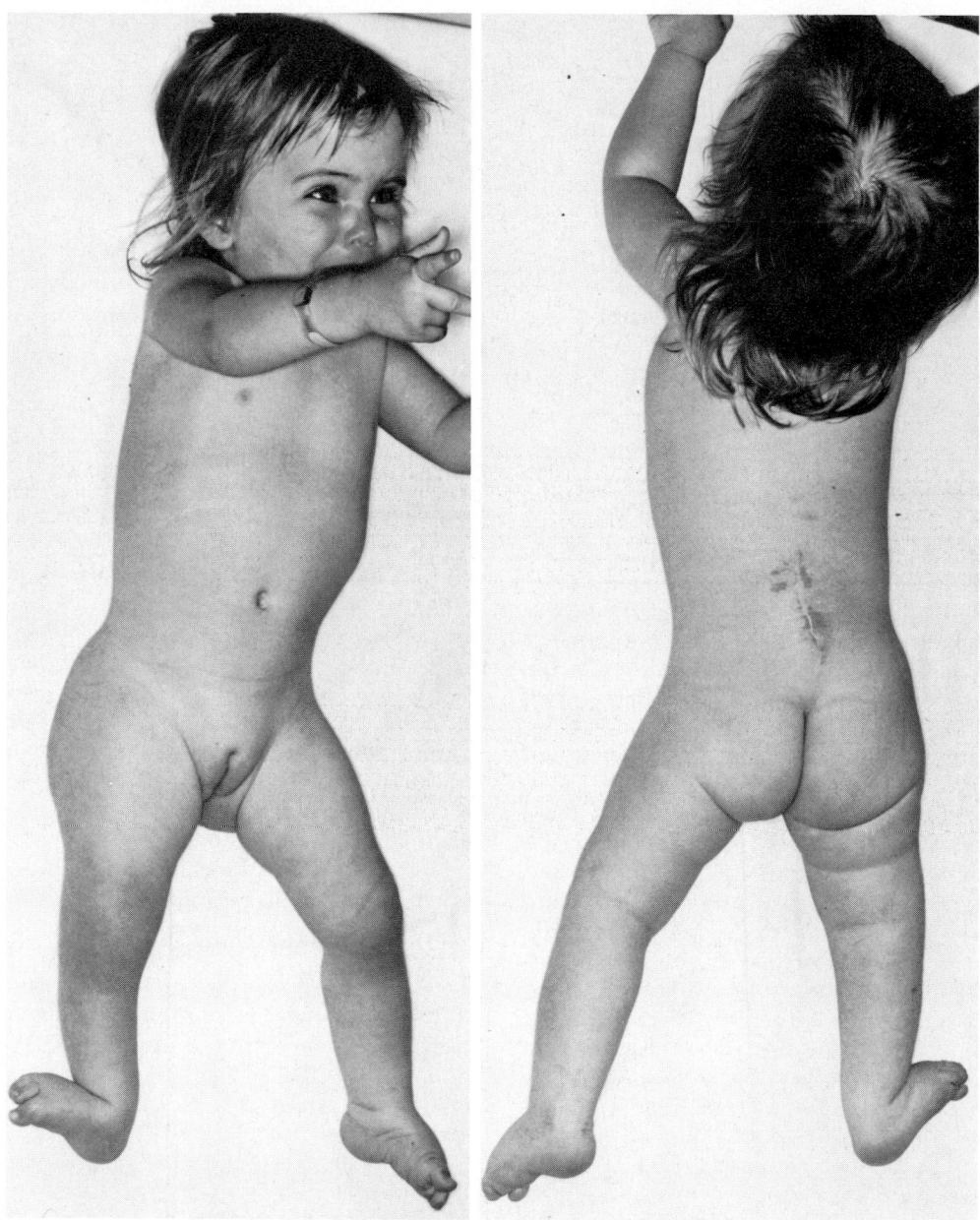

FIGURE 5–55. *A one-year-old infant with myelomeningocele.*

Note the calcaneovalgus deformity of the right foot caused by fibrosis of long toe extensors and peroneal muscles.

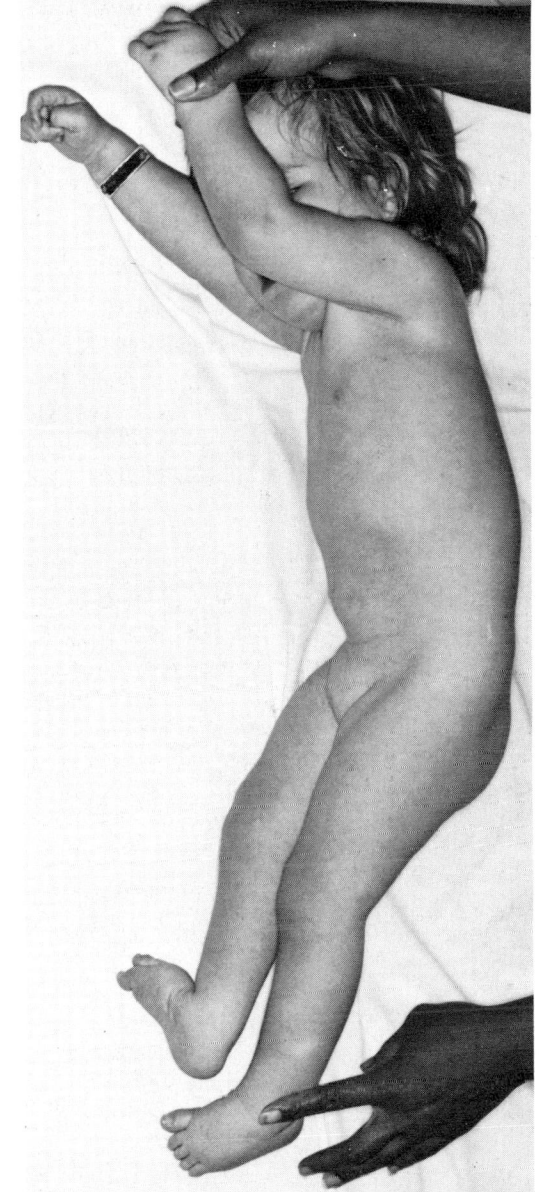

FIGURE 5–55 Continued. *A one-year-old infant with myelomeningocele.*

Note the calcaneovalgus deformity of the right foot caused by fibrosis of long toe extensors and peroneal muscles.

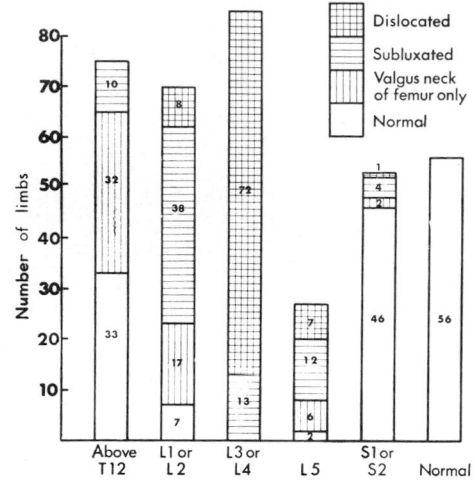

FIGURE 5-56. *Hip disorders in 183 children with lumbar myelomeningocele.*

Roentgenographic status of the hip joint at 12 months of age, related to the neurosegmental level of the lesion. (From Sharrard, W. J. W.: Posterior iliopsoas transplantation in the treatment of paralytic dislocation of the hip. J. Bone Joint Surg., *46-B*:427, 1964.)

factor in instability of the hip, it is corrected by derotation osteotomy. One may consider transfer of the external oblique muscle to restore power of hip abduction.

When a child is brought for orthopedic care late with an already dislocated hip, the problem is a difficult one and treatment should be individualized. An attempt at closed reduction following an initial period of traction should be made. If the femoral head cannot be brought down, it is best to leave these hips alone. If one attempt at open reduction fails, it is best to accept a dislocated hip, as it is mobile and more functional than a reduced but stiff hip. Every precaution should be taken to prevent development of a frozen hip.

FLEXION DEFORMITY

This develops when there is hip flexor power in the absence of hip extensor power. In the older child who is primarily a sitter, hip flexion deformity also results from static forces of malposture. Excessive lordosis of the spine will result in the presence of hip flexion contracture. In infancy, it is treated by passive stretching exercises. If it

is marked and does not respond to the exercise regimen, bilateral split Russell skin traction is applied to correct the deformity. With early posterior transfer of the iliopsoas muscle, progressive flexion deformity can be prevented. When the patient is seen late and flexion deformity is very severe, extension osteotomy of the proximal femur may be indicated.

In the armamentarium of the orthopedic surgeon there are two other procedures to increase hip extensor strength: posterior transfer of the hip adductor origin to the ischial tuberosity, thus converting the flexor action of the deforming anterior hip adductors into extension; and erector spinae transfer with fascia lata to the greater trochanter. The personal experience of the author with the preceding two procedures in patients with myelomeningocele has been disappointing. Hogshead and Ponseti reported the results of fascia lata transfer to the erector spinae in nine patients with myelomeningocele. The transfer provided a dynamic fasciodesis and relief of hip flexion contracture, stabilization of the hip, and relief of lumbar lordosis.[303]

Unilateral contracture of the iliotibial band will cause pelvic obliquity, with the contralateral hip gradually becoming dislocated. In such a case, following the Ober-Yount procedure, the subluxated hip is reduced and placed in wide abduction and some flexion, while the hip with iliotibial band contracture is placed in the position of extension and neutral adduction (Fig. 5-59). The operative technique of the Ober-Yount procedure is described in the section on poliomyelitis.

The Knee

EXTENSION OR HYPEREXTENSION CONTRACTURE OF THE KNEE

This disabling deformity may either be caused by dynamic imbalance of muscles resulting from normal strength of the quadriceps femoris muscle and paralyzed hamstrings (seen in lesions in which the level of involvement is distal to the third or fourth lumbar segment), or it may be due to fibrosis of the quadriceps muscles (which usually occurs in higher levels of involvement with a flail lower limb), or it may result from structural osseous deformity of the distal femur (such as that seen following malunited fractures). A stiff knee in extension will cause repeated fracture of the femur because of its levering action on the osteoporotic bone and will also cause difficulty in the proper fitting of orthotic appliances. The anesthetic aproprioceptive knee joint may develop arthrofibrotic and early degenerative changes under the abnormal stresses of body weight.

Treatment depends upon the type of extension contracture of the knee. In quadriceps femoris fibrosis, conservative methods such as wedging casts, passive stretching exercises, or traction are not ordinarily tolerated by the myelomeningocele child; however, for the very young infant, the author recommends a period of three weeks of conservative management, following which the knee joint is held in a night splint or bivalved cast in the maximal degree of flexion. Often conservative management proves to be unsuccessful, and when the child is over one year of age, open surgical lengthening of the fibrosed quadriceps femoris is performed.

When the quadriceps femoris muscle is normal in motor strength and the extension contracture is due to a dynamic imbalance between the knee flexors and extensors, management is more conservative. Genu recurvatum can usually be controlled by orthotic support and night splints. When hyperextension deformity of the knee is progressive and the hip flexors are normal in motor strength, one may consider in the older child a posterior tenodesis (Heyman-Herndon) or a myodesis by posterior transfer of the vastus lateralis muscle to the sectioned tendons of the semitendinosus and biceps femoris muscles. The vastus medialis, rectus femoris, and vastus intermedius muscles are lengthened and remain anteriorly to function as a knee extensor, whereas the vastus lateralis will provide posterior stability to the knee joint. Gravitational forces will assist knee flexion when the hip is flexed. It should be emphasized, however, that this is a split muscle transfer across a weight-bearing joint to gain stability.

FLEXION DEFORMITY

This is usually caused by contracture of the iliotibial band owing to malposture while sitting or in a supine position. Later on, with growth and persistence of malposture, contracture of the posterior capsule of the knee joint and permanent shortening and fibrosis of the hamstring muscles take place. These static soft-tissue deformities can be prevented by proper positioning and splinting of the limbs. If they do become fixed, however, soft-tissue release by open surgery is indicated.

Bony deformity due to malunited fractures may also cause flexion deformity of the knee, or angular and torsional deformities of the lower limb. These are corrected by osteotomy at the appropriate level.

The Spine

Deformities of the spine are common, as the vertebral column is the primary site of involvement in myelomeningocele. With improved medical and surgical care, more and more of these children are surviving into adolescence, and the progressive deformities of the spine present serious and challenging problems to the orthopedic surgeon.

Abnormal lordosis, scoliosis, and kyphosis are the deformities frequently encountered. These may be present in pure form or in varying combinations. It is imperative that all patients with myelomeningocele have anteroposterior and lateral roentgenograms of the spine taken periodically for early detection of spinal deformities.

LORDOSIS

The most common of the spinal deformities in myelomeningocele is abnormal lordosis. It is often compensatory in origin — for purposes of balance. In the presence of bilateral paralysis of the triceps surae and gluteus maximus muscles, but normal strength of the hip flexors and quadriceps femoris muscles, the patient stands with a characteristic calcaneus crouch posture, i.e., the hips and knees are flexed, the ankles are dorsiflexed, and the lower limbs are inclined forward. Stability is given by the action of a strong quadriceps femoris muscle. Compensation and balance are provided by holding the lumbar spine in severe lordosis (Fig. 5–60).

Hip flexion contracture will increase the

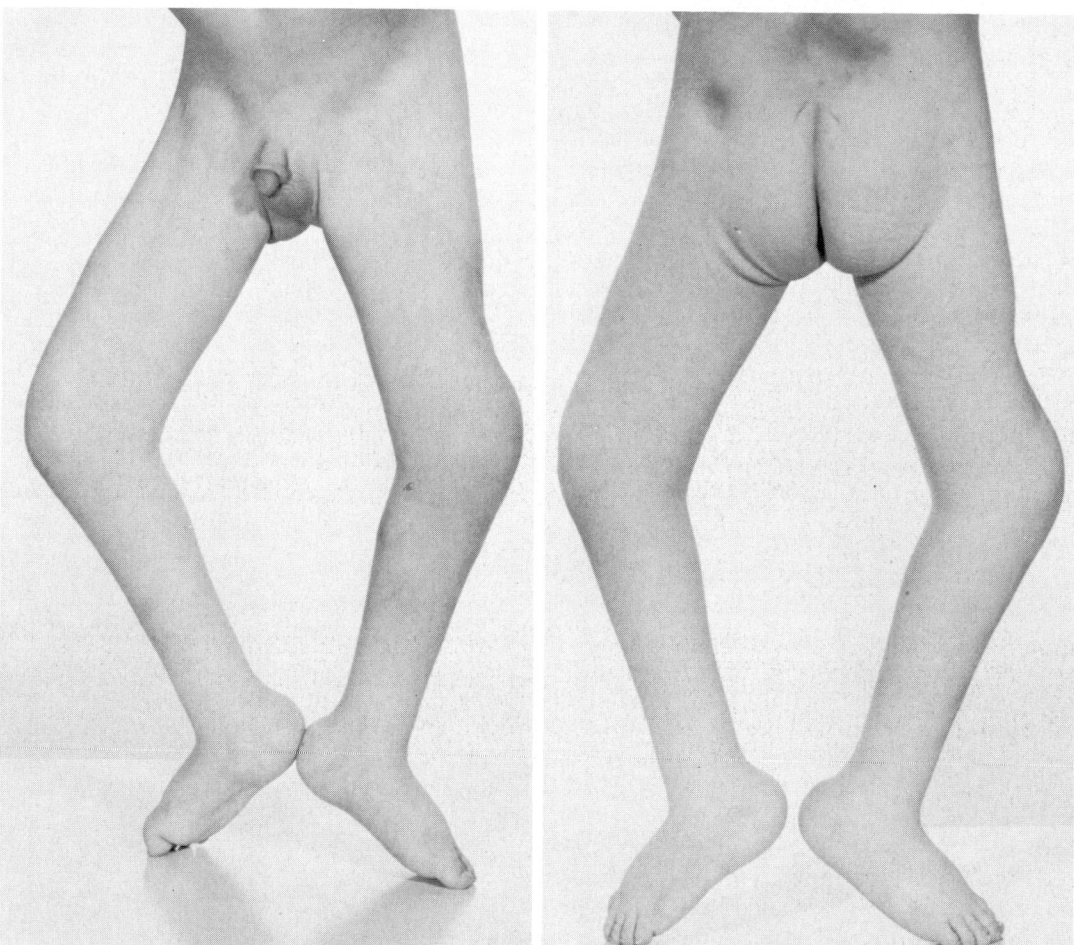

FIGURE 5–57. *A two-year-old child with myelomeningocele with paralysis below the twelfth thoracic level of innervation.*

Note the flexion, abduction, and external rotation contracture of both hips, flexion contracture of the knees, and bilateral pes equinus. These are static deformities produced by faulty posture in utero and in postnatal life. They can be prevented by positioning of the flail limbs of the paralyzed infant, by use of night splints, and by gentle passive stretching exercises.

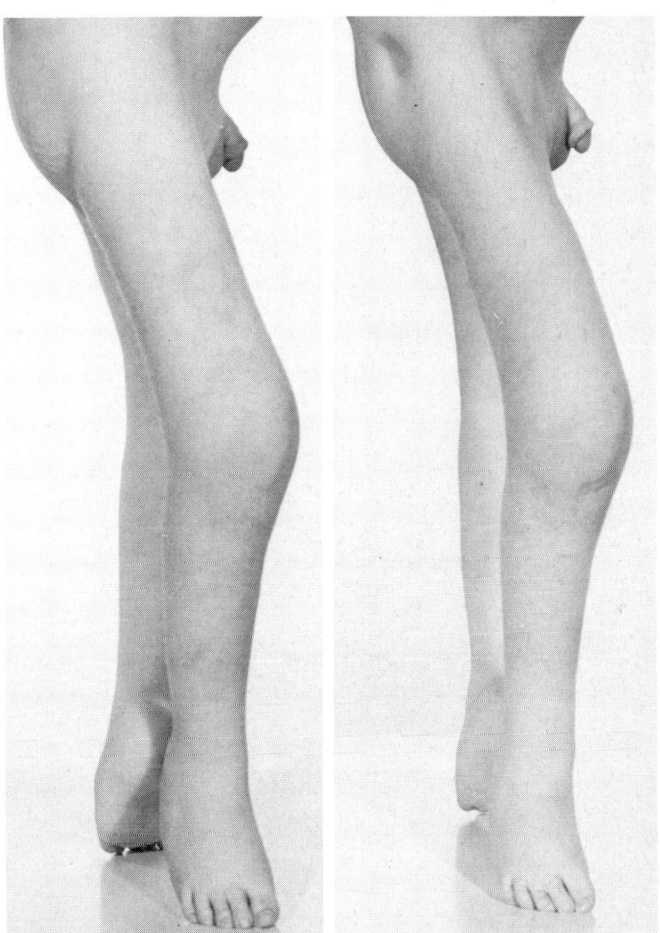

FIGURE 5–57 Continued.   A two-year-old child with myelomeningocele with paralysis below the twelfth thoracic level of innervation.

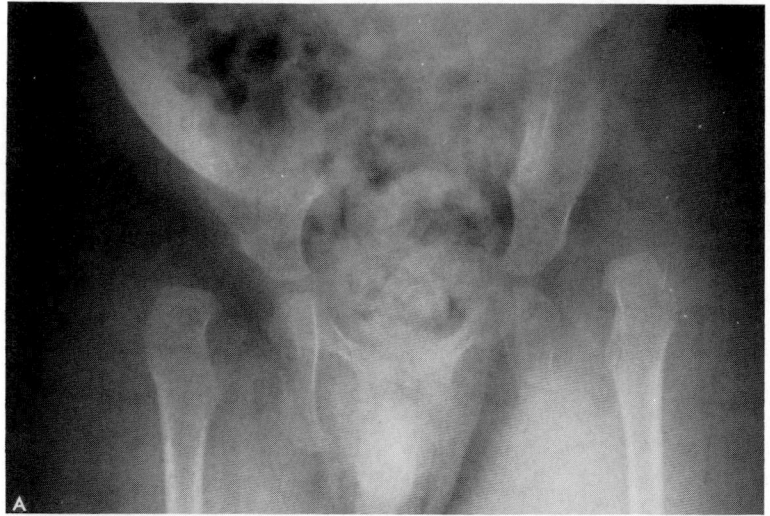

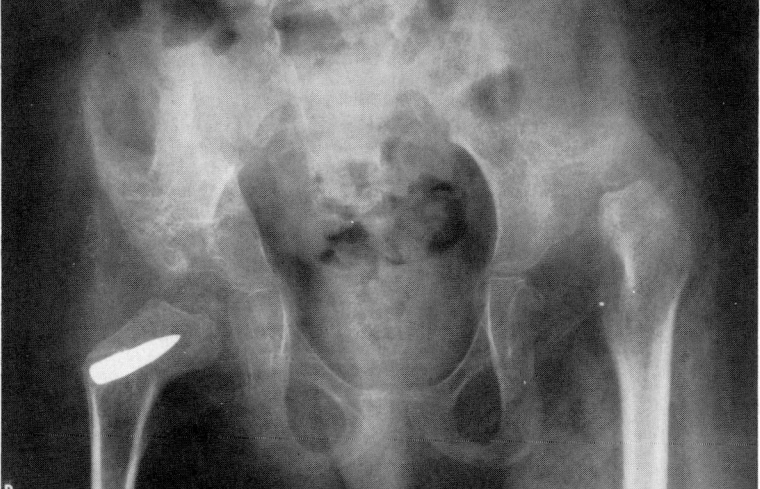

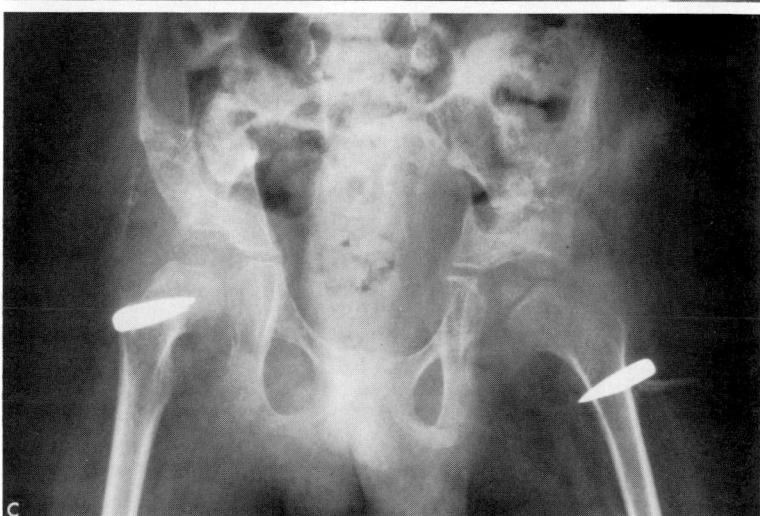

FIGURE 5-58. *Bilateral congenital dislocation of the hip in a child with myelomeningocele.*

The neurosegmental level of paralysis is distal to the third lumbar. The hip flexors and adductors are normal in motor strength, but the hip abductors and extensors are paralyzed. Bilateral open reduction, capsular plication, innominate osteotomy, and posterior iliopsoas transfer were performed in two stages. **A**. Preoperative roentgenogram. **B** and **C**. Postoperative roentgenograms. (The staples are used to fix the iliopsoas tendon to the subtrochanteric region of the femur.)

pelvic inclination and force the lumbar spine into excessive lordosis. Muscle imbalance between the hip flexors and extensors and contracture of the iliotibial band are common causes of flexion deformity of the hip. Posterior osseous defect of the lumbosacral spine and congenital spondylolisthesis are other etiologic factors.

Lordosis in myelomeningocele may be of two types: a *low type*, in which the proximal end of the exaggerated anterior curve is at or below the third lumbar vertebra, or a *high type*, in which lordotic curve extends from the second lumbar vertebra into the thoracic vertebrae, where lordosis is not normally present. The location and extent of lordosis usually corresponds with the level of paralysis. Compensation of abnormal lordosis takes place by the development of a commensurate posterior curve in the spine (kyphosis) above and flexion of the hip below. In stance, when the center of gravity of the body falls immediately in front of the ankle joint, the lordosis is *balanced* and minimum external support is required for standing; when the center of gravity falls in front of the toes but the patient is able to stand with crutches, lordosis is *partially balanced*; and when crutch-standing is impossible or impractical because of severity of lordosis, it is regarded as *off-balance* (Fig. 5–61).

The functional performance of patients with low type lordosis is better than that of those with high type lordosis. Most patients with high type lordosis are off-balance or only partially balanced, whereas, in low type lordosis, balance or partial balance of the spine is the rule.[321]

Treatment. Lordosis of the spine will progress with growth unless aggressive measures are taken to check it. Knee-chest exercises are performed several times a day to maintain flexibility of the lumbosacral spine. Passive stretching exercises are carried out to correct the hip flexion and iliotibial band contractures. A plastic body jacket may be used to support the trunk in sitting and in stance.

Surgical measures are directed toward elimination of deforming factors. If a strong iliopsoas muscle is causing the deformity, it is transferred posteriorly to the greater trochanter to function as a hip abductor and extensor. If iliotibial band contracture is

present to a significant degree and does not respond to passive stretching exercises, it is surgically released by the Ober-Yount procedure. Erector spinae transfer may improve trunk stability. Fascial transplants to reinforce abdominal musculature may be considered.

Spinal fusion is indicated when the preceding measures fail to improve or arrest the increasing lordosis and there is progressive loss of balance. The sacrum should be included in the fusion area, and Harrington instrumentation is used for internal fixation. Functional range of hip motion is a prerequisite for lumbosacral fusion; otherwise, the patient will be unable to sit.

SCOLIOSIS

In myelomeningocele, scoliosis may have several causes: It may be due to (1) *congenital deformities of the spine* such as hemivertebrae or unsegmented vertebral bars (Fig. 5–62), (2) *asymmetrical paralysis* of the erector spinae and quadratus lumborum and trunk muscles, (3) *fixed pelvic obliquity* as a result of dislocation of one hip or adductor-abduction contracture of the hips (Fig. 5–63), or (4) *static forces* of chronic malposture necessitated by paralysis or by a period of recumbency for care of frequently recurring ischial or greater trochanteric pressure sores.

In general, the severity of scoliosis is greater with higher levels of paralysis. Most of these patients are primarily sitters whose functional handicap is increased by the severe scoliotic deformity that makes sitting extremely difficult.

Treatment. A plastic body jacket will support the trunk effectively; however, it will not prevent progression of the scoliosis (Fig. 5–64). A Milwaukee brace, unfortunately, is not usually tolerated by the myelomeningocele child; however, it may be tried when the child is cooperative and the parents diligent. A pad may be placed under the high buttock to accommodate pelvic obliquity. Arm rests may be used for support in the wheel chair.

Surgical measures should be taken to correct the infrapelvic deforming forces. Spinal fusion should be considered early when the curve is flexible and can be corrected with minimal effort. When the surgeon is inex-

(*Text continued on page 936.*)

Iliopsoas Muscle Transfer for Paralysis of the Hip Abductors

THE PROCEDURE

The patient lies supine with a small sandbag under the sacrum and a larger sandbag under the ipsilateral scapula. The entire involved lower limb, the hip, the lower abdomen and chest, and the iliac and sacral regions are prepared sterile and draped so that the limb that is to be operated on can be freely manipulated and the incision extended to the posterior third of the iliac crest without contamination.

A. The skin incision extends forward from the junction of the posterior and middle thirds of the iliac crest to the anterior superior iliac spine; it is then carried distally into the thigh along the medial border of the sartorius muscle for a distance of 10 to 12 cm., ending 2 cm. distal to the lesser trochanter.

B. The deep fascia is incised over the iliac crest and the fascia lata is opened in line with the skin incision.

The lateral femoral cutaneous nerve is identified; it usually crosses the sartorius muscle 2.5 cm. distal to the anterior superior iliac spine and lies in close proximity to the lateral border of the sartorius. The nerve is mobilized by sharp dissection and protected by retracting it medially with a moist hernia tape. The wound flaps are undermined and retracted. The anterior medial margin of the tensor fasciae latae muscle is identified and, by blunt dissection, the groove between the sartorius and rectus femoris muscles medially and the tensor fasciae latae muscle laterally is opened. The dissection is carried deep through the loose areolar tissue that separates these structures, and the adipose tissue that covers the front of the capsule of the hip joint is exposed. The ascending branch of the lateral femoral circumflex artery and the accompanying vein cross the midportion of the wound; they are isolated, clamped, cut, and ligated.

The origin of the sartorius muscle from the anterior superior iliac spine is detached and the muscle is reflected distally and medially. The free end is marked with a silk whip suture for later reattachment. The origins of the two heads of the rectus femoris are divided and reflected distally. The femoral nerve and its branches to the sartorius and rectus femoris are identified. A moist hernia tape is passed around the femoral nerve for gentle handling. The femoral vessels and nerve are retracted medially.

C. The cartilaginous apophysis of the ilium is split and the dissection is deepened along the iliac crest down to bone. With a broad periosteal elevator the tensor fasciae latae and the gluteus medius and minimus muscles are stripped subperiosteally from the lateral surface of the ilium and reflected in one continuous mass laterally and distally to the superior margin of the acetabulum. Bleeding is controlled by packing the interval between the reflected muscles and ilium with laparotomy pads.

D. Then with a large periosteal elevator, the iliacus muscle is subperiosteally elevated and reflected medially, exposing the inner wall of the wing of the ilium from the greater sciatic notch to the anterior superior iliac spine.

By careful blunt dissection with a periosteal elevator, the iliacus muscle is freed, elevated, and mobilized from the inner wall of the ilium and the anterior capsule of the hip joint. It is important to stay lateral and deep to the iliacus muscle and work in a proximal to distal direction.

Plate 39.   Iliopsoas Muscle Transfer for Paralysis
of the Hip Abductors

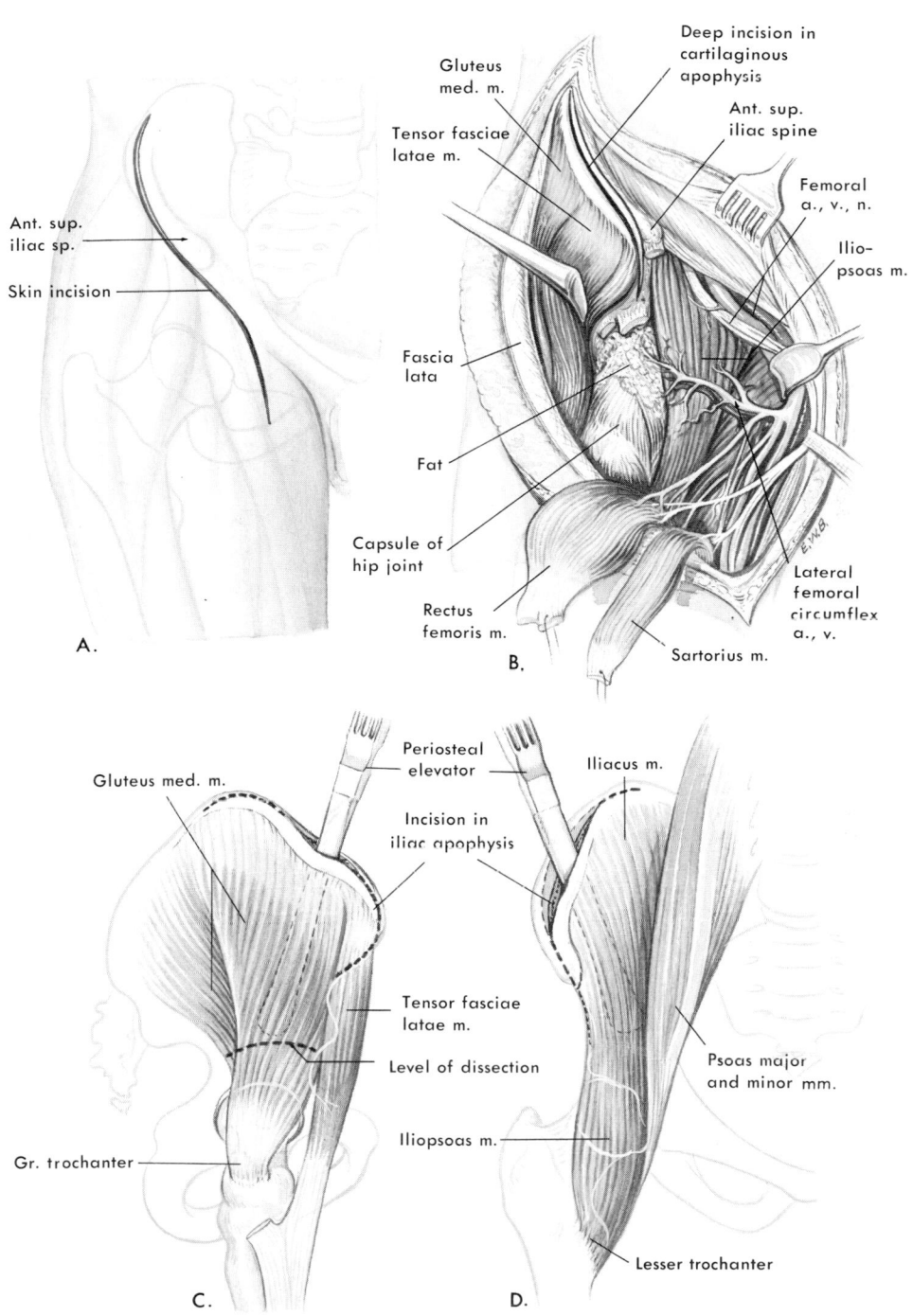

A.

Ant. sup. iliac sp.

Skin incision

B.

Gluteus med. m.

Tensor fasciae latae m.

Deep incision in cartilaginous apophysis

Ant. sup. iliac spine

Femoral a., v., n.

Iliopsoas m.

Fascia lata

Fat

Capsule of hip joint

Rectus femoris m.

Sartorius m.

Lateral femoral circumflex a., v.

C.

Gluteus med. m.

Gr. trochanter

Periosteal elevator

Incision in iliac apophysis

Tensor fasciae latae m.

Level of dissection

Iliacus m.

Psoas major and minor mm.

Iliopsoas m.

Lesser trochanter

D.

923

Iliopsoas Muscle Transfer for Paralysis of the Hip Abductors
(Continued)

E to **G.** Next, the hip is flexed, abducted, and externally rotated, and with the index finger, the lesser trochanter is cleared of soft tissues proximally, posteriorly, and distally. The index finger is then placed on the posteromedial aspect of the lesser trochanter and is used to direct a curved osteotome to the superior and deep aspect of the base of the lesser trochanter.

The lesser trochanter is osteotomized and the distal insertion of the iliacus muscle on the linea aspera of the femur is freed with a periosteal elevator.

H. The iliacus and psoas muscles are reflected proximally by sharp and dull dissection. It is very essential not to injure the nerve to the iliacus, which at times enters the muscle belly quite distally; also, the femoral nerve should not be damaged. The author finds the use of a nerve stimulator of great help. Circumflex vessels are clamped, cut, and ligated as necessary.

I. In the middle third of the wing of the ilium a rectangular hole, usually 1½ to 2 inches, is cut with drill holes and osteotomes. The hole should be large enough to accommodate the transferred muscle. It should be located as far posteriorly as possible to allow a more direct line of muscle action. The limiting factor is the nerve supply to the iliacus, which should not be stretched.

Plate 39. Iliopsoas Muscle Transfer for Paralysis of the Hip Abductors

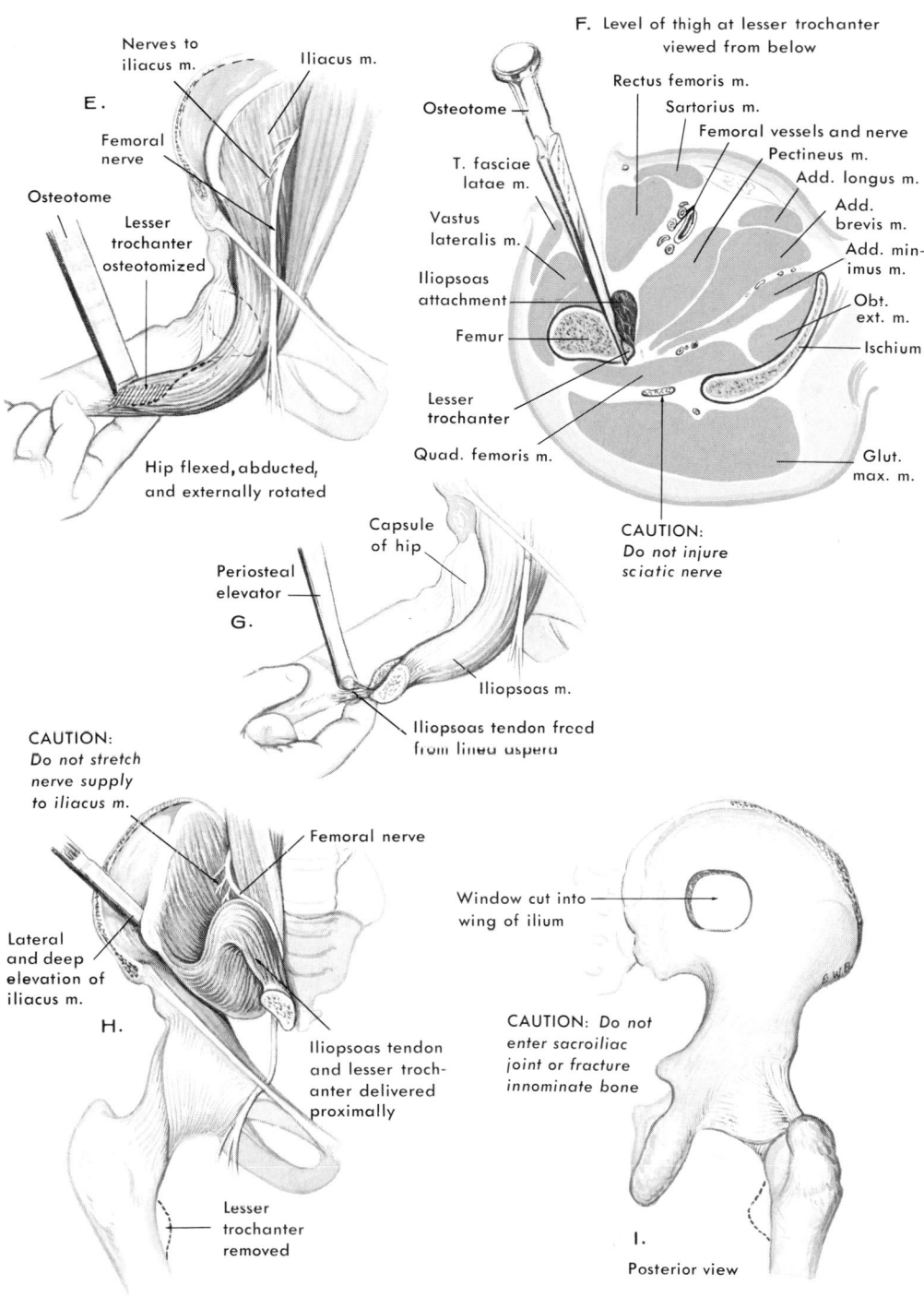

E.

Nerves to iliacus m.

Iliacus m.

Femoral nerve

Osteotome

Lesser trochanter osteotomized

Hip flexed, abducted, and externally rotated

F. Level of thigh at lesser trochanter viewed from below

Osteotome

Rectus femoris m.

Sartorius m.

Femoral vessels and nerve

Pectineus m.

Add. longus m.

Add. brevis m.

Add. minimus m.

Obt. ext. m.

Ischium

Glut. max. m.

T. fasciae latae m.

Vastus lateralis m.

Iliopsoas attachment

Femur

Lesser trochanter

Quad. femoris m.

CAUTION: *Do not injure sciatic nerve*

Capsule of hip

Periosteal elevator

G.

Iliopsoas m.

Iliopsoas tendon freed from linea aspera

CAUTION: *Do not stretch nerve supply to iliacus m.*

Femoral nerve

Lateral and deep elevation of iliacus m.

H.

Iliopsoas tendon and lesser trochanter delivered proximally

Lesser trochanter removed

Window cut into wing of ilium

CAUTION: *Do not enter sacroiliac joint or fracture innominate bone*

I.

Posterior view

925

Iliopsoas Muscle Transfer for Paralysis of the Hip Abductors
(Continued)

J. With the hip in extension and internal rotation, the greater trochanter is exposed by a longitudinal lateral incision. The vastus lateralis muscle is split and the lateral surface of the proximal 4 to 5 cm. of femor shaft is subperiosteally exposed.

K. It is important not to damage the greater trochanteric epiphyseal plate.

L. Next, a large Ober tendon passer is inserted through the hole in the wing of the ilium, directed deep to the glutei, and brought out in the greater trochanteric region by splitting the insertion of the fibers of the gluteus medius muscle.

M and **N.** The iliopsoas muscle is then transferred laterally by this route with the Ober tendon passer. The nerve supply to the iliacus is again checked to be sure it is not under great tension. Next, the hip is abducted at least 45 to 60 degrees and internally rotated 10 to 15 degrees. The site of insertion of the iliopsoas tendon on the femoral shaft is determined and is roughened with curved osteotomes. The muscle should be under proper tension.

Plate 39. Iliopsoas Muscle Transfer for Paralysis of the Hip Abductors

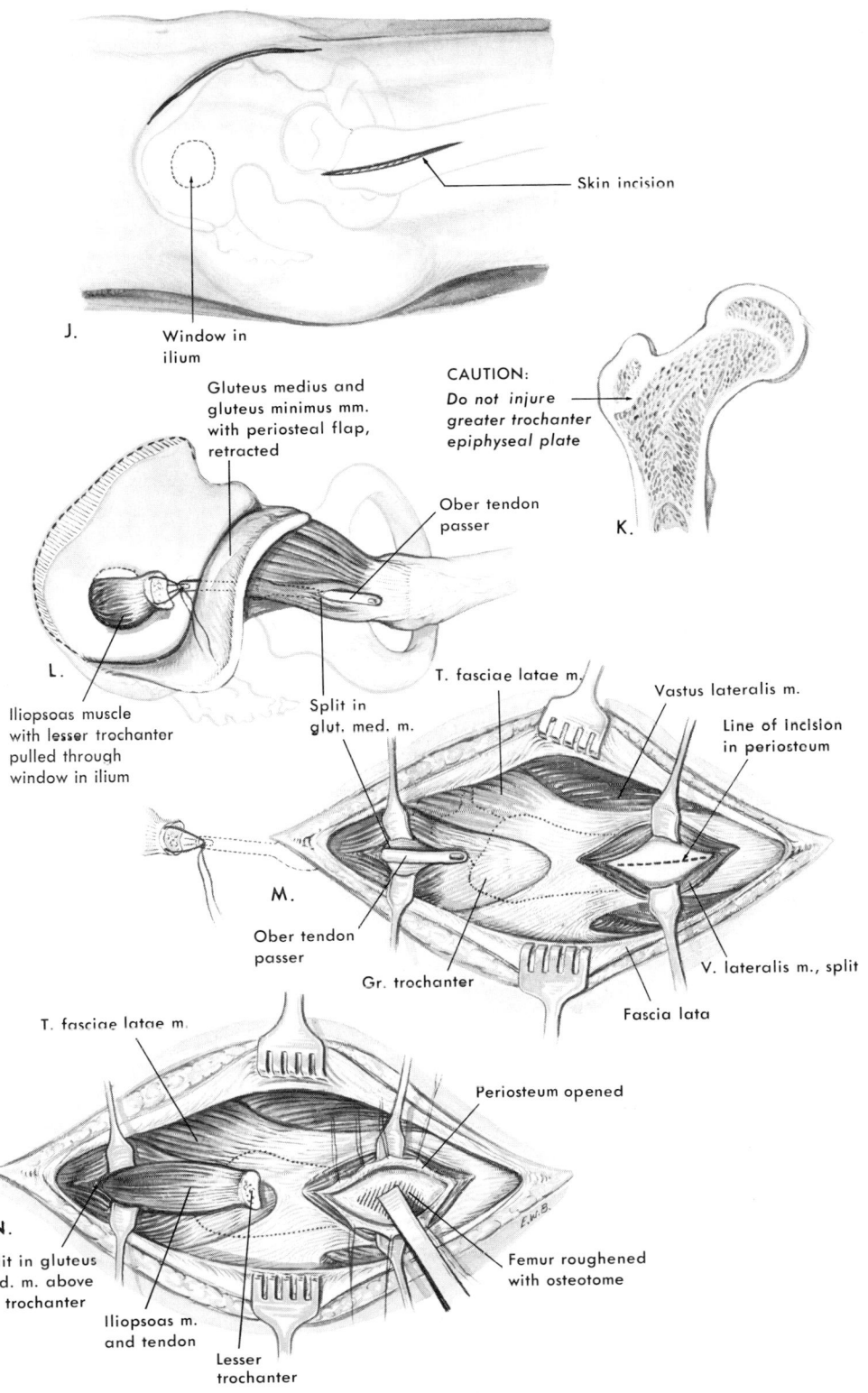

J.

Skin incision

Window in ilium

Gluteus medius and gluteus minimus mm. with periosteal flap, retracted

Ober tendon passer

CAUTION:
Do not injure greater trochanter epiphyseal plate

K.

L.

Iliopsoas muscle with lesser trochanter pulled through window in ilium

Split in glut. med. m.

T. fasciae latae m.

Vastus lateralis m.

Line of incision in periosteum

M.

Ober tendon passer

Gr. trochanter

V. lateralis m., split

Fascia lata

T. fasciae latae m.

Periosteum opened

N.

Split in gluteus med. m. above gr. trochanter

Iliopsoas m. and tendon

Lesser trochanter

Femur roughened with osteotome

E.W.B.

927

Iliopsoas Muscle Transfer for Paralysis of the Hip Abductors
(Continued)

O. The lesser trochanter is anchored to the proximal femur by one or two transversely placed small staples. Mustard recommends making a trap door in the femur into which the lesser trochanter is drawn and anchored by heavy wire sutures.

P. The periosteum and vastus lateralis muscle are sutured to the edges and over the iliopsoas tendon.

Q and **R.** The rectus femoris and sartorius muscles are sutured to the inferior and superior iliac spines, respectively. The tensor fasciae latae, the gluteus medius and minimus, and the abdominal muscles are sutured to the iliac crest. The wound is closed in layers in routine manner. A one and one half hip spica cast is applied, with the hip in 60 degrees of abduction, 10 to 15 degrees internal rotation, and slight flexion.

POSTOPERATIVE CARE

Four to six weeks following surgery, the patient is readmitted to the hospital and the cast is removed and a new bivalved hip spica cast made. This should be cut low on the lateral side so that hip abduction exercises can be performed in the posterior half of the cast. Roentgenograms of the hips are made to determine the stability of the hip joint. Great care should be exercised so that a pathologic fracture of the femur is not caused when the child is lifted out of the cast.

Training of the iliopsoas transfer follows the same general principles as those for training tendon transfers in poliomyelitis. In myelomeningocele, however, there is extensive paralysis of the lower limb, necessitating orthotic support, and the patient is much younger. Thus, as soon as the transferred iliopsoas has fair motor strength and the lower limbs can be adducted to neutral position, weight-bearing is permitted in bilateral above-knee orthoses. The butterfly pelvic band will keep the hips in 5 to 10 degrees of abduction during locomotion. At night, the hips and the transfer are protected in the bivalved hip spica cast.

*Plate 39.   Iliopsoas Muscle Transfer for Paralysis
of the Hip Abductors*

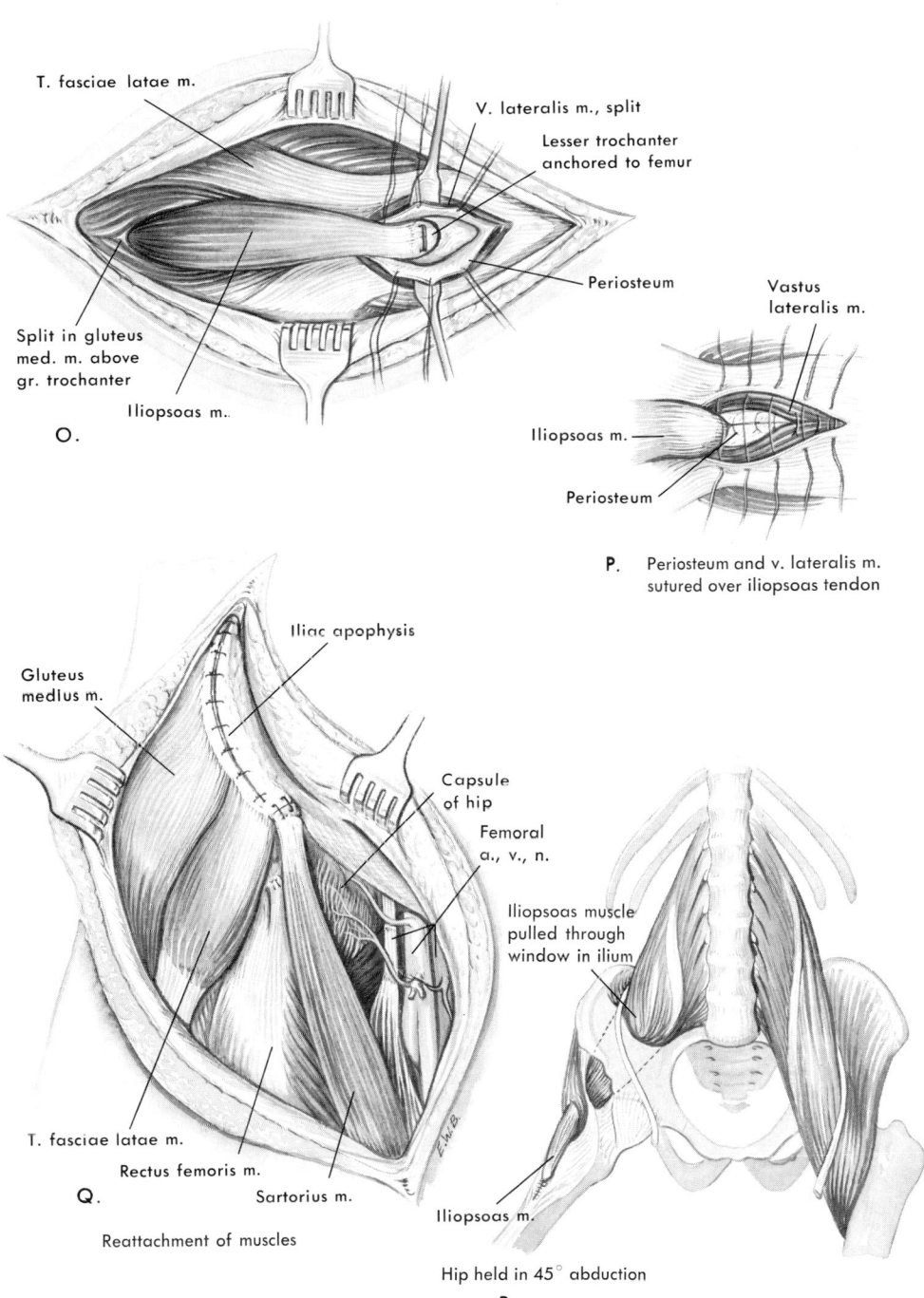

T. fasciae latae m.

V. lateralis m., split

Lesser trochanter
anchored to femur

Periosteum

Split in gluteus
med. m. above
gr. trochanter

Iliopsoas m.

O.

Vastus
lateralis m.

Iliopsoas m.

Periosteum

P.   Periosteum and v. lateralis m.
sutured over iliopsoas tendon

Iliac apophysis

Gluteus
medius m.

Capsule
of hip

Femoral
a., v., n.

Iliopsoas muscle
pulled through
window in ilium

T. fasciae latae m.

Rectus femoris m.

Sartorius m.

Q.

Reattachment of muscles

Iliopsoas m.

Hip held in 45° abduction

R.

929

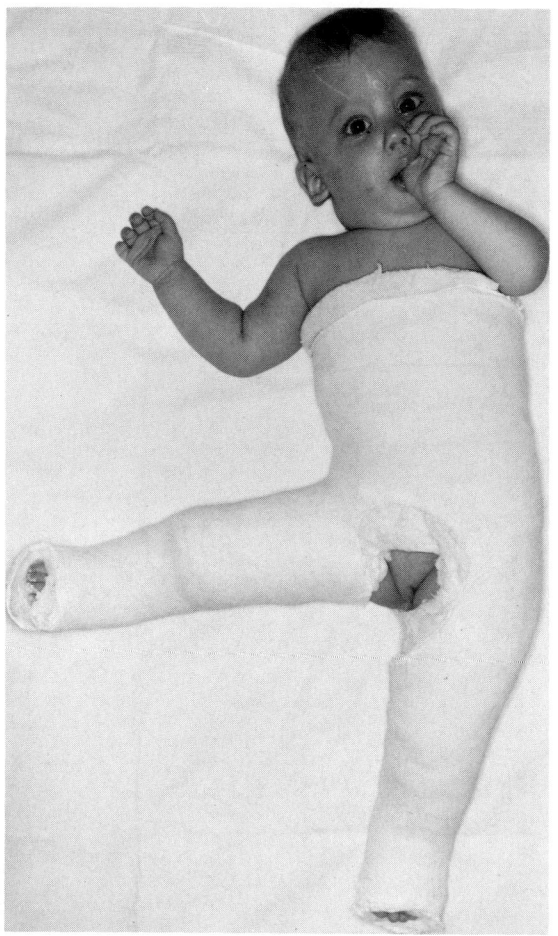

FIGURE 5–59. *An infant with lumbosacral myelomeningocele and pelvic obliquity due to unilateral contracture of the iliotibial band on the left.*

The right hip had become dislocated. The contracted iliotibial band on the left was released by the Ober-Yount procedure, and the right hip was reduced by closed manipulation. Note the position of immobilization of the hips in the hip spica cast—the left hip is in extension and neutral adduction, whereas the right hip is in wide abduction and in some flexion.

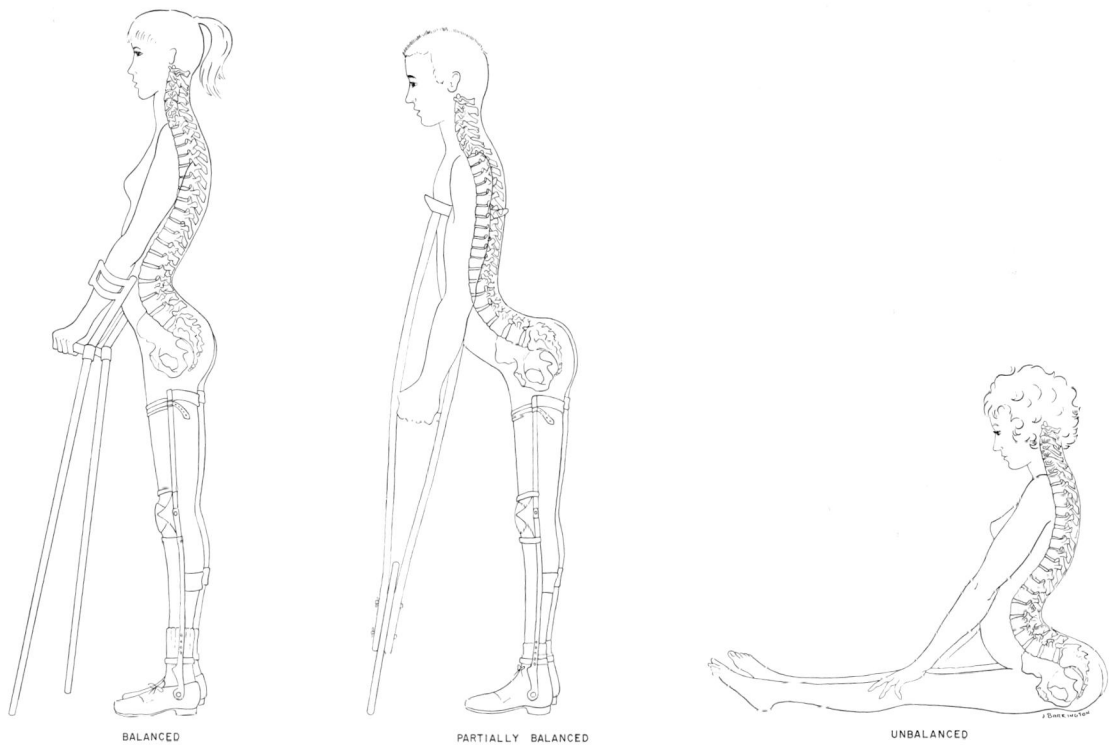

FIGURE 5-60. *Lordosis in myelomeningocele.*

A. Balanced. **B**. Partially balanced. **C**. Unbalanced. (From Kilfoyle, R. M., Foley, J. J., and Norton, P. L.: The spine and pelvic deformity in childhood paraplegia. J. Bone Joint Surg., *47-A*:661, 1965.)

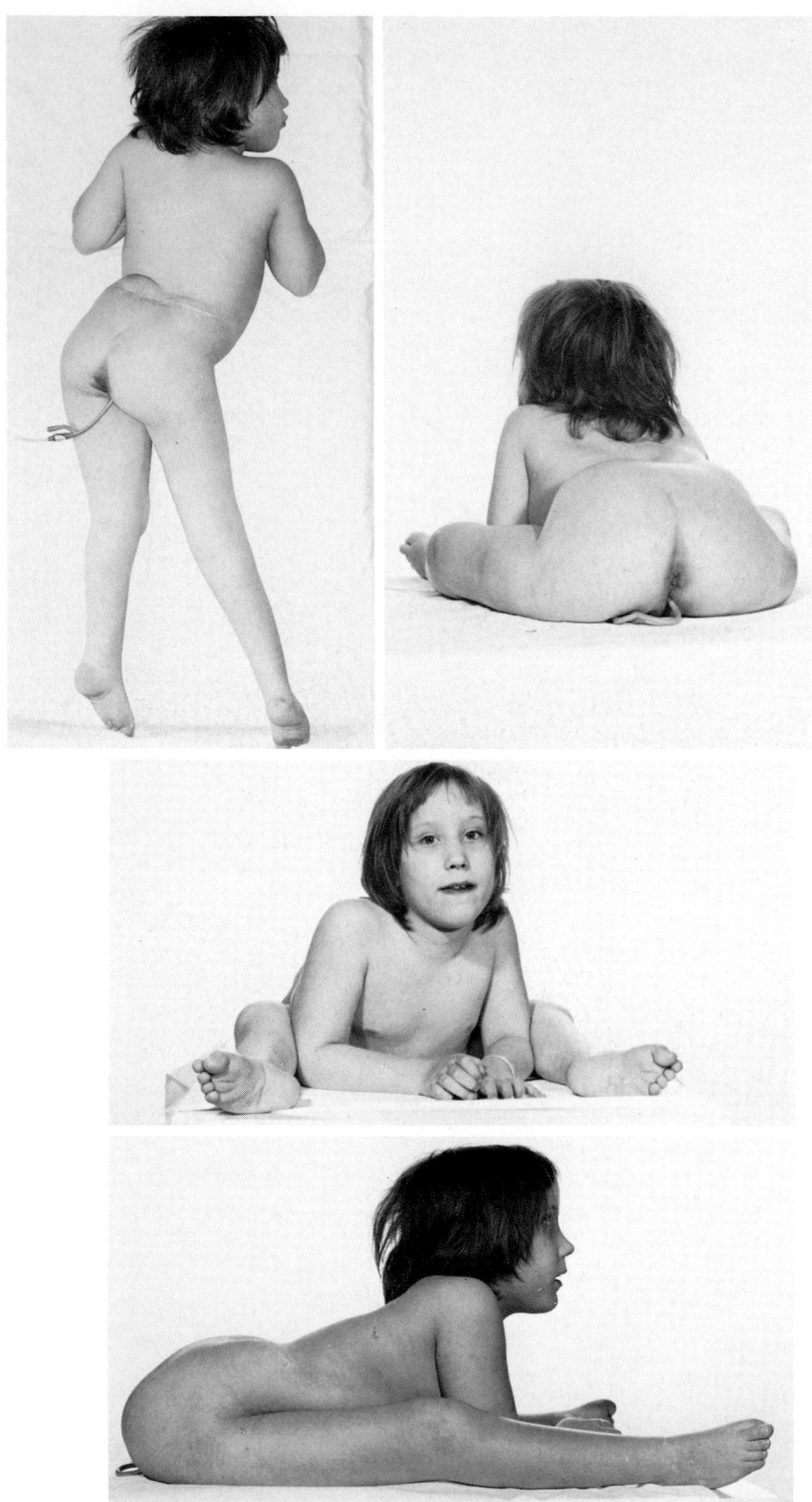

FIGURE 5–61. *A seven-year-old girl with myelomeningocele.*

Note the severe lordosis. The spine is decompensated and off-balance, making standing impossible. Sitting is assisted with support of hands.

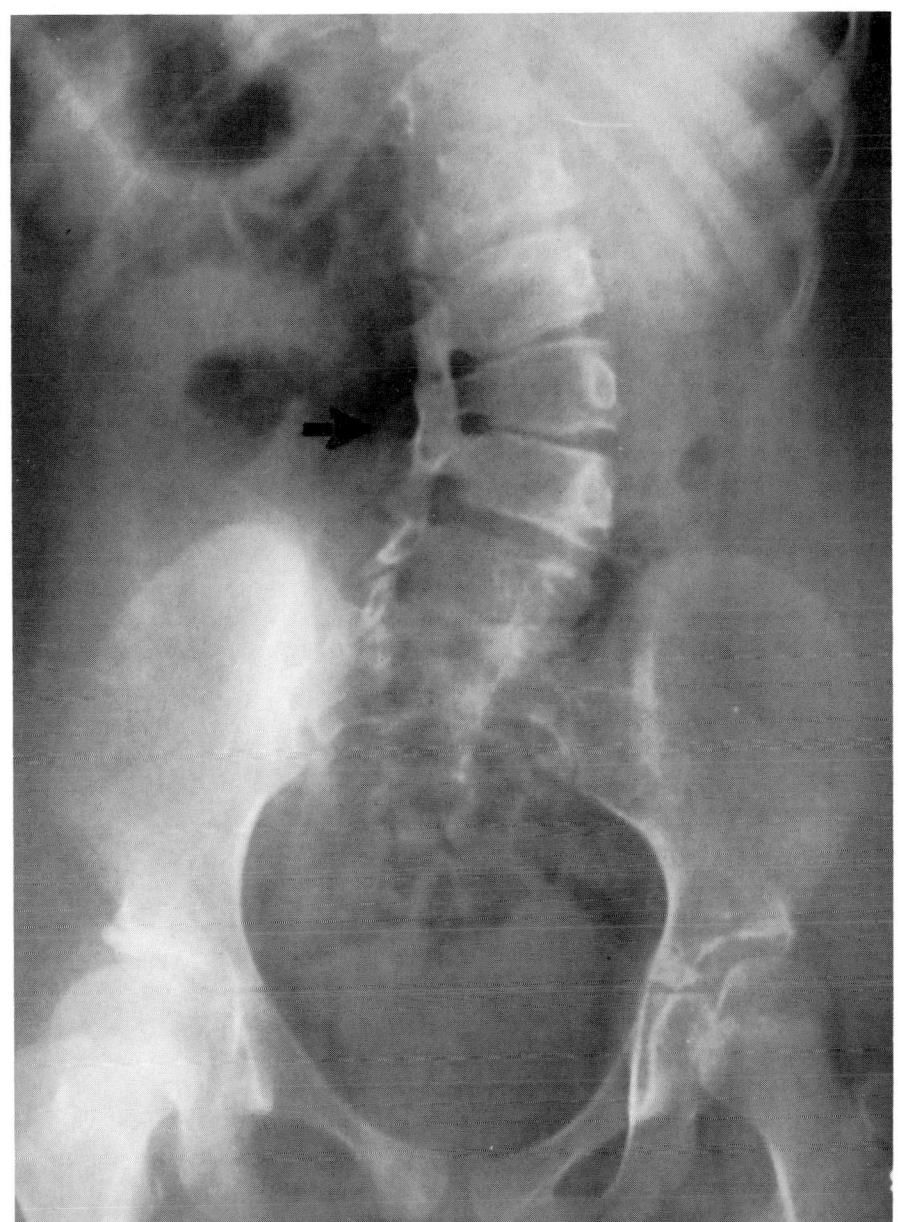

FIGURE 5–62. Congenital scoliosis in a child with myelomeningocele.

Note the unsegmented unilateral bar between the second and fourth lumbar vertebrae.

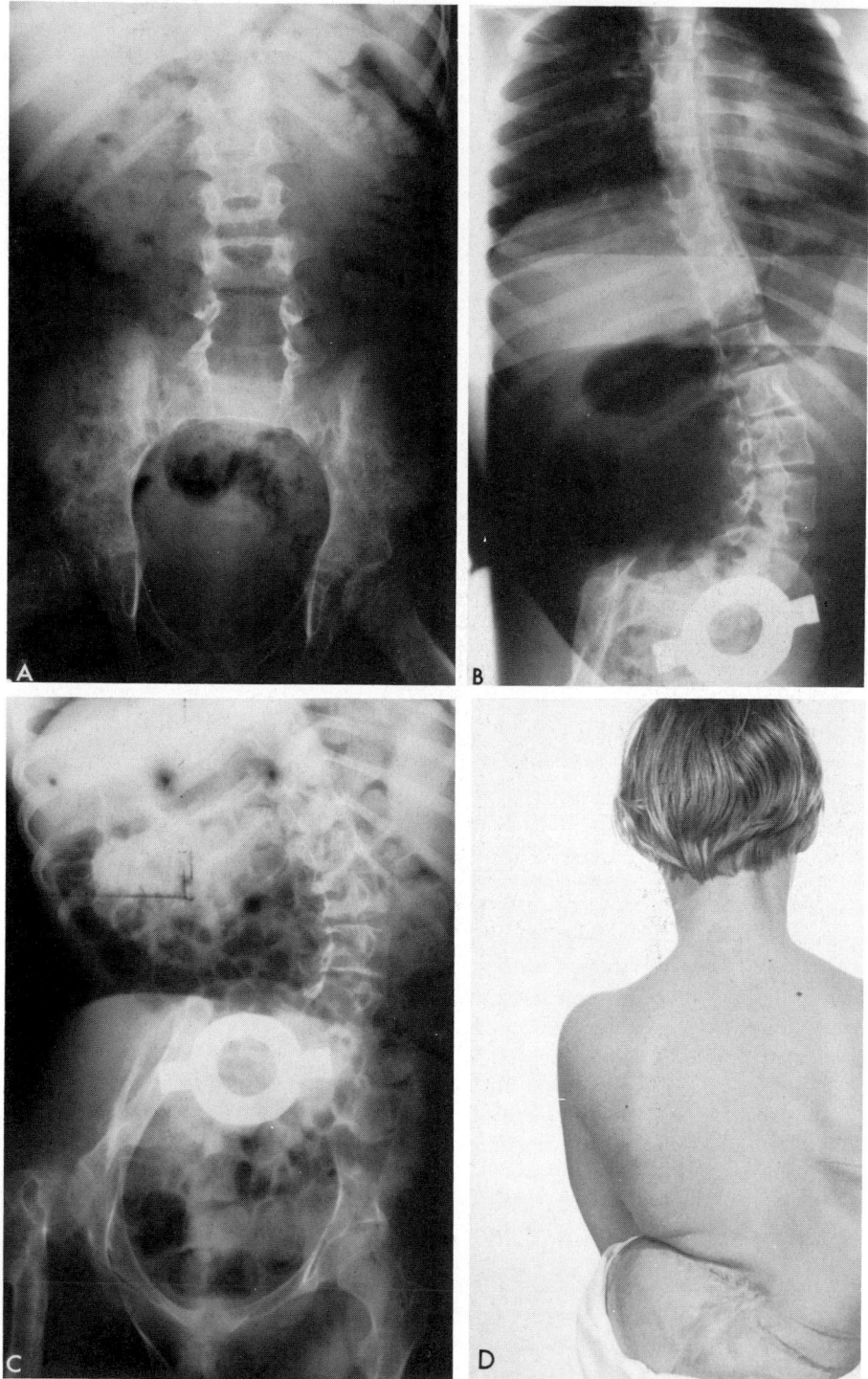

FIGURE 5-63.   *Paralytic scoliosis in a child with myelomeningocele.*

Note the progression of the scoliosis and the fixed pelvic obliquity. Roentgenograms of the spine at three years of age (**A**); (**B**) at five years of age; and (**C**) at ten years of age. **D**. Clinical appearance of patient.

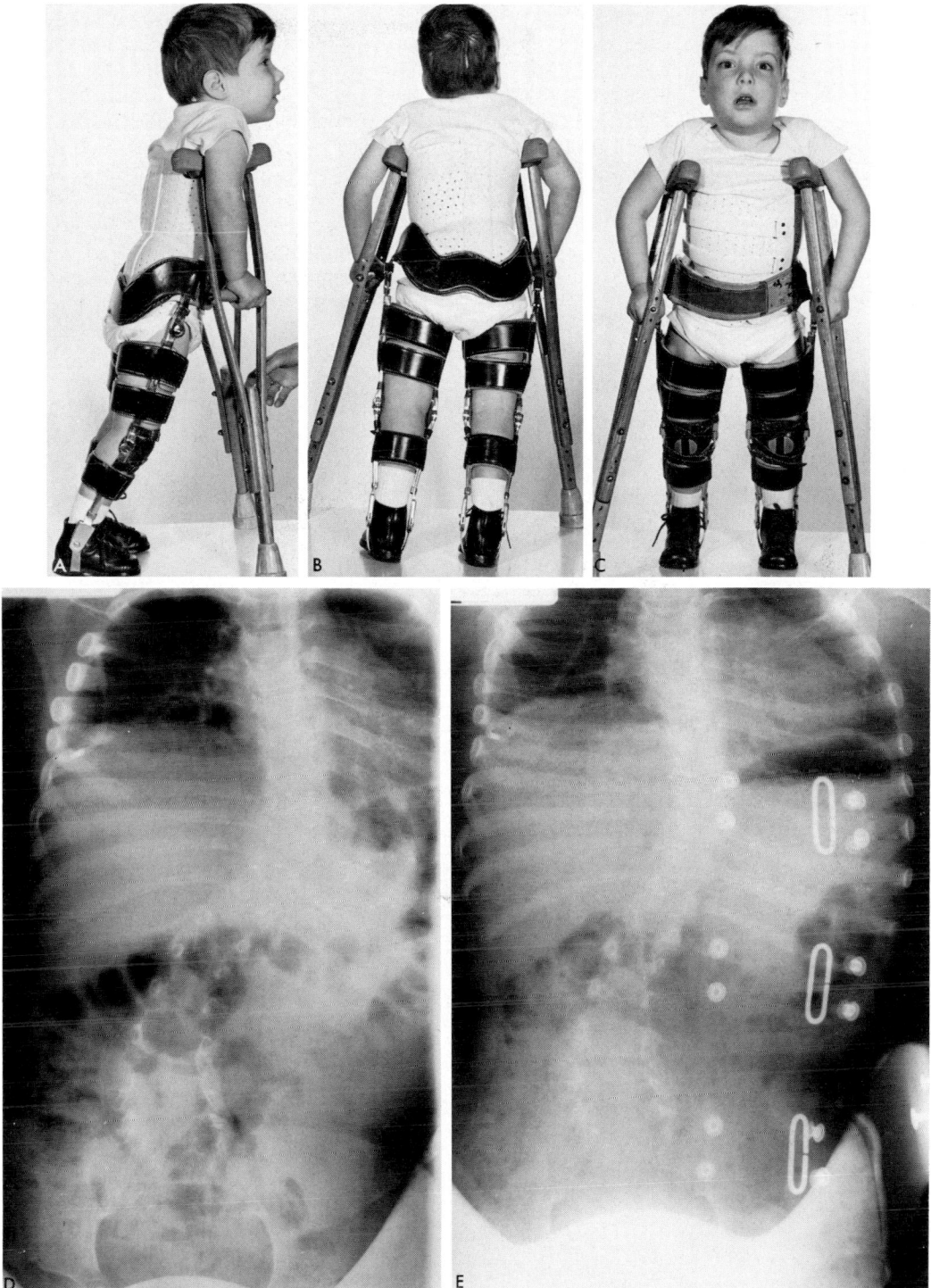

FIGURE 5 61.   *A five-year-old boy with myelomeningocele and paralytic scoliosis.*

A plastic body jacket will support the trunk effectively; however, it will not prevent progression of the scoliosis. **A** to **C.** Clinical appearance of patient with the body jacket and orthosis. **D**. Standing roentgenogram of the spine without the body jacket support. **F.** Roentgenogram with the body jacket—note balancing of the trunk.

perienced, it is recommended that this procedure be a combined neurosurgical and orthopedic one, as the engorged dural veins can often be a very troublesome source of bleeding. The entire paralyzed and scoliotic area should be fused, and the fusion should extend distally to include the sacrum. Harrington instrumentation with a sacral bar is inserted to provide secure internal fixation. The postoperative body cast should include both lower limbs.

KYPHOSIS

Kyphosis in myelomeningocele may be congenital or acquired in origin. Failure of segmentation of the vertebrae and wedge vertebrae are causes of congenital kyphosis. Mechanisms of compensation for abnormal kyphosis are the development of lordotic curves above and below the site of dorsal angulation, and hyperextension of the hip if the length of the spinal segment is not sufficient to form a lordosis. Kyphosis is *balanced* if the center of gravity of the body falls immediately anterior to the ankle joints; it is *partially balanced* when the center of gravity of the body falls behind the heels. Kyphosis is *unbalanced* when the patient is unable to stand or walk because of insufficient lordosis or hyperextension of the hip to compensate for the marked dorsal angulation of the spine (Fig. 5–65).

An entity that is uniquely found in myelomeningocele is *congenital lumbar kyphosis* in which there is rigid posterior angulation of the spine limited to the area of the osseous defect. Its incidence is reported by Hoppenfeld to be 12.5 per cent.[304] The cause of congenital lumbar kyphosis in association with myelomeningocele is unknown. Sharrard believes that in such instances the lesional defect is very wide, the erector spinae muscles are atrophic or absent, and the quadratus lumborum is displaced laterally, becoming a flexor of the lumbar spine. Thus the action of abdominal muscles is unopposed and the lumbar kyphosis develops in utero.

The kyphotic deformity is evident at birth. The pedicles in the lesional area are spread widely apart and project postero-

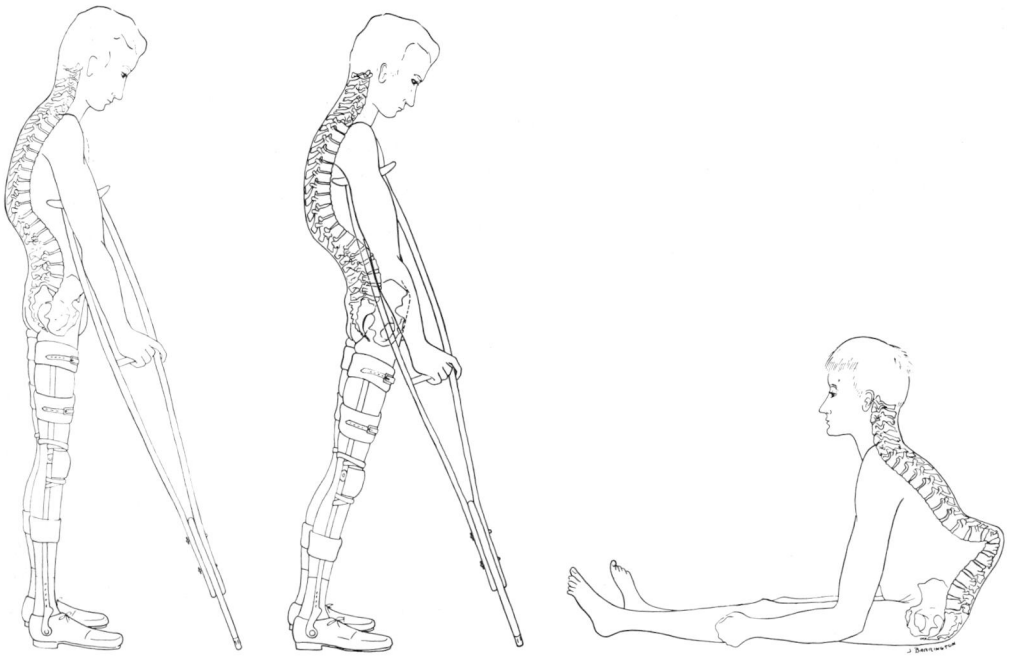

FIGURE 5–65.   Kyphosis in myelomeningocele.

A. Balanced. **B.** Partially balanced. **C.** Unbalanced. (From Kilfoyle, R. M., Foley, J. J., and Norton, P. L.: The spine and pelvic deformity in childhood paraplegia. J. Bone Joint Surg., *47–A*:668, 1965.)

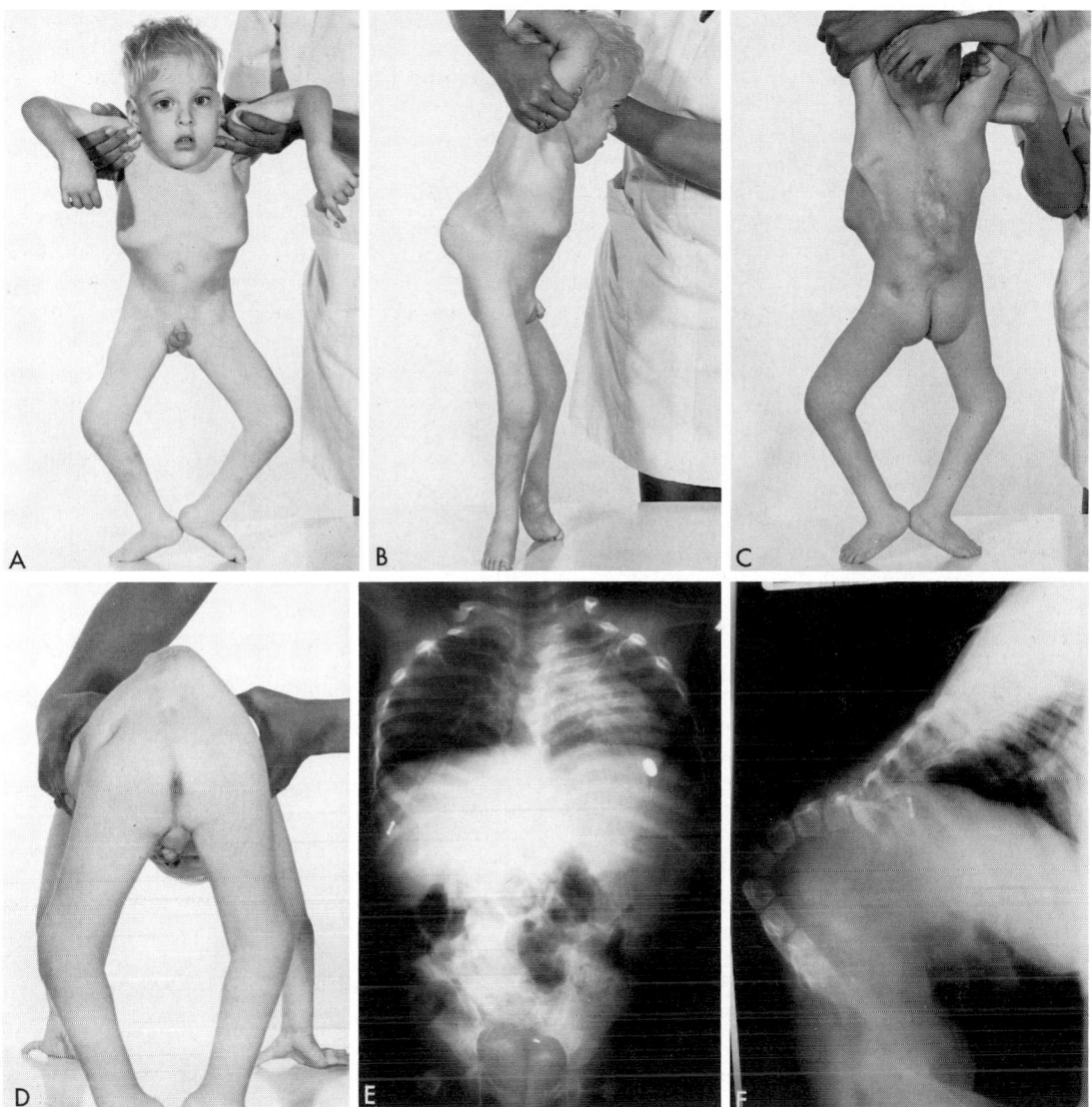

FIGURE 5–66. *Congenital lumbar kyphosis in a two-year-old child with myelomeningocele.*

A to **D**. Clinical appearance of patient. **E** and **F**. Roentgenograms of spine.

laterally, accentuating the kyphotic appearance and acting as pressure points over which the skin is blanched. The skin defect is extremely large, the open spinal cord being stretched over the kyphotic lumbar vertebrae. The pathologic anatomy has been reviewed by Hoppenfeld.[304]

The kyphos is fixed — it cannot be reduced by passive manipulation and is not altered by changing the position of the infant from supine to prone. Upon sitting and standing, the degree of kyphosis is increased by the incumbent body weight, and a compensatory thoracic lordosis develops above the kyphos. The pelvis will be markedly rotated, giving an apparent severe flexion deformity of the hips, with the plane of the lower limbs at right angles to the trunk (Fig. 5–66). This true congenital kyphosis should be distinguished from postural roundback, a condition characteristic of all infants who are placed in sitting posture. The postural kyphosis is flexible and can be corrected passively.

The deformity tends to increase with growth, and progressive neurologic deficit develops as a result of stretching of neural tissues over the kyphos. Skin necrosis and ulcers caused by pressure on the body prominences when the child is lying, sitting, or wearing an orthosis are common.

Roentgenograms demonstrate the characteristic findings. In the lesional area the spinous processes and laminae are absent and the interpedicular spaces markedly widened — these are common to all spina bifida cystica cases. In the lateral roentgenogram, the localized kyphotic deformity is easily seen. The vertebral bodies are wedged anteriorly, mostly at the apex of the curve. The intervertebral disc interspaces are usually narrowed. The pelvic inclination is markedly increased and the lower limbs seem to be elevated from their normal downward inclination to a more horizontal position (Fig. 5–66 F).

Treatment. Congenital lumbar kyphosis presents serious problems with operative closure of the extensive defect. Even with use of skin flaps and relaxing incisions, satisfactory skin closure without great tension is impossible. The skin closure breaks down, and secondary infection of the stretched neural tissues develops, causing complete paralysis of the lower limbs.

The kyphotic deformity is very rigid. Attempts at correction by traction in extension and corrective plaster casts are futile and are not tolerated by the anesthetic skin.

In the newborn, Sharrard has recommended correction of deformity by osteotomy of the spine with resection of one or more vertebral bodies at the apex of the kyphos. The vertebral bodies are removed laterally between the nerve roots to avoid injury to the large vessels running on the posterior abdominal wall and to the neural tissues (Fig. 5–67). Postoperatively, the spine is held in extension by suspension-traction with adhesive straps on the abdomen and lower limbs, with the infant lying on a small Bradford frame.

In the older child with severe fixed lumbar kyphosis and total paralysis of the lower limbs, Sharrard recommends transverse osteotomy, correction of deformity by overlapping of fragments, and internal fixation with four screws (Fig. 5–68). In the milder kyphotic deformity he recommends excision of the laterally directed prominent laminae and pedicles to prevent recurrent ulceration of the skin and to facilitate fitting of the orthosis for walking.

Orthotic Management

To stand and walk the myelomeningocele child will require the support of orthotic devices. As was stated previously, the primary purpose of orthopedic treatment is to keep these children free of deformity and to enable them to walk by one and one half years of age.

Prerequisites for orthotic support in myelomeningocele are normal control of the head and neck, good sitting balance, and functionally adequate upper limbs for the handling of crutches. The children should possess sufficient intelligence and motivation to walk, and the parents should be cooperative.

The type of orthosis used depends upon the distribution and extent of paralysis. In general, when the gluteus maximus is paralyzed, the following orthosis is prescribed: bilateral double upright above-knee orthosis with drop-lock knee and drop-lock hip, double-action ankle joint (plantar flexion and dorsiflexion assist), with a trunk extension unit attached to a butterfly pelvic band and pivoting thoracic band, and abdominal corset support (Fig. 5–69). Later on in childhood, if an ileal conduit is performed, the abdominal corset is modified with a padded opening to accommodate the conduit bag. The shoes should be high-top, open-toed, laced to the toes, and have a crepe nonskid sole. The counter of the heel should be softened. Occasionally, sheepskin padding of the heel is used to prevent pressure sores, or the shoe may be padded with felt to obliterate irregularities of the seam. A transparent heel is prescribed by some surgeons for double-checking the proper fit of the heel in the shoe.

The parents should be diligently instructed how to place the orthosis on the child. If there is limited flexion of the knee, it is imperative that one not force the knees into flexion and cause the femur to fracture.

The child is usually admitted to the hospital for extensive physical therapy and gait training. Initially he is instructed to ambu-

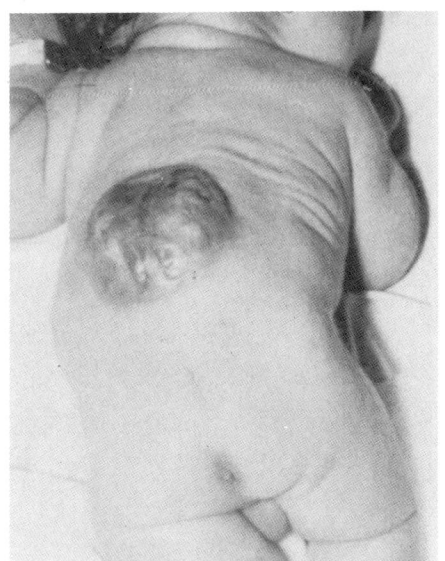
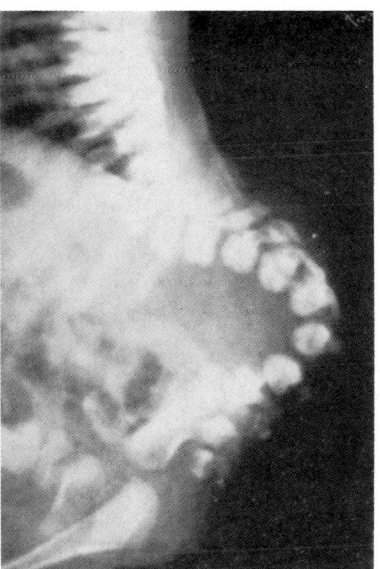

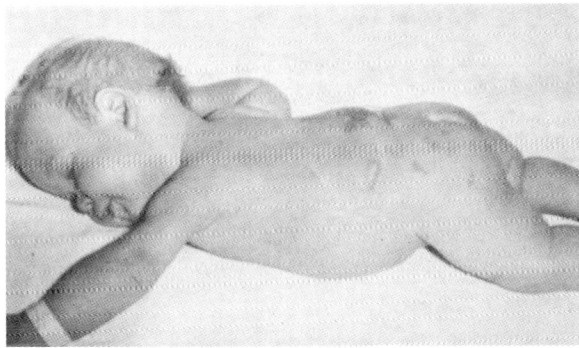

FIGURE 5-67. *Congenital kyphosis of lumbar spine in a newborn infant with myelomeningocele.*

A and **B**. Photograph of patient and lateral roentgenogram of the spine showing the deformity. The open spinal cord is stretched over the kyphotic lumbar vertebrae. **C** and **D**. Postoperative photograph and roentgenogram following neonatal osteotomy resection. Note improvement in the kyphotic deformity and the skin covering the spine. (From Sharrard, W. J. W.: Spinal osteotomy for congenital kyphosis in myelomeningocele. J. Bone Joint Surg., *50–B*:466, 469, 1968.)

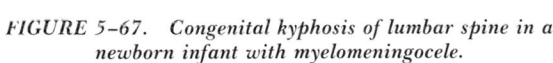

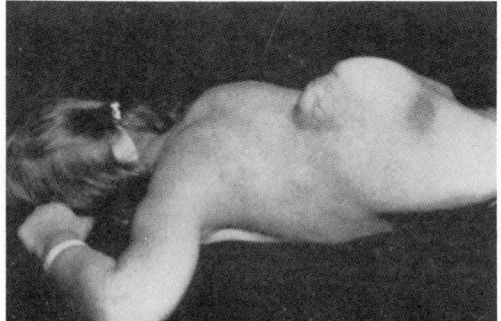

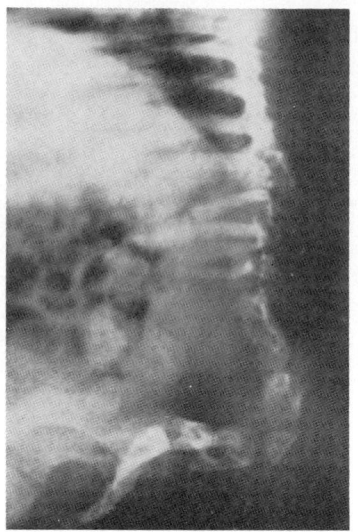

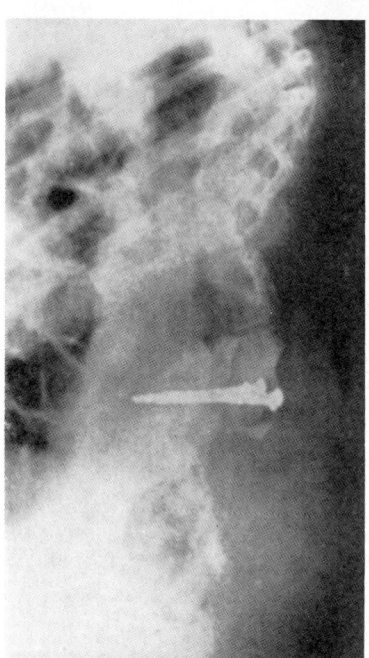

FIGURE 5–68. *A 12-year-old child with myelomeningocele and severe lumbar kyphosis.*

A. Photograph of patient showing the marked kyphos which had made it impossible to wear orthoses for ambulation. **B**. Lateral roentgenogram of the spine. The kyphotic deformity was corrected by transverse osteotomy, overlap of fragments, and internal fixation with four screws. Shortness of the anterior abdominal structures precludes wedge osteotomy. **C**. Postoperative roentgenogram showing the correction and realignment of the lower limbs, which permit fitting of orthoses for ambulation. (From Sharrard, W. J. W.: Spinal osteotomy for congenital kyphosis in myelomeningocele. J. Bone Joint Surg., *50-B:*470, 1968.)

late in parallel bars, but soon crutches are given. If the hip flexors are fair in motor strength, the patient is taught a four-point crutch gait; if the hip flexors are inactive, the gait pattern is ordinarily swing-through. The crutches should be of the regular type, not Canadian.

With growth and development the child gains balance and increases the motor strength of the upper limbs. The components of the orthosis are then removed cephalocaudally. The trunk extension unit is first discontinued and later the pelvic band. Control of rotation of the lower limbs is often a problem following removal of the pelvic band. In such an instance,

either an abdominal corset with twisters or an elastic rotational strap attached to the uppermost part of the thigh uprights is given. If both lower limbs are in external rotation, the elastic rotational strap is attached anteriorly to the lateral uprights. If both lower limbs are internally rotated, the elastic strap is anchored posteriorly.

When the quadriceps femoris, hip flexors, and hamstring muscles are fair or better in motor strength and the child is over three or four years of age, a below-knee orthosis is given for dynamic control and support of the ankle and foot. The type of ankle joint of the orthosis depends upon the motor picture: for example, when the leg is totally flail below the knee, a double-action ankle joint is given, whereas, if the toe extensors and anterior tibial are normal, but the triceps surae is paralyzed, a plantar flexion assist (reverse Klenzac) ankle joint is given. Varus and valgus straps and shoe wedges are added as indicated. Lifts to compensate for leg discrepancy are given as necessary.

Research is in progress to utilize plastic material to reduce the weight of the orthosis. A standing platform with reciprocating hip joints has been used to assist ambulation of children with free upper limbs.

Obesity will present a formidable handicap to the myelomeningocele child, as it increases the amount of effort required for physical activity. It should be avoided by strict dietary control.

Decubitus ulcers can be prevented by constant vigilance and meticulous skin care. All appliances should be adequately padded. Silicone-filled paddings are of great help.

The use of wheel chairs should be discouraged for routine activities of daily living. However, when long distances beyond the functional competence of the patient are to be traveled, a wheel chair may be used. A wheel chair is a practical necessity when the level of paralysis is at the twelfth thoracic or first lumbar neurosegmental level.

Fractures*

Spontaneous and painless fractures of the lower limbs are common in myelomeningocele, occurring in about 25 per cent of the patients. Their presence is usually discovered by the parents, the nurse, or the physical therapist, who will usually first note the increased local heat, swelling, gross deformity, and crepitation. Bruising and subcutaneous hematoma are characteristically absent. A healing fracture is occasionally found in roentgenograms taken for other reasons. It is often difficult to ascertain exactly when these fractures occur; the usual cause is injury sustained in a fall. They may also result from removal of a hip spica cast, or may occur during manipulation of the knee or hip while a heavy

patient is being turned, or may take place when the foot becomes entangled in the rails on the side of the bed.

Several underlying abnormalities and other factors are responsible for the incidence of pathologic fractures in myelomeningocele. The bone is osteoporotic, owing to muscular paralysis and disuse atrophy. Sensation is diminished or absent, with the result that these children are oblivious to the pain of trauma and do not have protective reflex mechanisms. Fixed deformities of the knee or hip increase susceptibility to undue stress on the atrophic bones during application of the orthoses or night support. The necessity for frequent and prolonged immobilization of the limbs in the cast for correction of associated deformities severely increases the already existing paralytic bone atrophy.

The femur and tibia are common sites of fractures, which are usually of the spiral or greenstick type. Epiphyseal displacement may occur. On occasion, bizarre skeletal changes may be seen in the area of the metaphysioepiphyseal junction; these include irregular, dense, slightly widened metaphyses, broadened epiphyseal plates, and subperiosteal new bone formation. These roentgenographic changes represent responses to multiple minute fractures and subsequent healing in the metaphysioepiphyseal junctions in insensitive limbs that are subjected to the stresses of weight-bearing. They should not be mistaken for osteomyelitis or a malignant bone tumor.

Neurotrophic joints usually do not develop in myelomeningocele, as weight-bearing is a prerequisite for the progressive changes of excessive bone production as well as the joint disintegration commonly seen in Charcot's joints.

Definite steps should be taken to prevent fractures. Parents, nurses, and attendant personnel should be informed of the danger of fracture and should exercise gentle care in the application of shoes, orthoses, or bivalved night casts, handling the child cautiously while performing passive exercises or while turning him, in routine bed care, and in daily activities. Stiff and rigid deformity of joints should be avoided; if present, the joints should be mobilized to functional range as a safeguard against fractures. As bone atrophy is an important

---

*See References 287, 290, 295, 319, 328.

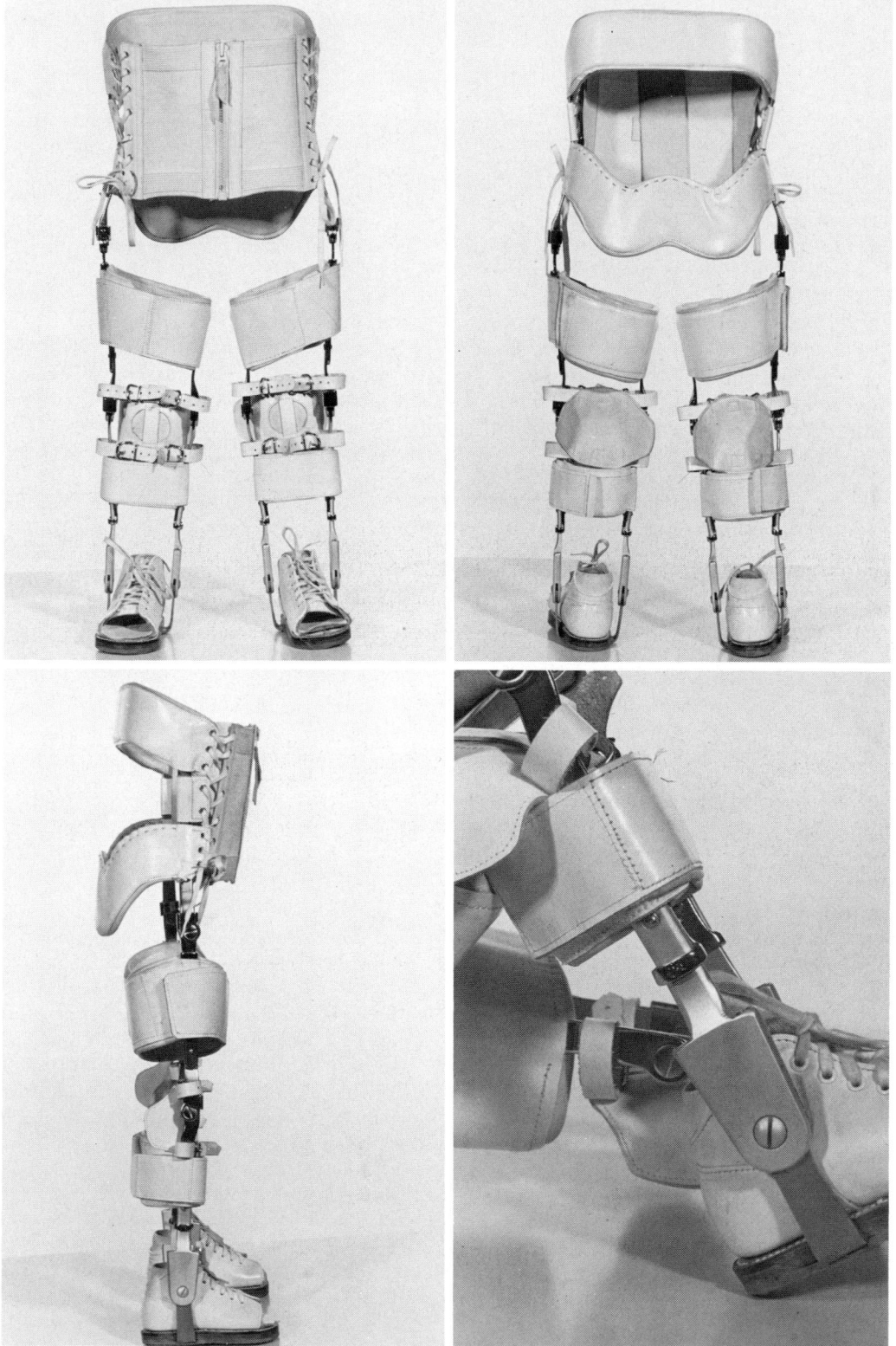

FIGURE 5–69.   *Orthosis used to support the child with myelomeningocele and assist him to walk.*

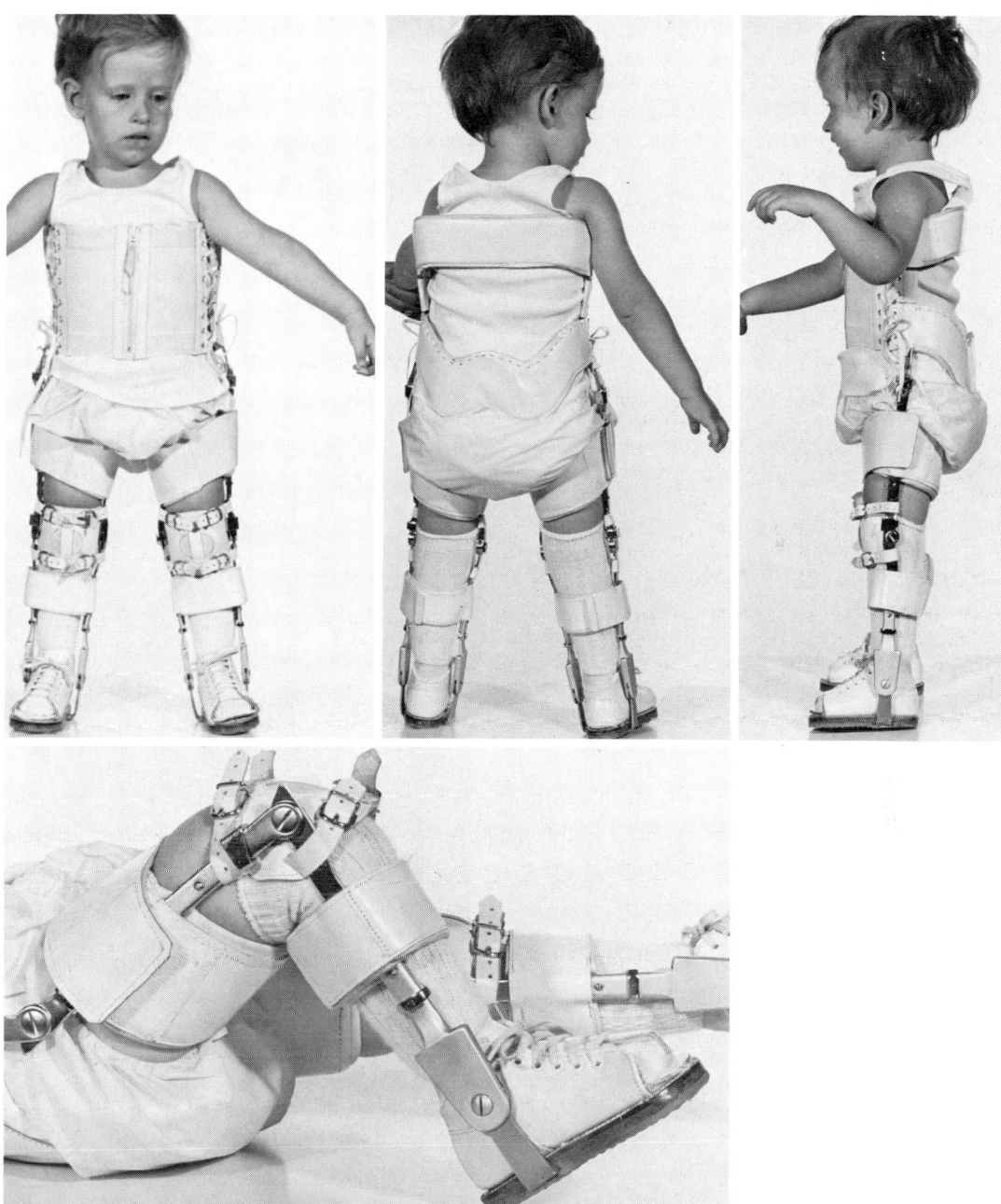

FIGURE 5–69 Continued.   Orthosis used to support the child with myelomeningocele and assist him to walk.

factor and increases susceptibility to fractures, the limbs should be immobilized as briefly as possible. A double, rather than a one and one half, hip spica cast should be applied when a hip joint is immobilized. Weight-bearing on a tilt table should be encouraged to stimulate osteogenesis.

When a fracture occurs, pre-existing deformities should be carefully assessed. If the site of the fracture is convenient and is discovered early enough, it can be utilized as an osteotomy to correct a rotational or angular deformity. For example, a supracondylar fracture of the femur is commonly associated with hyperextension contracture of the knee; in such an instance, the distal femoral fragment is tilted posteriorly to correct the genu recurvatum. With subtrochanteric fractures of the femur, the status of the hip should be analyzed; is there an indication for derotation or varization osteotomy of the proximal femur?

Fractures in myelomeningocele heal normally despite the absence of muscle tone. Ordinarily skeletal traction in femoral fractures is not tolerated. Pressure sores frequently develop, and the Kirschner wire in the osteoporotic bone will often migrate distally and cause injury to the physis. It is simpler and more effective to manipulate the fracture into the desired position and to maintain the reduction in a well-padded, snug bilateral hip spica cast. This also allows early weight-bearing with the support of the cast, minimizing disuse bone atrophy. Fractures of the tibia do not present any particular problem. Night bivalved casts or other orthotic appliances should not be used to treat these fractures, as such methods provide inadequate immobilization and frequently cause rotational and angular deformities or shortening.

POLIOMYELITIS

Poliomyelitis is an acute infectious disease caused by a group of neurotrophic viruses that initially invade the gastrointestinal and respiratory tracts and subsequently spread to the central nervous system through the hematogenous route. The poliomyelitis virus has a special affinity for the anterior horn cells of the spinal cord and for certain motor nuclei of the brain stem. These cells undergo necrosis with loss of innervation of the motor units that they supply.

The first description of paralytic poliomyelitis was given by Underwood, in 1789.[673]

Infection may be caused by Type I, II, or III poliomyelitis virus. There is no cross immunity between the various types of polio virus; thus infection may recur in the same individual.[573, 624] Polio virus is a member of the enterovirus group that includes the Coxsackie and the ECHO viruses. Paralytic disease that is clinically and pathologically indistinguishable from poliomyelitis can be produced by various other members of the enterovirus group. These viruses may be isolated on tissue culture.

In the past, poliomyelitis was an epidemic disease in the summer and fall months, with sporadic cases occurring throughout winter and spring. The development and widespread use of prophylactic vaccine has greatly reduced the incidence of poliomyelitis; however, sporadic cases still do occur and the continued rehabilitation of patients who have had the disease is still a concern of the orthopedic surgeon.[573, 625, 626, 630, 653]

This textbook deals with general principles of management of paralytic deformities of the musculoskeletal system resulting from poliomyelitis. These principles not only are applicable to treatment of poliomyelitis, but are fundamental to management of similar problems of flaccid paralysis due to other causes. For a detailed account of the disease and its medical aspects of management, the reader is referred to the voluminous literature on the subject.

Pathology

The polio virus has a definite predilection for the anterior horn cells of the spinal cord as well as for certain motor nuclei in the brain stem. The lumbar and cervical enlargements of the cord are the most commonly affected. The damaging action upon the motor neurons may be *direct*, i.e., by the toxic effects of the virus, or *indirect*, by ischemia, edema, and hemorrhage in their supportive glial tissue.[416]

The motor neurons swell and the Nissl substance in their cytoplasm undergoes chromatolysis. An inflammatory reaction ensues, with infiltration of polymorphonuclear and mononuclear cells into the gray matter, particularly in the perivascular areas. The necrotic bodies are subsequently replaced by scar tissue.

Involvement of the anterior horn cells varies from minimal injury with temporary inhibition of metabolic activity with rapid recovery to complete and irrevocable destruction.

Paralysis is of the flaccid type, with the individual motor units following the "all or none" law, because the virus affects the anterior horn cells rather than the muscle. The percentage of motor units destroyed varies, and the resultant muscle weakness is proportionate to the number of motor units that are lost; for example, a muscle with "poor" muscle strength will have 20 per cent of its motor units functioning, whereas a muscle with "good" motor strength will have 80 per cent of its motor units functioning. These remaining functional motor units are called *guiding neuromuscular units* and are of particular importance in retaining the patterns of motion of the individual muscles or muscle groups during the recovery stage. The recovery in muscle power is primarily dependent upon restitution of the anterior horn cells of the spinal cord that have been damaged but not destroyed.

Immediately following onset, it is difficult to give an accurate prognosis as to the rate and extent of spontaneous recovery. It is best to assume that the involved muscles will recover until that time when the subsequent course of the disease demonstrates otherwise. Muscle recovery is most marked in the first three to six months, with this potential ceasing at approximately 16 to 18 months after the onset.

The two primary factors to consider in the prognosis are the severity of initial paralysis and the diffuseness of its regional distribution. If total paralysis of a muscle persists beyond the second month, severe motor cell destruction is indicated, and the likelihood of any significant return of function is poor. If the initial paralysis is partial, the prognosis is better.

The condition of the neighboring muscles is another consideration. A weakened muscle surrounded by completely paralyzed muscles has less chance of recovery than a muscle of corresponding power that is surrounded by muscles that are strong. Muscle spasm, contracture of antagonist muscle groups, deformity, and inadequate early treatment are other factors that may interfere with recovery of muscle function.

The course of the disease is subdivided into the following stages:

The acute phase (lasting from five to ten days) is the period of acute illness when paralysis may occur. It is further subdivided into the *preparalytic phase* and the *paralytic phase*. The acute phase is ordinarily considered to terminate 48 hours following the return to normal temperature.

The convalescent phase encompasses the 16-month period following the acute phase; during this time a varying degree of spontaneous recovery in muscle power takes place. This phase is also further subdivided into the *sensitive phase* (lasting from two weeks to several months) characterized by hypersensitivity of muscles, which are tender and "in spasm," and the *insensitive phase*, in which the muscles are no longer sensitive but are still in the period of recovery.

The chronic or residual phase is the final stage of the disease after the recovery of muscle power has taken place. It encompasses the rest of the patient's life span following termination of the convalescent period.[566]

Treatment

The management of poliomyelitis varies with the stage of the disease and the severity and extent of paralysis.[492, 493] Treatment in the acute febrile stage is primarily the domain of the pediatrician or internist, with the patients being admitted to the services in infectious disease hospitals or isolation units of general hospitals. Care of the musculoskeletal system, however, is important from the first day of the disease. It is imperative that the orthopedic surgeon be called in consultation to examine a suspected case prior to performance of lumbar puncture. He should be responsible for all orders concerning the management of the musculoskeletal system. The pediatrician is responsible for general care of the patient, especially any problems of respiratory and bulbar involvement, should they develop. Once the patient has been afebrile for 48 hours (i.e., termination of the acute stage), he should be transferred to the service of the orthopedic surgeon, who assumes the dominant role. Such delineation and continuity of supervision is mandatory, as it stimulates early attention to deforming tendencies and prevents their development.

ACUTE PHASE.

During this initial febrile phase of the disease, the primary concern of the orthopedic surgeon is the comfort of the patient and prevention of deformity. It is best to place the patient at complete bed rest and restrict his physical activities to a minimum. The patient is irritable and apprehensive. It is important to reassure him and allay his fears.

General medical measures consist of administration of a varied diet with a relatively high fluid intake, attention to urinary retention and bladder paralysis, prevention of constipation and fecal impaction, and analgesia for pain. Opiates and other medications that have a depressing action on the central nervous system should not be given in the presence of impending paralysis of the muscles of respiration.

A detailed determination of the severity and extent of muscle paralysis is not warranted during this febrile period. By gentle handling of the limbs and trunk, however, an approximate assessment of the degree and distribution of motor weakness can be made without much distress to the patient. This initial muscle examination has its diagnostic and therapeutic implications. It will also provide the necessary information to prevent the development of potential deformities consequent to paralysis.

Ordinarily, paralysis develops two or three days after onset of fever and increases in severity for several days. Progressive involvement will cease only after return of elevated temperature to normal. Characteristically paralysis in poliomyelitis is asymmetrical. In the presence of symmetrical paralysis of the limbs and trunk, a paralytic disease other than poliomyelitis should be considered. In a large epidemic the care of patients will be much simplified if those with paralysis are separated from those without paralysis.

Patients with bulbar and respiratory involvement require specialized intensive care. An early appraisal of the distribution and extent of paralysis will help to detect muscle weakness in certain areas, which should alert the clinician to the possible development of such distressing complications. For example, a patient who cannot lift his head because of paralysis of anterior neck muscles or one who has a nasal intonation to his voice, difficulty in swallowing, and weakness of facial muscles should be watched carefully for bulbar involvement. Prompt diagnosis and treatment is essential to keep the patient's airways open, since the condition may be fatal. Aspiration of unswallowed secretions is a definite danger. The foot of the bed is elevated and the patient is placed in prone or lateral position. Frequent suction or postural drainage is usually required. Occasionally tracheostomy may be necessary.

Another anatomic area that should be observed for muscle weakness is the shoulder girdle. The nerve supply of the deltoid muscle is the fifth cervical root, which is adjacent to the fourth cervical root innervating the diaphragm. Consequently, progressive paralysis of the deltoid muscle is usually followed by paralysis of the intercostal muscles and the diaphragm. Is there an increased rate of breathing? Is the patient using accessory muscles of respiration? Is he restless, anxious, and disoriented? These are signs that should alert the physician to the possible need for a mechanical respirator. Paralysis of the diaphragm is easily detected on fluoroscopy. Abdominal muscle weakness is determined by asking the patient to lift his head and shoulder or the lower limbs. Asymmetry of power is shown by the Beevor's sign, which is the shift of the umbilicus toward the stronger muscles.

The patient should be positioned to provide correct anatomic alignment of the limbs and proper posture of the trunk. The aim is to prevent development of deformities. The bed should give adequate support and should not sag. A firm foam rubber mattress is preferable. Bedboards should be placed beneath the mattress and should be hinged to permit sitting in the later convalescent period. A padded footboard is used to maintain the ankles and feet in neutral position when the patient is lying supine or prone. By pulling the end of the mattress away from the footboard about 10 cm., an interspace is provided in which the heels are allowed to fall. Periods in the supine position should be alternated with periods of prone posture, the latter position being important for maintenance of good muscle tone of the gluteus maximus and erector spinae muscles.

When the patient is lying on his back, the knees should be held in slight flexion with padded rolls under them and behind the proximal ends of the tibiae in order to prevent genu recurvatum and posterior subluxation of the tibiae. A slightly flexed position of the knees will relax the sensitive hamstrings. Excessive flexion of the knees, however, should be avoided. Sandbags or rolled pads are placed on the lateral sides of the thighs and legs to prevent external rotation deformity of the lower limbs. Intermittent use of rolls between the scapulae will prevent hunching forward of the shoulders.

The limbs should not be maintained in rigidly fixed positions. Several times a day, the joints are carried passively through their range of motion; this will help to relieve muscle pain. Overstretching of muscles, however, should be avoided. The patient should be handled as gently as possible. Passive motion of the joints of a limb is imperative to prevent stiffness and myostatic contractures. At times, when there is severe spasm of the hip flexors, hamstrings, and gastrocnemius, the sensitivity and pain of muscles will be so great that anatomic alignment cannot be assumed without excessive discomfort.

Muscle Spasm. A principal manifestation of poliomyelitis in its early stages—the so-called muscle spasm—is characterized by protective contraction of the muscles to prevent a potentially painful movement. Muscle resistance to stretch is more descriptive of this reflex guarding action of the muscles, which resembles the muscle spasm associated with painful phenomena such as hamstring spasm in synovitis of the knee. True spasticity and signs of upper motor neuron involvement are absent. The exact cause of muscle pain and sensitivity is unknown. Most probably it is due to inflammatory changes in the posterior ganglia and meninges. Other possible causes are lesions in the reticular substance and lesions of the internuncial neurons in which inhibitory fibers to the anterior horn cells are affected.

The degree of muscle pain and sensitivity varies considerably. Some muscle discomfort is usually present in the preparalytic period. Nerve traction tests, such as those of Lasègue and Kernig, increase "muscle spasm" and pain. Spontaneous severe pain is rare, though it is occasionally seen in the adult patient. The important consideration is that the painful strong muscles tend to shorten during the sensitive phase; if they are maintained in their shortened position, myostatic contracture and fixed deformity will develop.

Moist Heat. In the acute and sensitive phase of convalescence, moist heat will serve to relieve sensitivity of the muscles and alleviate discomfort. Physiologically, heat will increase the local temperature and increase blood flow to the muscle. It has no specific therapeutic effect on the course of the paralysis and actual recovery of the involved nerve cells. Heat is more beneficial if applied for intermittent short periods.

In the acute phase, in order to minimize handling of the patient, a "lay-on wool pack" consisting of three layers, one of wool blanket material (wrung out of boiling water by passing it twice through a wringer), and one of waterproof material that, in turn, is covered by an outer layer of wool blanket. The number and duration of the use of these packs is individualized, depending upon the intensity of pain and spasm. In general, two moist heat packs are applied during a 20-minute period. Continuous and overzealous use of heat should be avoided, as it can be tiring and harmful to the patient. It is best used prior to physiotherapeutic measures in order to assist in developing greater range of joint motion and to facilitate the performance of active exercises. Warm tub baths are substituted for the "lay-on packs" within a few days after the patient's temperature has returned to normal and when his general condition permits. The buoyant effect of the water makes execution of motion in the weakened muscles easier. Active exercises in water should be closely supervised so that the patient does not substitute stronger muscles for the weaker ones. Again, the patient's comfort is the primary consideration. The temperature of the tub baths should be about 100° F., and the total period of immersion in the tub should not exceed 20 minutes. In cases with extensive paralysis, overhead cranes may be used to lower the patient directly into the tub from the stretcher.

CONVALESCENT PHASE

The objectives of treatment during the convalescent stage are: (1) the attainment of maximum recovery in individual muscles; (2) the restoration and maintenance of a normal range of joint motion; (3) the prevention of deformities and their correction if they occur; and (4) the achievement of as good a physiologic status of the neuromusculoskeletal system as is possible.[492]

In the early part of the convalescent stage, because muscle sensitivity and "spasm" are still present, the use of hot packs is continued for the comfort of the patient. Passive exercises are performed four to six times a day to prevent development of contractural deformity. When there is limitation of joint motion, gentle passive stretching exercises are added to the therapy program. This exercise regimen should not cause the patient discomfort; however, the threshold of pain may be very low in an apprehensive sensitive person. A firm but sympathetic attitude by the therapist is important, and the patient should be encouraged more each time to gain a greater degree of motion. Tendencies toward deformity should be observed, such as external rotation and abduction of the hips, plantar flexion of the feet, or adduction of the shoulders. Passive stretching exercises should be directed toward preventing and correcting deformity.

Several days after the onset of the convalescent stage, a complete muscle examination should be performed. Ordinarily it is done in stages in order not to fatigue or disturb the patient. This initial motor assessment provides a basis for comparison with subsequent examinations, and it also serves as a guide to the therapy regimen that is to be instituted. The rate and extent of muscle recovery is determined by repeating these muscle tests periodically, i.e., monthly during the first four months, bimonthly during the following eight months, and then quarterly during the second year of the disease. The prognostic value of the serial muscle tests is evident; when a muscle exhibits little or no improvement in power during a three-month period, it is unlikely that it will recover or gain strength of functional significance. In this case, the patient should be fitted with appropriate orthotic support and allowed greater activity. On the other hand, a muscle that shows steady improvement has a good possibility of recovery to a functional level; hence, it is unwise to apply an above-knee orthosis on this patient's weak limb and permit him to walk.

In the management of the convalescent stage of poliomyelitis, the following principles of neuromuscular function must be considered.[492]

Patterns of Motor Activity. Motions of a limb are complex and are not the result of isolated contraction of a single muscle. The functions of many muscles are integrated and coordinated in execution of a motion and are controlled by the automatic reflexes of the central nervous system. In dorsiflexion of the ankle, for example, the anterior tibial muscle, toe extensors, and the peroneus tertius are the prime movers that execute the desired movement, whereas the triceps surae and the toe flexors are the antagonist muscles that become relaxed because of the reciprocal innervation of the agonist and antagonist muscles. The synergist and fixation muscles also contract while the prime mover acts.

In the presence of muscle weakness, the tendency is to use a strong group of muscles that can perform the action more easily and readily, thus excluding the weaker muscles from the pattern of motor activity. A muscle that has been temporarily paralyzed will be left out of the pattern of motion permanently if other muscles substitute for its action during the period of its recovery. In the convalescent stage, these muscular substitutions and abnormal patterns of motor activity should be avoided.

Some neuromuscular units often remain

intact in the paralyzed muscles; these act as "guiding contractile units," and in performance of active exercises, these functioning neuromuscular units should be utilized to guide the part in execution of normal motion.

For example, in re-education of a poor anterior tibial muscle, the ankle joint is first passively dorsiflexed through its full arc of motion, stretching any contracture of the triceps surae muscle that is present. The limb is then placed in a side-lying position to eliminate force of gravity, and the ankle joint is again passively dorsiflexed in some inversion through its full range, assisting the patient to localize the action of the anterior tibial muscle and emphasizing that substitution by the toe extensors and peroneus tertius muscle be avoided.

Next the patient is asked to produce an active, sustained contraction of the anterior tibial throughout its full arc of motion, first with and then without assistance. As the muscle becomes stronger, the limb is placed in supine position to make the muscle work against gravity and gradually increasing manual resistance is applied. The active exercises are graduated on the basis of performance. Muscles that are overworked will lose strength.

In poliomyelitis, reciprocal innervation between agonist and antagonist muscles is often disturbed, with resultant loss of synergistic muscular action and normal pattern of motor activity.

Fatigue. A paralyzed muscle is easily fatigued. This is readily shown by its rapid loss of power and its inability to function following several effective contractions. Forcing such a weak muscle beyond its point of maximal action does not increase its strength; on the contrary, it will inhibit the recovery of the paralytic muscle. It is important to observe the level of functional activity of a weak muscle so that it is not forced to exceed its capability.

Contractural Deformity and Progressive Loss of Function. Flaccid paralysis is the chief cause of functional loss. Muscular action is also inhibited by pain, sensitivity, and "spasm." When a muscle is maintained in a shortened position for a prolonged period, it will develop myostatic contracture. Muscle imbalance and increased stress due to abnormal patterns of activity are other factors producing deformity. Growth is an important consideration in the management of poliomyelitis in children. The contour of bony structures is influenced by paralysis and dynamic muscle imbalance. For example, when the triceps surae muscle is weak, and the ankle dorsiflexors are of normal motor strength, progressive calcaneus deformity of the hindfoot will result. If the child is permitted to walk without support and protection, the loss of power of the triceps surae muscle will be greater, as it is working against gravity. Figure 5–70 presents the "vicious circle" of factors that cause progressive loss of function in poliomyelitis.

In the *asensitive stage*, proper alignment of the limbs and full range of joint motion must be restored and maintained. Passive stretching exercises are performed vigorously. In the presence of muscle imbalance and when there is a tendency to develop contracture, bivalved casts should be used at night to maintain the part in correct position. When a deformity is fixed, wedging casts or traction may be applied.

Active exercises are performed to integrate recovering motor units into the normal pattern of motion; their primary objective

FIGURE 5–70. *Diagram showing the principal factors concerned with progressive loss of function in the residual stage of poliomyelitis.*

(From Green, W. T., and Grice, D. S.: The management of chronic poliomyelitis. American Academy of Orthopedic Surgeons Instructional Course Lectures. Vol. 9, p. 86. Ann Arbor, Mich., J. W. Edwards, 1952.)

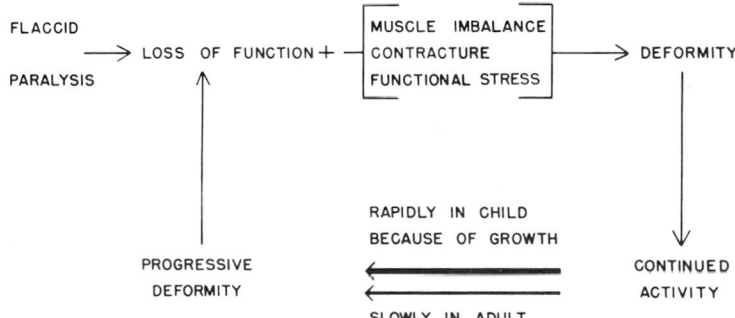

is not to produce hypertrophy of muscles that are already functioning normally. Hydrotherapy and active exercises in a pool are utilized for patients with extensive paralysis. Motion of the hips, shoulders, and trunk is greatly facilitated in the pool, as the buoyant effect of the water facilitates the coordinated motion of the parts. Strict supervision by the therapist is mandatory, however, to prevent substitution of strong muscles for those that are weak. Excessive exercises and overwork should be avoided. Patients with extensive paralysis are initially instructed to ambulate in the pool; when there is adequate control of the trunk and lower limbs, this is no longer necessary. Standing balance should be developed first and then walking with the help of crutches. The gait pattern should be reciprocal four-point gait, the amount of body weight borne depending upon the degree of paralysis. The physical therapist assists in locomotion, so that abnormal mechanisms shall not develop. During the convalescent period, use of an orthosis should be restricted to a minimum, as it increases the work load on the paralytic levels and tends to produce abnormal gait patterns. In severe paralysis of the lower limbs and trunk, however, locomotion may be impossible without the support of an adequate orthosis. General activities of the patient are gradually increased. During the first few minutes of locomotion the gait may be very effective, but with fatigue it may become very poor. Random, purposeless activity should be discouraged.

CHRONIC PHASE

The purposes of treatment in the residual stage are to enable the patient to attain maximal function and to obtain the greatest amount of productive activity in spite of residual weakness.[493] With continued growth and use of the limb, progressive deformities may develop, which will ultimately cause loss of function. Hence, an equally important task during the chronic stage is to prevent deformities, and to correct them, should they develop. The residual stage is a dynamic, not a static, period. Much can be done to improve the functional capacity of the patient. Aspects of treatment are discussed under the headings of Physical Ther-

apy, Orthoses and Apparatus, and Surgery.

Physical Therapy. In the residual stage the physical therapy regimen is directed toward (1) prevention or correction of deformity by passive stretching exercises; (2) increase of motor strength of muscles by active or hypertrophy exercises; (3) achievement of maximum functional activity.[561]

ACTIVE HYPERTROPHY EXERCISES. It is obvious there is little to be gained by exercising zero or trace muscles that remain so after 18 months, and the same is true of muscles that have a good or normal rating. Active hypertrophy exercises are performed primarily for the benefit of marginal muscles to elevate or maintain their functional level. For example, when the anterior tibial and toe extensor muscles are fair in motor strength and the triceps surae muscles are normal, it is important that active exercises of the ankle dorsiflexors be performed to maintain them at the antigravity functional level. The calf muscles should also be passively stretched to prevent the development of equinus deformity; this is implemented by the use of a night bivalved cast, which holds the foot out of equinus and in neutral position. Progressive resistance exercises utilize activity graded in proportion to the strength of the involved muscles; their use is recommended in the residual stage of poliomyelitis to increase the strength and improve the endurance of such individual muscles or groups of muscles as a fair quadriceps or triceps surae or a fair plus hip abductor muscle to the maximum capacity. Whether progressive resistive exercises are of any permanent value when the motor strength of a muscle is less than fair minus is doubtful; a poor quadriceps muscle cannot, by hypertrophy exercises, be improved to fair strength so that it can lift the leg against gravity. Correction of flexion deformity of the knee, however, may provide added strength by eliminating the need for the quadriceps muscle to work against deformity.

PASSIVE STRETCHING EXERCISES. Prevention of contractural deformity is much simpler than its correction. When a limb is continuously maintained in one position, contracture and fixed deformity will develop as a result of the effects of gravity and dynamic imbalance of muscles. An ankle joint held in plantar flexion because of weak dorsiflexors and strong triceps surae will develop progressive equinus deformity if the ankle is not passively stretched into dorsiflexion every day. Passive stretching exercises should be performed gently, several times a day. In the presence of muscle imbalance, however, they are not adequate to prevent deformity and other measures should be employed, such as the use of a removable bivalved long leg night cast, which holds the foot in neutral position, and the wearing of a below-knee dorsiflexion assist spring orthosis during the day. Later, during the chronic stage, muscle balance may be restored by transfer of muscles.

FUNCTIONAL TRAINING. The purpose of such a therapy program is to enable the patient to overcome the handicaps imposed by his physical disability. The residual deficit in function varies, depending upon the extent and severity of paralysis. The needs of a growing child progressively change. In the residual stage the patient is taught how to use all the available muscles in order to accomplish a task successfully. This is in contrast to the convalescent stage, when he is not allowed to substitute stronger muscles for weaker ones. For example, when the anterior tibial is poor in motor strength in the convalescent stage, the child is not permitted to use his toe extensors to dorsiflex the foot when active exercises are performed with the anterior tibial. In the chronic stage, when anterior tibial function is still poor, he is taught how to dorsiflex his foot by using his toe extensors and peroneal muscles.

At times, the activity of stronger muscles is suppressed in order to prevent the development of deformity. For example, an individual with normal sartorius, biceps femoris, and peroneal muscles, but poor iliopsoas, medial hamstring, and anterior tibial muscles will walk with marked external rotation deformity of the foot and leg. It is important to supervise his gait, teaching him to suppress the eversion power of the peroneals and the externally rotating power of the biceps femoris and the sartorius to prevent development of external rotation deformity of the lower limb.

To teach a child merely to walk with crutches and orthoses is not satisfactory. He should be instructed in activities of daily living, such as how to get in and out of chairs, to open doors, and to enter an automobile.

Orthoses and Other Apparatus. Use of an apparatus may be necessary during the asensitive period of the convalescent and residual stages of poliomyelitis. The primary purposes of the orthosis are: (1) to support the patient, enabling him to walk and increasing his functional activity; (2) to protect a weak muscle from overstretching; (3) to augment the action of weak muscles or to substitute for those completely lost; (4) to prevent deformity and malposition; and (5) to correct deformity by stretching certain groups of muscles that have been contracted.

The elements of support, substitution, and correction may be combined in a single apparatus. In general, dynamic splinting is more desirable than static splinting. For example, when the toe extensor and anterior tibial muscles are paralyzed and the triceps surae muscle is normal, a dorsiflexion assist spring orthosis (which acts as an active substitute for the weak ankle dorsiflexors) is preferable to a below-knee caliper orthosis with a posterior stop that prevents plantar flexion of the ankle beyond neutral position. In paralysis of the gastrocnemius and soleus muscles, a plantar flexion assist spring below-knee orthosis with a dorsiflexion stop at neutral position is prescribed (Fig. 5–71). In the presence of a flail ankle and foot, a double-action ankle joint (both plantar flexion and dorsiflexion assist) is given, and a varus or valgus T-strap added to the shoe, as necessary. Also, inside or outside wedges to the shoe are given, depending upon the deformity of the foot (see Chapter 7).

When the muscles controlling the knee are paralyzed, an above-knee orthosis with a drop-lock knee joint is prescribed. This type of orthosis will provide knee stability for walking and can be unlocked during sitting. If genu recurvatum results from paralysis of the triceps surae in the presence of some strength of the quadriceps femoris, it can be controlled by an above-knee orthosis with a free knee joint so constructed as to prevent complete extension of the orthosis at the knee. Proper positioning of the thigh and calf bands will also check genu recurvatum. Genu varum or knock-knee pads are added as necessary.

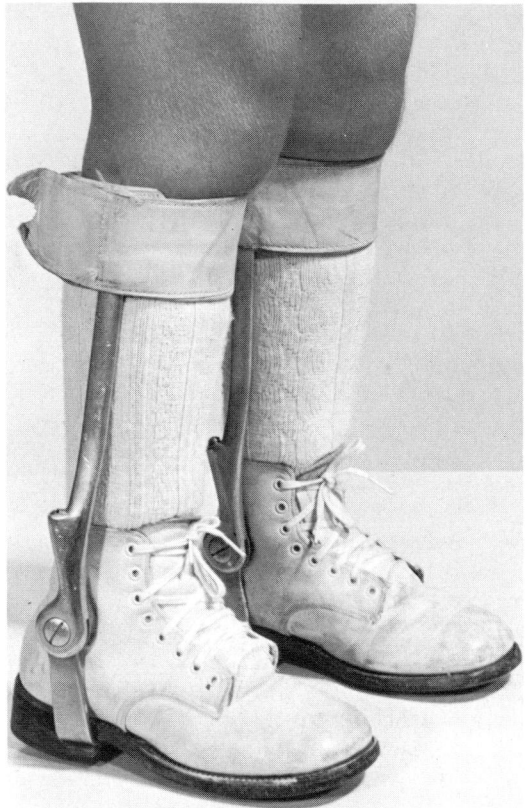

FIGURE 5–71. *Plantar flexion assist below-knee orthosis with a dorsiflexion stop at neutral position.*

When flexion deformity of the knee is present as a result of dynamic imbalance between the hamstrings and quadriceps femoris muscles, a well-padded anterior knee pad is given. An Engen extension knee orthosis is worn at night to correct flexion deformity of the knee.

When the muscles controlling the hip are weak, stability of the hip joint can be provided by an ischial weight-bearing thigh socket; crutches are used if necessary. Rotational alignment of the lower limbs is obtained by the addition of rotation straps or twisters. Ordinarily the patient does walk better without a pelvic band and drop-lock hips; however, in a young child with gluteus maximus paralysis, they may be used temporarily for balance. Often the spine will also require support. Upon resumption of upright posture, the abdominal muscles will overstretch, and severe lumbar lordosis and paralytic scoliosis will develop. Any asymmetrical involvement of the abdominal and trunk musculature should always be care-

fully noted. An abdominal corset support with metal stays often serves to control abdominal muscle paralysis. In the presence of weakness of the trunk extensors, a spinal orthosis with an abdominal corset is given. If the spine is unstable and collapsing, it may be supported by a molded plastic body jacket constructed from a plaster of Paris cast made with the patient standing with traction from a head sling. In paralytic scoliosis, usually a Milwaukee brace is worn, provided that the paralysis of the lower limbs is not very extensive and that the wearing of such an appliance does not prevent ambulation. In such instances, the Milwaukee brace is used intermittently during periods of recumbency or sitting, or both.

In the upper limb, the paralyzed shoulder muscles, particularly the deltoid, are best protected from the effects of gravity with a sling; this allows functional use of the forearm and hand. During the initial period of six to eight weeks, an abduction shoulder splint may be worn at night and during part of the day to prevent overstretching of the deltoid muscle; this is particularly indicated when there is associated paralytic subluxation or dislocation of the shoulder joint. A cock-up wrist splint is given when the wrist extensors are paralyzed, and an opponens splint when there is weakness of the opponens of the thumb. When there is paralysis of the intrinsic muscles of the hand, hyperextension of the metacarpophalangeal joints is prevented by a knuckle-bender dynamic splint.

Certain general principles should be followed in regard to use of an apparatus in poliomyelitis:

Whenever satisfactory recovery of function is expected, an orthosis should be used with caution in the lower limbs, since its use will tend to produce an abnormal gait pattern. Thus, during the early convalescent period, the use of an orthosis should be deferred until after maximum recovery of muscle function has taken place. Locomotion without an orthosis but with the support of crutches should be attempted, in order to stimulate active muscular function by the exercise derived from walking. Use of an orthosis should not, however, be postponed if deformities tend to develop incident to the stresses of weight-bearing. The needs of each patient are different, depending upon the severity of muscle weakness and the degree of dynamic imbalance of muscles. In the presence of extensive paralysis of the lower limbs, use of an orthosis may be the only means of stance and locomotion.

As a general principle, use of an orthosis should be as minimal as the condition permits. For example, when a patient with paralysis of both lower limbs is fitted with two above-knee orthoses, he will also require the use of two crutches to walk. If he is to use two crutches, he can do as well with an above-knee orthosis on one leg only, only minimal motor strength being required of the other leg to walk without an orthosis. During the stance phase on the leg without the orthotic support, the tripod base is completed by the two crutches; the knee is stabilized by locking it in hyperextension. Fair motor strength in the ankle dorsiflexors and hip flexor muscles will clear the lower limb in the swing phase. For prevention of fatigue, however, bilateral above-knee orthoses are used.

It is imperative to explain to the patient the reasons for the use of the orthosis. He should understand clearly that wearing the orthosis will help him at this stage of the disease, and that, at a later date, it may be discarded following training or reconstructive surgery. For example, the use of a dorsiflexion assist below-knee orthosis may be unnecessary following a successful anterior transfer of the peroneal tendons, or an opponens splint may be discarded after a satisfactory opponens tendon transfer; or when the child becomes an adult, he may no longer require the above-knee orthosis used to prevent genu recurvatum.

It is always wise to question at intervals whether the continued use of the orthosis is necessary. Before advising that use of an orthosis be discontinued, one should be quite certain that there is no possibility for development of progressive deformities and that the level and quality of functional performance will not deteriorate.

Surgery. A multitude of operative procedures may be employed both in the correction of paralytic deformities and in the total physical rehabilitation of the child with poliomyelitis. These procedures may include fasciotomy, capsulotomy, tendon transfers, osteotomy, and arthrodesis. Leg

length inequality commonly occurs in poliomyelitis as a result of shortening in the paralyzed leg. The various methods of equalizing leg lengths are presented in Chapter 7.

PRINCIPLES OF TENDON TRANSFER. Tendon transfer is the shifting of the insertion of a muscle from its normal attachment to another site to replace active muscular action that was lost by paralysis and to restore dynamic muscle balance. The procedure was originally described by Nicoladoni in 1882. Many surgeons have devised various types of tendon transfers and established their usefulness. Lange, Velpeau, Vulpius, Codivilla, Mayer, Biesalski, Goldthwait, Ober, Steindler, Bunnell, and Green are some who may be mentioned.[*] The term *tendon transplantation* should not be used interchangeably with the term *tendon transfer*, as the two are not synonymous. Tendon transplantation refers to the procedure of "excision of a tendon and its use as a free graft." In *muscle transplantation*, both the origin and insertion of a muscle are detached, and the entire muscle with its intact neurovascular supply is transplanted to a completely new site.

Basic principles of tendon transfers have been outlined by Green:

1. The muscle to be transferred must have adequate motor strength to carry out the new function. As a rule, the motor rating of the muscle should be good or normal to warrant transfer. The function that the transferred muscle is intended to perform is another consideration. In the lower limb, for example, in the presence of drop foot, anterior transfer of the peroneus longus is adequate to produce effective ankle dorsiflexion, whereas in calcaneus limp, posterior transfer of the peroneus longus alone to the os calcis is not sufficient to substitute for the gastrocnemius-soleus action, and the additional action of two or three motors such as the flexor digitorum communis and anterior tibial muscles is required. Ordinarily one grade of motor power is lost after a muscle is transferred.

2. The range of motion of muscles on contraction is an important consideration. This range must be similar to that of the

[*]See References 413, 427, 452, 488, 556, 578–580, 585, 597–603, 654–662, 679.

muscles for which they are being substituted; also, whenever muscles are transferred in combination, their range of contraction should not differ significantly. The transfer of antagonistic muscles ordinarily is not as effective as that of muscles having similar function or corollary activity. However, with meticulous postoperative care, antagonistic muscles may be transferred effectively with good results; the posterior transfer of the anterior tibial to the os calcis and of the hamstring muscles to the patella are common examples of such antagonistic transfers.

3. In choosing the muscles for transfer the loss of original function that will result from the tendon transfer must be balanced against the gains to be obtained. For example, in the presence of hip flexor weakness, the hamstring muscles should not be transferred to the patella for quadriceps paralysis, as loss of active knee flexion added to lack of hip flexion will be a greater disability. Whenever possible, muscle balance must be restored. Ideally, a deforming muscle force must be shifted so as to substitute for an essential weakness. In the foot and ankle, for example, the muscles of inversion and eversion and those of plantar flexion and dorsiflexion should be balanced. A common pitfall is transfer of the peroneus longus muscle posteriorly to the os calcis in the presence of a strong anterior tibial muscle. Normally, the anterior tibial muscle dorsiflexes the first metatarsal and the peroneus longus opposes this action. With posterior transfer of the peroneus longus, the unopposed anterior tibial gradually causes the first metatarsal to ride up, producing a dorsal bunion. Thus the peroneus longus should not be transferred to the os calcis unless the anterior tibial is shifted from its insertion on the first metatarsal to the midline of the foot.

4. The joints upon which the transferred muscle is to act should have functional range of motion. All contractural deformity should be corrected by wedging casts or soft-tissue release prior to tendon transfer. An anterior transfer for drop foot, for example, should not be performed in the presence of equinus deformity of the ankle.

5. A smooth gliding channel with adequate space must be provided for excursion of the tendon in its new location. The paratenon and synovial sheath are preserved over the tendon surface during dissection. It is preferable to pass the tendon beneath the deep fascia through tissues that permit free gliding rather than subcutaneously. A wide portion of the intermuscular septum is excised whenever muscles are passed from one muscle compartment to another. Sufficient space should be provided for the tendon so that adhesions will not form. An Ober tendon passer of appropriate size should be used to redirect the tendon to its new insertion: it spreads the tissues and prevents binding.

6. The neurovascular supply of the transferred muscle must not be damaged while transferring the tendon. One must be careful not to denervate the muscle while freeing it for redirection. When the tendon is pulled up from the distal wound into the proximal incision, traction should not be applied on the origin of the muscle. Stretching of the motor nerve is prevented by use of the double hand technique, i.e., with a moist sponge, the proximal segment of the tendon is held steady while, with another sponge, traction is applied on its distal segment. Acute angulation or torsion of the neurovascular bundle is another cause of injury. Gentle handling is imperative for preservation of innervation and function of the transferred muscle.

7. In the rerouting of the tendon a *straight line* of contraction must be provided between the origin of the muscle and its new insertion. Angular courses and passages over pulley systems should be avoided. In order to allow adequate freeing of the muscle toward its origin, the incision over the belly of the muscle must be long and proximally located.

8. The tendon should be reattached to its new site under sufficient tension so that the transferred muscle will have a maximal range of contraction. The transferred muscle should be tested at surgery to ensure that it will hold the part in optimal position. Ordinarily, in the lower limb, where weight-bearing forces are involved, the tendon is attached to bone; whereas in the upper limb, it is sutured to the tendon. An important technical detail is scarification of the distal segment of the tendon that is to be anchored to a bone or tendon; this is achieved by excision of the sheath and paratenon and

"roughening" of the tendon by scraping and crosshatching it with a knife. The position of immobilization in a plaster of Paris cast should allow the transferred tendon to be in a relaxed attitude in order to diminish any tension on the tendon while healing. For example, when the flexor carpi ulnaris is transferred to the extensor carpi radialis longus, the tension on the tendon should be sufficient to hold the wrist in 30 degrees of dorsiflexion. Yet when the cast is applied, the wrist is immobilized in the overcorrected position of 45 to 50 degrees of dorsiflexion.[491]

POSTOPERATIVE CARE AND TRAINING. These are fundamental in obtaining a good result. The following principles, given by Green, should be followed meticulously.

First, the age of the patient at the time of tendon transfer is an important preoperative consideration. The child should be old enough, preferably over four years of age, to cooperate in the training of the transfer. A delay in tendon transfer in the presence of muscle imbalance will lead to progressive deformity. Usually, conservative measures should be undertaken to control deforming factors, but in certain instances, early surgery is indicated when such a delay of tendon transfer results in increasing structural deformity. A common example is the rapid development of progressive calcaneus deformity of the foot with paralysis of the gastrocnemius-soleus muscles and strong ankle dorsiflexors. An early posterior transfer will prevent the development of a deformed foot.

Support of the part in overcorrected position should be continued until the muscle has assumed full function and until there is no tendency for the deformity to recur. Use of a bivalved cast will serve to hold the transferred tendon in a relaxed position.

It is best to teach the patient preoperatively to localize contracture in the muscle to be transferred. Active exercises are continued postoperatively as soon as the reaction to surgery and pain has subsided. The surgeon should assist the physical therapist during the initial exercises. When tendon transfer is combined with arthrodesis, muscle re-education is delayed until adequate bony union has taken place.

The patient is instructed to contract the transferred muscle voluntarily, moving the part through the arc of motion that was the original normal action of the muscle, while the therapist manually guides the part to move in the direction that is intended to be provided by the transfer. For example, when the peroneus longus muscle is transferred anteriorly to the base of the second metatarsal, the active motion called upon is eversion in combination with guided dorsiflexion, or if the anterior tibial muscle has been transferred posteriorly to the os calcis, active inversion is combined with guided plantar flexion of the ankle; in anterior transfer of the hamstrings to the patella for quadriceps femoris paralysis, the patient is placed in side-lying position and is asked to extend the hip actively (using the hamstrings) as the knee is guided into extension; or when the flexor carpi ulnaris is transferred to the extensor carpi radialis longus, the wrist is gently guided into extension as the patient deviates it ulnarward. With one hand, the therapist should palpate the belly and tendon of the transferred muscle to ensure its contraction. In the beginning, the exercises are performed in the bivalved cast. Motion of the concerned joint is executed slowly, steadily, and smoothly through as full a range as possible. Soon the limb is taken out of the plaster cast, is properly positioned, and measures are taken to prevent stretching of the tendon out of its resting position.

Occasionally the patient is unable to contract the transferred muscle actively and has difficulty in "finding" it. To enable him to use the transfer actively and to assist him in acquiring the feeling desired, one may exert gentle mild tension on the transferred tendon, shift positions while actively contracting it, or use corollary motions. If, after two weeks, such difficulty in "finding" the transfer persists, electrical stimulation may be employed to initiate contraction as the patient himself attempts to use the muscle. After a few sessions, the patient begins to "feel" the transfer and to contract it voluntarily.

As soon as the patient is able to contract the transferred muscle actively, exercises in the direction of the original action of the muscle are discontinued and only those motions in the new function provided by the transfer are performed.

When the transferred muscle develops poor motor strength, i.e., can carry the part through the full range of motion with gravity eliminated, the physical therapist instructs one of the parents to perform the exercises with the patient. The exercise regimen is supervised by the physical therapist and the surgeon, who check it at weekly or biweekly intervals.

In the beginning, the limb should be retained in the bivalved cast for support except during the exercise periods. As soon as the motor strength of the transfer becomes fair, the use of a bivalved cast during the day is gradually discontinued. Controlled activities are permitted to develop function. These are permitted sooner in the upper than in the lower limb. The age and dependability of the patient are other considerations. Resistive exercises to develop power are begun whenever the transfer has a normal range of action and is fair in strength. It is also important to exercise the antagonistic muscles to prevent disuse atrophy.

The next stage of training is the incorporation of the transfer into the new functional pattern. This is particularly important in the lower limb, in which the muscles are concerned with gait. For example, the action of the peroneus transfer may be good, dorsiflexing the ankle through full range and taking moderate resistance; yet, during locomotion, voluntary control over the transfer is "lost" and the patient walks with a drop-foot gait. The transition to walking requires diligent supervision. Of particular importance is the use of crutches—they serve to protect the limb from undue strain and at the same time allow the patient to be taught the use of the transfer and to become accustomed to it. First the patient is asked to take a single step, ensuring that the muscle contracts and dorsiflexes the ankle. As soon as the transfer functions throughout all the phases of a single step, the walking periods are gradually increased until the normal gait pattern becomes a conditioned reflex.

The use of orthoses in the postoperative period should be judicious and for specific reasons. Orthotic support protects the part and allows early activity. This is indicated particularly when paralysis is extensive, as in myelomeningocele. In a posterior transfer to the os calcis, for example, a plantar flexion assist orthosis with a dorsiflexion stop at right angles with crutches may be used to aid developing function in the transfers and prevent stretching. However, standing and walking exercises are also performed without the brace to stimulate function in the transfer.

Prolonged use of a bivalved night cast is very important to prevent development of contractural deformity that will oppose the action of the transfer, as for example, in the instance of anterior transfer for dorsiflexion, equinus deformity of the ankle. From the beginning, daily stretching exercises should be a part of the exercise regimen. Stretching and night support are continued over a long period of time, until the muscle has developed full strength and there is balanced function between the agonist and antagonist muscles with no tendency for recurrence of the original deformity. In fact, stretching and active exercises should be a simple rule of daily living.

Arthrodesis to provide stability and correct osseus deformity may be indicated, particularly in the foot. However, if dynamic balance is established prior to development of structural deformity, arthrodesis may be unnecessary. When it is necessary to combine arthrodesis with tendon transfer, muscle re-education must be delayed until adequate bony union has taken place.

The Hip

SOFT-TISSUE CONTRACTURE

The common deformity of the hip secondary to soft-tissue contracture is one of flexion, abduction, and external rotation. Several factors must be considered in its pathogenesis. During the acute and convalescent stages of poliomyelitis, the patient lies supine in the so-called "frog-leg" attitude with the hips flexed, abducted, and externally rotated, the knees flexed, and the feet in equinovarus posture. This position is assumed because of spasm of the hamstrings, hip flexors, tensor fasciae latae, and hip abductor muscles, and because of the forces of gravity acting on the flail lower limbs. Maintenance of the lower limbs in malposture results in permanent shortening of the soft tissues. Contracture of the intermuscular septae and enveloping fasciae takes place first. This fact can be easily observed at surgery. Upon sectioning of the contracted fasciae that cover normal muscle fibers, and 2 to 3 cm. retraction of the cut edges of the fascia, the underlying muscle tissue will be found to be in relaxed condition when it is elevated with tissue forceps. Partially paralyzed muscle becomes shortened because of contracture of the involved fibrosed muscle fibers scattered throughout the normal muscle tissue. Adaptive shortening of normal muscle occurs later. Structural bony deformity develops with growth in the presence of soft-tissue contracture and dynamic muscle imbalance.

The iliotibial band (or tract) is the thickened lateral portion of the fascia lata located along the entire lateral aspect of the thigh and extending from the greater trochanteric region to below the knee. Superiorly, the iliotibial band is attached to the iliac crest by three prongs: a middle one through the aponeurosis over the gluteus medius, an anterior one through the tensor fasciae latae; and a posterior one through the gluteus maximus (Fig. 5–72).

Throughout its extent on the lateral aspect of the thigh, the iliotibial tract is continuous on its deep surface with the lateral intermuscular septum through which it is firmly attached to the linea aspera on the posterior aspect of the femur. At the knee joint level, fascial expansions from the anterior border of the iliotibial tract join expansions that emanate from the quadriceps muscle to form the lateral patellar retinaculum. The lower end of the iliotibial band is attached to the lateral condyle of the tibia and the head of the fibula. Proximally the iliotibial band is located in a plane that is anterior and lateral to the axis of the hip joint, whereas distally, in a normal limb, the iliotibial tract inserts on the tibia in front of the axis of the knee joint. Irwin states, however, that the lower part of the iliotibial tract lies in a plane posterior and lateral to the axis of the knee joint.[541]

Contracture of the iliotibial band may contribute directly or indirectly to the development of the following deformities.[475, 479, 541, 544, 693]

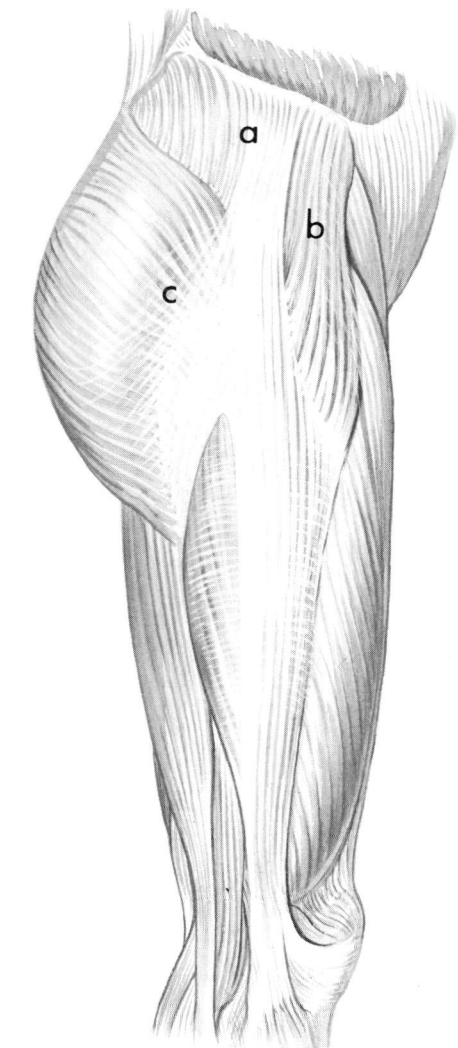

FIGURE 5–72. The three-pronged attachment of the upper part of the iliotibial band to the iliac crest.

There is a middle prong (a) through the aponeurosis over the gluteus medius, an anterior one (b) through the tensor fasciae latae, and a posterior one (c) through the gluteus maximus. Proximally, the location of the iliotibial tract is anterior and lateral to the axis of the hip, whereas inferiorly, in the normal knee, it inserts on the tibia well in front of the axis of the knee joint.

The Lower Limb

FLEXION, ABDUCTION, AND EXTERNAL ROTATION CONTRACTURE OF HIP. The shortened iliotibial band, which is in a plane anterior and lateral to the hip joint, will draw the femur into flexion and abduction at the hip with the pelvis as the fixed point. External rotation deformity is due to maintenance of the malposture of the "frog-leg" position. The related muscles, i.e., the tensor fasciae latae, reflected head of the rectus femoris, sartorius, and external rotators of the hip, undergo myostatic contracture if the fascial contracture is not corrected. The fixed soft-tissue contracture will cause anteversion of the proximal femur.

FLEXION AND VALGUS DEFORMITY OF KNEE AND EXTERNAL TORSION OF TIBIA. The iliotibial band crosses lateral to the axis of the knee. When it is contracted, a force is exerted on the lateral aspect of the joint and the tibia is gradually abducted on the femur. Its deforming action resembles that of a taut string on the concavity of an archer's bow. Irwin proposed that flexion deformity of the knee developed as a result of the location of the band in a plane posterior to the axis of motion of the knee joint.[541] However, subsequent studies have not supported this observation. The short head of the biceps takes its origin in part from the intermuscular septum, which in turn is attached to the iliotibial band. Flexion deformity of the knee will develop as a result of spasm and subsequent myostatic contracture of the short head of the biceps. Prolonged maintenance of the knee in flexion will cause contracture of the patellar retinacula and soft tissues behind the knee.

EXTERNAL TORSION OF THE TIBIA AND SUBLUXATION OF THE KNEE JOINT. The pull of the laterally located iliotibial band and the short head of the biceps femoris gradually rotates the tibia and fibula externally on the femur. When the contracture is not controlled, the deforming forces will cause posterolateral subluxation of the knee with displacement of the fibular head into the popliteal space.

POSITIONAL PES VARUS. This results from an ill-fitted orthosis that fails to compensate for the external tibial torsion. The axes of the knee and ankle joints do not occupy the same horizontal plane in external torsion of the tibia. When an above-knee orthosis manufactured with these joints in the same horizontal plane is fitted to a limb with external tibial torsion, the appliance will force the foot into varus position so that the ankle is in line with the knee joint. Initially the varus deformity is a purely functional one (the foot will assume

normal alignment when the lateral upright of the orthosis is allowed to rotate externally on the thigh); it will later become fixed due to permanent shortening of the soft tissues and adaptive osseous changes in the tarsal bones.

The Pelvis and Trunk

PELVIC DEFORMITY, LUMBAR SCOLIOSIS, SUBLUXATION OF CONTRALATERAL HIP. In abduction deformity of the hip due to iliotibial band contracture, the pelvis is level or is at a right angle to the vertical axis of the trunk as long as the affected hip is maintained in abduction; however, when it is brought parallel to the vertical axis of the body in the weight-bearing position, the pelvis is forced to assume an oblique position. This pelvic obliquity is due to contracture below the iliac crest. A lumbosacral scoliosis, convex to the low side of the pelvis, simultaneously develops. The contralateral hip will subluxate.

EXAGGERATED LUMBAR LORDOSIS. This is produced when there is bilateral flexion contracture of the hips. It is a compensatory response to the increased pelvic inclination when the trunk assumes an upright position.

Treatment. Static malpostural deformities of the lower limbs in the acute and subacute stages of poliomyelitis can be prevented by the use of bivalved casts, which maintain the joints in neutral position. A horizontal bar in the posterior half of the cast or a rotational strap will control malrotation at the hips. The knees should be in slight flexion to prevent genu recurvatum. Passive exercises are performed to maintain full range of joint motion.

Minimal contracture of the iliotibial band can be corrected by passive stretching exercises, which follow the same steps as the Ober test (See Figure 1–9). They can also be performed in the supine position with the hip that is to be stretched hanging away from the edge of the bed. In the older patient the iliotibial band can be stretched by the following exercise: The patient should stand sideways about 2 feet away from the wall with the hip that is to be stretched placed facing it. With the feet on the ground and the legs together, the hip is brought toward the wall to the count of 10 and is then returned to the original position. This exercise should be performed in sequences of 20 times, three times a day.

When the iliotibial band is contracted to such a degree that fixed deformity at the hip and knee with tilting of the pelvis has resulted, correction cannot be obtained by manipulative stretching or application of a series of plaster casts. The pelvis cannot be locked securely enough to permit stretching forces to be exerted on the shortened iliotibial band; instead, the pelvis will be tilted into an oblique and hyperextended position, stretching the lateral and anterior abdominal muscles on the side of the contracture.

Surgical intervention is the only way to correct the deformity. The shortened soft tissues must be sectioned proximally as well as distally by combining Ober's fasciotomy with Yount's procedure.[601, 693] As stated previously, the primary cause of the deformities is contracture of the intermuscular septa, the enveloping fascia, and the fibrosed muscular tissue in the patrially involved muscles. Normal muscle tissue should not be divided.

Ober's and Yount's fasciotomies are performed as follows:

Both lower limbs and hips are prepared and draped sterile. *Ober's fasciotomy* is performed through an incision that starts at the junction of the posterior and middle thirds of the iliac crest and then extends distally to the anterior superior iliac spine, where it swings posterolaterally for a distance of 10 cm. The wound flaps are mobilized to expose the sartorius, rectus femoris, tensor fasciae femoris, and the gluteus medius and minimus muscles. The enveloping fascia of these muscles, the intermuscular septa, the intervening fibrosed muscular tissue, and the iliotibial band are sectioned as far back as the greater trochanter. The Ober and Thomas tests are performed to determine by palpation the presence of any tight bands, which, if present, are divided. Normal muscle tissue and the anterior capsule of the hip joint should not be divided. The contracted fibers of the Bigelow ligament can be released without entering the hip joint. *Yount's procedure* consists of excision of a segment of the iliotibial band and of the lateral intermuscular septum in the distal thigh. A mid-lateral longitudinal incision is made beginning immediately above the knee joint line and extending cephalad for a distance of 10 cm. The subcutaneous tissue is divided and the wound flaps are mobilized by blunt dissection to expose the anterolateral aspect of the thigh in its distal one fourth. Next a 7 cm. block of the iliotibial band, the fascia lata covering the vastus lateralis muscle, and the lateral intermuscular septum are excised. It is important to divide the lateral intermuscular septum down to the femur. If it is contracted and contributes to flexion deformity of the knee, the lateral patellar retinaculum is also divided.

In severe cases with lateral rotatory subluxation of the knee, the biceps femoris muscle is lengthened by the fractional method, extreme care being taken not to injure the common peroneal nerve (see Plate 32). This can be performed through the same incision. Then an attempt at reduction is made by forcibly extending and internally rotating the knee. Often a Z-lengthening of the fibular collateral ligament will be necessary to achieve reduction.

Both the hip and thigh wounds are closed routinely. Bilateral long leg casts are applied holding the knees in full extension. Metal rings are anchored on the cast on both its anterior and posterior aspects so that the patient can be placed in suspension traction. One set of rings is placed in the distal one fourth of the leg and another set of rings in the proximal one fourth of the leg. Rotational straps can be added to the plaster cast if necessary. The patient is placed on two or three half mattresses so that his lower limbs can hang free at the edge of the mattress and his hips can be hyperextended or flexed by suspension (Fig. 5–73). An infant or small child can be placed on a bent hyperextended Bradford frame to achieve the same result. The opposite lower limb is flexed at the hip to obliterate the lumbar lordosis. The affected limb is gradually hyperextended, adducted, and internally rotated at the hip, stretching out all remaining contractural deformity. The same position of the hips can be accomplished with the patient prone or supine. In bilateral cases the hips are alternated several times a day. Manipulative stretching exercises are performed three times a day. Meticulous observation of circulation and sensation in the toes is imperative, especially if excessive shortening of neurovascular structures was observed at operation.

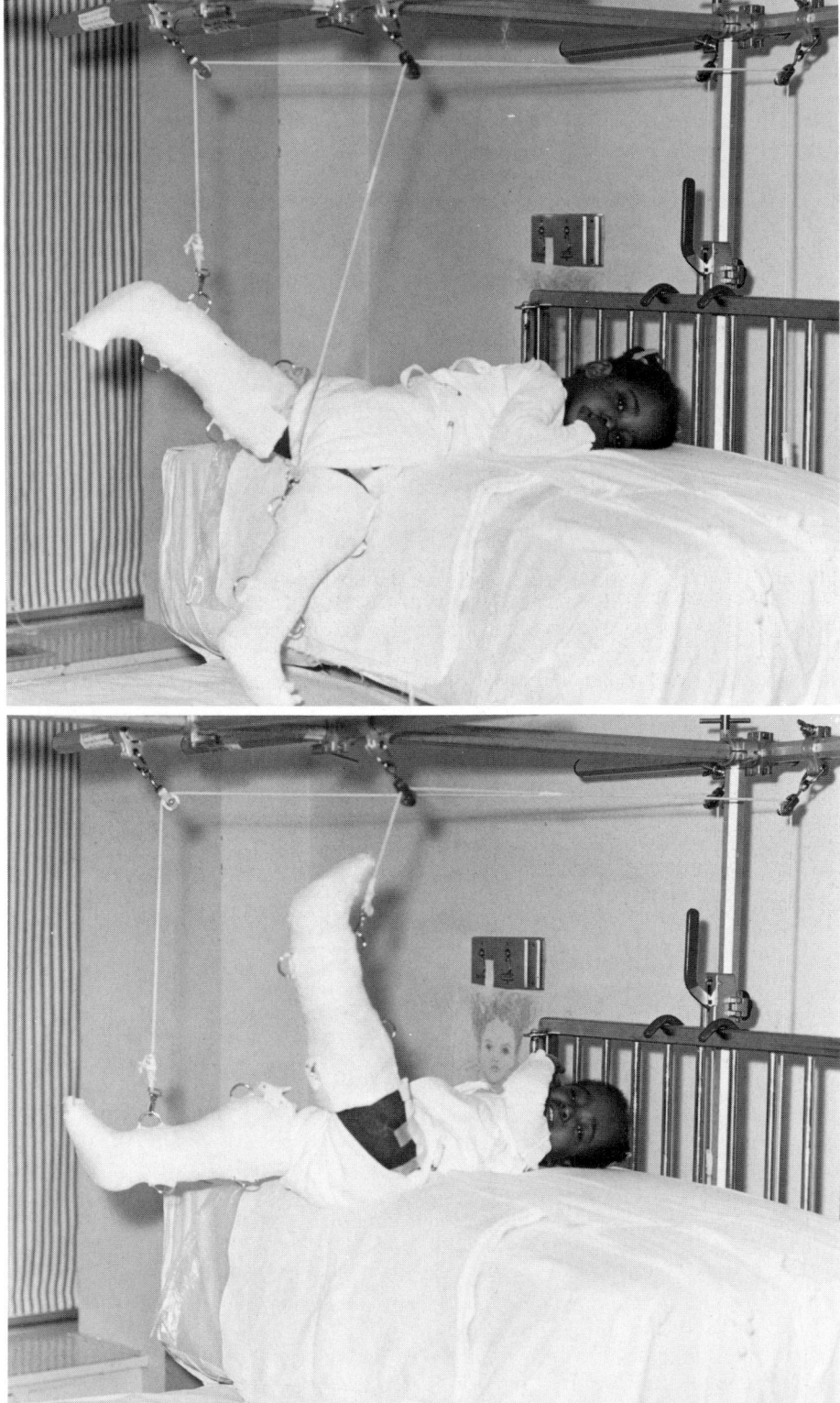

FIGURE 5–73.   Method of suspension-traction following Ober-Yount release of the iliotibial band.

In myelomeningocele patients with impaired sensation, stretching by the method described may cause pressure sores. Atrophied bones of these children may also be fractured easily by vigorous manipulations or stretching procedures.

Passive stretching by the preceding suspension-traction method is continued for a period of three weeks.

With progressive longitudinal growth of the femur, contracture of the iliotibial band will recur unless passive stretching exercises and proper positioning of the joints in bivalved casts are continued during periods of growth.

GLUTEUS MEDIUS PARALYSIS

When the hip abductor muscles are paralyzed, the trunk will sway toward the affected side and the contralateral side of the pelvis will drop during the weight-bearing phase of gait. Lateral stability of the hip joint is best provided by transferring the *iliopsoas muscle* from the lesser trochanter to the greater trochanter (see Plate 39). The author commonly performs the Sharrard modification of the Mustard iliopsoas transfer, making the hole in the ilium as far posteriorly as the nerve supply to the iliacus will allow.[592, 593] One cannot overemphasize the importance of using a nerve stimulator while transferring the iliopsoas muscle. Details of postoperative care following iliopsoas transfer are described in the section on myelomeningocele. The hip should be protected with crutches until the transferred iliopsoas is fair plus or good in motor strength and the Trendelenburg test is negative. During this period the patient should sleep in a bivalved hip spica cast, which maintains the hip in 40 to 60 degrees of abduction. Active hip abduction exercises should be performed diligently — graduating from the supine position to side-lying against gravity, and then to standing Trendelenburg.

The *external oblique abdominal muscle* can be used to restore hip abduction power. Lowman used part of the external oblique muscle and attached it to the greater trochanter with a strip of fascia lata.[567, 569] Thomas, Thompson, and Straub transferred the entire muscle belly of the external oblique.[666] The remaining abdominal muscles (rectus abdominis, internal oblique, and transversus muscles) will maintain integrity of the abdominal wall. The author has had no personal experience with external oblique muscle transfer for paralysis of hip abductors. Physiologically, the procedure is sound; for details of operative technique, the reader is referred to the original article.[666] Also, the tensor fasciae latae muscle may be transferred posteriorly on the iliac crest for increase of hip abduction strength.[559]

GLUTEUS MAXIMUS PARALYSIS

Instability of the hip and exaggerated lumbar lordosis result from paralysis of the gluteus maximus muscle. In gait, the trunk lurches backward when the body weight is borne on the affected side. When the hip flexor muscles are of normal strength, increasing flexion deformity of the hip will develop.

For motor evaluation of the gluteus maximus muscle, the patient is placed in prone position, with the lower limbs hanging off the examining table. The knee is in flexion to eliminate action of the hamstrings. The patient is asked to extend his hip against gravity and manual resistance. The position also serves to evaluate the degree of flexion deformity of the hip when it is extended passively. If the patient is unable to lift the thigh against gravity, he is placed in side-lying position to eliminate the force of gravity. Any abduction contracture is best determined by the Ober test, as the degree of hip abduction noted on maximal extension of the hip in prone position is not as accurate.

In gluteus maximus paralysis, stability of the pelvis may be provided by the addition of posterior gluteal crisscross straps between the pelvic band and the thigh band of the above-knee orthosis; an alternate method is to discard the pelvic band and fit an ischial weight-bearing quadrilateral socket to the upper thigh segment of the orthosis. Often, however, the additional support of one or two crutches is required.

Muscle transfers to restore gluteus maximus function are not always successful and should be undertaken only after considerable deliberation. Lange transferred the erector spinae muscle to the greater trochanter, using silk sutures to obtain length.[551, 556] Ober and Hey Groves used a strip of fascia lata to attach the erector spinae muscle to the greater trochanter.[500,597]

The technique of Ober was further improved by Barr, who used a wide strip of fascia lata, including the iliotibial tract and tensor fasciae latae muscle (Fig. 5–74).[406] Contractures about the hip, such as fascia and tight intermuscular septa, are released, particularly those that are anterior and lateral to the hip joint. Complete mobilization of the iliotibial tract and shift of its pull laterally to the greater trochanter removes a major deforming force. Release of contracted investing fascia about the shortened erector spinae muscle permits rotation of the pelvis to nearly normal position and diminishes the severity of fixed lumbar lordosis.

Malrotation of the limb is prevented and corrected by transfer of the insertion of the tensor fasciae latae into the greater trochanter. Stability of the hip is provided if there is power in the erector spinae and tensor fasciae latae muscles, which act in conjunction as a diagastric muscle transfer. The operation does not significantly improve the extensor or abductor power of the hip, but appears to produce a more dynamic fasciodesis. Stance and gait are improved by relief of hip flexion contracture, stabilization of the hip, and relief of lumbar lordosis.[644]

The operative technique, as advocated by Barr in 1964, is as follows:

Operative Technique [Barr]. The patient, under general anesthesia, is placed in the lateral position with both limbs flexed 90 degrees at the hip and knee; the affected limb is uppermost, abducted, and resting on pillows. The skin of the lumbar region, buttock, and limb is prepared from the ribs to the mid-calf. The operative field is draped so that the limb can be moved freely. The incision in the thigh begins just anterior to the head of the fibula and ends proximally just distal to the anterior superior iliac spine passing over the greater trochanter. The iliotibial band is exposed through its full length and breadth and is divided transversely at the level of the distal pole of the patella. A stout silk suture is passed through its free end and as wide a strip of fascia as it is possible to obtain is dissected upward and preserved as the tendon of insertion of the tensor fasciae latae muscle. Beginning at the trochanteric level, the dissection is carried toward the anterior iliac spine, mobilizing the distal half of the tensor fasciae latae muscle and preserving its neurovascular bundle. The intermuscular septa and other contracted fascial structures at the knee and anterior to the hip are divided as necessary while an assistant holds the hip and knee in as much extension as possible. The sartorius and rectus muscles are tenotomized if they are contracted and totally paralyzed. The iliopsoas tendon, if need be, may be divided at its insertion but should be transposed to a more proximal and anterior position in the intertrochanteric region. The anterior capsule of the hip may also be divided through the same incision if it prevents extension of the hip. The neurovascular bundle is preserved.

Subperiosteal anchorage of the fascial strip to the femur is accomplished by making two parallel longitudinal incisions, usually five to six centimeters long, through the origin of the vastus lateralis and the periosteum, one on the anterolateral, the other on the posterolateral aspect of the femur just below the greater trochanter and tunneling beneath the periosteum to join the two incisions. The strip of fascia is then passed through the tunnel and secured to the periosteum by silk sutures. This must be done with the hip held in as much extension as possible, without putting undue force on the tissues, and maintaining slight abduction and neutral position as regards rotation.

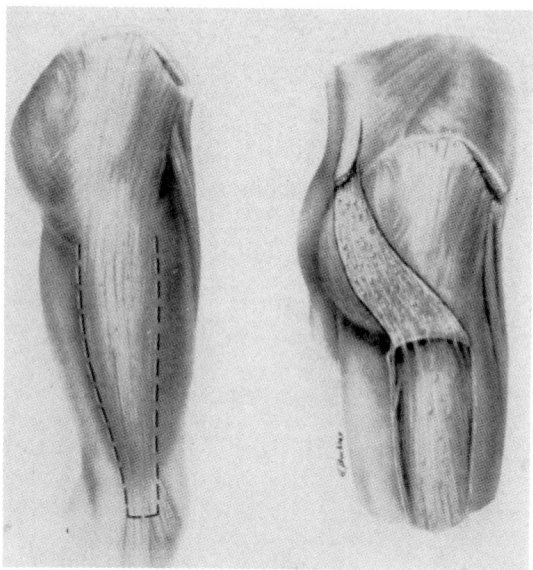

FIGURE 5–74. *Erector spinae transfer or fascia lata transfer to the greater trochanter.*

(From Hogshead, H. P., and Ponseti, I. V.: Fascia lata transfer to the erector spinae. J. Bone Joint Surg., *46-A*:1390, 1964.)

The lumbar incision is about fifteen centimeters long. It is made parallel to and five to eight centimeters lateral to the line of the spinous processes of the fourth and fifth lumbar and first sacral vertebrae. The inferior end of the incision is located medial to and about five centimeters distal to the posterior superior iliac spine. The incision is deepened through the lumbodorsal fascia, which is reflected to expose the underlying erector spinae muscle. By blunt dissection along a vertical line, the lateral two-thirds of this muscle mass is mobilized and freed from the medial one-third, which is left attached to the adjacent spinous processes and laminae. The mobilized muscle is freed by sharp dissection from its origin to the ilium and sacrum. Since the nerve and blood supply to this muscle is segmental and enters from its ventral surface, it may be necessary to sacrifice one or two of the most distal neurovascular bundles in order to mobilize a ten-centimeter length of muscle mass.

By means of a long tendon carrier, the free end of the fascia lata is passed within the gluteal muscle compartment entering the lumbar incision just medial to the posterior superior iliac spine. The tunnel at its point of emergence is carefully dilated by the surgeon's finger so that the fascia can glide freely. The gliding deep surface of the fascia should be placed as it lies ventrally. With the hip held in extension, the fascia is attached, under moderate tension, to the free end of the mobilized erector spinae muscle. This is best done by laying the ventral surface of the muscle on the subcutaneous surface of the fascial strip, passing the suture in the end of the fascia through the muscle, as far proximally as possible, and then fixing the edges of the fascia to the edges of the muscle flap by a series of interrupted sutures. The distal end of the muscle is thus covered on its deep surface by the fascia lata. The lumbar incision is closed in layers; it is usually possible to close the lumbodorsal fascia over the transplant partially. The thigh incision is closed in a routine manner. No attempt should be made to close the defect in the fascia of the thigh. After application of sterile dressings, the extremity is immobilized by elastic bandages and long plaster splints which extend from the ribs to the toes. The hip is immobilized in as much extension as can be obtained comfortably. No attempt is made to correct the hip-flexion contracture completely at this time.

Technique for Correction of Remaining Contractures in Poliomyelitic Deformities

After ten days to two weeks, when the incisions have healed, the remaining contractures are gradually stretched out. The lumbar spine and the opposite lower extremity are immobilized in a spica with that hip in sufficient flexion to obliterate the lumbar lordosis. A separate toe-to-groin cast is applied to the affected limb with the knee preferably in almost complete extension. With the patient supine the affected limb in its plaster cast is suspended from an overhead frame. The contracture can then be stretched gradually and completely by lowering the limb in day-to-day increments until the hip comes into hyperextension. During this procedure, the circulation and sensation in the toes should be watched carefully, especially if excessive shortening of the femoral vessels and nerves was observed at operation.

If a knee-flexion deformity is present it may be corrected simultaneously by wedging the cast.

As a rule the deformity is satisfactorily corrected in two to three weeks. The apparatus is then removed and assistive muscle re-education exercises are begun with the patient in recumbency. Underwater exercises are of value. A bivalved long spica to hold the hip in the corrected position should be worn at night for several months. Walking with crutches is permitted as soon as the transplant functions satisfactorily, usually about six weeks postoperatively.

Many patients require bilateral transplants and should undergo operation in two stages, four to six weeks apart. Careful gait training is essential if the best results are to be obtained.*

Hogshead and Ponseti found the formation of an erector spinae flap in myelomeningocele to be difficult. The procedure was bloody and the ramifications of the meningocele sac were inadvertently entered, with the result that there was troublesome drainage of cerebrospinal fluid through the wound. Since, in their experience, erector spinae transfer did not provide active power of hip extension or abduction, they recommended attachment of the distal end of the fascia lata band to the freed lumbodorsal fascia at the level of the third or fourth lumbar vertebra (Fig. 5–75). They term the operative procedure fascia lata transfer to the erector spinae.[527] The route of the transfer should be subfascial, and its direction from the greater trochanter to the region of the posterior superior iliac spine should be as far posterior as possible.

Caution should be exercised in the anterior release of soft-tissue contracture of the hip. Every effort should be made to preserve viable muscles and their nerve and blood supply. The anterior capsule of the

*From Barr, J. S.: Discussion. J. Bone Joint Surg., 46–A:1402, 1964. Reprinted with permission.

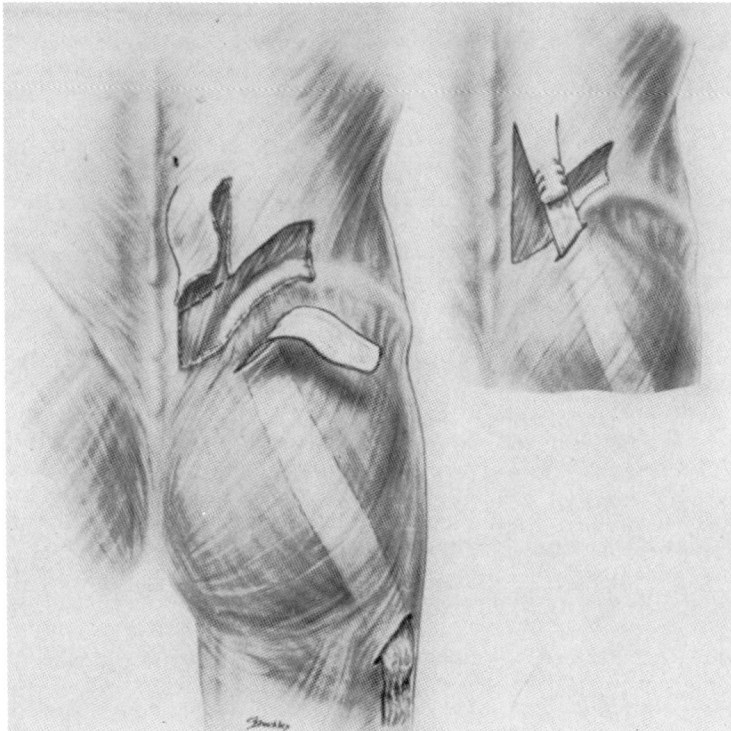

FIGURE 5-75. *Fascia lata transfer to lumbodorsal fascia to provide posterior stability to the hip joint.*

(From Hogshead, H. P., and Ponseti, I. V.: Fascia lata transfer to the erector spinae. J. Bone Joint Surg., *46-A:*1404, 1964.)

hip should not be sectioned, in order to prevent anterior dislocation of the femoral head. When contracture of the anterior capsule is fixed and it limits extension of the hip, it is *lengthened.*

In the Sharrard modification of the Mustard operation a hole is made in the posterior part of the ilium and the iliacus muscle is sutured to the lateral surface of the ilium (see Plate 39). The operation was designed to provide power of hip extension as well as hip abduction. Unfortunately the motor nerve supply of the iliacus muscle is frequently distal in its location, limiting the degree of posterior positioning of the iliac hole. In the author's experience, Sharrard iliopsoas transfer has not been successful in providing active power of hip extension against gravity in the presence of complete paralysis of the gluteus maximus muscle. When the hamstring muscles are normal in motor strength and the gluteus maximus is only partially paralyzed, it will restore functional strength of hip extension and give substantial improvement in gait.

PARALYTIC DISLOCATION OF THE HIP

Hip dislocation in poliomyelitis is an acquired deformity caused by flaccid paralysis and the resulting muscular imbalance that develops. When, in a young child, the gluteus maximus and medius muscles are paralyzed and the hip flexors and adductors are of normal strength, eventual luxation of the hip is almost inevitable. Loss of hip abductor power causes retardation of growth from the greater trochanteric apophysis. Disparity of relative growth from the capital femoral epiphysis and the greater trochanteric apophysis causes increasing valgus deformity of the femoral neck. In severe cases, the angle between the neck and shaft of the femur increases to 180 degrees. Excessive anteversion of the femoral neck may also develop. When the angle between the femoral neck and the horizontal plane of the pelvis approaches 90 degrees, the hip joint becomes mechanically unstable. Gradually, under the forces of body weight, the capsule becomes lax and the femoral head rides out of the acetabulum. The empty acetabulum retains an adequate depth for several years following paralytic dislocation. With lack of concentric pressure of the femoral head in the acetabulum, however, progressive shallowness and obliquity of the acetabular roof develop. Thus, factors in the pathogenesis of true paralytic dislocation are muscle imbalance, coxa valga, and laxity of the capsule. In treatment, it is important to remember that coxa valga precedes subluxation and shallowness of the acetabulum.[545, 546, 646]

Acquired hip dislocation does not usually occur in a totally flail lower limb, particularly if the patient has been walking with the support of an orthosis. If inadequately treated, however, the flail hip may develop abduction–flexion–external rotation contracture due to shortening of the iliotibial band. When the lower limbs are aligned parallel to the vertical axis of the body in the weight-bearing position, the pelvis will be forced into an oblique position. The contralateral hip, i.e., the one on the high side of the pelvis, is in a markedly functional valgus position and will become dislocated eventually. Pelvic obliquity may result also from the foregoing factors; another cause may be severe structural scoliosis in the suprapelvic region. This type of scoliosis should be distinguished from positional scoliosis that is produced by pelvic obliquity due to contractural deformities below the pelvis.

Treatment. Dislocation of the hip in poliomyelitis may be prevented by restoration of dynamic balance about the hip; this is achieved by appropriate muscle transfers. If the age of onset of paralysis and muscle imbalance is less than two years, iliopsoas transfer to restore power of hip abduction is performed when the child is four or five years old. If the coxa valga deformity is less than 150 degrees, a preliminary varization osteotomy is unnecessary; the valgus deformity will correct itself with growth once hip abductor power is restored. If the coxa valga deformity is greater than 150 degrees, it is best to correct the deformity and obtain a femoral neck-shaft angle of 110 degrees prior to iliopsoas transfer.

If, at the time of paralysis, the patient is more than two years of age, iliopsoas transfer may be postponed and the stability of the hip followed by taking periodic roentgenograms. When the coxa valga exceeds 160 degrees and the femoral head starts to subluxate laterally, varization osteotomy is performed. In patients under six years of age, the femoral neck-shaft angle is reduced to 105 degrees; in older patients, the angle is corrected to 125 degrees. Often, if dynamic muscle imbalance persists, valgus deformity will recur with growth. The procedure should be followed in six months to a year with an iliopsoas transfer.

The operative technique of varization osteotomy follows the same principles as that of valgus osteotomy. First, if there is any adduction contracture of the hip, it should be passively stretched and corrected by split Russell traction, gradually bringing the hips into wide abduction. Adductor myotomy of the hip should be avoided whenever possible. The anterolateral surface of the subtrochanteric region of the femur is subperiosteally exposed, as described in Plate 6 on page 186. The line of osteotomy is shaped like a modified dome with a lateral buttress of cortical bone in the proximal segment to lock the upper end of the distal segment while the femoral shaft is adducted. This procedure is the reverse of valgus osteotomy. Rotational malalignment can be corrected at the same time. The author uses Crow pins or threaded Steinmann pins and Roger Anderson apparatus to fix the fragments together. Others may use a bone plate with four screws, a blade plate, or two staples. It is a matter of personal preference and depends upon past experience. Blundell Jones exposes the trochanteric region of the proximal femur posterolaterally with the patient in prone position and corrects the valgus deformity by excision of a wedge of bone with its base medially.[545, 546]

When the hip is completely dislocated, the hip joint capsule is stretched out and lax. Paralytic hip dislocation is very easily reduced. In the beginning the femoral head can be relocated into the acetabulum by simple abduction of the hip. Later on, however, soft-tissue contracture may develop and an initial period of skin or skeletal traction will then be indicated. Prolonged immobilization of the hip following reduction in a spica cast is not recommended. Following removal of the cast, the dislocation will recur. The use of a solid hip spica cast does not correct the etiologic factors; it also has the additional disadvantage of causing disuse atrophy of muscles and bone. To stimulate normal growth of the proximal femur, weight-bearing should be restored as soon as possible.

Reefing and repair of the capsule is very essential. It is described and illustrated in Plate 4, page 157. An iliopsoas transfer is performed at the same time to restore power of hip abduction and muscle balance about the hip. If the acetabulum is shallow and maldirected, the procedure may be combined with a Salter innominate osteotomy.

Arthrodesis of the Hip. Stabilization of the hip in poliomyelitis may result in increased ability to walk and eliminate the necessity for use of orthotic support. The procedure does have serious disadvantages, however, which should be carefully considered. Sharp et al. reported a series of 16 hip fusions performed in children for paralysis caused by poliomyelitis.[640] There was a high percentage of fractures (eight of the femur and one of the tibia). In addition, there were three cases of pseudar-

throsis and one of slipped capital femoral epiphysis. In three patients, the hip was fused and subsequently required correction by femoral osteotomy. One patient had marked limitation of knee motion following prolonged immobilization in the cast; in another, amputation was indicated because of excessive shortening of the limb.

A stiff hip burdens the spine and knee with abnormal stress and strain. Thus, ligamentous instability of the knee, progressive lumbosacral scoliosis, and trunk instability due to extensive paralysis of abdominal muscles are absolute contraindications to hip fusion in poliomyelitis. A functional quadriceps femoris is desirable but not absolutely necessary, provided there is no flexion deformity of the knee, and stability of the foot and ankle is provided by a strong triceps surae muscle or by pantalar arthrodesis in a 15 degree equinus position. Stability of the flail knee is achieved as the body weight falls on the ball of the foot by forcing the heel on the ground and driving the knee into hyperextension (Fig. 5–76).

Hallock, in 1942, 1950, and 1958, reported an enlarging series of hip fusions

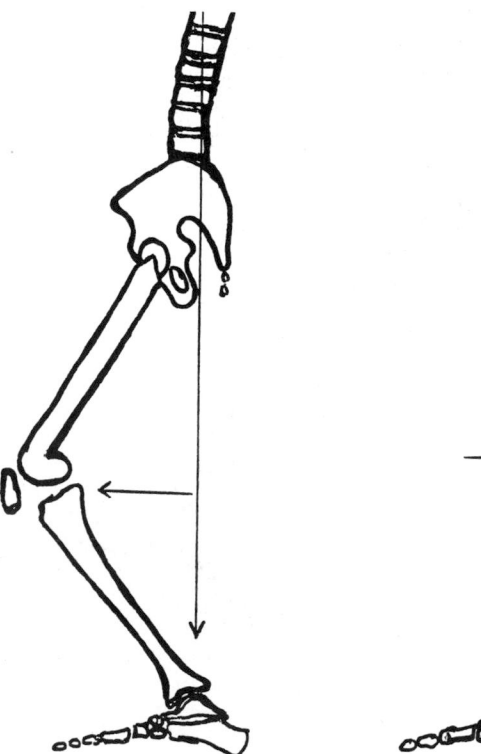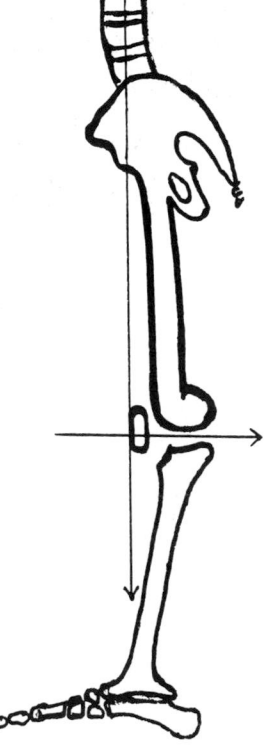

FIGURE 5–76. *The principle of dynamic knee stabilization when the hip is fused and the ankle is fixed in slightly equinus position.*

On the left is shown the collapsible knee when the hip and ankle are flail; on the right, stability of the knee is achieved when the body weight falls on the ball of the foot, forces the heel to the ground, and locks the knee, driving it into hyperextension. (From Sharp, N., Guhl, J. F., Sorenson, R. I., and Voshell, A. F.: Hip fusion in poliomyelitis children. J. Bone Joint Surg., *46-A:*122, 1964.)

being performed in patients with flail lower limbs resulting from poliomyelitis.[506-508] In the beginning, the procedure was employed only in those instances in which there was painful arthritic subluxation or dislocation of the hip, or when previous reconstructive operations such as open reduction, shelf stabilization, or muscle transfers failed. Later, Hallock extended his indications to include several individuals with severe hip lurch from extensive hip muscle paralysis without dislocation. He found his results to be most gratifying: the arthrodesis relieved pain, achieved stability, and decreased the limp. Hallock recommended that the optimum position of fusion be 35 degrees of flexion, neutral rotation, and neutral abduction-adduction position, except in girls or when considerable shortening is present, in which cases 10 or 15 degrees of abduction is advised for biologic reasons and to compensate in some measure for the inequality of leg length.[507]

When there is marked shortening of the flail limb, making equalization impractical, hip fusion should not be performed. The age of the patient is another consideration; it is imperative that he be mature enough to understand the disadvantages of a stiff hip. Hip fusion in a paralytic flail lower limb is controversial and should be considered only after thorough and meticulous assessment of the patient.

The Knee

QUADRICEPS FEMORIS PARALYSIS

The quadriceps is commonly affected by poliomyelitis. When there is slight genu recurvatum and adequate strength of the triceps surae and hamstring muscles, the knee is stabilized by locking it in hyperextension (Fig. 5-77) These patients are able to walk quite satisfactorily. During the stance phase of gait, quadriceps weakness is compensated by tilting the trunk and center of gravity of the body forward. The only functional disabilities are difficulty in climbing steps and running. In the presence of knee flexion deformity, however, the knee joint becomes unstable because it cannot be locked in hyperextension.

When the hamstring muscles are normal,

they can be transferred anteriorly to the patella and the ligamentum patellae so as to provide extension and stability of the knee. This procedure is advised when instability of the knee interferes with ordinary walking or when with such a transfer the patient will be able to dispense with his orthosis. Each case, however, must be individually considered. When the hip flexors are less than fair in motor strength, anterior transfer of hamstrings is absolutely contraindicated. Following surgery, the patient will be unable to clear his limb from the floor; consequently, his disability will be greater. The triceps surae muscle must be at least fair in strength; if not, with loss of all dynamic posterior knee support, marked genu recurvatum will develop. It is preferable to have adequate strength of the gluteus maximus and hip abductor muscles. Prior to tendon transfer, any flexion contracture of the knee and equinus deformity of the ankle should be fully corrected by wedging casts. The mechanics of patellofemoral articulation should be normal. Any significant malalignment of the lower limb, such as marked genu valgum, should also be corrected preoperatively.

A number of muscles have been transferred to restore knee extension power, namely, the biceps femoris, semitendinosus, sartorius, tensor fasciae latae, and adductor longus.*

The transfer of both the biceps femoris and the semitendinosus muscle is the procedure of choice. The strength of the tensor fasciae latae and sartorius muscles is not sufficient to substitute for the quadriceps. In an electromyographic study of 21 patients with paralysis of the lower limb due to poliomyelitis, in whom 39 muscle transfers for quadriceps paralysis were performed, Sutherland, Bost, and Schottstaedt reported the following results: 10 to 14 hamstring transfers achieved conversion from swing phase to stance phase activity (roughly comparable to that of the normal quadriceps femoris); two of 11 sartorius transfers and 4 of 12 tensor fasciae latae transfers achieved stance phase activity.[665]

The operative technique of transfer of the biceps femoris and semitendinosus

_____

*See References 422, 429, 456, 519, 550, 552, 608, 619, 636, 671.

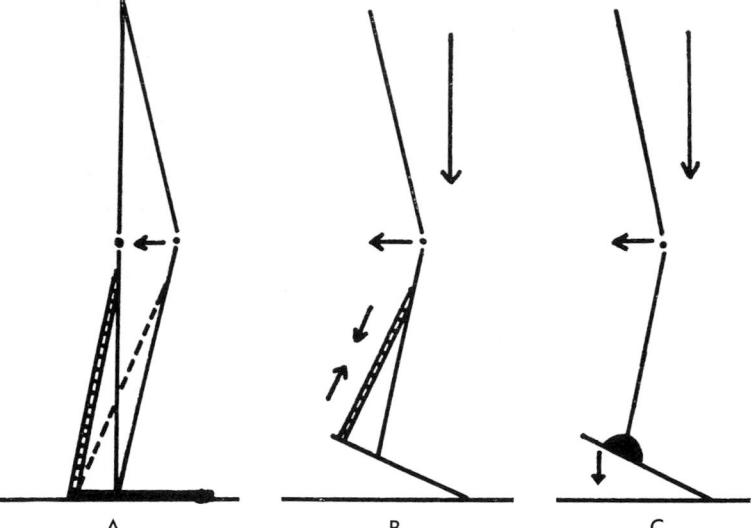

FIGURE 5–77.   *The effect of muscle-controlled or fixed talipes equinus upon extension of the knee.*

A. Normal action of soleus as an extensor of the knee with the foot on the ground. **B**. Soleus as a fixator of the foot in equinus position. **C**. Rigid equinus foot, showing effect of body weight in extending the knee. (Vertical arrows represent body weight. Horizontal arrows indicate direction of movement of the knee joint.) (From Robins, R. H. C.: The ankle joint in relation to arthrodesis of the foot in poliomyelitis. J. Bone Joint Surg., *41-B*:340, 1959; modified from Steindler, after von Baeyer.)

A   B   C

muscles, as described by Crego and Fischer, and Schwartzmann and Crego, is as follows (Fig. 5–78):[456, 636]

The patient is placed supine with a large sandbag under the ipsilateral hip so that he is tilted 45 degrees to the opposite side and the knee to be operated on is in semiflexion. A longitudinal incision is made over the posterolateral aspect of the thigh, starting immediately above the head of the fibula and extending proximally to terminate at the junction of the proximal and middle thirds of the thigh. The subcutaneous tissue and deep fascia are incised in line with the skin incision. The common peroneal nerve, located posteromedial to the biceps tendon, is identified and gently retracted posteriorly with a moist umbilical tape. The biceps femoris tendon is dissected free of its surrounding soft tissues and is retracted anterolaterally. At its point of attachment the lateral collateral ligament to the fibular head is quite adherent to the biceps tendon; great caution is exercised to protect it and not to divide it. Next, the biceps tendon is detached from its insertion to the head of the fibula. By sharp and dull dissection, the muscle bodies of the short and long heads of the biceps muscle are freed proximally as high as possible, care being taken to preserve their nerve and blood supply. The new direction of the line of pull of the transfer must be as nearly vertical as pos-

sible; if they run horizontally, the muscles will pull the patella in a posterior direction.

Next, a transverse incision is made over the anterior aspect of the knee, centering over the distal third of the patella. The subcutaneous tissue and deep fascia are divided. The wound flaps are undermined to expose the patella and patellar tendon. With a large Ober tendon transfer, a wide subcutaneous tunnel is made, extending from the patellar incision to the one on the lateral thigh. A 10 to 15 cm. long segment of the intermuscular septum and the iliotibial band is excised to allow free gliding of the transferred muscle belly.

Next, the sandbag is removed and placed under the opposite hip so that the patient is positioned semilaterally, being turned to the ipsilateral side. A longitudinal incision is made over the posteromedial aspect of the thigh, beginning 3 cm. proximal to the popliteal crease and extending to the junction of the middle and proximal thirds of the thigh. The subcutaneous tissue and deep fascia are divided. The semitendinosus tendon is isolated and through a separate small incision over the anteromedial aspect of the proximal leg, it is detached from its insertion on the tibia. It is easy to identify the semitendinosus tendon in the distal leg wound by pulling on it in the proximal thigh wound; anatomically, at its insertion, the semitendinosus tendon is located posterior to the sartorius tendon and inferior to the tendon of the gracilis. Next, the semitendinosus tendon is delivered into the proximal wound and dissected free to the middle third of the thigh. Through a wide subcutaneous tunnel from the anterior transverse knee incision to the postero-medial thigh incision, the semitendinosus tendon is rerouted and delivered into the prepatellar area. Again, the deep fascia is widely incised to avoid angulation and to permit free gliding of the semitendinosus tendon.

Next, the prepatellar bursa is reflected and retracted to one side and an I-shaped incision is made through the quadriceps tendon and periosteum over the anterior surface of the patella. These tissues are stripped and reflected medially and laterally. With a ⁹⁄₆₄ inch drill two oblique longitudinal tunnels are made through the patella, starting at the superolateral and superomedial poles of the patella and emerging at each side of the patellar tendon. The tunnels are enlarged with progressively increasing sizes of hand drills and curets. One should be cautious so that the articular surface of the patella is not damaged.

With braided silk whip sutures on their ends, the biceps femoris tendon and the semitendinosus tendon are each pulled through their respective tunnels in the

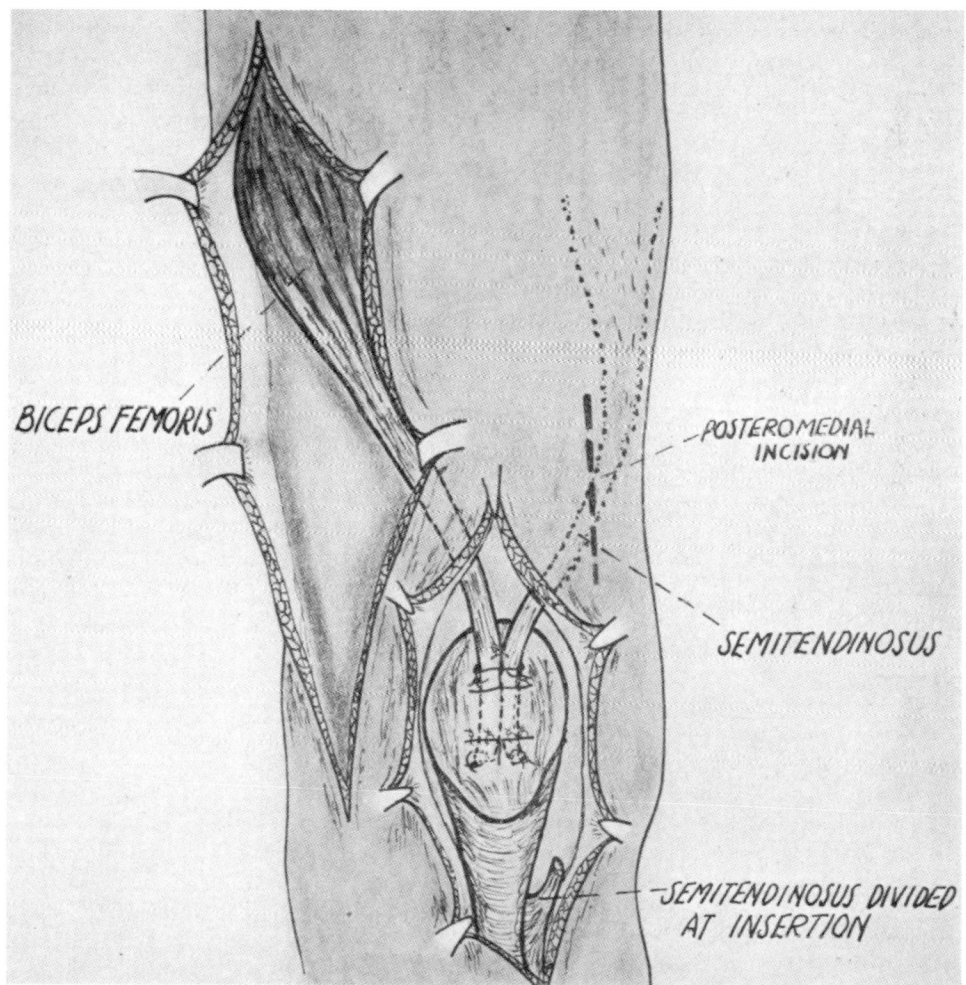

FIGURE 5-78. *Transfer of semitendinosus and biceps femoris tendons to patella to restore knee extension.*

(From Schwartzmann, J. R., and Crego, C. H.: Hamstring tendon transplantation for the relief of quadriceps femoris paralysis in residual poliomyelitis. J. Bone Joint Surg., *30-A:*545, 1948.)

patella and sutured to the patellar tendon under tension. Additional interrupted sutures are placed proximally and distally, fixing the biceps and semitendinosus tendons to the rectus femoris and patellar tendons. The soft tissues are sutured over the anterior aspect of the patella and the wounds are closed. A long leg cast is applied, which holds the knee in neutral position, but not in hyperextension.

Meticulous postoperative care is very important to obtain a satisfactory result. Tension on the transferred hamstring is prevented by avoiding flexion of the hip. The patient is kept supine in bed for a period of three weeks, and it should be strongly emphasized to personnel that he is not to sit.

Functional training of the transfer is begun three to five days following surgery, or as soon as the patient is comfortable. The patient is placed on his side to eliminate the force of gravity. The knee and hip are slightly flexed, and the patient is asked to extend his hip and knee. Active contraction of hamstrings as knee extensors is initiated by having them execute their former action of hip extension. Then active guided knee extension exercises are performed from starting positions of greater knee flexion and decreasing hip flexion; the patient should soon be encouraged to divorce the two movements of knee and hip extension. The active exercise of knee extension is performed with the hip in the partially flexed position of the normal pattern of locomotion without, however, extending the hip.

The function of the antagonist muscles should not be ignored. Active knee flexion exercises are carried out (through a limited range initially), making sure that the transferred muscle is not used in both extensor and flexor functions.

As soon as the transferred muscle is fair minus in motor strength, the patient, while still supine in bed, is asked to go slowly through the motions of walking; namely, ankle-foot dorsiflexion and hip flexion, followed by knee extension (using the transfer), hip extension, and ankle plantar flexion. The same exercises are performed standing, first in parallel bars, and then in crutches. During the stance phase, hyperextension of the knee should be avoided. A night bivalved cast is worn for 8 to 12 months to prevent stretching of the transferred muscles. Orthotic devices to support the knee are not usually necessary, unless their use is indicated for control of the foot and ankle.

Genu recurvatum is a not infrequent complication; it occurs in 10 to 20 per cent of the reported cases, being a natural consequence of an operation in which the hamstring muscles that normally provide dynamic support to the knee posteriorly are removed and transferred anteriorly. Other contributory factors in its pathogenesis are: (1) pes equinus, (2) selection of patients with inadequate (less than fair) strength in the triceps surae muscle, (3) immobilization of the knee in hyperextension in the postoperative period, (4) lack of an adequate and diligent postoperative exercise regimen with the resultant failure to develop active knee flexion against gravity, and (5) improper use of orthotic support following surgery. The development of genu recurvatum can be minimized if the preceding combination of factors is circumvented.

Lateral instability of the knee often results from inadvertent operative division of the tibial or fibular collateral ligaments while detaching the semitendinosus and biceps tendons from their insertion.

Lateral dislocation of the patella commonly occurs when the biceps femoris alone is transferred; this complication can be prevented by transfer of both the biceps and semitendinosus muscles.

Failure of transfer may be due to denervation of the muscles during proximal dissection, inadequate postoperative training, or by binding down of the transfer by adhesions in sharp angular pathways to the patella.

FLEXION DEFORMITY OF THE KNEE

Contracture of the iliotibial band due to static forces of malposture of a flail lower limb will cause flexion contracture of the knee along with flexion–abduction–external rotation deformity of the hip, genu valgum, and external tibial torsion. This deformity is preventable, and if minimal, it can be corrected by passive exercises and wedging casts.[455,513] When it is marked, Ober-Yount open surgical release of the contracted iliotibial band will be required.

Flexion contracture of the knee may also result from a dynamic imbalance between the quadriceps femoris and hamstring muscles (Fig. 5–79). As stated previously, when there is flexion deformity of the knee,

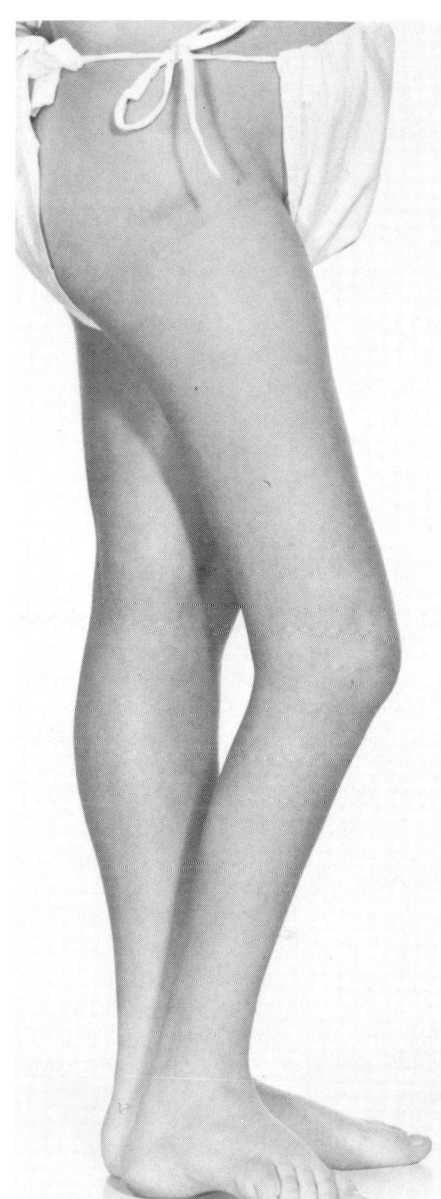

FIGURE 5–79. *Flexion deformity of the right knee in poliomyelitis.*

Dynamic imbalance between quadriceps femoris and hamstring muscles caused the deformity. Note also the calcaneovalgus deformity of the right foot.

paralysis of the quadriceps muscle cannot be compensated by locking the knee in hyperextension and the knee will then be unstable. Thus it is imperative that knee flexion deformity be fully corrected.

It is important to understand the pathomechanics of a knee that has become fixed in flexion. In the normal knee, the last 5 degrees of extension are accompanied by medial rotation of the femur on the tibia — a movement that tightens the collateral ligaments and oblique posterior ligament, thus locking the knee in extension. As the axis of knee motion does not pass through the joint line, but through the upper attachments of the collateral ligaments, the tibial plateau has to glide forward on the femoral condyles. In fixed flexion deformity of the knee this normal gliding movement does not take place; instead, a simple rocking motion occurs. When the knee is forced into extension, the tibia subluxates posteriorly, and the knee joint becomes incongruous and painful. In correction of fixed flexion deformity of the knee, it is important to preserve joint congruity by pulling the tibial plateau forward on the femoral condyles. This is accomplished by skeletal traction through a pin in the proximal tibia, following section of the contracted iliotibial band and patellar retinacular expansions that are usually adherent to the joint capsule and that obliterate the lateral recesses. Posterior capsulotomy of the knee is usually not required.

Supracondylar osteotomy may be indicated in cases in which fixed flexion deformity is very marked and there are structural bony changes in the femoral condyles. Osteotomy is also indicated to align the lower limb when significant genu valgum persists following correction of soft-tissue contracture.[504]

GENU RECURVATUM

Hyperextension of the knee in poliomyelitis may develop as a result of stretching of the soft tissues in the back of the knee or may be due to structural bone changes with depression and downward sloping of the anterior portion of the tibial plateau.

The first type occurs when there is extensive paralysis of the lower limb with marked weakness of the hamstrings, triceps surae, and quadriceps femoris muscles (Fig. 5–80). There is often calcaneus deformity of the foot. With continued weight-bearing, the hamstring and triceps surae muscles and the capsule and ligaments in the posterior aspect of the knee will stretch and elongate. The degree of genu recurvatum rapidly increases with loss of the support normally provided by the muscles and ligaments. Functional disability is usually great; an above-knee orthosis with a posterior knee strap is frequently required to support the knee. Heyman recommends the use of peroneal tendons to construct posterior check ligaments to prevent hyperextension of the knee.[522-524] When there is associated excessive lateral instability of the knee, the collateral ligaments are also reinforced. The tendons are passed through drill holes that are superior to the epiphyseal plate at the lower end of the femur, and inferior to the epiphyseal plate of the upper end of the tibia, thus avoiding any injury to the epiphyseal plate. The tendons are firmly anchored with the knee in 30 degrees of flexion. A long leg cast is worn for six weeks. The knee is then further protected for three months in an above-knee orthosis that limits extension of the knee at 5 degrees less than neutral. In a long term follow-up note, Heyman reported complete and lasting correction in five cases, with extension of the knee limited to a point just short of neutral. In the experience of the author, however, under the forces of body weight, the tendons and shortened soft tissues eventually become stretched and the deformity recurs. The author recommends the Heyman tenodesis operation for genu recurvatum in a patient under ten years of age in whom osseous structural changes in the tibial plateau have not yet taken place. To prevent deformity from recurring until skeletal growth has been completed, the patient sleeps in a night bivalved cast, which holds the knee in 40 degrees of flexion. For walking, the knee is held in 5 to 10 degrees of flexion in an above-knee orthosis.

The second type of genu recurvatum develops when there is equinus deformity of the ankle with normal triceps surae and hamstring muscles but a weak quadriceps femoris muscle. The paralyzed quadriceps muscle is unable to lock the knee in neutral extension, and on heel-strike the proximal end of the tibia is forced into hyperextension with limited dorsiflexion of the ankle. With continued walking and stresses of weight-bearing, the anterior portion of the tibial plateau becomes depressed and is tilted inferiorly. The bony deformity is corrected either by open-up wedge osteotomy or by close-up wedge osteotomy of the proximal tibia.[539, 663] It is usually performed at the subcondylar level distal to the proximal tibial tubercle. It is best to delay surgery until completion of skeletal growth. The technique described by Irwin is simple and very satisfactory (Fig. 5–81 A and B).[539] A modified dome-shaped osteotomy will achieve the same result (Fig. 5–81 C and D).

The author, however, prefers an open-up wedge osteotomy (Fig. 5–81 E and F). The operative technique is as follows:

A curved transverse incision is made

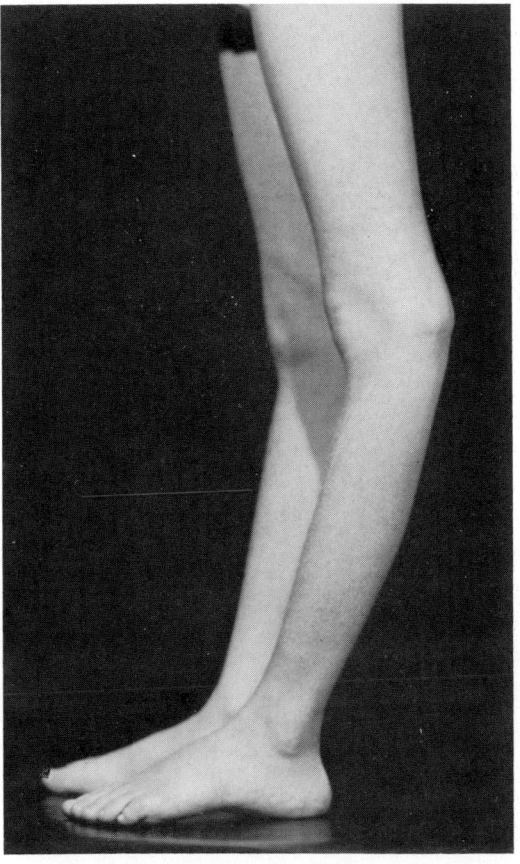

FIGURE 5–80. *Genu recurvatum in a patient with chronic poliomyelitis.*

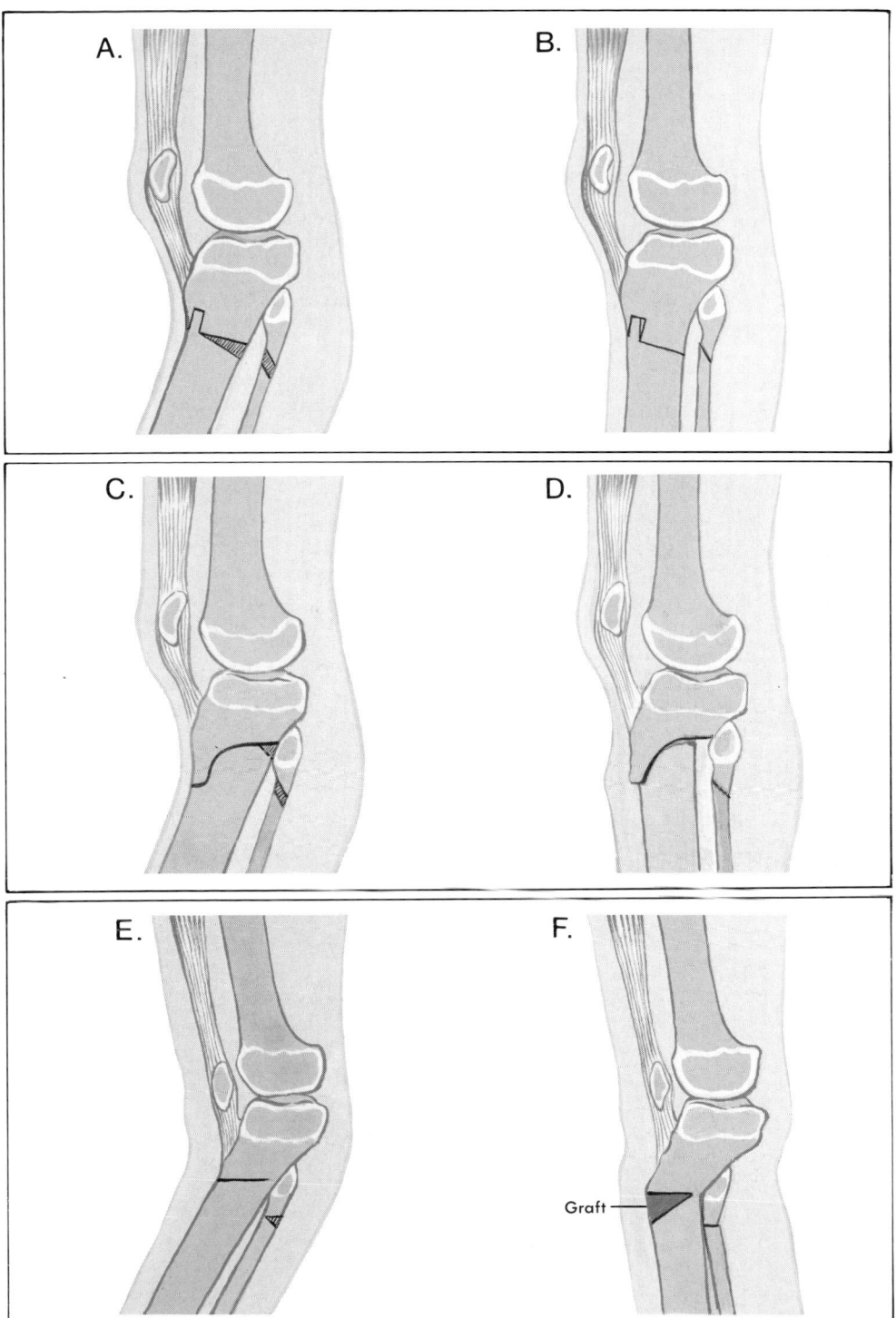

FIGURE 5–81. *Surgical method of correction of genu recurvatum.*

A and **B.** Irwin technique. **C** and **D.** Modified dome osteotomy. **E** and **F.** Open-up wedge osteotomy.

across the anterior aspect of the leg, centering 1.5 cm. distal to the proximal tibial tubercle. The lateral limb of the incision is continued proximally to terminate immediately superior and posterior to the upper end of the fibula. Subcutaneous tissue and fasciae are divided in line with the skin incision, and the wound flaps are mobilized and retracted. First, the neck and 2 cm. of the proximal shaft of the fibula are extraperiosteally exposed. Meticulous attention must be paid to avoiding damage to the common peroneal nerve and proximal fibular epiphyseal plate (if open). With drill holes and a sharp thin osteotome, a simple short oblique osteotomy of the proximal shaft of the fibula is performed. Often it is desirable to excise a wedge of bone from the proximal fibula with its base posteriorly.

Next, a T-shaped incision is made in the periosteum over the anteromedial surface of the proximal tibia. The growing apophysis of the proximal tibial tubercle and the upper epiphyseal plate of the tibia should not be disturbed by stripping the periosteum. The level of osteotomy is immediately distal to the proximal tibial tubercle; its line is marked with a starter, and then drill holes are made through the anteromedial and lateral cortices, leaving the posterior cortex of the tibia intact.

Next, three large threaded Steinmann pins are chosen and their fit in the Roger Anderson apparatus is double-checked. Starting from the medial side, the first threaded Steinmann pin is placed transversely through the distal portion of the proximal fragment. The pin should just engage in the lateral cortex of the tibia (avoiding injury to the common peroneal nerve), and it should be more posterior in position away from the proximal tibial tubercle. The second and third Steinmann pins are placed transversely through the distal fragment of the tibia 5 and 10 cm. distal to the osteotomy site. Then the tibia is divided with an osteotome, leaving the posterior cortex intact. By keeping the proximal tibial fragment in maximal hyperextension by forward pull on the first Steinmann pin and by manual pressure on the anterior surface of the knee and distal thigh, the leg and the distal segment of the tibia are forced posteriorly, creating a wedge-shaped defect at the osteotomy site with its

base anteriorly. A lamina spreader may be used effectively to open up the wedge.

Osteotomes of different widths are placed into the osteotomy site to determine the size of the iliac bone graft wedges, which are taken in routine manner with both cortices intact. It is best to take roentgenograms with the proper osteotome placed at the osteotomy site to double-check the correction. The degree of angulation at the osteotomy site should be approximately 10 degrees greater than that of the genu recurvatum, and the longitudinal axis of the distal fragment of the tibia should be parallel with that of the femur. The proximal tibial fragment should be in hyperextension.

Next, two iliac bone graft wedges are placed at the osteotomy site (one is medial, the other lateral to the tibial crest) these are locked in place with an impactor. The surrounding spaces are firmly packed with bone graft chips. The lateral bars of the Roger Anderson apparatus are tightened to provide additional stability to the osteotomy site. The correction obtained is then rechecked with roentgenograms. The wound is closed in the usual manner. The Roger Anderson apparatus is padded with petrolatum gauze in order to prevent its incorporation in the cast. A long leg cast is applied with the knee in extension.

FLAIL KNEE

A flail knee is unstable (Fig. 5–82). For weight-bearing it requires the support of an above-knee orthosis with a drop-lock knee. With such an orthosis, the patient is able to flex his knee while sitting. Arthrodesis of the knee should not be performed in children; it is best postponed until adult life when the patient is mature enough to understand and assess the advantages and disadvantages of a fused stiff knee. In unilateral involvement the author does not recommend arthrodesis of the knee, especially if there is associated muscle weakness of the hip and foot. When both lower limbs are paralyzed, however, one limb can be supported in an above-knee orthosis and the other knee stabilized by fusion, provided the hip has normal musculature and the foot is fixed in slightly equinus posture. For technical details of arthrodesis

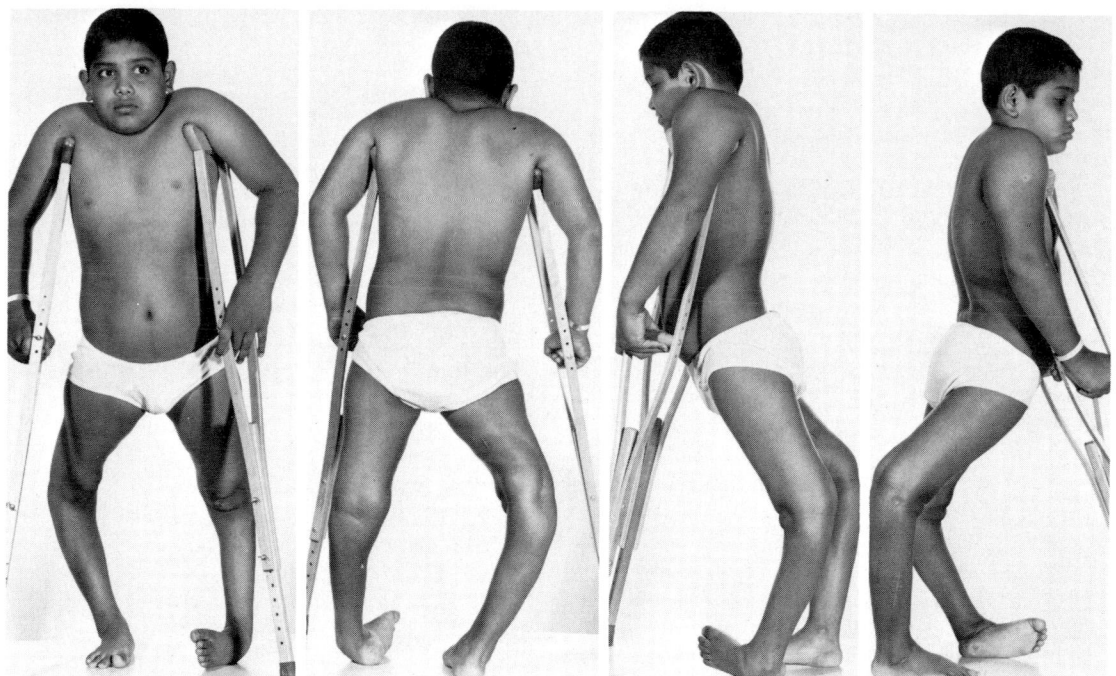

FIGURE 5–82. *Bilateral unstable flail knees in a patient with chronic poliomyelitis.*

of the knee, the reader is referred to the references.[449,588]

The Foot and Ankle

Paralysis of the muscles acting on the foot may result in various deformities and functional disability of the foot, depending upon the particular muscle or muscles involved and the strength of the remaining musculature.

The stability of the foot is dependent on several factors: the contour of the bones and the articular surfaces, the integrity of the ligamentous and capsular support, and the motor strength of the muscles.

The combined mobility of the foot and ankle is equal to that of a universal joint. Motions of the ankle, subtalar, and midtarsal joints are related to each other. In inversion of the hindfoot, for example, the os calcis is displaced forward, producing adduction and inversion of the forefoot; when the hindfoot is everted, the os calcis moves backward and the forefoot is abducted and everted. When the ankle joint is plantar flexed, the hindfoot inverts,

whereas, in dorsiflexion of the ankle, the hindfoot everts. The foot is most stable in eversion and dorsiflexion and least stable in equinus position and inversion.

The muscles that produce *plantar flexion* are the gastrocnemius-soleus, flexor hallucis longus, flexor digitorum longus, peroneus longus, peroneus brevis, and posterior tibial. *Dorsiflexor muscles* are the anterior tibial, extensor hallucis longus, extensor digitorum communis, and peroneus tertius. The muscles that produce *inversion* are the posterior tibial, flexor hallucis longus, anterior tibial; the *evertors* of the foot are the peroneus brevis, peroneus tertius, extensor digitorum communis, and extensor hallucis longus. The muscles that plantar flex the ankle and foot provide the force for forward propulsion of the body during locomotion. The dorsiflexor muscle group clears the foot during the swing phase of gait.

About two thirds of the total musculature of the leg is constituted by the triceps surae—one of the strongest muscles in the body. It acts on the foot as a first-class lever with the ankle joint as a fulcrum. The working capacity of the triceps surae is 6.5

kg.-m., whereas that of the dorsiflexors of the ankle joint is only 1.4 kg.-m., or a relative ratio of 4:1. This gross discrepancy of muscle mass between the plantar flexors and dorsiflexors of the ankle is the result of developmental and mechanical factors. The strength of the calf muscles is a necessary antigravitational force against the elevated center of body gravity in the upright posture. Also, since the center of gravity of the human body falls anterior to the ankle joint, it has a strong rotatory component of ankle dorsiflexion that the triceps surae must counteract. The muscles that provide lateral stability to the foot in plantar flexion are the posterior tibial and peroneals; whereas in dorsiflexion it is given by the action of the anterior tibial and extensor digitorum communis.

Muscle imbalance will produce progressive deformity. This is flexible in the beginning, but with skeletal growth fixed soft-tissue and structural osseous deformity will develop. The deformities of the foot and loss of function produced by muscle imbalance are predictable. The *dynamic imbalance* from paralysis of the major muscle groups, the resultant deformity, and its treatment are presented in Table 5–11.

PARALYSIS OF PERONEAL MUSCLES

When the peroneus longus and brevis muscles are paralyzed, the os calcis is pulled into inversion by the strong posterior tibial muscle. The forefoot adducts following inversion of the hindfoot and also by the unopposed action of the anterior tibial muscle. Gradually, a varus deformity of the foot is produced (Fig. 5–83). Normally, the peroneus longus depresses the first metatarsal and the anterior tibial raises it. When the peroneus longus muscle is paralyzed, the first metatarsal becomes dorsiflexed by the unopposed action of the anterior tibial, and a dorsal bunion will result. The opposing actions of the peroneus longus and anterior tibial muscles on the first metatarsal should always be considered whenever there is a dynamic imbalance between the two.

Treatment consists of lateral transfer of the anterior tibial to the base of the second metatarsal bone. Lateral stability of the foot will be adequate; arthrodesis is not required.

PARALYSIS OF PERONEALS, EXTENSOR DIGITORUM LONGUS, AND EXTENSOR HALLUCIS LONGUS

The resultant deformity will be moderately varus and somewhat equinus. Dynamic balance of the foot is restored by lateral transfer of the anterior tibial muscle to the base of the third metatarsal bone. Pes valgus deformity may result if the anterior tibial is transferred to the fourth or fifth metatarsal bones. The operative technique of lateral transfer of the anterior tibial tendon is as follows:

A longitudinal incision is made over the medial aspect of the foot; it begins at the base of the first metatarsal bone and extends proximally parallel to the course of the anterior tibial tendon for a distance of 3 cm. The anterior tibial tendon is detached from its insertion into the base of the first metatarsal bone and the medial and under surface of the first cuneiform bone. A silk whip suture is inserted into the distal end of the tendon. By sharp dissection, the tendon is mobilized over the dorsum of the foot. The dorsalis pedis artery, lying between the tendon of the extensor hallucis longus and the first tendon of the extensor digitorum longus, should not be divided.

Then a second 8 to 10 cm. long longitudinal incision is made over the anterior tibial compartment in the distal third of the leg, beginning at the upper border of the transverse crural ligament. The subcutaneous tissue and deep fascia are divided. The anterior tibial tendon is located immediately on the fibular side of the anterior crest of the tibia. The anterior tibial vessels lie between the anterior tibial and extensor hallucis longus muscles in the middle third of the leg. At the ankle, the extensor hallucis longus tendon crosses the anterior tibial vessels from the lateral to the medial side. The deep peroneal nerve is located on the lateral side of the anterior tibial vessels in the upper third of the leg, in front of the artery in the middle third and then again lateral in the distal third. Caution should be exercised in order not to injure the deep peroneal nerve and the anterior tibial vessels. The anterior tibial sheath is divided and by gentle traction, using the two-hand technique, the tendon is delivered into the proximal wound. Transfer of the anterior tibial tendon on the dorsum of the foot distal to the transverse crural ligament from the medial to the lateral side will not correct the varus action of the muscle.

Next, an incision 3 cm. long is made over the dorsum of the foot with its center over the base of the third metatarsal bone. With an Ober tendon passer, the anterior tibial tendon is delivered into the dorsum of the foot, passing deep to the transverse crural ligament to produce straight dorsiflexion. It is securely fixed to the base of the third metatarsal bone with the ankle joint in neutral or 5 degrees dorsiflexed position (see Plate 40). The muscle should be under physiologic tension. The wounds are closed in routine fashion and a long leg cast is applied, with the ankle in 5 degrees of dorsiflexion and the knee in 45 degrees of flexion.

PARALYSIS OF ANTERIOR TIBIAL MUSCLE

Dorsiflexor and inversion power of the foot is lost when the anterior tibial muscle is paralyzed, and equinovalgus deformity of the foot will develop (Fig. 5-84). The toe extensors are overactive in an attempt to substitute for the action of the anterior tibial in dorsiflexion of the ankle. The proximal phalanges of the toes become hyperextended and depress the metatarsal heads, causing cock-up deformity of the toes. Equinus deformity of the ankle gradually results from contracture of the triceps surae. Occasionally cavovarus deformity of the foot may result because of the action of the peroneus longus muscle, which acts as a depressor of the first metatarsal. On active dorsiflexion of the ankle, the forefoot is everted, but on weight-bearing it goes into inversion to permit horizontal contact of all metatarsal heads on the ground. The heel will invert following the forefoot inversion.

Treatment. During the convalescent phase of poliomyelitis, aggressive measures should be taken to retain passive range of dorsiflexion of the ankle joint. Passive heel cord stretching exercises are performed every day. At night, a bivalved cast is used to hold the ankle in neutral position, and during the day a below-knee dorsiflexion assist orthosis supports the ankle.

If proper treatment is neglected, fixed equinus deformity may develop. In such an instance, the heel cord should not be lengthened, and every effort should be made to retain function of the triceps surae muscle. Range of dorsiflexion of the ankle may be obtained by a wedging cast or a short-leg walking cast with an anterior heel. In severe fixed equinus deformity, posterior capsulotomy of the ankle and subtalar joints is performed and the heel cord is stretched with skeletal traction through a Steinmann pin in the os calcis. Functional disability is great following loss of plantar flexion power.

Dorsiflexion power of the ankle is restored by anterior transfer of the peroneus longus tendon to the base of the second metatarsal bone. The peroneus brevis is sutured to the distal stump of the peroneus longus. The operative technique and postoperative care of anterior transfer of the peroneus longus is described and illustrated in Plate 40. The peroneus longus tendon should not be attached to the base of the first metatarsal since it will displace the bone upward and cause a dorsal bunion. If there is a cock-up deformity of the toes, the long toe extensors are transferred to the heads of the metatarsals. If both peroneals are transferred, lateral instability of the foot will develop, necessitating stabilization of the hindfoot by extra-articular subtalar arthrodesis or triple arthrodesis.

PARALYSIS OF ANTERIOR TIBIAL, TOE EXTENSORS, AND PERONEALS

Equinovarus deformity of the foot will develop from the unopposed action of the posterior tibial and triceps surae muscles (Fig. 5-85). Treatment consists of anterior transfer of the posterior tibial tendon through the interosseous space to the base of the third metatarsal (Plate 41). Preoperatively, equinovarus deformity should be fully corrected by a stretching cast. Soft-tissue release may be indicated for correction of the fixed pes varus.

The flexor digitorum longus or flexor hallucis longus may be transferred anteriorly through the interosseous route to reinforce the strength of dorsiflexion power of the posterior tibial transfer. Anterior

Table 5–11.   *Tendon Transfers for Paralytic Deformities of the Foot and Ankle*

Dynamic Imbalance Paralyzed or Weak	*Normal or Strong*	**Deformity of Foot**	**Tendon Transfer**	**Remarks**
Peroneus longus Peroneus brevis	*Anterior tibial* Extensor hallucis longus Extensor digit. communis Posterior tibial Gastrocnemius-soleus Flexor hallucis longus Flexor digit. longus	Varus

Dorsal bunion (first metatarsal dorsi-flexed because of unopposed action of anterior tibial) | Lateral transfer of anterior tibial to base of second metatarsal | Perform transfer before fixed deformity develops Lateral stability will be retained Do not transfer more lateral than second metatarsal in presence of strong extensor digit. communis (will cause pes valgus) |
| Peroneus longus Peroneus brevis Extensor digit. communis Extensor hallucis longus | *Anterior tibial* Posterior tibial Gastrocnemius-soleus Flexor hallucis longus Flexor digit. longus | Varus, some equinus | Lateral transfer of anterior tibial to base of third metatarsal | Do not transfer further lateral than base of third metatarsal (will cause pes valgus) |
| Peroneus longus Peroneus brevis Extensor digit. communis Extensor hallucis longus Anterior tibial | *Posterior tibial* Gastrocnemius-soleus Flexor hallucis longus Flexor digit. longus | Equinovarus | Anterior transfer of posterior tibial tendon through interosseous space to base of third metatarsal | Preoperatively, equinovarus deformity should be fully corrected by stretching cast or soft-tissue surgery May consider reinforcing posterior tibial transfer by adding flexor hallucis longus or flexor digit. longus to anterior transfer through interosseous space; anterior tenodesis to prevent dropping down of foot is another choice Postoperatively, support transfer by dorsi-flexion assist below-knee orthosis |
| Anterior tibial | *Peroneus longus* Peroneus brevis Extensor hallucis longus Extensor digit. communis Gastrocnemius-soleus Posterior tibial Flexor hallucis longus Flexor digit. longus | Equinovalgus

Cock-up deformity of toes (over-activity of toe extensors displaces proximal phalanges of toes into hyperextension and depresses metatarsal heads Occasionally cavovarus deformity of foot results (unopposed peroneus longus acts as depressor of first metatarsal) | Anterior transfer of peroneus longus to base of second metatarsal (suture peroneus brevis to distal stump of peroneus longus) | Do not attach peroneus longus to first metatarsal (will displace it upward and cause dorsal bunion) Transfer long toe extensors to heads of metatarsals if cock-up deformity of toes is present If both peroneals are transferred, lateral instability of foot will develop, necessitating stabilization by subtalar extra-articular or triple arthrodesis |
| Gastrocnemius-soleus (motor strength zero or trace) | *Peroneus longus* *Peroneus brevis* *Flexor hallucis longus* *Posterior tibial*

Flexor digit. longus *Anterior tibial* Extensor hallucis longus Extensor digit. communis | Calcaneus or Calcaneocavus | Posterior transfer (to os calcis) of both peroneals, posterior tibial, and flexor hallucis longus | *Caution* — Prevent development of dorsal bunion by lateral transfer of anterior tibial to base of second metatarsal within a year In adolescent patient with fixed calcaneus deformity, before tendon transfers, perform triple arthrodesis with posterior shift of os calcis to correct bony deformity In young child, calcaneus deformity will correct with subsequent growth; however, subtalar extra-articular arthrodesis may be required for lateral stability |

Table 5–11. *Tendon Transfers for Paralytic Deformities of the Foot and Ankle (Continued)*

Dynamic Imbalance Paralyzed or Weak	Normal or Strong	Deformity of Foot	Tendon Transfer	Remarks
Gastrocnemius-soleus (motor strength poor)	As above	Calcaneus or Calcaneocavus	Posterior transfer (to os calcis) of posterior tibial and peroneus longus	Suture distal stump of peroneus longus to peroneus brevis Watch closely for possible development of dorsal bunion; lateral transfer of anterior tibial to base of second metatarsal may be indicated
Gastrocnemius-soleus Posterior tibial Peroneus longus Peroneus brevis	*Anterior tibial* *Flexor hallucis longus* Extensor hallucis longus Extensor digit. communis Flexor digit. longus	Calcaneovarus	Posterior transfer (to os calcis) of anterior tibial and flexor hallucis longus	Suture distal stump of flexor hallucis longus to flexor hallucis brevis Interphalangeal joint fusion of great toe may be necessary
Anterior tibial Gastrocnemius-soleus	*Peroneus longus* *Peroneus brevis* *Posterior tibial* Flexor hallucis longus Flexor digitorum longus Extensor hallucis longus Extensor digitorum longus	Calcaneovarus	Posterior transfer (to os calcis) of both peroneals and posterior tibial	Perform triple arthrodesis in adolescence to provide lateral stability to hindfoot.
Gastrocnemius-soleus Posterior tibial Peroneus longus Peroneus brevis Flexor hallucis longus Flexor digit. longus	*Anterior tibial* Extensor hallucis longus Extensor digit. communis	Calcaneovarus	Posterior transfer (to os calcis) of anterior tibial	Protect transfer with plantar flexion assist orthosis until skeletal maturity Consider tendo Achillis tenodesis In adolescence, if adequate function exists in transferred anterior tibial, foot is stabilized by triple arthrodesis If anterior tibial function is inadequate, Chuinard type ankle fusion is performed (will provide stability and gait will improve considerably)
Gastrocnemius-soleus Posterior tibial Peroneus longus Peroneus brevis Flexor hallucis longus Flexor digit. longus Anterior tibial	Extensor hallucis longus Extensor digit. communis	Calcaneovalgus (minimal)	Ankle fusion (Chuinard type)	Stability and muscle control of knee should be adequate Full knee extension and functioning hamstrings are prerequisite
Flail ankle and foot (all muscles paralyzed)	None except short toe flexors and intrinsic muscles of foot	Flexion of toes and metatarsus varus Hindfoot neutral or valgus (may be in inversion due to contracture of plantar fascia)	Pantalar arthrodesis Resect motor branches of plantar nerves	As above
Anterior tibial Extensor hallucis longus Extensor digit. communis Peroneus longus Peroneus brevis Posterior tibial	Gastrocnemius-soleus Flexor digit. longus Flexor hallucis longus	Equinus	Anterior transfer of flexor digit. longus and flexor hallucis through interosseous space Anterior tenodesis	Do not lengthen tendo Achillis (will produce calcaneus deformity) Disability is little (patient must lift leg to clear toes) Stretch triceps surae, use night support to prevent fixed equinus deformity

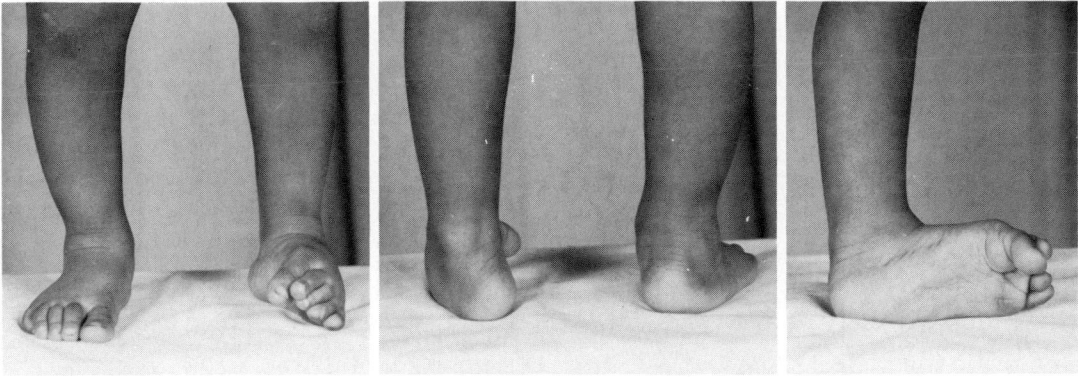

FIGURE 5–83.   Paralytic pes varus.

The deformity is the result of paralysis of the peroneus longus and brevis muscles. The hindfoot is inverted by the pull of the strong posterior tibial muscle, and the forefoot is adducted and inverted by the unopposed action of the anterior tibial muscle. Note that the first metatarsal is dorsiflexed and a dorsal bunion is produced.

tenodesis is another method of preventing the foot from dropping down in plantar flexion. In the postoperative period, the anterior transfer and tenodesis should be supported in a below-knee dynamic dorsiflexion assist orthosis during the day and a bivalved cast at night.

PARALYSIS OF TRICEPS SURAE MUSCLE

When the gastrocnemius and soleus muscles are weak or paralyzed, the patient will walk with a calcaneus limp, i.e., there is weakness or lack of push-off. The tibia is displaced posteriorly on the talus by the forward thrust of the trunk, and the foot is forced into excessive dorsiflexion at the ankle joint.

The tendo Achillis inserts into the posterior aspect of the apophysis of the os calcis. Normally, the force exerted by the triceps surae muscle elevates the heel, depresses the anterior end of the os calcis, and pushes the body forward. The longitudinal arch is flattened as the head of the talus plantar-flexes with the anterior end of the os calcis. In paralysis of the gastrocnemius and soleus muscles, the head of the talus and anterior end of the os calcis are displaced upward to a more vertical position. This results in the disappearance of the normal prominence of the heel and an increase in the range of dorsiflexion of the ankle. When the accessory plantar flexor

muscles (i.e., the posterior tibial, flexor hallucis longus, flexor digitorum longus, and peroneals) are strong, the forefoot is forced into equinus position, producing a cavus deformity. The foot is shortened by plantar flexion of the metatarsals and by rotation of the os calcis into a vertical position. Soon the plantar fascia and short flexors of the toes will develop contracture and act as a bowstring, pulling together the metatarsal heads and the os calcis, and increasing the cavus deformity (Fig. 5–86). The calcaneocavus deformity progressively increases with every step. With paralysis of the triceps surae, growth of the apophysis of the os calcis is retarded. This is particularly important in a young child in whom, following an early and successful posterior tendon transfer to the os calcis, the calcaneus deformity of the heel may be restored to normal.

Treatment. As stated previously, the triceps surae muscle is the strongest muscle of the foot. Therefore, it is desirable to transfer three or four muscles posteriorly to the os calcis, depending upon their availability and the degree of weakness of the triceps surae. Plantar flexion at the ankle is more important functionally than dorsiflexion.

When the motor strength of the triceps surae muscle is zero, both peroneus longus and brevis, the posterior tibial, and flexor hallucis longus are transferred to the os calcis. The anterior tibial is transferred laterally to the base of the second metatarsal
(Text continued on page 986.)

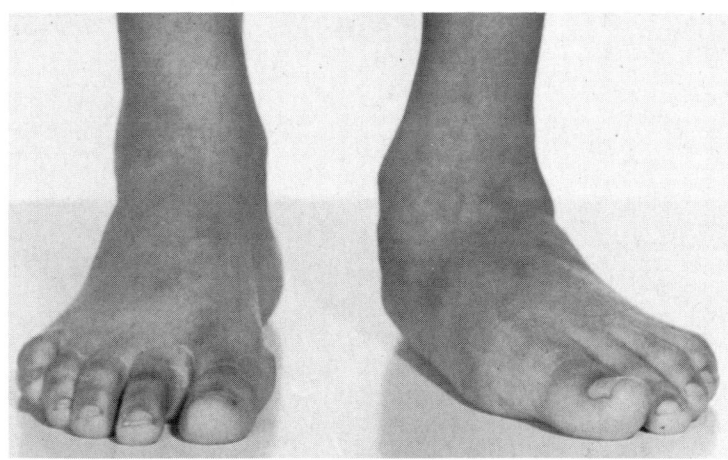

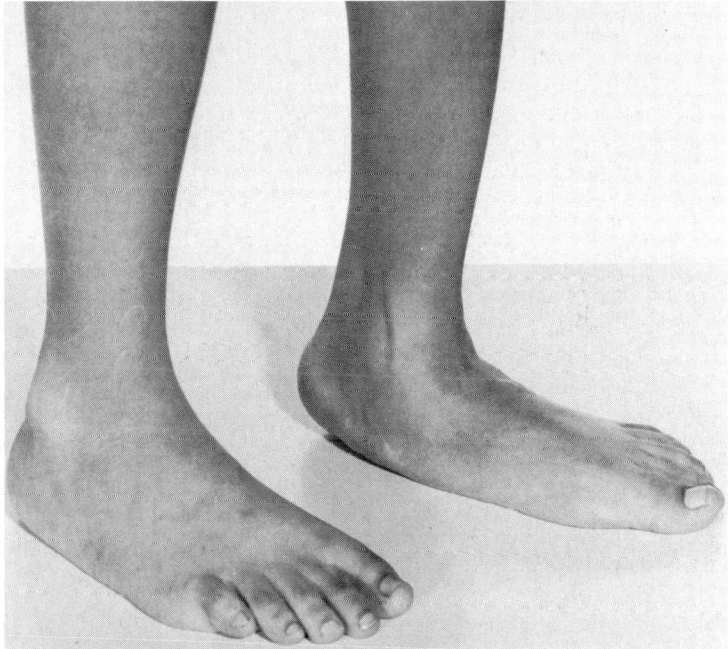

FIGURE 5–84. Equinovalgus deformity of the foot as a result of paralysis of the anterior tibial muscle.

Anterior Transfer of Peroneus Longus Tendon to Base of Second Metatarsal

The patient is placed in semilateral position with a sandbag under the hip on the affected side.

A. A 3 to 4 cm. long incision is made over the lateral aspect of the foot, extending from the base of the fifth metatarsal to a point 1 cm. distal to the tip of the lateral malleolus. Subcutaneous tissue is divided and the tendons of the peroneus longus and brevis are exposed. Then a second incision is made over the fibular aspect of the leg; it begins 3 cm. above the lateral malleolus and extends proximally for a distance of 7 cm. Subcutaneous tissue and deep fascia are incised, and the peroneal tendons are exposed by dividing their sheath. The peroneus longus tendon lies superficial to that of the peroneus brevis. The muscle is inspected to ensure that it is of normal gross appearance.

B. Next, the peroneus brevis muscle is detached from the base of the fifth metatarsal and a whip suture is inserted into its distal end.

C and **D.** The peroneus longus tendon is divided as far distally as possible. The peroneus brevis is sutured to the distal stump of the peroneus longus to preserve the longitudinal arch and depression of the first metatarsal.

Plate 40. *Anterior Transfer of Peroneus Longus Tendon to Base of Second Metatarsal*

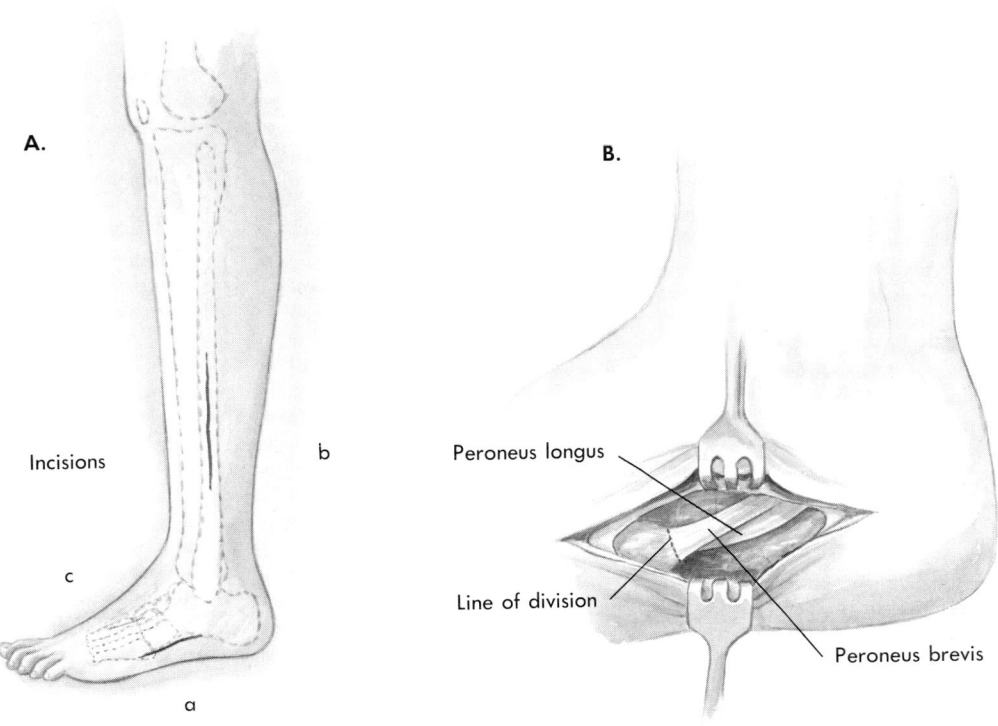

A.

Incisions

b

c

a

B.

Peroneus longus

Line of division

Peroneus brevis

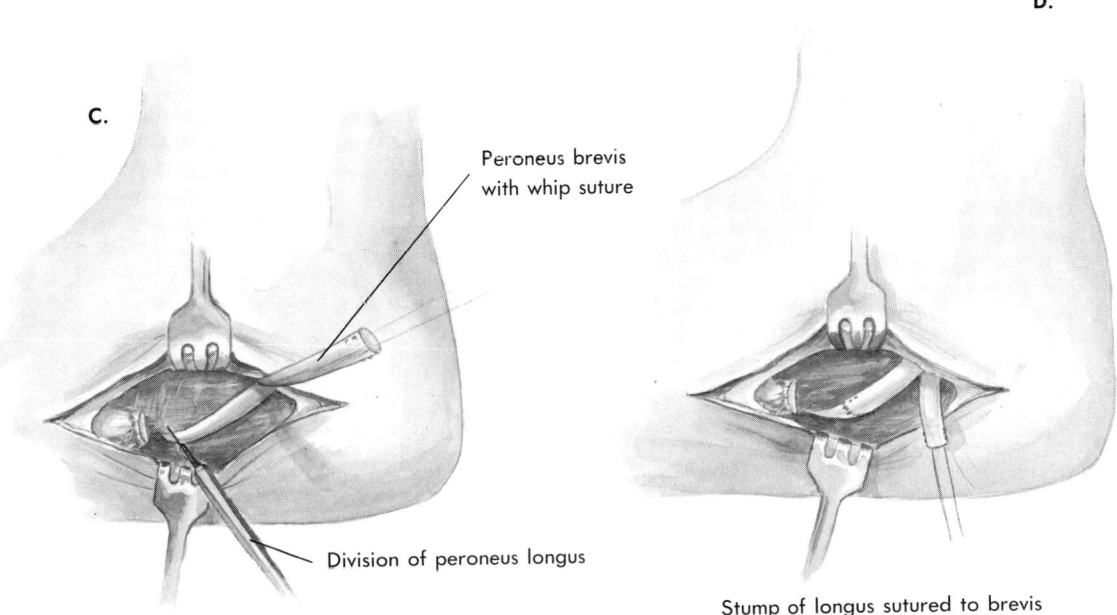

C.

Peroneus brevis
with whip suture

Division of peroneus longus

D.

Stump of longus sutured to brevis

983

Anterior Transfer of Peroneus Longus Tendon to Base of Second Metatarsal *(Continued)*

E and **F.** The peroneus longus tendon is mobilized, and with the two-hand technique, it is gently pulled into the proximal wound in the leg. The origin of the peroneus brevis from the fibula should not be disrupted.

An adequate opening is made in the intermuscular septum, taking care not to injure neurovascular structures.

G and **H.** A 2 to 3 cm. long longitudinal incision is made over the dorsum of the foot, centering over the base of the second metatarsal bone. The deep fascia is divided and the extensor tendons are retracted to expose the proximal one fourth of the second metatarsal bone. The periosteum is divided longitudinally and the cortex of the recipient bone is exposed.

With an Ober tendon passer, the peroneus longus tendon along with its sheath is passed into the anterior tibial compartment, deep to the cruciate crural and tarsal ligaments, and delivered into the incision on the dorsum of the foot. The author does not recommended a subcutaneous route. It should be ensured that there is a direct line of pull of the peroneus longus tendon from its origin to its insertion.

I and **J.** A drill hole is made in the base of the second metatarsal. A star-head hand drill is used to enlarge the hole to receive the tendon adequately. The peroneus longus tendon is passed through the recipient hole and sutured on itself under correct tension. If the peroneus longus tendon is not of adequate length, two small holes are made 1.5 cm. distal to the large hole at each side of the metatarsal shaft. The silk sutures at the end of the tendon are passed from the large central hole to the lateral distal small holes and the tendon is securely sutured to the bone. The ankle joint should be in neutral position or 5 degrees of dorsiflexion. The pneumatic tourniquet is released and hemostasis is obtained. The wounds are closed in routine manner. A long leg cast is applied with the ankle in 5 degrees of dorsiflexion and the knee in 45 degrees of flexion. Postoperative care follows the guidelines outlined in the section on principles of tendon transfer.

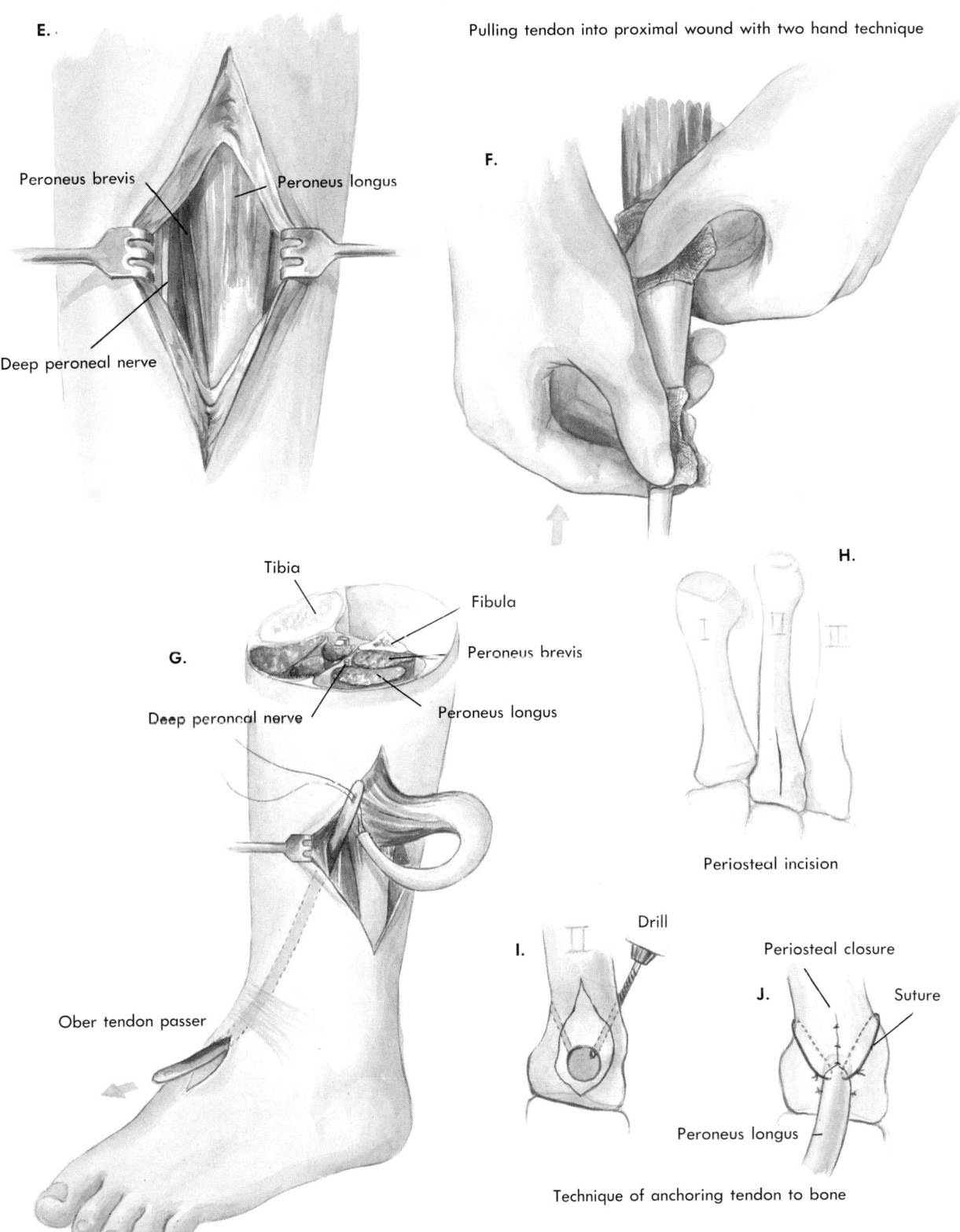

E.

Peroneus brevis

Peroneus longus

Deep peroneal nerve

Pulling tendon into proximal wound with two hand technique

F.

G.

Tibia

Fibula

Peroneus brevis

Deep peroneal nerve

Peroneus longus

Ober tendon passer

H.

I

II

III

Periosteal incision

Drill

I.

J.

Periosteal closure

Suture

Peroneus longus

Technique of anchoring tendon to bone

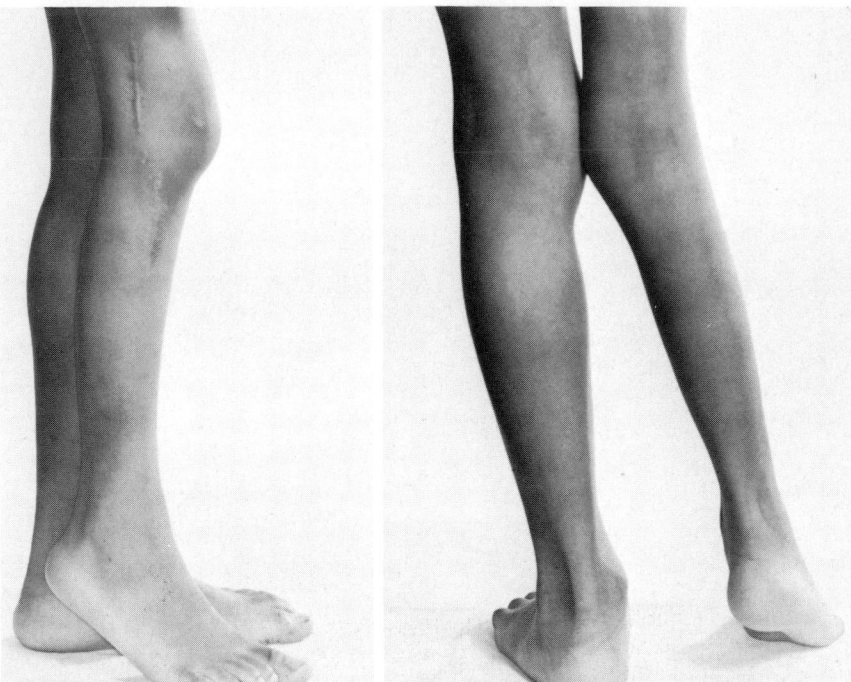

FIGURE 5–85. *Equinovarus deformity of right ankle and foot caused by unopposed action of the triceps surae and posterior tibial muscles.*

within a year to prevent formation of a dorsal bunion. In adolescents with fixed calcaneus deformity, the hindfoot is stabilized by triple arthrodesis, the bony deformity is corrected, and the os calcis is shifted posteriorly. In a young child, calcaneus deformity will be corrected by subsequent growth if the posterior transfer is successful; however, a subtalar extra-articular arthrodesis may be required later for lateral stability.

When the gastrocnemius-soleus muscles are poor in motor strength, only the peroneus longus and posterior tibial muscles are transferred. The distal stump of the peroneus longus is sutured to the peroneus brevis. If a dorsal bunion tends to develop, lateral transfer of the anterior tibial to the base of the second metatarsal may again be indicated.

When the posterior tibial and peroneal muscles are paralyzed along with the triceps surae, the muscles available for posterior transfer are the anterior tibial and flexor hallucis longus. The flexor digitorum longus may be added if necessary. The interphalan-geal joints, particularly that of the great toe, are fused.

When the anterior tibial muscle is paralyzed with the triceps surae, posterior transfer of both peroneals and the posterior tibial is performed; lateral stability of the hindfoot is provided by triple arthrodesis.

When all the plantar flexor muscles are paralyzed, the anterior tibial muscle is transferred to the os calcis. The posterior transfer is protected with a plantar flexion assist below-knee orthosis until skeletal maturity. Tendo Achillis tenodesis may be performed to provide posterior stability to the ankle joint. In adolescence, if plantar flexion function of the transferred anterior tibial is adequate, the hindfoot is stabilized by triple arthrodesis. When the anterior tibial function is inadequate, Chuinard type ankle fusion is performed.

When only the toe extensors are functioning, there will be no muscles available for posterior transfer. An ankle fusion is performed, provided there is adequate stability and muscle control of the knee.

The operative technique and postoperative care of posterior tendon transfer to the os calcis is presented in Plate 38, and Chuinard type distraction-compression bone graft arthrodesis of the ankle in Plate 44. Dorsal bunion is treated by open-up wedge osteotomy of the base of the first metatarsal and transfer of the flexor hallucis longus to the head of the first metatarsal (Plate 42).

ARTHRODESIS OF THE FOOT AND ANKLE

In the operative treatment of the paralyzed foot, a multitude of surgical procedures have been developed to provide stability, to correct deformity, and to improve function.

The history of the evolution of stabilizing operations of the foot and ankle is given in Table 5–12. The reader is referred to the original contributions and to Hart, Hallgrimson and Schwartz for comprehensive historical reviews.[505, 514, 635]

In general, stabilizing operations on the foot and ankle can be subdivided into the following: (1) triple arthrodesis, (2) extra-articular subtalar arthrodesis, (3) ankle fusion, and (4) anterior or posterior bone blocks to limit motion at the ankle joint. These procedures may be performed alone or in combination.

Triple Arthrodesis. This procedure was devised by Ryerson in 1923 and consists of fusion of the subtalar, calcaneocuboid, and talonavicular joints.[623] The operation is designed to provide lateral stability, and it will also correct deformity if the articular surfaces are resected by pattern. In locomotion, the essential motions of the foot and ankle are plantar flexion and dorsiflexion. In the presence of muscle weakness, triple arthrodesis will stabilize the hindfoot and diminish the functional demand on the remaining active muscles by reducing the number of joints that they control.

The operative technique of triple arthrodesis is described and illustrated in Plate 43.

The subtalar and midtarsal joint motions are particularly important for balance when an individual is walking upon rough or uneven terrain. The loss of lateral mobility of the hindfoot following triple arthrodesis may result in difficulty in locomotion on an irregular surface.

Triple arthrodesis may exert excessive ligamentous strain on the ankle joint. It is imperative to determine the stability of the body of the talus in the ankle mortise. This is done clinically by testing passive lateral motion of the ankle. If ankle stability is questionable, weight-bearing anteroposterior roentgenograms of the ankle with the hindfoot first in forced maximal eversion and abduction and then in forced inversion and adduction are taken. Normally, there is no lateral motion of the body of the talus in the ankle mortise except when the ankle is in marked plantar flexion; then it may be present in minimal amount. When there is marked instability of the ankle joint, varus or valgus deformity of the hindfoot may recur following triple arthrodesis, and stabilization of the ankle joint may be indicated.

Anterior subluxation of the ankle joint may be present in severe equinus deformity; this should be ruled out by making lateral roentgenograms of the ankle with the foot in maximal plantar flexion and forced dorsiflexion.

Alignment and weight-bearing lines of the lower limb should be carefully studied. The presence of genu varum, knock-knee, or any excessive internal or external tibial torsion should be noted. External tibial torsion and genu valgum are common deformities in poliomyelitis. In stance, does the center of gravity of the body fall on the second metatarsal bone? Failure to recognize malalignment of the leg will result in improper positioning of the foot. During surgery, it is mandatory that the knee be draped sterile in the operative field. The foot should be aligned with the ankle mortise and not with the knee (Fig. 5–87). If there is significant torsional or angular deformity of the leg, it is corrected at a subsequent operation.

The growth of the foot in a young child should not be disturbed. The tarsal bones grow concentrically at their periphery and resection of their articular surfaces will inhibit their growth. Triple arthrodesis should be deferred until the foot has achieved skeletal maturity, which in girls is 10 to 12 years; in boys, 12 to 14 years.

The osseous deformity of the foot should be carefully analyzed in the preoperative roentgenograms. These should include

(*Text continued on page 992.*)

Anterior Transfer of Posterior Tibial Tendon Through
Interosseous Membrane

A. A 4 cm. long incision is made over the medial aspect of the foot, beginning posterior and immediately distal to the tip of the medial malleolus and extending to the base of the first cuneiform bone. A second longitudinal incision is made 1.5 cm. posterior to the subcutaneous medial border of the tibia, beginning at the center of the middle third of the leg and ending 3 cm. from the tip of the medial malleolus.

B. The posterior tibial tendon is identified at its insertion and its sheath is divided. The tendon is freed and sectioned at its attachment to the bone, preserving maximal length. The peritenon of the distal 3 cm. of the tendon is excised and a 00 silk whip suture is inserted in its distal end.

C. The posterior tibial muscle is identified in the leg incision and its sheath opened and freed. Traction on the stump in the foot incision will aid in its identification. Moist sponges and the two-hand technique are used to deliver the posterior tibial tendon into the proximal wound. The muscle belly is freed well up the tibia. One should be careful to preserve the nerve and blood supply to the posterior tibial muscle.

D. Next, a longitudinal skin incision is made anteriorly, one fingerbreadth lateral to the crest of the tibia, starting at the proximal margin of the cruciate ligament of the ankle and extending 7 cm. proximally. Then a 4 cm. long longitudinal incision is made over the dorsum of the foot, centering over the base of the second metatarsal.

Plate 41. Anterior Transfer of Posterior Tibial Tendon Through Interosseous Membrane

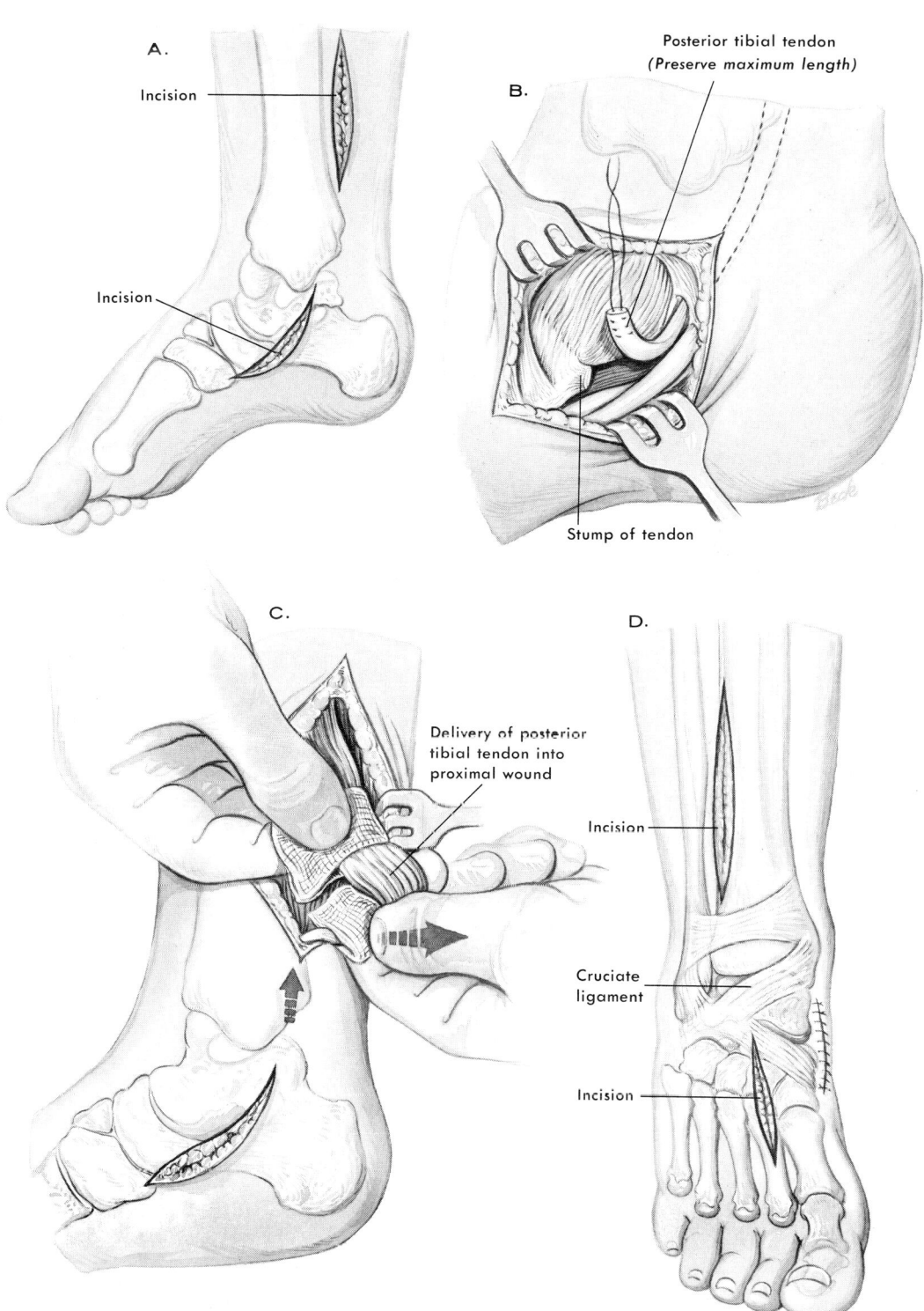

A.

Incision

Incision

B.

Posterior tibial tendon
(Preserve maximum length)

Stump of tendon

C.

Delivery of posterior
tibial tendon into
proximal wound

D.

Incision

Cruciate
ligament

Incision

Anterior Transfer of Posterior Tibial Tendon Through Interosseous Membrane (Continued)

E. The anterior tibial muscle is exposed, and elevated from the anterolateral surface of the tibia together with the anterior tibial artery and extensor hallucis longus muscle. It is retracted laterally, exposing the interosseous membrane. Next, a large rectangular window is cut in the interosseous membrane. One should avoid stripping the periosteum from the tibia or fibula.

F and **G.** Then, with an Ober tendon passer, the posterior tibial tendon is passed through the window in the interosseous membrane from the posterior into the anterior tibial compartment. One should be careful not to twist the tendon or to damage its nerve or blood supply. Next, with the aid of an Ober tendon passer, the posterior tibial tendon is passed beneath the cruciate ligament and the extensors and delivered into the wound on the dorsum of the foot. It is anchored to the base of the second metatarsal bone according to the method described in anterior transfer of peroneal tendons (Plate 40). The wounds are closed in layers in the usual manner. A long leg cast is applied, holding the foot in neutral position at the ankle joint and the knee in 45 degrees of flexion.

The principles of postoperative care are the same as for any tendon transfer.

Plate 41. Anterior Transfer of Posterior Tibial Tendon Through Interosseous Membrane

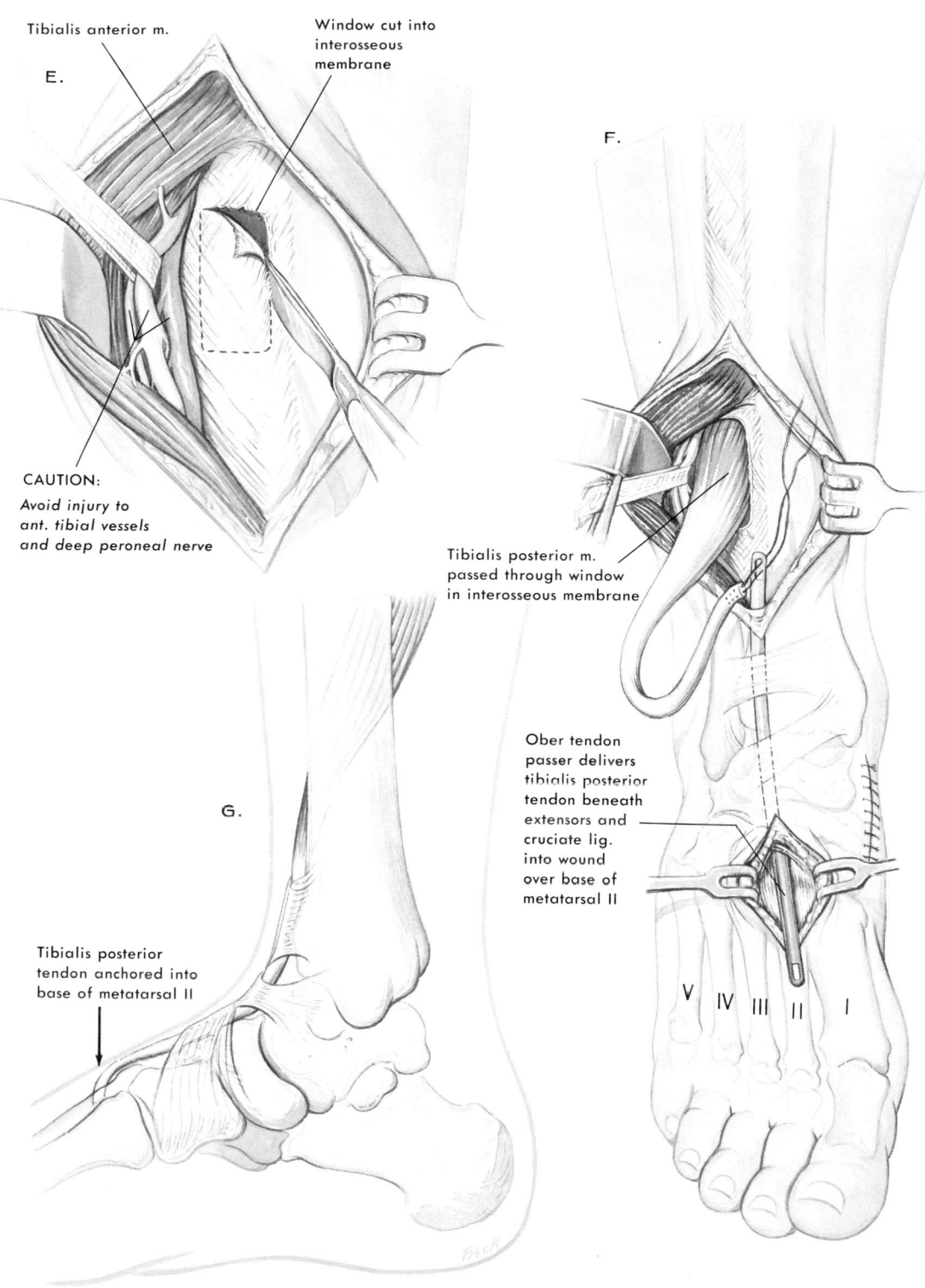

Tibialis anterior m.

Window cut into interosseous membrane

E.

CAUTION:
Avoid injury to ant. tibial vessels and deep peroneal nerve

F.

Tibialis posterior m. passed through window in interosseous membrane

Ober tendon passer delivers tibialis posterior tendon beneath extensors and cruciate lig. into wound over base of metatarsal II

G.

Tibialis posterior tendon anchored into base of metatarsal II

V IV III II I

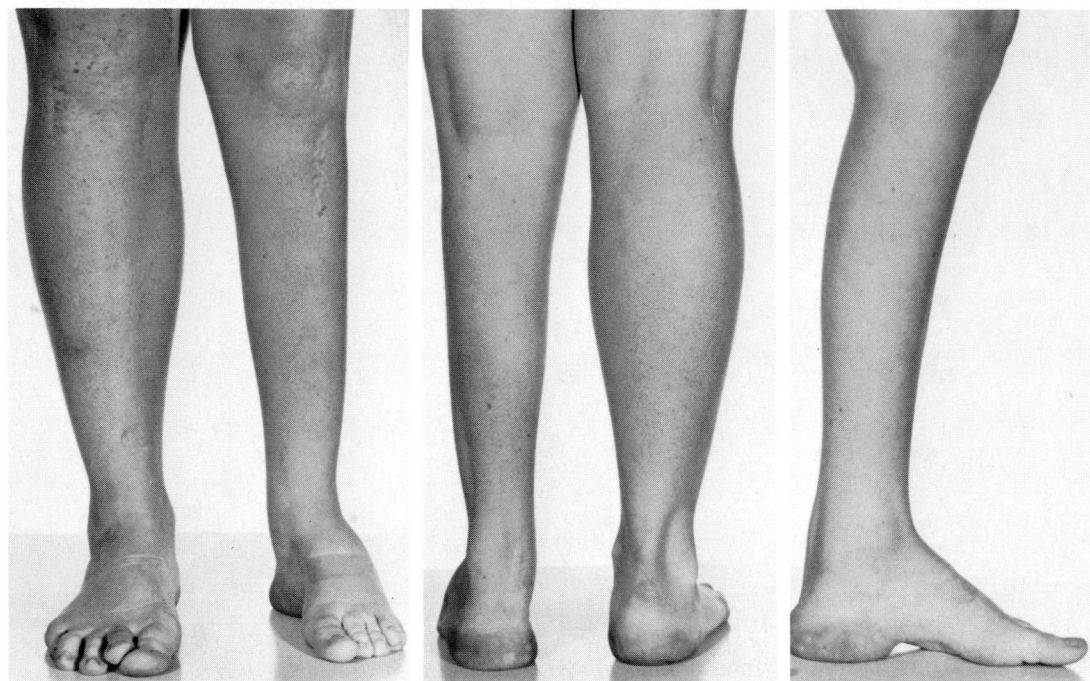

FIGURE 5–86.   Calcaneocavus deformity of the left foot and ankle.

anteroposterior and mediolateral weight-bearing views of the foot and ankle. It is important to make the roentgenograms with the foot held in the positions of maximum correction. Tracings of the foot are made on x-ray negative films. The foot and ankle are divided into three segments, according to function: (1) the talus with the tibia and ankle joint; (2) the os calcis; and (3) the tarsal bones, the joints distal to the midtarsal joint, the metatarsals and phalanges. The talus is the only tarsal bone that transmits the entire body weight; thus, the importance of double-checking the stability of the body of the talus in the ankle mortise cannot be overemphasized.

The pattern of osteotomies and the plane of resection of the articular surfaces of each joint should be carefully and precisely planned. It is best to draw these lines on tracings of the preoperative lateral roentgenograms of the foot.

In the correction of varus deformity a wedge of bone with its base lateral is resected from the talonavicular and calcaneocuboid joints (Fig. 5–88). Lateral displacement of the forefoot is often prevented by the "beak" of the navicular bone, which projects posteriorly along the medial side of the head of the talus. It is important to excise this "beak" flush with the main body of the navicular—through a separate incision if necessary. The planes of osteotomies of the talonavicular and calcaneocuboid joints should be parallel to each other in the vertical axis in order to have close apposition of bones. To correct varus deformity of the heel, a wedge with its base lateral is resected from the subtalar joint. Most of the bone should be removed from the superior surface of the calcaneus. Only a minimal amount of bone should be excised from the talus. A slight valgus position of the heel will provide stability; however, the hindfoot should not be placed in more than 5 to 10 degrees of eversion, as it will cause difficulty in the proper wearing of shoes and is not cosmetically satisfactory. A varus position of the heel should not be accepted.

Valgus deformity of the foot is corrected by excision of a wedge from the midtarsal area with its base medial, and a wedge from the subtalar region, also with its base medial. The use of a laminectomy spreader in the subtalar joint will adequately expose the medial side of the hindfoot. Great care should be exercised not to injure the posterior tibial nerves and artery, which lie adjacent and superficial to the flexor hallucis longus tendon. In the valgus foot, the os calcis is everted and the head of the talus is plantar-flexed over the medial aspect of the foot. The common tendency is to excise a large wedge in order to reduce the calcaneus medially beneath the talus. This should be avoided, as it will reduce the height of the hindfoot and lower the malleoli, resulting in a wide ankle contour and extreme difficulty in fitting shoes. When correcting severe valgus, varus, or calcaneus deformity of the foot, it is best to add bone graft wedges rather than to excise too much bone. Resection of excessive bone from the talus and navicular may also cause avascular necrosis of these tarsal bones with subsequent degenerative arthritis of the ankle and pseudarthrosis of the talonavicular joint.

For restoration of alignment of the calcaneus foot, a wedge of bone based posteriorly is resected from the subtalar joint (Fig. 5-89). Often there is associated cavus deformity, which is corrected by excising a wedge based dorsally from the talonavicular and calcaneocuboid joints. It is imperative to displace the os calcis posteriorly to provide a longer lever arm. When contracted, the anterior capsule of the ankle joint is stretched out preoperatively by passive manipulation and corrective casts. Soft-tissue contracture release may be indicated when the contracture is very fixed. It is imperative to obtain normal range of plantar flexion of the ankle.

In severe talipes calcaneus, the bony deformity and soft-tissue contracture are rigid, fixing the talus and os calcis in marked dorsiflexion. The associated cavus deformity will be marked, with severe contracture of the plantar fascia and osseous changes in the midtarsal bones. Correction of deformity by wedge resections will result in appreciable reduction in the height and length of the foot.

Plantar fasciotomy is performed first. The anterior capsule of the ankle joint is released through an anterolateral approach. Next, the articular surfaces of the subtalar and talonavicular and calcaneocuboid joints are minimally resected, exposing raw cancellous bone. The calcaneus deformity is corrected by inserting a wedge of bone graft

with its base anterior in the subtalar joint. Forefoot equinus deformity can be corrected by excising a wedge of bone based dorsally from the talonavicular and calcaneocuboid joints. Frequently, the author postpones surgical correction of the cavus deformity until solid healing of the triple arthrodesis has taken place. During the application of the long leg cast, however, it is important to immobilize the heel in moderate plantar flexion and the forefoot in maximal dorsiflexion. The common pitfall is to hold the forefoot in equinus position, permitting the cavus deformity to increase. The metatarsal heads should be well padded to prevent skin slough. Three to four months later, the metatarsals are osteotomized at their base and elevated into dorsiflexion, correcting the forefoot equinus deformity. In this way, some degree of mobility of the naviculocuneiform and cuneiform metatarsal joints is preserved.

Talectomy will correct the severe calcaneus deformity.[531, 570, 668, 686, 687] However, it reduces the height of the foot, lowers the malleoli, and causes great difficulty in fitting shoes. This is particularly disturbing to women. Fibroarthrosis and degenerative arthritis of the ankle joint will often develop in later years. For these reasons, astragalectomy is not recommended.

In classic triple arthrodesis, it is difficult to displace the os calcis backward. Dunn described a method of excising the navicular and part of the head and neck of the talus to permit posterior displacement of the calcaneus.[468, 469] Hoke had previously resected the navicular and head and neck of the talus; after subtalar joint resection and posterior displacement of the foot, he recommended reshaping and reimplantation of the head and neck of the talus.[530] The Hoke and Dunn procedures, however, shorten the foot and increase the likelihood of pseudarthrosis of the talonavicular joint. For these reasons, the author prefers correction of calcaneus deformity by bone graft wedges.

In correction of pes equinus, fixed contracture of the posterior capsule of the ankle and subtalar joints and the triceps surae muscle must be preoperatively corrected. As stated previously, function of the gastrocnemius-soleus muscles should be maintained as much as possible. Wedging

Treatment of Dorsal Bunion by Open-Up Osteotomy of Base of First Metatarsal

A. A longitudinal incision is made over the dorsomedial aspect of the foot, starting at the first cuneiform bone and extending distally to the first metatarsal head, where it is curved plantarward.

B. The base of the first metatarsal is exposed. A dorsal capsulotomy of the tarso-metatarsal and navicular-cuneiform joint may be necessary to bring the first metatarsal bone into plantar flexion. With a starter and drill, the line of open-up osteotomy on the dorsal aspect of the base of the first metatarsal is marked. The plantar cortex should be left intact. Next, with a scalpel, a U-shaped flap of capsule is raised from the dorsum of the metatarsophalangeal joint with its base attached to the proximal phalanx. If necessary, any abnormally prominent bone on the meta-tarsal head is excised. If the flexion contracture of the great toe is not corrected by manipulation, capsulotomy of the plantar aspect of the first metatarsophalangeal joint is performed. Next the flexor hallucis longus tendon is divided near its insertion and delivered into the proximal part of the wound. A tunnel is drilled in the head of the first metatarsal from its dorsal to its plantar aspect.

C. Next the osteotomy of the dorsal, medial, and lateral parts of the base of the first metatarsal is completed. The distal part of the metatarsal is manipulated into plantar flexion, taking due care not to break the plantar cortex. A wedge of autogenous bone graft from the tibia or fibula is obtained and inserted at the osteotomy site, correcting the dorsiflexion deformity of the first metatarsal. The flexor hallucis longus tendon, with a whip suture in its distal end, is brought from plantar to dorsal aspect through the tunnel in the first metatarsal head and sutured to itself; this makes the flexor hallucis longus muscle a plantar-flexor of the first metatarsal instead of the great toe.

D. The dorsal U-flap of the capsule is sutured to the flexor hallucis longus tendon on the dorsum of the metatarsal head, holding the great toe in neutral position. The wound is closed in the usual fashion. A below-knee walking cast is applied and is worn for five to six weeks.

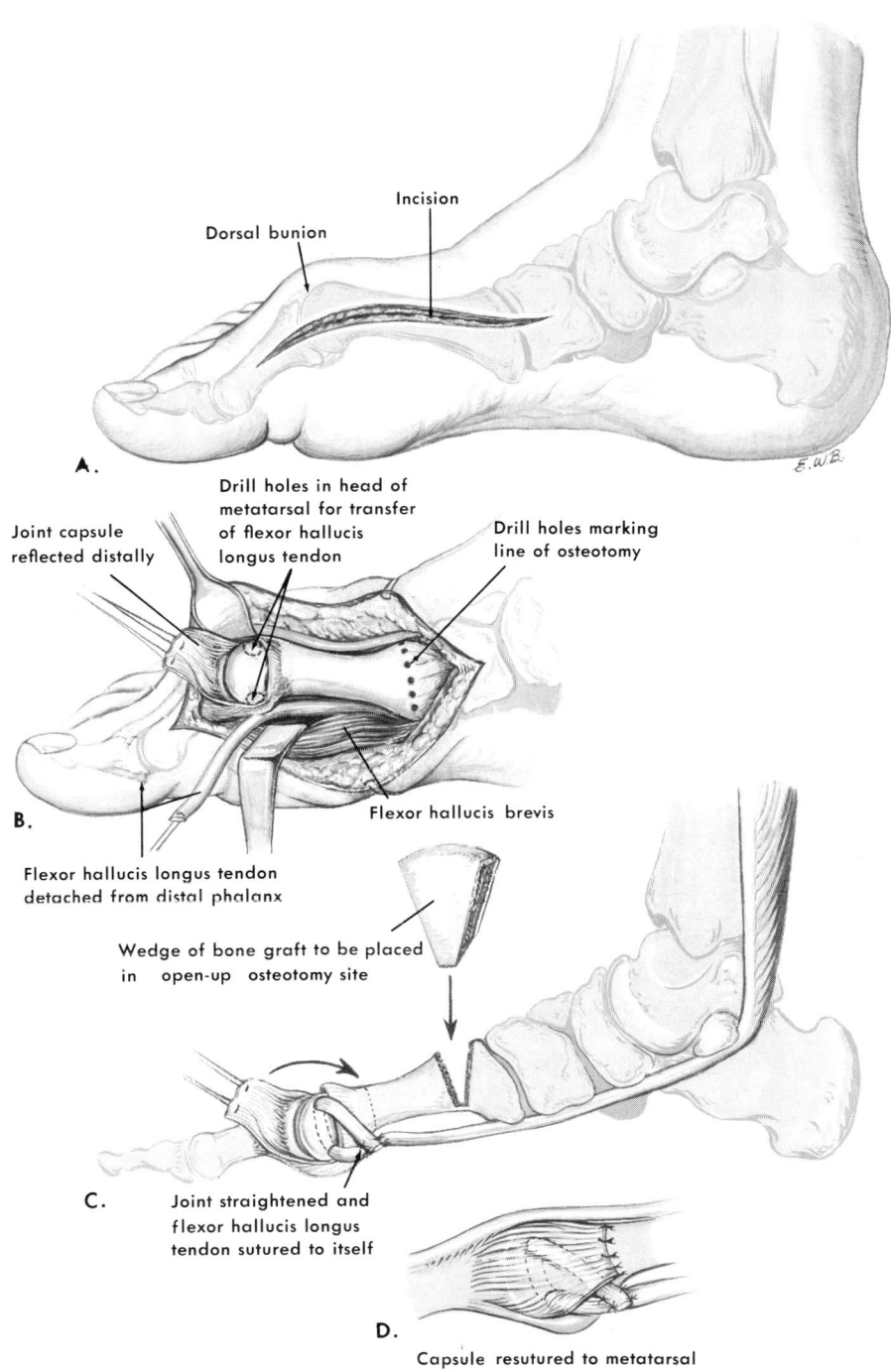

Incision

Dorsal bunion

A.

Drill holes in head of
metatarsal for transfer
of flexor hallucis
longus tendon

Joint capsule
reflected distally

Drill holes marking
line of osteotomy

Flexor hallucis brevis

B.

Flexor hallucis longus tendon
detached from distal phalanx

Wedge of bone graft to be placed
in open-up osteotomy site

C. Joint straightened and
flexor hallucis longus
tendon sutured to itself

D.

Capsule resutured to metatarsal

Table 5–12.   *History of Stabilizing Operations of the Foot and Ankle*

1879	Albert	Tibiotarsal or ankle joint arthrodesis
1879	Von Lesser	Tibiotarsal or ankle joint arthrodesis
1884	Samster	Ankle and subtalar joint arthrodesis
1901	Whitman	Talectomy and posterior displacement of the foot
1905	Nieny	Talocalcaneal and talocalcaneonavicular or subtalar arthrodesis
1908	Jones	Talocalcaneal and talocalcaneonavicular or subtalar arthrodesis
1908	Goldthwait	Supratalar and infratalar arthrodesis
1911	Lorthioir	Pantalar arthrodesis (temporary removal of the talus)
1911	Ombredanne	Surgical approach for exposure of the subtalar and midtarsal joints
1912	Soule	Talonavicular arthrodesis
1912	Soule	Talonavicular and subtalar arthrodesis
1913	Davis	Subtalar arthrodesis (transverse horizontal section of the tarsus) with posterior displacement of the foot
1915	Albee	Talonavicular arthrodesis with bone graft peg
1916	Davis	Subtalar or calcaneotalar and calcaneotalonavicular arthrodesis
1919	Dunn	Midtarsal tarsectomy and calcaneotalar arthrodesis
1920	Toupet	Posterior bone check
1921	Hoke	Calcaneotalonavicular arthrodesis resection, reshaping and reimplantation of head and neck of the talus, and posterior displacement of the foot.
1922	Dunn	Excision of navicular bone, calcaneotalocuneiform and calcaneocuboid arthrodesis with posterior displacement of the foot
1922	Putti	Anterior bone check
1922	Steindler	Pantalar arthrodesis (talus not temporarily removed)
1923	Ryerson	Triple (subtalar and calcaneocuboid) arthrodesis
1923	Ryerson	Lateral arthrodesis (cuneonavicular, first and fifth tarsometatarsal arthrodesis)
1923	Campbell	Posterior bone block
1925	Smith and von Lackum	Calcaneotalonavicular and calcaneocuboid arthrodesis, excision of head and neck of talus with posterior displacement of the foot
1927	Lambrinudi	Resection of wedge of bone from plantar aspect of head and neck of talus to lock the talus in equinus position at the ankle while the rest of the foot is in the desired degree of dorsiflexion
1933	Brewster	Calcaneonaviculocuneiform arthrodesis, excision of head and neck of the talus, posterior displacement of the foot and countersinking of the body of the talus in the os calcis
1935	Girard	Arthrodesis of subtalar and calcaneocuboid joints; shortening of the neck of the talus; posterior displacement of foot; construction of ankle joint mortise
1952	Grice	Extra-articular arthrodesis of subtalar joint
1963	Chuinard and Peterson	Distraction-compression bone graft arthrodesis of the ankle

casts are tried first, followed by posterior capsulotomy and skeletal traction through the os calcis. In severe equinus deformity, limited heel cord lengthening may have to be performed, but it is preferable to leave some tightness of the triceps surae. It is imperative that the foot be dorsiflexed to neutral position; otherwise a rocker-bottom deformity of the foot will result. In cerebral palsied patients, the author maintains reduction with a large Kirschner wire. One pin is placed through the os calcis into the talus and across the ankle joint into the tibia, while the other transfixes the talonavicular joint. When equinus posture is due simply to drop foot and the foot can be passively dorsiflexed beyond neutral position, it is preferable to perform tendon transfer anteriorly to provide power of active dorsiflexion. If adequate muscles are not available for anterior transfer, the triple arthrodesis may be modified to prevent the foot from dropping down into plantar flexion. Lambrinudi, in 1927, described a method of triple arthrodesis in which a wedge of bone is excised from the plantar aspect of the head and neck of the talus and the distal sharp margin of the body of the talus is inserted into a prepared trough in the navicular. Thus the talus is locked in equinus position at the ankle joint, whereas the rest of the foot is maintained in the desired degree of dorsi-flexion.[553]

The Lambrinudi operation is not recommended by the author, as his experience with it has been unsatisfactory. For adequate correction of equinus deformity, too much bone has to be resected from the talus, with consequent development of avascular necrosis of the talus, talonavicular pseudarthrosis, flattening of the superior surface of the talus, and painful arthritis of the ankle.[411, 476, 515, 554, 572, 577, 606]

Extra-articular Subtalar Arthrodesis.

Grice, at the suggestion of William T. Green, developed a method of fusion of the subtalar joint by insertion of autogenous bone grafts in the sinus tarsi in the lateral aspect of the foot for correction of paralytic pes valgus and restoration of the height of the longitudinal arch.[496, 498] Any interference with subsequent normal growth of the foot is minimal, at most, because the procedure is extra-articular. The operative technique is described and illustrated in plate 30.

With paralysis of the posterior tibial and anterior tibial muscles, and with unopposed action of the strong peroneal and triceps surae muscles, the os calcis becomes everted and displaced laterally and posteriorly. The talus moves forward and on weight-bearing, its head drops into equinus position, projecting on the plantar and medial aspects of the instep of the foot. The forepart of the foot is displaced laterally. In the beginning, the deformity is flexible and the normal anatomic relationship of the talus and calcaneus can be restored by passive inversion of the os calcis and the placing of its anterior portion medially and forward beneath the head of the talus. With growth over a period of several years, the deformity becomes fixed; the capsules of the tibiotalar and midtarsal joints contract, the triceps surae shortens permanently, and secondary structural changes take place. All these factors prevent the repositioning of the anterior part of the calcaneus beneath the head of the talus. Preoperatively it is imperative to determine if the calcaneus can be restored to its normal position beneath the talus by making lateral roentgenograms of the foot after it has been passively manipulated into an equinus position and inversion.

When there is contracture of the triceps surae muscle, it is essential to make a lateral roentgenogram of the foot and ankle with the foot in inversion and the ankle in maximal forced dorsiflexion. Equinus deformity should be corrected by diligent use of wedging casts prior to the subtalar extra-articular arthrodesis. If correction cannot be obtained with a wedging cast alone, posterior capsulotomy of the tibiotalar joint and skeletal traction through the os calcis is carried out. In severe equinus deformity, limited heel cord lengthening may be indicated as a last resort.

Failure to correct equinus deformity of the talus will result in fusion of the os calcis to the talus, with the heel in fixed equinus position and eversion and the forefoot in abduction. Upon weight-bearing the talus will be tilted into valgus deviation within the ankle mortise. If it is impossible to place the calcaneus in a normal position beneath the talus, the Grice procedure should not be performed.

A valgus ankle joint may also be caused by shortening of the fibula. In paralyzed limbs the fibula is frequently underdeveloped, with the distal fibular epiphyseal plate being at the same or at a more proximal level than that of the tibia.[574] Removal of a bone graft from the ipsilateral tibia will definitely accelerate growth of that bone and further increase the disparity in length between the fibula and tibia.[604] It is best to use fibular bone graft from the involved limb, as it will stimulate growth of the shortened fibula.[444] Too long a segment of the fibula should not be excised, however, and its periosteum should be meticulously closed to ensure union. When bilateral extra-articular subtalar arthrodesis is performed, an autogenous fibular bone graft should be taken from each leg. A common tendency is to take a long segment of the fibula from one leg to use for both feet; this, however, will result in nonunion of the fibula, a high-riding lateral malleolus, and valgus deformity of the ankle.

When there is marked valgus deformity of the ankle, correction by supramalleolar osteotomy of the tibia may be required. A growth arrest of the medial side of the distal tibial epiphyseal plate performed at the appropriate age will also correct the deformity; however, it should not be performed when the involved leg is short, since it will further increase the leg length discrepancy. It

(*Text continued on page 1002.*)

Triple Arthrodesis

A pneumatic tourniquet is placed on the proximal thigh, and the patient is positioned semilaterally with a large sandbag under the hip on the affected side.

A. A curvilinear incision is made, centering over the sinus tarsi. It starts one fingerbreadth distal and posterior to the tip of the lateral malleolus and extends anteriorly and distally to the base of the second metatarsal bone.

B. Skin flaps should not be developed. The incision is carried to the floor of the sinus tarsi. By sharp dissection, with scalpel and periosteal elevator, the periosteum of the calcaneus, the adipose tissue contents of the sinus tarsi, and the tendinous origin of the exterior digitorum brevis are elevated in one mass from the calcaneus and lateral aspect of the neck of the talus and retracted distally. It is essential to provide a viable soft-tissue pedicle to obliterate the dead space remaining at the end of the operation.

Next, an incision is made superiorly over the periosteum of the talus, and the head and neck of the talus are carefully exposed. The upper flap of the skin, subcutaneous tissue, and periosteum should be kept as thick as possible to avoid necrosis. Traction sutures are placed on the periosteum. At no time are the skin edges to be retracted. It is not necessary to divide the peroneal tendons or their sheaths. By subperiosteal dissection, the peroneal tendons are retracted posteriorly for exposure of the subtalar joint.

C and **D.** The capsules of the calcaneocuboid, talonavicular, and subtalar joints are incised. These joints are opened and their cartilaginous surfaces clearly visualized by turning the foot into varus position. A laminar spreader placed in the sinus tarsi will aid in exposure of the posterior subtalar joint. Before excision of articular cartilaginous surfaces, one should review the deformity of the foot and decide on the wedges of bone to be removed to correct the deformity (Figs. 5–88 and 5–89). Circulation of the talus and the complications of avascular necrosis of the talus and arthritis of the ankle following triple arthrodesis should always be kept in mind. The height of the foot is another consideration. A low lateral malleolus will cause difficulty with wearing shoes. At times, it is best to add a bone graft rather than resect wedges of bone. With a sharp osteotome, the cartilaginous surfaces of the calcaneocuboid joint are excised. Next, the articular cartilage surface of the talonavicular joint is exposed, the plane of osteotomy being perpendicular to the long axis of the neck of the talus and parallel to the calcaneocuboid joint. When the beak of the navicular is unduly prominent medially, or when, in a varus foot, one cannot obtain adequate exposure of the talonavicular joint without excessive retraction, a second dorsomedial incision may be used to expose the talonavicular joint.

Plate 43. Triple Arthrodesis

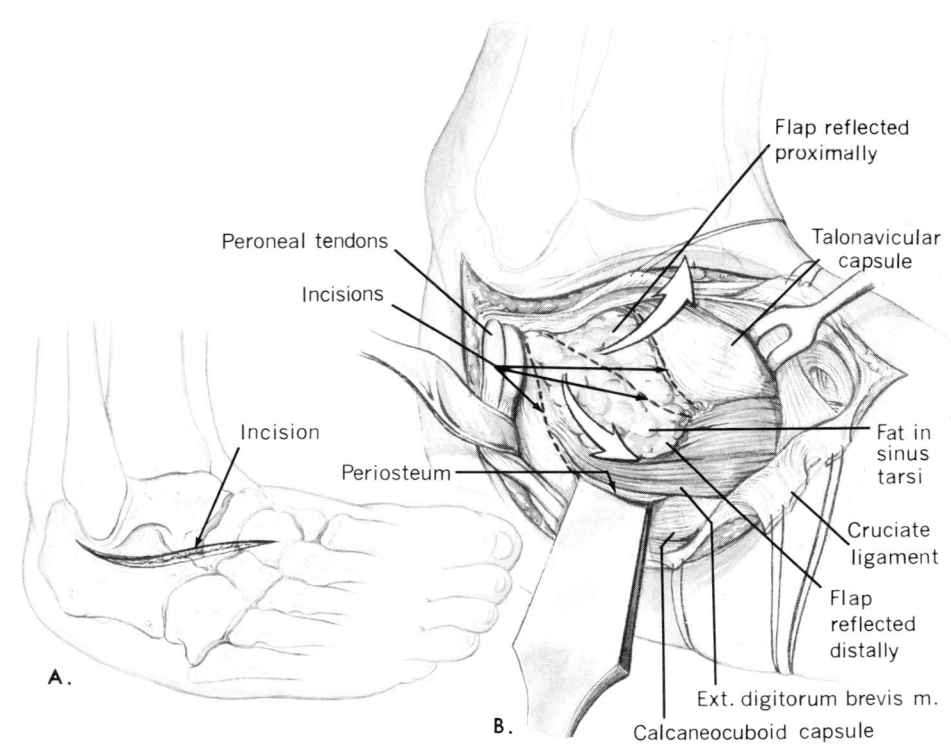

Flap reflected proximally

Talonavicular capsule

Peroneal tendons

Incisions

Incision

Periosteum

Fat in sinus tarsi

Cruciate ligament

Flap reflected distally

Ext. digitorum brevis m.

Calcaneocuboid capsule

A.

B.

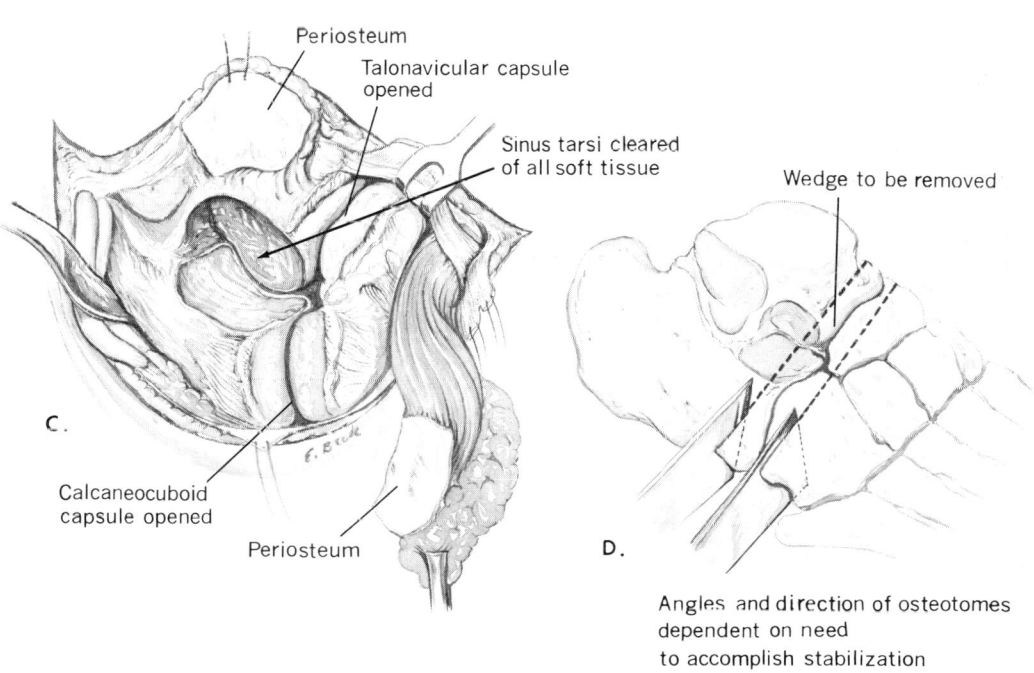

Periosteum

Talonavicular capsule opened

Sinus tarsi cleared of all soft tissue

Wedge to be removed

C.

Calcaneocuboid capsule opened

Periosteum

D.

Angles and direction of osteotomes dependent on need to accomplish stabilization

Triple Arthrodesis *(Continued)*

E to **H.** With a laminar spreader in the sinus tarsi, the subtalar joint is widely exposed and the cartilage of the anterior and posterior joints are excised. One should keep in mind the neurovascular structures behind the medial malleolus. The wedges of bone that must be removed to correct the deformity are excised in one mass with the articular cartilage. It is of great help to leave the osteotome used on the opposing articular surface in place and held steady by the assistant as a second osteotome or gouge is used to take contiguous cartilage and bone. The divided articular surfaces of the joints to be arthrodesed are "fish-scaled" for maximum raw cancellous bony contact.

The skin is closed with interrupted stutures. A well-molded long leg cast is applied, holding the foot in the desired position. The author has not found necessary and does not recommend fixation of the joints by staples. In foot stabilization in children with cerebral palsy, especially in the severely athetoid or spastic, secure criss-cross Kirschner wires are used to maintain position. These are removed in six to eight weeks.

Plate 43.   Triple Arthrodesis

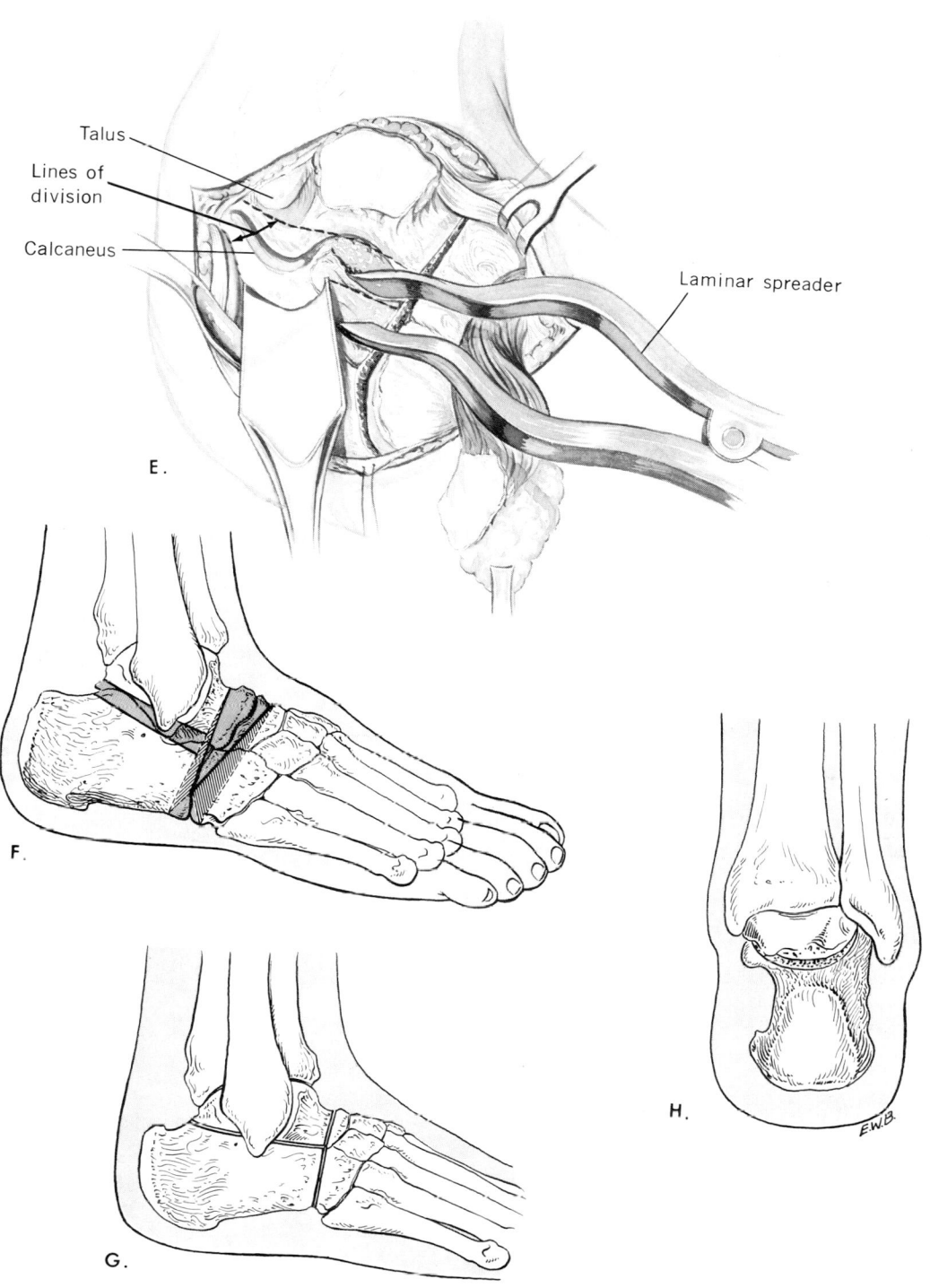

Talus

Lines of
division

Calcaneus

Laminar spreader

E.

F.

G.

H.

E.W.B.

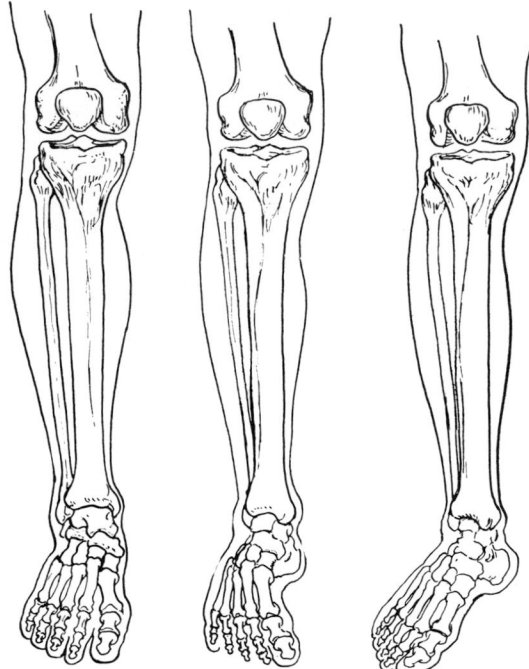

FIGURE 5–87.   Alignment of the foot.

A. Normal foot, ankle, and knee alignment without tibial torsion. **B**. *Incorrect.* Foot is aligned with knee, not ankle, in the presence of external tibial torsion. **C**. *Correct.* Foot is aligned with ankle joint in the presence of external tibial torsion. (From Patterson, R. L., Parrish, F. F., and Hathaway, E. N.: Stabilizing operations on the foot. J. Bone Joint Surg., *32-A:3,* 1950.)

should also be remembered that normally at birth the plane of the ankle mortise is 10 degrees valgus in relation to the longitudinal axis of the tibia, and with growth, this normal valgus obliquity of the ankle joint decreases. Around 10 years of age, the plane of the ankle mortise is horizontal and at right angles to the longitudinal axis of the tibia. In assessing valgus ankle, one should compare the involved limb with the opposite normal side.

Failure to recognize deformity in the midtarsal region is another pitfall. The Grice procedure will *not* correct fixed valgus or varus deformity of the forepart of the foot, nor will it improve ligamentous relaxation of the talonavicular or navicular-cuneiform joints. In such instances, triple arthrodesis is indicated when the foot is skeletally mature.

Overcorrection will cause varus deformity;

its prevention is ensured at the time of surgery. After the graft is placed in the sinus tarsi, the position of the heel is carefully inspected clinically and on roentgenographic views. The hindfoot should never be fused in varus position.*

The dynamic balance of the muscles that act on the foot should be restored by appropriate tendon transfers. Overzealous correction of invertor-evertor muscle imbalance of the foot is another pitfall that causes varus deformity of the foot. Transfer of both peroneals in the presence of normally functioning flexor hallucis longus and flexor digitorum longus muscles (secondary invertors of the foot) and the addition of a bone block to prevent pes valgus is an open invitation to the development of pes varus in the growing foot. Only one peroneal muscle should be transferred and never more medially than the midline of the foot, which is the second ray. The dynamic balance between the anterior tibial and peroneus longus muscles on the first metatarsal should always be considered. Transfer of the peroneus longus in the presence of a normally acting anterior tibial will result in a dorsal bunion.

Malposition or shifting of the bone graft in the sinus tarsi should also be recognized and corrected in the operating room. Other possible complications include: failure of the bone graft to unite to the talus or calcaneus, pseudarthrosis in its midportion, or resorption of the entire graft. The incidence of pseudarthrosis has been greatly reduced by the use of autogenous fibular or iliac bone graft, rather than homologous bone bank bone; however, it will still develop in a certain percentage of cases, and it is important that it be detected and revised or corrected by reinsertion of another graft, as necessary. Otherwise the correction will be lost and the os calcis will be united to the talus with the foot in fixed planovalgus position.

Ankle Fusion and Pantalar Arthrodesis†
When surgical reconstruction is being considered for a flail foot and ankle, their relationship to the lower limb as a whole

*See References 405, 422, 533, 576, 604, 611, 622, 639, 645, 684, 695.
†See References 399, 407, 414, 434, 440, 490, 509, 534, 549, 563, 606.

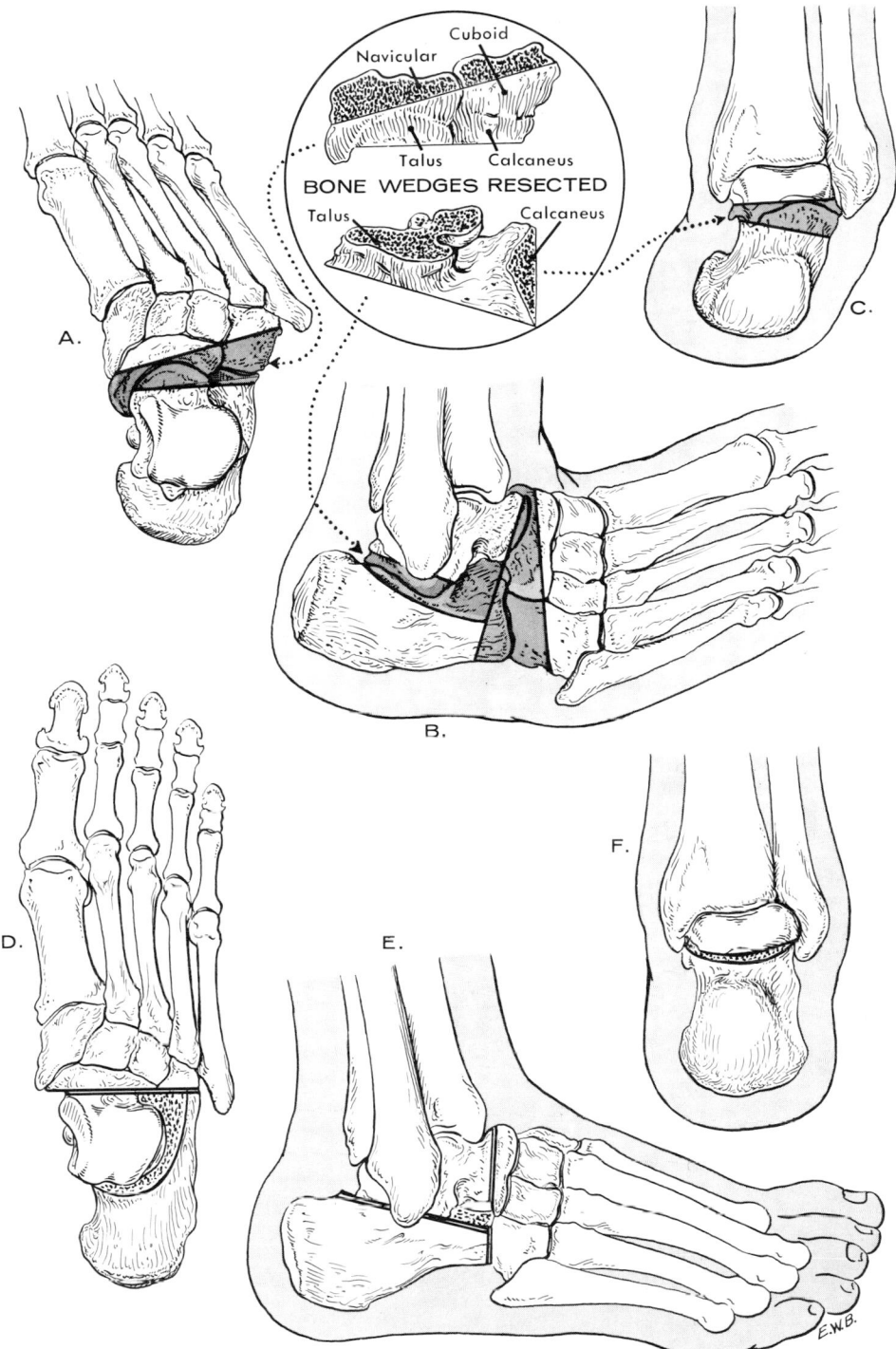

FIGURE 5–88. Wedges of bone to be resected for correction of pes varus.

A to **C.** Three views of the varus deformity. Shaded areas show amount of bone wedges to be resected. **D** to **F.** Corrected positions of the bones postoperatively.

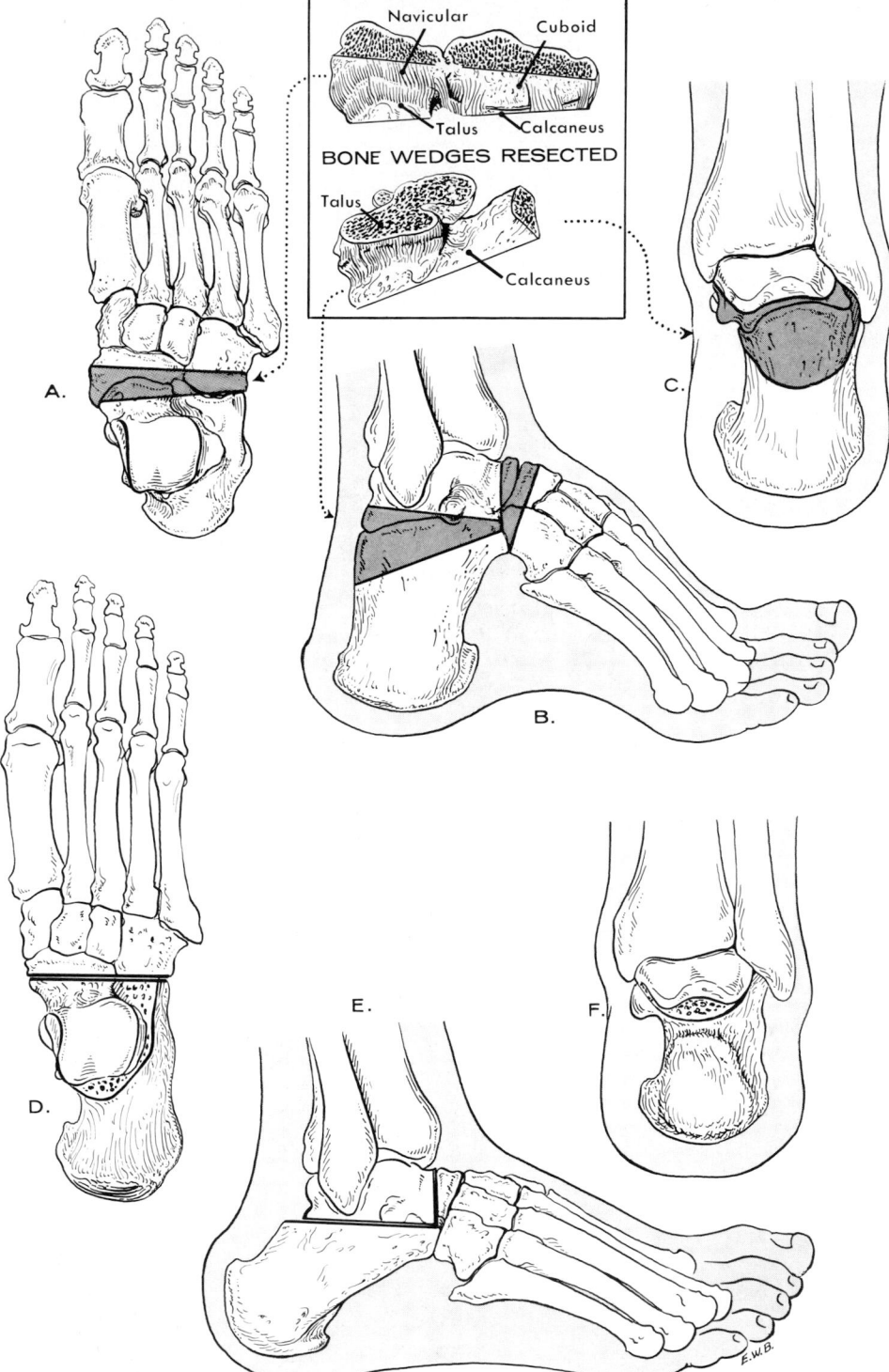

Navicular　　Cuboid

Talus　　Calcaneus

BONE WEDGES RESECTED

Talus

Calcaneus

FIGURE 5–89. *Wedges of bone to be resected for correction of calcaneocavus deformity.*

A, B, and **C.** Dorsal, lateral, and posterior views show the deformity. Shaded areas indicate amount of bone removed. **D** to **F**. Positions of the bones after correction of deformity by triple arthrodesis. Note the posterior displacement of the hindfoot.

should be carefully assessed, since there is often associated paralysis of the muscles throughout the lower limb.

Pantalar arthrodesis is surgical fusion of the joints around the talus, i.e., the ankle, subtalar, and talonavicular joints; the calcaneocuboid joint (which is not an articulation of the talus) is also included in the stabilization, thus making the procedure a combination of triple arthrodesis and ankle fusion.

Lorthioir, as he originally reported the procedure in 1911, extirpated and replaced the talus as an autogenous bone graft.[565] In 1922, Steindler advised against the temporary removal of the talus from the wound because of the danger of avascular necrosis; he also included the calcaneocuboid joint in the fusion to provide stability and to maintain correction.[657]

When the muscles below the knee are paralyzed, pantalar arthrodesis will provide stability to the ankle and hindfoot, thus eliminating the need for orthotic support, provided the gluteus maximus is of adequate strength and the knee is stable. Extensor strength of the knee is desirable but not imperative. When the quadriceps muscle is paralyzed, stability of the knee joint is provided by shifting forward the center of gravity of the body anterior to the plane of the knee joint. To lock the knee in extension, the tibia should not be allowed to come forward through a dorsiflexion movement of the ankle, either by a strong triceps surae muscle or by a fixed equinus ankle joint. A good gluteus maximus muscle will transmit push-off power to the ball of the foot when the ankle is rigid and the knee is locked in extension.

Position of ankle fusion is an important consideration. In arthrodesis of the ankle, excessive plantar flexion to stabilize the knee in extension during the stance phase of gait or to compensate for a short limb will result in increased pressure on the metatarsal heads. Callosities will form and eventually the skin will ulcerate. Consequently, in later adult life, pain in the forefoot will be a constant complaint. Unequal heel heights are another cause of patient dissatisfaction; often they would rather accept shortening and a full sole build-up. It is imperative that the position of ankle fusion be 5 to 10 degrees equinus. Lateral roentgenograms of

the foot and ankle should be made at the time of surgery, and the position of stabilization of the ankle accurately measured with a goniometer.

Pronation or supination of the forefoot results in unequal pressure on its sides and may also cause painful callosities and ulceration. When the forefoot is in supination, callosities develop over the fifth metatarsal head, whereas in pronation they develop over the first and second metatarsal heads; and when in excessive equinus inclination, over the first and fifth metatarsal heads.

The plantar surface of the foot should be in the normal weight-bearing position, with no pronation or supination or pressure under the metatarsal heads. The lateral border of the foot should be equally distributed, with the heel in neutral or slightly valgus position and the ankle in less than 10 degrees of plantar flexion.

Waugh, Wagner, and Stinchfield reported the results of 116 pantalar arthrodeses in 97 patients with a mean follow-up of five years and an average follow-up of 6.9 years. In general, pantalar arthrodesis was found to be an effective and satisfying procedure. About 80 per cent of the patients had no complaints referable to their pantalar arthrodesis. Adequate compensatory motion developed in the forepart of the foot, so that rigidity of the feet was not a problem, despite fusion of the ankle and hindpart of the foot. Of the 52 patients who had used an orthosis preoperatively, 47 were able to discard it following fusion. Pseudarthrosis occurred in 14.7 per cent of the cases.[682]

When the foot has normal alignment and adequate bony and ligamentous stability, the author recommends ankle fusion only, using the distraction-compression bone graft arthrodesis described by Chuinard and Peterson (Plate 44).[466] In the paralyzed limb, there are no compressional forces to maintain the tibia and talus in close apposition, and the weight of the cast pressing on the dorsum of the foot may distract them.[408]

Anterior or Posterior Bone Blocks to Limit Motion at Ankle. In pes calcaneus, construction of a bone buttress anteriorly in the talus will limit dorsiflexion of the ankle by impinging upon the anterior lip of the distal tibia, whereas in equinus deformity of the foot, plantar flexion of the ankle may be

Arthrodesis of Ankle Joint Through Anterior Approach Without Disturbing Distal Tibial Growth Plate

THE PROCEDURE

A and **B.** A longitudinal skin incision is made, beginning 7 cm. proximal to the ankle joint between the extensor digitorum longus and extensor hallucis longus tendons; it extends distally across the ankle joint in line with the third metatarsal and ends 4 cm. distal to the ankle joint.

The subcutaneous tissue is divided and the skin flaps are mobilized and retracted to their respective sides. The veins crossing the field are clamped, divided, and coagulated. The intermediate and medial dorsal cutaneous branches of the superficial peroneal nerve are identified and protected by retraction to one side of the wound.

C. The deep fascia and transverse crural and cruciate crural ligaments are divided in line with the skin incision. The ligaments are marked with 00 silk suture for accurate closure later.

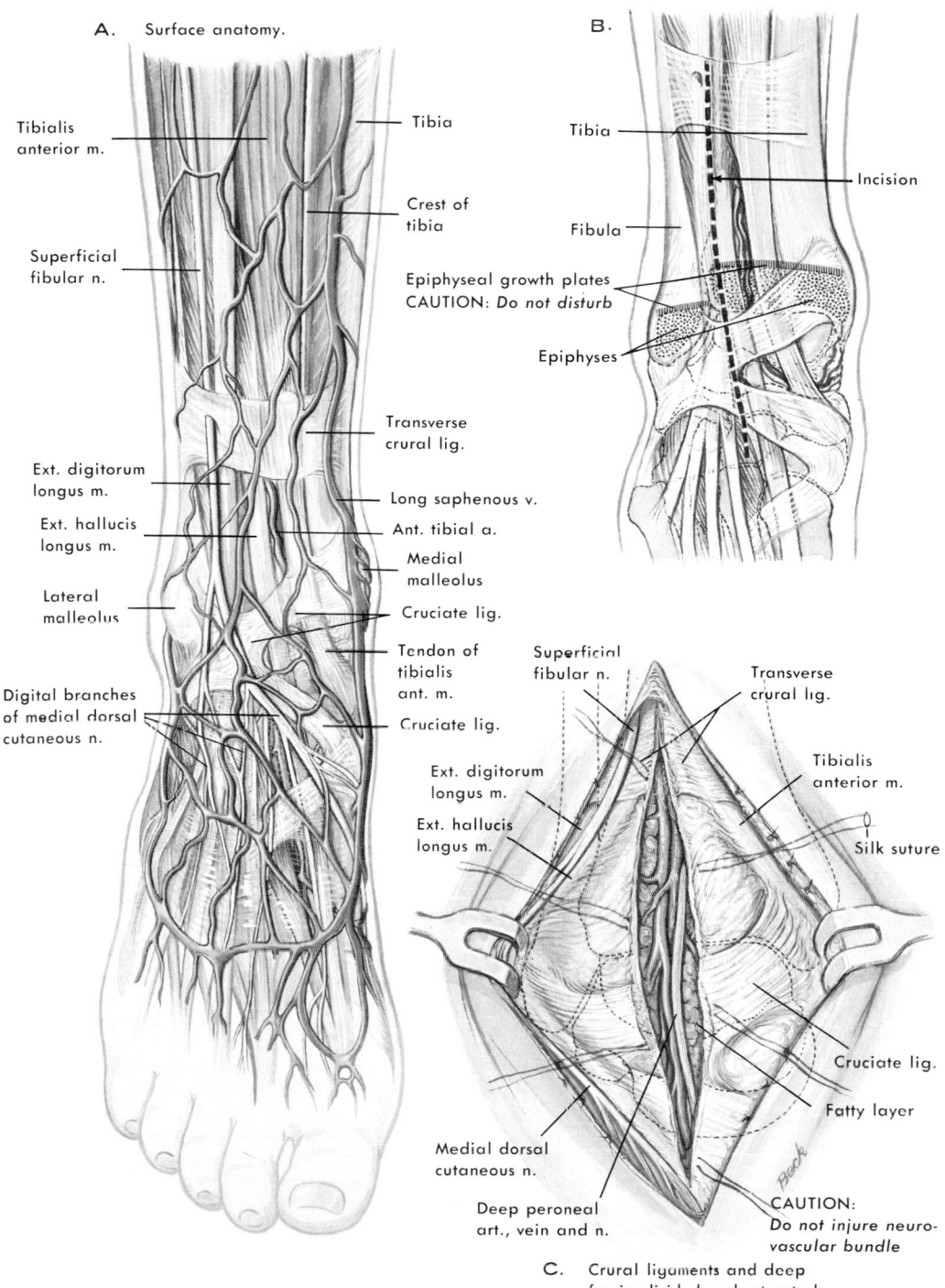

A.   Surface anatomy.

Tibialis
anterior m.

Tibia

Crest of
tibia

Superficial
fibular n.

Transverse
crural lig.

Ext. digitorum
longus m.

Long saphenous v.

Ext. hallucis
longus m.

Ant. tibial a.

Medial
malleolus

Lateral
malleolus

Cruciate lig.

Digital branches
of medial dorsal
cutaneous n.

Tendon of
tibialis
ant. m.

Cruciate lig.

B.

Tibia

Tibia

Incision

Fibula

Epiphyseal growth plates
CAUTION: *Do not disturb*

Epiphyses

Superficial
fibular n.

Transverse
crural lig.

Ext. digitorum
longus m.

Tibialis
anterior m.

Ext. hallucis
longus m.

Silk suture

Cruciate lig.

Fatty layer

Medial dorsal
cutaneous n.

Deep peroneal
art., vein and n.

CAUTION:
*Do not injure neuro-
vascular bundle*

C.   Crural ligaments and deep
fascia divided and retracted
with silk sutures

1007

Arthrodesis of Ankle Joint Through Anterior Approach Without Disturbing Distal Tibial Growth Plate (Continued)

D. The neurovascular bundle (deep peroneal nerve, anterior tibial–dorsalis pedis vessels) is identified, isolated, and retracted laterally with the extensor hallucis longus, extensor digitorum longus, and peroneus tertius tendons. The anterolateral malleolar and lateral tarsal arteries are isolated, clamped, divided, and ligated. The distal tibia, ankle joint, and talus are identified. A transverse incision is made in the capsule of the talotibial joint from the posterior tip of the medial malleolus to the lateral malleolus. The edges of the capsule are marked with 00 silk suture for meticulous closure later.

E to **G.** The capsule is reflected and retracted distally on the talus and proximally on the tibia. The periosteum of the tibia should not be divided. The distal tibial and fibular epiphyseal plates should not be disturbed in growing children. With thin curved and straight osteotomes, the cartilage and subchondral bone are removed from the opposing articular surfaces of the distal tibia and proximal talus down to raw bleeding cancellous bone. Cartilage chips should not be left posteriorly.

H. Next, a large piece of bone for grafting is taken from the ilium and fashioned to fit snugly in the ankle joint. The graft should have both cortices intact and should be thicker at one end, wedge-shaped. The cortices of the graft are perforated with multiple tiny drill holes. The ankle joint is held in the desired position and the bone graft is firmly fitted into the joint with an impacter. If any space is left on each side of the graft, it is packed with cancellous bone from the ilium. The graft in the ankle joint gives compressional force to the arthrodesis and adds to the height of the foot and ankle. The capsule of the ankle joint and the transverse crural and cruciate crural ligaments are closed carefully in layers. The deep fascia and the wound are closed in the usual manner. Roentgenograms are obtained in anteroposterior and lateral views to ensure that the ankle joint is in the desired position.

I. A long leg cast is applied with the ankle joint in the desired position of plantar-flexion (boys, 10 degrees; girls, 15 to 20 degrees) and the knee in 45 degrees of flexion.

POSTOPERATIVE CARE

Periodic roentgenograms are obtained to determine the position of the graft and the extent of healing. Eight to ten weeks after surgery, the solid cast is removed and roentgenograms are obtained with the cast off. Ordinarily, by this time, the fusion is solid and the patient is gradually allowed to be ambulatory. Full weight-bearing is begun two to three weeks later.

Plate 44. Arthrodesis of Ankle Joint Through Anterior Approach Without Disturbing Distal Tibial Growth Plate

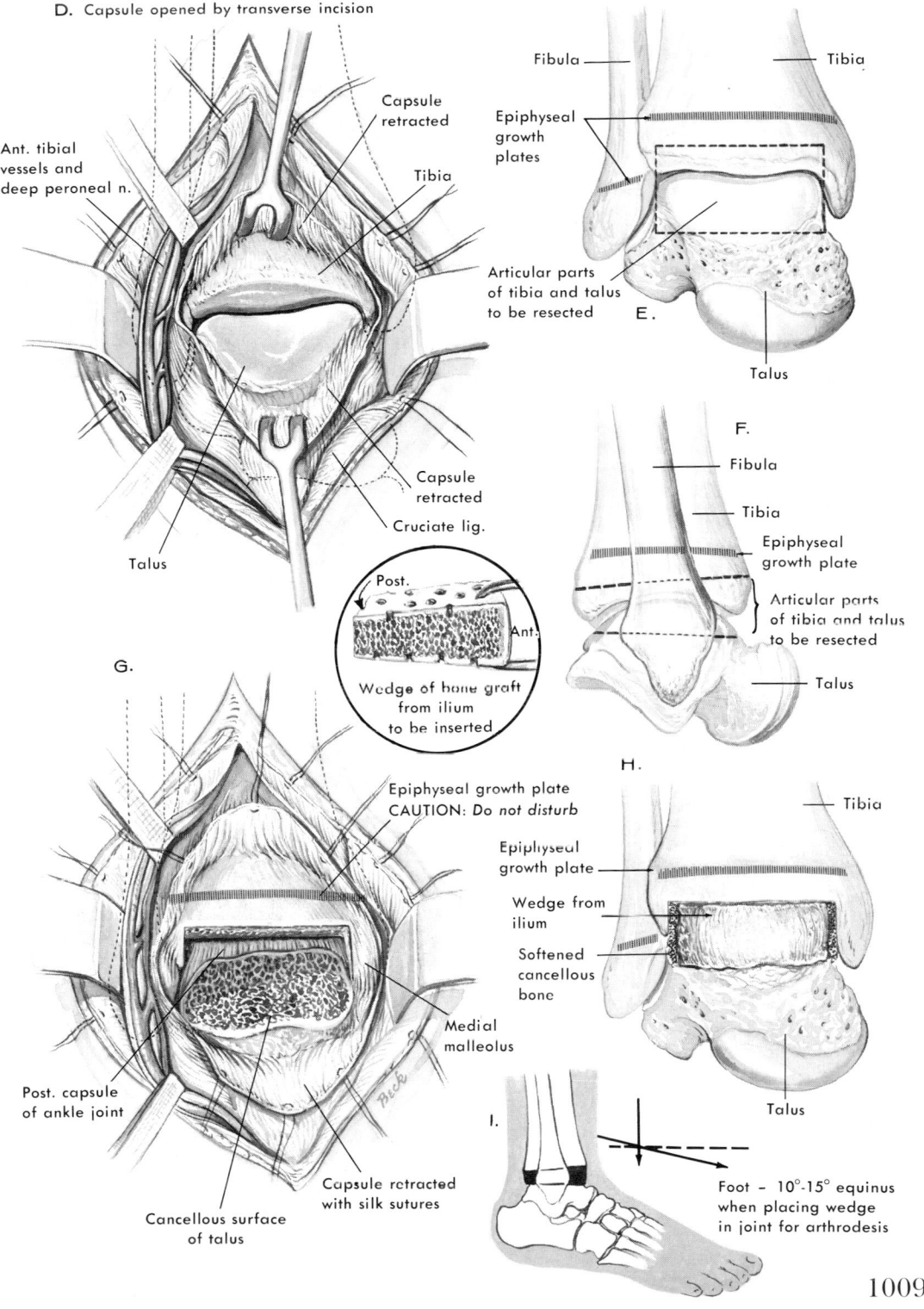

D. Capsule opened by transverse incision

Ant. tibial vessels and deep peroneal n.

Capsule retracted

Tibia

Capsule retracted

Cruciate lig.

Talus

Fibula

Tibia

Epiphyseal growth plates

Articular parts of tibia and talus to be resected

E.

Talus

F.

Fibula

Tibia

Epiphyseal growth plate

Articular parts of tibia and talus to be resected

Talus

Post.

Ant.

Wedge of bone graft from ilium to be inserted

G.

Epiphyseal growth plate CAUTION: *Do not disturb*

Medial malleolus

Post. capsule of ankle joint

Capsule retracted with silk sutures

Cancellous surface of talus

H.

Tibia

Epiphyseal growth plate

Wedge from ilium

Softened cancellous bone

Talus

I.

Foot – 10°-15° equinus when placing wedge in joint for arthrodesis

1009

restricted by bone block construction on the posterior aspect of the talus.[431, 432, 484, 485] These procedures were developed for use in cases of paralytic calcaneus or drop foot, when there is no musculature available for transfer to provide plantar flexion or dorsiflexion power. Long term follow-up studies of bone block operations have disclosed a high incidence of recurrence of deformity and fibrous ankylosis or painful degenerative arthritis of the ankle joint. The author does not recommend bone blocks to limit motion at the ankle, as the procedure has all the disadvantages of arthrodesis of the ankle without providing the pain-free stability of the latter.

The only indication for a posterior bone block is a female patient who desires to wear shoes with heels of varying height and who has fair strength of the triceps surae muscle but no dorsiflexor power. Following triple arthrodesis, small subarticular grafts are placed posteriorly to lift the articular surface of the posterior aspect of the talus and limit plantar flexion. Massive bone grafts that abut the posterior aspect of the tibia should not be used. These small blocks placed beneath the articular surface of the talus are just as effective, heal rapidly, can be performed in combination with triple arthrodesis, and are less likely to cause pain.[495]

The Trunk

The etiology and treatment of pelvic obliquity is discussed in the section on contracture of the iliotibial band. Pelvic obliquity may also be caused by unilateral paralysis of the quadratus lumborum muscle. Paralysis of the abdominal muscles will result in exaggeration of the anterior pelvic tilt and an increase in lumbar lordosis. Lowman has described fascial transplants to substitute for the paralyzed abdominal muscles. For indications and operative technique the reader is referred to Lowman, Dickson, Clark and Axer, Mayer, and Williamson, Moe, and Bascom.[402, 448, 464, 567-569, 584, 690]

The treatment of postpolio paralytic scoliosis follows the same principles as that of idiopathic scoliosis (see Chapter 6).

The Shoulder

The shoulder joint is a multiaxial one. On full abduction of the shoulder, the scapulothoracic motion contributes 60 degrees and the glenohumeral movements, 120 degrees, in a ratio 1:2. When the arm is abducted to 90 degrees, the arm should rotate externally to allow full abduction. Full 180 degree forward flexion is permitted by internal rotation of the arm. Extension of the shoulder joint is limited to 80 degrees by the mechanical block of the acromion process and the adjacent spine of the scapula. Normal scapulohumeral rhythm is imperative for execution of graceful motions and strength of the shoulder joint.[627]

Functional classification of the muscles acting at the shoulder joint, as given by Saha, is as follows:[628, 629]

Prime Movers. These are the deltoid and clavicular head of the pectoralis major. They provide the greatest amount of active power in shoulder abduction, exerting force in three directions. Their insertion is most distal from the shoulder joint, at the juncture of the middle and upper thirds of the humeral diaphysis. When these prime movers are paralyzed, natural automatic substitution of function with adjacent motors is not feasible. To restore active shoulder abduction, muscle transfer is required.

Steering Group. This group consists of the subscapularis, supraspinatus, and infraspinatus muscles. Their force is exerted at the junction of the head-neck and shaft of the humerus, their primary function being to stabilize the humeral head in the glenoid cavity by steering, i.e., by rolling and gliding movement. Secondarily, they also assist in shoulder abduction.

The infraspinatus muscle acts primarily as a posterior glider of the humeral head during the final stages of full abduction. The supraspinatus and subscapularis muscles are indispensable for shoulder abduction, steering the head of the humerus during abduction in different planes through an arc of 150 degrees. The scapula moves anteriorly and posteriorly and rotates vertically through the extremes of the arc (about 30 degrees on either side). In general, vertical gliding of the humeral head is accomplished by the muscle fibers acting in the plane of motion, whereas the muscle fibers that are anterior and posterior to these act to glide the humeral head in the horizontal plane at succeeding stages of shoulder abduction.

Depressor Group. This consists of the sternal head of the pectoralis major, the latissimus dorsi, and the teres major and teres minor. (Teres minor is included in this group, as electromyographic evidence has shown that it participates in this motion, though anatomically it is classified as belonging to the short rotator group.) The function of these muscles is to rotate the shaft of the humerus during abduction and to depress the humeral head, assisting in the last few degrees of full abduction. The steering action that they exert on the humeral head is minimal, however.

Scapular rotation takes place through its body in an anteroposterior axis and contributes about 60 degrees of total shoulder abduction. Fixation of the scapula is equally important during abduction provided by gravity and the lower fibers of the serratus.

When the deltoid and clavicular head of the pectoralis major are paralyzed, it is important to determine the action of the steering group of muscles when performing tendon transfers to restore shoulder abduction. If the latter are paralyzed, transfer of a single muscle (such as the trapezius) or several muscles to a common attachment to restore function will give at best only 90 degrees of shoulder abduction and scapulohumeral rhythm will still be disturbed. According to Saha, if there is paralysis of any two of the steering group of muscles, appropriate tendon transfers should be performed to restore their function. This is as imperative as trapezius transfer for paralysis of the deltoid.

Table 5–13 gives Saha's recommendations for possible tendon transfers to restore power at the shoulder joint.

The Saha trapezius transfer for paralysis of the deltoid is shown in Figure 5–90. The upper and middle trapezius is completely mobilized from its insertion, providing an additional 5 cm. of length without disturbing the nerve and blood supply to the muscle. The detached portion of the trapezius with the distal end of the clavicle, the capsule of the acromioclavicular joint, the acromion process, and the adjoining portion of the posterior border of the spine of the

Table 5–13. *Possible Tendon Transfers to Restore Power at the Shoulder Joint**

Muscle Requiring Replacement or Reinforcement	Action	Choice of Muscles for Transfer (in Order of Preference)
Deltoid and clavicular head of pectoralis major	Prime mover (abduction)	1. Trapezius (as far down as possible on shaft)
Supraspinatus	Superior glider	1. Levator scapulae (first choice because of direction and length of its fibers) 2. Sternocleidomastoid 3. Scalenus anterior 4. Scalenus medius 5. Scalenus capitis (All act from above and are good substitutes)
Infraspinatus	Posterior glider (acting from behind)	1. Latissimus dorsi 2. Teres major
Subscapularis	Posterior glider	1. Upper two digitations of serratus anterior 2. Pectoralis minor 3. Pectoralis major (whole or part) (These muscles act in almost same direction as fibers of subscapularis)

*Modified from Saha, A. K.: Surgery of the paralyzed and flail shoulder. Acta Orthop. Scand., Suppl. 97, p. 40, 1967.

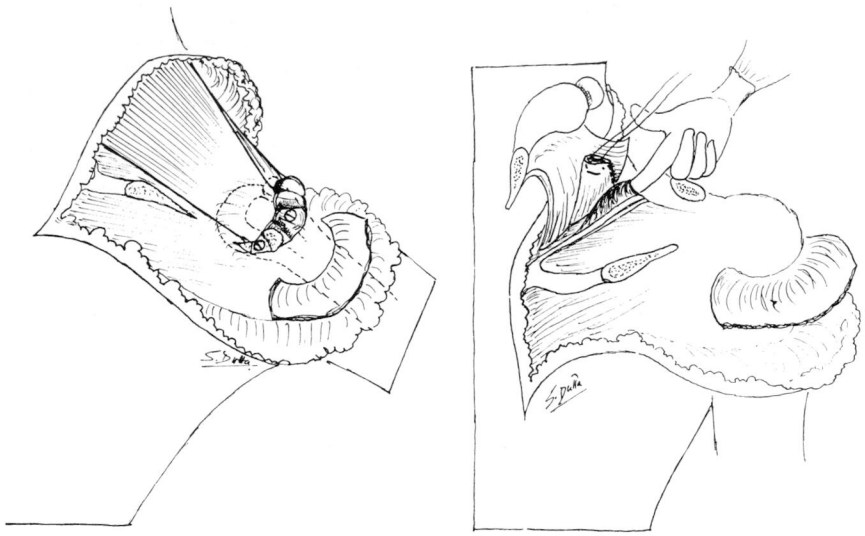

FIGURE 5-90. *Trapezius muscle transfer (Saha) for paralysis of deltoid muscle.*

(From Saha, A. K.: Surgery of the paralyzed and flail shoulder. Acta Orthop. Scand., Suppl. 97, p. 57, 1967.)

scapula are rerouted and attached by two screws to the humeral shaft as far distally as possible. The acromion is crushed to aid coaptation with the curve of the shaft of the humerus.

Transfer of the upper two digitations of the serratus anterior for paralysis of the subscapularis is shown in Figure 5-91. Levator scapulae transfer for paralysis of the supraspinatus is shown in Figure 5-92; pectoralis minor transfer for paralysis of the subcapularis in Figure 5-93; sterno-cleidomastoid transfer for paralysis of the supraspinatus in Figure 5-94; and either latissimus dorsi or teres major transfer, or both, for paralysis of the subscapularis in Figure 5-95. For technical details the reader is referred to the original paper of Saha.[629]

ARTHRODESIS OF THE SHOULDER

This is indicated when there is paralytic subluxation of dislocation of the shoulder and extensive paralysis of the scapulo-humeral muscles. Because scapulothoracic motion will serve as a substitute for that of the glenohumeral joint, it is important that the motor strength of the tapezius and ser-ratus anterior be normal. The direct action of the scapula will move the arm. Normal

function of the hand, however, is a primary requisite. It is best to delay shoulder arthro-desis until after epiphyseal closure has taken place.

The optimum position for shoulder fu-sion, as recommended by the Research Com-mittee of the American Orthopedic Asso-ciation, is 50 degrees of abduction, 20 degrees of flexion, and 25 degrees of in-ternal rotation. This position is very functional, allowing the patient to reach his face and the top of his head with the elbow flexed.[409]

It is wise, however, to consider the sex and occupation of the patient, and the regional muscle power and functional status of the opposite limb. In general, office workers require more abduction than do laborers. In females, the degree of abduc-tion should be less, since this permits the scapula a better resting position in relation to the trunk. For cosmetic reasons, girls strongly object to the winging of the scapula. The lesser degree of abduction is function-ally compensated by fusing it in greater internal rotation. The most acceptable posi-tion of shoulder arthrodesis in girls is 30 degrees of glenohumeral abduction, 5 to 10 degrees of flexion, and 45 degrees of internal rotation. The shoulder should never be fused in external rotation, as the limb will be positioned in an awkward and functionally poor position. It should be explained to the patient that following surgery, extension and rotation of the shoulder will be limited and that he will have difficulty in lying on the side of the arthrodesis to sleep. Fusion of both shoulders should never be performed because of the loss in range of motion. Arthrodesis of the shoulder will increase the power of both flexion and extension of the elbow and will provide adduction power to the shoulder, enabling the patient to grip an object between his arm and body.

For technical details of shoulder fusion, the reader is referred to the original papers in the references.* It should be emphasized, however, that the position of fusion should be calculated according to the angle between the humerus and scapula rather than that of the arms and thorax. Internal fixation is imperative; otherwise, the angle will be changed in the shoulder spica cast.

The Elbow

Loss of elbow flexion results from paralysis of the biceps brachii and the brachialis

---

*See References 409, 410, 420, 425, 426, 440–442, 483, 548, 681.

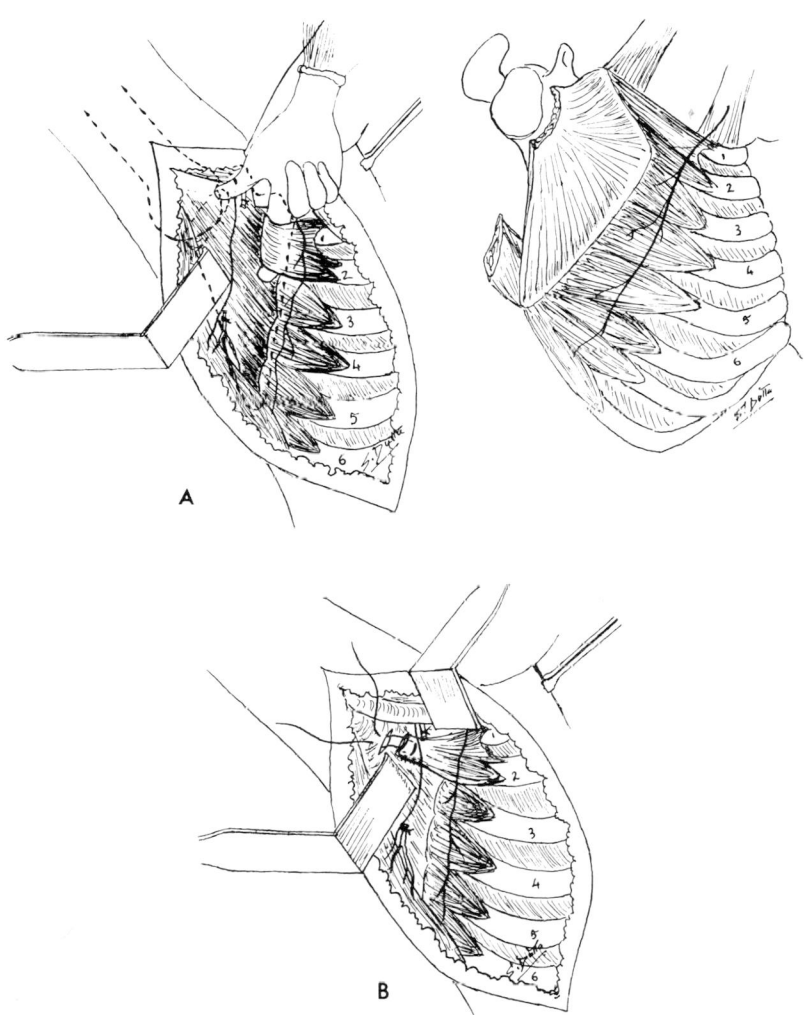

FIGURE 5–91. *Transfer of upper two digitations of serratus anterior for paralysis of subscapularis muscle.*

(From Saha, A. K.: Surgery of the paralyzed and flail shoulder. Acta Orthop. Scand., Suppl. 97, p. 59, 1967.)

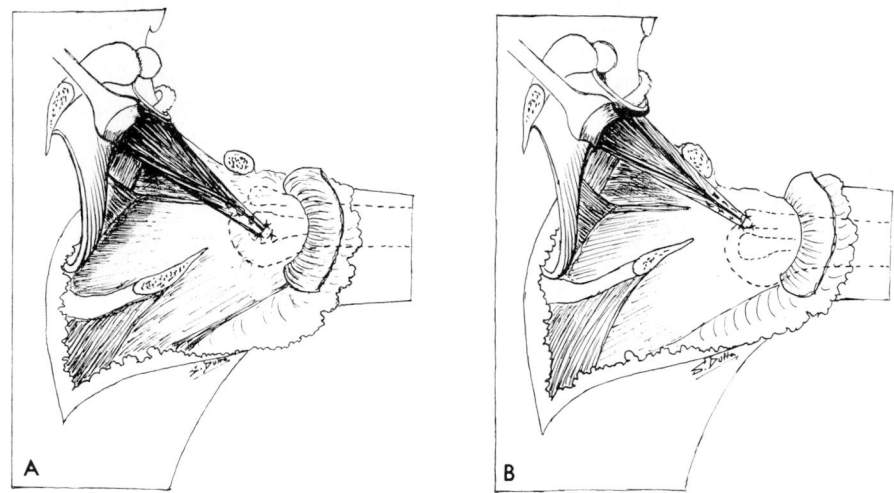

FIGURE 5-92. *Levator scapulae transfer for paralysis of supraspinatus.*

(From Saha, A. K.: Surgery of the paralyzed and flail shoulder. Acta Orthop. Scand. Suppl. 97, p. 60, 1967.)

muscles. The resultant functional deficit is considerable, as the patient is unable to bring his hand to his head, mouth, or trunk.

A number of operative procedures have been devised to restore elbow flexion: (1) Steindler flexorplasty;[654] (2) Transfer of the distal third of the pectoralis major muscle (Clark);[447] (3) Transfer of the pectoralis major tendon (Brooks and Seddon);[424] (4) Transfer of the sternocleidomastoid muscle (Bunnell);[427] (5) Transfer of latissimus dorsi (Hovnanian);[532] (6) Transfer of pectoralis minor (Spira);[650] (7) Anterior transfer of the triceps brachii tendon to the biceps

insertion on the radial tuberosity (Bunnell and Carroll).[427, 435]

Prior to the selection of a specific procedure, it is imperative to assess carefully the motor strength of the muscles of the entire upper limb and the functional status of the opposite limb. With paralysis of the elbow flexors, there is often a varying degree of paresis of the muscles of the scapulo-humeral joint, forearm, and hand.

Function of the hand is of primary concern. Restoration of elbow flexion is only one step in total functional reconstruction of the upper limb, and procedures on the

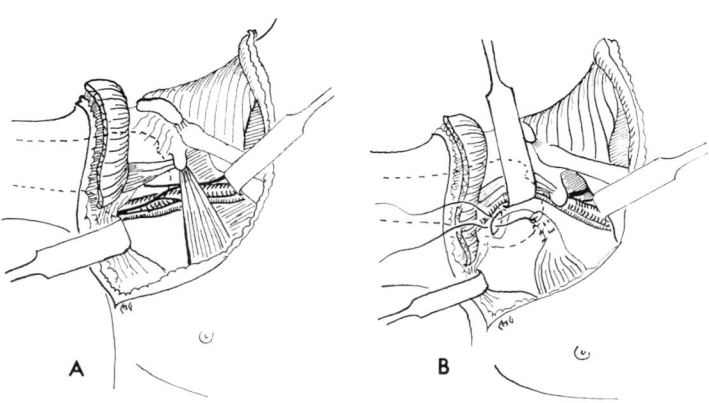

FIGURE 5-93. *Pectoralis minor transfer for paralysis of subscapularis.*

(From Saha, A. K.: Surgery of the paralyzed and flail shoulder. Acta Orthop. Scand., Suppl. 97, p. 61, 1967.)

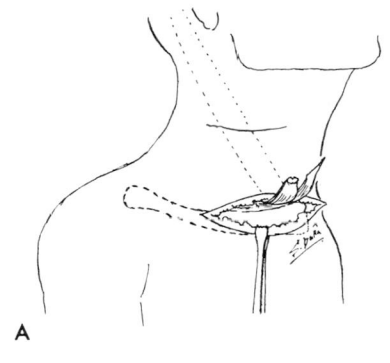

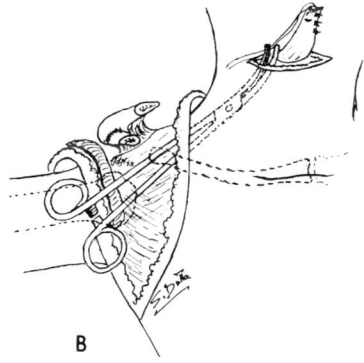

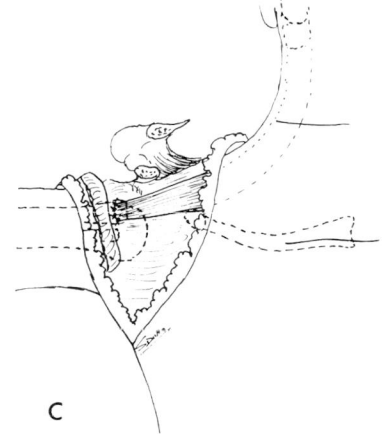

FIGURE 5–94. Sternocleidomastoid transfer for paralysis of supraspinatus muscle.

(From Saha, A. K.: Surgery of the paralyzed and flail shoulder. Acta Orthop. Scand., Suppl. 97, p. 62, 1967.)

hand should precede those on the elbow. In the absence of a functional hand, flexorplasty of the elbow should not be performed.

STEINDLER FLEXORPLASTY

Steindler, in 1918, described a procedure in which the humeral origins of the flexor carpi radialis, the palmaris longus, the pronator teres, the flexor digitorum sublimis, and the flexor carpi ulnaris are transferred to a more proximal site on the humerus, thereby changing the leverage of these muscles across the elbow joint and enhancing their flexor action at the elbow.[654] Later, he reviewed the results of flexorplasties of the elbow and pointed out that the disadvantage of this transfer was an increase in the pronatory action of these muscles on the forearm.[658–660, 662] Bunnell modified the Steindler flexorplasty by attaching the transferred muscles

to the lateral border of the humerus to decrease their tendency to cause pronation. In order to reach the lateral border of the humerus, the common flexor muscles had to be elongated with a fascial graft (Fig. 5–96).[427] This method of fascial lengthening is technically difficult if one is to obtain secure fixation and maximum strength of the flexorplasty. Mayer and Green attached the transferred muscles on the anterior surface of the humerus through holes drilled in bone.[586] This direct fixation to bone ensured firm healing of the transferred muscle. The operative technique of Steindler flexorplasty as modified by Mayer and Green is described and illustrated in Plate 45.

Carroll and Gartland reported the results of Steindler flexorplasty in 27 patients.[437] Kettlekamp and Larson evaluated the results of Steindler flexorplasty in 15 patients, determining the maximum strength of the

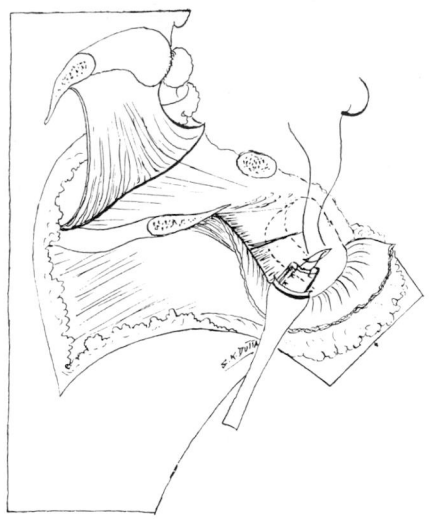

FIGURE 5–95. *Latissimus dorsi or teres major transfer for paralysis of subscapularis muscle.*

(From Saha, A. K.: Surgery of the paralyzed and flail shoulder. Acta Orthop. Scand., Suppl. 97, p. 64, 1967.)

flexorplasty through a useful range of flexion. Nine of the fifteen patients were able to lift a weight of 1 pound or greater to 110 degrees of flexion. Upon correlating the strength of the flexorplasty with the degree of flexion contracture of the elbow, they found the average strength of the flexorplasty to be 2 pounds to 110 degrees of flexion when the degree of flexion contracture was between 30 and 60 degrees. The mechanical advantage and strength of the transfer were increased in the presence of flexion contracture of the elbow.[547] When there is marked paralysis of the opposite limb, the strength restored by flexorplasty is a greater consideration than is cosmetic appearance.

Mayer and Green, however, emphasize the importance of the appearance of the arm, preferring that the flexion position of the elbow not exceed 15 degrees. They recommend that a turnbuckle extension orthosis be worn at night to prevent the development of flexion contracture of the elbow. As soon as the strength of the transfer is fair or fair plus, a night splint is used and passive stretching exercises of the elbow flexors are performed.[586]

The motor strength of the triceps is another important factor in the develop-

ment of flexion contracture of the elbow, as this contracture represents the residuum of flexorplasty and the end result of dynamic imbalance between elbow flexors and extensors over the years. A flexion deformity of the elbow greater than 30 degrees will usually develop when the triceps brachii is less than fair in motor strength. In the presence of a weakened triceps brachii, the period of postoperative immobilization should be short, and assisted active exercises should be started on the fifth to seventh postoperative day, taking precautions to prevent the transfer from being stretched away from the bone. There should be an extensive period of postoperative splinting at night with the elbow in extension.

Loss of supination is an inherent complication of Steindler flexorplasty. The attachment of the transferred muscles as far laterally on the humerus as possible minimizes the severity of pronation contracture; however, even with this precaution a varying degree of pronation deformity of the forearm results in the presence of dynamic imbalance between a strong pronator teres

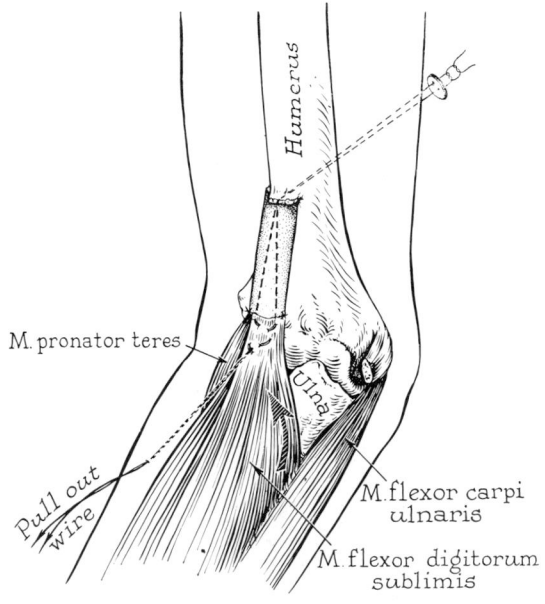

FIGURE 5–96. *Bunnell's modification of Steindler flexorplasty of the elbow.*

The common flexor muscles are elongated by a fascial graft. (From Bunnell, S.: Restoring flexion to the paralytic elbow. J. Bone Joint Surg., *33-A*:566, 1951.)

and a paralyzed biceps brachii—its chief supinator opponent. The strength of the flexorplasty is not influenced by the degree of pronation contracture; however, it does impair the position of the hand and impedes its functional use. If the motor strength of the supinators of the forearm is poor, flexor carpi ulnaris transfer to the dorsum of the radius is performed to enhance supinator function and to prevent development of pronation contracture of the forearm.

In poliomyelitis, paralysis of the elbow without paralysis of the muscles that control the scapulohumeral joint is rarely seen. A flail shoulder will greatly impede the effectiveness of the flexorplasty. In the abducted position of the shoulder, the force of gravity assists elbow flexion and the amount of strength required to flex the elbow is decreased. Arthrodesis of the shoulder will markedly improve the results of flexorplasty.

Overestimation of the motor strength of the common flexor muscle group is a common pitfall, and accounts for poor results in some patients. For the transfer to function effectively, these muscles must rate at least good in motor strength. If they are weaker, other reconstructive methods must be employed. The flexor digitorum sublimis may be strong and the flexor carpi ulnaris and carpi radialis weak; in such an instance, following Steindler flexorplasty, flexion of the elbow is only accomplished by clenching the fingers, and any relaxation of the grip will allow the elbow to extend. This interferes with function of the hand, which is the primary interest of the patient.

PECTORALIS MAJOR TRANSFER TO RESTORE ELBOW FLEXION

A portion of the pectoralis major transfer was used by Clark to restore active elbow flexion.[447] The nerve supply of the distal third of the pectoralis major muscle (from branches of the medial thoracic nerve) is separate from that of its proximal part. This inferior strip of the pectoralis major muscle, which is 5 to 7 cm. in width, is freed from the chest wall and mobilized toward the axilla as far as its nerve and blood supply will allow. The muscle is then passed subcutaneously down the arm and sutured

to the biceps tendon. The reader is referred to Clark's original description for the specific technical details.[547] Clark's operation is particularly indicated in patients with traction injury of the upper trunk of the brachial plexus, in which the clavicular head of the pectoralis major is paralyzed but whose sternal head is normal in motor strength. Seddon reported satisfactory results in 15 of 16 of Clark's pectoralis major transfers.[637] In a more recent report by Segal, Seddon and Brooks, the results of Clark's operation in 17 patients were graded excellent or good in 47 per cent and fair or failure in 53 per cent.[638]

Brooks and Seddon devised a technique in which the entire pectoralis major muscle is transferred to restore elbow flexion.[424] The gap between the distal end of the pectoralis major tendon and the tuberosity of the radius is bridged by the long head of the biceps, which is detached from its origin and completely mobilized. Reducing the blood supply of the biceps brachii induced conversion of the muscle into tendon. The procedure was recommended by Brooks and Seddon in either those patients in whom the lower part of the pectoralis major is paralyzed (or too weak for the Clark transfer) but the clavicular head is strong, or the entire muscle is of such weakness that it is desirable to use all the active muscle. They reported the results as excellent or good in six; fair in two; and failure in two (one patient had arthrogryposis multiplex congenita, and the other poliomyelitis).

The operative technique of the Brooks-Seddon procedure is described and illustrated in Plate 46. The author recommends its use when the Steindler flexorplasty is not applicable; of course, it should be employed only when the biceps brachii is completely and permanently paralyzed. The procedure does restore some degree of active supination of the forearm and rarely limits passive extension of the elbow.

One disadvantage of the pectoralis major transfer is that in the presence of weak scapulohumeral muscles, active flexion of the elbow is often accompanied by shrugging, adduction, and internal rotation of the shoulder. These undesirable motions, with the hand hitting the chest wall, seriously impair the result of the operation. If

(*Text continued on page 1028.*)

Flexorplasty of the Elbow (Steindler)

A. With the elbow in extension, a curved longitudinal incision is made over the anteromedial side of the elbow, beginning approximately 3 inches above the flexion crease of the elbow joint over the medial intermuscular septum and extending distally to the anterior aspect of the medial epicondyle. At the joint level it turns anterolaterally on the volar surface of the forearm along the course of the pronator teres muscle for a distance of approximately 2½ inches.

B. The subcutaneous tissue and fascia are divided in line with the skin incision and the skin flaps are widely mobilized and retracted. Next, the ulnar nerve is located posterior to the medial intermuscular septum and lying in a groove on the triceps muscle. It is isolated and a moist hernia tape is passed around it for gentle handling. The ulnar nerve is traced distally to its groove between the posterior aspect of the medial epicondyle of the humerus and the olecranon process. The fascial roof over the ulnar nerve is carefully divided under direct vision over a grooved director.

C. The ulnar nerve is dissected free distally to the point where it passes between the two heads of the flexor carpi ulnaris muscle. Inadvertent damage to the branches of the ulnar nerve to the flexor carpi ulnaris muscle should be avoided. A second hernia tape is passed around the ulnar nerve in the distal part of the wound, and the nerve is retracted posteriorly.

Plate 45. *Flexorplasty of the Elbow (Steindler)*

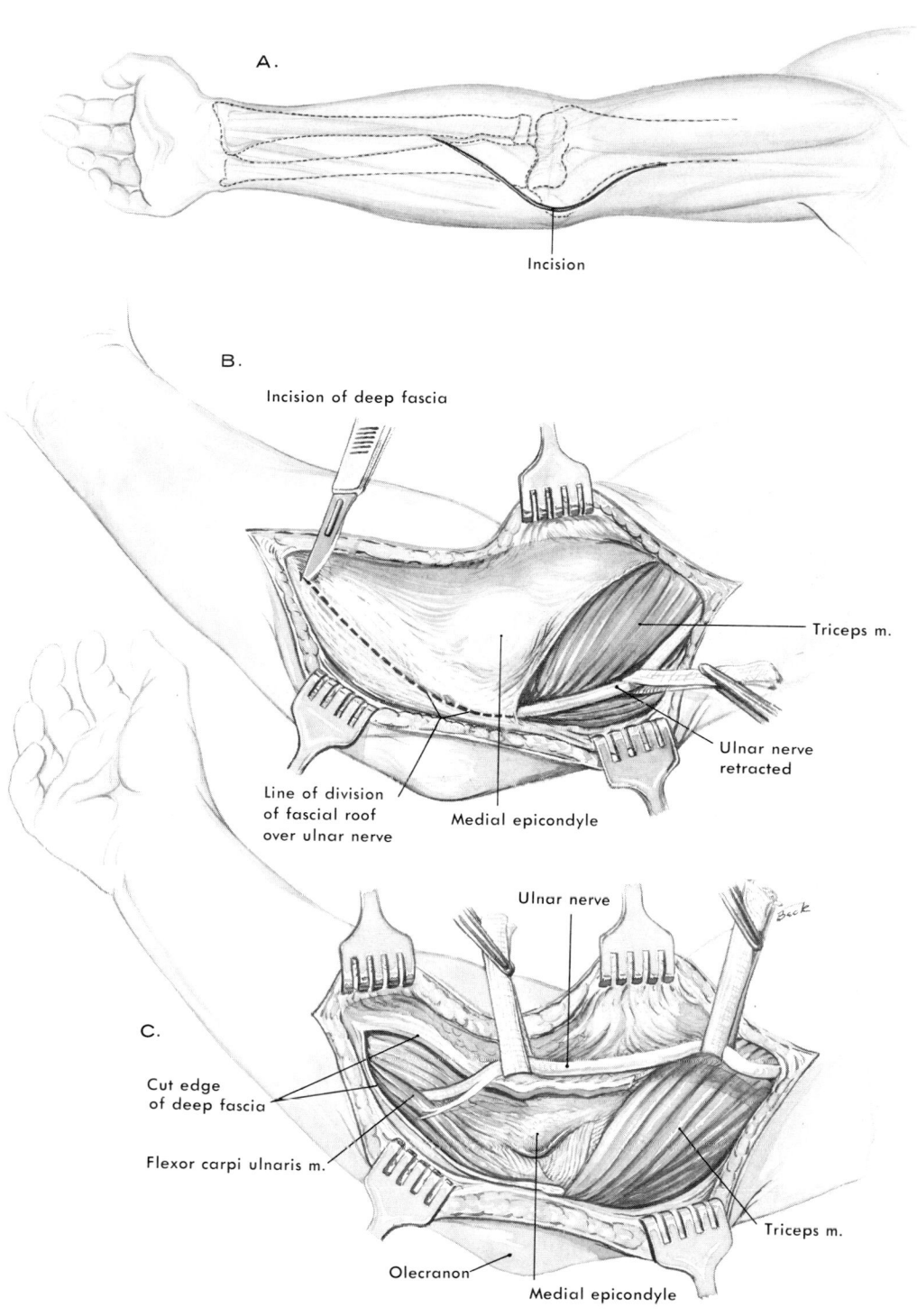

A.

Incision

B.

Incision of deep fascia

Triceps m.

Ulnar nerve retracted

Line of division of fascial roof over ulnar nerve

Medial epicondyle

C.

Ulnar nerve

Cut edge of deep fascia

Flexor carpi ulnaris m.

Triceps m.

Olecranon

Medial epicondyle

1019

Flexorplasty of the Elbow (Steindler) (Continued)

D. Next, the biceps tendon is identified over the anterior aspect of the elbow joint. The deep fascia and the lacertus fibrosus are divided along the medial aspect of the biceps tendon.

E. By digital palpation, the interval between the biceps and pronator teres muscles is developed. The brachial artery with its accompanying veins runs along the medial side of the biceps tendon. The median nerve, lying medial to the brachial artery, is dissected free of the surrounding tissues and gently retracted anteriorly with a moist hernia tape. The branches of the median nerve to the pronator teres muscle must be identified and protected from injury.

F. Next, with an osteotome, the common flexor origin of the pronator teres, flexor carpi radialis, palmaris longus, flexor digitorum sublimis, and flexor carpi ulnaris is detached en bloc with a flake of bone from the medial epicondyle.

Plate 45. *Flexorplasty of the Elbow (Steindler)*

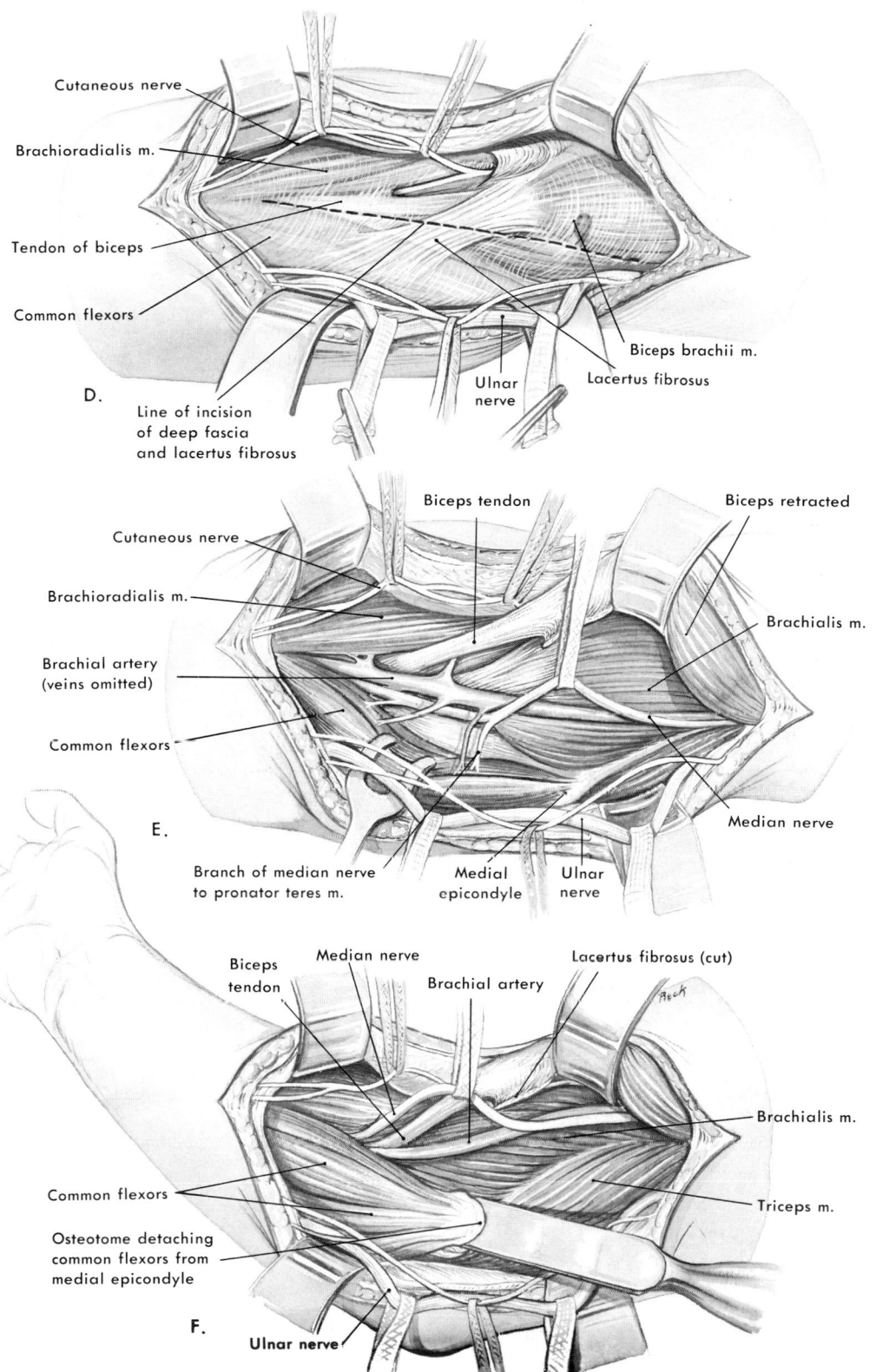

D.

Cutaneous nerve

Brachioradialis m.

Tendon of biceps

Common flexors

Biceps brachii m.

Lacertus fibrosus

Ulnar nerve

Line of incision of deep fascia and lacertus fibrosus

E.

Biceps tendon

Biceps retracted

Cutaneous nerve

Brachioradialis m.

Brachial artery (veins omitted)

Common flexors

Brachialis m.

Median nerve

Branch of median nerve to pronator teres m.

Medial epicondyle

Ulnar nerve

F.

Biceps tendon

Median nerve

Brachial artery

Lacertus fibrosus (cut)

Brachialis m.

Common flexors

Triceps m.

Osteotome detaching common flexors from medial epicondyle

Ulnar nerve

Flexorplasty of the Elbow (Steindler) (Continued)

G. By sharp and blunt dissection, the flexor muscle mass is freed and mobilized distally away from the joint capsule and the ulna as far as the motor branches of the median nerve and ulnar nerve will permit. A No. 1 silk whip suture is placed in the proximal end of the common flexors.

H. The biceps muscle, brachial vessels, and median nerve are retracted laterally, and the atrophied brachial muscle is split longitudinally. The periosteum is incised and stripped, exposing the anterior aspect of the distal humerus.

The elbow is then flexed to 120 degrees to determine the site of attachment of the transfer (usually 2 inches proximal to the elbow). With a drill, a hole is made on the anterior surface of the humerus. The opening is enlarged with progressively larger diamond-head hand drills to receive the transferred muscle. The action of the transfer as a pronator of the forearm is decreased by transferring it laterally on the humerus. With smaller size drill points, two tunnels are made from the lateral and medial cortices of the humerus and are connected to the larger hole for passing the suture.

I and **J.** Because the elbow will be immobilized in acute flexion, it is best to close the distal half of the wound before anchoring the transplant to the humerus. The ends of the whip suture are brought out through the tunnels, and the common flexors and the origin are firmly secured in the larger hole. The periosteum is closed with interrupted sutures over the transferred tendon, thus reinforcing its anchorage. The proximal half of the wound is closed and a long arm cast is applied with the elbow in acute flexion and the forearm in full supination.

For postoperative care, see the guidelines outlined in the text on principles of tendon transfer.

Plate 45. Flexorplasty of the Elbow (Steindler)

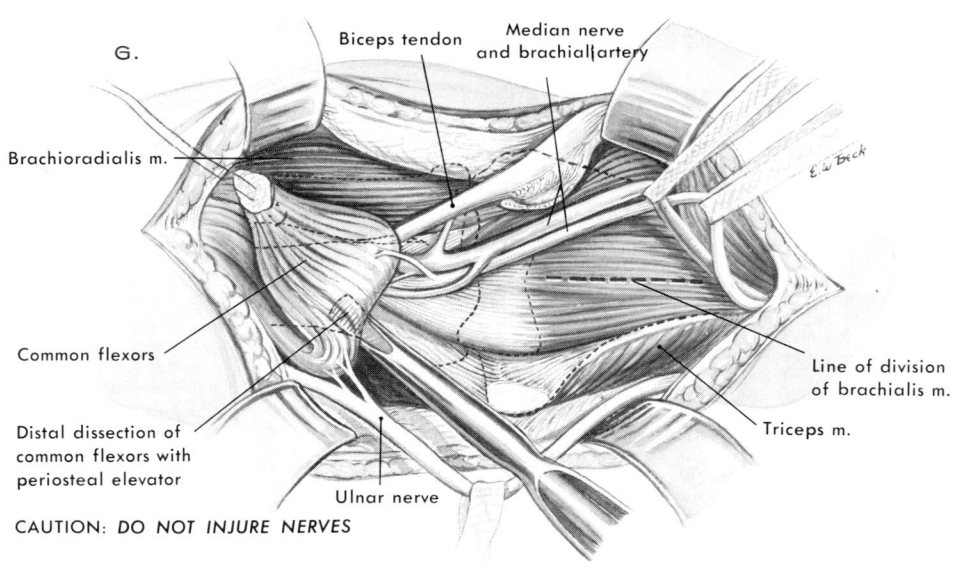

G.

Biceps tendon

Median nerve and brachial artery

Brachioradialis m.

Common flexors

Distal dissection of
common flexors with
periosteal elevator

Ulnar nerve

Line of division
of brachialis m.

Triceps m.

CAUTION: DO NOT INJURE NERVES

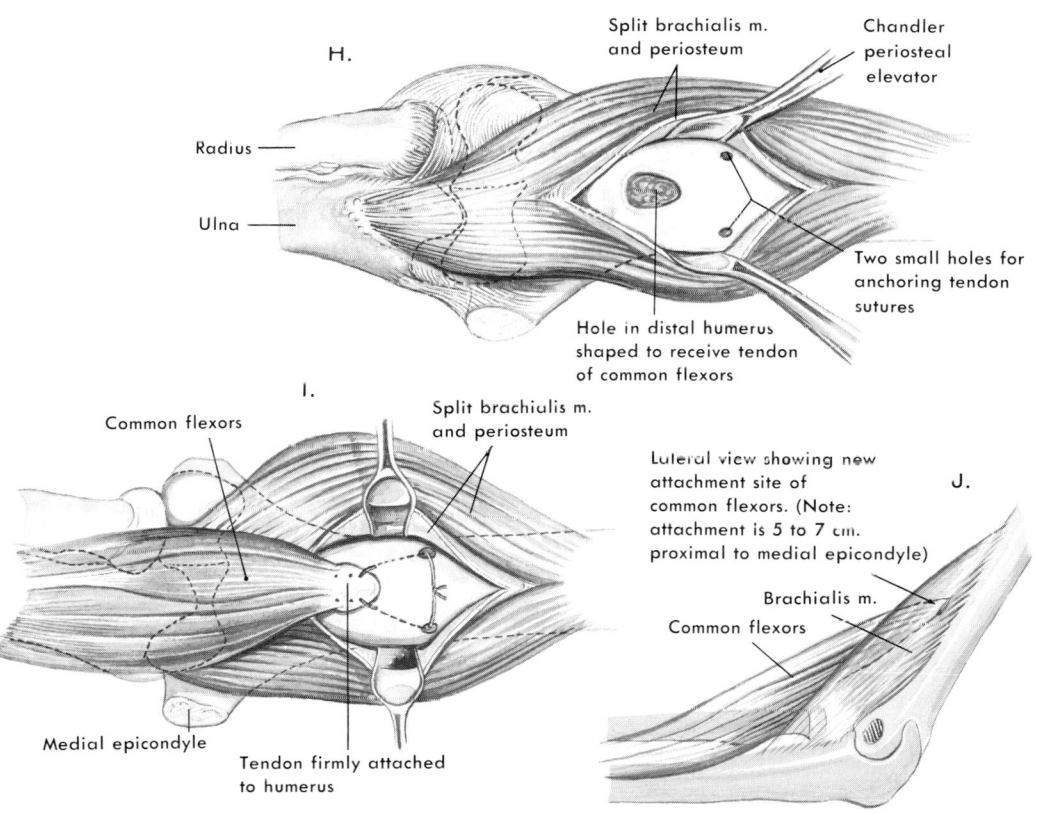

H.

Split brachialis m.
and periosteum

Chandler
periosteal
elevator

Radius

Ulna

Two small holes for
anchoring tendon
sutures

Hole in distal humerus
shaped to receive tendon
of common flexors

I.

Common flexors

Split brachialis m.
and periosteum

Lateral view showing new
attachment site of
common flexors. (Note:
attachment is 5 to 7 cm.
proximal to medial epicondyle)

J.

Brachialis m.

Common flexors

Medial epicondyle

Tendon firmly attached
to humerus

Pectoralis Major Transfer for Paralysis of Elbow Flexors

THE PROCEDURE

A. The patient is positioned supine with the upper limb supported on a hand table with the shoulder in 45 degrees of abduction and 30 degrees of external rotation. Two incisions are made, the first one following the deltopectoral groove extending from the clavicle down to the junction of the upper and middle thirds of the arm. The second incision is centered over the anteromedial aspect of the elbow.

B. Through the first incision the subcutaneous tissue and deep fascia are divided, and the cephalic vein is ligated if necessary.

C. The pectoralis major tendon is identified and divided at its insertion, as close to the bone as possible. By blunt dissection, the muscle is mobilized from the chest wall toward the clavicle. The deltoid muscle is then retracted laterally and the tendon of the long head of the biceps exposed running upward toward the shoulder joint. It is severed at the upper end of the bicipital groove and pulled distally into the wound.

Plate 46. *Pectoralis Major Transfer for Paralysis of Elbow Flexors*

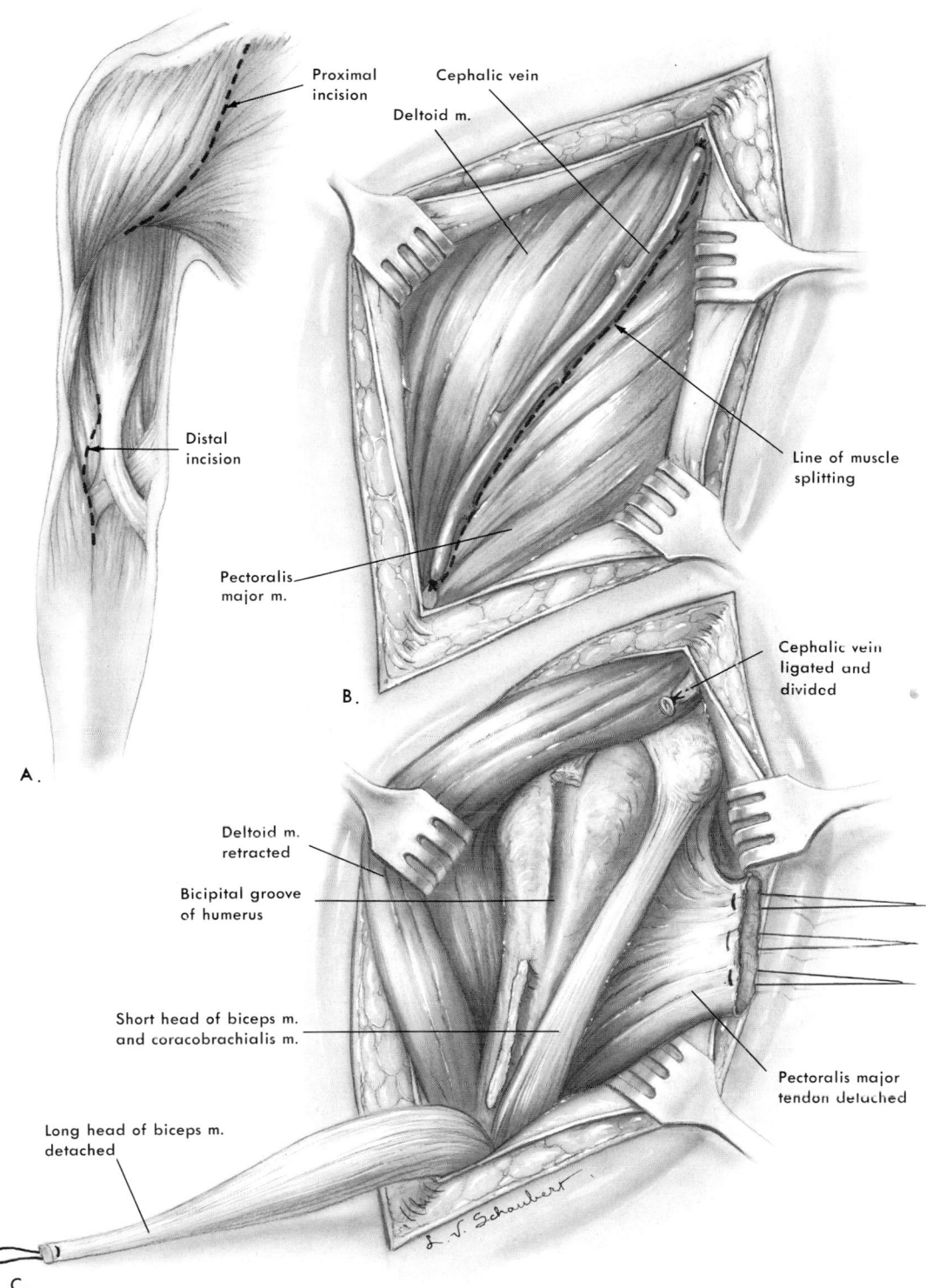

Proximal incision

Cephalic vein

Deltoid m.

Distal incision

Line of muscle splitting

Pectoralis major m.

A.

B.

Cephalic vein ligated and divided

Deltoid m. retracted

Bicipital groove of humerus

Short head of biceps m. and coracobrachialis m.

Pectoralis major tendon detached

Long head of biceps m. detached

C.

L. V. Schaubert

1025

Pectoralis Major Transfer for Paralysis of Elbow Flexors
(Continued)

D. By blunt and sharp dissection, the muscle belly of the long head of the biceps is mobilized to the lowest third of the arm by freeing it from the short head. The vessels and nerves entering the muscle belly are divided and ligated as necessary. The tendon and muscle of the long head are delivered into the distal second incision and freed down to the tuberosity of the radius. Often, freeing the muscle from adhesions to the overlying fascia requires sharp dissection. After complete mobilization of the long head of the biceps by traction on its proximal end, one should be able to flex the elbow.

E. The long head of the biceps is pulled into the upper wound. Two slits are made in the tendon of the mobilized pectoralis major through which the tendon of the long head is passed, looped on itself, and brought down again into the distal wound. With the elbow acutely flexed, the proximal end of the tendon is sutured to its own tendon of insertion through a slit in the distal tendon. Silk sutures are also inserted at the level of the tendon of the pectoralis major. The incisions are then closed in the routine manner. A plaster of Paris reinforced Velpeau bandage is applied with the elbow acutely flexed.

POSTOPERATIVE CARE

Plaster of Paris immobilization is continued for three weeks. At the end of this time active flexion and extension exercises of the elbow are started, first with gravity eliminated and then against gravity. A sling is used to protect the transferred tendon from stretching. Care should be taken to extend the elbow gradually so that active flexion above the right-angle position is maintained. Extension of the elbow is regained slowly.

Plate 46.   Pectoralis Major Transfer for
Paralysis of Elbow Flexors

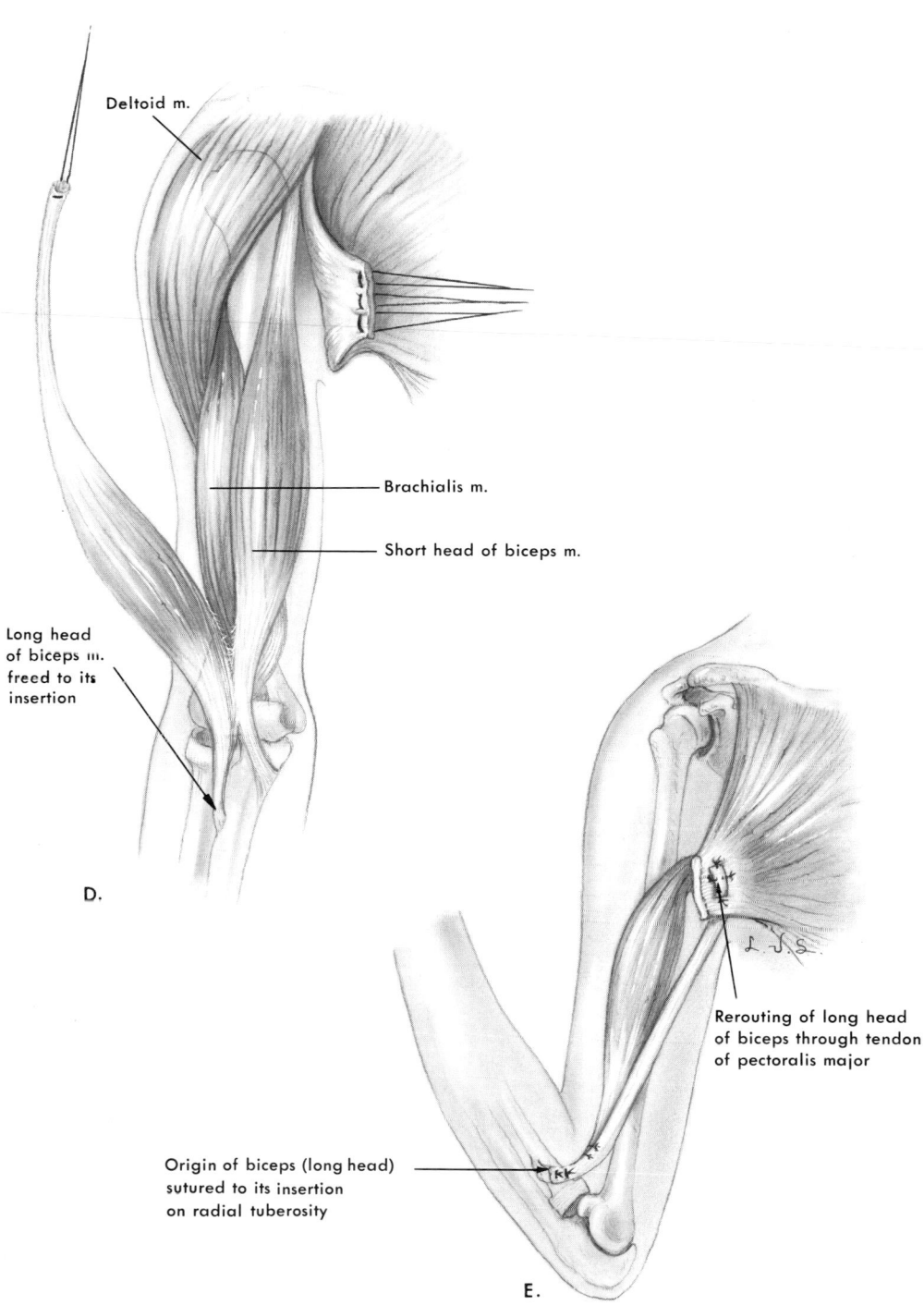

Deltoid m.

Brachialis m.

Short head of biceps m.

Long head
of biceps m.
freed to its
insertion

D.

Rerouting of long head
of biceps through tendon
of pectoralis major

Origin of biceps (long head)
sutured to its insertion
on radial tuberosity

E.

there is appreciable paralysis of the shoulder muscle, the pectoralis major transfer must be followed by arthrodesis of the scapulo-humeral joint.

PECTORALIS MINOR TRANSFER

Spira, in 1957, reported the successful use of the pectoralis minor as a motor to restore elbow flexion. The patient had complete paralysis of the pectoralis major, biceps brachii, and brachialis muscles. A tube of fascia lata was used to bridge the gap between the detached origin of the pectoralis minor and the paralyzed biceps tendon.[650]

STERNOCLEIDOMASTOID TRANSFER

Bunnell utilized the sternocleidomastoid muscle as a motor to restore active elbow flexion.[427] The sternoclavicular insertion of the sternocleidomastoid muscle is detached and by gentle blunt dissection the distal half of the muscle is mobilized. A long tube of fascia lata is used to bridge the gap, extending from the distal end of the sterno-cleidomastoid muscle and then passing forward subcutaneously in the arm to the elbow where the graft is attached to the tuberosity of the radius (Fig. 5–97).

Carroll reported the results of 15 cases of sternocleidomastoid transfer with satisfactory results in 80 per cent. He stressed the importance of placing the transferred muscle under maximal tension at the time of operation.[436]

In the personal experience of the author with seven patients, the strength of elbow flexion following Bunnell's sternocleidomastoid transfer is excellent; however, the aesthetic appearance of the procedure is very grotesque and is objectionable, particularly in girls. It should be used in cases in which it is the only method available, but must be limited to the male patient only, in whom function is the primary consideration and the resultant deformity can be hidden by the buttoned collar of a shirt.

ANTERIOR TRANSFER OF TRICEPS BRACHII

This was described by Bunnell in 1948 and in 1951, and later by Carroll, who

showed the feasibility and effectiveness of the procedure without the use of the fascial graft that was recommended by Bunnell.[427, 435] In 1970 Carroll reported the results of triceps transfer in 15 patients (8 with arthrogryposis multiplex congenita, and 7 with post-traumatic and paralytic loss of elbow flexion). The criteria of success were the inability to flex the elbow against gravity and to bring the hand to the mouth before surgery and the ability to do so postoperatively. The results of Carroll were as follows: In the post-traumatic and paralytic group there were five successes, one limited result, and one failure; in the arthrogrypotic group, there were five successes, one limited result, and two failures.[438]

The operative technique described by Carroll is as follows:

The patient is placed in lateral position. A midline incision is made on the posterior aspect of the arm, beginning in its middle half and extending distally to a point lateral to the olecranon process; then the incision is carried over the subcutaneous surface of the shaft of the ulna for a distance of 5 cm. The subcutaneous tissue is divided, and the wound flaps are mobilized. The ulnar nerve is identified and mobilized medially to protect it from injury. The intermuscular septum is exposed laterally. The triceps tendon is detached from its insertion with a long tail of periosteum. Then the triceps muscle is freed and mobilized proximally as far as its nerve supply permits. The motor branches of the radial nerve to the triceps enter the muscle in the interval between the lateral and medial heads as the radial nerve enters the musculospiral groove. The distal portion of the detached triceps is then sutured to itself to form a tube. Through a curvilinear incision in the antecubital fossa, the interval between the brachioradialis and the pronator teres is developed. With an Ober tendon passer, the triceps tendon is passed into the anterior wound subcutaneously, superficial to the radial nerve. With the elbow in 90 degrees of flexion and the forearm in full supination, the triceps tendon is either sutured to the biceps tendon or anchored to the radial tuberosity by a suture passed through a drill hole (Fig. 5–98). The wound is closed in routine fashion. A long arm cast is applied with the

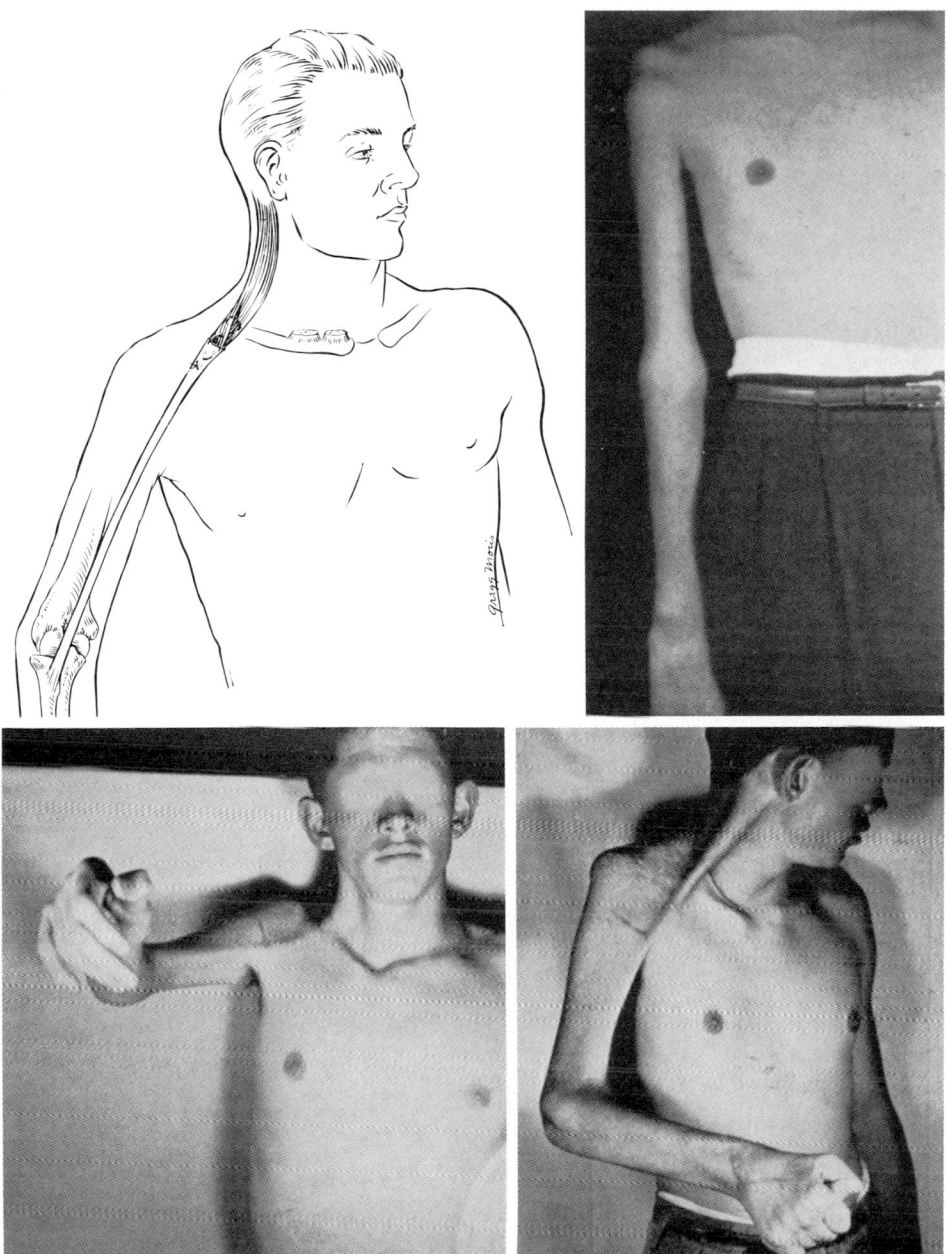

FIGURE 5-97. *Bunnell's sternocleidomastoid transfer to restore active flexion of the elbow.*

A. Drawing showing the sternocleidomastoid muscle transfer. **B.** Preoperative photograph of patient with flail shoulder and elbow and partially paralyzed hand. The shoulder was fused; the sternocleidomastoid muscle was transferred; the wrist was arthrodesed in functional position. **C** and **D.** Postoperative photographs show the result. Function of the useless right upper limb was greatly improved. (From Bunnell, S.: Restoring flexion to the paralytic elbow. J. Bone Joint Surg., *33-A*:569, 1951.)

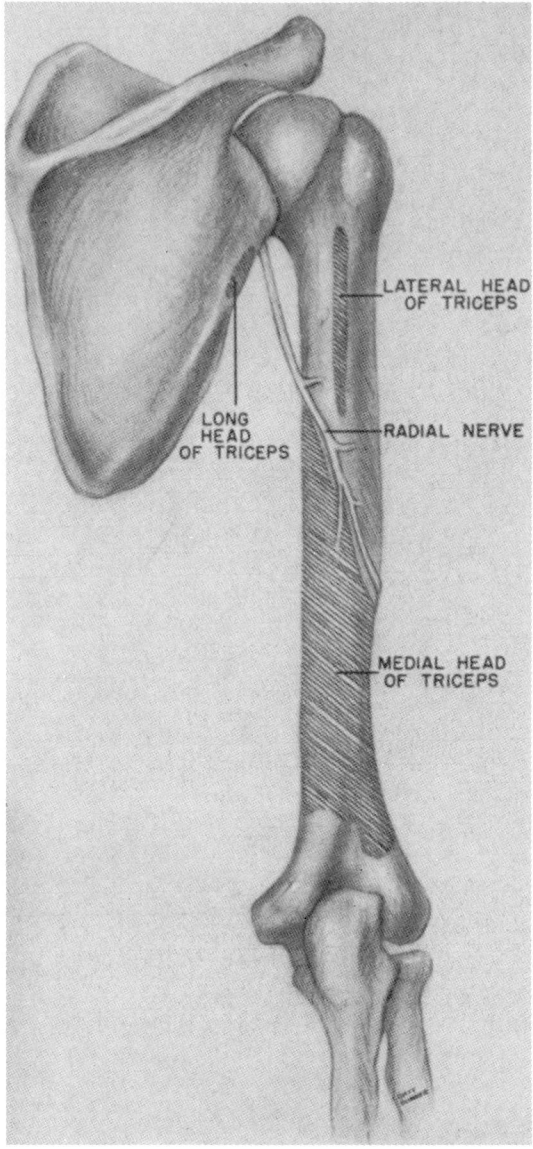

A

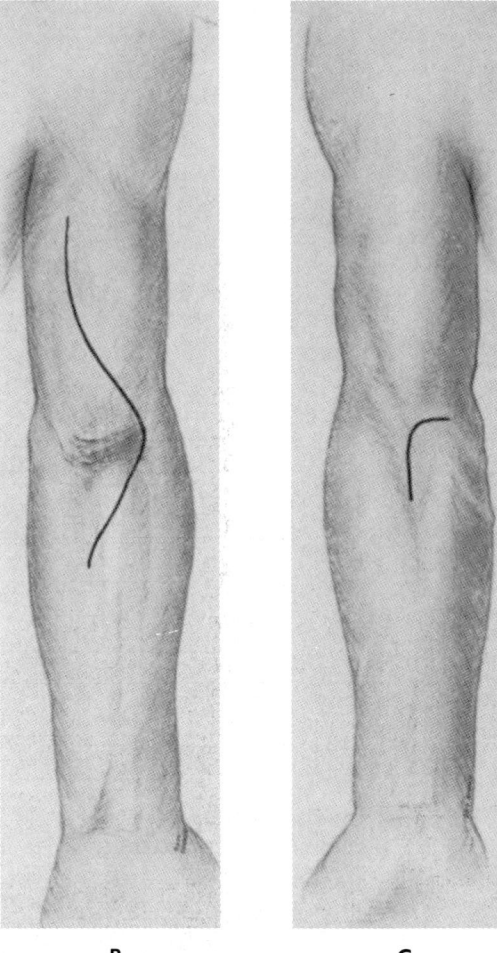

B   C

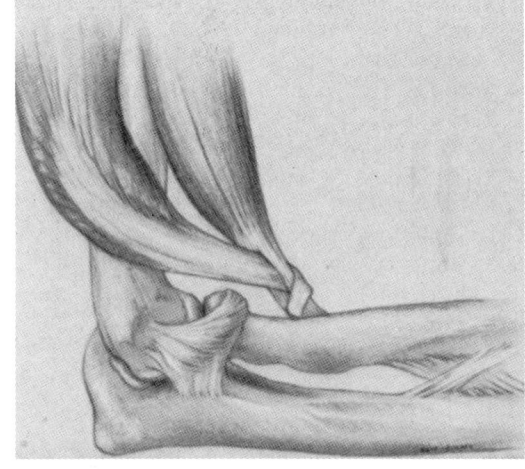

D

*FIGURE 5–98.   Carroll's modification of
Bunnell's anterior transfer of triceps for
paralysis of biceps.*

A. The motor branches of the radial nerve are given
off in the area between the medial and lateral heads of
the triceps muscle. **B.** The long curvilinear incision
avoids pressure points of the elbow and gives adequate
exposure. **C.** Only a small incision is necessary to expose
the ulnar aspect. **D.** The tendon of the mobilized
triceps brachii is woven through the biceps tendon with
the elbow in flexion. It may be anchored directly to the
radial tuberosity. (From Carroll, R. E.: Restoration of
flexor power to the flail elbow by transplantation of
the triceps tendon. Surg. Gynec. Obstet., 95:686, 1952.)

elbow in 90 degrees of flexion and full supination for four weeks, at which time immobilization is discontinued and active exercises begun. Gravity provides extension to the elbow.[438]

Loss of active extension against gravity is a definite disadvantage of anterior transfer of the triceps. The operation should be restricted to exceptional cases in which restoration of elbow flexion is imperative and in which no other tendon transfer is possible. Another indication for anterior transfer of the triceps is that of brachial plexus injuries, in which simultaneous contraction of the triceps (the antagonistic muscle) occurred on active flexion of the elbow, and the action of the pectoralis major transfer was impaired. This simultaneous flexion-extension mass action can be successfully overcome by anterior transfer of the triceps into the flexor apparatus.

LATISSIMUS DORSI TRANSFER

Hovnanian described a method of transfer of the origin and belly of the latissimus dorsi muscle into the arm.[532] This is feasible because the nerve supply of the latissimus dorsi (the thoracodorsal nerve) is a long nerve (12 to 17 cm. in length) and is highly mobile and easily identified; also, the blood supply of the latissimus dorsi muscle enters from a wide zone in its proximal third. Thus the latissimus dorsi can be mobilized without denervating or devascularizing the muscle. Active elbow flexion is restored by anchoring the origin of the latissimus dorsi muscle into the biceps tendon near the radial tuberosity; active extension of the elbow is given by suturing it to the olecranaon (Fig. 5–99).

PARALYSIS OF TRICEPS BRACHII MUSCLE

Loss of active extension of the elbow due to paralysis of the triceps muscle seldom causes significant disability because the elbow will extend passively under the force of gravity. A strong triceps is not essential for crutch walking, provided good shoulder depressors are present. A triceps strap or band is added to the crutch and with the elbow locked in slight hyperextension, the patient can ambulate quite well. If there is marked paral-

ysis of both lower limbs and trunk, however, a functional triceps is desirable in order to lock the elbow in extension in daily activities such as arising from a bed or chair, or reaching for objects overhead.

Various operative procedures have been devised to restore active extension of the elbow. Trapezius muscle transfer was used in 1930 by Lange, who detached it from the acromion and joined it by long silk sutures to the olecranon.[556] Ober and Barr described a technique for transferring the brachioradialis muscle by rerouting it at the elbow to a more posterior position.[603] Extensor carpi radialis longus muscle was added to the brachioradialis muscle transfer if greater strength was necessary. The transfer of flexor carpi radialis and ulnaris muscles was proposed by Hohmann.[528, 529] Friedenberg transferred the biceps brachii for triceps paralysis.[482] The posterior part of the deltoid was proposed by d'Aubigné.[400, 401] Latissimus dorsi was used for transfer to restore elbow extension by Hohmann, Lange, Harmon, Schottstaedt, Larsen and Bost, Hovnanian, and DuToit and Levy.[466, 511, 528, 529, 532, 556, 634]

The relative merits and shortcomings of the various procedures are not discussed here as the author has had no personal experience with them. The Hovnanian transfer of the origin of the latissimus dorsi to the olecranon, leaving its insertion intact is recommended, as the procedure is physiologically sound and has been successful in the author's experience.

The Forearm

Fixed supination and pronation contractures of the forearm are deformities in flaccid paralysis that require surgical treatment.

Supination contracture of the forearm is rare but disabling. It results from selective paralysis of the four muscles that originate from the medial epicondyle of the humerus (the pronator teres, flexor carpi ulnaris, palmaris longus, and flexor carpi radialis) in the presence of a strong biceps brachii muscle. Contracture of the interosseous membrane soon develops. With growth and under the influence of unopposed action of the biceps brachii muscle, osseous changes take place,

(*Text continued on page 1036.*)

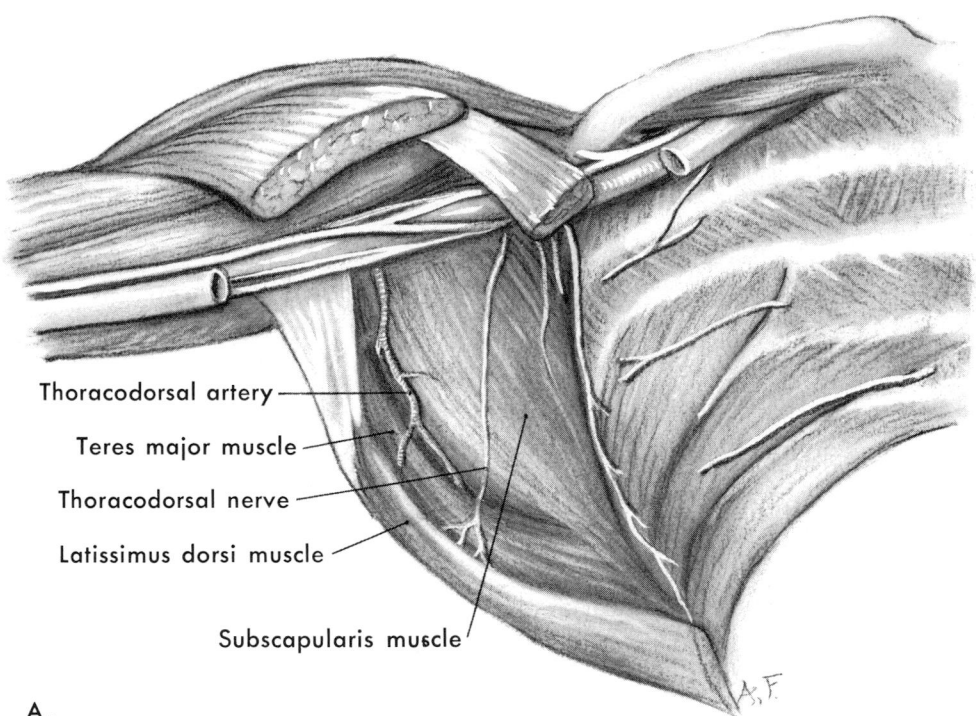

Thoracodorsal artery

Teres major muscle

Thoracodorsal nerve

Latissimus dorsi muscle

Subscapularis muscle

A.

FIGURE 5-99. *Latissimus dorsi transfer to restore flexion or extension at the elbow (Hovnanian operation).*

A. The anatomy of the axilla and the latissimus dorsi muscle. (From Hovnanian, A. P.: Latissimus dorsi transplantation at the elbow. Ann. Surg., *143*:493, 1956.)

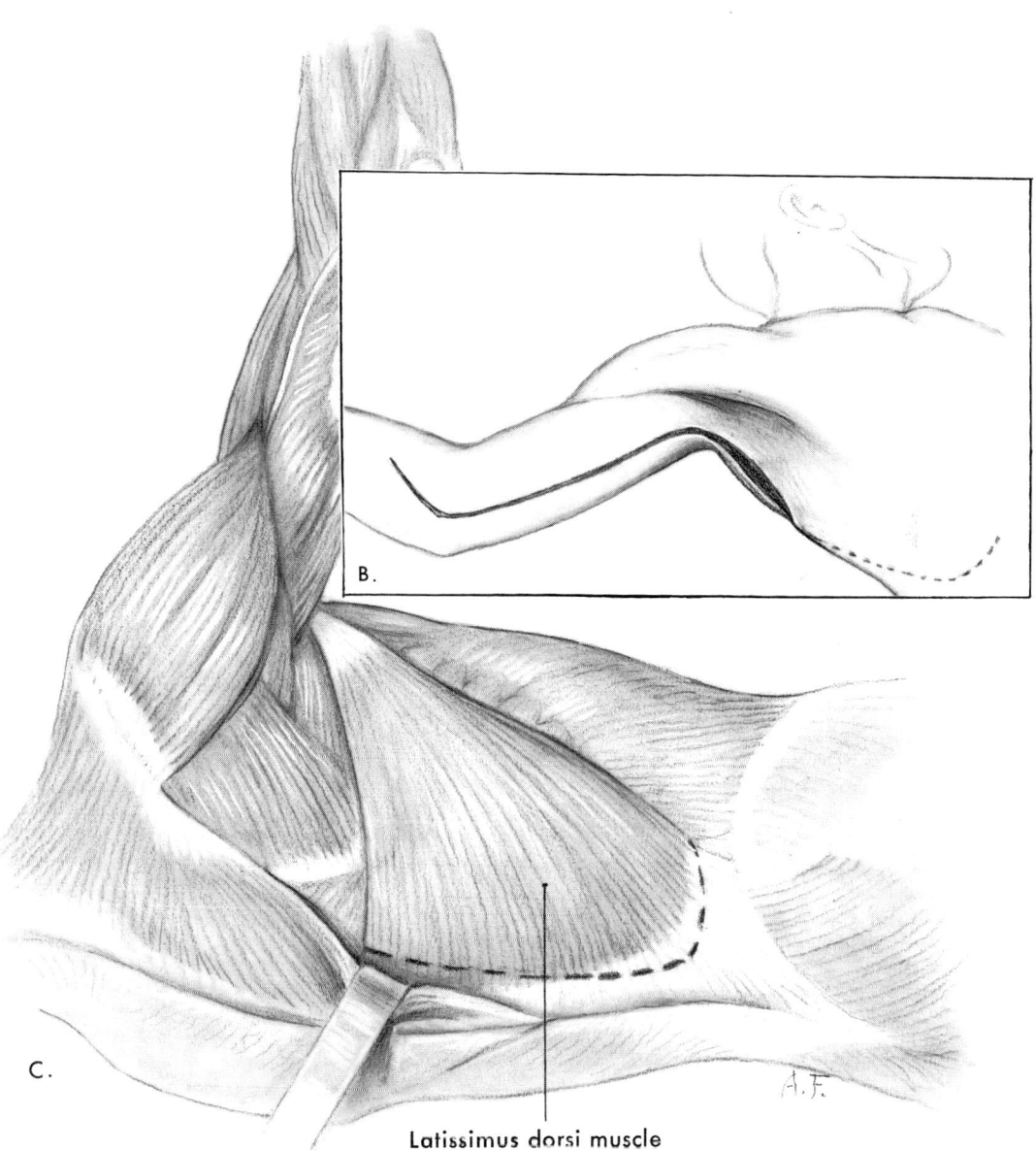

Latissimus dorsi muscle

FIGURE 5-99 Continued. *Latissimus dorsi transfer to restore flexion or extension at the elbow (Hovnanian operation).*

B. Skin incision used to restore elbow flexion. The lumbar extension of the skin incision is shown by dotted lines. **C.** The line of section of latissimus dorsi muscle across its musculofascial portion inferiorly and its muscle fibers superiorly. (From Hovnanian, A. P.: Latissimus dorsi transplantation at the elbow. Ann. Surg., *143*:493, 1956.)

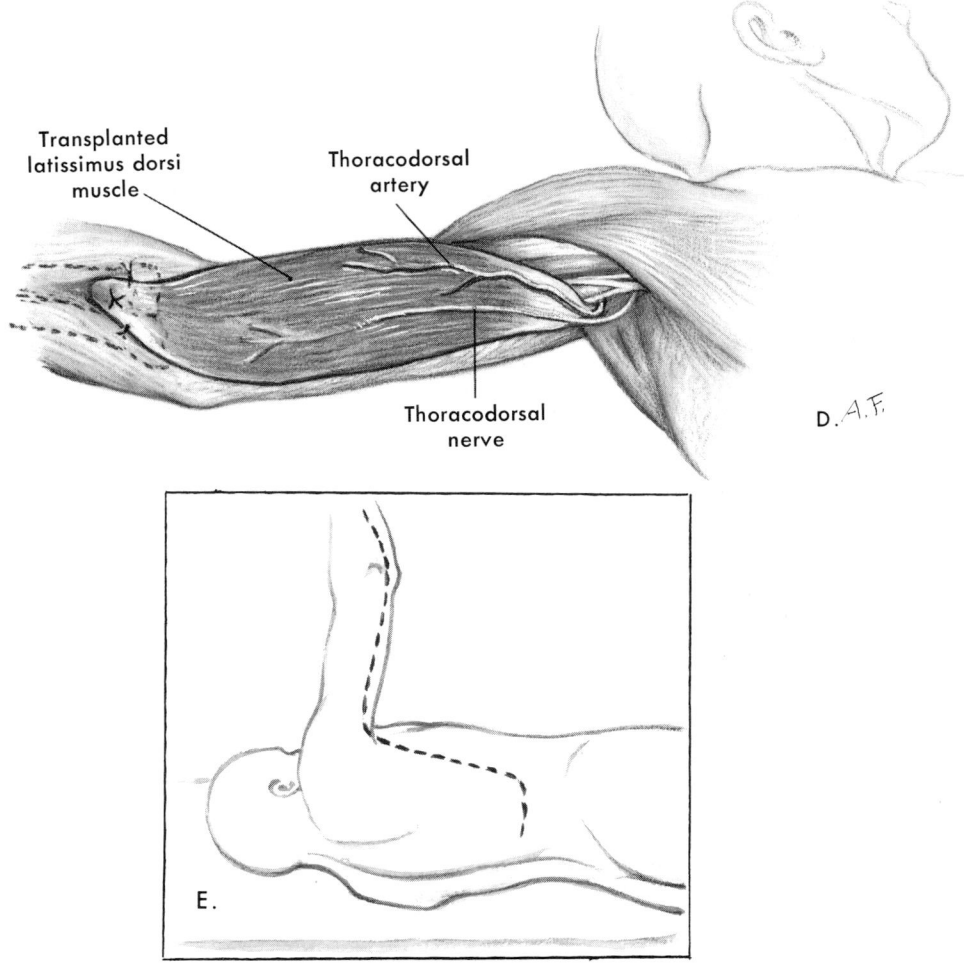

FIGURE 5–99 Continued.   *Latissimus dorsi transfer to restore flexion or extension at the elbow (Hovnanian operation).*

D. To restore elbow flexion, the belly and origin of the latissimus dorsi is transferred into the anteromedial aspect of the arm, and its origin is anchored into the biceps tendon near the radial tuberosity. **E.** Skin incision used to restore elbow extension. (From Hovnanian, A. P.: Latissimus dorsi transplantation at the elbow. Ann. Surg., *143*: 493, 1956.)

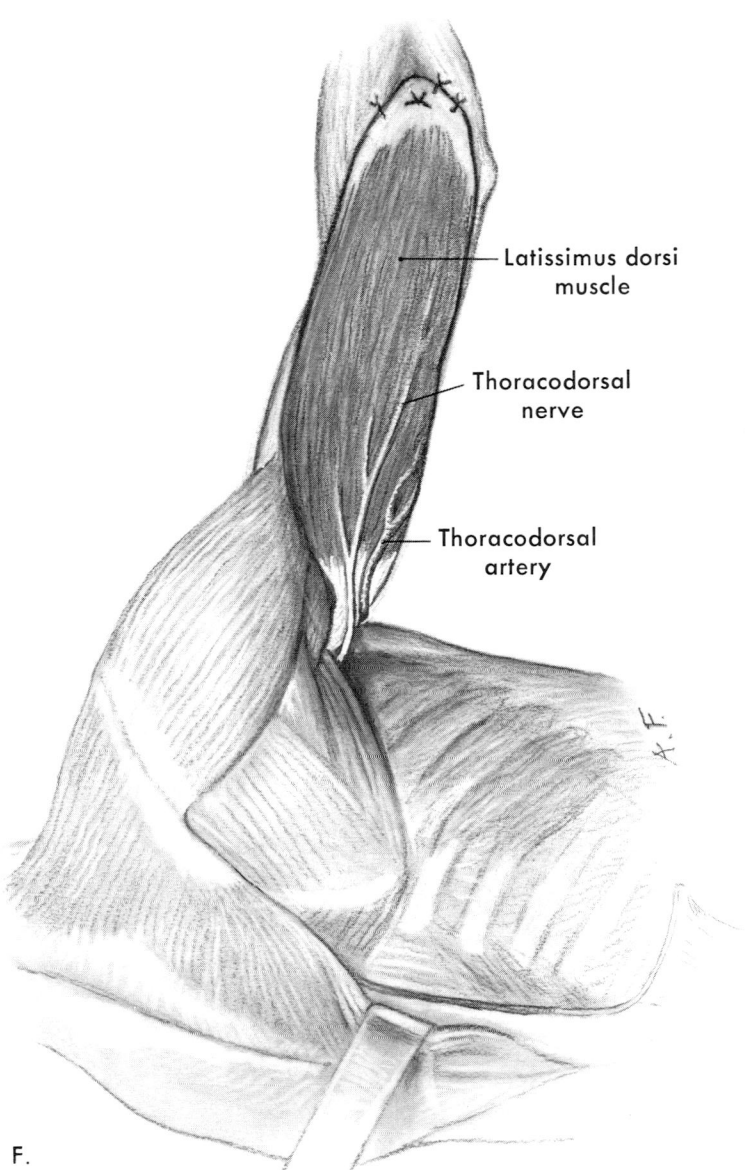

Latissimus dorsi muscle

Thoracodorsal nerve

Thoracodorsal artery

F.

FIGURE 5–99 Continued. *Latissimus dorsi transfer to restore flexion or extension at the elbow (Hovnanian operation).*

F. The latissimus dorsi muscle is transferred to the posterior aspect of the arm and anchored to the olecranon and triceps tendon. (From Hovnanian, A. P.: Latissimus dorsi transplantation at the elbow. Ann. Surg., *143*: 493, 1956.)

causing the radius to become curved and spiral around the ulna. If deformity remains uncorrected and there is still muscle imbalance, progressive fixed deformity will develop, with permanent shortening of the soft tissues, primarily the interosseous membrane, biceps brachii, and supinator muscles. The radius becomes markedly bowed and the radioulnar joints may subluxate. In children under 12 years of age, closed osteoclasis of the middle third of both bones of the forearm is recommended by Blount.[415] Because of recurrence of deformity, which can occur with further growth, he advises overcorrection. In two of the nine reported cases, osteoclasis was later repeated because of recurrence of supination contracture.

Zaoussis corrected the fixed supination deformity by open osteotomy near the tuberosity of the radius.[697] He found more or less permanent "blocking" of the forearm rotation following surgery, but the synostosis of the proximal radius and ulna did not seem to impair the functional result. As internal fixation was not used by Zaoussis, angulation, displacement, and delayed union of the osteotomy occurred; however, these complications did not affect the cosmetic and functional result.

The transfer of the biceps brachii to the side of the radial tuberosity opposite its normal insertion was mentioned by Schottstaedt, Larsen, and Bost.[634] A year later Grilli described the operative technique of rerouting the biceps tendon insertion to the radial side of the neck of the radius to convert its function from a supinator to that of pronator.[499]

Zancolli included surgical release of the contracted soft tissues in biceps transfer, especially the interosseous membrane.[696] He reported satisfactory results in 14 patients with supination contracture of the forearm (eight patients had obstetrical brachial plexus paralysis, four patients had poliomyelitis, and two patients, traumatic quadriplegia). Correction was maintained in all 14 patients. Active pronation (measuring 10 to 60 degrees and using the transferred biceps brachii muscle) was achieved in eight patients. Active supination (measuring 20 to 80 degrees) was retained in eight patients. The procedure permits a more normal anatomic relationship of the radius and ulna to develop, resulting in nearly normal shape of the forearm. For details of operative technique, the reader is referred to the original paper of Zancolli.[696]

Affections of the Peripheral Nerves

Traumatic Disorders

OBSTETRICAL BRACHIAL PLEXUS PALSY

Paralysis of the upper limb resulting from traction injury to the brachial plexus at birth has decreased with the advent of improved obstetrical techniques. The entity was first mentioned by Smellie, in 1764.[726]

Etiology and Classification

The mechanism of trauma is that of forced stretching of one or more components of the brachial plexus by traction. The affected babies are large, their birth weight averaging 2 pounds heavier than normal.[698] Delivery is usually difficult. In breech delivery traction is applied on the brachial plexus at the stage when the head is extracted by strong lateral flexion of the trunk and neck, while in vertex presentation the brachial plexus is injured when the shoulders are delivered by forced lateral flexion of the head and neck.

In experimental studies on the tensile strength of the brachial plexus, Wickstrom found that disruption of the lower plexus components occurred with approximately half the force required to disrupt the components of the upper plexus and that the soft-tissue structures surrounding the plexus contributed to the resistance to stretch of the tissues. Most of the disruptions occurred at the foramen or within the groove of the transverse process. Avulsion of the nerve roots from the spinal cord and cord disruption accounted for the upper motor neuron lesion findings often present in brachial plexus injuries.[731, 732]

Obstetrical brachial plexus palsy may be classified according to the severity of damage and according to the components of the plexus that are injured.

Injury to nerves by increased traction on the plexus may vary from slight stretching (neurapraxia or axonotmesis) to complete rupture (neurotmesis). In *mild* lesions failure of conduction results from simple stretching of the nerve fibers and associated perineural edema and hemorrhage. In this type of injury, usually complete and early recovery takes place with absorption of the edema and hemorrhage. On occasion, however, cicatricial fibrosis occurs and recovery is slow and incomplete. In *moderate* lesions, some of the nerve fibers are stretched and others are torn, with associated intraneural and extraneural bleeding. Depending upon the severity of involvement, recovery of nerve conduction and function is slow and incomplete in this type. In *severe* lesions, there is almost complete rupture of the trunks of the plexus, or actual avulsion of the roots from the spinal cord. In this type, recovery is very poor.

According to the components of the plexus injured, obstetrical brachial plexus paralysis may be grouped into (1) *the upper arm paralysis of Erb-Duchenne,* in which the fifth and sixth cervical nerve roots or their derivatives are principally involved; (2) *the lower arm paralysis of Klumpke,* in which the eighth cervical and first thoracic roots are affected; and (3) *paralysis of the entire arm* in which there is some involvement of all components of the plexus.[705, 706, 711]

Clinical Features

Immediately following birth the injury is evident. The affected limb lies motionless at the side of the trunk with the elbow in extension (Fig. 5–100). The Moro reflex is absent on the involved side (Fig. 5–101). In the lower arm and whole arm types of paralysis, there is loss of the grasp reflex. In the Klumpke type, the cervical sympathetic fibers in the first dorsal root may be involved, producing an ipsilateral Horner's syndrome characterized by enophthalmos, miosis, and ptosis. Avulsion of the nerve roots from the spinal cord may produce hematomyelia, which accounts for the presence of the transient spastic paralysis in the opposite upper limb and both lower limbs. In some instances there may be supraclavicular swelling and tenderness due to hemorrhage, or the nerve injury may be accompanied by a fractured clavicle, traumatic separation of the upper humeral epiphysis, or a fracture of the humeral shaft. Passive movements of the affected limb may be painful owing to associated "neuritis."

The distribution of motor paralysis depends upon the site of nerve injury. In the upper arm or Erb-Duchenne type, the deltoid muscle, the external rotator muscles of the shoulder (supraspinatus, intraspinatus, and teres minor), the biceps brachii, brachialis, supinator, and brachioradialis muscles are usually paralyzed. The fingers and wrist have normal active motion. There may be slight sensory deficit. The upper arm paralysis is the most frequent type.

In the lower arm paralysis of Klumpke, the wrist flexors, the long flexors of the fingers, and the intrinsic muscles of the hand are affected. The muscles controlling the shoulder and elbow are not involved. This is the rarest type. Sensation is ordinarily normal. When the entire arm is paralyzed, the upper limb is almost completely flaccid and there is often extensive sensory loss.

Residual Deformities

SHOULDER

Fixed internal rotation and adduction deformity of the shoulder is commonly present. Both active and passive abduction and external rotation of the shoulder are limited (Figs. 5–101 and 5–102). It is caused by paralysis of the deltoid, supraspinatus, infraspinatus, and teres minor muscles and asynergy (dyskinesia) of the muscles controlling the shoulder. The strong pectoralis major, subscapularis, teres

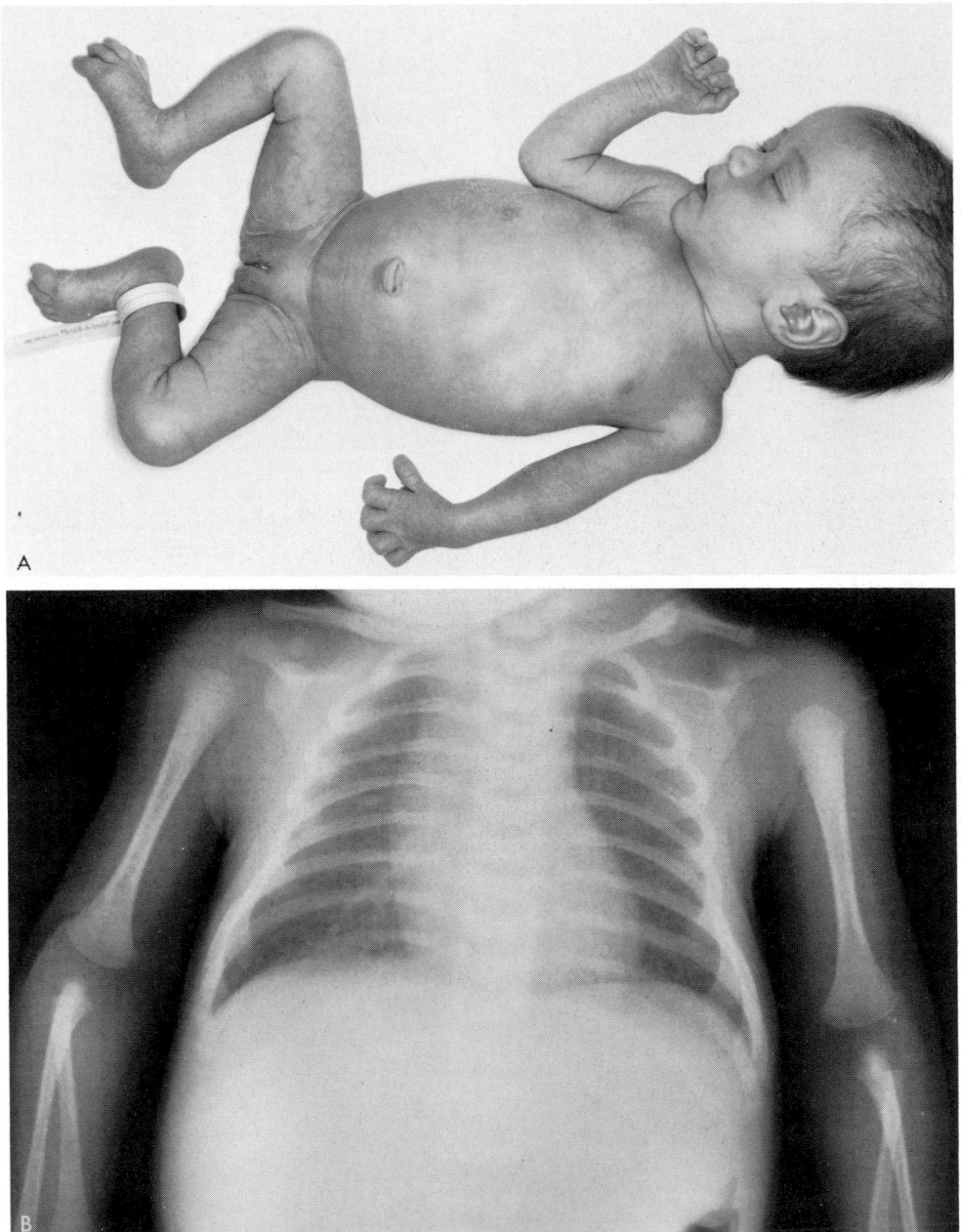

FIGURE 5–100.   *Obstetrical brachial plexus paralysis on the left in a newborn infant.*

A. Clinical appearance of patient. The left upper limb lies at the side of the trunk with the elbow in extension. **B.** Roentgenogram shows healing fracture of left clavicle.

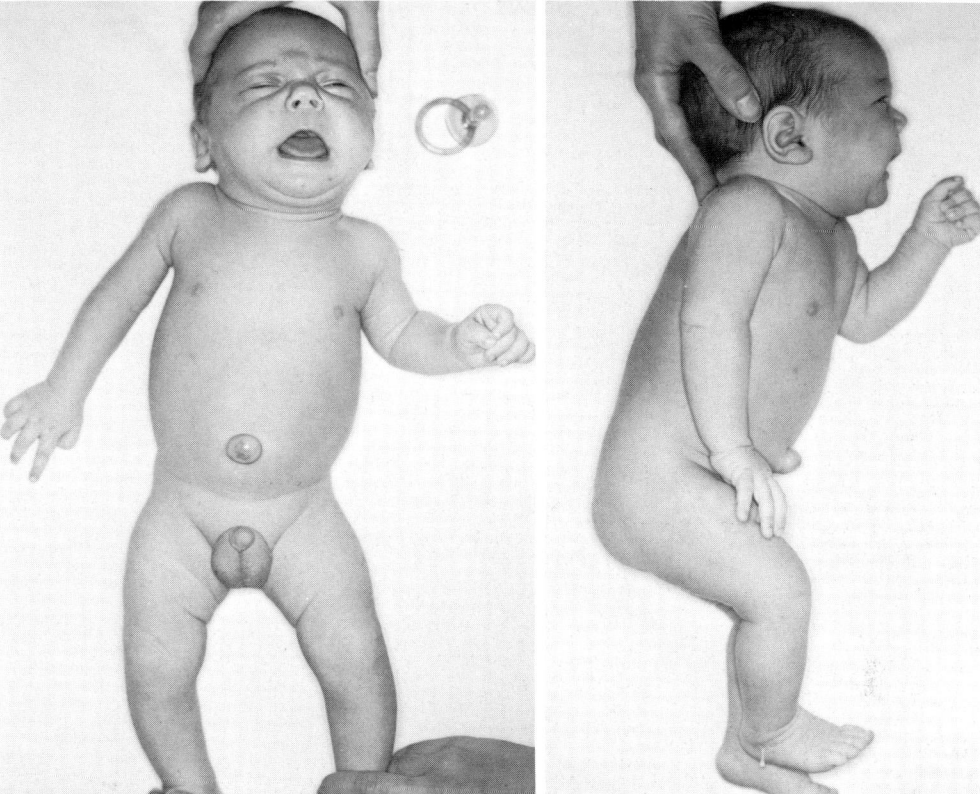

FIGURE 5–101. *Obstetrical brachial plexus paralysis on the right in a one-month-old infant.*

Note the lack of active motion in response to testing of asymmetrical tonic and Moro reflexes.

major, and lattismus dorsi muscles develop myostatic contracture (Fig. 5–103). With the shoulder in the adducted and internally rotated position, dysplasia with broadening and flattening of the glenoid fossa of the scapula develops and the humeral head tends to be dislocated posteriorly. The coracoid process becomes elongated, hooks downward and laterally, and comes to rest in the position formerly occupied by the humeral head, and in fact, interferes with the return of the humeral head to its normal position. The acromion beaks downward as a result of lack of shoulder abduction (Fig. 5–103). These secondary bony abnormalities tend to obstruct external rotation and abduction of the shoulder. In obstetrical brachial plexus paralysis, the scapula tends to be smaller than normal, lies higher in position, and develops shortening of its neck.

Abduction contracture of the scapulohumeral articulation is commonly seen, probably as a result of the constant abduction required to compensate for the limited external rotation of the shoulder. Another etiologic factor is the improper use of splints in the "Statue-of-Liberty" position in the early paralytic phase of the disease. Abduction contracture of the scapulohumeral joint causes winging of the scapula when the arm is held at the side of the trunk.

Asynergy (or dyskinesia) of the muscles controlling the shoulder is a prominent feature. The normal scapulohumeral rhythm is disturbed. During attempted abduction, the scapula moves initially, and the greater part of the combined action at the shoulder is scapulocostal rather than scapulohumeral. When active shoulder abduction is attempted, hypertonicity of the flexor muscle groups is triggered and the shoulder and elbow joints simultaneously go into automatic flexion. The holding motor power of the deltoid muscle in abducted position is strong, but when the

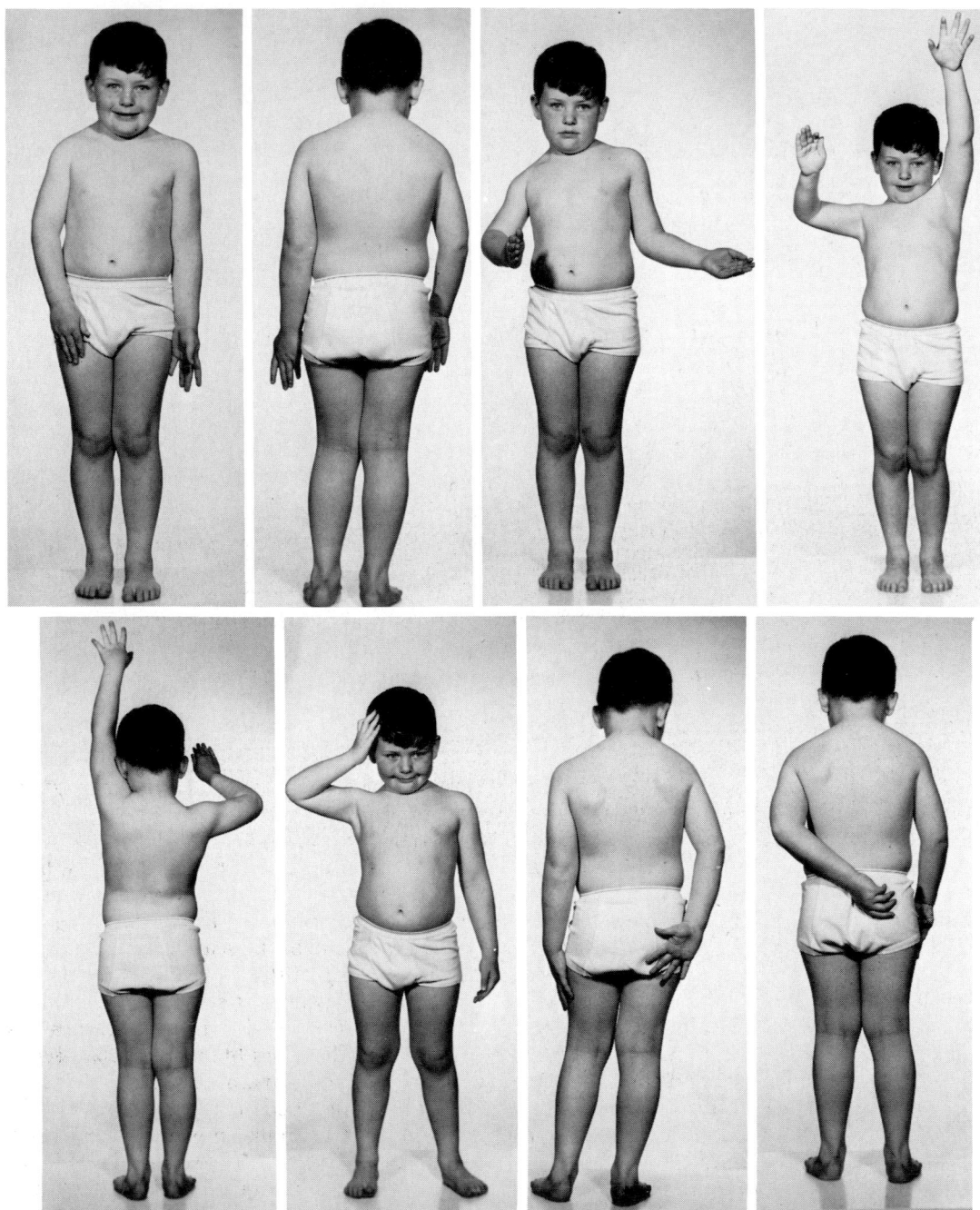

FIGURE 5–102. *Obstetrical brachial plexus paralysis of the right upper limb in a six-year-old boy.*

Note the limitation of active abduction and external rotation of the shoulder, and also the pronation contracture of the forearm.

MUSCLE IMBALANCE

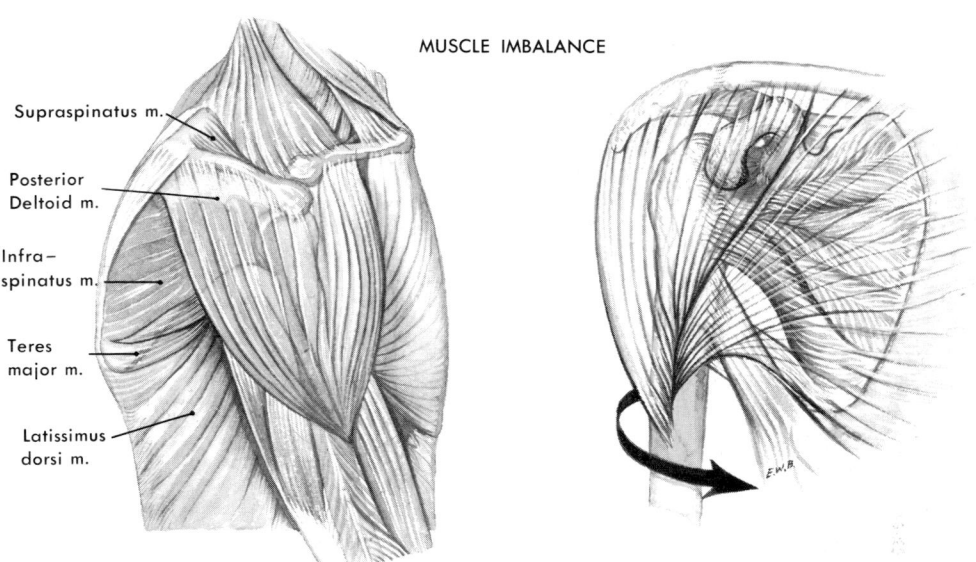

Supraspinatus m.

Posterior
Deltoid m.

Infra-
spinatus m.

Teres
major m.

Latissimus
dorsi m.

External rotators and abductors (supraspinatus, infraspinatus, posterior and
middle deltoid) are weak.

Adductors and internal rotators are normal
in motor strength (pectoralis major, coracobrachialis, pectoralis minor, subscapularis,
teres major, and latissimus dorsi).

BONY DEFORMITIES

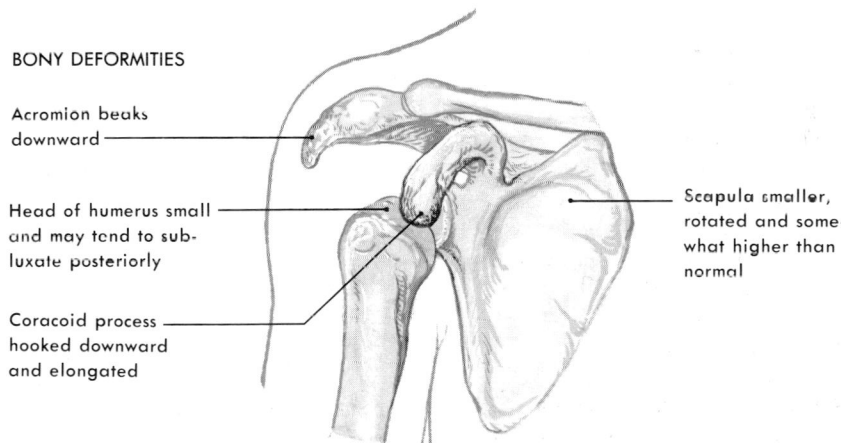

Acromion beaks
downward

Head of humerus small
and may tend to sub-
luxate posteriorly

Coracoid process
hooked downward
and elongated

Scapula smaller,
rotated and some-
what higher than
normal

FIGURE 5-103. *The muscle imbalance and residual bony deformities of the shoulder in obstetrical*
brachial plexus paralysis.

arm is in adducted position, the deltoid muscle is weak (usually fair minus) in motor strength. There are two possible etiologic factors in the pathogenesis of dyskinesia: the presence of retrograde upper motor neuron changes in the spinal cord as a result of avulsion of nerve roots from the cord, and the lack of development of functional cerebral motor patterns of coordination caused by paralysis occurring at birth.

Functional use of the upper limb is greatly handicapped as a result of limited abduction, external rotation, and extension of the shoulder. The asynergy of the muscles controlling the shoulder is an added factor in functional disability. The patient has difficulty in moving the hand to the mouth, to the top of the head, or to the back of the neck. Associated deformities of the forearm and paralysis of the hand compound the functional deficit. If the hand is normal, however, restoration of active external rotation and abduction of the shoulder serve to improve function of the limb immeasurably. In total involvement, the problem is that of a severe flaccid paralysis or flail limb.

ELBOW

Flexion contracture of the elbow joint frequently develops as a result of overaction of the flexors—the biceps and the brachialis. Another possible factor in its pathogenesis is constant use of the elbow in hyperflexed position because of limited abduction at the shoulder. Development of secondary bony changes, such as hypertrophy of the olecranon and coronoid process, further block extension of the elbow. In untreated cases in adolescence, the elbow joint may be in 45 to 90 degrees of flexion and can be very disturbing cosmetically.

Posterior dislocation of the radial head is a common deformity. Aitken, in a survey of 107 cases of Erbs palsy, found 27 instances (25.5 per cent) of incipient or actual posterior dislocation of the radial head.[699] This is acquired, produced by muscle imbalance and improper rigid splinting over a long period of time. Diagrammatic illustration of the progressive changes leading to posterior dislocation of the radial head is shown in Figure 5–104. Aitken proposes that when the paralyzed limb is rigidly immobilized over an unduly prolonged period

in a Fairbank's splint, bowing of the ulna is produced as a result of forced flexion of the elbow against the pull of the spastic triceps in the absence of a balancing biceps and brachialis pull (Fig. 5–105). Increased pressure is produced in the axis of the upper radius by forced supination against the pull of the spastic pronator teres muscle. This increased pressure of the proximal radial epiphysis against the capitellum causes abnormal bone growth and progressive osseous changes, namely, "clubbing," flattening, and anterior notching of the upper end of the radius, which begins to subluxate posteriorly and eventually becomes dislocated. Contracture of the pronator teres and interosseous membrane is also a contributory force.

FOREARM AND HAND

The distribution and extent of paralysis determine the type of residual deformity at this level. Pronation deformity of the forearm is common. When the entire arm is paralyzed in the whole arm type of obstetrical brachial plexus paralysis, supination contracture of the forearm may develop (Fig. 5–106). Paralysis of muscles of the hand is often present in the lower arm type.

Differential Diagnosis

In the neonatal period, in the differential diagnosis, one should consider fracture of the humerus, separation of the proximal humeral epiphysis, fracture of the clavicle, acute osteomyelitis of the humerus, and septic arthritis of the shoulder. Roentgenograms of the upper limb, clavicle, and cervical spine should be routinely obtained in all suspected cases of obstetrical brachial plexus paralysis. A cervical myelogram is not indicated. When a patient is seen later in infancy, the possibility of a spinal cord tumor, cerebral palsy, and unrecognized poliomyelitis should be considered.

Prognosis

The degree and rate of recovery varies with the type and severity of paralysis. It is difficult to estimate the end point of

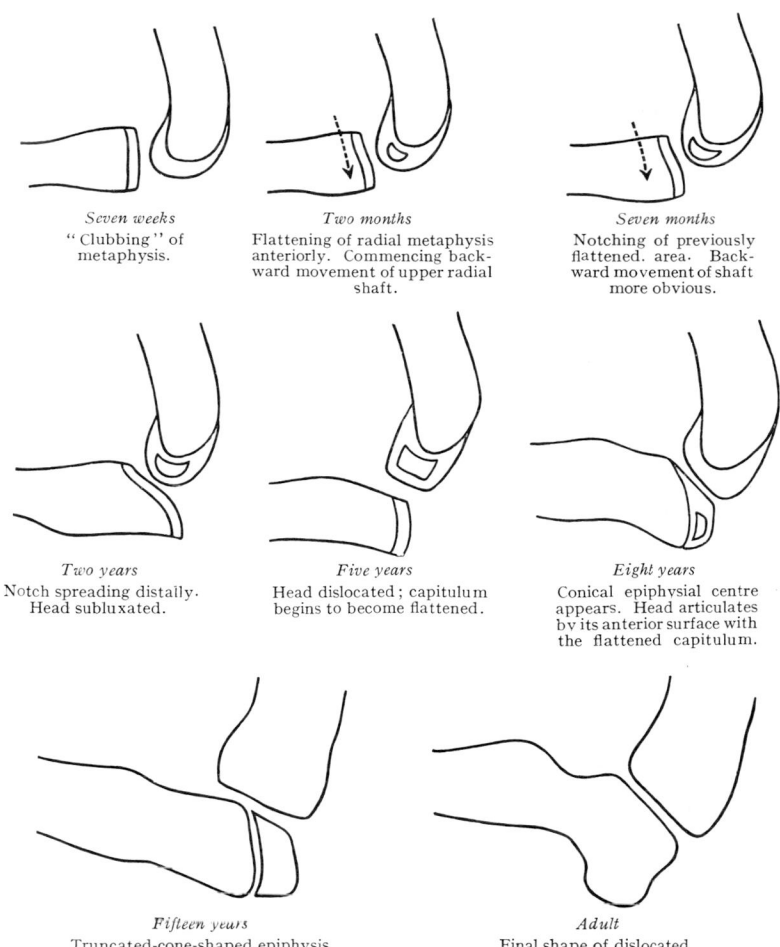

Seven weeks "Clubbing" of metaphysis.	*Two months* Flattening of radial metaphysis anteriorly. Commencing back- ward movement of upper radial shaft.	*Seven months* Notching of previously flattened. area. Back- ward movement of shaft more obvious.
Two years Notch spreading distally. Head subluxated.	*Five years* Head dislocated ; capitulum begins to become flattened.	*Eight years* Conical epiphysial centre appears. Head articulates by its anterior surface with the flattened capitulum.

Fifteen years
Truncated-cone-shaped epiphysis
about to fuse with shaft.

Adult
Final shape of dislocated
head.

FIGURE 5–104. *Diagrammatic illustration of the progressive changes leading to posterior dislocation of the radial head in obstetrical brachial plexus paralysis.*

(From Aitken, J.: Deformity of the elbow joint as a sequel to Erb's obstetrical paralysis. J. Bone Joint Surg., 34-B:361, 1952.)

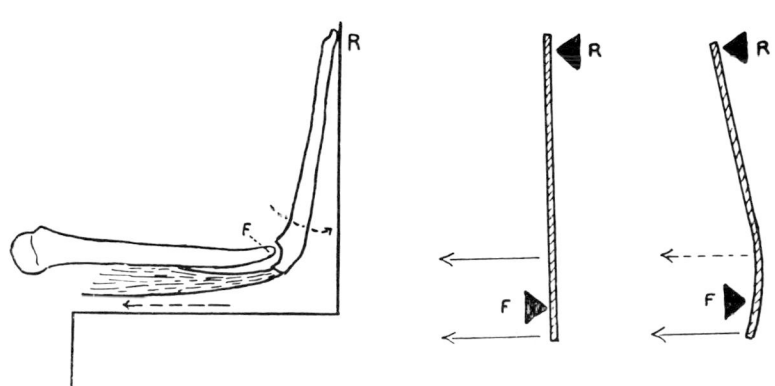

FIGURE 5–105. *The bowing of the ulna in obstetrical brachial plexus paralysis.*

The deformity results from imbalance between the spastic triceps and the paralyzed biceps and brachialis combined with firm corrective splinting. (From Aitken, J.: Deformity of the elbow joint as a sequel of Erb's obstetrical paralysis. J. Bone Joint Surg., 34-B:361, 1952.)

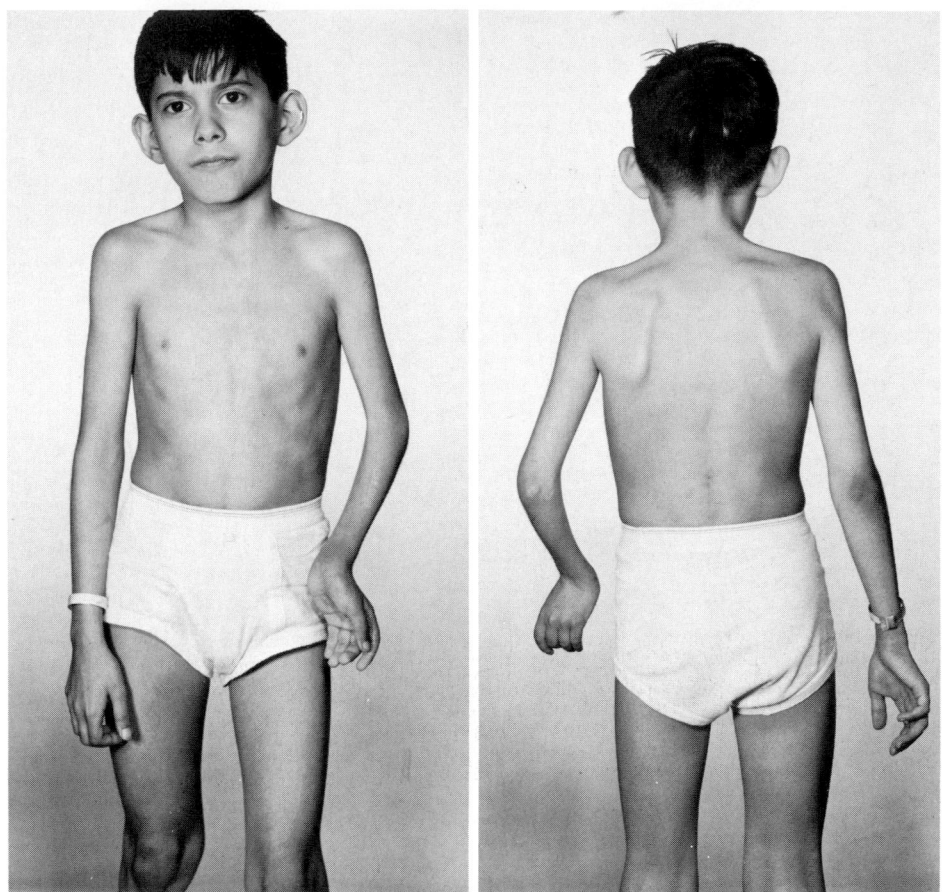

FIGURE 5–106.   *Supination contracture of the left forearm and flexion deformity of the elbow in the whole arm type of obstetrical brachial plexus paralysis.*

maximum spontaneous recovery, as it may vary from 1 to 18 months. In general, those patients with involvement of the entire plexus or lower plexus have a slower and more incomplete return than do those with only upper plexus involvement. Two other findings that herald a poor recovery are the presence of Horner's syndrome and paralysis of the parascapular muscles; both these findings indicate involvement of the roots before they form the trunks of the brachial plexus—a level of poor repair following nerve injury.

Treatment

The early management is conservative. Attempts at surgical repair of injured nerves have proved to be fruitless and are not justified. In the early stages, the nerve roots are frayed and friable, and there is absence of a suitable nerve sheath in the infant; later, the marked perineural fibrosis and proximal level of the lesion preclude any improvement.

Conservative care is aimed at preventing contractural deformities during the period of spontaneous recovery. In the nursery, the arm may be pinned in abduction and external rotation with the help of a diaper; however, it is imperative to take precautions that the infant not be inadvertently lifted from the bed, which will cause dislocation of the shoulder. As soon as is feasible, a light splint is made that holds the shoulder in about 70 degrees of abduction, 10 degrees of forward flexion, 90 degrees external rotation, with the elbow in 60 degrees of flexion, the forearm in midpronation, and the wrist in neutral position.

Improper and rigid immobilization in a splint is dangerous. Too much forward flexion at the shoulder will cause posterior dislocation of the humeral head. Forced full supination of the forearm against the pull of the tight pronator teres may cause bowing of the ulna and posterior dislocation of the radial head.

Three times a day, the splint should be removed and passive exercises performed by the parents, putting all joints of the upper limb through their full range of motion. Abduction contracture of the shoulder and other contractural deformities should not be permitted to develop (either because of shortened muscles or because of improper use of the orthosis). Guided active exercises are performed to develop normal cerebral motor patterns. The orthosis is used for gradually decreasing periods as recovery takes place. Within three months, its use is discontinued during the day; it is usually needed for night use for an additional two to four months, depending upon the rate of recovery. Because of dangers inherent in the orthosis, some authors condemn use of the so-called "Statue-of-Liberty" splint. Experience of the author has demonstrated that proper and intermittent support of the affected limb prevents contractural deformity and enhances the rate of maximal recovery. It is the improper and rigid use of the orthosis that is to be condemned.

Passive and active exercises should be performed during the period of growth. If residual deformity persists after five years of age, surgical correction may be indicated.

Various operations have been proposed to improve the fixed deformities of the shoulder. Fairbank corrected internal rotation-adduction deformity of the shoulder by sectioning the upper portion of the pectoralis major, the subscapularis, and the anterior capsule of the shoulder.[707] Sever modified the Fairbank procedure; he performed a complete division of the pectoralis major and the subscapularis, but did not open the joint capsule (as the latter caused anterior dislocation of the shoulder).[722] L'Episcopo described transfer of the teres major to a lateral position, making it an external rotator of the shoulder.[713] Zachary added the latissimus dorsi to the transfer, a modification subsequently adopted by L'Episcopo.[734] To assist in external rotation of the shoulder, Moore suggested posterior transfer of the origin of the anterior deltoid.[717, 718] Rotation osteotomy of the humerus to place the distal segment in external rotation has been advocated by many.[730, 731]

The purpose of the preceding operative procedures is to place the arm in a better functional position, to release any fixed contracture that hinders effective action of the weakened muscles, and to reinforce the weaker muscles when feasible. The Sever procedure compromises the appearance of the individual, creating a large defect due to the retraction of the muscle and its subsequent scarring. Furthermore, when the pectoralis major and the subscapularis are detached and the remaining internal rotators (latissimus dorsi and teres major) are transferred, there is marked weakness of internal rotation of the shoulder. For these reasons, Green adopted a technique in which he lengthened the pectoralis major and the subscapularis and balanced it with the active external rotation of the transferred latissimus dorsi and teres major.[710] As a part of the procedure, the coracoid process is excised when it is long and hooked, and the lateral portion of the acromion is resected if indicated. The operative technique of this modified Sever-L'Episcopo procedure is described and illustrated in Plate 47.

When the shoulder is luxated posteriorly, a posterior capsuloplasty is performed and the long head of the triceps is transferred to the posterior acromion and the spine of the scapula.

Ordinarily when there is structural instability of the shoulder joint with subluxation or dislocation, the author advocates derotation osteotomy of the humerus instead of tendon transfer. The level of osteotomy is usually proximal above the insertion of the deltoid and distal to the attachment of the pectoralis major through an anteromedial approach, and it is combined with lengthening of the pectoralis major tendon. When there is significant flexion deformity of the elbow, the osteotomy is performed through the distal hu-

(Text continued on page 1056.)

Modified Sever-L'Episcopo Procedure (After Green)

THE PROCEDURE

A sandbag is placed under the upper part of the chest for proper exposure. The entire upper limb, the front and back of the shoulder, and the lateral half of the chest are prepared and draped sterile. An adequate amount of whole blood should be available for transfusion.

A. An anterior incision is made, beginning over the coracoid process and extending distally along the deltopectoral groove for 12 cm. When exposure of the acromion is indicated, the incision extends superiorly and laterally.

B. The cephalic vein is identified. It may be ligated or retracted out of the way with a few fibers of deltoid muscle. By blunt dissection, the interval between the pectoral and deltoid muscles is developed and the coracobrachialis, the short head of the biceps, the coracoid process, the insertion of the tendinous portion of the subscapularis, and the insertion of the pectoralis major are exposed by adequate retraction.

C. The short head of the biceps and coracobrachialis are detached from their origin from the coracoid process and reflected downward. In the distal part of the wound, the insertion of the pectoralis major is exposed at its humeral attachment. Both its anterior and posterior surfaces are well-defined and separated from the adjacent tissues.

Plate 47. *Modified Sever-L'Episcopo Procedure (After Green)*

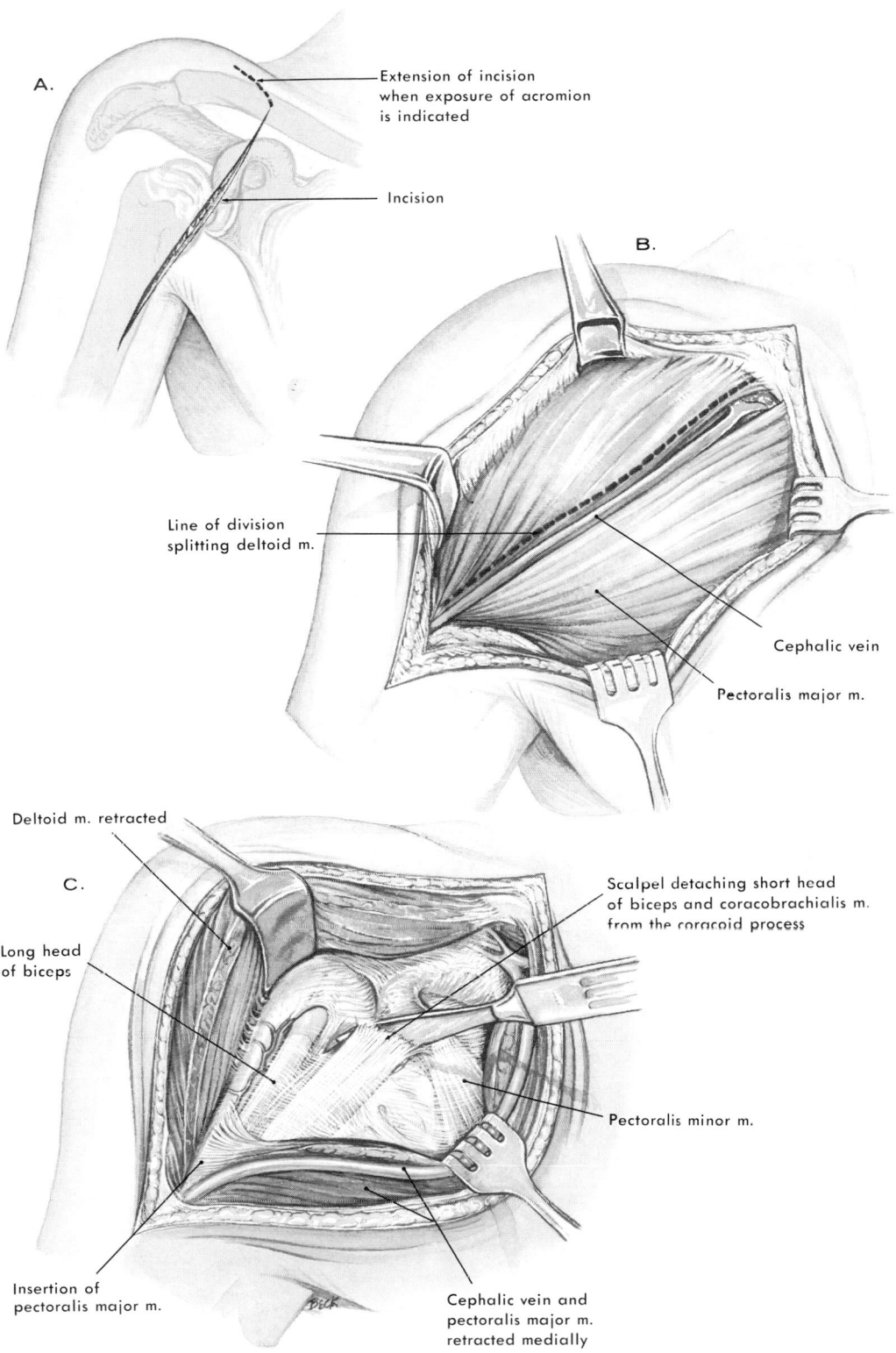

A.

Extension of incision when exposure of acromion is indicated

Incision

B.

Line of division splitting deltoid m.

Cephalic vein

Pectoralis major m.

Deltoid m. retracted

C.

Long head of biceps

Scalpel detaching short head of biceps and coracobrachialis m. from the coracoid process

Pectoralis minor m.

Insertion of pectoralis major m.

Cephalic vein and pectoralis major m. retracted medially

Modified Sever-L'Episcopo Procedure (After Green) (Continued)

D to **F.** With a periosteal elevator, the muscle fibers of the pectoralis major are reflected medially in order to expose as much as possible the tendinous portion of its insertion. Z-lengthening is obtained by dividing the distal half of the tendinous insertion of the pectoralis major immediately on the humeral shaft. The upper half of the tendinous portion of the pectoralis major is divided as far medially as good aponeurotic tendinous material exists, usually 4 to 5 cm. from its insertion. Later, the distal tendon stump is to be attached to the proximal tendon left inserted on the humerus, thus providing further length to the pectoralis major. The re-attachment of the tendon more proximally permits a greater degree of shoulder abduction, but still allows rotary function. At this time whip sutures are applied to the tendon still attached to the shaft and to the portion of the tendon attached to the muscle.

Plate 47.   Modified Sever-L'Episcopo Procedure
(After Green)

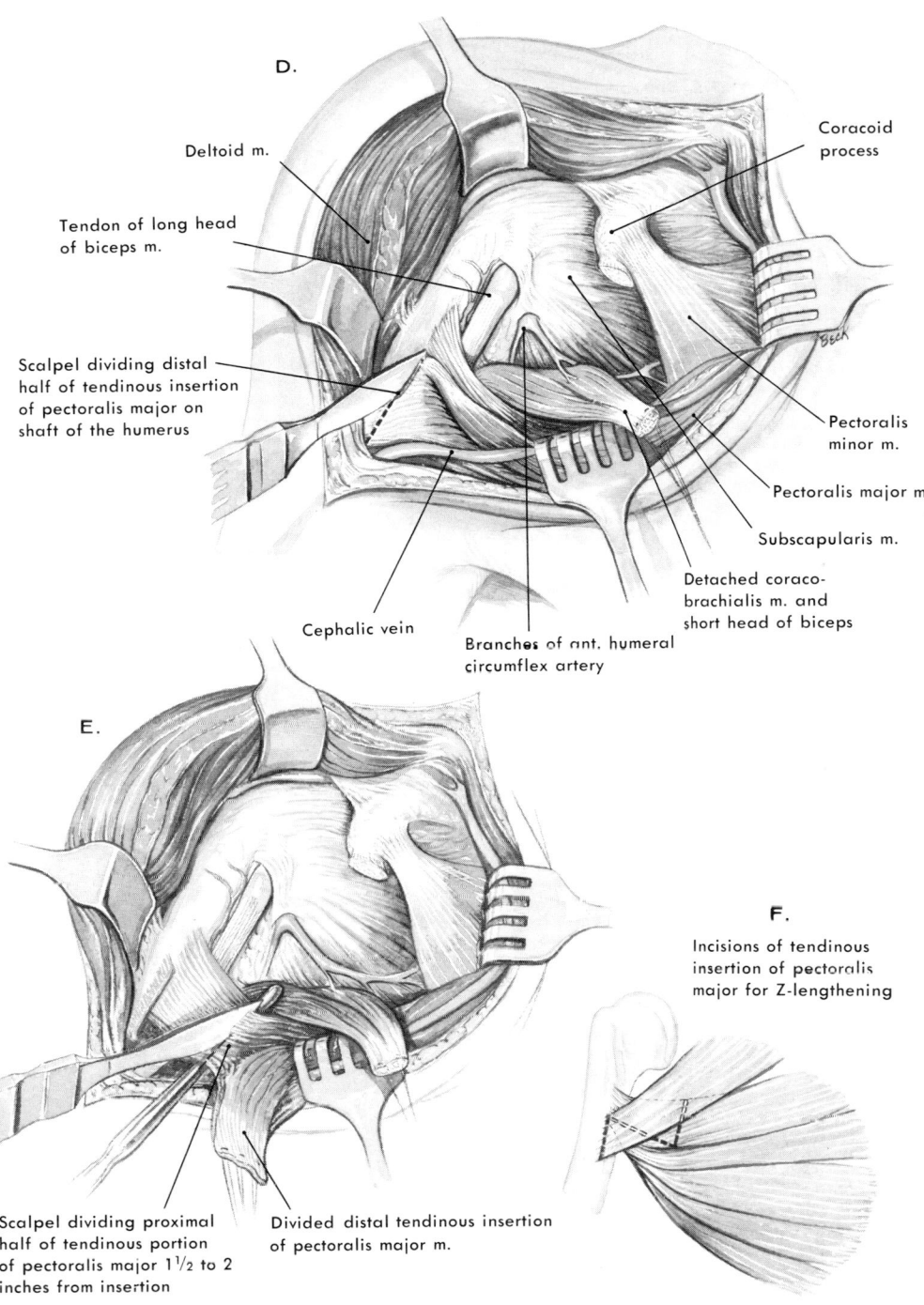

D.

Deltoid m.

Coracoid process

Tendon of long head of biceps m.

Scalpel dividing distal half of tendinous insertion of pectoralis major on shaft of the humerus

Pectoralis minor m.

Pectoralis major m.

Subscapularis m.

Detached coraco-brachialis m. and short head of biceps

Cephalic vein

Branches of ant. humeral circumflex artery

E.

F.

Incisions of tendinous insertion of pectoralis major for Z-lengthening

Scalpel dividing proximal half of tendinous portion of pectoralis major 1½ to 2 inches from insertion

Divided distal tendinous insertion of pectoralis major m.

Modified Sever-L'Episcopo Procedure (After Green) (Continued)

G. Next, the subscapularis muscle is exposed over the head of the humerus. Starting medially with a blunt instrument, the subscapularis muscle is separated and elevated from the capsule. The shoulder capsule should not be opened; if, inadvertently, it is incised, it should be repaired.

H. With a knife, the subscapularis tendon is lengthened on the flat by an oblique cut starting medially, splitting the tendon into anterior and posterior halves, becoming more superficial laterally, and completing the division at the insertion of the subscapularis into the humerus. Again, meticulous care should be taken not to open the capsule. Ordinarily, once the subscapularis is divided, the shoulder joint will abduct and externally rotate freely. The coracoid process is excised to its base if it is elongated, hooked downward and laterally, and limits external rotation. The acromion process is partially resected if it is beaked downward, obstructing shoulder abduction.

I. Next, the insertions of the latissimus dorsi and teres major are identified and exposed by separating them from adjacent tissues both anteriorly and posteriorly. The attachment of the latissimus dorsi is superior and anterior to that of the teres major. Both tendons are divided immediately on bone, and into each tendon 0 silk is sutured by a whip stitch.

Plate 47. *Modified Sever-L'Episcopo Procedure (After Green)*

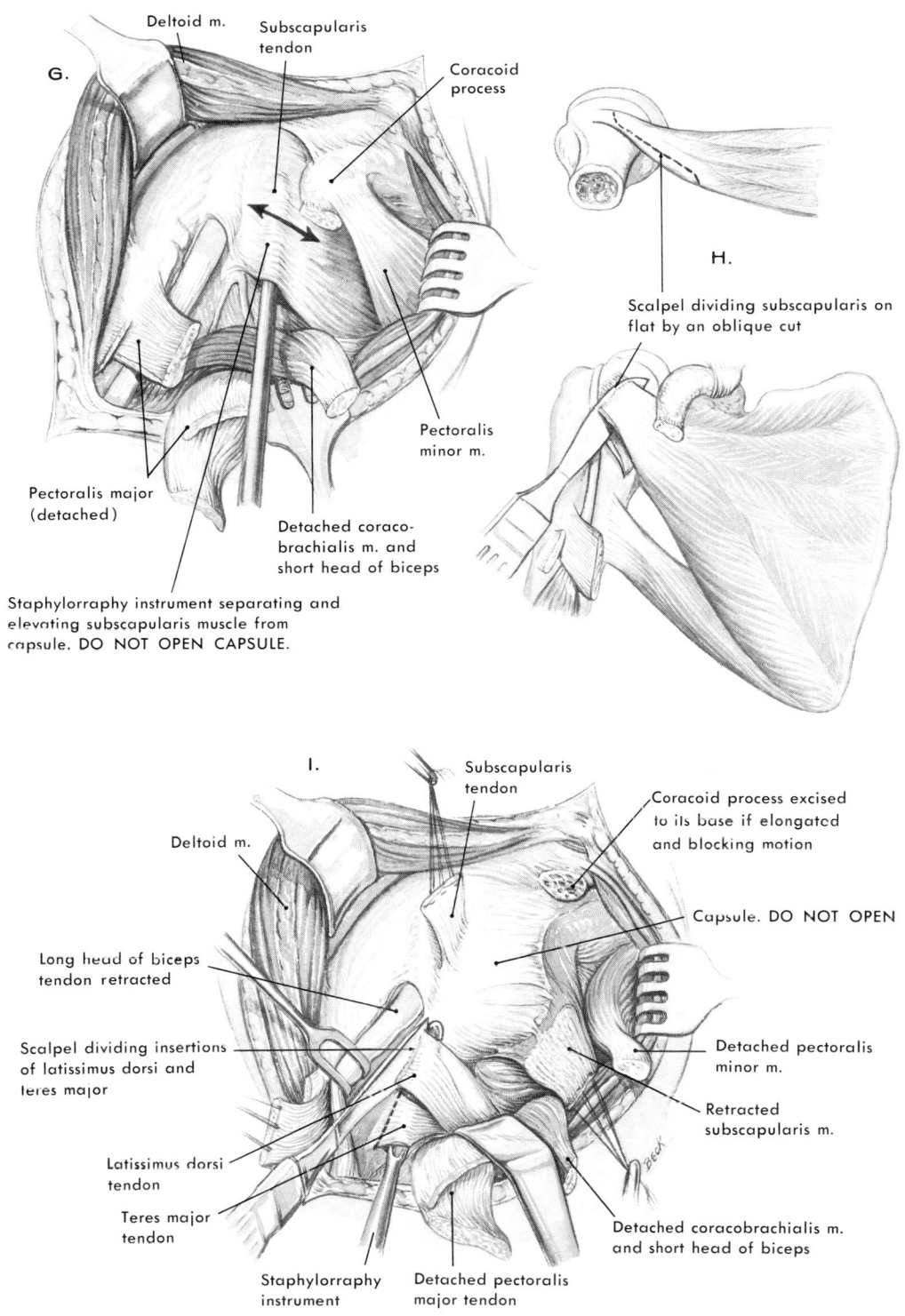

G.

Deltoid m.

Subscapularis tendon

Coracoid process

Pectoralis minor m.

Pectoralis major (detached)

Detached coraco-brachialis m. and short head of biceps

Staphylorraphy instrument separating and elevating subscapularis muscle from capsule. DO NOT OPEN CAPSULE.

H.

Scalpel dividing subscapularis on flat by an oblique cut

I.

Subscapularis tendon

Coracoid process excised to its base if elongated and blocking motion

Capsule. DO NOT OPEN

Deltoid m.

Long head of biceps tendon retracted

Scalpel dividing insertions of latissimus dorsi and teres major

Latissimus dorsi tendon

Teres major tendon

Staphylorraphy instrument

Detached pectoralis major tendon

Detached pectoralis minor m.

Retracted subscapularis m.

Detached coracobrachialis m. and short head of biceps

Modified Sever-L'Episcopo Procedure (After Green) *(Continued)*

J. Then, with the patient turned over on his side and his arm adducted across the chest, a 7 to 8 cm. long incision is made over the deltoid-triceps interval.

K. The deltoid muscle is retracted anteriorly and the long head of the triceps, posteriorly. One should be careful not to damage the radial and axillary nerves. The lateral surface of the proximal diaphysis of the humerus is subperiosteally exposed. A 5 cm. long longitudinal cleft is made, using drills, osteotome, and curet.

L to N. Four drill holes are made from the depth of the cleft coming out on the medial surface of the humeral shaft at the site of the former insertion of the teres major and latissimus dorsi muscles. The tendons of the latissimus dorsi and teres major are identified in the anterior wound and are delivered into the posterior incision so that their line of pull is straight from their origins to the proposed site of attachment on the lateral humerus. The latissimus dorsi and teres major tendons are drawn into the slot in the humerus and tied securely in position with 0 silk sutures in the front.

Plate 47. Modified Sever-L'Episcopo Procedure
(After Green)

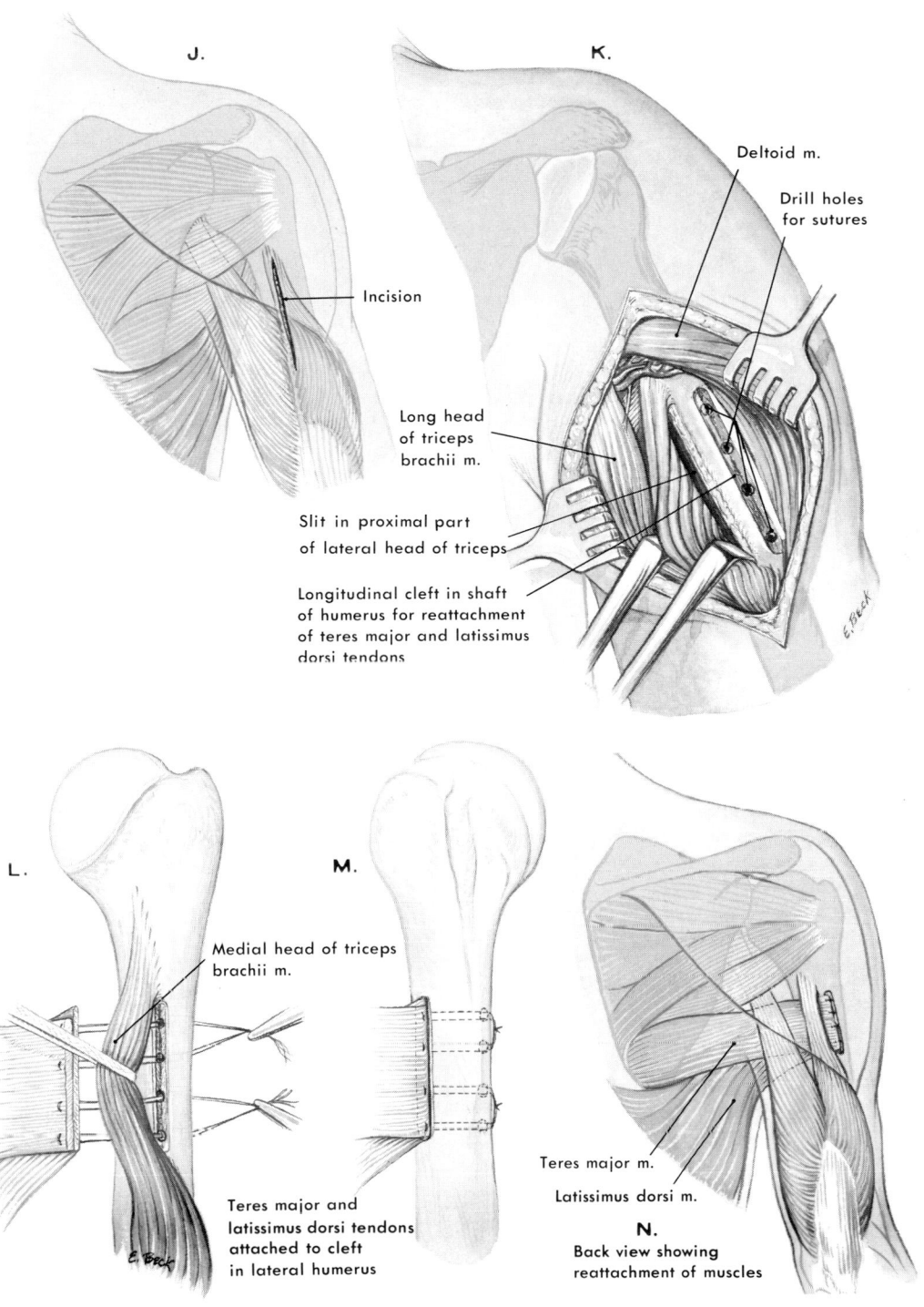

J.

K.

Incision

Deltoid m.

Drill holes
for sutures

Long head
of triceps
brachii m.

Slit in proximal part
of lateral head of triceps

Longitudinal cleft in shaft
of humerus for reattachment
of teres major and latissimus
dorsi tendons

L.

M.

Medial head of triceps
brachii m.

Teres major and
latissimus dorsi tendons
attached to cleft
in lateral humerus

Teres major m.

Latissimus dorsi m.

N.
Back view showing
reattachment of muscles

Modified Sever-L'Episcopo Procedure (After Green) *(Continued)*

O to **Q.** The subscapularis tendon, which is lengthened "on the flat," is sutured at its divided ends so as to provide maximal lengthening. The pectoralis major is reconstituted in a similar way. The coracobrachialis and short head of the biceps are reattached to the coracoid process at its base. If the coracobrachialis and short head of the biceps are short, they are lengthened by a turnover type of lengthening on the flat. The lengthened muscles should be of sufficient length to permit complete external rotation in abduction without undue tension. The wound is closed in the usual manner and the upper limb is immobilized in a previously prepared bivalved shoulder spica cast that holds the shoulder in 90 degrees of abduction, 90 degrees of external rotation, and 20 degrees of forward flexion. The elbow is in 80 to 90 degrees of flexion. The forearm and hand are placed in a functional neutral position.

An alternate method is to utilize a single anterior incision. The teres major and latissimus dorsi tendons, after detachment at their insertion, are passed posteriorly about the humerus from the anterior incision and reattached to the humerus immediately lateral to the course of the long head of the biceps lateral to the bicipital groove. Another variation in technique is employed when the teres major is markedly contracted; in such an instance, the teres major tendon may be attached to the latissimus dorsi tendon in a recessed position, which, in turn, is attached to the humerus. This allows greater scapulohumeral motion.

POSTOPERATIVE CARE

About three weeks after surgery, exercises are begun to develop abduction and external rotation of the shoulder, as well as shoulder adduction and internal rotation. Particular emphasis is given to developing function and strength of the transferred muscles. When the arm adducts satisfactorily, a sling is used during the day and the bivalved shoulder spica cast at night. The night support is continued for three to six more months. Exercises are performed for many months or years to preserve functional range of motion of the shoulder and to maintain muscle control.

Plate 47.   Modified Sever-L'Episcopo Procedure
(After Green)

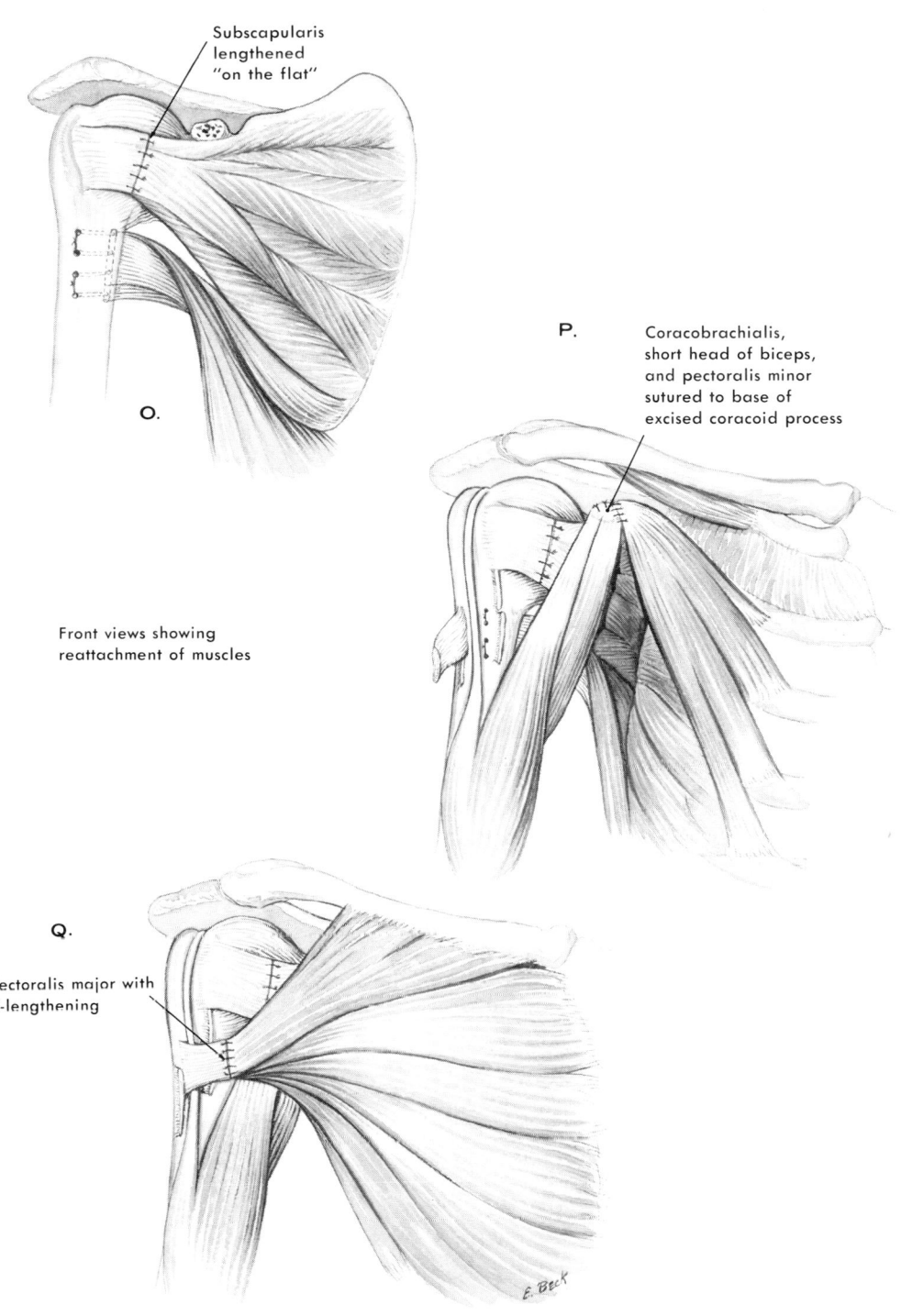

Subscapularis
lengthened
"on the flat"

O.

P.   Coracobrachialis,
short head of biceps,
and pectoralis minor
sutured to base of
excised coracoid process

Front views showing
reattachment of muscles

Q.

Pectoralis major with
Z-lengthening

E. Beck

1055

meral diaphysis, tilting the distal segment into hyperextension as it is externally rotated.

Flexion deformity of the elbow is managed by passive stretching exercises and active exercises to strengthen the triceps brachii. Persistent physical therapy by the parents will usually check progression of the deformity beyond 20 to 25 degrees, which is both cosmetically and functionally acceptable.

In the more severe deformities, a night bivalved cast is used, which serves to hold the elbow in maximal extension. The wearing of a cast or extension orthosis ordinarily has its problems, as it keeps sliding and coming off the arm. This can be prevented by anchoring the cast to shoulder straps and putting the wrist in extension. On occasion, a turnbuckle cast is applied, stretching the elbow into extension; the degree of correction obtained is then maintained in a bivalved cast.

When flexion deformity of the elbow exceeds 40 to 50 degrees and does not respond to the foregoing conservative measures, surgical correction is indicated. Correction of shoulder deformities should precede elbow surgery, as mentioned previously. Hyperflexion of the elbow is often a mechanism to compensate for limited shoulder abduction. The hypertrophied portion of the olecranon process blocking extension is resected. The brachialis muscle is fractionally lengthened by transverse division of its tendinous portion at two levels. It is best to avoid damage to the muscle fibers of the brachialis and the periosteum in order to prevent myositis ossificans. The biceps tendon is lengthened, if indicated; power of elbow flexion, however, should be preserved, as the functional deficit will be greater if the patient loses functional range and strength of elbow flexion. On occasion, the pronator teres and common flexor muscle mass are lengthened at their tendinous origin from the medial epicondyle of the humerus.

Posterior dislocation of the radial head presents a difficult problem. It is best to await completion of growth, at which time the radial head is resected, if so indicated.

Pronation contracture of the forearm is managed by a corrective cast. When full supination cannot be obtained, the pronator teres is lengthened by division of its tendinous fibers. This is usually combined with a flexor carpi ulnaris transfer to give power of active supination. If the wrist dorsiflexors are normal in motor strength, a Steindler procedure is performed, i.e., the flexor carpi ulnaris tendon is attached to the distal radius (in growing children it is anchored to the tendon of the brachioradialis at its insertion to the radial styloid); whereas, if there is weakness of wrist dorsiflexion, the Green modification is utilized, i.e., the flexor carpi ulnaris tendon is attached to the extensor carpi radialis brevis. On occasion, bony deformity of the ulna and radius is present to such a degree that there is a bony block to rotation of the forearm; in such an instance, osteotomy of both bones of the forearm is performed and the forearm is placed in neutral position.

Supination contracture of the forearm is usually encountered in the whole arm type of paralysis. This deformity requires closed osteoclasis or open osteotomy of the radius and ulna to place the forearm in neutral functional position. Depending upon the muscle picture, tendon transfers can be performed for dynamic balance of muscles controlling rotation of the forearm after the osteotomy is healed.

Surgical procedures for correction of paralytic deformities of the hand depend upon the distribution and extent of paralysis.

In the severe flaccid paralysis of the whole arm type, if there is adequate sensation of the hand, elbow flexion is obtained by Bunnell's sternocleidomastoid transfer or Clark's pectoralis major transfer. Shoulder fusion is performed if there is muscular control of the scapula, and an automatic hinge hand is given. If sensory loss of the upper limb is extensive, functional improvement is best obtained by an above-elbow amputation and fitting the patient with a prosthetic limb.

SCIATIC NERVE PALSY*

The common cause of sciatic nerve injury in infants and children is intramuscular

---

*See References 737–748.

injection of antibiotics or other medications into the gluteal region. The noxious agent is placed directly in or immediately adjacent to the nerve trunk as it emerges from the sciatic notch and is crossed by the piriformis muscle. The unfortunate victim may be an emaciated and sick child with marked gluteal atrophy, or he may be a robust uncooperative infant who is crying and kicking around at the time of inoculation. Such a mishap can also occur when the site of injection is inadequately exposed in an anesthetized patient covered by surgical drapes or when the nurse or physician is simply careless and ignorant.

Parenteral administration of therapeutic agents through the umbilical vessels in a newborn may cause thrombosis of the inferior gluteal arteries and damage to both sciatic nerves. The skin over the buttocks may slough in such an instance. The sciatic nerve may stretch and become paralyzed during closed or open reduction of congenital dislocation of the hip or during femoral lengthening. Posterior traumatic dislocation of the hip is very rare in children; however, when it does occur, it can cause sciatic nerve palsy. The sciatic nerve may also be injured during Salter innominate osteotomy.

Of the two components of the sciatic nerve, the common peroneal nerve is the most frequently injured, as its superficial and more lateral location at the level of the piriformis muscle makes it more susceptible to the iatrogenic insult of the needle. It is rare that the posterior tibial component of the sciatic nerve is solely involved; if this does occur, its prognosis for recovery is good. Mechanical trauma of the needle, intraneural hemorrhage, and the toxic effects of the high local concentration of the chemical agents are all factors to consider in the pathogenesis of injection palsy. Pathologically, an acute inflammation of the intraneural and perineural tissues develops first, followed by destruction of the axons and disappearance of the myelin sheaths and eventual fibrosis of the nerve.

On exploration, one may find a 2 to 3 cm. long segment of the nerve trunk shrunk to a fibrous band. Characteristic features of injection palsy are the marked local hypervascularity and adhesion of the nerve to neighboring areolar and muscular tissues.

Loss of motor and sensory function in the sciatic nerve distribution is present immediately following injection. This is usually accompanied by intense local and referred pain that can only be controlled by strong analgesics. After several days, the hypersensitivity radiating along the course of the involved nerves gradually subsides. On deep palpation of the gluteal region there may be local tenderness. If the paresis involves the common peroneal nerve, the patient will be unable to dorsiflex and evert the foot actively, and the lateral aspect of the leg and foot will be anesthetic; whereas if the entire sciatic nerve is paralyzed, the foot and ankle will be flail, with anesthesia of the sole of the foot, the lateral aspect of the leg, and the dorsum of the foot. The ankle jerk will be absent. The neurologic deficit is maximal immediately following injury. The paresis may either improve or remain static, but it will not increase. Destruction of nerve tissue is not progressive.

A thorough assessment of neurologic deficit is made initially and repeated at monthly intervals. Prognosis for satisfactory recovery is good if paralysis is incomplete at the beginning and if some improvement of motor function is shown by the repeated examinations. Prognosis is poor, however, if there is total paralysis at the onset and periodic examination does not disclose any return of neurologic function.

If, within three months following injury, there is no improvement, the sciatic nerve should be surgically explored. During this period of observation, it is important to perform passive stretching and active exercises to maintain the ankle and foot in neutral position in a bivalved cast at night, and to support the ankle in a below-knee orthosis during the day. Every effort should be made to prevent the development of contractural deformity. If there is progressive improvement of function, observation for 12 months is recommended, at the end of which time the residual motor and sensory picture is assessed. If adequate function is not restored, exploration of the sciatic nerve is again indicated.

The patient is placed in prone position and the entire lower limb and gluteal region is prepared and draped sterile in order to permit evaluation of function by electrical stimulation during surgery. Beginning over the posterior superior iliac spine, the incision extends toward the greater trochanter and then distally over the posterior aspect of the thigh to terminate 5 cm. above the popliteal crease. The subcutaneous tissue and deep fascia are divided in line with the skin incision. The gluteus maximus and gluteus medius muscles are detached from their insertions and reflected medially to expose the sciatic nerve. This surgical approach permits exposure of the entire sciatic nerve from the sciatic notch to the popliteal space. The status of the nerve is determined by gross inspection and by direct electrical stimulation. If the pathologic change is simple perineural scarring, a meticulous neurolysis is carried out. In the presence of total destruction of the nerve, however, the damaged segment is resected and end-to-end anastomosis is performed. Relative length of the sciatic nerve is obtained by mobilizing it subcutaneously and by placing the hip in hyperextension and the knee in flexion. A magnifying glass is of great assistance for accurate anastomosis. Following closure of the wound, the patient is placed in a bivalved hip spica cast, which is made preoperatively with the hip in hyperextension and the knee in 90 degrees of flexion and the ankle in neutral position. Immobilization in the cast is continued for a period of eight weeks, at which time gentle range of motion exercises of the hip and knee are instituted. Care of muscles in the recovery period follows the principles outlined in poliomyelitis.

Measures to prevent sciatic nerve injury in infants and children include the following: (1) Give intramuscular injections in the anterior and lateral portions of the midthigh (quadriceps femoris muscle). (2) If multiple intramuscular injections are to be administered, rotate them from the left to the right side. (3) Inject into the upper and outer quadrant of the buttocks if the gluteal muscle is to be used. (4) Expose the site of injection adequately and have an assistant securely immobilize the child in prone position. (5) Always have both hands free, "picking up" the muscle with one hand and introducing the needle with the other. (6) Do not use a long intramuscular needle and always control the depth of needle penetration. (7) Make it a routine habit to double-check the point of the needle both before and following injection. (8) If repeated parenteral medications are to be given to a sick child, use the intravenous route through an indwelling catheter.

Developmental and Degenerative Disorders

PERONEAL MUSCULAR ATROPHY
(Charcot-Marie-Tooth Disease)

Peroneal muscular atrophy of Charcot-Marie-Tooth may be defined as a hereditary and familial degenerative disorder of the peripheral nerves, motor nerve roots, and frequently, of the spinal cord. The process is slowly progressive and begins in the feet and legs and spreads to the hands and forearms after a lapse of several years. It is characterized by atrophy of certain muscle groups, particularly the peroneals and the intrinsic musculature of the hands and feet.

The condition was described in 1886, almost simultaneously, by Charcot and Marie of France and Tooth of England.[755, 788] It was first considered to be a myopathy; however, Tooth and later Hoffman emphasized its neuritic features.[771, 788] The radicular pathology was pointed out by England and Denny-Brown, who showed the pattern of sensory loss.[766] Herringham, in 1888, reported a study of four generations in one family in which only males were affected, stressing the hereditary aspects.[770]

Incidence

Its incidence is highly variable. In some geographic areas it is rare, with only one or two cases per year seen in large neurologic clinics, whereas in others it is one of the commoner of the degenerative diseases of the peripheral nervous system. Boys are more frequently affected than girls. According to Jacobs and Carr, the Negro race appears to be exempt from Charcot-Marie-Tooth disease.[773]

Genetic Factors

The disease has a variable pattern of heredity. It may be inherited as an autosomal dominant, an autosomal recessive, or a sex-linked recessive trait.[749, 758, 765, 767, 770, 777, 784] A positive family history is usually present, but on occasion, there may be none. The hereditary pattern determines the age of onset and the severity of the clinical course. When the inheritance is by a simple recessive gene, peroneal atrophy begins before the age of eight, and by the second decade the patient becomes totally disabled. The intensity of the disease is very severe because a defective gene is supplied by each parent and there are no factors to ameliorate the condition. In the sex-linked mode of inheritance the patient receives one defective gene from the mother, with no corresponding normal gene from the father. Atrophy becomes apparent about the middle of the second decade of life, and by the age of 25 years the patient is bedridden or on crutches. Those with the heterozygous pattern of inheritance have the mildest form of the disease, as they receive a normal gene from one parent and a defective gene from the other. The atrophy becomes apparent after the age of 25 years. Pes cavus deformity and motor weakness are only moderate.[749]

Pathology

The peripheral nerves and motor nerve roots show degenerative changes with loss of myelin and fragmentation of axis cylinders. In the spinal cord, there may be secondary loss of anterior horn cells and degeneration of posterior roots and posterior columns. There is disagreement as to whether other spinal tracts are involved. Occasionally degenerative changes occur in the lateral funiculi, which are not explainable on the basis of changes secondary to primary nerve root or peripheral nerve degeneration. The muscle fibers show neural atrophy, with blastic proliferation and infiltration of fat cells.[769]

Clinical Picture

The onset of symptoms is usually between 5 and 15 years, but may be deferred until the third decade. The presenting complaints may include difficulty in walking or in wearing shoes, muscle cramps, and paresthesia in the legs.

The muscular atrophy is symmetrical and distal in distribution. The peroneals and intrinsic muscles of the feet are affected first. As a result of muscular imbalance, pes varus is the early deformity. Later, the atrophy spreads to the anterior compartment, involving the anterior tibial and the toe extensor muscles (Fig. 5–107). The patient walks with a toe-heel gait. Soon cavovarus deformity of the feet and claw toes develop (Fig. 5–108). With steady progression of the disease, the gastrocnemius and other calf muscles are eventually atrophied.

The upper limbs are involved at a later stage. In most cases, by the time there is atrophy of the calves, symmetrical atrophy of the intrinsic muscles of the hand and the forearm develops. The characteristic deformity of the hands is one of mild clawing, which becomes quite marked in severe cases. Opposition of the thumb may be lost. The pelvic and shoulder girdle musculatures and the muscles of the arms and thighs are usually not affected, and the face and trunk musculatures are practically always spared. Therefore, in the moderately advanced case, the legs, feet, forearms, and hands are wasted and very slender, whereas there is normal development of the thighs and upper arms. The contrast between the plump thighs and the slender legs with their claw toes gives the characteristic appearance of an inverted champagne bottle, which has been termed "ostrich legs."

The motor weakness is essentially a flaccid paralysis with fascicular twitchings often present in the wasting muscles. Contractural deformity, particularly equinus deformity of the ankle, may develop. The deep tendon

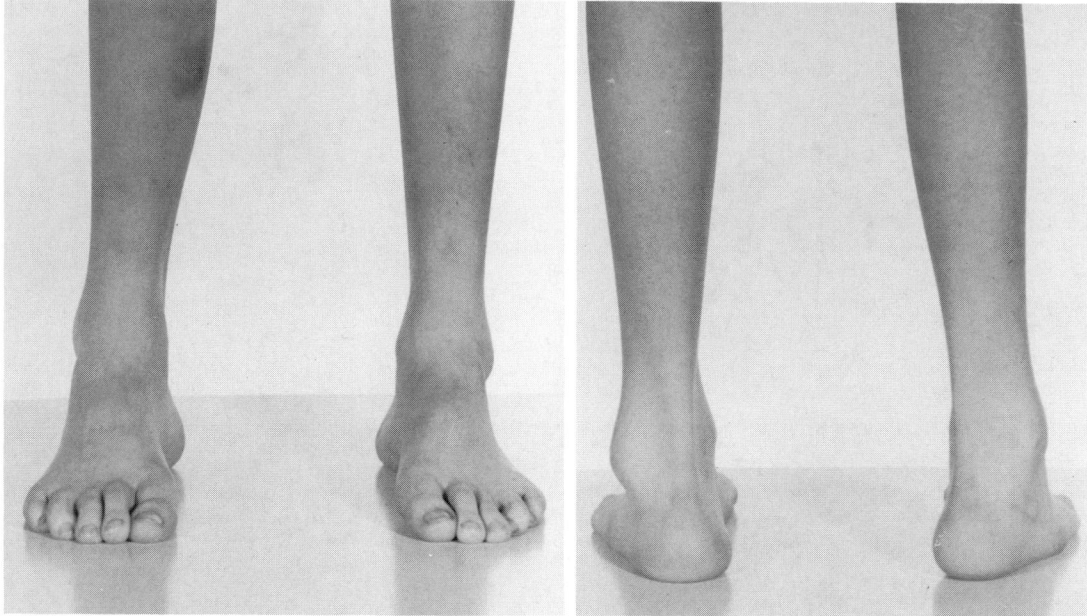

FIGURE 5–107.   Charcot-Marie-Tooth disease.

Moderate varus and slight equinus deformity of both feet result from atrophy of peroneal, anterior tibial, and toe extensor muscles.

reflexes are decreased or absent. The ankle jerk is the first to be involved, followed by the radial periosteal reflex when the upper limbs are affected. The patellar, biceps, and triceps reflexes are usually preserved.

Sensory examination may reveal diminution in vibration and position senses, and in some cases, definite areas of hypoesthesia. Ataxia is not present. Sphincter tone is normal. Intelligence is not affected. The condition progresses slowly with normal life expectancy. The patients are often ambulatory, and in many instances, remain remarkably free of serious disability until well past the fourth decade of life.

Diagnosis

Peroneal muscular atrophy of Charcot-Marie-Tooth disease is suggested by the findings of: (1) weakness and atrophy that begin in the peroneal group of muscles and extend slowly to other muscles of the anterior tibial compartment, intrinsic muscles of the foot, and later to the intrinsic mus-

cles of the hand and muscles of the forearm, with the relative sparing of the muscles of the thigh and upper arm; (2) the slow course of the disease; and (3) the positive family history.

The conduction velocity of the peripheral motor nerves is low in Charcot-Marie-Tooth disease.[764, 768] Dyck, Lambert, and Mulder studied a total of 157 members of a family with peroneal muscular atrophy; 103 of these had neurologic examinations and studies of nerve conduction. Each of the 16 persons who showed definite evidence of Charcot-Marie-Tooth disease on clinical examination also had low conduction velocity of the peripheral motor nerves. In addition, seven persons who showed no certain clinical evidence of the disease had low conduction velocity. They concluded that determination of conduction velocity was a valuable method for identifying carriers of the disease trait, at least in this family.[762]

The cerebrospinal fluid findings are normal, although occasionally the protein content may be slightly elevated. The electromyogram will disclose reduction of electrical reactions.

In the differential diagnosis, one should consider distal muscular dystrophy, various forms of chronic polyneuritis, hypertrophic interstitial neuritis of Déjerine-Sottas, Roussy-Lévy syndrome, and Friedreich's ataxia. These conditions may be variants of the same disease process.[750, 785, 789]

Roussy-Lévy syndrome, characterized by familial bilateral pes cavus and absence of deep tendon reflexes, is very similar to peroneal muscular atrophy.[775, 780, 781, 790] Symonds and Shaw expressed the view that it is a forme fruste of Charcot-Marie-Tooth disease.[787] Conduction velocity is low in both conditions. Static tremor of the hands is the distinguishing feature of Roussy-Lévy syndrome. Friedreich's ataxia is characterized by the presence of cerebellar signs, speech disturbance, nystagmus, and positive Babinski response.

Treatment

In the early stages, treatment consists of passive stretching exercises and splinting at night in an overcorrected position to prevent the development of fixed deformities

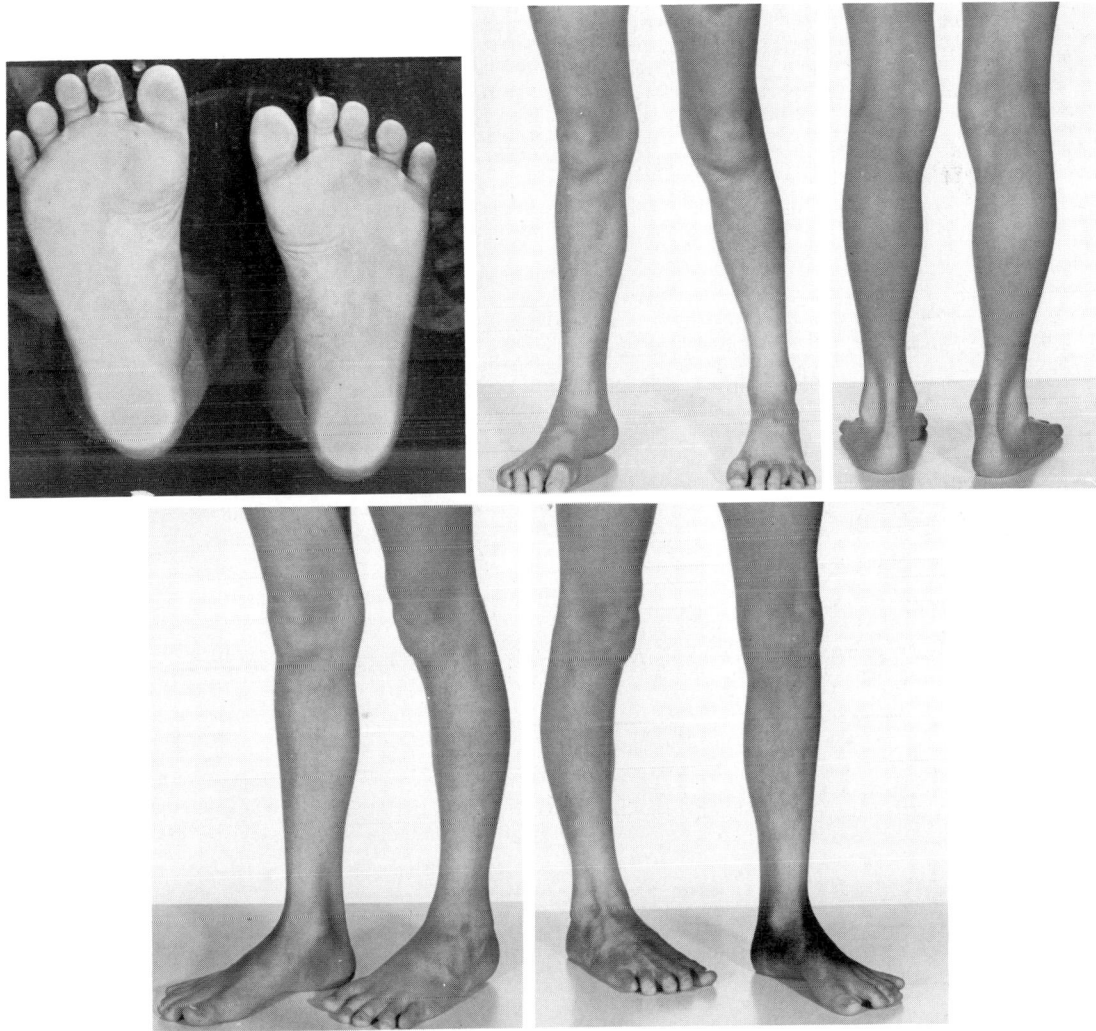

FIGURE 5–108.   *Charcot-Marie-Tooth disease.*

There is moderate pes cavus deformity. Note the beginning of development of claw toes.

of pes varus, equinovarus, or cavus. Active exercises to maintain the strength of the weakened peroneals, toe extensors, and anterior tibial muscles are in order. Muscle testing at regular intervals is essential to record the progress of the disease.

In the advanced case, properly chosen surgical procedures can correct and prevent deformities. Often functional disability can be substantially diminished.[773, 774] The type of operation depends upon the muscle picture and the severity of foot deformity. When the peroneal muscles are of trace or zero strength, the anterior tibials are fair plus or good, and the posterior calf muscles are good or normal, the indicated procedure is anterior transfer of the posterior tibial tendon through the interosseous route to the base of the third metatarsal and the lateral transfer of the anterior tibial to the base of the second metatarsal. Triple arthrodesis is performed to stabilize the hindfoot and to correct the cavovarus deformity. Percutaneous plantar fasciotomy is performed if the fascia is contracted. It is best to correct equinus deformity by wedging casts rather than by lengthening the tendo Achillis. If the anterior tibial is weaker than fair in motor strength, the posterior tibial muscle only is transferred anteriorly through the interosseous route to the base of the third metatarsal.

HYPERTROPHIC INTERSTITIAL NEURITIS

Déjerine and Sottas, in 1893, described a chronic familial polyneuropathy of childhood and adolescence.[796] This condition had been previously described by Gombault and Mallet, in 1889, as a pathologic variant of tabes dorsalis.[797] The original cases described by Déjerine and Sottas were in siblings with presumably unaffected parents. Later reports, however, traced the disorders through three to five generations.[792, 793, 795, 800] The disease is believed to be inherited as a dominant trait.

The etiology of the condition is unknown. Disturbance of pyruvate metabolism was proposed by Joiner et al.; subsequent studies, however, have failed to show evidence of any thiamine deficiency. Allergic factors may play a role in the pathogenesis.[794, 799]

Pathology

Peripheral nerves are enlarged as a result of the proliferation of perineural and endoneural connective tissue. The axis cylinders gradually decrease in size and eventually disappear. On cross section of nerve fibers, concentrically laminated structures are found about the nerve fibers—the so-called "onion bulb formation." This characteristic finding is caused by proliferation of the Schwann cells. Muscles show atrophy of neural origin.

Clinical Features

Difficulty in locomotion is the usual presenting complaint. Walking is delayed. The child is unsteady, falls frequently, and has difficulty in going up and down stairs. He is unable to run and to "keep up" with his playmates. His feet are weak and floppy. The abnormality of gait is similar to that of steppage gait. Subjective sensory disturbances such as paresthesias and lightning type pains of the limbs may occur. Pes cavus and muscle weakness in the lower limbs, which is distal in distribution, develop early, antedating the more florid findings by several years. Paralysis of the intrinsic muscles of the hand appears later. Flexion contracture of the fingers and wrist is usually present toward the end of the first decade. Scoliosis develops during the rapid growth of the spine in early adolescence.

The deep tendon reflexes are diminished or absent. Superficial skin reflexes such as abdominal and cremasteric reflexes are lost later. Sensory loss involves all modalities of sensation. Anesthesia to light touch and pinprick is of the "stocking-glove" type. Proprioceptive sensory disturbance is shown by the loss of sensation of position and vibration and by the presence of a positive Romberg sign. Abnormalities of the pupil, such as the Argyll Robertson phenomenon, result from involvement of the cranial nerves. Nystagmus and slurred speech occur in some cases. Incoordination and motor deficit result from the combination of muscle weakness and sensory deficit.

Enlargement of the peripheral nerves is a late manifestation; it first develops in the proximal segments of the nerves.

Laboratory Findings

The total protein level in the cerebrospinal fluid is elevated abnormally. On manometric tests there is no block to cerebrospinal fluid circulation. Total and differential cell counts are within normal range.

Serum aldolase and creatine phosphokinase levels are not increased. The serologic test for syphilis should be performed to rule out luetic infection of the central nervous system.

Roentgenograms of the entire spine should be obtained to rule out the possibility of an intraspinal tumor. Spinal nerve root enlargement may be demonstrated by myelography; it should not, however, be performed routinely.

Pyruvate metabolism may be studied by determination of concentration of pyruvate in whole blood before and at intervals after the administration of glucose by mouth. Excessive accumulation of pyruvate in the blood, occurring as a response to a glucose load, is an indication that effective levels of thiamine are lacking in the body. In interstitial hypertrophic neuritis, there is no evidence of thiamine deficiency and the hydrochloric acid concentration of gastric contents is normal. Levels of blood glucose are determined to rule out diabetes. Lead or arsenic poisoning should also be ruled out.

Electromyography may disclose evidence of muscle atrophy of neural origin with reduced interference pattern, the presence of fibrillation potentials, and action potentials that are prolonged with normal or polyphasic potentials. Nerve conduction studies should be performed; evoked sensory and mixed nerve potentials will be absent, diminished in amplitude, or will disclose a prolonged conduction time.

Muscle and nerve biopsies should be performed to confirm the diagnosis by histologic examination of the tissues.

Prognosis and Treatment

The course of the disease is one of slow progression with remissions and exacerbations. In mild cases, the disease may reach a plateau and life expectancy may be normal.

There is no specific treatment. Adrenal steroids are reported to improve the condition and may be tried in severe cases or during acute exacerbations.[791] Orthopedic management consists of passive stretching exercises and use of night splints to prevent development of contractural deformity. In advanced cases, orthotic support to the lower limbs and spine may be indicated. Pes cavus may require surgical correction.

REFSUM'S DISEASE (Heredopathia Atactica Polyneuritiformis)*

Heredopathia atactica polyneuritiformis is an extremely rare condition caused by a disorder of lipid metabolism. The basic defect appears to be in the enzyme that catalyzes the alpha-oxidative process by which phytanic acid is shortened by one carbon atom. Endogenous synthesis of phytanic acid is minimal, and the metabolic defect is one of degradation. In the serum and lipid deposits of the liver, kidney, and other organs is found an unusual fatty acid, 3,7,11,15-tetramethyl-hexadecanic acid. In patients with Refsum's disease, exogenous phytol is radily converted to phytanic acid. The disease is transmitted by a recessive gene.

Pathologic findings consist of interstitial hypertrophic polyneuritis and degenerative changes in the anterior horn cells and olivocerebellar tracts.

In children, clinical symptoms are usually manifest between four and seven years of age. The cardinal features of the disease are chronic polyneuritis, retinitis pigmentosa, and signs of cerebellar involvement. The gait is unsteady, and the limbs show weakness and atrophy of the distal musculature. Romberg's sign may be present, and vibration and position sense in the legs may be disturbed. Ichthyosis (especially on the limbs), night blindness, and retinal pigmentary changes are common. Some patients also complain of nerve deafness, anosmia, and nystagmus.

Electrocardiographic changes, e.g., lengthening of the systolic period, are

---

*See References 801–810.

present in most patients. The protein level in the cerebrospinal fluid may be elevated.

In the differential diagnosis, one should consider Friedreich's ataxia, peroneal muscular atrophy, and Roussy-Lévy syndrome. Retinitis pigmentosa is the distinguishing feature of Refsum's disease.

Treatment consists of a diet that is free of chlorophyll and those foods that might contain phytol, phytanic acid, or their precursors. With such a diet, the level of phytanic acid in the blood can be reduced and clinical improvement effected.[802] Pes cavus and other deformities of the limbs are managed according to the principles outlined in the section on Friedreich's ataxia.

CONGENITAL ANALGIA (Congenital Indifference to Pain, Familial Dysautonomia [Riley-Day Syndrome], and Congenital Sensory Neuropathy)

Congenital indifference to pain is a rare disorder characterized by absence of normal subjective and objective responses to noxious stimuli in patients with intact central and peripheral nervous systems.*

The condition was first reported by Dearborn, who described a "human pin cushion" performing vaudeville acts in which spectators thrust sterile needles into his limbs. The stage performance of this actor terminated with a special "crucifixion stunt" in which a lady in the audience fainted when spikes were driven through his palms. The neurologic examination of this person was entirely within normal limits except for the absence of pain sensation.[818]

The etiology of the condition is unknown. There is no sex predilection.

Clinical and Pathologic Features

Although life without pain sounds ideal, in actuality the lack of protective reflexes handicaps the afflicted children in various ways.

---

*See References 811–818, 821–828, 830–838, 841–846, 848, 849.

As soon as the eruption of teeth takes place, the condition is first evidenced by biting of the tongue, lips, or fingers. Burns and multiple bruises are common occurrences. The infant often fails to cry when hurt. Dental sepsis causes early loss of teeth. Corneal opacity may result from trauma or foreign bodies in the eye. The intelligence of these patients is normal.

Skeletal manifestations vary, depending upon the nature of the injury and the age of the patient. Severe trauma causes ordinary fractures of the long bones, the skull, and the short tubular bones of the hands and feet. The bones are not unduly fragile (Fig. 5–109). However, delayed diagnosis and failure to treat these fractures result in gross deformities of the long bones and pseudarthrosis. Repeated injury to the same limb compounds fracture upon fracture. In infancy, epiphyseal separations occur; in early childhood the fractures take place at the metaphysis, and in later childhood, in the diaphysis. In adolescence and adult life, the incidence of acute fractures decreases, as with maturity and increasing awareness of analgia, the patient learns how to prevent injury. Aseptic necrosis of the talus and of the femoral head occurs frequently.

In the infant and the young child, widening of the epiphyseal plate develops from repeated minimal traumata, causing rachitic type changes in the roentgenogram. Direct injury and subperiosteal hemorrhage result in cortical thickening of long bones. Growth disturbances are produced by epiphyseal injury.

Joints respond to multiple injuries by effusion, hemarthrosis, synovial thickening, and ligamentous laxity. With continued chronic trauma, neuropathic arthropathy develops. Weight-bearing joints, especially the ankle, are common sites. The presence of Charcot's joints in a child should arouse suspicion of congenital indifference to pain.

Osteomyelitis of long bones is a common incidental finding in the roentgenogram, and is seen as an area of rarefaction in the metaphysis. The bone infection is usually discovered in its chronic stage, as it is indolent. Neglected foci of infection (such as infected teeth, burns, or bitten fingers) and local trauma are predisposing factors. Whenever a child is suspected of having congenital indifference to pain, a roent-

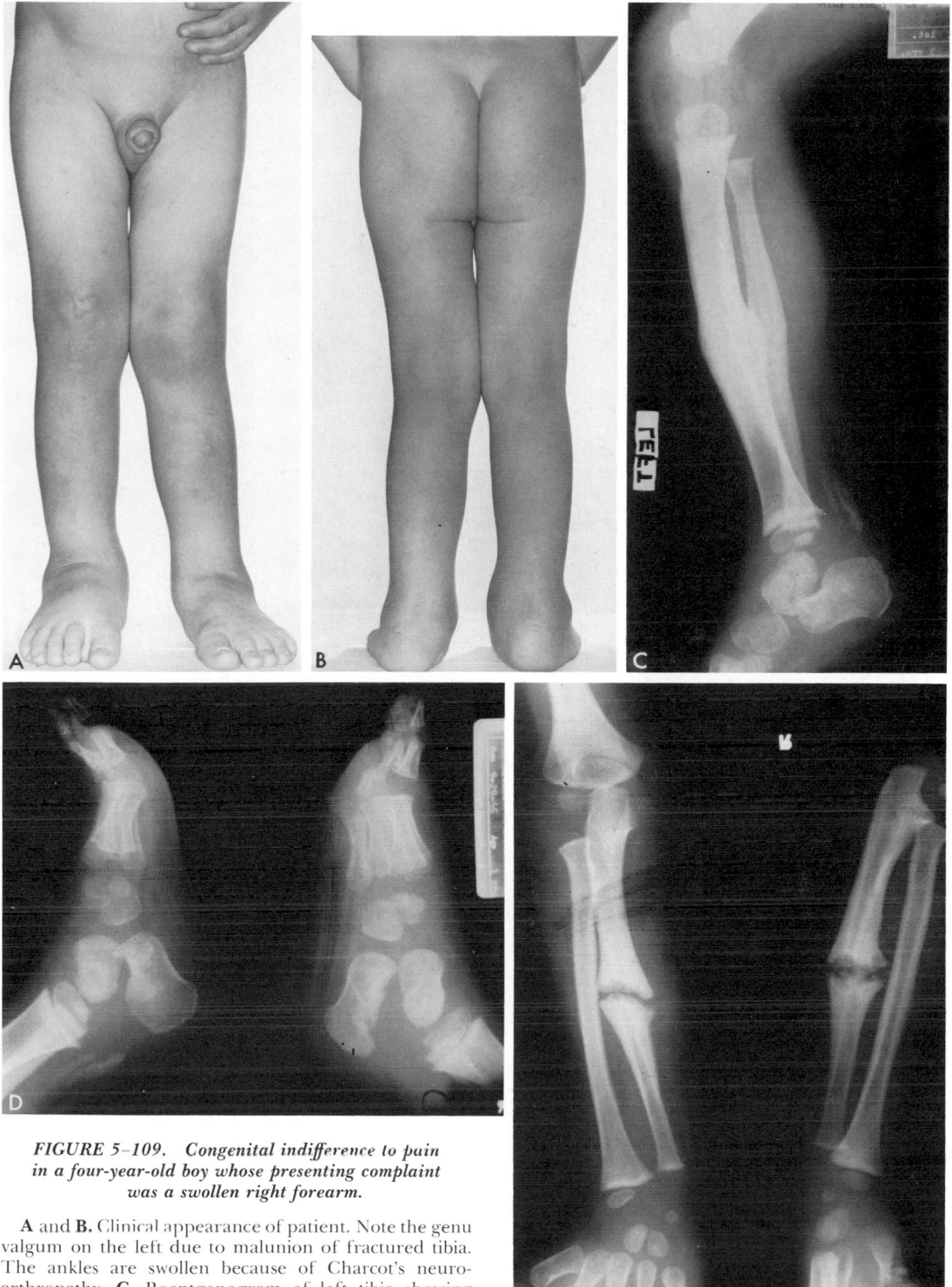

***FIGURE 5–109.   Congenital indifference to pain
in a four-year-old boy whose presenting complaint
was a swollen right forearm.***

A and **B.** Clinical appearance of patient. Note the genu
valgum on the left due to malunion of fractured tibia.
The ankles are swollen because of Charcot's neuroarthropathy. **C.** Roentgenogram of left tibia showing
healing fracture. **D.** Roentgenogram of both feet and
ankles. Note the early Charcot's joints, particularly on the right. **E.** X-ray views of right forearm showing nonunion
of fracture in the middle third of the ulna. After immobilization in a long arm cast for a period of three months
there was no evidence of healing. Thus, an open reduction, intramedullary fixation with a Steinmann pin, and
onlay bone grafting was performed.

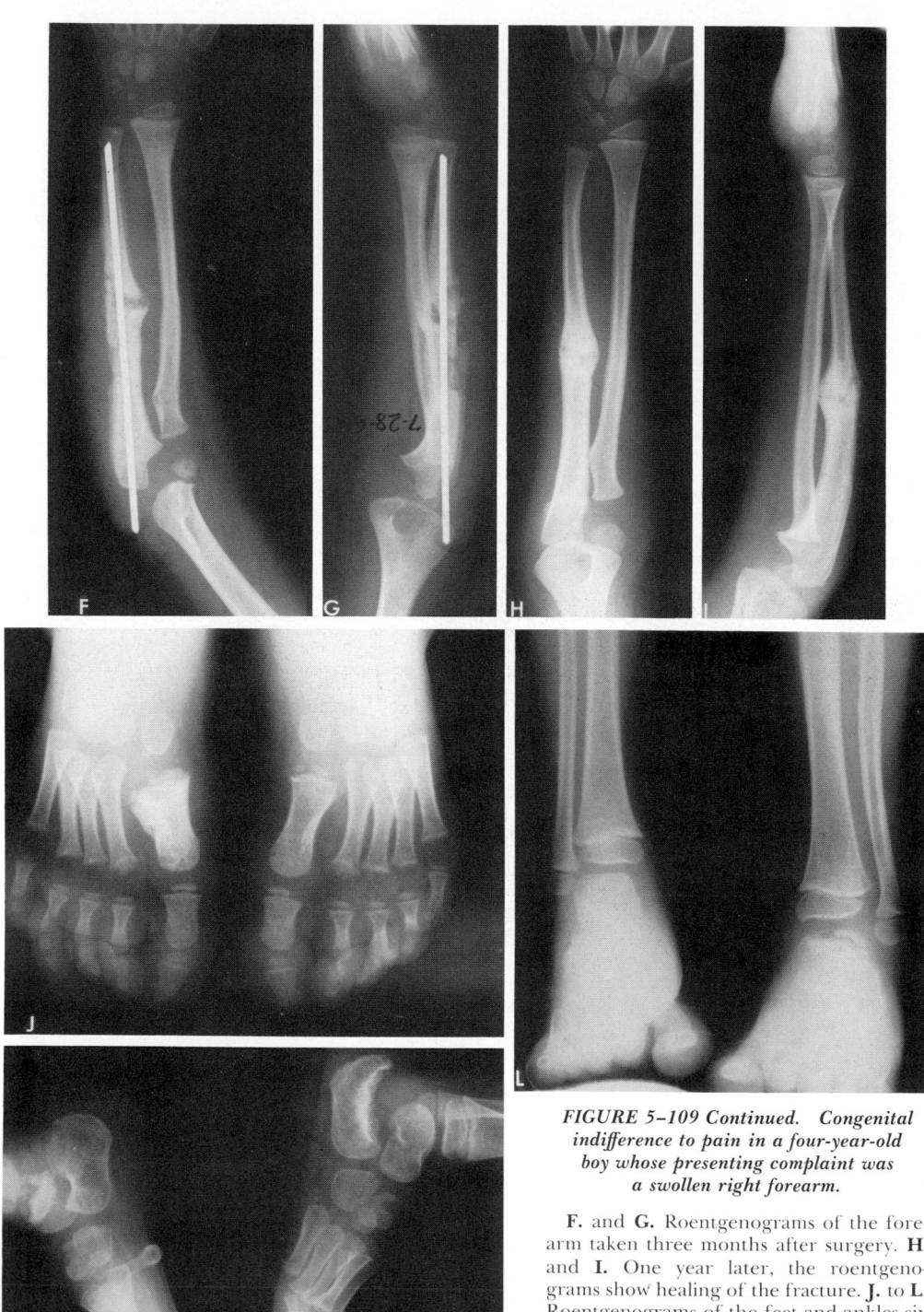

FIGURE 5–109 Continued. *Congenital indifference to pain in a four-year-old boy whose presenting complaint was a swollen right forearm.*

F. and **G.** Roentgenograms of the forearm taken three months after surgery. **H.** and **I.** One year later, the roentgenograms show healing of the fracture. **J.** to **L.** Roentgenograms of the feet and ankles six months later. Note the progression of neuroarthropathic changes in the subtalar and ankle joints, and extensive subperiosteal new bone formation of the right first metatarsal. Patellar tendon weight-bearing orthosis was given to protect the ankles and hindfeet.

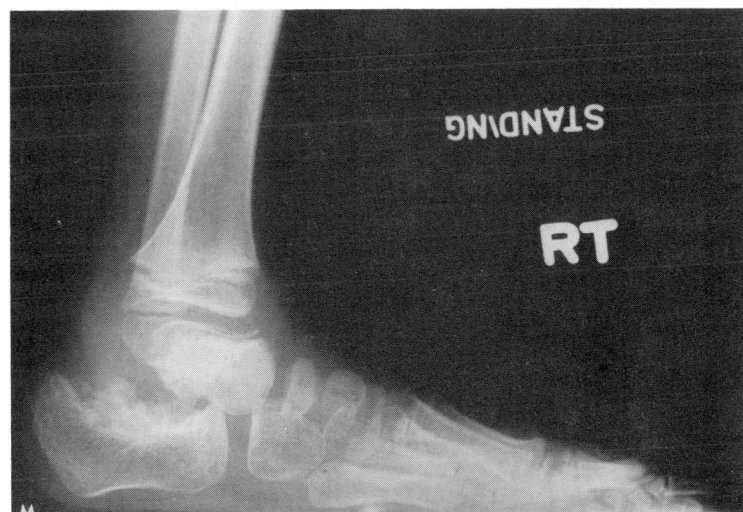

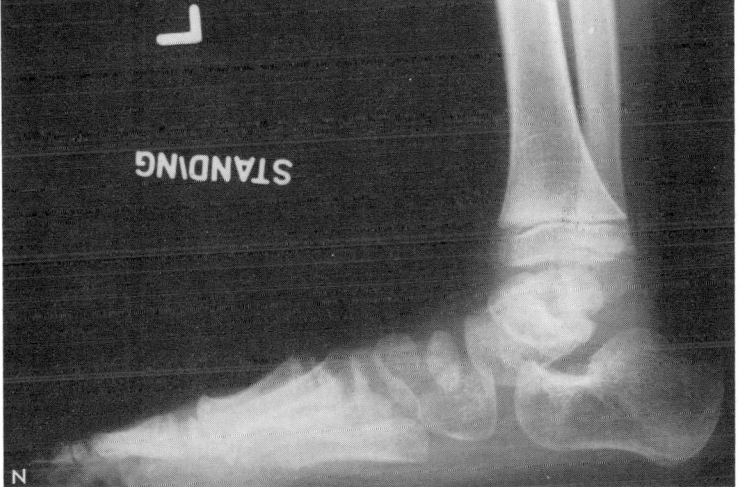

FIGURE 5–109 Continued.
Congenital indifference to pain in a
four-year-old boy whose presenting
complaint was a swollen
right forearm.

M. and **N.** Lateral roentgenograms
of the feet and ankles taken a year
later show some improvement in
the Charcot's joints.

genographic skeletal survey should be obtained to rule out silent bone lesions and fractures. Electroencephalograms and psychological and intelligence test scores are normal. There are no abnormalities of cutaneous nerve endings in the skin or periosteum, and the central, peripheral, and autonomic nervous systems are intact.

Diagnosis

General analgesia is classified by Winkelmann et al. as follows:[849]

I. Cerebral level
   A. Without lesions
      1. Congenital indifference to pain
      2. Oligophrenia
      3. Psychic states (hysteria, etc.)
   B. With lesions
      1. Asymbolia
      2. Postleukotomy state
II. Spinal cord level
   A. Syringomyelia
   B. Syringobulbia
III. Peripheral nerve
   A. Congenital sensory neuropathy
   B. Familial progressive neuropathy
   C. Acquired peripheral neuropathy (toxic or infectious)

When a patient is suspected of having loss of pain sensation, a systematic investigation of pain reaction should be made. Winkelmann et al. perform this test in three sections: (1) a study of affective reaction or perception of the stimulus, (2) demonstration of the state of the peripheral receptors and pathways for pain appreciation, and (3) demonstration of integrated involuntary reflex responses to painful stimuli.

Intelligence and psychometric tests are performed. A thorough neurologic examination, though difficult in a child, is essential. The neurologist possesses many devices to elicit pain in the examination; however, a sharp pin is as satisfactory as any sophisticated device such as the square-wave electric pulse generator that gives shock at a definite milliamperage. Deep pain is tested by pressure on muscles or bones and by deep insertion of hypodermic needles. Various objectively recognizable physiologic responses to pain stimuli are studied: these include pupillary dilatation, blood pressure elevation, and a rise in the respiratory and pulse rate. The important determination is

whether there is a lack of sensation when a painful stimulus is applied or whether sensation is present but the patient is indifferent and does not recognize it as being a noxious one.

The integrity of peripheral nerves is assessed by nerve conduction studies. Sometimes a cutaneous nerve biopsy may be indicated. The presence of normal sudomotor and vasomotor reactions in the skin demonstrates an intact autonomic nervous system. Is the axon reflex response to histamine normal? A skin biopsy is performed to demonstrate whether the nerve end organs are intact and also the presence or absence of nonspecific cholinesterase activity in them. Electromyography may be helpful to rule out the presence of lower motor neuron disease or the possibility of a myopathy. When cerebral organic disease is suspected, an electroencephalogram should be obtained.

The differential diagnosis between the major sensory syndromes with absence of pain perception is given in Table 5–14.

The two principal entities that must be distinguished from congenital indifference to pain are familial dysautonomia and congenital sensory neuropathy. *Familial dysautonomia (Riley-Day syndrome)* is very rare and is seen specifically in persons of Jewish ancestry. It is inherited as an autosomal recessive trait with varying expressivity. The disease manifests itself at birth with lack of lacrimation, excessive perspiration, and poor temperature control. The corneal reflex and the normal axon reflex responses to histamine are absent. There is a characteristic lack of fungiform papillae on the tongue. The afflicted children are emotionally unstable, and development of speech is abnormally delayed. The intelligence level is usually subnormal. Temperature perception is diminished, but touch perception is normal. There is lack of objective physiologic response to painful stimuli. The distribution of sensory loss is incomplete.[829, 839, 840, 846, 847]

In *congenital sensory neuropathy* the sensations of touch, temperature, and pain are lost. Distribution of sensory loss is diffuse, but islands of normal sensation are usually present. Myelinated nerve fibers and dermal nerve networks are absent. The brain and spinal cord are intact. Motor nerve conduction is normal, but conduction over sensory

Table 5–14.*

Parameter	Congenital Indifference	Familial Dysautonomia	Congenital Sensory Neuropathy	Hereditary Sensory Radicular Neuropathy	Familial Sensory Neuropathy with Anhidrosis	Acquired Sensory Neuropathy (Toxic, Infectious)	Syringomyelia
Heredity	None	Recessive	None, occasionally dominant	Dominant	Recessive	None	None
Age of onset	Birth	Birth	Birth	Early adolescence	Birth	Adult	Young adult
Physiologic pain reactions	Present	Absent	Absent	Absent	Absent	Absent	Absent
Touch perception	Normal	Normal	Lost	Lost	Normal	Normal	Normal
Temperature perception	Normal	Diminished	Lost	Lost	Diminished	Normal	Normal
Distribution of sensory loss	Universal	Incomplete	Islands of normal sensation	Legs and feet, occasionally hands	Islands of normal sensation	Legs and feet, occasionally hands	Arms and hands
Axon reflex	Normal	Absent	Absent	Absent	Absent	Absent	Normal
Nerve conduction	Normal	Normal	Sensory absent; Motor present	Sensory absent; Motor normal	Sensory absent; Motor normal	Motor and sensory abnormal	Normal or slightly reduced
Motor strength	Normal	Normal	Normal	Normal	Normal	Weak (atrophied)	Weak (atrophied)
Sensory nerve biopsy	Normal	Absence of fungiform papillae on tongue	No myelinated fibers	No myelinated fibers	Myelinated fibers present	Loss of myelinated fibers	Normal
Skin biopsy	Normal	Normal	No nerve endings; No cholinesterase	———	Normal	Degeneration of nerve, normal cholinesterase	Normal
Brain and other	Normal	Normal *Autonomic N.S.* Lack of lacrimation Excessive perspiration Poor temperature control	Normal	Normal	Normal Absence of Lissauer's tract and small dorsal root axon	Normal	Normal
Intelligence	Normal	Dull to average	Dull to average	Normal	Defective	Normal	Normal

*Modified from Winkelmann, R. K., Lambert, E. H., and Hayles, A. B.: Congenital absence of pain. Report of a case and experimental studies. Arch. Derm., 85:334, 1962.

cutaneous nerves is absent. Physiologic responses to pain stimuli cannot be elicited. The condition occurs sporadically, but is sometimes inherited as a dominant trait.[819, 820]

Treatment

The patient and his parents should be educated to prevent injury. Early diagnosis and immediate treatment are important. Fractures ordinarily heal without difficulty. With delayed diagnosis and neglected treatment, pseudarthrosis may develop, necessitating a bone graft. A patellar bearing orthosis is used to protect the talus with aseptic necrosis and the neuropathic ankle joint. Osteomyelitic lesions are treated in the usual manner.

ACUTE POLYRADICULONEURITIS (Guillain-Barré Syndrome)*

In this rare syndrome there is symmetrical motor and sensory paresis of the limbs and, in some cases, of the trunk. The paralysis, characteristically, ascends centripetally and may involve the cranial nerves. The etiology of the condition is unknown; most probably it is the result of a disturbance of the immune mechanism. A direct viral etiology has not been demonstrated. The syndrome is known by the eponyms *Guillain-Barre syndrome* and *Landry's paralysis.*

The posterior nerve roots and ganglia, the proximal portion of the peripheral nerves, and the anterior nerve roots are involved. Initially, pathologic changes consist of edema, followed by degeneration of axons and myelin, with some lymphocytic infiltration. In severe cases the peripheral nerves undergo wallerian degeneration.

Clinical Features

There is great variation in the mode of onset, the severity of motor and sensory involvement, and the distribution of paresis. Ordinarily, the distal part of the limbs is involved initially and the paresis ascends.

Paralysis is usually symmetrical and is more marked distally than proximally. The deep tendon reflexes are absent or diminished. The motor weakness is accompanied by some degree of sensory disturbance, which may vary from minimal hypoesthesia to total loss of all modalities of sensation. In severe cases, sphincter disturbances and inability to urinate or defecate may be seen. Cranial nerves may be involved, usually the seventh or eleventh. On occasion, papilledema may be present. Autonomic disturbance is manifest as persistent tachycardia. Mentality is usually normal.

The course of the disease varies with the severity of the condition. In minimally involved cases, complete recovery may occur within one to two months; whereas in the severe forms it may take one to two years and varying grades of residual paralysis may persist. In the acute stage, paralysis of the limbs and trunk may be total, with the exception of some eye movement. In such cases, death may occur from cardiorespiratory collapse. Recurrent attacks may be encountered in an occasional patient.

Diagnosis

The cerebrospinal fluid shows an increase of proteins with a normal cellular picture. The concentration of cerebrospinal fluid proteins reaches its maximal level in two to four weeks and starts to decline to normal values. Occasionally it may be abnormally high for several months.

Conduction in the motor and sensory fibers is slowed, as shown by nerve conduction studies; and evoked sensory potentials are absent or decreased in amplitude.

In the differential diagnosis, one should consider acute poliomyelitis, acute myelitis, acute porphyria, tick paralysis, and toxic neuropathy.

Treatment

Corticosteroids may be given during the acute paralytic phase; however, the results of such therapy are hard to assess.

Paralysis of the limbs is treated by supporting the parts in appropriate splints and passive and active assisted exercises to maintain range of motion of joints. When-

---

*See References 850–888.

ever the antigravity weight-bearing muscles have regained fair motor strength, the patient is allowed to be ambulatory with the help of crutches. Orthotic devices are used as indicated. In the severely involved cases in which some degree of residual paralysis persists, orthopedic operations such as arthrodesis or tendon transfers are required for stabilization of joints and re-establishment of dynamic balance of muscles. In such instances, it is advisable to wait for two years to be sure that the paralysis is permanent.

Respiratory paralysis is a serious complication that occurs during the acute stage of the disease. It is treated by immediate tracheostomy and by the use of either tank type respirators or positive pressure systems.

HERPES ZOSTER

Herpes zoster, commonly known as shingles, is an acute viral infection of one or more dorsal root ganglia or sensory ganglia of the cranial nerves. It is accompanied by a painful vesicular rash of the skin or mucous membrane that is distributed in the corresponding dermatome along the course of the peripheral sensory nerves arising in the affected ganglia. Herpes zoster and varicella appear to be caused by the same virus. Weller et al. have been able to propagate the etiologic agent in vitro in cultures of human tissues.[911, 912] The viral bodies from vesicles of varicella and zoster are identical in appearance, size, and serologic reactions. Infection with one disease may occur after contact with a patient suffering from the other. It seems herpes zoster results from neurogenous spread of reactivated latent varicella virus in a partially immune individual, whereas varicella is caused by hematogenous spread of the virus in a nonimmune individual.[893]

Herpes zoster commonly occurs in individuals over 40 years of age; it is not, however, rare in children, in whom it is most frequently encountered in association with malignant neoplasms such as leukemia, lymphomas, or neuroblastoma. Other predisposing factors are poisoning with arsenic or other drugs, and trauma affecting the nerve roots, in which case herpes zoster develops in the involved dermatome.

Pathology

The lesions in the nervous system may be categorized as (1) inflammation of the spinal posterior root ganglia or the sensory ganglia of the cranial nerves (in the acute stage, there is a marked lymphocytic reaction with a varying degree of cell necrosis, followed by secondary degeneration of the afferent fibers and eventual gliosis), (2) a "poliomyelitic-like" lesion involving both the anterior and posterior horns and roots, (3) a relatively mild localized leptomeningitis, and (4) true peripheral mononeuritis.[894]

The involvement of the anterior horn cells of the spinal cord accounts for the motor manifestations of the disease. Broadbent is credited as being the first to describe paralysis of the upper limb due to herpes zoster, in 1866.[891] Upper motor neuron involvement with hemiplegia was reported by Duncan in 1868; and a description of lower limb paralysis was published by Hardy in 1876.[895, 900]

The epithelial layer of the skin is markedly inflamed, and acidophilic intranuclear inclusion bodies will be found in the epithelial cells of the vesicles.

Clinical Features

The manifestations of the disease are milder in children than in adults, and the face is less frequently involved. There may be generalized malaise, low-grade fever, burning dysesthesia in the involved dermatome, or pain in the underlying muscles during the prodromal period, which may last three or four days. The regional lymph nodes may be enlarged. Neck stiffness and headache are occasional complaints.

The eruptions develop suddenly, with characteristic distribution along the course of the sensory nerve. It is first papular, then vesicular, and eventually becomes crusted. The rash may form a complete girdle or "cingulum," from which the name shingles is derived. The common site of the skin lesions is the trunk or face; it occurs less frequently on the limbs, where it is more proximal than distal in location. Involvement is more often unilateral than bilateral.

Paralysis of the limbs occurs in about 5 per cent of cases. Gupta et al. have found limb paralysis in 15 of the 274 patients with zoster referred to the hospital—seven of the upper limbs, seven of the lower limbs, and one of both the upper and lower limbs on the same side (lower motor neuron type).[897] Grant and Rowe reported five patients with paralysis of the limbs among 101 patients admitted to Massachusetts General Hospital (two of the upper and three of the lower limbs).[896] Herpetic eruption frequently precedes the paralysis, the time interval between the two incidents being one to six days; however, it may take three and a half months for the paralysis to develop following the herpetic eruption. Occasionally the eruption and paralysis occur simultaneously.

The prognosis for full recovery is good in paralysis of the limbs in herpes zoster. Gupta et al. reported complete recovery in two thirds of the patients within a year. Permanent paralysis occurred in one sixth of the patients studied.[897] Permanent paralysis usually takes place in muscles that are mainly or wholly supplied from single segments of the spinal cord, such as the hemidiaphragm, muscles of the anterior tibial compartment, and the intrinsic muscles of the hand.

The motor paralysis may suggest intraspinal tumor. The presence of herpetic rash should aid in the differential diagnosis.

Treatment

There is no specific remedy for herpes zoster. Relief of pain is afforded by analgesics. Therapy of paralysis of limbs follows the principles outlined in poliomyelitis.

MISCELLANEOUS AFFECTIONS OF PERIPHERAL NERVES

Neuropathy Associated with Diabetes Mellitus

In severely diabetic children, neuropathy may develop as early as ten years of age. It may be manifest in several forms.[915, 919, 921] In *Type I*, the lower limbs are primarily involved, with loss of deep tendon reflexes and a variable degree of anesthesia. Motor weakness and disability are minimal. In *Type II* the autonomic system is predominantly affected. The presenting symptoms are incontinence of urine, diarrhea, orthostatic hypotension, and anhidrosis. *Type III* is characterized by sudden onset of asymmetrical cranial nerve palsy (commonly of the third and seventh) and complete or partial paralysis of one or several of the lumbar nerve roots. Nerve conduction studies will disclose a diminution of the conduction rate in both motor and sensory fibers or absence of evoked potentials. There is no specific therapy. Vitamin B_{12} injections are often given. Good control of diabetes mellitus is imperative.

Acute Intermittent Porphyria

This disorder of porphyrin metabolism usually has its onset in adult life, but it may occur in children. The symptoms are acute. Colicky abdominal pain, constipation, mental confusion varying from neurosis to psychosis, and polyneuropathy characterize the condition. Sensory loss and paresthesia are uncommon. Involvement is predominantly motor, with paralysis of the proximal muscle groups and cranial nerves. The clinical picture may simulate polyradiculoneuritis. The urine contains excessive amounts of uroporphyrins and coproporphyrins, Types I and III. The freshly voided urine is normal in color but turns reddish brown on standing. The proteins may be increased in cerebrospinal fluid. Death may occur from respiratory paralysis.

Toxic Neuropathy

Toxic neuropathy may result from the administration of various drugs such as isoniazid and nitrofurantoin, or from accidental poisoning with toxins such as arsenic, insecticides, lead, and mercury. Neuropathy may also follow prophylactic inoculations.[913, 914, 918, 920] In the differential diagnosis, the preceding conditions should be considered.

Affections of Muscles

Congenital Anomalies of Muscles

CONGENITAL ABSENCE OF MUSCLES

Developmental abnormalities in the fetus may lead to hypoplasia or aplasia of various skeletal muscles. Any of the voluntary muscles may be congenitally absent in whole or in part, but certain muscles are deficient more frequently than others. The pectoralis, particularly the sternocostal part of the pectoralis major, is most commonly involved.[924, 927] Next in order of frequency are the trapezius, quadratus femoris, serratus magnus, omohyoideus, semimembranosus, brachioradialis, abdominis, deltoid, latissimus dorsi, sternocleidomastoid, rhomboid, supraspinatus and intraspinatus, biceps brachii, thenar or hypothenar of the hand, and quadriceps femoris.[922, 926]

Usually the abnormality is discovered at birth or soon afterward. It tends to be unilateral and may involve a single muscle or a related group of muscles. The resulting functional disability remains stationary.

Congenital absence of a muscle may be combined with congenital abnormalities of other organs. Some of the best known examples of these are agenesis of the pectoral muscles in conjunction with syndactyly or microdactyly and malformations of the genitourinary and alimentary tracts associated with congenital absence of the abdominal musculature (prune belly).[923, 925, 928, 929]

ACCESSORY MUSCLES

Supernumerary muscles are rare. In the limbs, they often simulate soft-tissue tumors, and because of the possibility of malignancy, surgical exploration is carried out. Dunn reports two cases of soleus accessorius muscles, both of which appeared bilaterally as a mass anteromedial to the Achilles tendon (Fig. 5–110).[931] An anomalous accessory hamstring muscle may be manifest as a popliteal swelling (Fig. 5–111). This usually originates from the linea aspera of the femur and passes medially to insert into the dorsal part of the capsule of the knee joint.[931, 933]

In the hand, Lipscomb described a duplication of the hypothenar muscle that was explored on the assumption that it was a tumor.[938] Anomalies of the extensor indicis muscle have been described.[930] When it is a short muscle and arises from the distal end of the radius, proximal carpal bones, or related ligaments, it is called extensor digitorum brevis manus. This usually is mistaken for a ganglion or other soft-tissue tumor.

An accessory palmaris muscle may present clinically as a mass that produces symptoms by compression of the subjacent nerves and tendons.[939] This anomalous muscle usually arises from the palmaris longus tendon and inserts into the ulnar border of the hand. The mass will enlarge on flexion and ulnar deviation of the wrist, and will decrease in size or disappear on wrist extension.

IDIOPATHIC FIBROSIS OF MUSCLES

Progressive Fibrosis of Quadriceps Muscle

In this rare affliction of early childhood there is insidious development of extension contracture of the knee due to progressive fibrosis of one or more components of the quadriceps muscle. The condition is preponderant in girls. Its exact cause is unknown. Hněvkovský, who first described the entity in 1961, believed the fibrosis to be the result of muscular dysplasia of congenital origin.[950] Because of the resemblance of its histologic picture to that of contracture of the sternocleidomastoid muscle in congenital muscular torticollis, a similar path-

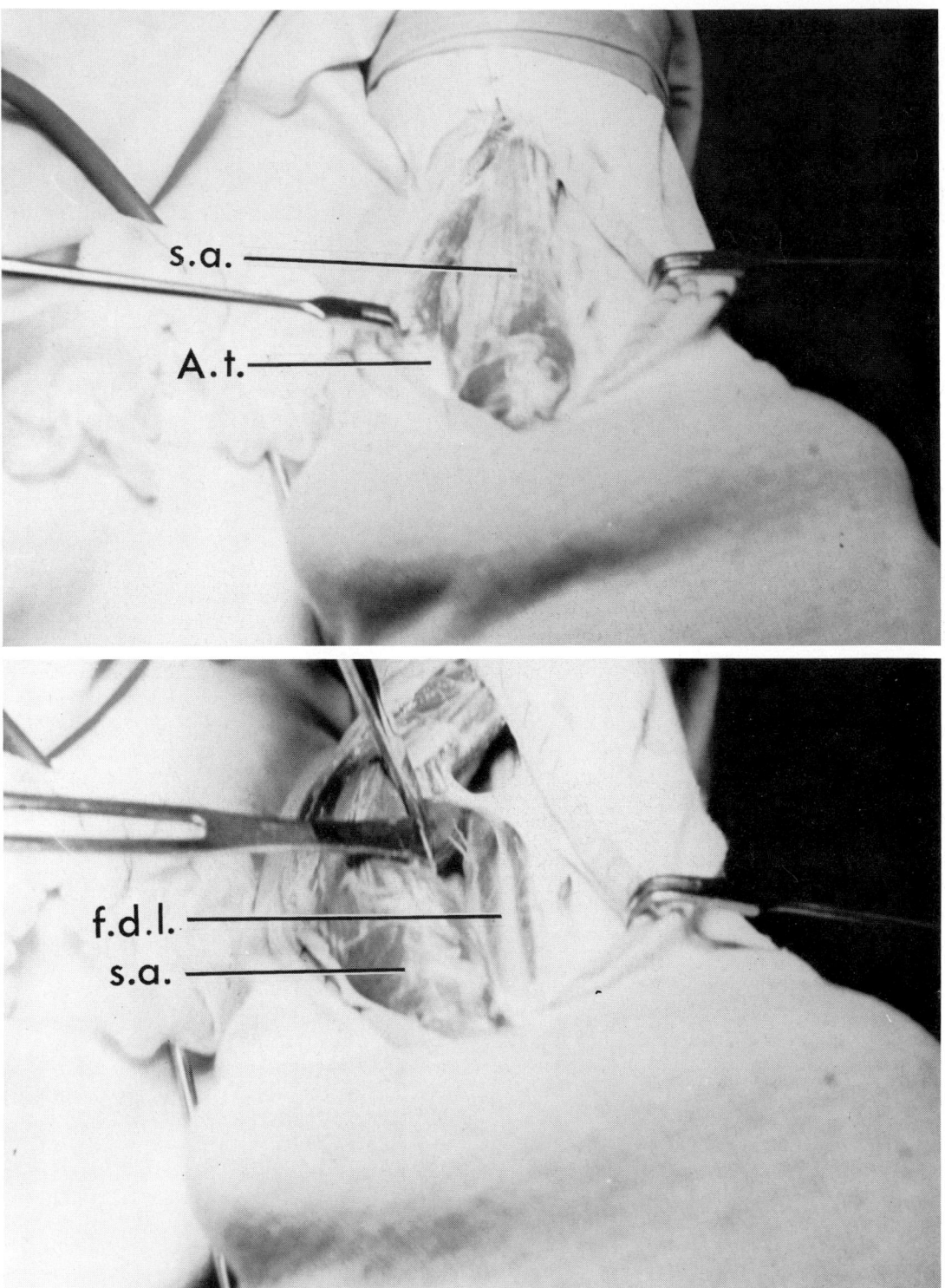

FIGURE 5–110. *Soleus accessorius muscle stimulating a soft-tissue tumor.*

Gross appearance at surgery. s.a., Soleus accessorius muscle; A.t., Achilles tendon; f.d.l., flexor digitorum longus muscle and tendon. (From Dunn, A. W.: Anomalous muscles simulating soft tissue tumors in the lower extremities. J. Bone Joint Surg., *47-A*:1398, 1965.)

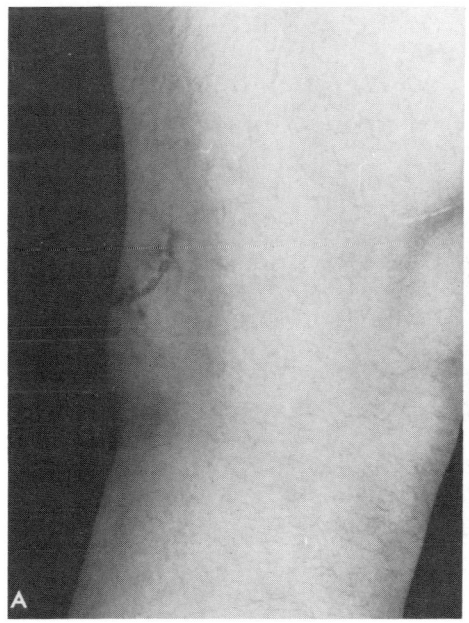 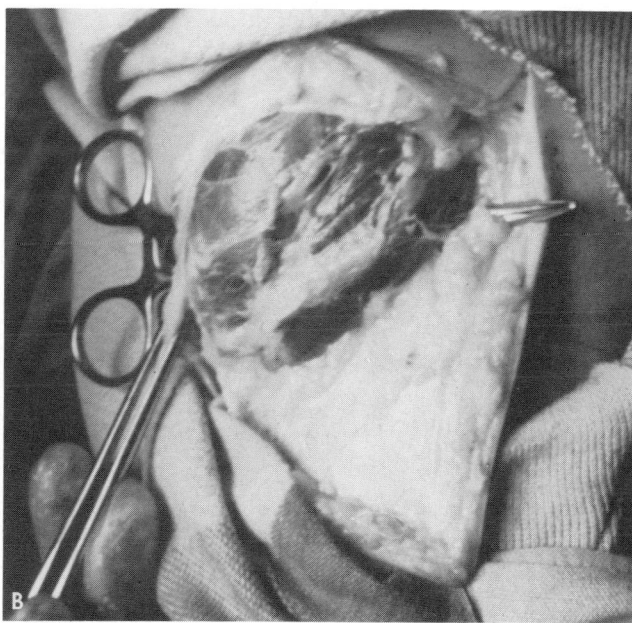

FIGURE 5–111. *Anomalous hamstring muscle presenting as a popliteal mass.*

A. Clinical appearance. **B.** Findings at operation. Note that muscle crosses the popliteal fossa from the lateral to the medial side. The thumb forceps is pulling the semitendinosus tendon medially. (From Dunn, A. W.: Anomalous muscles simulating soft tissue tumors in the lower extremities. J. Bone Joint Surg., *47-A*:1399, 1965.)

ogenesis for the two conditions has been suggested by others.[942, 944, 945] A number of authors have proposed the cause to be multiple injections of antibiotics into the thigh muscles in early infancy.[948, 953, 955]

The distal portion of the quadriceps muscle is principally involved, the vastus intermedius being affected most frequently. There is fibrosis within and in between the muscle fibers. The subcutaneous adipose tissue may be decreased over the affected area. A dimple in the skin produced by the rigid fibrous septa that extend between the skin and deep fascia may be present and will deepen on forced flexion of the knee. Painless and progressive limitation of knee flexion is the principal clinical finding (Figs. 5–112 and 5–113). The patella will be high-riding.

The contracture does not respond to passive stretching exercises or to other conservative measures. Treatment is by surgical division and lengthening of the fibrotic portion of the quadriceps muscle. Postoperatively the knee is immobilized in 90 degrees of flexion for three weeks. Active and passive exercises are then performed to obtain full range of knee motion.

The author has seen one case of idiopathic fibrosis of the proximal part of the rectus femoris muscle. The resultant deformity was flexion contracture of the hip and limited flexion of the knee.

Deltoid Muscle

A similar condition occurring in the deltoid muscle has been described by several authors.[940, 941, 946, 952, 954] Abduction contracture of the shoulder is produced when the intermediate part of the deltoid muscle is fibrosed, whereas fibrosis of the anterior part of the deltoid muscle will result in flexion contracture of the shoulder. Treatment is by surgical division of the fibrous band.

FIBRODYSPLASIA OSSIFICANS PROGRESSIVA (Myositis Ossificans Progressiva)

This rare congenital affection, first described by Guy Patin in 1692, is charac-

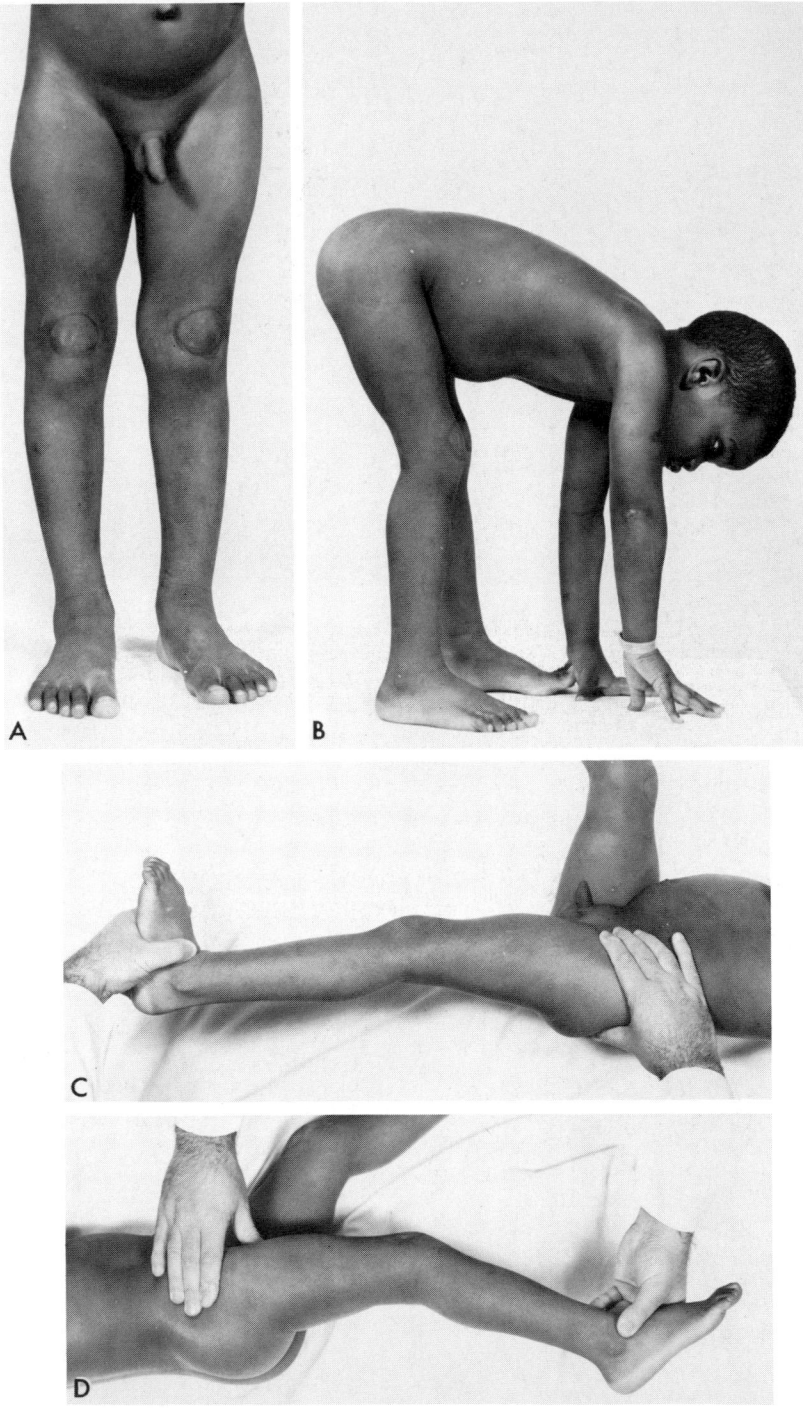

FIGURE 5–112. *Progressive fibrosis of quadriceps muscle of both thighs in a three-year-old boy.*

In early infancy this child had multiple injections of antibiotics in both thighs for treatment of pneumonia. **A.** Standing view showing the high-riding patellae. **B.** He cannot flex his knees to squat. **C** and **D.** These demonstrate the maximum range of passive flexion of both knees. At surgery, fibrosis of the vastus intermedius and vastus lateralis muscles was found.

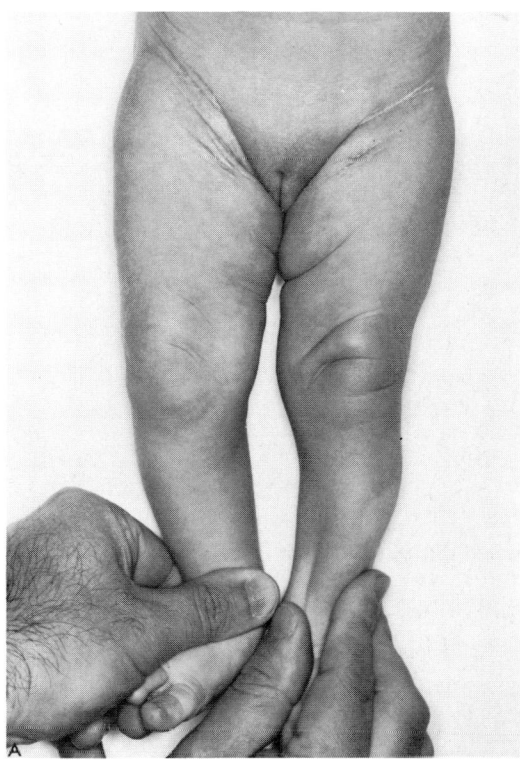

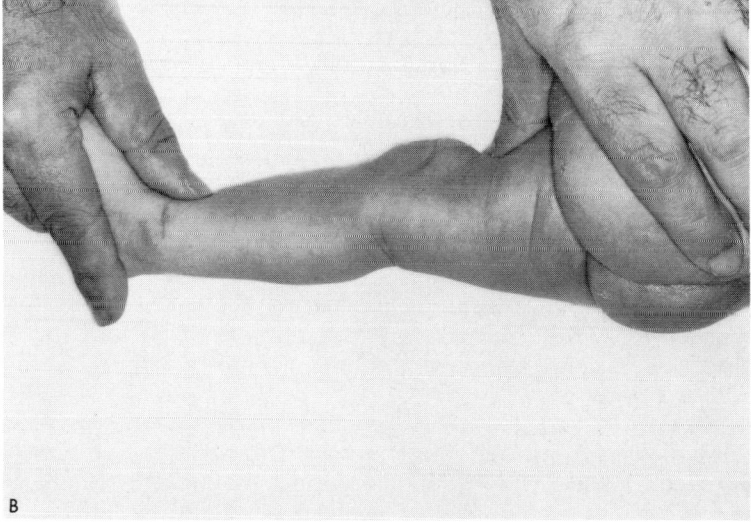

FIGURE 5–113.   *Progressive fibrosis of left quadriceps muscle in a five-month-old child who was the product of a premature birth.*

A. Note the scars of bilateral femoral vein cut downs for infusion. She also received multiple antibiotic injections in her thighs. **B.** The maximum range of passive flexion of the left knee. Passive exercises and corrective casts failed to improve range of left knee motion. At surgery, the vastus lateralis, vastus intermedius, and rectus femoris were found to be fibrosed.

terized by microdactyly and progressive ossification of the fasciae, aponeuroses, ligaments, tendons, and connective tissue in interstitial tissues of skeletal muscles. The skeletal muscles are fundamentally normal; the basic defect resides in connective tissue. Thus, the term *myositis ossificans progressiva* is a misnomer and the name *fibrodysplasia ossificans progressiva* is better used to describe the condition.[976] Rosenstirn, in 1918, collected 119 cases from the literature and added one of his own.[988] Other comprehensive reviews include those of Lutwak, McKusick and Nutt.[975, 976, 982] Helferich was first to observe the constant association of microdactyly with fibrodysplasia ossificans progressiva.[971]

The condition is most probably inherited as a mendelian dominant trait with irregular penetrance.[976] It has been reported in homozygotic twins.[964, 995] There is a preponderance in the male sex, the male to female ratio being 4:1 according to Ryan, and 3:2 according to Fairbank.[965, 989] Rosenstirn found 62 per cent of the cases in the male.[988]

The exact etiology of the disease is unknown.[957] The basic pathogenetic factor appears to be a hereditary defect of some element of connective tissue, leading to secondary calcification and ossification. High alkaline phosphatase activity is found in areas of heterotopic ossification.[996] A congenital deficiency of an inhibitor material or a relative excess of an inhibitor-destroying mechanism was postulated by Lutwak.[975]

Pathology

The early lesions are characterized by marked interstitital edema and connective tissue proliferation. The muscle fibers undergo secondary atrophic and degenerative changes. Later calcification and ossification of the involved mesodermal tissues take place. On occasion, it may be difficult to distinguish fibrodysplasia ossificans progressiva from osteogenic sarcoma.

Clinical Features

Manifestations of the disease usually develop before the age of ten years; on occa-

sion, however, the abnormalities in the fasciae and tendons may be present at birth, indicating onset of the pathologic process in fetal life.[972, 978, 988] Microdactyly definitely has a prenatal origin.

In a typical case, swellings first appear in the neck, the dorsal aspect of the trunk, the shoulder girdle, and eventually in the proximal parts of the limbs. The site of involvement may also be determined by local injury. These swellings are usually small in size, although at times, they may be as large as an egg or an apple. In the early acute phase they are painful, locally tender, slightly warm, and associated with low-grade fever. Swellings may be cystlike and fluctuant, or they may be firm from onset. Often they are attached to the deep fascia, and the overlying skin is normal and loose; but on occasion, they may be ill-defined and not adherent to the deep fascia.

Torticollis is a common presenting complaint; the head is tilted to one side, with painful swellings in the region of the sternocleidomastoid muscle. Flexion of the neck is limited when the ligamentum nuchae is involved. Motion of the temporomandibular joint is diminished, with affection of the masseters (about 20 per cent of the cases). Restriction of the shoulder, elbow, hip, and knee eventually develops. The soft swellings subside within a few days or weeks, whereas the indurated swellings usually persist.

Involvement of the limbs distal to the knees and elbows is rare. The tongue, heart, larynx, diaphragm, and sphincters are exempt from involvement.

In this early stage the finding of *microdactyly* will be of great help in diagnosis. Stunting of growth of the great toe (due to the reduced length of its phalanges) is present in almost all cases of true fibrodysplasia ossificans progressiva. The proximal phalanx may be diminished to a mere wedge-shaped fragment. Rarely is the first metatarsal bone shortened. Hallux valgus is common. The thumbs are shortened less frequently (about 50 per cent of cases). On occasion other digits may be reduced in length. Other rare deformities include absence of a phalanx, fusion of a metacarpal or metatarsal to the proximal phalanx, and volar-radial deviation of the distal phalanx of the little finger.

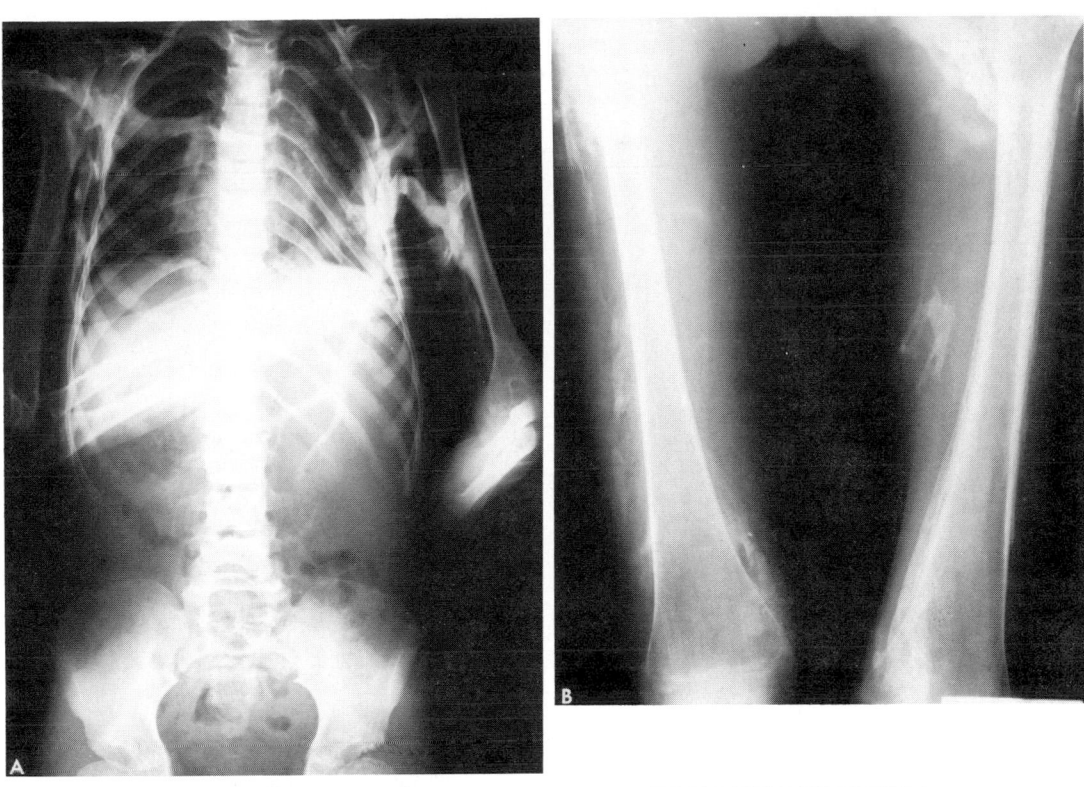

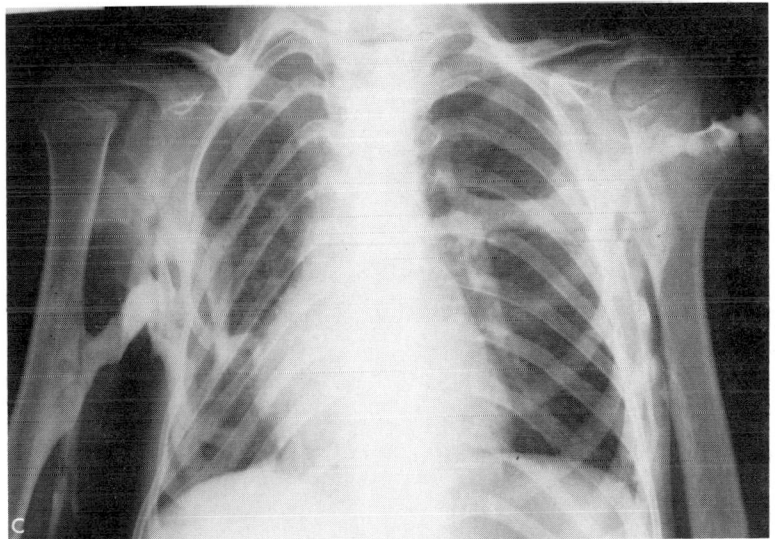

FIGURE 5–114. Fibrodysplasia ossificans progressiva.

A. Initial roentgenogram. **B** and **C.** Roentgenograms taken one year later, showing progression of the disease. Note the columns and plaques of ectopic bone.

Advanced ossification of the epiphyses and widening of the femoral necks may be present. Dystrophic calcification and ossification develop gradually in the involved areas. If a swelling is firm and persistent, ossification will usually take place within a period of two to eight months. The ossific areas may be arranged in columns, lying along the course of muscles, tendons, or ligaments; or they may be seen in the form of irregular masses in the fasciae or aponeuroses. The skin may ulcerate over a protruding mass of bone. The spine and the joints in the vicinity of ossified areas become progressively stiff and then completely rigid. Eventually, the patient may be unable to sit.

Roentgenographic Findings

The columns and irregular masses of extraskeletal bone have varying densities in the roentgenogram. They may be connected to skeletal bone, or they may be entirely free (Figs. 5–114 and 5–115). The skeleton as a whole discloses disuse atrophy.

The microdactyly and digital anomalies are self-evident.

In the *differential diagnosis* several entities should be considered. In infancy and early childhood, the condition may be mistaken for *congenital muscular torticollis;* however, the findings of microdactyly and the progressive nature of the disease should determine the diagnosis of fibrodysplasia ossificans progressiva. Prior to the stage of advanced ossification, the swellings may suggest *Weber-Christian syndrome* or *relapsing nodular nonsuppurative panniculitis.* The latter condition is very rare and is characterized by the appearance of crops of painful subcutaneous nodules of degenerating and inflamed adipose tissue on the trunk, thighs, and arms. It is commonly associated with fever, leukopenia, and an elevated sedimentation rate. Within one or two weeks, the nodules regress, leaving behind a pigmented depression. The etiology of this disease is unknown and there is no specific therapy.

Fibrodysplasia ossificans progressiva should also be distinguished from calcinosis universalis and dermatomyositis. In *calci-*

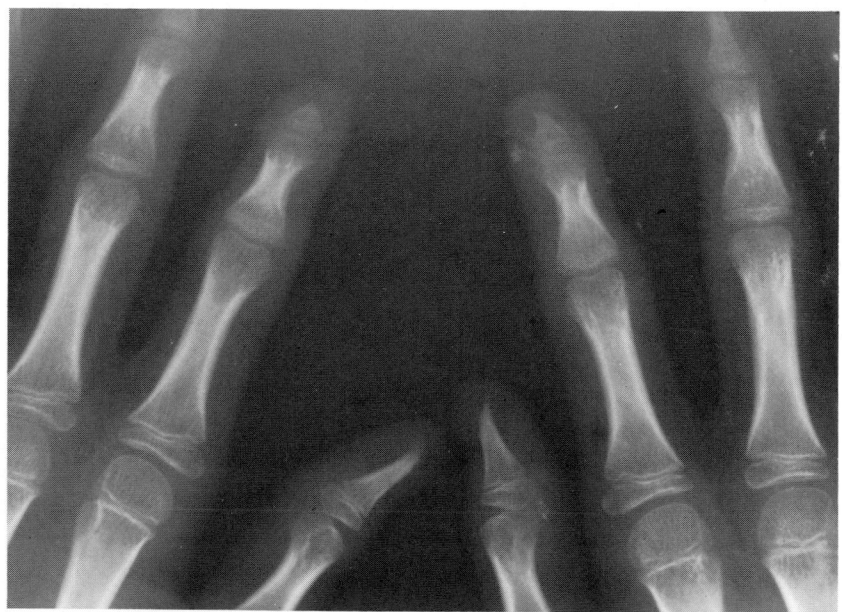

FIGURE 5–115. *Fibrodysplasia ossificans progressiva.*

Roentgenograms of the hands, showing microdactyly of the thumbs and index fingers. Note the tapered ends of the distal phalanx of the thumb.

nosis universalis the calcification will cast a granular and fragmentary shadow in the roentgenogram. The lesions are more common in the limbs, beginning in the subcutaneous tissues and later extending to involve the ligaments, tendons, and connective tissue of the muscles. *Dermatomyositis* also initially affects the limbs and later involves the trunk. The skin and underlying muscle are inflamed, with local tenderness, induration, swelling, and weakness. The necrotic foci in the muscle and subcutaneous fat may calcify and be visible on the roentgenogram.

Prognosis and Treatment

The course of the disease is one of steady progression, with periods of remission and acute exacerbations. Eventually the patient becomes totally disabled.

There is no specific therapy. A trial of treatment with adrenocortical hormones has given dubious results. Beryllium has been tried and found to be of doubtful benefit.[993] Roentgen therapy will aggravate the condition. The progress of the disease is not arrested by treatment with disodium ethylenediamine tetraacetate (EDTA). Operative excision of the bony columns to relieve ankylosis has been disappointing, as the surgical trauma has aggravated the condition and more extensive bone has re-formed.

PROGRESSIVE MUSCULAR DYSTROPHY

Definition and Classification

Progressive muscular dystrophy is a genetically determined primary degenerative disease of skeletal muscle. It is generally classified as a *myopathy*, a broad term that encompasses diseases caused by pathologic, biochemical, or electrical changes in the muscle fibers or in the interstitial tissues of the voluntary musculature, and in which there is no abnormality of the innervation of the affected muscles.

The classification of muscular dystrophy that is most adequate from the clinical and genetic standpoints is the one given by Walton:

1. The "pure" muscular dystrophies
   (a) The Duchenne type muscular dystrophy
       Sex-linked recessive variety
       Autosomal recessive variety
   (b) Limb-girdle muscular dystrophy
       Autosomal recessive or rarely dominant
       Sporadic variety
   (c) Facioscapulohumeral muscular dystrophy
       Autosomal dominant
           (rarely recessive)
   (d) Distal muscular dystrophy
   (e) Ocular myopathy
   (f) Congenital muscular dystrophy

2. Cases with myotonia
   (a) Myotonia congenita
   (b) Dystrophia myotonica
   (c) Paramyotonia congenita[1056]

Adams et al. classified muscular dystrophy into five main groups; namely, severe generalized familial muscular dystrophy, mild restricted muscular dystrophy, progressive dystrophic ophthalmoplegia, dystrophia myotonica, and late distal muscular dystrophy.[997]

Probably the first true observation of muscular dystrophy as such was made by Meryon, in 1852, who described several families whose members had developed progressive atrophy and weakness of muscles in childhood; in two of these patients, pathologic examination at autopsy disclosed the spinal cord and nerves to be normal, but the muscles showed a form of "granular degeneration." Meryon unfortunately still confused the condition with progressive neural muscular atrophy.[1027]

In 1868, Duchenne published his important treatise on "pseudohypertrophic or myosclerotic paralysis," in which he observed the increase of connective tissue and fat cells in the affected muscles, and also the preservation of striation. In later postmortem studies he demonstrated that the pathologic findings were present only in the interstitial tissues of muscles and that there were no changes in the nervous system.[1009]

Both Leyden and Mobius, in 1876 and 1879 respectively, described a familial form of dystrophy of the pelvic girdle musculature.[1025, 1029] Landouzy and Déjerine, in

1884, gave a classic description of the facioscapulohumeral form; Erb later published a report on the juvenile or scapulohumeral form of the disorder.[1011, 1023]

Gowers, in 1879, in an excellent treatise on pseudohypertrophic dystrophy in young boys, already recognized that muscular hypertrophy and atrophy could occur in variable proportions in the same family, and in 1902 he described another form of the disease in which the distal muscles of the limbs were primarily affected.[1015, 1016]

Batten, in 1909, suggested that the simple atrophic variety of muscular dystrophy could simulate amyotonia congenita.[1000] Hutchinson and Fuchs reported involvement of the external ocular muscles.[1013, 1021]

During this period, another disorder of skeletal muscles, myotonia, was recognized. Myotonia is characterized by a delay in muscular relaxation. Thomsen, in 1876, described individuals in whom all the skeletal muscles were affected from birth; this condition is now known as *myotonia congenita* or *Thomsen's disease.*[1042] Eulenberg, in 1886, described a condition in which myotonia occurred from exposure to cold and there were associated attacks of disabling muscle weakness.[1012] Another more common condition known as dystrophia myotonica was reported later, in which there is progressive atrophy and weakness of the distal muscles of the limbs and of the facial muscles associated with myotonia, which is less severe and localized to only a few muscles.[1001, 1018, 1039]

Etiology

The cause of muscular dystrophy is unknown. It is a hereditary disease. Genetic aspects of the various specific forms are mentioned in the section on clinical features. For a more thorough discussion of the subject, the reader is referred to Kloepfer.[1022]

Several abnormalities in the chemistry of dystrophic muscle have directed research efforts toward a search for a fundamental biochemical defect or defects in muscular dystrophy. To date, a specific relationship between the biochemical aberrations and the dystrophic process has not been established. By analogy with other hereditary diseases, the basic defect in muscular dystrophy caused by a genetic aberration may be the complete or partial failure to synthesize a particular enzyme, the activity of which is essential for the maintenance of normal cell structure.

Pathology

Histopathologic examination does not distinguish reliably between the various types of muscular dystrophy. Essential changes in the muscles are the same in all types. The subdivision of dystrophic diseases is based upon the type of inheritance, the pattern of muscle involvement, the age of onset, and the pace of the disease.

Gross appearance depends on the relative amounts of fat and fibrous tissue that replace the muscle fibers. In pseudohypertrophic muscular dystrophy, the enlarged calf muscles look like a fatty tumor at autopsy. Other affected muscles show varying degrees of atrophy and range in color from yellowish to pinkish-gray.

The most important histologic feature of muscle dystrophy is the loss of muscle fibers, which appears to result from atrophy and the eventual fragmentation of fibers.

The following histologic changes are found in varying degrees (Fig. 5–116):

Great variation in the size of individual muscle fibers. The largest fibers may reach a size of 230μ and the smallest fibers may be as narrow as 10μ. These large and small muscle fibers, along with the normal sized ones, are scattered in haphazard arrangements throughout the muscle in all stages of the disease. The enlargement of fibers may be simply due to work hypertrophy, or it may represent the primary change of dystrophy.[997, 1011]

Retraction of the muscle fibers from the endomysial sheaths.

Forking or branching of fibers.[1060] A common feature in all dystrophies is actual splitting of muscle fibers into daughter fibers, each with distinct sarcolemma within the same endomysial tube. This could represent a regenerative response.

Necrosis of single fibers or groups of fibers with signs of phagocytosis. Recent degeneration of muscle fibers is represented by clusters of histiocytes. There is diminution in the complement of muscle fibers.

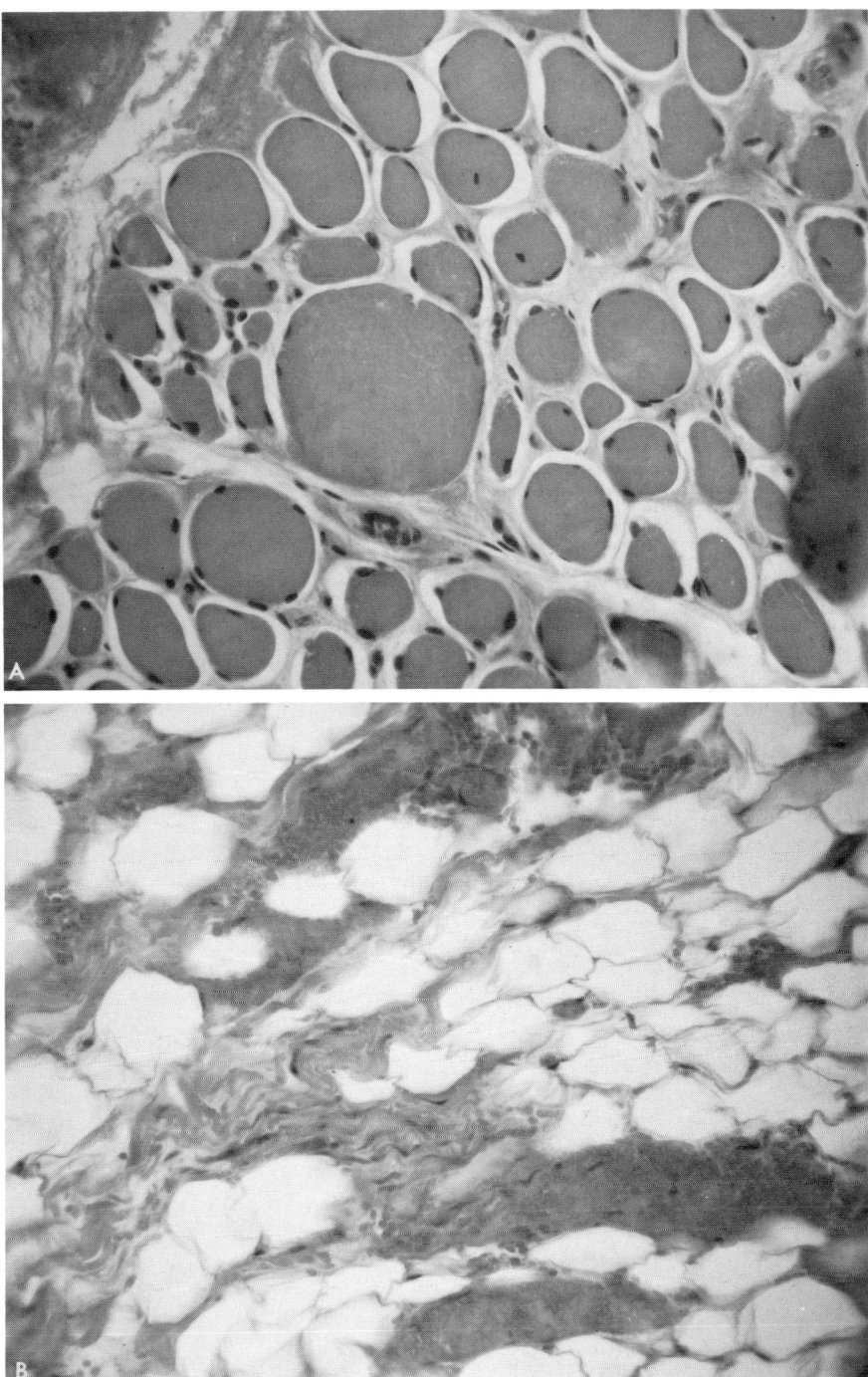

FIGURE 5–116.   *Histologic changes in progressive muscular dystrophy.*

A. Transverse section taken from vastus lateralis muscle of seven-year-old boy. Early stage (× 400, hematoxylin and eosin stain). Note the great variation in the size of individual muscle fibers and retraction of the muscle fibers from the endomysial sheaths. **B.** Longitudinal section from enlarged gastrocnemius muscle. Note the accumulation of adipose tissue and the reduction in number of muscle fibers (× 250, hematoxylin and eosin stain).

Increase in size of sarcolemmal nuclei with prominent nucleation. There is central nucleation in some muscle fibers. Long chains of central nuclei are more characteristic of myotonic dystrophy.

Increase in endomysial connective tissue. This fibrosis could be secondary to loss of muscle fibers.

Hyperplasia of adipose tissue in the form of fat cells. Fat cell infiltration may be due to reduced volume and number of muscle fibers. In the severely involved muscle one will see a few scattered atrophic muscle fibers in a vast field of fatty and connective tissue. Thus, in the terminal stage of muscular dystrophy, there is disappearance of muscle fibers; muscle is reduced to fat and connective tissue, with a few stray surviving fibers. This is the basis for paralysis.

There are no significant changes in the motor and sensory peripheral nerve fibers nor in the central nervous system.

In the cardiovascular system, fibrosis of the myocardium is the most striking finding, varying from finely diffused sclerosis to large areas of scarring. There is no evidence of a specific inflammatory reaction.

The prominent histologic findings in the various types of muscular dystrophy are reflected by the pace of the disease and the age of onset. For example, in the Duchenne pseudohypertrophic type, the rapid progression of the disease is evidenced by the prominent necrosis, phagocytosis, abortive regeneration, and forking of fibers. Enlargement of fibers is also a prominent feature of the pseudohypertrophic type; whereas, in the slowly advancing general adolescent and adult types (Landouzy-Déjerine facioscapulohumeral, limb girdle, and distal), there is little necrosis—the usual findings are variation in fiber size, central nucleation, and fibrosis and fat cell infiltration—and enlargement of fibers is less frequent than that seen in the Duchenne type. In the late adult and restricted muscular dystrophies (such as the ocular form) necrosis is rare; the dominant findings are variation in size of muscle fibers, fibrosis, and increase in fat cells. In myotonic dystrophy, the distinctive features are the rows of central nuclei and annulets (Ringbinden) and peripheral masses of clear sarcoplasm devoid of myofibrils. Electron microscopic findings reported

in the literature thus far have been nonspecific and even conflicting.[1031] Difficulties arise because of lack of knowledge of an acceptable variable in normal material and difficulty in determining the time sequence of various changes.

Clinical Features of Specific Forms of Muscular Dystrophy

The principal types of muscular dystrophy differ with respect to heredity, age of onset, groups of muscles involved by the disease process, and the rate of progression of muscular weakness.

DUCHENNE TYPE MUSCULAR DYSTROPHY

This is the most common type of the disorder and is characterized by predominant occurrence in males. The onset is usually in early childhood, with transmission generally by a sex-linked recessive gene with a high mutation rate (in less than 10 per cent it is transmitted as an autosomal recessive trait). There is symmetrical involvement of the pelvic girdle musculature initially, followed after three to five years by affection of the muscles of the shoulder girdle. A predominant feature of the condition is pseudohypertrophy, which is caused by accumulation of fat. The disease progresses rapidly, resulting in inability to walk within ten years, and death in the latter part of the second decade or sometimes in middle life from respiratory infection, cardiac arrest, or inanition.

The initial symptoms of the disease are usually apparent within the first three years of life, and are manifest as slowness in learning to walk or run at the usual age, proneness to fall frequently, and difficulty in climbing stairs and rising from the floor. In a few cases, the disease may commence between the third and sixth years, and rarely, in early or late adolescence. Symptoms due to weakness of the shoulder musculature appear in the later stages.

On examination, the child stands with a protuberant abdomen and excessive lumbar lordosis. The shoulders are carried behind the pelvis. The calf muscles are enlarged. The shoulders have a sloping appearance because of the weakness of the shoulder girdle musculature.

The gait is waddling, with a gluteus maximus, gluteus medius, and quadriceps limp. If the anterior tibial and peroneal muscles are weak and there is contracture of the triceps surae, the child will have a toe-heel or toe-toe gait. When caught off balance he will tend to fall because his knees give way. He may walk and stand by placing his feet wide apart to increase his base of support, and often will utilize trick movements to maintain equilibrium.

The difficulty in climbing stairs or in rising from the floor is due to bilateral weakness of the gluteus maximus and the quadriceps muscles. The affected child "climbs up on his legs" when rising from the floor, i.e., he first puts his hands on his knees (to keep them extended), and then pushes his trunk upward by working the hands up the thighs, a finding referred to as *Gowers' sign* (Fig. 5–117).

The muscle weakness is proximal in distribution; it is usually first evident in the gluteus maximus, hip abductors and ad-

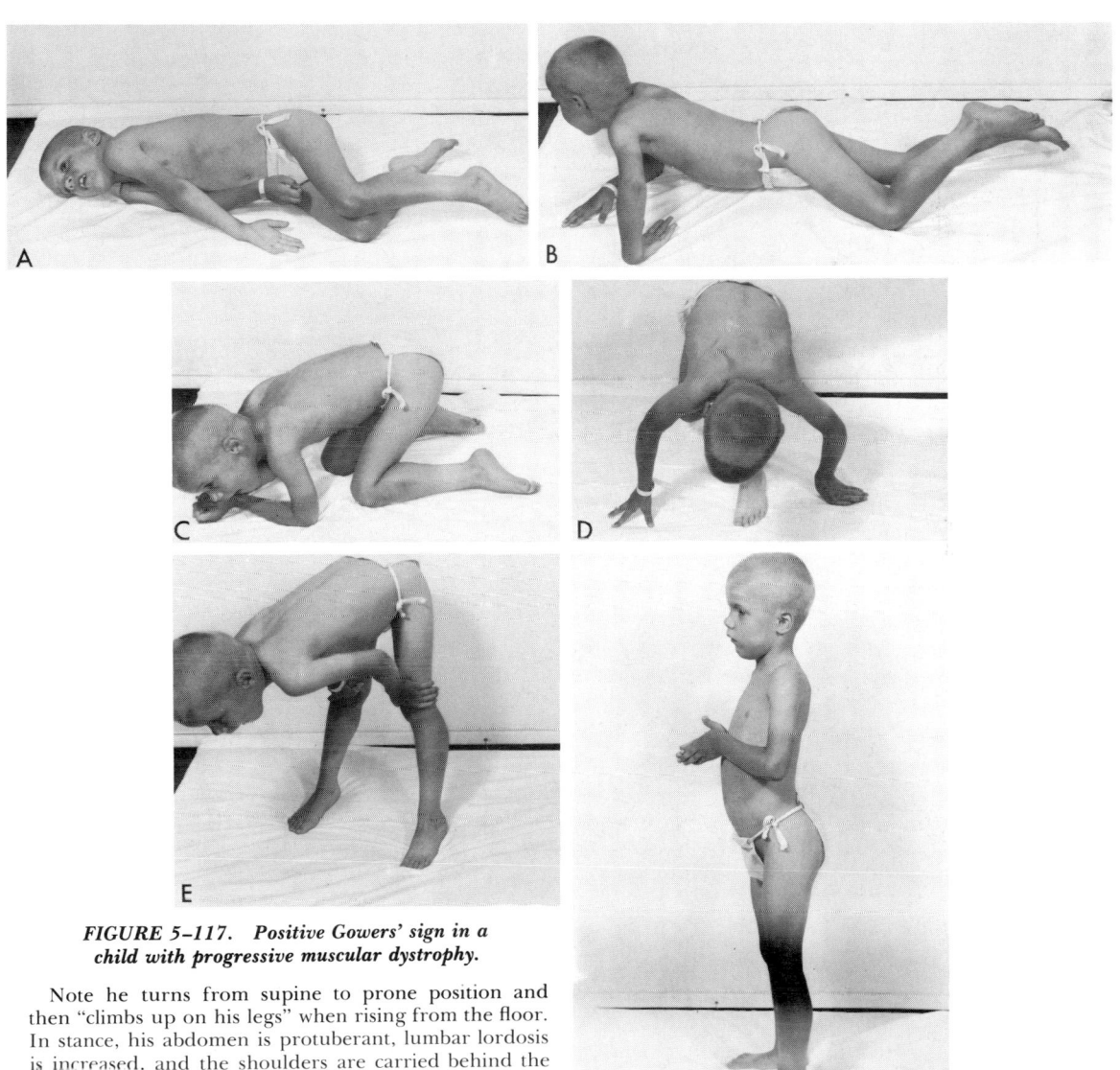

FIGURE 5–117. *Positive Gowers' sign in a child with progressive muscular dystrophy.*

Note he turns from supine to prone position and then "climbs up on his legs" when rising from the floor. In stance, his abdomen is protuberant, lumbar lordosis is increased, and the shoulders are carried behind the pelvis.

ductors, iliopsoas, anterior abdominal, and quadriceps muscles; and eventually involves the anterior crural group. The muscles of the neck and upper limbs involved in the early stages include the lower and middle parts of the trapezius, the rhomboids, the latissimus dorsi, and the inward rotators. Later, the biceps and brachioradialis are affected. The neck muscles are involved comparatively late in the course of the disease, and the gastrocnemius-soleus, tibialis posterior, and toe flexors may remain comparatively strong for several years. The intercostal muscles are eventually affected. With progression of the disease, muscle weakness spreads to the periphery of the limbs with ultimate loss of the entire motor strength of the hip, knee, shoulder, elbow, and ankle joints. The hamstring muscles in the lower limb and the muscles of the hand, face, jaw, pharynx, larynx, and eyes are relatively spared to the end. Diaphragmatic movement is usually normal. Complete manual muscle tests should be performed on all patients with muscular dystrophy and should be repeated at regular intervals to determine the course of muscle weakness.

The affected muscles may be increased or decreased in size. Pseudohypertrophy caused by accumulation of fat attracts attention first and is present in about 80 per cent of cases. It is frequently seen in the calf muscles, but sometimes also in the quadriceps and deltoid muscles. The pseudohypertrophied muscles have a typical firm rubbery texture and are not as strong as healthy muscles of the same size.

Muscular atrophy eventually sets in during the course of the disease. It usually begins near the insertion of the muscles and then spreads proximally. Excessive deposition of subcutaneous fat may hide the muscle atrophy and tend to preserve the contour of the limbs. In the terminal stages of the disease, all the muscles of the limbs, pelvic and shoulder girdles, and of the trunk become atrophic, giving the appearance of severe inanition.

The deep tendon reflexes are normal or hypoactive early in the disease, but later disappear as the muscles concerned become too weak to respond to the stimuli. Superficial reflexes are usually present. With loss of muscle tone, venous insufficiency develops, causing mottling and cyanosis of the limbs.

Early in the disease the joints have full range of motion and the limbs are loose and flaccid. Weakness of one group of muscles but not of its antagonists results in permanent shortening of the stronger muscles and subsequently the development of contractures. These are commonly seen in the triceps surae muscle, with equinus deformity of the ankles and feet. Later in the course of the disease, when the affected children are confined to a wheel chair or bed, contractures develop because of remaining in one position for prolonged periods; these are commonly seen in the hamstrings, the hip flexors, and the iliotibial band.

Scoliosis and kyphoscoliosis are common in the late stages of muscular dystrophy. Changes in the skeleton develop as a result of disuse and the maintenance of abnormal postures of the trunk and limbs. The bones undergo demineralization, with narrowing of the shafts and rarefaction of the ends of long bones. The appearance of the centers of ossification is delayed. Fractures as a result of minimal trauma are not rare.

Myocardial degeneration with fatty infiltration and fibrosis eventually develops. Cardiomegaly and persistent tachycardia are frequently present in the late stages. The electrocardiogram will disclose prolongation of the PR interval, slurring of the QRS complex, bundle branch block, elevation or depression of the ST segment, and other changes, indicating conduction defects or myocardial degeneration. Sudden death may occur from myocardial failure.

Intellectual impairment is common in patients with the Duchenne type of muscular dystrophy, the mean intelligence quotient being approximately 15 to 20 per cent lower than that of normal peers. The personality pattern of these children is characterized by dependency, withdrawal, passivity, and lack of ambition and spontaneity.

The course of Duchenne type muscular dystrophy is one of steady and rapid progression. In general, the cases of autosomal recessive origin run a more benign course than do the sex-linked recessive ones; hence, the Duchenne type of muscular dystrophy is less severe in girls than it is in boys. Periods of bed rest, necessitated by febrile illness or surgical procedures, will result in rapid deterioration. The child is usually confined to a wheelchair between the ages of 10 and 15 years, which leads to the development of severe flexion contractures of the hips, knees, and elbows. Scoliosis results from weakness of the trunk and abdominal muscles. Eventually the patient is unable to sit and is confined to bed with little or no residual active movement in his limbs, except some weak grasp with his hands and flexion of his toes and feet. The muscles of the face and those involved in respiration and swallowing are relatively spared. Survival beyond the age of 20 years is a rarity. Most patients die from sudden cardiac failure or from pulmonary infection. A few in whom the onset of disease was comparatively late may survive until the fourth or fifth decade.

LIMB GIRDLE MUSCULAR DYSTROPHY

This generally less severe form of muscular dystrophy is less common than the Duchenne type, but it is not infrequent. There is great variability in its age of onset. It usually begins in the second decade of life, and less often in the third; occasionally its onset may occur in the latter part of the first decade or between the ages of 30 and 50 years.

The disease is expressed in either sex and is transmitted usually as an autosomal recessive trait, but in rare instances as an autosomal dominant; many cases of the sporadic variety occur.

The initial symptoms develop slowly. Depending on where the disease begins, the early symptoms consist of hunched shoulders and difficulty in lifting the arms above the head or difficulty in climbing stairs and rising from the floor or low chairs. Usually if the shoulder girdle is affected initially, the pelvic girdle musculature will not be involved for quite some time. However, if the dystrophy begins in the muscles of the pelvic girdle, the shoulder girdle muscles will be affected soon.

Pseudohypertrophy of the calf and anterior thigh muscles occurs in less than a third of these patients. Enlargement of the muscles of the upper limbs, particularly the deltoid muscle, is rare. The pattern of muscle weakness is proximal, but not unique, as it is also seen in Duchenne dystrophy. In the upper extremity, the muscles most commonly affected early include the lower and middle parts of the trapezius, rhomboids, latissimus dorsi, and medial rotators of the shoulder. In the lower limb, the gluteus maximus, iliopsoas, hip adductors, and quadriceps are usually involved early in the course of the disease. The disease spreads distally, affecting the anterior tibial and peroneal muscles. The calf muscles are usually spared until later in the course. On occasion, there is comparatively early involvement of the muscles of the forearm and hand. Contractures and skeletal changes develop late and are similar to, but less severe than, those of the Duchenne type. The knee jerk and biceps and radial periosteal reflexes are often diminished or absent, but the Achilles tendon and triceps reflexes remain normal until late in the disease.

The intellectual level is normal in this type of muscular dystrophy. Cardiac involvement is very rare.

There is considerable variation in severity and rate of progression. Severe disability is usually present 20 years after the onset, and most patients die before normal age. In general, the course of the disease is slower in cases in which the shoulder muscles are first affected than in those in which the disease begins in the pelvic girdle musculature. In some there may be periods of remission, but in others there is steady progression resulting in grave disability.

FACIOSCAPULOHUMERAL MUSCULAR DYSTROPHY OF LANDOUZY AND DÉJERINE

This form of muscular dystrophy affects males and females in equal frequency. It is usually transmitted as an autosomal dominant character, occasionally with apparent sex limitation in some families; on very rare occasions, it may be inherited as an autosomal recessive trait.

Partially affected or abortive cases are common in this type of muscular dystrophy.[1019, 1020, 1022] In the mild form, the patient may even be unaware that he is suffering from the disease; in the abortive forms, the disease may remain limited to one or two muscles or muscle groups.

The condition begins at any age from early childhood until adult life, but usually the onset is in the second decade. Initially the face and shoulder girdle muscles are affected, but later on it spreads to the pelvic girdle.

The characteristic appearance of the face is due to weakness of the facial muscles (Fig. 5–118). Wrinkles are often absent from the forehead and around the eyes. The patient cannot close the eyes properly, whistle, or pout the lips. There may be a transverse smile. As muscle weakness progresses, speech becomes indistinct.

The pattern of muscle involvement in the early stages of facioscapulohumeral dystrophy is quite unique. The upper part of the pectoralis major in the neck and shoulder area and the anterior tibial in the lower limb are affected early, while the back extensors, iliopsoas, gluteus medius, tensor fasciae latae, and quadriceps are spared. This pattern is somewhat similar to that of the limb girdle type.

Pseudohypertrophy is rare, but on occasion it is seen in the calf musculature and the deltoids.

Contractural and bony deformities are mild and occur late. The intelligence level is normal, and cardiac involvement is rare.

The disease progresses insidiously with prolonged periods of apparent arrest. Occasionally, however, there is unusually rapid progression. Most patients survive and remain ambulatory to a normal age.

DISTAL MUSCULAR DYSTROPHY

First described by Gowers in 1902, this is distinguished from the limb girdle type by initial involvement of the distal limb muscles rather than the proximal ones. Welander's extensive experience, in Sweden, of 250 cases of distal muscular dystrophy is unique, as the disorder is considered to be very rare.[1058] It is inherited as a dominant character and affects both sexes. The age of onset varies from 20 to 77 years, with a mean of 47 years. The small muscles in the hand are affected first; in the lower limb, the condition begins in the anterior tibial and calf muscles. Later the weakness slowly spreads proximally. The course of the disease is comparatively benign. Distal muscular dystrophy should be differentiated from dystrophia myotonica.

OCULAR MYOPATHY OR PROGRESSIVE DYSTROPHIA OPHTHALMOPLEGIA

This is a rare and very slowly progressive myopathy involving primarily and usually limited to the external ocular muscles and levators of the eyelids. The disease may develop at any age from infancy to over 50 years and begins with ptosis or with diplopia. It slowly progresses to complete bilateral ophthalmoplegia in most cases. In some cases, the pattern of facial weakness may resemble facioscapulohumeral dystrophy; however, it may be distinguished by the absence of the pouting appearance that is characteristic of the former.

It is inherited as a simple dominant or simple recessive trait, equally affecting males and females. There is a history of familial incidence in approximately half the cases.

CONGENITAL MUSCULAR DYSTROPHY

This type of muscular dystrophy is present at birth or soon afterward. The course of the disease is one of steady progression. The child with congenital muscular dystrophy presents one example of the "floppy infant" syndrome that must be distinguished from the more benign myopathies and spinal muscular atrophy.

The pattern of muscle involvement is proximal. The deep tendon reflexes are depressed or absent. The pharyngeal muscles are not affected. The muscles of respiration are affected last. Diagnosis is made on the histologic appearance of the muscle, serum enzyme and electromyographic findings, and the clinical course of the disease.

DYSTROPHIA MYOTONICA (MYOTONIC DYSTROPHY)

This is a steadily progressive familial disease in which a myopathy involving the face, jaw, eye, neck, and distal limb muscles is associated with myotonia. The onset is usually in late adolescence or early adult life. The condition is usually transmitted as a mendelian dominant character (Fig. 5–119). In the second generation, the dys-

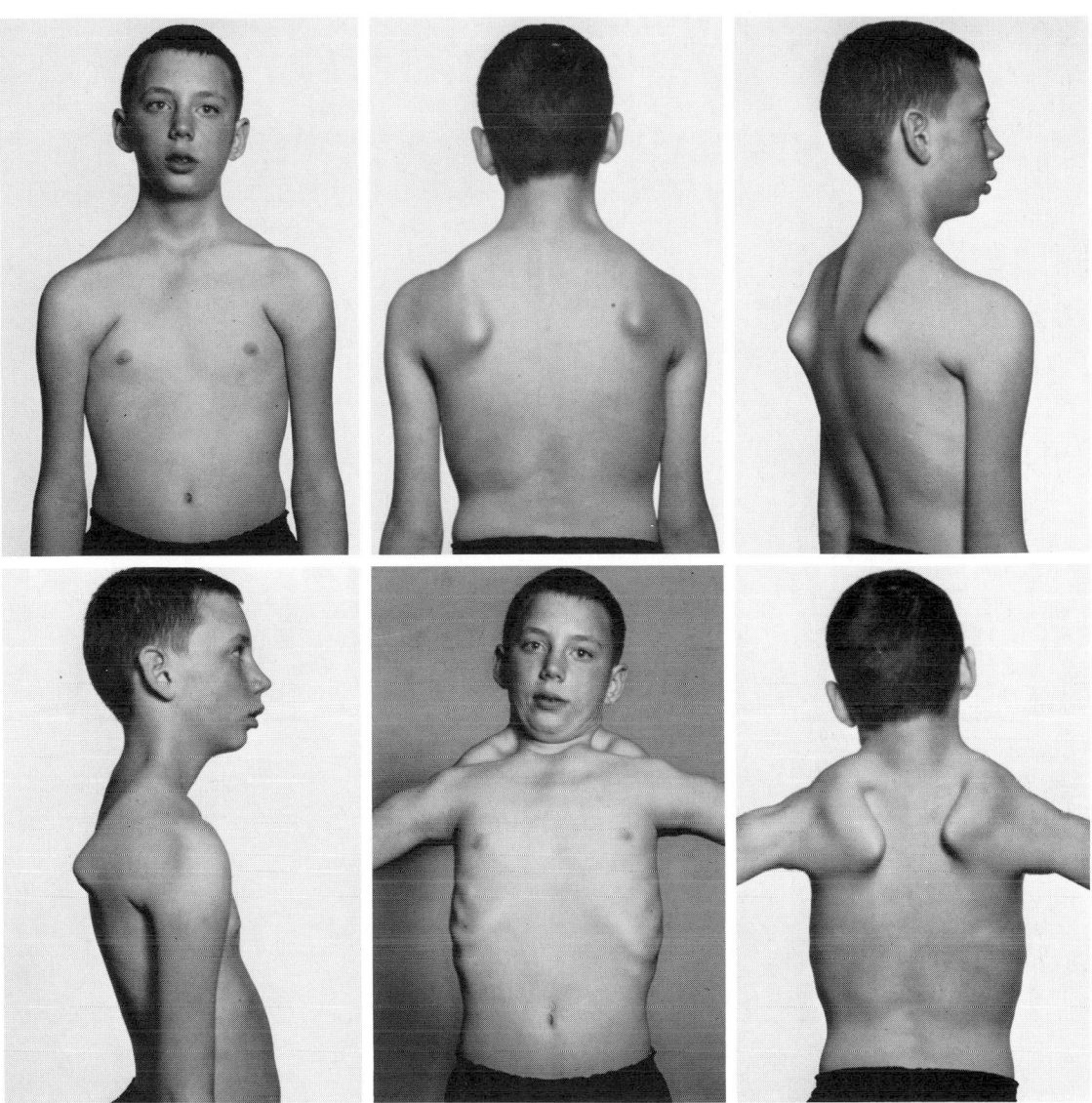

FIGURE 5–118. *An adolescent boy with facioscapulohumeral muscular dystrophy of Landouzy and Déjerine.*
Appearance of the face and weakness of scapulohumeral muscles are characteristic.

trophia myotonica is much more severe and begins at an earlier age, commonly in childhood.

Myotonia, the striking feature of the disease, is characterized by failure of the voluntary muscle to relax immediately and persistence of contraction following voluntary movement or mechanical or electrical stimulation. Myotonia is evidenced clinically by apparent slowness in relaxation of the hand grip and is best demonstrated as a persistent dimpling after a sharp blow on a muscle belly, such as the thenar eminence, tongue, or deltoid (Fig. 5–120).

There is great variation in the clinical picture. The muscles affected by myotonia are those of the hands, the face and tongue, and occasionally the limbs. Upon tight closure of the eyes, there is a long delay in relaxation. The degree of myotonia is lessened with repetition of motion. Tripping,

falling, and difficulty in walking are other manifestations of the disease.

The pattern of muscle weakness in the limbs, in contrast to most myopathies, is distal in distribution rather than proximal. The long flexors and extensors of the fingers, small muscles of the hand, tibialis anterior and peroneal muscles are involved early. Soon the disease affects the calf muscles, and later spreads proximally to involve the quadriceps and hamstrings. The deep tendon reflexes are diminished or absent. Contractural deformities are mild and occur late (Fig. 5–121).

The face is expressionless (Fig. 5–122). Ptosis is invariable. The patient has difficulty in closing the eyes, in pursing the lips, and in whistling. The voice is monotonous and nasal owing to involvement of the laryngeal muscles. Dysarthria is common.

The characteristic facial appearance,

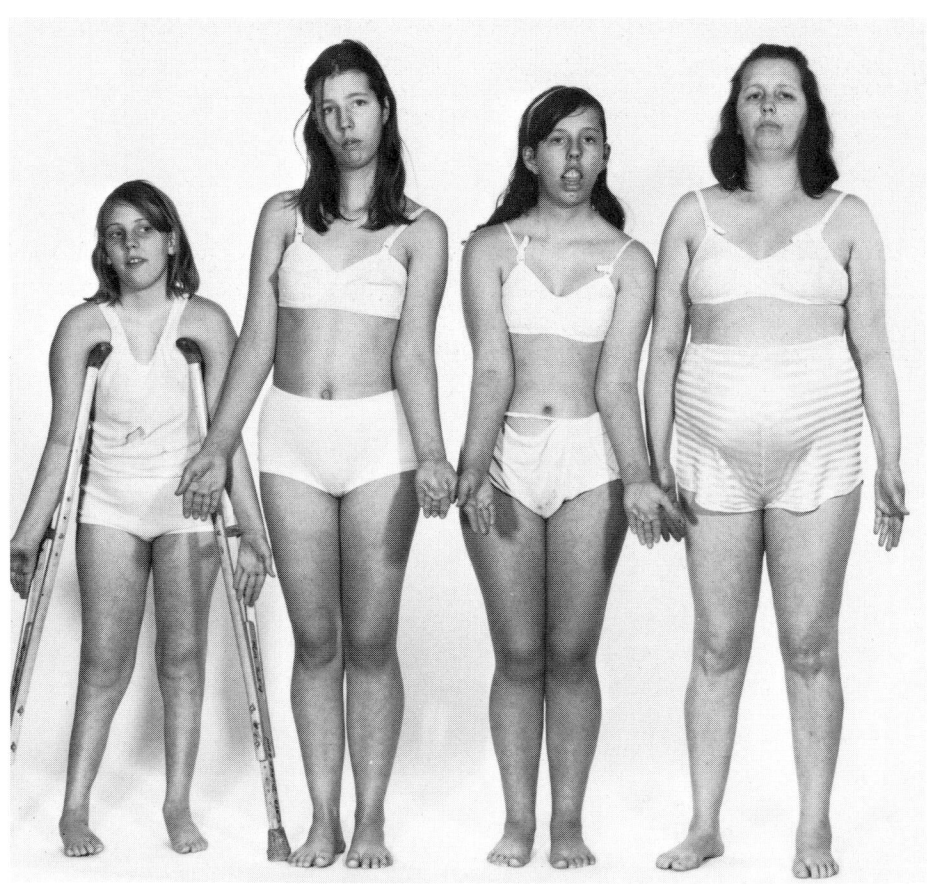

FIGURE 5–119. *Dystrophia myotonica in a mother and her three daughters.*

The condition is transmitted as a mendelian dominant character.

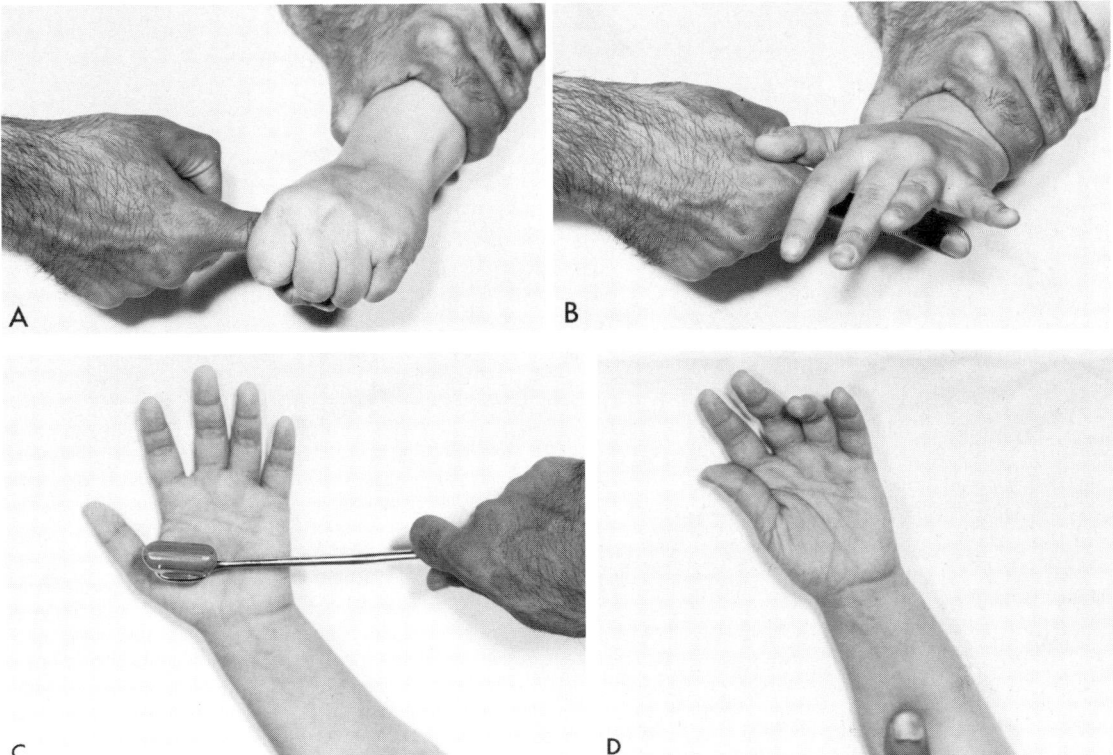

FIGURE 5-120. *Clinical signs of myotonia in an adolescent girl with myotonic dystrophy.*

A and **B.** Relaxation of the hand grip is slow. **C** and **D.** After a sharp blow on the belly of the thenar muscles in the thenar eminence a dimple is formed and the thumb is adducted.

called "myopathic facies," is haggard, being produced by atrophy of the masseters, narrowing of the lower half of the face and mandible, bilateral ptosis, and general weakness of the facial musculature. The sternocleidomastoids are frequently wasted, resulting in increased cervical lordosis ("swan neck").

Most patients with dystrophia myotonica develop cataracts, frontal baldness (in the male), and gonadal atrophy. Mental retardation is not uncommon.

The course of the disease is one of steady progression; within 20 years of the onset of symptoms, most patients are severely disabled and unable to walk. The majority die before the normal age.

MYOTONIA CONGENITA AND PARAMYOTONIA CONGENITA

There is some controversy about whether dystrophia myotonica and myotonia con-genita are separate diseases or clinical variants of the same disease.[1041] Intermediate cases do occur, however, but they are generally regarded as different clinical syndromes. Myotonia congenita (Thomsen's disease) and paramyotonia congenita (Eulenberg's disease) are not associated with dystrophy and are discussed later.[1042]

The differential diagnosis of the principal types of muscular dystrophy is presented in Table 5-15.

Biochemical Considerations

CHANGES IN BODY FLUID

Creatine and Creatinine. Historically, the first biochemical defect observed in muscular dystrophy was a decrease in urinary creatinine excretion reported by Rosenthal in 1870.[1034] Levine and Kristeller, in 1909, noted an increase in urinary excretion of

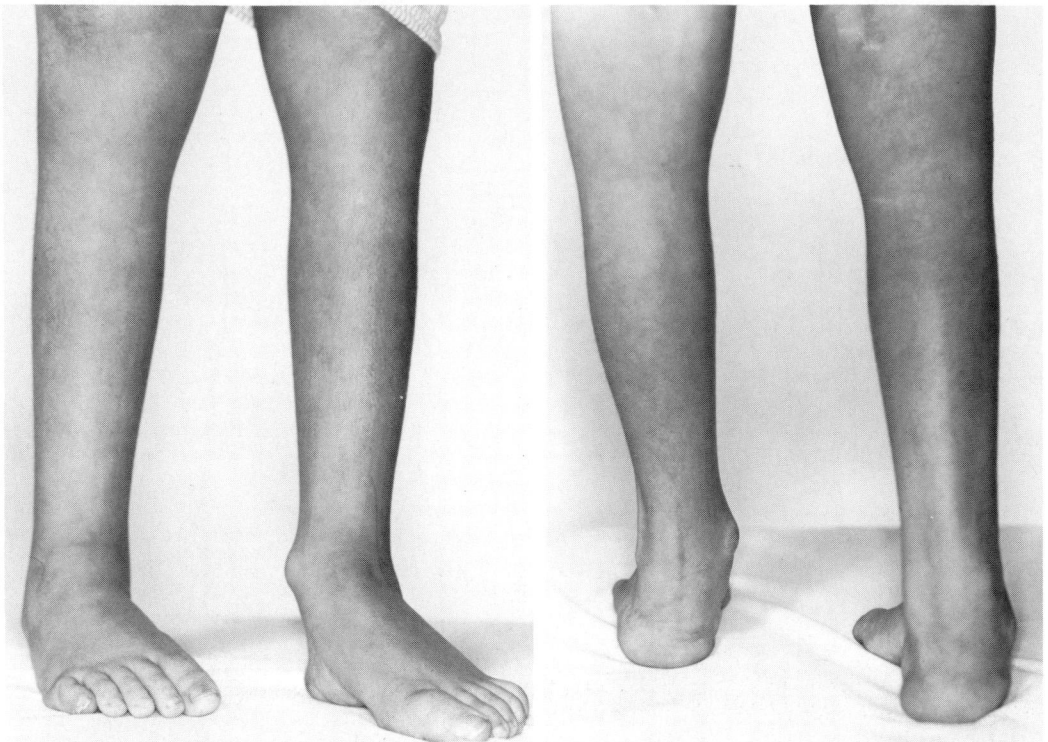

FIGURE 5–121.   Calcaneovarus deformity of the right foot in a 12-year-old girl with myotonic dystrophy.

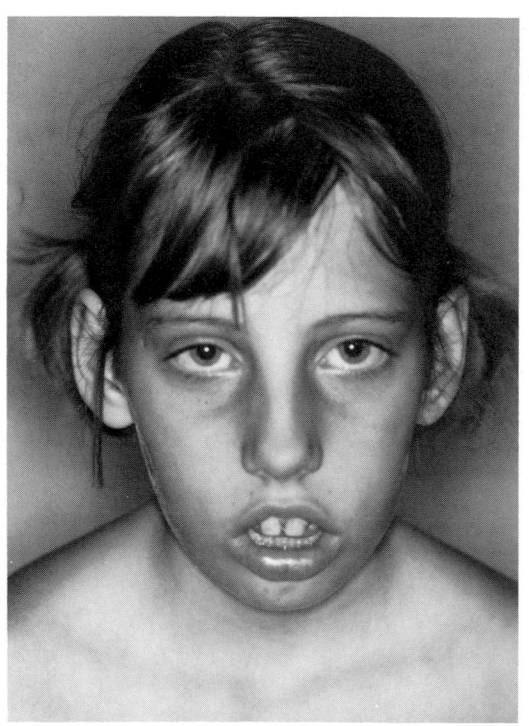

FIGURE 5–122.   Expressionless face in dystrophia myotonica.

The patient has difficulty in pursing the lips, closing the eyes, and whistling.

Table 5–15. *Differential Diagnosis of the Principal Types of Muscular Dystrophy*

Clinical Features	Duchenne Type Muscular Dystrophy	Limb Girdle Muscular Dystrophy	Facioscapulo-humeral Muscular Dystrophy	Distal Muscular Dystrophy	Progressive Dystrophia Ophthalmoplegia	Congenital or Infantile Muscular Dystrophy
Incidence	Commonest	Less common, but not infrequent	Not common	Rare	Rare	Rare
Age at onset	Usually prior to 3 yr., some between 3 and 6 yr.	Variable (usually by second decade, occasionally later)	Variable (usually in second decade)	20–77 yr. (mean 47 yr.)	At any age (infancy to over 50 yr.)	At or soon after birth
Sex preponderence	Male	Either sex	Male and female equally affected	Either sex	Either sex	Not yet determined
Inheritance	Sex-linked recessive, autosomal less than 10 per cent	Autosomal recessive, on rare occasions autosomal dominant	Autosomal dominant usually, autosomal recessive very rarely	Autosomal dominant	Simple dominant or simple recessive	Unknown
Pattern of muscle involvement	Proximal (pelvic and shoulder girdle muscles affected early, spreads to periphery of limbs late in course)	Proximal (shoulder and pelvic girdle, spreads to periphery late)	Face and shoulder girdle; later spreads to pelvic girdle	Distal (hand first, anterior tibial, and calf in leg)	Usually limited to external ocular muscles	Generalized
Muscles spared until late	Gastrocnemius, toe flexors posterior tibial, hamstrings, hand muscles, upper trapezius, biceps, triceps, face, jaw pharyngeal, laryngeal, and ocular	In upper extremity brachioradialis and hand, calf muscles	Back extensors, iliopsoas, hip abductors, quadriceps	Proximal until late	See above	– – – –
Pseudohypertrophy	80 per cent of cases (calf muscles)	Less than 33 per cent of cases	Rare	Not seen	Not seen	Not seen
Myotonia	Absent	Absent	Absent	Absent	Absent	Absent
Contractural deformities	Common	Develop late in course, less severe than Duchenne	Mild, occur late	Mild, late	– – –	Severe
Scoliosis and kyphoscoliosis	Common in late stage	Mild, in late stage	Mild, occur late	– – –	– – –	?
Heart involvement	Hypertrophy and tachycardia common; in late stages widespread degeneration, fibrosis, and fatty infiltration	Very rare	Very rare	Very rare	Not seen	Not observed
Endocrine changes	Not seen	Not seen	Not seen	Not seen	Not seen	?
Intellectual level	Commonly decreased	Normal	Normal	Normal	Normal	?
Course	Steady rapid progression	Slow progression, considerable variation in pace of disease	Progresses insidiously	Comparatively benign	Slow progression	Steady progression

creatine in addition to a diminished creatinine output.[1024]

Creatine, an amino acid, is synthesized from glycine, arginine, and methionine, largely in tissues other than muscle; the liver, kidney, and pancreas are probably the most important sites. Skeletal muscle contains the largest amount of creatine (more than any other organ or tissue). Most of the creatine formed is delivered to the muscle. In the muscle cell, creatine is phosphorylated by the action of creatine kinase, with the help of adenosine triphosphate, to form creatine phosphate, which represents an important reserve of energy for muscular contraction.

Creatinine, an anhydride of creatine, is a degradation product of it. Creatinine content of muscle is low (about 5 mg. per 100 gm.) since it is readily diffused from the muscle fiber into serum and is then completely disposed of by the kidneys. The normal serum values for creatinine range from 0.8 to 1.4 per cent and are increased only in kidney failure. The daily excretion of creatinine in the urine is considerable and constant (1 to 2 gm. per day).

The normal serum values for creatine are 0.2 to 0.6 mg. per 100 ml. in the adult male and 0.4 to 0.9 mg. per 100 ml. in the adult female. The renal threshold for creatine is about 0.5 mg. per 100 ml.; hence, the urine of normal adults contains little or no creatine (the average 24 hour urine excretion of creatine is 60 to 150 mg. in the adult male, and 120 to 300 mg. in the adult female).

In muscular dystrophy there is a disturbance in creatine and creatinine excretion; namely, (1) a decrease in creatinine content in the urine, (2) an increase in urinary creatine, and (3) often a mild hypercreatinemia. In the past, it was speculated that muscular dystrophy was caused by a disturbance of creatine metabolism; however, these claims have now been abandoned and it is generally accepted that decreased urinary output of creatinine and hypercreatinuria is a nonspecific manifestation of muscle atrophy. If the amount of muscular bulk is diminished because of atrophy, creatine will be removed less rapidly from the blood, the blood level will be higher, and excretion by the kidneys will be increased.

Van Pilsum and Wolin reported the following mean figures for creatine excretion (in milligrams per kilogram of body weight per day) in various conditions:[1048]

Normal adults	0
Pseudohypertrophic muscular dystrophy	18
Adult muscular dystrophy	18
Poliomyelitis	14
Amyotonia congenita	9
Paraplegia	5
Quadriplegia	5
Polymyositis	9
Disuse atrophy	4
Charcot-Marie-Tooth peroneal atrophy	4
Amyotrophic lateral sclerosis	4
Dermatomyositis	14
Myotonia dystrophica	3
Myasthenia gravis	0
Progressive muscular dystrophy	8

These figures demonstrate that an increase in creatine excretion is found in almost all types of muscle disease.

Creatine tolerance is decreased in muscular dystrophy.[1005] This finding is nonspecific and indicates a reduction in functional muscle mass. If a test dose (1 to 3 gm.) is given orally to a normal subject, most of the creatine will be taken up by skeletal muscle and little or no creatinuria will result. In muscular dystrophy or in muscle diseases in which the muscle mass is decreased, the creatine tolerance is disturbed because the remaining musculature is not capable of absorbing all the creatine and some spills out into the urine.

Serum Enzymes

CREATINE KINASE. A very pronounced increase in creatine kinase activity in the serum of patients with muscular dystrophy was reported by Ebashi, Toyokura, Momoi, and Sugita in 1959.[1010] It is known that creatine kinase reversibly transfers a phosphate group from creatine phosphate to adenosine diphosphate, forming creatine and adenosine triphosphate. The average serum level of creatine kinase in normal persons is about 2 units, i.e., μ moles of creatine formed per hour per milliliter of serum. In children with the early Duchenne type of muscular dystrophy, values up to several hundred units have been found. In fact, the increase may occur long before any overt clinical signs of the disease are apparent. To a varying degree, elevation of the serum creatine kinase level is found in the great majority of mothers who transmit the Duchenne type of dystrophy; this demonstrates that clinically normal carriers of the abnormal gene may show biochemical abnormalities characteristic of the disease to a minor degree. Normal values of creatine kinase do not rule out the possibility that the mother is a carrier, for only two thirds of probable or known carriers have an abnormally high level of creatine kinase.[1031] Creatine kinase is a more specific indicator than aldolase, as it does not appear to increase in liver disease.

Another practical advantage of measuring creatine kinase is that erythrocytes contain very little of this enzyme and serum assays are not disturbed by hemolysis of the sample. Its disadvantages are the requirement that the blood specimens reach the laboratory for freezing more quickly and also the possibility of greater pitfalls due to certain technical difficulties. However, these are outweighed by its advantages of specificity and sensitivity.

ALDOLASE. High levels of serum aldolase in muscular dystrophy were reported by Sibley and Lehninger in 1949[1035] The enzyme aldolase is found in most tissues and catalyzes one of the steps in the breakdown of glucose—the splitting of fructose 1:6-diphosphate. The normal serum values are less than 10 (expressed in the most commonly used Bruns units). In the Duchenne type of muscular dystrophy, values of over 100 are frequently found. In adult types of muscular dystrophy and in myotonic dystrophy, the elevation in serum aldolase is much less and is often absent.

The increase of serum aldolase and creatine kinase is most marked in the early stages of the disease. Their serum values decline as the disease progresses and in fact, in the end stages of the disease, they may be just above the normal range.[1004, 1043] One can often correlate the level of the enzymes with the duration of the disease.

A rise in serum aldolase is often seen in polymyositis and dermatomyositis, but in neural atrophies, elevated levels have been only very rarely encountered. The real value of the test is in the diagnosis of primary myopathy.

Other enzymes may appear in increased amounts in the blood in muscular dystrophy. Of these, lactate dehydrogenase and the two aminotransferases–aspartate aminotransferase and alanine aminotransferase—GOT and GPT—have been studied most extensively.[1032] The source of increased amounts of the aforementioned serum enzymes is largely or wholly the muscle tissue itself; they leak out of the fibers as the latter are disturbed and damaged by the disease.

There are other reported changes in body fluids in muscular dystrophy. Increased amino-aciduria is often present and seems to result from protein breakdown associated with muscle wasting. Another significant change is an increase in serum α_2 globulin, for further discussion of which the reader is referred to Oppenheimer and Milhorat.[1030]

CHANGES IN MUSCLE

There is, as yet, little information on biochemical changes in diseased muscle itself. Research in this area is proceeding at an increasing pace.[1032] A decrease, relative to noncollagen nitrogen, in the amount of the main contractile protein, myosin, in dystrophic muscle was found by Vignos and Lefkowitz.[1051] A fall in the myoglobin content of dystrophic muscle was reported by Hughes in 1961.[1020] There is evidence that there are qualitative alterations in myoglobin in muscular dystrophy.[1059] An elevated sodium and decreased potassium content has been found in dystrophic muscles.[1019]

Studies of the activity of various enzymes in dystrophic muscles have been carried out. Dreyfus et al. found a decrease in the rate of glycolysis in specimens of the transversus abdominis muscle from patients with muscular dystrophy on comparing them with corresponding normal muscles obtained during appendectomy, using noncollagen protein as a reference base. The extent of the decrease paralleled the severity of the disease.[1007, 1008] Other workers, using histochemical techniques, have shown increased activity of dephosphorylating enzymes in dystrophic muscle.[1014] Elevated levels of cathepsins (intracellular proteolytic enzymes) in muscle biopsies from boys with the Duchenne type of dystrophy are reported by Pennington.[1032]

Diagnosis

The established case of muscular dystrophy with its characteristic pattern of muscular weakness rarely presents a diagnostic problem. It is in the early stages of the disease, when the complaints are clumsiness of gait and difficulty in climbing stairs, that diagnosis is more difficult. Often the patient has consulted a number of physicians and has been treated for unrelated conditions such as retarded development before the correct diagnosis is made. A careful analysis of the physical, genetic, biochemical, electromyographic, and histologic findings is essential to make the diagnosis of muscular dystrophy.

When a child is presented with muscle weakness, it should first be determined whether this is caused by a primary myopathic or by a neuropathic disease. The distinguishing clinical and laboratory features of disorders of the anterior horn cells, peripheral nerves, and muscles is presented in Table 5-1.

A manual muscle test is performed to localize the specific pattern of muscle involvement. Distal weakness is the first indication of neurogenic disease, in contrast to proximal involvement, which is characteristic of the various types of muscular dystrophy; however, one must be cautious about too rigid categorization of diseases solely on the basis of distal or proximal involvement. Distal myopathy and dystrophia myotonica should be distinguished from peroneal muscular atrophy. The loss of vibratory sense at the ankles in Charcot-Marie-Tooth disease, and the associated cataracts, frontal baldness, and sternocleidomastoid weakness in dystrophia myotonica are valuable distinguishing findings.

Other diagnostic signs of neuropathic disease are the presence of fasciculation (rarely, if ever, seen in muscular dystrophy), and changes in deep tendon reflexes (which are usually preserved until late in the course of muscular dystrophy).

The differential diagnosis between muscular dystrophy and polymyositis is sometimes a difficult one. The diagnostic criteria that are of value in differentiating the two diseases are listed in Table 5-16.

Histologic examination of muscle obtained by open biopsy is important in establishing the diagnosis of muscular dystrophy. A muscle biopsy clamp will maintain the length of the muscle as it is being fixed (Fig. 5-123.)

Treatment

There is no specific treatment for muscular dystrophy. Glycine, adenosinetriphosphatase, alpha-tocopherol-phosphate, corticosteroids, digitalis, thyroid, and many other medicinal agents have been tried without benefit.

Though progressive muscular dystrophy almost always results in complete loss of ambulation, there is reason to believe that its loss is premature in many cases. It is imperative that independent ambulation be maintained as long as possible. Progressive muscle weakness eventually leads to the inevitable wheelchair and bed confinement; there is no specific remedy for it. However, there are a variety of contributory factors that can be controlled to delay this loss of independence as much as possible.

In view of these facts, patients with muscular dystrophy are assessed as to their total motor performance on the basis of the degree of functional capacity they still possess. Vignos has given a functional classification graded on a scale of 1 through 10, with the higher classifications representing progressively severer involvement:

1. Obvious defect in posture and walking stance, but walks and climbs stairs without assistance.
2. Walks, but climbs steps only with aid of railing.
3. Walks, but climbs eight standard steps with aid of railing in over 25 seconds.
4. Walks, but cannot climb steps.
5. Walks unassisted, but cannot climb steps or get out of chair.
6. Walks only with assistance of braces.
7. In wheelchair. Sits erect, can roll chair and perform bed or chair activities of daily living.
8. In wheelchair. Sits erect, unable to perform bed and chair activities without assistance.

Table 5–16. *Differential Diagnosis of Progressive Muscular Dystrophy and Polymyositis*

Features	Duchenne Type Progressive Muscular Dystrophy	Polymyositis
Sex preponderance	Males	Females
Inheritance	Sex-linked recessive Autosomal recessive less than 10 per cent	None
Pattern of muscle involvement	Proximal, much more selective	Proximal, sometimes distal
Facial muscle weakness	May be present in some forms	Almost never
Weakness of neck and back extensors	Rare except very late	Common
Dysphagia	Very rare except terminally	Frequent
Muscular atrophy	Severe	Mild (with tenderness)
Pseudohypertrophy	Common	Rare
Deep tendon reflexes	Preserved until late	Preserved longer
Skin changes	Not observed	Present
Electromyography	Short low amplitude potentials	Short low amplitude potentials Fibrillations
Serum enzymes (creatine kinase and aldolase)	Elevated	Elevated
Muscle biopsy	Variable fiber size degeneration	Degeneration and inflammatory cells
Specific treatment	None	Steroids (definite clinical response if given early in high dosage)
Course	Steady progression	More rapid progression
Prognosis	Usually death within 20 years	Spontaneous remission in 80%

9. In wheelchair. Sits erect only with support. Able to do only minimal activities of daily living.

10. In bed, can do no activities of daily living without assistance.[1049]

Of the multiple factors involved in the loss of ambulation, *muscle power* is the most important. The antigravity muscles essential for independent locomotion are the gluteus maximus, quadriceps, and triceps surae. When these muscles become poor in motor strength, some external support such as long leg braces is usually necessary to maintain independent ambulation.

Contractural deformity is another important factor affecting walking. In muscular dystrophy, contractures result from a dynamic imbalance of the agonist-antagonist muscles and from maintenance of limbs in faulty postures for prolonged periods. The most common contractural deformity is an equinus deformity of the foot and ankle, caused by permanent shortening of the triceps surae muscle. As the motor strength of the posterior tibial muscle persists until later in the course of the disease, the foot often tends to assume a varus posture. The equinovarus deformity of the feet interferes with locomotion, as it is difficult to balance oneself on one's toes.

Flexion contracture of the knee, another serious deformity, causes instability and impedes mechanical efficiency of the quadriceps muscle, thus weakening it further. It is usually minimal during the walking phase; however, when the patient is confined to a wheelchair, it becomes progressively severe.

Hip flexion contracture results in anterior shifting of the center of gravity of body weight, making standing balance precarious, particularly in the presence of poor gluteus maximus muscles.

The development of contractures can be prevented or minimized through passive stretching exercises and the use of light-

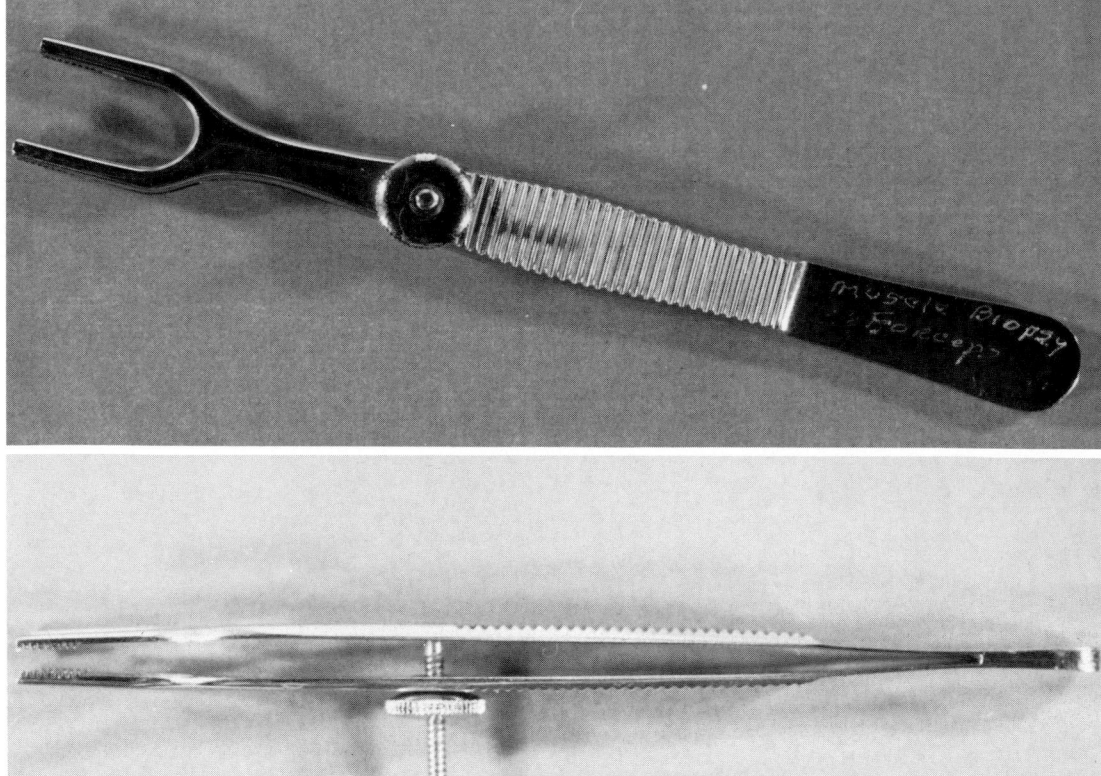

FIGURE 5–123. *Muscle biopsy clamp used to maintain the length of the muscle as it is being fixed.*

weight night bivalved casts or orthotic splints.

Inactivity is detrimental, as it will cause disuse atrophy of the muscles. Patients with muscular dystrophy should be encouraged to walk and use their limbs as much as possible. When the dystrophic child suffers a fracture or has a febrile illness, he should not remain in bed any longer than is absolutely necessary. A fractured tibia should be treated in a walking cast. Prolonged bed rest will result in marked loss of motor strength, eventually leading to permanent wheelchair or bed confinement.

A sizeable weight gain greatly increases the difficulties in ambulation. Because of inactivity and decreased energy needs, the caloric intake should be limited and carefully controlled. This is a difficult problem, however, owing to a combination of psychic overeating and pampering.

Many *emotional factors* influence the re-

gression of locomotion. Most children with muscular dystrophy are withdrawn and exhibit extreme passivity and dependency. A fear of falling produces increased anxiety. A restrained optimism and positive encouragement will boost the morale of these children and motivate walking. Parents and teachers not infrequently are responsible for a too hurried transition from ambulatory to wheelchair status. This premature confinement is a definite deterrent to the child's psychological and intellectual development.

ORTHOTIC SUPPORT

Orthotic devices should be used judiciously, as their cumbersome weight interferes with trick movements to maintain balance. They should be used toward the end of independent ambulation, i.e., when the child reaches the stage at which he walks less and less and uses furniture and walls for support in getting from place to place. Above-knee orthoses should be used before the child is confined to the wheelchair and prior to development of flexion contractures of the hips and knees. One should not expect a child who has been nonambulatory for more than a month to begin walking after contractural deformities are corrected and he is braced. Miller states that orthoses, when used at the appropriate stage in the disease, improve the functional capacity of the dystrophic child and extend the period of ambulation.[1028] When the patient is not able to walk even with the help of braces, he can stand with assistance, thus preventing the development of flexion contractural deformities of the knees and hips, as well as improving his general stamina. Below-knee orthoses do not contribute to functional improvement; their only value lies in preventing contractural deformities of the foot and ankle by supporting them in a functional position.

A *wheel chair* is required for mobility in the later stages of the disease when the patient becomes incapable of independent ambulation. It should be of the folding type, with brakes, extensible leg rests, and seat belt (to obviate falls). Hyperextension of the neck may be prevented with an extended back and head rest. With progressive weakness of the shoulder and arm muscles, a lapboard or overhead devices can be added to the wheelchair to assist in bringing the hands to the mouth, as hand function usually persists until very late in the course of the disease.

Adequate support should be provided to the trunk, as paralytic scoliosis usually develops late in the disease, with the spine collapsing under the strain of body weight. A well-molded plastic body jacket is ordinarily adequate to support and balance the trunk. On occasion, with high thoracic curves, a special head piece is required or a Milwaukee brace is used to check progression of the scoliosis.

SURGICAL MEASURES

Soft-tissue surgery for release of contractural deformities followed by immediate support in orthoses and ambulation has proved to be of some value. Percutaneous heel cord lengthening with a sharp Ryerson tenotome is indicated in equinus deformity; however, lengthening of the heel cord should only be performed when the patient is to be placed in above-knee orthoses. He will not be able to walk without the orthoses following heel cord lengthening, for they are important in stabilizing the knees. It is best to fit them to the child on the day of operation and start ambulation immediately. If orthoses are not available, long leg casts with walking heels are applied and the patient is placed upright on a tilt table. Casts are removed as soon as the braces are ready, and the child starts ambulation.

Spencer recommends anterior transfer of the posterior tibial muscle while performing heel cord lengthening, as posterior tibial muscle function persists until late in the course of the disease. This procedure removes a deforming force and gives power of dorsiflexion.[1036]

Hip and knee flexion contractures are usually slight during the walking phase, but become severe when the child is confined to a wheelchair—a stage in the course of the disease when there is no reason to perform surgical release.

MYOTONIA CONGENITA (Thomsen's disease)

Myotonia congenita is a congenital affliction characterized by myotonia of the entire voluntary musculature—a state of delayed relaxation of the muscle following voluntary contraction or mechanical or electrical stimulation. The condition is extremely rare. It was first described by Julius Thomsen, who himself suffered from the disease and could trace it through five generations of his family. About one fourth of the reported cases are inherited by autosomal dominant transmission.[1063] A recessive pattern of inheritance has been reported.[1078] Males and females are equally affected.

Etiology and Pathology

The cause of Thomsen's disease is unknown. The basic defect resides in the sarcoplasm of the muscle itself. The myotonic response may be the result of blockage of potassium transfer across the cell membrane, or it may be produced by defective formation or utilization of energy rich phosphates.

The only significant pathologic finding is hypertrophy of the muscle fibers. There is no evidence of degenerative or dystrophic changes. The central nervous system is found to be normal at autopsy.[1068, 1073] Mytonia occurs independently of the nerve supply to the muscle or its motor end plate.

Clinical Features

Myotonia, the cardinal feature of Thomsen's disease, may be noted in infancy or early childhood. Often a history of delay in motor development is given by the parents. The presenting complaints are difficulty and stiffness in initiating any active movement following rest, difficulty in walking or running after prolonged sitting, frequent falling, and clumsiness. Myotonia is usually more marked in the lower limbs. It is also worse with the initial motion; after repetitive movements, the myotonia decreases and successive movements are executed with greater ease. Repetitive movement of one group of muscles, however, does not prevent myotonia from taking place in a separate group of adjacent muscles. Thus, limbering of the legs by walking does not prevent myotonia when attempting to ascend a flight of stairs.

The characteristic physical finding is myotonia, which can be observed when the surface of any muscle is sharply percussed with a reflex hammer or pencil. The stimulated area of the muscle will contract and will remain contracted for several seconds

Table 5–17.   *Differential Diagnosis of Myotonia in Children*

	Myotonia Congenita (Thomsen's Disease)	Paramyotonia Congenita (Paramyotonia of Eulenberg)	Myotonic Dystrophy
Age at onset	Childhood or infancy	Infancy or early childhood	Childhood to adulthood
Inheritance	Autosomal dominant ($\frac{1}{4}$ of cases) Recessive gene often (Becker)	Autosomal dominant	Autosomal dominant
Sex incidence	Males and females equally affected	Males and females equally affected	Males and females equally affected
Precipitating factors	Voluntary movement after prolonged sitting or inactivity	Exposure to cold	Voluntary movement
Clinical findings Muscle group involved	Generalized	Proximal muscles of limbs, eyelids, and tongue	Muscles in face, tongue, and distal limbs, particularly upper
	Difficulty in walking or running after prolonged sitting	Intermittent attacks of weakness may last from few minutes to 24 hr.	
	Clumsiness	Myotonia precedes weakness	
Response to activity	Improves myotonia	Aggravates myotonia	Aggravates myotonia and fatigues affected muscles.
Muscle hypertrophy	Present ("Herculean appearance")	Absent	Muscle atrophic

before relaxing (see Fig. 5–120 C and D). Another way to demonstrate myotonia is to ask a patient to open a tightly clenched fist rapidly (see Fig. 5–120 A and B). Muscle weakness and endocrine abnormalities are not found in myotonia congenita. Neurologic examination is normal. As the child grows older, diffuse hypertrophy of the muscles develops, giving the patient a so-called "Herculean appearance."

Laboratory Findings

The electromyogram will disclose a rapid volley of action potentials. The sound of rhythmic myotonic discharges emanating from the electromyographic loudspeaker exhibits a crescendo and decrescendo quality that has been likened to that of a diving airplane. These electromyographic findings are similar in all myotonic disorders.[1072]

The levels of serum enzymes, creatine phosphokinase and aldolase, are normal. In myotonia congenita, however, creatine clearance is increased, reflecting the increased metabolism and greater production of creatinine by hypertrophic muscles. Creatine is not excreted in urine.

Differential Diagnosis and Treatment

Myotonia congenita should be distinguished from myotonic dystrophy and paramyotonia congenita of Eulenberg (Table 5–17).

Quinine sulfate (300 mg. orally two or three times a day) or procaine amide will

Table 5–17. *Differential Diagnosis of Myotonia in Children* (Continued)

	Myotonia Congenita (Thomsen's Disease)	Paramyotonia Congenita (Paramyotonia of Eulenberg)	Myotonic Dystrophy
Endocrine, cardiac, other abnormalities	None	None	Testicular atrophy, EKG changes Frontal baldness, mental retardation
Laboratory findings Serum potassium level	Normal	High normal or elevated	Normal
Creatine phosphokinase, aldolase levels	Normal	Normal	Elevated
Creatine clearance	Increased	Normal	Decreased
EMG	Rapid volley of action potentials on insertion of electrode in myotonic muscle	Rapid volley of action potentials on insertion of electrode in myotonic muscle	Rapid volley of action potentials of varying amplitude on insertion of electrode in myotonic muscle
Histologic	Hypertrophy of muscle fibers No dystrophic changes	Similar to myotonic dystrophy	Dystrophic changes (see text)
Treatment	Quinine hydrochloride and procaine amide effective	Not available Calcium gluconate may abort an attack	No specific treatment
Prognosis	Disability minimal Condition remains stationary	Improves with age Nonprogressive	Progressive, moderate disability over a period of many years

ameliorate the myotonia. Prednisone is equally effective in relieving myotonia; however, it should be used with caution because of its side effects.

Disability is minimal, and often patients learn how to live satisfactorily with the disease by "warming up" to limber the muscles before activity. Drug therapy should be reserved for use only in severe cases.

TRAUMATIC MYOSITIS OSSIFICANS
(Myositis Ossificans Conscripta)

Traumatic myositis ossificans is characterized by heterotopic calcification and ossification in muscle tissue; it may or may not be associated with periosteum. Injury is an important factor in its pathogenesis. Most likely the process represents metaplasia of fibroblasts at the site of injury. There seems to be an individual diathesis for the abnormal ossification in soft tissues.

The condition may be subdivided into (1) the traumatic myositis ossificans that follows a severe single injury such as that seen following dislocation and fractures at the elbow (this is the most common form seen in children) and (2) the myositis ossificans that follows repeated minor injuries and occupational strain of certain muscles. This type usually occurs in adolescents and young adults. Common examples are heterotopic bone formation in the soleus muscle in ballerinas (toe dancer's bone), in the brachialis anticus in fencers, or in the thigh adductors in equestrians.

Pathology

Ackerman has reviewed the pathologic findings, emphasizing the presence of four histologic zones: (1) a central, undifferentiated zone, which is highly cellular, with mitotic figures and with extreme variation in the size and shape of the cells (cytologic differentiation of this zone from sarcoma is extremely difficult; (2) an adjacent zone in which there are well-oriented zones of cellular osteoid separated by loose cellular stroma; (3) a more peripheral zone showing new bone formation with osteoblasts and

fibrous tissue undergoing trabecular organization; and (4) an outermost zone of well-delimited and oriented bone encapsulated by fibrous tissue.[1087] The benign nature of the lesion is established by the presence of the zone phenomenon, i.e., the innermost undifferentiated area merging into oriented osteoid formation and finally into well-formed bone in the periphery. As the bone matures, the area involved becomes smaller.

Clinical Features

Physical findings consist of tenderness over the area, palpable swelling, and pain on motion. Often in children a history of acute trauma is obtained with symptoms and signs of the injury that gradually regress over a period of 7 to 14 days, only to recur with increasing severity in the third week. Persistence of local discomfort and marked limitation of joint motion noted at three weeks following posterior dislocation of the elbow is suggestive of the possibility of myositis ossificans. In this early stage, roentgenograms disclose discrete calcification of delicate texture in the mass. After a variable interval, the acuteness of symptoms and signs subsides, the mass tends to regress, and the calcification becomes smaller and of greater density (Fig. 5–124). The process is self-limited, with the period of acute activity lasting from a few weeks to several months.

In the neurogenic form, the process is likely to be much more extensive and often no history of trauma is obtained. In the absence of normal innervation of the part, trauma may occur without its being appreciated.

Myositis ossificans must be distinguished from calcifying hematoma, interstitial calcinosis, and osteogenic sarcoma. Calcification in myositis ossificans is diaphyseal in location, lying parallel to the surface of the bone and often separated from it by a distinct area in which the cortex and periosteum have a normal appearance; whereas osteogenic sarcoma is likely to show some evidence of involvement of the cortex and periosteum, and it is metaphyseal in location. In doubtful cases, serial roentgenograms taken at short intervals should

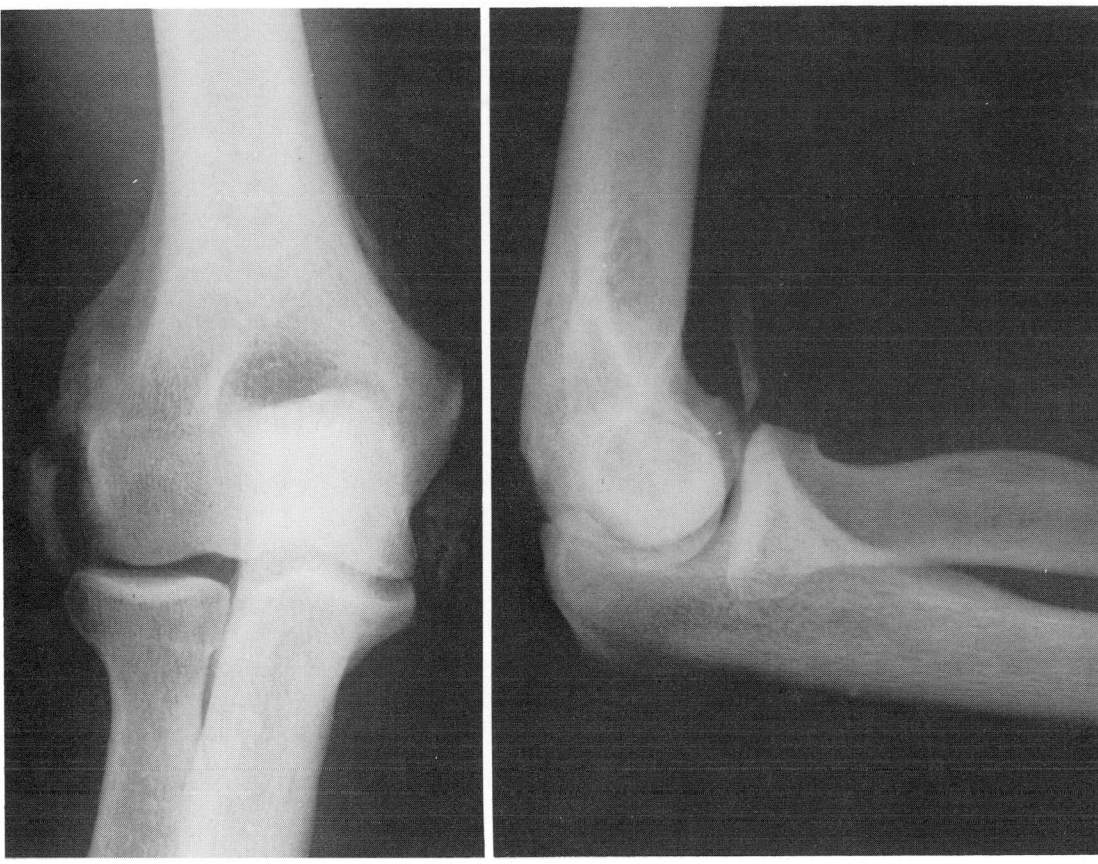

FIGURE 5-124. Traumatic myositis ossificans following posterior dislocation of the elbow joint.

Note the new bone formation in the brachialis muscle and in the capsule.

demonstrate the difference between the two processes. Occasionally, the differentiation is difficult and even the histologic examination may be misinterpreted.

Treatment

Rest of the affected part during the period while the process is active is the basic principle of treatment. All physiotherapeutic measures should be avoided. Immobilization to a greater or lesser degree is desirable, with gradual resumption of motion and activity as the acute phase subsides. Myositis ossificans about the elbow is greatly ag-

gravated by strenuous attempts to develop motion; prophylactically, all physiotherapeutic measures to increase motion of the elbow should be minimal and consist of only gentle active assisted exercises. Once the process has matured, it may be excised if the location or the size of the residual mass interferes with function; otherwise, it is left alone.

Excision is not performed until a year or so after the acute stage at a time when, as judged from the roentgenograms, the bone is fully mature. Roentgenotherapy in the acute stage has been advocated by some surgeons, but is not recommended by the author.

Myositis

Myositis is a general term used to describe several inflammatory conditions of

muscles, such as suppurative myositis, traumatic myositis, parasitic infestation of muscles (trichinosis), and polymyositis. Often what may be interpreted as myositis is due to a spasm or sensitivity in the muscles arising from lesions in other tissues in related structures such as adjacent joints or from the nervous system.

POLYMYOSITIS AND RELATED DISORDERS

Polymyositis is a nonsuppurative inflammation of muscles associated with motor weakness. It was first described by Wagner, in 1863.[1125] When it occurs in conjunction with nonsuppurative inflammation of the skin, the term *dermatomyositis* is used to describe the condition. Unverricht (1887) is credited as being the first to delineate the subgroup of dermatomyositis.[1124]

The etiology of polymyositis and dermatomyositis is unknown. It most probably is an autoimmune disorder. The hypersensitivity may be due to an "altered" muscle protein or to a tumor antigen. Some cases of polymyositis may be the result of an as yet unrecognized infectious, toxic or metabolic cause.

About one sixth of the cases of polymyositis occur in children, and the condition is twice as common in females as in males.

Pearson has subdivided polymyositis into six types: polymositis in adults (Type I), typical dermatomyositis in adults (Type II), typical dermatomyositis (occasionally polymyositis) with malignancy (Type III), childhood dermatomyositis (Type IV), acute myolysis (Type V), and polymyositis in Sjögren's syndrome (Type VI).

It should be noted that dermatomyositis is the more common form observed in children. Acute myolysis is frequently a disease of childhood, although it may occur in adults.

In adults there is a significant association between malignant tumors and polymyositis or dermatomyositis. The overall incidence of the disease found in the combined form is reported to be 20 per cent; simultaneous occurrence of these two pathologic conditions is not found in children. Arundell et al. state that an adult male over 40 years of age with dermatomyositis has a 50 per cent chance of eventually developing a neoplasm.[1106]

Pathology

The involved skeletal muscles may be pale red, grayish red, or yellowish in color, and on palpation their consistency is either soft and friable or rubbery and firm, depending on the duration of the disease. The principal histologic abnormalities are widespread degeneration of muscle fibers with some regenerative activity, perivascular collections of chronic inflammatory cells, and phagocytosis of necrotic muscle fibers. In the later stages of the disease, interstitial fibrosis takes place. Vasculitis with hyperplasia of the intima of the arteries and veins may be present.[1105, 1126]

In order to observe typical histologic changes, it is essential to choose the site carefully for muscle biopsy; the muscle should be neither markedly weakened and atrophic nor of normal strength.

In dermatomyositis, the epidermis is thinned, and there is edema and vasculitis in the dermis.

Clinical Features

Polymyositis is a kaleidoscopic disease with great diversity in its symptoms, variable modes of onset and rate of progression, with exacerbation and remissions. It is difficult to portray a unified clinical picture of the disease.

The symptoms may become manifest following exposure to sunlight, an exanthem, febrile illness, or injury, and following ingestion of drugs such as the sulphonamides or penicillin. Often a precipitating cause cannot be found, and most likely the preceding "inciting factors" are coincidental, occurring during the subclinical stage of the disease. In dermatomyositis, however, photosensitivity is common, with sunlight initiating or aggravating the eruption on the face, upper limbs, and trunk.

Dermatomyositis in children may have a sudden onset and acute course, or an insidious beginning and chronic course.

Muscle weakness of varying severity is present in all cases. In its absence, the diagnosis of polymyositis should not be made. In the subacute and chronic forms of the disease, muscular weakness develops insidiously, similarly to that seen in progressive muscular dystrophy. The muscles of the pelvic and shoulder girdles are first affected. Initial symptoms consist of difficulty in arising from the floor or in climbing up steps without holding the hand rails. Soon the patient is unable to comb his hair and cannot abduct the shoulders to 90 degrees. As the disease progresses and the sternocleidomastoid muscles become affected, he is unable to flex his neck and lift his head against gravity while supine. Involvement of the muscles of the pharynx and deglutition causes dysphagia and dif-

ficulty in eating. In severe cases, weakness may extend to involve all the muscles of the body. The patient becomes confined to a wheelchair or to bed. Progressive involvement of the respiratory muscles may lead to death in some cases.

The affected muscles become tender, brawny, and indurated. Pain is more prominent about the shoulders, upper back, arms, and thighs.

The skin lesions of dermatomyositis are quite characteristic. The rash consists of a dusky or faint erythema over the bridge of

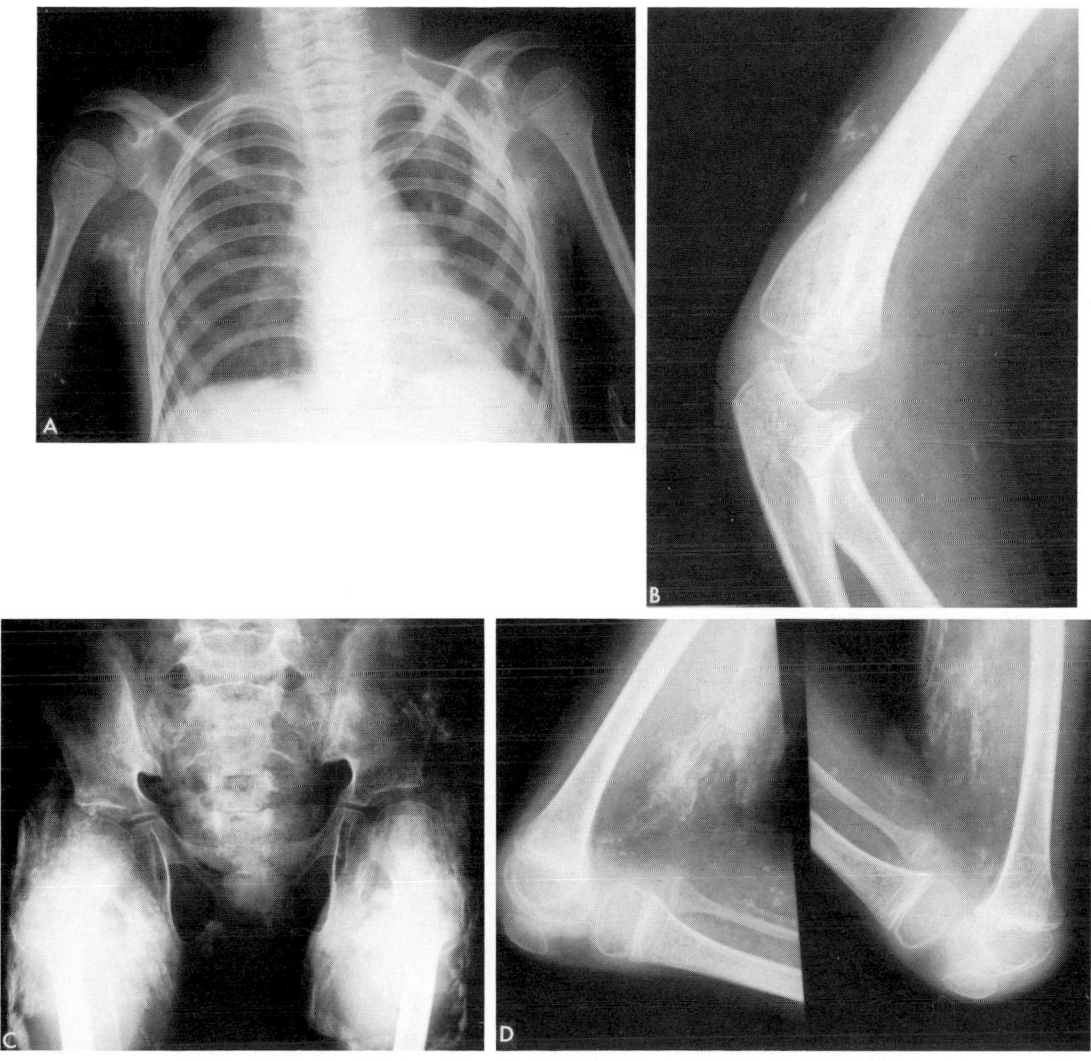

FIGURE 5–125. Dermatomyositis in a child.

A and **B.** Roentgenograms of shoulders and elbow showing calcification of subcutaneous tissues. **C** and **D.** Roentgenograms of hips and knees. Note the progression of calcification involving the muscles of the proximal thigh and pelvic girdle.

the nose and the malar areas in the butterfly distribution. A violaceous discoloration of the upper eyelids can be seen, which is called heliotrope eyelids and is pathognomonic for dermatomyositis. The skin on the extensor surfaces of the elbows, knees, and metacarpophalangeal joints and on the medial malleoli often becomes erythematous, atrophic, and scaly. These may be linear hyperemic streaks on the dorsum of the hands and fingers. In the acute stage of the disease, the skin and subcutaneous tissue frequently develop nonpitting edema. Later, the skin over the involved parts becomes tight and glossy. During the chronic stage, the skin becomes atrophic and adherent to underlying structures. Calcium deposits eventually develop in the subcutaneous tissues, muscles, and fasciae (Fig. 5–125).

Mild transient nonspecific synovitis of the knees, wrists, and metacarpophalangeal and interphalangeal joints occurs in about 40 per cent of cases. Occasionally, articular manifestations are present prior to the appearance of muscle weakness. Raynaud's phenomenon may be present, with the fingers becoming cyanotic or blanched following emotional stress or exposure to cold temperature. Visceral manifestations of polymyositis are rare. Dysphagia results from weakness of the pharyngeal muscles and hypotonicity of the esophagus. Occasionally there may be associated pneumonitis, myocarditis, pericarditis, and nephritis.

Laboratory Findings

In acute polymyositis the serum levels of the various enzymes that normally reside in voluntary muscle are elevated. Of particular value are creatine phosphokinase, aldolase, and glutamic and pyruvic transaminases. The biochemical changes are not pathognomonic for polymyositis, but serial determinations of these enzyme levels are of definite diagnostic and prognostic help. When the acute inflammation of the muscle responds to corticosteroid therapy, the elevated levels of serum enzymes decline toward normal, and within 4 to 6 weeks the muscles gradually recover motor strength. In muscular dystrophy serum creatine phosphokinase and aldolase values are increased,

but they do not decrease following any form of treatment. In neural atrophy, these serum enzymes remain normal. In the late stages of polymyositis, when the muscle fibers have degenerated and are replaced by fibrous tissue, the serum enzyme levels are normal or slightly elevated.

Nonspecific changes reflecting the underlying myopathic process are elevation of α and γ globulins of serum proteins and abnormal levels of creatine and creatinine in the serum and urine. The sedimentation rate is elevated. Rheumatoid factor is sometimes present, but lupus erythematosus (L.E.) cells are usually not found.

The electromyogram will disclose the following abnormalities: (1) sponteneous fibrillation and positive or saw-tooth potentials at complete rest or after mild mechanical irritation; (2) complex polyphasic or short-duration potentials of low amplitude, which occur on voluntary contraction; and (3) salvos of repetitive potentials of high frequency occurring after mechanical stimulation or use of the electrode.[1117–1121] According to Pearson these changes in the electromyogram are quite characteristic but not absolutely specific for polymyositis.[1120]

Diagnosis

In the typical form of dermatomyositis, biopsy is usually not indicated, as the muscle weakness, characteristic rash, elevated serum enzyme levels, and electromyographic findings are diagnostic. In doubtful cases and in polymyositis, muscle biopsy is performed for definitive histologic diagnosis. In the differential diagnosis one should consider muscular dystrophy, various polyneuropathies, systemic lupus erythematosus, juvenile rheumatoid arthritis, and scleroderma.

Treatment

In the acute stage of polymyositis and dermatomyositis when the muscles are painful, tender, and edematous, the patient is put to bed and moist heat is applied over the sore muscles to alleviate the discomfort. Corticosteroids (prednisone [Meticorten]) are usually given, though their effect on the course of the myopathy is debatable.[1127] They ameliorate the acute inflammatory reaction and diminish pain. Serum enzyme levels are determined at regular intervals; their return to normal is a good prognostic sign, indicating good chance of recovery of motor strength. The dosage of corticosteroids is slowly reduced until an effective maintenance dosage is reached. In children, dermatomyositis runs a self-limited course and the value of corticosteroid therapy seems to be primarily for symptomatic relief.[1119]

Active and passive exercises are performed gently to preserve normal range of joint motion. If contractural deformities develop, the affected limbs are supported in functional position in well-padded splints.

In the later stages of the disease, when contracture and calcification of the deep fascia, intermuscular septa, and subcutaneous tissue have taken place, William T. Green recommends excision of these thickened calcified tissues. The author has found the procedure to be very satisfactory; it will increase the circulation and function of the muscles and improve nutrition of the skin.

SUPPURATIVE MYOSITIS

This is rare and is usually seen in patients with severe septicemia and diffuse involvement of the muscles with bacterial emboli, or it may arise by direct extension from an adjacent infectious process. Wounds infected with *Clostridium welchii* lead to more severe types of muscle infection with resultant necrosis of muscle and gas gangrene.

Clinical findings of suppurative myositis consist of acute pain that is aggravated by motion, local tenderness, swelling, induration, followed by fluctuation. Erythema is not common in the early stages. Often there is associated high fever and leukocytosis.

Most infections that are suspected of being myositis are in reality osteomyelitis, particularly in the infant; the pus perforates the cortex at the metaphysis and breaks through the periosteum to lie in the soft tissues. Acute osteomyelitis must always be the first consideration in the differential diagnosis when myositis is suspected.

Treatment of suppurative myositis should follow the same principles of treatment as any similar soft-tissue infection. The part should be immobilized with splints. Local heat in the form of poultices or packs should be applied, and appropriate antibiotics should be administered. As the process localizes, if it does not regress and fluctuation is present, simple incision and drainage are indicated.

Tetanus must be considered as a possible complication in all traumatic wounds, particularly in those that are grossly contaminated and in which debridement and cleaning are delayed. Appropriate measures against tetanus must be adopted as indicated.

TRAUMATIC MYOSITIS, "MUSCLE CRAMPS"

Fibrillary tears of muscles and contusions of muscle are often sustained by healthy active youngsters, but usually they are of little significance. A "charley horse" represents a hemorrhage into the muscle belly arising from a tear of fibers or from contusion. The clinical findings are swelling, sensitivity to palpation, and pain on use of the muscle. Fluctuation is present if the hematoma is large. Treatment is by rest and immobilization. Elevation of the part and application of ice packs for the first few hours after the injury will reduce the inflammation. As the symptoms subside, function should be resumed gradually. If the hematoma is large, it may require aspiration. Usually little treatment is necessary except for protection until the symptoms subside.

A muscle working at a mechanical disadvantage because of faulty body mechanics, whether in the back, foot, or elsewhere, is subject to abnormal fatigue. If the handicap to function is sufficient, the muscle atrophies rather than hypertrophies, with the result that the strain may be progressive.

Persistent abnormal muscle function in a growing child tends to produce permanent structural abnormality. Such alterations are promoted not only by mechanical factors but also by factors of general health that contribute to muscular fatigue.

Muscle cramps and "growing pains" seem to be a manifestation of chronic muscle strain and fatigue. The most common site of muscle cramps is in the calves and in the intrinsic muscles of the feet. These are usually associated with pronated feet and foot strain with "tight heel cords" in which there is myostatic contracture of the triceps surae muscle. Tight posterior structures, including contracted hamstrings, are often present. Muscle cramps are probably initiated by overexertion of muscle with tissue anoxia; it has been asserted that they are associated with "the accumulation of nitrogenous wastes." The exact relation of vasospasm to the phenomenon has not been clarified.

Treatment is aimed at correcting the mechanical abnormality and adapting the structures to better functional position. In instances, for example, in which foot strain is the factor, the child should be given support for his feet and the contracted triceps surae muscles should be stretched.

Metabolic Diseases of Muscle

PERIODIC PARALYSIS

Transient and recurring weakness or paralysis of skeletal muscles may occur in familial or sporadic forms. The plasma level of potassium may be either low (hypokalemia), elevated (hyperkalemia), or normal (normokalemia).

Familial or Hypokalemic Periodic Paralysis

This rare disorder is usually inherited as an autosomal dominant trait, with complete penetrance in the male and variable penetrance in the female. Sporadic cases, autosomal recessive, or sex-linked recessive forms may occur on occasion.

The exact etiology of the disease is unknown. During an attack the plasma potassium falls as a result of shift of potassium from the extracellular to the intracellular compartments.[1148] There is no loss of potassium from the body.[1129, 1134] During paralysis the potassium moves into the muscle cells and during spontaneous recovery it is rereleased into the plasma. The basis of pathogenesis appears to be an enzyme defect that causes an excessive accumulation of indiffusable intermediates of carbohydrate metabolism, with the resultant passage of potassium and water into the cell.[1140] This theory is supported by the finding of hyperdilatation of the endoplasmic reticulum on microscopy. During paralysis neuromuscular transmission is blocked and there is failure of spread of electrical action potential along muscle fibers. This was originally ascribed to hyperpolarization or to an increase in potential of the muscle fiber membrane; however, direct measurements of the resting membrane potential in patients with familial periodic paralysis during attacks of paralysis revealed this to be normal.[1131, 1137, 1145] Why the membrane potential does not rise with sharp reduction in the extracellular potassium concentration has not been explained.

The onset of periodic attacks of paralysis is usually in early adolescence; they tend to decrease in number and severity with advancing years, and may completely disappear after 40 years of age.

The paralytic episodes are usually induced by prolonged inactivity following vigorous exercise or after a meal largely consisting of carbohydrates. Anxiety, emotional stress, and exposure to extreme cold may be other predisposing factors. The patient awakes in the night to find himself paralyzed. The proximal muscles of the lower limbs are affected first, followed by those of the upper limbs. Next, paralysis of the muscles of the neck, trunk, and face occurs. The respiratory and ocular muscles are rarely involved. The spincters are not affected. The mentation is normal. Attacks are usually self-limited, lasting several hours. Severe paralysis in a child, however, may last two or three days, and very occasionally, a patient may die because of total paralysis.

Urinary output is decreased and thirst increased during paralysis; abnormal sweating and diuresis follow during recovery. These symptoms most probably result from the concomitant shift of water and potassium in and out of the cells. The muscles of the paralyzed limbs appear enlarged during an attack and fail to respond to direct mechanical or electrical stimulation. The deep tendon reflexes are absent. The heart may be enlarged, and bradycardia and cardiac arrhythmia occasionally occur. In later life, permanent muscle weakness and atrophy may develop in the severe case.

The electrocardiogram during a paralytic episode will show findings characteristic of hypokalemia—prominent U waves, flattening of the T waves, prolongation of the PR, QRS, and QT intervals with depression of the RST segment. The plasma potassium level falls during an attack, usually to about 2 to 2.5 mEq. per liter.

TREATMENT

Potassium will abort or control a hypokalemic paralytic attack. It is usually administered orally in water in doses of 0.2 gm. per kilogram of body weight, up to a maximum dose of 10 gm. If, within one to two hours, there has been no improvement, half of the preceding dose may be repeated. When attacks are frequent, preventive measures should be taken in the form of a prophylactic dose of potassium at night, restriction of sodium intake, and avoidance of excessive exercise and heavy intake of carbohydrates. Spironolactone in doses of 100 to 200 mg. each day orally may be effective in controlling the attacks. If cardiac arrhythmia develops, the attacks are controlled by infusion of 50 mg. of potassium. Digitalis should not be given.

Hyperkalemic Periodic Paralysis

Gamstorp gave the name *adynamia episodica hereditaria* to a rare disease characterized by periodic attacks of paralysis of the limbs and trunk in which the serum potassium concentration is increased during an attack.[1135] Tyler et al. previously had investigated a family in which the serum potassium did not fall during attacks and in which paralysis failed to respond to potassium.[1146]

The condition is inherited as an autosomal dominant trait. Its exact etiology is unknown. Paralysis is due to an abnormally low resting muscle membrane potential.[1131] Potassium leaks from the muscle during attacks, with resultant lowering of the concentration of potassium in the muscle, and an increase in that of the sodium chloride.[1141] The serum potassium level is increased to as much as 7.0 mEq. per liter during an attack, with concomitant increase of urinary output of potassium. In normal individuals, muscle weakness does not develop until the serum potassium is elevated to 8.0 mEq. per liter, indicating an undue susceptibility in the affected patients.

The attacks usually start in infancy and early childhood. They are induced by rest after heavy exercise. The muscles involved first are the gluteals, lower erector spinae, the quadriceps, and triceps surae. Gradually, the paralysis spreads to the musculature of the upper limb. The neck muscles may be affected in severe attacks. The muscles supplied by the cranial nerves are occasionally involved; transient blurring of vision and diplopia have been noted. Bulbar and respiratory paralysis rarely occur.

The paralytic attacks occur during the day, and are frequent and short, lasting from 20 to 60 minutes. Exercise accelerates recovery; rest following exercise induces paralysis. During the attacks, especially in mild cases, myotonia may be elicited by direct percussion of a muscle. When the attack is severe, the muscles fail to respond to direct stimulation and the deep tendon reflexes are diminished or absent. The presence of myotonia in some families links the condition with paramyotonia congenita.

During an attack, the serum potassium level is elevated and electromyography shows action potential change indicating loss of both individual fibers and whole motor units. Hyperirritability of the myotonic type may be present in some fibers.

The mild or moderate attacks usually do not require any treatment, for they are very short. If they are too frequent, their incidence can be reduced or they can be prevented by administering diuretics that promote excretion of potassium and sodium. Dichlorphenamide in 50 to 100 mg. daily dosage is usually very effective in preventing attacks. The severe and prolonged episodes are treated by intravenous administration of calcium gluconate (1 to 2 gm.). The attacks usually abate and disappear with increasing age.

Normokalemic Periodic Paralysis

In this very rare type of periodic paralysis, the attacks are severe and may last for days or even weeks, occurring mainly at night. The serum concentration of potassium is normal, even during the most severe attack. Potassium is retained rather than lost. Attacks are neither provoked nor made worse by administration of potassium; they may be improved by large doses of sodium chloride and prevented by daily administration of a combination of 250 mg. of acetazolamide and 0.1 mg. of 9α-fluorohydrocortisone.

McARDLE'S SYNDROME (Myophosphorylase Deficiency)

This rare disorder of muscle glycogen metabolism is characterized by muscular pain, stiffness, and weakness following exercise. The symptoms are relieved by rest. It was described first by McArdle, in 1951.[1150] The condition is transmitted by an autosomal recessive gene and is caused by absence in muscles of myophosphorylase—an enzyme that splits off the terminal glucose molecule from the arborizations of glycogen.

Any muscle in the body may be affected. The muscles that are exercised most develop the most severe symptoms; for example, in walking, the calf and thigh muscles are involved; and upon chewing, the masseter muscles. The affected muscles are abnormally stiff and remain in a contracted state for varying periods (the more strenuous the exercise, the longer the duration of affection). Muscular ischemia induces the symptoms more rapidly.

A characteristic laboratory finding is failure of the level of blood lactate and pyruvate to rise following exercise. Muscle glycogen is increased. Diagnosis is confirmed by biochemical study, which shows absence of myophosphorylase activity. On occasion, the condition may be associated with myo-

globinuria, in which case the prognosis must be more guarded. The disease, when not associated with myopathy, does not appear to be progressive.

Treatment consists of limitation of physical activity. Oral administration of glucose, or preferably fructose, prior to strenuous activity will increase the tolerance to exercise.

IDIOPATHIC PAROXYSMAL MYOGLOBINURIA

This rare condition was first described by Meyer-Betz, in 1911.[1163] It is characterized by recurrent transient acute attacks of severe pain and cramping in the muscles associated with weakness or paralysis, and followed within a few hours by myoglobinuria. The muscles of the lower limbs are more frequently affected. With rest, the attack subsides within a few days. In severe cases, oliguria and anuria may be present owing to renal damage from myoglobin.

In myoglobinuria, the urine is reddish brown and does not contain erythrocytes; the urine becomes burgundy in color on exposure to light. The presence of myoglobin in the urine is confirmed by spectrophotometric examination.

Paroxysmal myoglobinuria is differentiated into two types. In the first, the attacks occur primarily in childhood, often following an acute infectious disease, and are frequently accompanied by fever, leukocytosis, and renal insufficiency. Familial incidence is low. In the other type, symptoms usually begin between the second and third decade. The attacks are induced by exercise. There is a high familial incidence, and recurrent severe attacks may result in permanent muscle atrophy.

Treatment is symptomatic, consisting of rest and alkalization of urine. Kidney function should be carefully observed, as uremia and death may occur in the childhood form.

STIFF-MAN SYNDROME*

This extremely rare entity of unknown etiology occurs primarily in the adult. It is

*See References 1168–1170.

characterized by stiffness and rigidity of skeletal muscles induced by a sudden stimulus or a voluntary movement. A neurologic and metabolic abnormality has not been found. Quinine and procaine are not effective in relieving the muscle spasm.

MYASTHENIA GRAVIS

Myasthenia gravis is a disease affecting transmission of impulses at the myoneural junction. It is characterized by excessive fatigability and apparent paralysis of voluntary muscles following repetitive activity or prolonged tension, with a marked tendency to recovery of motor power after a period of inactivity or diminution of muscular tension.[1192] The first case was described by Willis in 1672.[1197] The characteristics of the disease were fully described by Erb (1879) and Goldflam (1893); hence the eponym Erb-Goldflam disease.[1173, 1174] Jolly applied the term myasthenia gravis.[1178] A historical review of myasthenia gravis from 1672 to 1900 is given by Viets.[1191] Walker noted the similarity of a myasthenic patient to a curarized normal individual, and knowning the antagonism of physostigmine for curare, demonstrated the remarkable therapeutic effect of neostigmine (a synthetic analogue of physostigmine) on a myasthenic patient.[1194, 1195] Viets and Schwab devised a definitive neostigmine test.[1193]

The incidence of myasthenia gravis is variously reported as from 1 in 50,000 to 1 in 10,000 of the population. The disease may become manifest at any age. About 10 per cent of the patients have symptoms in infancy and childhood.[1181, 1182] There is a preponderance of the disease in the female, the female to male ratio being 4.5:1 in the first decade but reversing in later life.

The exact cause is unknown. Myasthenia gravis is considered to be an autoimmune disorder in which an antibody is produced against an end plate protein antigen, which is alleged to interfere with normal neuromuscular transmission. The thymus gland is thought to be the site of this antibody production. The muscles appear normal to the naked eye; however, lymphocytic infiltrations of muscles (termed lymphorrhages) are found in some muscles on histologic examination. Recently, "dystrophic" and "dysplastic" type changes have been observed in the motor end plates.[1187]

Abnormalities of the thymus gland, such as benign tumors, hyperplasia, and persistence of the gland, are frequently found in patients with myasthenia gravis, but the relation of these changes to the disease is uncertain.

Clinical Features

Myasthenia gravis in children has been subdivided into three groups by Millichap and Dodge. Depending upon the age at onset and features of the disease, they are: (1) neonatal transient, (2) neonatal persistent (congenital), and (3) juvenile myasthenia gravis.[1181]

NEONATAL TRANSIENT MYASTHENIA GRAVIS

In this type, all infants are born to mothers with myasthenia gravis. Symptoms begin soon after birth. They consist of generalized muscular weakness with little spontaneous movement, weak Moro response, weak suck, facial weakness, ptosis, respiratory weakness, and dysphagia. These symptoms are transient, lasting less than four weeks. It seems the antibody passed through the placenta to the fetus is slowly excreted or destroyed by the neonate. Death may occur if the infant is untreated. Therapy with prostigmine will result in recovery.

NEONATAL PERSISTENT (CONGENITAL) MYASTHENIA GRAVIS

In this form the mothers do not suffer from myasthenia gravis. The clinical features consist of ptosis, weak cry, and generalized weakness. In later life, external ophthalmoplegia develops. Involvement of the bulbar musculature and respiratory difficulty are uncommon, and in general, the symptoms are of mild degree. The disease runs a protracted course and is somewhat resistant to drug therapy, but prostigmine will relieve symptoms in most cases.

JUVENILE MYASTHENIA GRAVIS

Symptoms usually begin after 10 years of age. A family history of myasthenia gravis is usually not obtained. Ptosis is the commonest presenting sign, and is usually bilaterally symmetrical; however, it may be unilateral or bilaterally asymmetrical. Weakness in the upper and lower limbs occurs commonly. The child is unable to walk for long distances without rest. He has difficulty in climbing stairs and falls frequently because his knees collapse. There may be bilateral gluteus maximus and gluteus medius limp. The Trendelenburg test may be positive.

Weakness of the facial muscles gives a sad expression to the face, often out of line with the true emotional state. Weakness in mastication results from easy fatigability of the jaw muscles. Weakness of the tongue muscles causes dysarthria. The patient will pronounce several sentences clearly, and then complain that his tongue feels thick, talking as though he had a mouthful of food. Difficulty of deglutition arises from weakness of the voluntary muscles of the upper pharynx. Respiratory difficulty is not uncommon. Involvement of the bulbar muscles and respiratory failure may occur in myasthenia gravia and cause sudden death.

Fatigability of the voluntary muscles is always less in the morning, but as the day progresses, the weakness becomes more marked. Neurologic examination will disclose normal sensation and deep tendon reflexes. Pathologic reflexes are absent.

The course of the disease is extremely variable. There may be periods of remission that last for several months or even years.

Diagnosis

The cardinal feature of myasthenia gravis is a history of muscular weakness that is precipitated by activity. A positive edrophonium chloride (Tensilon) test will confirm the diagnosis. Edrophonium chloride is an analogue of prostigmine (neostigmine). Of the two agents, Tensilon is preferred because of its shorter duration of action and rapid excretion. The intravenous test dose is 1 mg. (in children up to 75 lb.) and 2 mg. (in children above 75 lb.); when administered intramuscularly, the test dose is 2 mg. (in children up to 75 lb.) and 5 mg. for children above this weight. In normal individuals edrophonium chloride has no effect on muscle strength, but has marked cholinergic side effects, such as excessive perspiration and salivation, lacrimation, and fasciculations. In the myasthenic patient, however, within the first minute after injection there is marked improvement in motor strength of weak muscles and cholinergic side reactions are minimal. Five minutes following administration of the drug the beneficial effects disappear.

Faradic stimulation will produce brisk, strong muscle contractions initially, but on repeated stimulation the contractions diminish and eventually disappear (the so-called "myasthenic reaction of Jolly").[1178]

This easy fatigability of voluntary muscles can also be demonstrated in the electromyogram in which the action potentials from the repeatedly stimulated muscles show a gradual diminution in amplitude as the stimulation is continued.

In the differential diagnosis, various conditions should be considered such as brain tumor, poliomyelitis, encephalitis, tuberculous meningitis, chronic barbiturate or bromide intoxication, muscular dystrophy, polyneuropathy, tumors of the larynx or esophagus, and psychoneurosis, particularly globus hystericus and the so-called "nervous fatigue syndrome." Myasthenia gravis is distinguished from these disorders by the positive Tensilon test and progressive weakness of voluntary muscles following activity or faradic stimulation.

Treatment

Prostigmine bromide (neostigmine), pyridostigmine bromide (Mestinon), and ambenonium chloride (Mytelase) are of great value as therapeutic agents, affording partial or complete relief from symptoms. The dosage of these drugs is variable, depending upon the age of the patient, the severity of the disease, and the response to medication.

Thymectomy or irradiation of the thymus should be reserved for those patients in whom drug therapy is ineffective and for those in whom an abnormally large thymus gland suggests the presence of thymoma.

When the muscles of respiration are involved, the assistance of a mechanized respirator may be required. Tracheostomy is indicated when there is marked pooling of secretions due to weakness of the pharyngeal muscles.

Prognosis

The outlook for children and adolescents with myasthenia gravis is generally favorable, although myasthenia crises may occur in about one of six patients, necessitating the use of a mechanical respirator. Occasionally the outcome may be fatal.[1181] Complete remission may be expected in about one fourth of the patients, possibly occurring more often in response to thymectomy than to medical therapy alone. At present, the value of thymic irradiation is difficult to assess.

Affections of Bursae

Bursae are thin-walled sacs lined by synovial membrane that are usually located about joints and serve to decrease function. Some of them communicate with the articular cavity. The synovial membrane of bursae is subject to the same pathologic processes that affect the synovial membrane of joints. Adventitious bursae develop secondarily from friction, as occurs in a bunion over the first metatarsal head.

BURSITIS

Bursitis may be traumatic, suppurative, tuberculous, gouty, or rheumatoid. Various tumorous processes, such as villonodular synovitis, osteochondromatosis, or synovioma may involve the bursae. Nonspecific bursitis secondary to calcified tendonitis does not occur in children.

Traumatic Bursitis

Injury usually affects bursae that are superficial in location, such as those over the olecranon or over the patella. The onset of symptoms is sudden following a direct injury such as a fall on the knee. There is distention of the bursa with hemorrhage, local pain, tenderness, and restriction of motion in the adjacent joint. If the bursa is deep in relation to tendons, pain on motion is the principal symptom, with protective muscle spasm restricting the motion. If the bursa is subcutaneous, tenderness to pressure is the salient finding.

Traumatic bursitis may be associated with ligamentous injury of neighboring joints. Roentgenograms should be taken to rule out fracture of adjacent bones. Treatment consists of aspiration of the fluid, compression bandage, and rest to the part in a splint or sling. If the condition is very acute, hot packs may be applied intermittently to enhance absorption. Local injection of hydrocortisone is usually not indicated. In "adventitious" bursitis, the underlying cause must be determined, and if possible corrected, for instance, by improving the fit of the shoe or orthosis that is causing undue irritation, using protective pads, or excision of the subjacent bony protuberance.

Chronic bursitis may follow an acute process but frequently develops insidiously. It occurs in children very occasionally; in the adult, however, chronic bursitis is a common disease, occurring in several specific and familiar locations, such as subdeltoid bursitis, olecranon bursitis, prepatellar bursitis, (housemaid's knee), ischial bursitis (weaver's or tailor's bottom), iliopectineal bursitis and pes anserinus bursitis. It is beyond the scope of this textbook to discuss calcareous tendonitis.

Infectious or Suppurative Bursitis

These are common in the superficial bursae, such as the prepatellar and olecranon bursae. They commonly occur in children. Pyogenic organisms are implanted within the bursal sac as a result of direct inoculation from a penetrating wound or by hematogenous metastatic spread. Local pain and tenderness on direct pressure and marked swelling of the affected bursa are the outstanding findings. There may be systemic signs of infection. The condition should be distinguished from pyogenic arthritis of a subjacent joint.

The exudate from the swollen bursa is aspirated and the pathogenic organism and sensitivity to antibiotics determined by cultural studies. (During aspiration of the bursa care should be taken not to contaminate the subjacent joint). Systemic antibiotics are administered. Antibiotics may be injected locally. The affected part of the limb is splinted and hot packs are applied. Often incision and drainage are necessary. If the process becomes chronic, excision of the bursa may be indicated.

References

CEREBRAL PALSY

1. Albaugh, C. H.: Congenital anomalies following maternal rubella in early weeks of pregnancy with special emphasis on congenital cataract. J.A.M.A., *129*:719, 1945.
2. Andersen, B.: Cerebral palsy. J. Oslo City Hosp., *4*:65, 1954.
3. Anthonsen, W.: Treatment of hip flexion contracture in cerebral palsy patients. Acta Orthop. Scand., *37*:387, 1966.
4. Aschenheim, E.: Shädigung einer menshlichen Frucht durch Röntgenstrahlen. Arch. Kinderheilk., *68*:131, 1920.
5. Asher, P., and Schonell, F. E.: A survey of 400 cases of cerebral palsy in childhood. Arch. Dis. Child., *25*:360, 1950.
6. Baker, L. D.: Triceps surae syndrome in cerebral palsy. Surgery, *68*:216, 1954.
7. Baker, L. D.: Surgery in cerebral palsy. Arch. Phys. Med., *36*:88, 1955.
8. Baker, L. D.: A rational approach to the surgical needs of the cerebral palsy patient. J. Bone Joint Surg., *38–A*:313, 1956.
9. Baker, L. D., and Dodelin, R. A.: Extra-articular arthrodesis of the subtalar joint (Grice procedure); results in seventeen patients with cerebral palsy. J.A.M.A., *168*:1005, 1958.
10. Baker, L. D., and Hill, L. M.: Foot alignment in the cerebral palsy patient. J. Bone Joint Surg., *46–A*:1, 1964.
11. Baker, L. D., Dodelin, R. A., and Bassett, F. H., III.: Pathological changes in the hip in cerebral palsy, incidence, pathogenesis, and treatment—preliminary report. J. Bone Joint Surg., *44–A*:1331, 1962.
12. Balf, C. L., and Ingram. T. T. S.: Problems in the classification of cerebral palsy. Brit. Med. J., *2*:163, 1955.
13. Balmer, G. A., and MacEwen, G. D.: The incidence and treatment of scoliosis in cerebral palsy. J. Bone Joint Surg., *52–B*:134, 1970.
14. Banks, H. H., and Green, W. T.: The correction of equinus deformity in cerebral palsy. J. Bone Joint Surg., *40–A*:1359, 1958.
15. Banks, H. H., and Green, W. T.: Adductor myotomy and obturator neurectomy for the correction of adduction contracture of the hip in cerebral palsy. J. Bone Joint Surg., *42–A*:111, 1960.
16. Barnett, H. E.: Orthopedic surgery in cerebral palsy. J.A.M.A., *150*:1396, 1952.
17. Barr, J. S.: Muscle transplantation for combined flexion–internal rotation deformity of the thigh in spastic paralysis. Arch. Surg., *46*:605, 1943.
18. Bassett, F. H., III, and Baker, D.: Equinus deformity in cerebral palsy. *In* Adams, J. P. (ed.): Current Practice in Orthopaedic Surgery, Vol. 3. St. Louis, C. V. Mosby Co., 1966, p. 59.
19. Beals, R. K.: Spastic paraplegia and diplegia. An evaluation of non-surgical and surgical factors influencing the prognosis for ambulation. J. Bone Joint Surg., *48–A*:827, 1966.
20. Berenberg, W., and Ong, B. H.: Cerebral spastic paraplegia and prematurity. Pediatrics, *33*:496, 1964.
21. Bertrand, P.: Correction du genu flexum chez les spastiques. Rev. Chir. Orthop., *45*:416, 1959.
22. Bleck, E. E.: The management of hip deformities in cerebral palsy. *In* Adams, J. P. (ed.): Current Practice in Orthopaedic Surgery, Vol. 3. St. Louis, C. V. Mosby Co., 1966.
23. Bleck, E. E., and Holstein, A.: Iliopsoas tenotomy for spastic paralytic deformities of the hip. Paper delivered at the Annual Meeting of the American Academy of Orthopaedic Surgeons, Chicago, 1963.
24. Blumel, J., Eggers, G. W. N., and Evans, E. B.: Genetic, metabolic, and clinical study on one hundred cerebral palsied patients. J.A.M.A., *174*:860, 1960.
25. Bobath, K., and Bobath, B.: Control of motor function in the treatment of cerebral palsy. Physiotherapy, *43*:295, 1957.
26. Bobath, K., and Bobath, B.: The facilitation of normal postural reactions and movements in the treatment of cerebral palsy. Physiotherapy, *1*:3, 1964.
27. Bobath, K., and Bobath, B.: The treatment of spastic paralysis by the use of reflex inhibition. Brit. J. Phys. Med., *13*:1, 1965.
28. Bobath, B., and Finnie, N.: Re-education of Movement Patterns in Everyday life in the treatment of cerebral palsy. Occup. Ther., *21*:23, 1958.
29. Bradford, E. H.: The surgical treatment of spastic paralysis in children. Trans. Amer. Orthop. Ass., *3*:7, 1890. (Boston Med. Surg. J., *73*:485, 1890.)
30. Braun, R. M., Mooney, V., and Nickel, V. L.: Flexor-origin release for pronation-flexion deformity of the forearm and hand in the stroke patient. J. Bone Joint Surg., *52–B*:907, 1970.
31. Broms, J. D.: Sub-talar extra-articular arthrodesis—follow-up study. Clin. Orthop., *42*:139, 1965.
32. Brooks, M., and Wardle, E. N.: Iliopsoas-muscle action and the shape of the femur. J. Bone Joint Surg., *44–B*:398, 1962.
33. Brown, A.: A simple method of fusion of the subtalar joint in children. J. Bone Joint Surg., *50–B*:2, 369, 1968.
34. Buchwald, E.: Physical Rehabilitation for Daily Living. New York, McGraw-Hill, 1952.
35. Burman, M. S.: Spastic intrinsic-muscle imbalance of the foot. J. Bone Joint Surg., *20*:145, 1938.
36. Byers, R. K.: Evolution of hemiplegias in infancy. Amer. J. Dis. Child., *61*:915, 1941.
37. Carroll, R. E.: The treatment of cerebral palsy in the upper extremity. Bull. N.Y. Orthop. Hosp., *3*:1958.
38. Carroll, R. E., and Craig, F. S.: The surgical treatment of cerebral palsy—the upper extremity. Surg. Clin. N. Amer., *31*:385, 1951.
39. Carruthers, D. G.: Congenital deaf mutism as sequela of rubella-like infection during pregnancy. Med. J. Aust., *1*:315, 1945.
40. Chambers, E. F. S.: An operation for correction of flexible flat feet of adolescents. West. J. Surg., *54*:77, 1946.
41. Chandler, F. A.: Re-establishment of normal leverage

of patella in knee flexion deformity in spastic paralysis. Surg. Gynec. Obstet., *57*:523, 1933.

42. Chandler, F. A.: Patellar advancement operation: Revised technic. J. Int. Coll. Surg., *3*:433, 1940.

43. Cooper, I. S.: Relief of juvenile involuntary movement disorders by chemopallidectomy. J.A.M.A., *164*:1297, 1957.

44. Cooper, I. S.: Neurosurgical alleviation of intention tremor of multiple sclerosis and cerebellar disease. New Eng. J. Med., *263*:441, 1960.

45. Cooper, I. S.: Clinical and physiologic implications of thalamic surgery for dystonia and torticollis. Bull. N.Y. Acad. Med., *41*:870, 1965.

46. Cooper, W.: Surgery of the upper extremity in spastic paralysis. Quart. Rev. Pediat., *7*:139, 1952.

47. Courville, C. B.: Cerebral Palsy. Los Angeles, San Lucas Press, 1954.

48. Courville, C. B.: Structural changes in the brain in cerebral palsy. *In* Illingworth, R. (ed.): Recent Advances in Cerebral Palsy. London, J. & A. Churchill, 1958.

49. Crothers, B., and Paine, R. S.: The Natural History of Cerebral Palsy. Cambridge, Mass., Harvard University Press, 1959.

50. Denhoff, E., and Robinault, I. P.: Cerebral Palsy and Related Disorders. A Developmental Approach to Dysfunction. New York, McGraw-Hill, 1960.

51. Denny-Brown, E.: The Basal Ganglia and Their Relation to Disorders of Movement. London, Oxford University Press, 1962.

52. Doman, R. J., Spitz, E. B., Zucman, E., Delacato, C. H., and Doman, G.: Children with Severe Brain Injuries. Neurological Organization in Terms of Mobility. J.A.M.A., *174*:257, 1960.

53. Dowd, C. N.: Tendon transfer for correction of spastic hand deformity. Med. Rec., *78*:175, 1910.

54. Duncan, W. R.: Release of rectus femoris in spastic paralysis. Presented at the Meeting of the American Academy of Orthopaedic Surgeons, Los Angeles, 1955.

55. Durham, H. A.: A procedure for the correction of internal rotation of the thigh in spastic paralysis. J. Bone Joint Surg., *20*:339, 1938.

56. Eggers, G. W. N.: Surgical division of the patellar retinacula to improve extension of the knee joint in cerebral spastic paralysis. J. Bone Joint Surg., *32–A*: 80, 1950.

57. Eggers, G. W. N.: Transplantation of hamstring tendons to femoral condyles in order to improve hip extension and to decrease knee flexion in cerebral spastic paralysis. J. Bone Joint Surg., *34–A*:827, 1952.

58. Eggers, G. W. N.: Selective surgery for the cerebral palsy patient. A.A.O.S. Instructional Course Lectures. Vol. 12. Ann Arbor, J. W. Edwards, 1955, p. 221.

59. Eggers, G. W. N., and Evans, E. B.: Surgery in cerebral palsy. An instructional course lecture. J. Bone Joint Surg., *45–A*:1275, 1963.

60. Evans, E. B.: The status of surgery of the lower extremities in cerebral palsy. Clin. Orthop., *47*:127, 1966.

61. Fay, T.: The use of pathological and unlocking reflexes in rehabilitation of spastics. Amer. J. Phys. Med., *33*: 347, 1954.

62. Ferreri, J. A.: Intensive Stereognostic Training. Amer. J. Occup. Ther., *16*:141, 1962.

63. Ford, F. R.: Diseases of the Nervous System in Infancy, Childhood, and Adolescence. 4th Ed. Springfield, Ill., Charles C Thomas, 1966.

64. Freud, S.: Infantile Cerebrallahmung. Nothnagel's specielle Pathologie und Therapie 9. Vol. 2. Vienna, 1897.

65. Gillette, H. E.: Kinesiology of Cerebral Palsy. Clin. Orthop., *47*:31, 1966.

66. Goldner, J. L.: Reconstructive surgery of the hand in cerebral palsy and spastic paralysis resulting from injury to the spinal cord. J. Bone Joint Surg., *37–A*: 1141, 1955.

67. Goldner, J. L.: Reconstructive surgery of the upper extremity affected by cerebral palsy or brain or spinal cord trauma. *In* Adams, J. P. (ed.): Current Practice in Orthopaedic Surgery, Vol. 3. St. Louis, C. V. Mosby Co., 1966.

68. Goldner, J. L., and Fertic, D. C.: Upper Extremity Reconstructive Surgery in Cerebral Palsy or Similar Conditions. A.A.O.S. Instructional Course Lectures. Vol. 18. St. Louis, C. V. Mosby Co., 1961, p. 169.

69. Green, W. T.: Tendon transplantation of the flexor carpi ulnaris for pronation-flexion deformity of the wrist. Surg. Gynec. Obstet., *75*:337, 1942.

70. Green, W. T., and McDermott, L. J.: Operative treatment of cerebral palsy of spastic type. J.A.M.A., *118*: 434, 1942.

71. Green, W. T., and Banks, H. D.: Flexor carpi ulnaris transplant and its use in cerebral palsy. J. Bone Joint Surg., *44–A*:1343, 1962.

72. Gregg, N.: Congenital cataract following German measles in the mother. Trans. Ophthal. Soc. Aust., *3*:35, 1942.

73. Gregg, N.: Further observations on congenital defects in infants following maternal rubella. Trans. Ophthal. Soc. Aust., *4*:119, 1946.

74. Hellebrandt, F. A.: Trends in the management of cerebral palsy. Lectures in Medical College of Virginia (unpublished manuscript). 1950–1951.

75. Henderson, J. L.: Cerebral Palsy in Childhood and Adolescence. A Medical, Psychological, and Social Study. Edinburgh, E. & S. Livingstone, Ltd., 1961.

76. Heyman, C. H.: The surgical treatment of spastic paralysis. *In* Dean Lewis: Practice of Surgery. Hagerstown, Prior, 1945, Vol. III.

77. Hohman, L. B.: Intelligence levels in cerebral palsied children. Amer. J. Phys. Med., *32*:282, 1953.

78. Hohman, L. B., Reed, R., and Baker, L. D.: Sensory disturbances in children with infantile hemiplegia, triplegia, and quadriplegia. Amer. J. Phys. Med., *37*:1, 1958.

79. Holt, K. S.: Hand function in young cerebral palsied children. Develop. Med. Child Neurol., *5*:635, 1963.

80. Holt, K. S.: Deformity and disability in cerebral palsy. Develop. Med. Child Neurol., *5*:629, 1963.

81. Holt, K. S.: Assessment of Cerebral Palsy. London, Lloyd Duke, 1965.

82. Hood, P. N., and Perlstein, M. A.: Infantile spastic hemiplegia. V. Oral language and motor development. Pediatrics, *17*:58, 1956.

83. Illingworth, R.: Recent Advances in Cerebral Palsy. London, J. & A. Churchill, 1958.

84. Illingworth, R. S.: The Development of Infants and Young Children, Normal and Abnormal. 3rd Ed. Edinburgh, E. & S. Livingstone, Ltd., 1964.

85. Inglis, A. E., and Cooper, W.: Release of the flexor-pronator origin for flexion deformities of the hand and wrist in spastic paralysis. A study of eighteen cases. J. Bone Joint Surg., *48–A*:847, 1966.

86. Ingraham, F. D., and Matson, D. D.: Subdural haematomas in infancy. Advances Pediat., *4*:231, 1949.

87. Ingram, A. J., Withers, E., and Speltz, E.: Role of intensive physical and occupational therapy in the treatment of cerebral palsy: Testing and results. Arch. Phys. Med., *40*:429, 1959.

88. Ingram, T. T. S.: A study of cerebral palsy in the childhood population of Edinburgh. Arch. Dis. Child., *30*:85, 1955.

89. Ingram, T. T. S.: Pediatric Aspects of Cerebral Palsy. Baltimore, Williams & Wilkins Co., 1964.

90. Jensen, G. D., and Alderman, M. E.: The prehensile grasp of spastic diplegia. Pediatrics, *31*:470, 1963.

91. Jones, A. R.: William John Little. J. Bone Joint Surg., *31–B*:123, 1949.

92. Jones, G. B.: Paralytic dislocation of the hip. J. Bone Joint Surg., *36–B*:375, 1954.

93. Jones, G. B.: Paralytic dislocation of the hip. J. Bone Joint Surg., *44–B*:573, 1963.

94. Kabat, H., and Knott, M.: Principles of neuromuscular re-education. Phys. Ther. Rev., 28:107, 1948.

95. Keats, S.: Combined adductor-gracilis tenotomy and selective obturator nerve resection for correction of adduction deformity of the hip in children with cerebral palsy. J. Bone Joint Surg., 39–A:1087, 1957.

96. Keats, S.: Surgery of the extremities in treatment of cerebral palsy. J.A.M.A., 174:1266, 1960.

97. Keats, S.: An evaluation of surgery for the correction of knee-flexion contractures in children with cerebral spastic paralysis. J. Bone Joint Surg., 44–A:1146, 1962.

98. Keats, S.: Surgical treatment of the hand in cerebral palsy: Correction of thumb-in-palm and other deformities. Report of nineteen cases. J. Bone Joint Surg., 47-A:274, 1965.

99. Keats, S.: Cerebral Palsy. Springfield, Charles C Thomas, 1965.

100. Keats, S.: A simple anteromedial approach to the lesser trochanter of the femur for the release of the iliopsoas tendon. J. Bone Joint Surg., 49–A:632, 1967.

101. Keats, S.: Operative Orthopedics in Cerebral Palsy. Springfield, Ill., Charles C Thomas, 1970.

102. Keats, S., and Kambin, P.: An evaluation of surgery for the correction of knee flexion contracture in children with cerebral spastic paralysis. J. Bone Joint Surg., 44–A:1146, 1962.

103. Keats, S., and Kouten, J.: Early surgical correction of the planovalgus foot in cerebral palsy. Extra-articular arthrodesis of the subtalar joint. Clin. Orthop., 61:223, 1968.

104. Keats, S., and Morgese, A. N.: Excessive lumbar lordoses in ambulatory spastic children. Clin. Orthop., 65:130, 1969.

105. Kendall, P. H., and Robson, P.: Lower limb bracing in cerebral palsy. Clin. Orthop., 47:73, 1966.

106. Kennard, M. A.: Age and other factors in motor recovery from pre-central lesions in monkeys. Amer. J. Physiol., 115:138, 1936.

107. Kennard, M. A.: Re-organization of motor function in cerebral cortex of monkeys deprived of motor and pre-motor areas in infancy. J. Neurophysiol., 1:477, 1938.

108. Khalili, A. A., and Benton, J. G.: A physiologic approach to the evaluation and management of spasticity with procaine and phenol nerve block. Clin. Orthop., 47:97, 1966.

109. Knott, M., and Voss, D. E.: Proprioceptive neuromuscular facilitation. New York, Hoeber-Harper, 1956.

110. Lamb, D. W., and Pollock, G. A.: Hip Deformities in Cerebral Palsy and Their Treatment. Develop. Med. Child Neurol., 4:488, 1962.

111. Legg, A. R.: Transplantation of tensor fasciae femoris in cases of weakened gluteus medius. J.A.M.A., 80:242, 1923.

112. Legg, A. T.: Transplantation of tensor fasciae femoris in cases of weakened gluteus medius. New Eng. J. Med., 209:61, 1933.

113. Levitt, S.: Physiotherapy in Cerebral Palsy. Springfield, Charles C Thomas, 1962.

114. Lewis, F. R., Samilson, R. R., and Lucas, D. B.: Femoral torsion and coxa valga in cerebral palsy. Develop. Med. Child Neurol., 6:591, 1964.

115. Little, W. J.: The deformities of the human frame. Lancet, 1:5, 1843.

116. Little, W. J.: On the Nature and Treatment of Deformities of the Human Frame (with Notes and Additions). London, Longmans, 1853.

117. Little, W. J.: On the influence of abnormal parturition, difficult labours, premature birth and asphyxia neonatorum on the mental and physical condition of the child, especially in relation to deformities. Trans. Obstet. Soc. Long., 3:293, 1862.

118. McCarroll, H. R., and Schwartzman, J. P.: Spastic paralysis and allied disorders. J. Bone Joint Surg., 25:747, 1943.

119. McCue, F. C., Honner, R., and Chapman, W. C.: Transfer of the brachioradialis for hands deformed by cerebral palsy. J. Bone Joint Surg., 52–A:1171, 1970.

120. McIvor, W., and Samilson, R. L.: Fractures in patients with cerebral palsy. J. Bone Joint Surg., 48–A:858, 1966.

121. Martz, C. D.: Talipes equinus correction in cerebral palsy. J. Bone Joint Surg., 42–A:769, 1960.

122. Massie, P., and Audic, B.: Critical evaluation of Eggers' procedure for the relief of knee flexion spasticity. Develop. Med. Child Neurol., 10:159, 1968.

123. Masse, P., Baron, P., Cahuzac, M., Lacheretz, M., Martin, C. H., Queneau, P., and Roullet, J.: La chirurgie de l'infirmité motrice cérébrale chez l'enfant. Rev. Chir. Orthop., 53:729, 1967.

124. Mathews, S. M., Jones, M. H., and Sperling, S. C.: Hip derangements seen in cerebral palsied children. Amer. J. Phys. Med., 32:213, 1953.

125. Meyer, R.: Historical background and personal experiences in surgical relief of hyperkinesia and hypertonus. In Fields, W. S. (ed.): Pathogenesis and Treatment of Parkinsonism. Springfield, Ill., Charles C Thomas, 1958.

126. Michele, A. A.: Iliopsoas. Springfield, Ill., Charles C Thomas, 1962.

127. Minear, W. L.: A classification of cerebral palsy. Pediatrics, 18:841, 1956.

128. Mortens, J.: Orthopaedic operations in the treatment of children with cerebral palsy. Danish Med. Bull., 12:22, 1965.

129. Mortens, J., Moller, H., and Salmonsen, L.: Early stabilizing operation for spastic talipes equino-valgus by Grice's extra-articular osteoplastic subtalar arthrodesis. Acta Orthop. Scand., 32:485, 1962.

130. Murphy, D. P.: Ovarian irradiation and the health of the subsequent child; a review of more than 200 previously unreported pregnancies in women subjected to pelvic irradiation. Surg. Gynec. Obstet., 48:766, 1929.

131. Murphy, D. P.: Congenital Malformations. 2nd Ed. Philadelphia, J. B. Lippincott Co., 1947.

132. Nashold, B. S.: Recent advances in the neurosurgical treatment of cerebral palsy and related disorders. Clin. Orthop., 47:85, 1966.

133. Page, C. M.: An operation for the relief of flexion-contracture in the forearm. J. Bone Joint Surg., 5:233, 1923.

134. Paine, R. S.: Neurological examination of infants and children. Pediat. Clin. N. Amer., 7:471, 1960.

135. Paine, R. S.: Cerebral palsy: Symptoms and signs of diagnostic and prognostic significance. In Adams, J. P. (ed.): Current Practice in Orthopedic Surgery, Vol. 3. St. Louis, C. V. Mosby Co., 1966, p. 39.

136. Pendergast, J. J.: Congenital cataract and other anomalies following rubella in mother during pregnancy. Med. J. Aust., 1:315, 1945.

137. Perlstein, M. A.: Neurologic sequelae of erythroblastosis fetalis. Amer. J. Dis. Child., 79:605, 1950.

138. Perlstein, M. A.: Infantile cerebral palsy. In Levine, S. Z., Anderson, J. A., et al. (eds.): Advances in Pediatrics, Vol. 7. Chicago, Year Book Medical Publishers, Inc., 1955.

139. Perlstein, M. A., and Barnett, H. E.: Nature and recognition of cerebral palsy in infancy. J.A.M.A., 148:1389, 1952.

140. Perlstein, M. A., and Hood, P. N.: Infantile spastic hemiplegia. J. Phys. Med., 34:391, 1955; Pediatrics, 15:676, 1955.

141. Peterson, L. T.: Tenotomy in the treatment of spastic paraplegia with special reference to the iliopsoas. J. Bone Joint Surg., 32–A:875, 1950.

142. Phelps, W. M.: Care and treatment of cerebral palsies. J.A.M.A., 111:1, 1938.

143. Phelps, W. M.: Treatment of cerebral palsies. Clinics, 2:981, 1943.

144. Phelps, W. M.: Classification of athetosis with special reference to the motor classification. Amer. J. Phys. Med., *35*:24, 1956.

145. Phelps, W. M.: Long-term results of orthopedic surgery in cerebral palsy. J. Bone Joint Surg., *39–A*:53, 1957.

146. Phelps, W. M.: Prevention of acquired dislocation of the hip in cerebral palsy. J. Bone Joint Surg., *41–A*: 440, 1959.

147. Phelps, W. M.: Complications of orthopedic surgery in the treatment of cerebral palsy. Clin. Orthop., *53*:39, 1967.

148. Pollock, G. A.: Treatment of adductor paralysis by hamstring transfer. J. Bone Joint Surg., *40–B*:534, 1958.

149. Pollock, G. A.: Surgical treatment of cerebral palsy. J. Bone Joint Surg., *44–B*:68, 1962.

150. Pollock, J. H., and Carrell, B.: Subtalar extra-articular arthrodesis in the treatment of paralytic valgus deformities. A review of 112 procedures in 100 patients. J. Bone Joint Surg., *46–A*:533, 1964.

151. Pollock, G. A., and English, T. A.: Transplantation of the hamstring muscles in cerebral palsy. J. Bone Joint Surg., *49–B*:80, 1967.

152. Rembolt, R. R.: Emotional factors in residential care. Clin. Orthop., *47*:65, 1966.

153. Roberts, W. M., and Adams, J. P.: The patellar advancement operation in cerebral palsy. J. Bone Joint Surg., *35–A*:958, 1953.

154. Robson, P.: The prevalence of scoliosis in adolescents and young adults with cerebral palsy. Dev. Med. Child Neurol., *10*:447, 1968.

155. Samilson, R. L.: Principles of assessment of the upper limb. Clin. Orthop., *47*:105, 1966.

156. Samilson, R. L.: Surgery of the upper limbs in cerebral palsy. Develop. Med. Child Neurol., *9*:109, 1967.

157. Samilson, R. L., and Morris, J. M.: Surgical improvement of the cerebral palsied upper limb—electromyographic studies and results of 128 operations. J. Bone Joint Surg., *46–A*:1203, 1964.

158. Seymour, N., and Evans, D. K.: A Modification of the Grice subtalar arthrodesis. J. Bone Joint Surg., *50–B*: 372, 1958.

159. Seymour, N., and Sharrard, W. J. W.: Bilateral proximal release of the hamstrings in cerebral palsy. J. Bone Joint Surg., *50–B*:274, 1968.

160. Sharrard, W. J. W.: Paralytic deformity in the lower limb. J. Bone Joint Surg., *49–B*:731, 1967.

161. Silver, C. M., and Simon, S. D.: Gastrocnemius-muscle recession (Silfverskiöld operation) for spastic equinus deformity in cerebral palsy. J. Bone Joint Surg., *41–A*: 1021, 1959.

162. Silver, C. M., Simon, S. D., Spindell, E., Lichtman, H. M., and Scala, M.: Calcaneal osteotomy for valgus and varus deformity of the foot in cerebral palsy. J. Bone Joint Surg., *49–A*:232, 1967.

163. Silfverskiöld, N.: Reduction of the uncrossed two-joint muscles of the leg to one-joint muscles in spastic conditions. Acta Chir. Scand., *56*:315, 1923–24.

164. Stamp, W. G.: Bracing in cerebral palsy. J. Bone Joint Surg., *44–A*: 1457, 1962.

165. Steindler, A.: Pathokinetics of cerebral palsy. A.A.O.S. Instructional Course Lectures. Vol. 9. Ann Arbor, J. W. Edwards, 1952, p. 118.

166. Stelling, F. H., and Meyer, L. C.: Cerebral palsy. The upper extremity. Clin. Orthop., *14*:70, 1959.

167. Stöffel, A.: The treatment of spastic contractures. Amer. J. Orthop. Surg., *10*:611, 1913.

168. Strayer, L. M., Jr.: Recession of the gastrocnemius, an operation to relieve spastic contracture of the calf muscles. J. Bone Joint Surg., *32–A*:671, 1950.

169. Strayer, L. M., Jr.: Gastrocnemius recession. Five-year report of cases. J. Bone Joint Surg., *40–A*:1019, 1958.

170. Svirsky, H. S.: The severely involved child: Maternal backache. Clin. Orthop., *47*:57, 1966.

171. Swanson, A. B.: Surgery of the hand in cerebral palsy and the swan-neck deformity. J. Bone Joint Surg., *42–A*:951, 1960.

172. Swanson, A. B.: Surgery of the hand in cerebral palsy and muscle release procedures. Surg. Clin. N. Amer., *48*:5:1129, 1968.

173. Swinyard, C. A.: Reflections about reflex therapy in cerebral palsy. Phys. Ther. Rev., *39*:103, 1959.

174. Tachdjian, M. O., and Minear, W. C.: Hip dislocation in cerebral palsy. J. Bone Joint Surg., *38–A*:1358, 1956.

175. Tachdjian, M. O., and Minear, W. C.: Sensory disturbances in the hands of children with cerebral palsy. J. Bone Joint Surg., *40–A*:85, 1958.

176. Thibodeau, A. A., Wagner, L. C., and Carr, F. J., Jr.: The evaluation of surgical procedures on bones, muscles and peripheral nerves in spastic paralysis. Amer. J. Surg., *43*:822, 1939.

177. Tizard, J. P. M.: Sensory defects in cerebral palsy. Cerebr. Palsy Bull., *2*:40, 1960.

178. Tizard, J. P. M., Paine, R. S., and Crothers, B.: Disturbances of sensation in children with hemiplegia. J.A.M.A., *155*:628, 1954.

179. Tohen, A. Z., Carmona, J. P., and Barrera, J. R.: The utilization of abnormal reflexes in the treatment of spastic foot deformities. Clin. Orthop., *47*:77, 1966.

180. Twitchell, T. E.: The neurologic examination in infantile cerebral palsy. Develop. Med. Child Neurol., *5*:271, 1963.

181. Vulpius, O., and Stöffel, A.: Orthopaedische Operationslehre. Ed. 2. Stuttgart, Ferdinand Enke, 1920.

182. Walker, J.: Oxygen levels in human umbilical cord blood. *In* Cross, K. W., Lelong, M., and Smith, C. A. (eds.): Anoxia of the New-Born Infant. Oxford, Blackwell, 1953.

183. Walshe, F. M. R.: On certain tonic or postural reflexes in hemiplegia with special reference to so-called "associated movements." Brain, *46*:1, 1923.

184. White, J. W.: Torsion of the Achilles tendon: Its surgical significance. Arch. Surg., *46*:784, 1943.

185. Woods, G.: Cerebral Palsy in Childhood. Bristol, Wright, 1957.

186. Wyllie, W. G.: The cerebral palsies of infancy. Modern Trends in Neurology, *1*:125, 1951.

187. Zancolli, E.: The Structural and Dynamic Bases of Hand Surgery. Philadelphia, J. B. Lippincott Co., 1968.

188. Zappert, J.: Ueber ein gehauftes Auftreten gutartiger Facialislämungen beim Kinde. Z. Kinderheilk., *38*:139, 1924.

189. Zausmer, E.: Locomotion in cerebral palsy. Clin. Orthop., *47*:49, 1966.

190. Zervas, N. T., Horner, F. A., and Pickren, K. S.: The treatment of dyskinesia by stereotactic dentatectomy. Confin. Neurol., *29*:93, 1967.

INTRACRANIAL TUMORS

191. Bailey, P., Buchanan, D. N., and Bucy, P. C.: Intracranial Tumors of Infancy and Childhood. Chicago, University of Chicago Press, 1939.

192. Bodian, M., and Lawson, D.: Intracranial neoplastic disease of childhood. Brit. J. Surg., *40*:368, 1953.

193. Cuneo, H. M., and Rand, C. W.: Brain Tumors of Childhood. Springfield, Ill., Charles C Thomas, 1952.

194. Ingraham, F. D., and Matson, D. D.: Neurosurgery of infancy and childhood. New Eng. J. Med., *259*:330, 1958.

195. Matson, D. D.: Cerebellar astrocytoma in childhood. J. Pediat., *18*:150, 1956.

196. Matson, D. D.: Benign intracranial tumors of childhood. New Eng. J. Med., *259*:330, 1958.

197. Matson, D. D.: Intracranial tumors. *In* Farmer, T. W. (ed.): Pediatric Neurology. New York, Hoeber Medical Division, Harper & Row, 1964, p. 443.

198. Walker, A. E., and Hopple, J. L.: Brain tumors in children. General considerations. J. Pediat., *35*:671, 1949.

INTRASPINAL TUMORS

199. Elsberg, C. A., and Dyke, C. G.: The diagnosis and localization of tumors of the spinal cord by means of measurements made on the x-ray films of the vertebrae, and the correlation of clinical and x-ray findings. Bull. Neurol. Inst. New York, *3*:359, 1934.
200. Haworth, J. B., and Keillor, G. W.: Use of transparencies in evaluation of the width of the spinal canal in infants, children, and adults. Radiology, *79*:109, 1962.
201. Hinck, V. C., Hopkins, C. E., and Savara, B. S.: Sagittal diameter of the cervical spinal canal in children. Radiology, *79*:97, 1962.
202. Matson, D. D., and Tachdjian, M. O.: Intraspinal tumors in infants and children. Postgrad. Med., *34*:279, 1963.
203. Simril, W. A., and Thurston, D.: The normal interpediculate space in the spines of infants and children. Radiology, *64*:340, 1955.
204. Tachdjian, M. O., and Matson, D. D.: Orthopaedic aspects of intraspinal tumors in infants and children. J. Bone Joint Surg., *47–A*:223, 1965.

FRIEDREICH'S ATAXIA

205. Boyer, S. H., Chisholm, A. W., McKusick, V. A.: Cardiac aspects of Freidreich's ataxia. Circulation, *25*:493, 1962.
206. Duchenne, G. B.: Physiologie des Mouvements. Paris, J. B. Ballière et Fils, 1867.
207. Friedreich, N.: Über degenerative Atrophie der spinalen Hinterstränge. Virchow. Arch. Path. Anat., *26*:391, and *27*:1, 1863.
208. Hartman, J. M., and Booth, R. W.: Friedreich's ataxia. A neurocardiac disease. Amer. Heart J., *60*:716, 1960.
209. Heck, A. F.: A study of neural and extraneural findings in a large family with Friedreich's ataxia. J. Neurol. Sci., *1*:226, 1964.
210. Hewer, R. L.: Study of fatal cases of Friedreich's ataxia. Brit. Med. J., *3*:649, 1968.
211. LaPresle, J.: Contribution à l'étude de la dystasie aréflexique héréditaire. Etat actuel de quatre des sept cas princeps de Roussy et Mlle. Lévy, trente ans après la première publication de ces auteurs. Sem. Hôp. Paris, *32*:2473, 1956.
212. Makin, M.: The surgical treatment of Friedreich's ataxia. J. Bone Joint Surg., *35–A*:425, 1953.
213. Podolsky, S., Pothier, A., Jr., and Krall, L. P.: Association of diabetes mellitus and Friedreich's ataxia. A study of two siblings. Arch. Intern. Med., *114*:533, 1964.
214. Robinson, N.: An enzyme study of the myocardium in Friedreich's ataxia. Neurology (Minneap.), *16*:1135, 1966.
215. Rombold, C. R., and Riley, H. A.: The abortive type of Friedreich's disease. Arch. Neurol. Psychiat., *16*:301, 1926.
216. Roth, M.: On a possible relationship between hereditary ataxia and peroneal muscular atrophy. With a critical review of the problems of "intermediate forms" in the degenerative disorders of the central nervous system. Brain, *71*:416, 1948.
217. Roussy, G., and Lévy, G.: Sept cas d'une maladie familiale particulaire: Troubles de la marche, pieds, bots er aréfléxie tendineuse généralisée, avec accessoirement, légère maladresse des mains. Rev. Neurol. (Paris), *45*:427, 1926.
218. Saunders, J. T.: Etiology and treatment of clawfoot. Arch. Surg., *30*:179, 1935.
219. Spillane, J. D.: Familial pes cavus and absent tendon jerks. Its relationship with Friedreich's disease and peroneal muscular atrophy. Brain, *63*:275, 1940.
220. Sylvester, P. E.: Some unusual findings in a family with Friedreich's ataxia. Arch. Dis. Child., *33*:217, 1958.
221. Symonds, C. P., and Shaw, M. E.: Familial claw-foot with absent tendon jerks. Brain, *49*:387, 1926.

222. Thilenius, O. G., and Grossman, B. J.: Friedreich's ataxia with heart disease in children. Pediatrics, *27*:246, 1961.
223. Yudell, A., and Dyck, P. J., and Lambert, E. H.: A kinship with Roussy-Lévy syndrome. Arch. Neurol., *13*:432, 1965.

**INFANTILE MUSCULAR ATROPHY
(WERDNIG-HOFFMANN DISEASE)**

224. Batten, F. E.: Progressive spinal muscular atrophy of infants and young children. Brain, *33*:433, 1911.
225. Brandt, S.: Werdnig-Hoffman's Infantile Progressive Muscular Atrophy. Copenhagen, E. Munksgaard, 1950.
226. Buchanan, D.: Some Disorders of the Motor Unit in Infancy and Childhood. Med. Clin. N. Amer., *34*:147, 1950.
227. Byers, R. K., and Banker, B. Q.: Infantile muscular atrophy. Arch. Neurol. (Chicago), *5*:140, 1961.
228. Greenfield, J. G., and Stern, R. O.: The anatomical identity of the Werdnig-Hoffmann and Oppenheim forms of infantile muscular atrophy. Brain, *50*:652, 1927.
229. Greenfield, J. G., Cornman, T., and Shy, G. M.: The prognostic value of the muscle biopsy in the "floppy infant." Brain, *81*:461, 1958.
230. Grinker, R. R.: The pathology of amyotonia congenita. A discussion of its relation to infantile progressive muscular atrophy. Arch. Neurol. Psychiat., *18*:982, 1927.
231. Hardman, R.: The floppy infant. Amer. J. Dis. Child., *101*:145, 1961.
232. Hoffman, J.: Ueber chronische spinale Muskelatrophie im Kindsalter, auf familiärer Basis. Deutsch. Z. Nervenheilk., *3*:427, 1893.
233. Kugelberg, E., and Welander, L.: Heredo-familial juvenile muscular atrophy simulating muscular dystrophy. A.M.A. Arch. Neurol. Psychiat., *75*:500, 1956.
234. Levesque, J., LePage, F., Boeswillwald, M., and Gruner, J.: Congenital familial muscular dystrophy simulating Werdnig-Hoffmann-Oppenheim disease. Arch. Franc. Pediat., *13*:202, 1956.
235. Millichap, J. G.: The hypotonic child. *In* Brennemann-Kelley Practice of Pediatrics. Vol. IV, Chapter 16. Hagerstown, Maryland, W. G. Prior Co., 1966.
236. Oppenheim, H.: Ueber allgemeine und localisierte Atonie der Muskulatur (Myatonie) im frühen Kindesalter. Mschr. Psychiat. Neurol., *8*:232, 1900.
237. Sandifer, P. H.: The differential diagnosis of flaccid paralysis. Proc. Roy. Soc. Med., *48*:186, 1955.
238. Shy, G. M., and Magee, K. R.: A new congenital nonprogressive Myopathy. Brain, *79*:610, 1956.
239. Thieffry, S., Arthus, M., and Bargeton, E.: Werdnig-Hoffman: 40 cases with 11 autopsies. Rev. Neurol., *93*:621, 1955.
240. Turner, J. W. A.: On amyotonia congenita. Brain, *72*:25, 1949.
241. Walton, J.: Amyotonia congenita. Lancet, *1*:1023, 1956.
242. Walton, J. N.: The "floppy" infant. Cerebr. Palsy Bull., *2*:10, 1960.
243. Werdnig, G.: Zwei frühinfantile hereditäre Fälle von progressiver Muskelatrophie unter dem Bilde der Dystrophie, aber auf neurotischer Grundlage. Arch. Psychiat. Nervenkr., *22*:437, 1891.
244. Woolf, A. L.: Muscle biopsy in the diagnosis of the "floppy baby": infantile hypotonia. Cerebr. Palsy Bull., *2*:19, 1960.

DIASTEMATOMYELIA

245. Bremer, J. L.: Dorsal intestinal fistula: accessory neureuteric canal; diastematomyelia. Arch. Path., *54*:132, 1952.
246. Cohen, J., and Sledge, C. B.: Diastematomyelia. Em-

bryologic interpretation. Amer. J. Dis. Child., *100*: 257, 1960.

247. Cowie, T. N.: Diastematomyelia with vertebral column defects. Brit. J. Radiol., *24*:156, 1951.

248. Cowie, T. N.: Diastematomyelia: Tomography in diagnosis. Brit. J. Radiol., *25*:263, 1952.

249. Matson, D. D., Woods, R., Campbell, J., and Ingraham, F. D.: Diastematomyelia (Congenital clefts of the spinal cord): Diagnosis and surgical treatment. Pediatrics, 6:98, 1950.

250. Maxwell, H., and Bucy, P.: Diastematomyelia. J. Neuropath. Exp. Neurol., 5:165, 1946.

251. Neuhauser, E. B. D., Wittenborg, M. H., and Dehlinger, K.: Diastematomyelia. Radiology, 54:659, 1950.

252. Perret, G.: Diagnosis and treatment of diastematomyelia. Surg. Gynec. Obstet., *105*:69, 1957.

253. Perret, G.: Symptoms and diagnosis of diastematomyelia. Neurology (Minneap.), *10*:51, 1960.

254. Sands, W. W., and Clark, W. K.: Diastematomyelia. Amer. J. Roentgen., *72*:64, 1954.

MYELOMENINGOCELE

255. Alter, M.: Anencephalus, hydrocephalus, and spina bifida. Arch. Neurol., 7:411, 1962.

256. Badell-Ribera, A., Shulman, K., and Paddock, N.: The relationship of non-progressive hydrocephalus to intellectual functioning in children with spina bifida cystica. Pediatrics, *37*:787, 1966.

257. Badell-Ribera, A., Swinyard, C. A., Greenspan, L., and Deaver, G. G.: Spina bifida with myelomeningocele: Evaluation of rehabilitation potential. Arch. Phys. Med., *45*:443, 1964.

258. Barr, J. S.: Poliomyelitic hip deformity and the erector spinae transplant. J.A.M.A., *144*:813, 1950.

259. Bergman, N. A.: Problems in anesthetic management in Patients with Meningocele and Spina Bifida. Anesth. Analg. (Cleveland), *36*:60, 1957.

260. Bluestone, S. S., and Deaver, G. G.: Habilitation of the child with spina bifida and myelomeningocele. J.A.M.A., *161*:1248, 1956.

261. Boris, M.: Increased Incidence of Meningomyeloceles J.A.M.A., *84*:768, 1963.

262. Brocklehurst, G., Gleave, J. R. W., and Lewin, W. S.: Early Closure of Myelomeningocele with Especial Reference to Leg Movement. Develop. Med. Child. Neurol., *13*:51, 1967.

263. Butler-Smythe, A. C.: Spina bifida and hydrocephalus occurring in the same family. Lancet, *1*:272, 1889.

264. Cameron, A. H.: The spinal cord lesion in spina bifida cystica. Lancet, 2:171, 1956.

265. Cameron, A. H.: Arnold-Chiari and other neuro-anatomical malformations associated with spina bifida. J. Path. Bact., *73*:195, 1957.

266. Campbell, J. B.: Congenital anomalies of the neural axis. Surgical management based on embryological considerations. Amer. J. Surg., *75*:231, 1948.

267. Carr, T. L.: Orthopaedic aspects of one hundred cases of spina bifida. Postgrad. Med. J., *32*:201, 1956.

268. Chrystal, M., and Hershey, L. S.: Total rehabilitation in relation to spina bifida. Phys. Ther. Rev., *31*:357, 1951.

269. Colonna, P. C.: An arthroplastic operation for congenital dislocation of the hip. A two-stage procedure. Surg. Gynec. Obstet., *63*:777, 1936.

270. Doran, P. A., and Guthkelch, A. N.: Studies in spina bifida cystica. J. General survey and reassessment of the problem. J. Neurol. Neurosurg. Psychiat., *24*: 331, 1961.

271. Dunn, H. G., and Salter, J. G.: Recurrent anencephaly; case report with note on aetiology of anencephaly and allied malformations. J. Obstet. Gynaec. Brit. Emp., *51*:529, 1944.

272. Eckstein, H. B., and MacNab, G. H.: Myelomeningocele and hydrocephalus. The impact of modern treatment. Lancet, *1*:842, 1966.

273. Eder, D.: Anterior sacral meningocele: Survey of literature and report of a case. Bull. Los Angeles Neurol. Soc., *14*:104, 1949.

274. Edwards, J. H.: Congenital malformations of the central nervous system in Scotland. Brit. J. Prev. Soc. Med., *12*:115, 1958.

275. Eskelund, V., and Bartels, E. D.: Spina bifida umbalis in uniovular twins. Nord. Med., (Hospitalstid), *11*: 2075, 1941.

276. Faber, L. A., and Ericksen, L. G.: Prenatal Diagnosis of Spina Bifida. J. Iowa Med. Soc., *26*:359, 1936.

277. Fawcitt, J.: Some radiological aspects of congenital anomalies of the spine in childhood and infancy. Proc. Roy. Soc. Med., *52*:331, 1959.

278. Fisher, R. G., Uihlein, A., and Keith, H. M.: Spina bifida and cranium bifidum: Study of 530 cases. Proc. Staff Meet. Mayo Clin., *27*:33, 1952.

279. Floyd, W., Lovell, W., and King, R. E.: The neuropathic joint. Southern Med. J., *52*:563, 1959.

280. Ford, F. R.: Diseases of the Nervous System in Infancy, Childhood, and Adolescence. 5th Ed. Springfield, Ill., Charles C Thomas, 1966, pp. 84–88, 159–166.

281. Fowler, I.: Responses of the chick neural tube in mechanically produced spina bifida. J. Exp. Zool., *123*:115, 1953.

282. Fry, A.: Spina bifida in binovular twins. Brit. Med. J., *1*:131, 1943.

283. Gardner, W. J.: Anatomic anomalies common to myelomeningocele of infancy and syringomyelia of adulthood suggesting a common origin. Cleveland Clin. Quart., *26*:118, 1959.

284. Gardner, W. J.: Myelomeningocele, the result of rupture of the embryonic neural tube. Cleveland Clin. Quart., *27*:88, 1960.

285. Gardner, W. J.: Rupture of the neural tube. A.M.A. Arch. Neurol., *4*:1, 1961.

286. Gillespie, H. W.: The significance of congenital lumbosacral abnormalities. Brit. J. Radiol., *22*:270, 1949.

287. Gillies, C. L., and Hartung, W.: Fracture of tibia in spina bifida vera. Radiology, *31*:621, 1938.

288. Gillman, J., Gilbert, C., and Gillman, T.: A preliminary report on hydrocephalus, spina bifida and other anomalies in the rat produced by trypan blue. Significance of these results in interpretation of congenital malformations following maternal rubella. S. Afr. J. Med. Sci., *13*:47, 1948.

289. Gillman, J., Gilbert, C., Spence, I., and Gillman, T.: A further report on congenital anomalies in the rat produced by trypan blue. S. Afr. J. Med. Sci., *16*:125, 1951.

290 Golding, C.: Spina bifida and epiphyseal displacement. J. Bone Joint Surg., *42-B*:387, 1960.

291. Greeley, P. W., Oldberg, E., and Curtin, J. W.: Plastic surgical repair of lumbar myelomeningocele. Ann. Surg., *142*:552, 1955.

292. Gross, H. P.: Myelomeningocele in one identical twin. J. Neurosurg., *20*:439, 1963.

293. Gunberg, D. L.: Spina bifida and the Arnold-Chiari malformation in the progeny of trypan blue injected rats. Anat. Rec., *126*:343, 1956.

294. Guthkelch, A. N.: Studies in spina bifida cystica. II. When to repair the spinal defect. J. Neurol. Neurosurg. Psychiat., *25*:137, 1962.

295. Gyepes, M. T., Newbern, D. H., and Neuhauser, E. B. D.: Metaphyseal and physeal injuries in children with spina bifida and meningomyelocele. Amer. J. Roentgen., *95*:168, 1965.

296. Haddad, F. S.: Anterior sacral meningocele. Report of two cases and review of the literature. Canad. J. Surg., *1*:230, 1958.

297. Hagberg, B., Sjögren, I., Bensch, K., and Hadenius, A. M.: The incidence of infantile hydrocephalus in Sweden. Acta Paediat. (Stockholm), *52*:588, 1963.

298. Hamburgh, M.: The embryology of trypan blue induced abnormalities in mice. Anat. Rec., *119*:409, 1954.

299. Haslam, E. T.: The orthopedic problem of spina bifida. Bull. Tulane Med. Fac., *12*:12, 1952.

300. Hayes, J. T., and Gross, H. P.: Orthopedic implications of myelodysplasia. J.A.M.A., *184*:762, 1963.

301. Hayes, J. T., Gross, H. P., and Dow, S.: Surgery for paralytic defects secondary to myelomeningocele and myelodysplasia. J. Bone Joint Surg., *46-A*:1577, 1964.

302. Hewitt, D.: Geographical variations in the mortality attributed to spina bifida and other congenital malformations. Brit. J. Prev. Soc. Med., *17*:13, 1963.

303. Hogshead, H. P., and Ponseti, I. V.: Fascia lata transfer to the erector spinae for the treatment of flexion abductor contractures of the hip in patients with poliomyelitis and myelomeningocele. J. Bone Joint Surg., *46-A*:1389, 1964.

304. Hoppenfeld, S.: Congenital kyphosis in myelomeningocele. J. Bone Joint Surg., *49-B*:276, 1967.

305. Ingalls, T. H., Pugh, T. F., and MacMahon, B.: Incidence of anencephalus, spina bifida, and hydrocephalus related to birth rank and maternal age. Brit. J. Prev. Soc. Med., *8*:17, 1954.

306. Ingraham, F. D., and Fowler, F.: Lumbar myelomeningocele. Surg. Clin. N. Amer., *36*:6, 1956.

307. Ingraham, F. D., and Hamlin, H.: Spina Bifida and Cranium Bifidum. Surgical Treatment. New Eng. J. Med., *228*:361, 1943.

308. Ingraham, F. D., and Matson, D. D.: Neurosurgery in infancy and Childhood. Springfield, Ill., Charles C Thomas, 1954.

309. Ingraham, F. D., and Swan, H.: Spina bifida and cranium bifidum. I. A survey of five hundred and forty-six cases. New Eng. J. Med., *228*:559, 1943.

310. Ingraham, F. D., Swan, H., et al.: Spina Bifida and Cranium Bifidum. Cambridge, Harvard University Press, 1944.

311. Irwin, C. E.: Iliotibial band. Its role in producing deformity in poliomyelitis. J. Bone Joint Surg., *31-A*: 141, 1949.

312. Jaeger, R.: Congenital spinal meningocele. J.A.M.A., *153*:792, 1953.

313. James, C. C. M., and Lassman, L. P.: Spinal dysraphism. The diagnosis and treatment of progressive lesions in spina bifida occulta. J. Bone Joint Surg., *44-B*:828, 1962.

314. Jelsma, F., and Ploetner, E. J.: Painful spina bifida occulta. With review of the literature. J. Neurosurg., *10*:19, 1953.

315. Jones, G. B.: Paralytic dislocation of the hip. J. Bone Joint Surg., *36-B*:375, 1954.

316. Jones, G. B.: Paralytic dislocation of the hip. J. Bone Joint Surg., *44-B*:573, 1962.

317. Jones, J. D. L., and Evans, T. G.: Anterior sacral meningocele. J. Obstet. Gynaec., *66*:477, 1959.

318. Josephson, J. F., and Waller, K. B.: Anencephaly in identical twins. Canad. Med. Ass. J., *29*:34, 1933.

319. Katz, J. F.: Spontaneous Fractures in Paraplegic Children. J. Bone Joint Surg., *35-A*:220, 1953.

320. Kilfoyle, R. M.: Myelodysplasia. Pediat. Clin. N. Amer., *14*:419, 1967.

321. Kilfoyle, R. M., Foley, J. J., and Norton, P. L.: The spine and pelvic deformity in childhood and adolescent paraplegia. J. Bone Joint Surg., *47-A*:659, 1965.

322. Laurence, K. M.: The natural history of spina bifida cystica. Proc. Roy. Soc. Med., *53*:1055, 1960.

323. Laurence, K. M.: New thoughts on spina bifida and hydrocephalus. Develop. Med. Child Neurol., *5*:68, 1963.

324. Laurence, K. M.: The natural history of spina bifida cystica: Detailed analysis of 407 cases. Arch. Dis. Child., *39*:41, 1964.

325. Laurence, K. M.: The survival of untreated spina bifida cystica. Develop. Med. Child Neurol., *8*:Suppl. 11, 10, 1966.

326. Lawrence, K. M., and Tew, B. J.: Follow-up of 65 survivors from the 425 cases of spina bifida born in South Wales between 1956 and 1962. Develop. Med. Child Neurol., *13*:1, 1968.

327. Lichtenstein, B.: "Spinal dysraphism"; spina bifida and myelodysplasia. Arch. Neurol. Psychiat., *44*:792, 1940.

328. Lodge, T.: Bone, joint, and soft tissue changes following paraplegia. Acta. Radiol., *46*:435, 1956.

329. Long, C., II, and Lawton, E. B.: Functional significance of spinal cord lesion level. Arch. Phys. Med., *36*:249, 1955.

330. Lorber, J.: The family history of spina bifida cystica. Pediatrics, *35*:589, 1965.

331. Lorber, J.: Incidence and Epidemiology of Myelomeningocele. Clin. Orthop., *45*:81, 1966.

332. Lorber, J.: Neurologic assessment of neonates with spina bifida. Clin. Pediat., *7*:676, 1968.

333. Lorber, J., and Levick, K.: Spina bifida cystica: Incidence of spina bifida occulta in parents and in controls. Arch. Dis. Child., *42*:171, 1967.

334. MacMahon, B., Pugh, T. F., and Ingalls, T. D.: Anencephalus, spina bifida, and hydrocephalus. Brit. J. Prev. Soc. Med., *7*:211, 1953.

335. Matson, D. D.: Surgical treatment of birth defects involving the central nervous system. J. Chron. Dis., *10*:131, 1959.

336. Matson, D. D.: Surgical repair of myelomeningocele. J. Neurosurg., *27*:180, 1967.

337. Matson, D. D.: Neurosurgery of Infancy and Childhood. Springfield, Ill., Charles C Thomas, 1969.

338. Mayer, L.: Further studies of fixed pelvic obliquity. J. Bone Joint Surg., *18*:87, 1936.

339. Menelaus, M. B.: Dislocation and deformity of the hip in children with spina bifida cystica. J. Bone Joint Surg., *51-B*:238, 1969.

340. Menelaus, M. B.: The Orthopedic Management of Spina Bifida Cystica. Edinburgh, E. & S. Livingstone, 1971.

341. Milham, S.: Increased incidence of anencephalus and spina bifida in siblings of affected cases. Science, *138*:593, 1962.

342. Morales, P. A., Deaver, C. C., and Hotchkiss, R. S.: Urological complications of spina bifida in children. J. Urol., *75*:537, 1956.

343. Morris, J. V.: Familial spina bifida. J. Irish Med. Ass., *40*:154, 1957.

344. Murphy, D. P.: The duplication of congenital malformations in brothers and sisters and among relatives: A study of sibling defects in 40 consecutive families. Surg. Gynec. Obstet., *63*:443, 1936.

345. Mustard, W. T.: Iliopsoas transfer for weakness of the hip abductors. J. Bone Joint Surg., *34-A*:647, 1952.

346. Mustard, W. T.: A follow-up study of iliopsoas transfer for hip instability. J. Bone Joint Surg., *41-B*:289, 1959.

347. Nash, D. F. E.: Meningomyelocele. Proc. Roy. Soc. Med., *56*:506, 1963.

348. Nathanson, L., and Lewitan, A.: Dislocation of the hip associated with spina bifida. Amer. J. Roentgen., *51*:635, 1944.

349. Norton, P. L., and Foley, J. J.: Paraplegia in children. J. Bone Joint Surg., *41-A*:1291, 1959.

350. O'Hare, J. M.: Progress Report in the Study of Congenital Paraplegics. Proceedings of Seventh Annual Clinical Paraplegia Conference, 1958.

351. Patten, B. M.: Embryological stages in the establishing of myeloschisis with spina bifida. Amer. J. Anat., *93*:365, 1953.

352. Peach, B.: Arnold-Chiari malformation. Arch. Neurol., *12*:613, 1965.

353. Von Recklinghausen, F.: Untersuchungen über die Spina bifida. Arch. Path. Anat., *105*:243, 1886.

354. Record, R. G., and McKeown, T.: Congenital malformations of the central nervous system. I. A survey of 930 cases. Brit. J. Soc. Med., *3*:183, 1949.

355. Record, R. G., and McKeown, T.: Congenital malfor-

mations of the central nervous system. III. Risk of malformation in siblings of malformed individuals. Brit. J. Soc. Med., *4*:217, 1950.

356. Russell, D. S., and Donald, C.: Mechanism of internal hydrocephalus in spina bifida. Brain, *58*:203, 1935.

357. Salter, R. B.: Innominate osteotomy in the treatment of congenital dislocation and subluxation of the hip. J. Bone Joint Surg., *43-B*:518, 1961.

358. Saunders, R. L. deC. H.: Combined anterior and posterior spina bifida in living neonatal human female. Anat. Rec., *87*:255, 1943.

359. Schwidde, J. T.: Spina bifida. Survey of two hundred twenty-five encephaloceles, meningoceles, and myelomeningoceles. Amer. J. Dis. Child., *84*:35, 1952.

360. Sharrard, W. J. W.: Congenital paralytic dislocation of the hip in children with myelo-meningocele. J. Bone Joint Surg., *41-B*:622, 1959.

361. Sharrard, W. J. W.: The mechanism of paralytic deformity in spina bifida. Develop. Med. Child Neurol., *4*:310, 1962.

362. Sharrard, W. J. W.: Posterior iliopsoas transplantation in the treatment of paralytic dislocation of the hip. J. Bone Joint Surg., *46-B*:426, 1964.

363. Sharrard, W. J. W.: Spina bifida. Physiotherapy, *50*:44, 1964.

364. Sharrard, W. J. W.: Paralytic deformity in the lower limb. J. Bone Joint Surg., *49-B*:731, 1967.

365. Sharrard, W. J. W.: Spinal osteotomy for congenital kyphosis in myelomeningocele. J. Bone Joint Surg., *50-B*:466, 1968.

366. Sharrard, W. J. W., and Grosfield, I.: The management of deformity and paralysis of the foot in myelomeningocele. J. Bone Joint Surg., *50-B*:456, 1968.

367. Sharrard, W. J. W., Zachary, R. B., Lorber, J., and Bruce, A. M.: A controlled trial of immediate and delayed closure of spina bifida cystica. Arch. Dis. Child., *38*:18, 1963.

368. Shulman, B. H.: Spina bifida with meningocele. Occurrence in two children of the same family. Arch. Neurol. Psychiat., *47*:474, 1942.

369. Shulman, K., and Ames, M.: Intensive treatment of fifty children born with myelomeningocele. New York J. Med., *68*:265, 1969.

370. Smith, E. D.: Spina Bifida and the Total Care of Spinal Myelomeningocele. Springfield, Ill., Charles C Thomas, 1965.

371. Smith, R. S.: Orthopedic considerations in the treatment of spina bifida. Surg. Gynec. Obstet., *62*:218, 1936.

372. Solovay, J., and Solovay, H. U.: Paraplegic neuroarthropathy. Amer. J. Roentgen. *61*:475, 1949.

373. Somerville, E. W.: Paralytic dislocation of the hip. J. Bone Joint Surg., *41-B*:279, 1959.

374. Soutter, F. E.: Spina bifida and epiphyseal displacement: Report of two cases. J. Bone Joint Surg., *44-B*:106, 1962.

375. Soutter, R.: A new operation for hip contracture in poliomyelitis. Boston Med. Surg. J., *170*:380, 1914.

376. Stark, G. D., and Baker, G. C. W.: The neurological involvement of the lower limbs in myelomeningocele. Develop. Med. Child Neurol., *9*:732, 1967.

377. Stoyle, T. F.: Prognosis for paralysis in myelomeningocele. Develop. Med. Child Neurol., *8*:755, 1966.

378. Sugar, M., and Kennedy, C. M.: The use of electrodiagnostic techniques in the evaluation of the neurological deficit in infants with meningomyelocele. Neurology, *15*:787, 1965.

379. Sutherland, C. G.: A roentgenographic study of developmental anomalies of the spine. J. Radiol. Iowa City, *3*:357, 1922.

380. Sutow, W. W., and Pryde, A. W.: Incidence of spina bifida occulta in relation to age. Amer. J. Dis. Child., *91*:211, 1956.

381. Swinyard, C. A.: Comprehensive Care of the Child with Spina Bifida Manifesta. Rehabilitation Monograph No. 31. New York, Institute of Rehabilitation Medicine, 1966.

382. Teng, P., and Papatheodoron: Arnold-Chiari malformation with normal spine and cranium. Arch. Neurol., *12*:622, 1965.

383. Tzimas, N., and Badell-Ribera, A.: Orthopedic and habilitation management of patients with spina bifida and myelomeningocele. Med. Clin. N. Amer., *53*:502, 1969.

384. Wallace, H. M., Baumgartner, L., and Rich, H.: Congenital malformations and birth injuries in New York City. Pediatrics, *12*:525, 1953.

385. Warkany, J., Wilson, J. G., and Geiger, J. F.: Myeloschisis and myelomeningocele produced experimentally in the rat. J. Comp. Neurol., *109*:35, 1958.

386. Warthen, R. O., Lo Presti, J. M., and Burdick, W. F.: Spina bifida cystica: Review of seventy cases with report of a case of cervical meningocele. Med. Ann. D.C., *18*:298, 1949.

387. Weissman, S. L., Torok, G., and Khermosh, O.: Intertrochanteric osteotomy in fixed paralytic obliquity of the pelvis. A preliminary report. J. Bone Joint Surg., *43-A*:1135, 1961.

388. Wiener, A. S.: Pathogenesis of spina bifida and related congenital malformations. New York J. Med., *47*:985, 1947.

389. Williams, P. F.: Surgical advances in the management of deformities of the spine and lower limbs in spina bifida. Aust. New Zeal. J. Surg., *34*:250, 1965.

390. Wilner, I. A.: Familial repetition of myelomeningocele. J. Mich. Med. Soc., *48*:727, 729, 1949.

391. Wilson, C. B., and Llewellyn, R. C.: The surgical management of meningocele and meningomyelocele. J. Pediat., *61*:595, 1962.

392. Wilson, M. A.: Multidisciplinary problems of myelomeningocele and hydrocephalus. J. Amer. Phys. Ther. Ass., *45*:1139, 1965.

393. Yen, S., and MacMahon, B.: Genetics of anencephaly and spina bifida. Lancet, *2*:623, 1968.

394. Young, B. H.: The orthopaedic surgeon takes a closer look at congenital paraplegia. Bull. Tulane Med. Fac., *20*:33, 1960.

395. Yount, C. C.: The role of the tensor fasciae femoris in certain deformities of the lower extremities. J. Bone Joint Surg., *8*:171, 1926.

POLIOMYELITIS

396. Albert, E.: Zur Resektion des Kniegelenkes. Wien. Med. Presse, *20*:705, 1879.

397. Albert, E.: Chirurgische Mittheilungen. Zbl. Chir., *8*:766, 1881.

398. Alldredge, R. H., and Riordan, D. C.: The use of staples and bone-chip grafts for internal fixation in foot-stabilization operations. J. Bone Joint Surg., *35-A*:951, 1953.

399. Ansart, M. B.: Pan-arthrodesis for paralytic flail foot. J. Bone Joint Surg., *33-B*:503, 1951.

400. d'Aubigné, R. M.: Treatment of residual paralysis after injuries of the main nerves (superior extremity). Proc. Roy. Soc. Med., *42*:831, 1949.

401. d'Aubigné, R. M.: Chirurgia Orthopedique des Paralysis. Paris, Masson, & Cie, 1959.

402. Axer, A.: Transposition of gluteus maximus, tensor fasciae latae and ilio-tibial band for paralysis of lateral abdominal muscles in children after poliomyelitis. A preliminary report. J. Bone Joint Surg., *40-B*:644, 1958.

403. Axer, A.: Into-talus transposition of tendons for correction of paralytic valgus foot after poliomyelitis in children. J. Bone Joint Surg., *42-A*:1119, 1960.

404. Baker, A. B., and Cornwell, S.: Poliomyelitis; the spinal cord. A.M.A. Arch. Path., *61*:185, 1956.

405. Baker, L. D., and Dodelin, C. D.: Extra-articular arthrodesis of the subtalar joint (Grice procedure). J.A.M.A., *168*:1005, 1958.

406. Barr, J. S.: Poliomyelitic hip deformity and the erector spinae transplant. J.A.M.A., *144*:813, 1950.

406a. Barr, J. S.: Discussion. J. Bone Joint Surg., *46-A*: 1402, 1964.

407. Barr, J. S., and Record, E. E.: Arthrodesis of the ankle for correction of foot deformity. Surg. Clin. N. Amer., 27:1281, 1947.

408. Barr, J. S., Stinchfield, A. J., and Reidy, J. A.: Sympathetic ganglionectomy and limb length in poliomyelitis. J. Bone Joint Surg., *32-A*:793, 1950.

409. Barr, J. S., Freiberg, J. A., Colonna, P. C., and Pemberton, P. A.: A survey of end-results on stabilization of the paralytic shoulder. Report of the research committee of the American Orthopaedic Association. J. Bone Joint Surg., *24*:699, 1942.

410. Bateman, J. E.: The shoulder and environs. St. Louis, C. V. Mosby Co., 1954.

411. Benyi, P.: A modified Lambrinudi operation for drop foot. J. Bone Joint Surg., *42-B*:333, 1960.

412. Bickel, W. H., and Moe, J. H.: Translocation of the peroneus longus tendon for paralytic calcaneus deformity of the foot. Surg. Gynec. Obstet., *78*:627, 1944.

413. Biesalski, K., and Mayer, L.: Die Physiologische Sehnenverpflanzung, Vol. 14. Berlin, Julius Springer, 1916.

414. Bingold, A. C.: Ankle and subtalar fusion by a transarticular graft. J. Bone Joint Surg., *38-B*:862, 1956.

415. Blount, W. P.: Osteoclasis for supination deformities in children. J. Bone Joint Surg., *22*:300, 1940.

416. Bodian, D.: Poliomyelitis: Neuropathologic observations in relation to motor symptoms. J.A.M.A., *134*: 1148, 1947.

417. Bradford, E. H., and Lovett, R. W.: Treatise on Orthopedic Surgery. London, Baillière, Tindall & Cox, 1915, p. 486.

418. Brewster, A. H.: Countersinking the astragalus in paralytic feet. New Eng. J. Med., *209*:71, 1933.

419. Brittain, H. A.: Architectural principles in arthrodesis. 2nd Ed. Edinburgh, E. & S. Livingstone, Ltd., 1952.

420. Brockway, A.: An operation to improve abduction power of the shoulder in poliomyelitis. J. Bone Joint Surg., *21*:451, 1939.

421. Broderick, T. F., Reidy, J. A., and Barr, J. S.: Tendon transplantations in the lower extremity. A review of end results in poliomyelitis. II. Tendon transplantations at the knee. J. Bone Joint Surg., *34-A*:909, 1952.

422. Broms, J. D.: Subtalar extra-articular arthrodesis. Follow-up study. Clin. Orthop., *42*:139, 1965.

423. Brooks, D. M.: Symposium on reconstructive surgery of paralyzed upper limb; tendon transplantation of the forearm and arthrodesis of the wrist. Proc. Roy. Soc. Med., *42*:838, 1949.

424. Brooks, D. M., and Seddon, H. J.: Pectoral transplantation for paralysis of the flexors of the elbow. A new technique. J. Bone Joint Surg., *41-B*:36, 1959.

425. Brooks, D. M., and Zaoussis, A.: Arthrodesis of the shoulder in reconstructive surgery of paralysis of the upper limb. J. Bone Joint Surg., *41-B*:207, 1959.

426. Buck-Gramcko, H.: Zur technik der intratrikulären Schultergelenksarthrodese. Z. Orthop., *91*:198, 1959.

427. Bunnell, S.: Restoring flexion to the paralytic elbow. J. Bone Joint Surg., *33-A*:566, 1951.

428. Burman, M.: Paralytic supination contracture of the forearm. J. Bone Joint Surg., *38-A*:303, 1956.

429. Caldwell, G. D.: Transplantation of the biceps femoris to the patella by the medial route in poliomyelitic quadriceps paralysis. J. Bone Joint Surg., *37-A*:347, 1955.

430. Caldwell, G. D.: Correction of paralytic footdrop by hemigastrosoleus transplant. Clin. Orthop., *11*:81, 1958.

431. Campbell, W. C.: An operation for the correction of "drop-foot." J. Bone Joint Surg., 5:815, 1923.

432. Campbell, W. C.: End results of operation for correction of drop-foot. J.A.M.A., *85*:1927, 1925.

433. Carayon, A., Bourrel, P., Bourges, M., and Touze, M.: Dual transfer of the posterior tibial and flexor digitorum longus tendons for drop foot. Report of thirty-one cases. J. Bone Joint Surg., *49-A*:144, 1967.

434. Carmack, J. C., and Hallock, H.: Tibiotarsal arthrodesis after astragalectomy, a report of eight cases. J. Bone Joint Surg., *29*:476, 1947.

435. Carroll, R. E.: Restoration of flexor power to the flail elbow by transplantation of the triceps tendon. Surg. Gynec. Obstet., *95*:685, 1952.

436. Carroll, R. E.: Restoration of elbow flexion by transplantation of the sternocleidomastoid muscle. *In* Proceedings of the American Society of Surgery of the Hand. J. Bone Joint Surg., *44-A*:1039, 1962.

437. Carroll, R. E., and Gartland, J. J.: Flexorplasty of the elbow. An evaluation of a method. J. Bone Joint Surg., *35-A*:706, 1953.

438. Carroll, R. E., and Hill, N. A.: Triceps transfer to restore elbow flexion. J. Bone Joint Surg., *52-A*:239, 1970.

439. Chambers, E. F. S.: Operation for correction of flexible flat feet in adolescents. Western J. Surg., *54*:77, 1946.

440. Charnley, J.: Compression arthrodesis of the ankle and shoulder. J. Bone Joint Surg., *33-B*:180, 1951.

441. Charnley, J.: Compression Arthrodesis. London, E. & S. Livingstone, Ltd., 1953.

442. Charnley, J., and Houston, J. K.: Compress on arthrodesis of the shoulder. J. Bone Joint Surg., *46-B*:614, 1964.

443. Chaves, J. P.: Pectoralis minor transplant for paralysis of the serratus anterior. J. Bone Joint Surg., *33-B*: 228, 1951.

444. Chigot, P. L., and Sananes, P.: Arthrodèse de Grice. Variente technique. Rev. Chir. Orthop., *51*:53, 1965.

445. Cholmeley, J. A.: Elmslie's operation for the calcaneus foot. J. Bone Joint Surg., *33-B*:228, 1951.

446. Chuinard, E. G., and Peterson, R. E.: Distraction-compression bone-graft arthrodesis of the ankle. A method especially applicable for children. J. Bone Joint Surg., *45-A*:481, 1963.

447. Clark, J. M. P.: Reconstruction of biceps brachii by pectoral muscle transplantation. Brit. J. Surg., *34*:180, 1946.

448. Clark, J. M. P., and Axer, A.: A muscle-tendon transposition for paralysis of the lateral abdominal muscles in poliomyelitis. J. Bone Joint Surg., *38-B*:475, 1956.

449. Cleveland, M.: Operative fusion of the unstable or flail knee due to anterior poliomyelitis. A study of late results. J. Bone Joint Surg., *14*:525, 1932.

450. Clippinger, F. W., Jr., and Irwin, C. E.: The opponens transfer, analysis of end results. Southern Med. J., *55*:33, 1962.

451. Close, J. R., and Todd, F. N.: The phasic activity of the muscles of the lower extremity and the effect of tendon transfer. J. Bone Joint Surg., *41-A*:189, 1959.

452. Codivilla, A.: Meine Erfahrugen über Schnenverpflanzungen. Z. Orthop. Chir., *12*:221, 1904.

453. Conner, A. N.: The treatment of flexion contractures of the knee in poliomyelitis. J. Bone Joint Surg., *52-B*: 138, 1970.

454. Coonrad, R. W., Irwin, C. E., Gucker, T., III, and Wray, J. B.: The importance of plantar muscles in paralytic varus feet. The results of treatment by neurectomy and myotenotomy. J. Bone Joint Surg., *38-A*:563, 1956.

455. Cravener, E. K.: Device for overcoming non-bony flexion contractures of the knee. J. Bone Joint Surg., *12*: 437, 1930.

456. Crego, C. H., Jr., and Fischer, F. J.: Transplantation of the biceps femoris for the relief of quadriceps femoris paralysis in residual poliomyelitis. J. Bone Joint Surg., *13*:515, 1931.

457. Crego, C. H., Jr., and McCarroll, H. R.: Recurrent de-

formities in stabilized paralytic feet. A report of 1100 consecutive stabilizations in poliomyelitis. J. Bone Joint Surg., 20:609, 1938.

458. Davidson, W. D.: Traumatic deltoid paralysis treated by muscle transplantation. J.A.M.A., 106:2237, 1936.

459. Davis, G. G.: Wedge-shaped resection of the foot for the relief of old cases of varus. New York J. Med., 56:379, 1892.

460. Davis, G. G.: The treatment of hollow foot (pes cavus). Amer. J. Orthop. Surg., 11:231, 1913.

461. Davis, J. B., and Cotrell, G. W.: A technique for shoulder arthrodesis. J. Bone Joint Surg., 44–A:657, 1962.

462. Dehne, E., and Hall, R. M.: Active shoulder motion in complete deltoid paralysis. J. Bone Joint Surg., 41–A: 745, 1959.

463. Dickson, F. D.: An operation for stabilizing paralytic hips; a preliminary report. J. Bone Joint Surg., 9:1, 1927.

464. Dickson, F. D.: Fascial transplants in paralytic and other conditions. J. Bone Joint Surg., 19:405, 1937.

465. Dickson, F. D., and Diveley, R. L.: Operation for correction of mild claw foot, the result of infantile paralysis. J.A.M.A., 87:1275, 1926.

466. duToit, G. T., and Levy, S. J.: Transposition of latissimus dorsi for paralysis of the triceps brachii. Report of a case. J. Bone Joint Surg., 49–B:135, 1967.

467. Drew, A. J.: The late results of arthrodesis of the foot. J. Bone Joint Surg., 33–B:496, 1951.

468. Dunn, N.: Stabilizing operations in the treatment of paralytic deformities of the foot. Proc. Roy. Soc. Med. (Section on Orthopaedics), 15:15, 1922.

469. Dunn, N.: Suggestions based on ten years' experience of arthrodesis of the tarsus in the treatment of deformities of the foot. In Robert Jones Birthday Volume. London, Oxford University Press, 1928, p. 395.

470. Durman, D. C.: An operation for paralysis of the serratus anterior. J. Bone Joint Surg., 27:380, 1945.

471. Eaton, G. O.: Results of abdominal stabilizations. Southern Med. J., 34:443, 1941.

472. Elkins, E. C., Janes, J. M., Henderson, E. D., and McLeod, J. J., Jr.: Peroneal translocation for paralysis of plantar flexor muscles. Surg. Gynec. Obstet., 102: 469, 1956.

473. Elmslie, R. L.: In Turner, G. G. (ed.): Modern Operative Surgery. 2nd Ed. London, Cassell & Co., Ltd., 1934.

474. Emmel, H. E., and LeCoco, J. F.: Hamstring transplant for the prevention of calcaneocavus foot in poliomyelitis. J. Bone Joint Surg., 40–A:911, 1958.

475. Fitchet, S. M.: "Flexion deformity" of the hip and the lateral intermuscular septum. New Eng. J. Med., 209:74, 1933.

476. Fitzgerald, F. P., and Seddon, H. J.: Lambrinudi's operation for drop-foot. Brit. J. Surg., 25:283, 1937.

477. Flexner, S., and Lewis, P. A.: Transmission of acute poliomyelitis to monkeys. J.A.M.A., 53:1639, 1909.

478. Flint, M. H., and MacKenzie, I. C.: Anterior laxity of the ankle. A cause of recurrent paralytic drop foot deformity. J. Bone Joint Surg., 44–B:377, 1962.

479. Forbes, A. M.: The tensor fasciae femoris as a cause of deformity. J. Bone Joint Surg., 10:579, 1928.

480. Fried, A., and Hendel, C.: Paralytic valgus deformity of the ankle. Replacement of the paralyzed tibialis posterior by the peroneus longus. J. Bone Joint Surg., 39–A:921, 1957.

481. Friedenberg, Z. B.: Arthrodesis of the tarsal bones. A study of failure of fusions. Arch. Surg., 57:162, 1948.

482. Friedenberg, Z. B.: Transposition of the biceps brachii for triceps weakness. J. Bone Joint Surg., 36–A:656, 1954.

483. Gill, A. B.: A new operation for arthrodesis of the shoulder. J. Bone Joint Surg., 13:287, 1931.

484. Gill, A. B.: An operation to make a posterior bone block at the ankle to limit foot-drop. J. Bone Joint Surg., 15:166, 1933.

485. Girard, P. M.: Ankle joint stabilization with motion. J. Bone Joint Surg., 17:802, 1935.

486. Goldner, J. L.: Paralytic equinovarus deformities of the foot. Southern Med. J., 42:83, 1949.

487. Goldner, J. L., and Irwin, C. E.: Paralytic deformities of the foot. In A.A.O.S. Instructional Course Lectures. Vol. 5. Ann Arbor, J. W. Edwards, 1948.

488. Goldthwait, J. E.: Tendon transplantation in the treatment of deformities resulting from infantile paralysis. Boston Med. Surg. J., 133:447, 1895.

489. Goldthwait, J. E.: The direct transplantation of muscles in the treatment of paralytic deformities. Five cases of transplantation of the sartorius muscle. Boston Med. Surg. J., 137:489, 1897.

490. Goldthwait, J. E.: An operation for the stiffening of the ankle joint in infantile paralysis. Amer. J. Orthop. Surg., 5:271, 1908.

491. Green, W. T.: Tendon transplantation in rehabilitation. J.A.M.A., 163:1235, 1957.

492. Green, W. T., and Grice, D. S.: The treatment of poliomyelitis: Acute and convalescent stages. A.A.O.S. Instructional Course Lectures. Vol. 13. Ann Arbor, J. W. Edwards, 1951, p. 261.

493. Green, W. T., and Grice, D. S.: The management of chronic poliomyelitis. A.A.O.S. Instructional Course Lectures. Vol. 9. Ann Arbor, J. W. Edwards, 1952.

494. Green, W. T., and Grice, D. S.: The surgical correction of the paralytic foot. A.A.O.S. Instructional Course Lectures. Vol. 10. Ann Arbor, J. W. Edwards, 1953, pp. 343–363.

495. Green, W. T., and Grice, D. S.: The management of calcaneus deformity. A.A.O.S. Instructional Course Lectures. Vol. 13. Ann Arbor, J. W. Edwards, 1956, pp. 135–149.

496. Grice, D. S.: An extra-articular arthrodesis of the subastragalar joint for correction of paralytic flat feet in children. J. Bone Joint Surg., 34–A:927, 1952.

497. Grice, D. S.: Further experience with extra-articular arthrodesis of the subtalar joint. J. Bone Joint Surg., 36–A:246, 1955.

498. Grice, D. S.: The role of subtalar fusion in the treatment of valgus deformities of the feet. A.A.O.S. Instructional Course Lectures. Vol. 16. St. Louis, C. V. Mosby Co., 1959, p. 127.

499. Grilli, F. P.: Il trapianto del bicipite brachiale in funzione pronatoria. Arch. Putti, 12:359, 1959.

500. Groves, E. W. H.: Some contributions to the reconstructive surgery of the hip. Brit. J. Surg., 14:486, 1926–1927.

501. Guildal, P., and Sodeman, T.: Results of 256 tri-articular arthrodeses of the foot in sequelae of infantile paralysis. Acta Orthop. Scand., 1:199, 1930–1931.

502. Gunn, D. R., and Molesworth, B. D.: The use of tibialis posterior as a dorsiflexor. J. Bone Joint Surg., 39–B: 674, 1957.

503. Haas, S. L.: The treatment of permanent paralysis of the deltoid muscle. J.A.M.A., 104:99, 1935.

504. Haas, S. L.: Correction of extreme flexion contracture of the knee joint. J. Bone Joint Surg., 20:839, 1938.

505. Hallgrimsson, S.: Studies on reconstructive and stabilizing operations on the skeleton of the foot, with special reference to subastragalar arthrodesis in treatment of foot deformities following infantile paralysis. Acta Chir. Scand. Suppl. 78, 88:1, 1943.

506. Hallock, H.: Surgical stabilization of dislocated paralytic hips; end-result study. Surg. Gynec. Obstet., 75:742, 1942.

507. Hallock, H.: Arthrodesis of the hip for instability and pain in poliomyelitis. J. Bone Joint Surg., 32–A:904, 1950.

508. Hallock, H.: Hip arthrodesis in poliomyelitis. Bull. N.Y. Hosp., 2:18, 1958.

509. Hamsa, W. R.: Panastragaloid arthrodesis. A study of end-results in eighty-five cases. J. Bone Joint Surg., 18:732, 1936.

510. Harmon, P. H.: Anterior transplantation of the posterior deltoid for shoulder palsy and dislocation in poliomyelitis. Surg. Gynec. Obstet., 84:117, 1947.

511. Harmon, P. H.: Technic of utilizing latissimus dorsi

muscle in transplantation for triceps palsy. J. Bone Joint Surg., *31–A*:409, 1949.

512. Harmon, P. H.: Surgical reconstruction of the paralytic shoulder by multiple muscle transplantation. J. Bone Joint Surg., *32–A*:583, 1950.

513. Hart, V. L.: Corrective cast for flexion-contracture deformity of the knee. J. Bone Joint Surg., *16*:970, 1934.

514. Hart, V. L.: Arthrodesis of the foot in infantile paralysis. Surg. Gynec. Obstet., *64*:794, 1937.

515. Hart, V. L.: Lambrinudi operation for drop-foot. J. Bone Joint Surg., *22*:937, 1940.

516. Henderson, M. S.: Reconstructive surgery in paralytic deformities of the lower leg. J. Bone Joint Surg., *11*: 810, 1929.

517. Henry, A. H.: An operation for slinging a dropped shoulder. Brit. J. Surg., *15*:95, 1927.

518. Henry, A. H.: Extensile Exposure Applied to Limb Surgery. 2nd Ed. Baltimore, Williams & Wilkins Co., 1957.

519. Herndon, C. H.: Tendon transplantation at the knee and foot. A.A.O.S. Instructional Course Lectures. Vol. 18. St. Louis, C. V. Mosby Co., 1961.

520. Herndon, C. H., Strong, J. M., and Heyman, C. H.: Transposition of the tibialis anterior in the treatment of paralytic talipes calcaneus. J. Bone Joint Surg., *38–A*:751, 1956.

521. Herzmark, M. H.: Traumatic paralysis of the serratus anterior relieved by transplantation of the rhomboidei. J. Bone Joint Surg., *33–A*:235, 1951.

522. Heyman, C. H.: A method for the correction of paralytic genu recurvatum. Report of a bilateral case. J. Bone Joint Surg., *6*:689, 1924.

523. Heyman, C. H.: Operative treatment of paralytic genu recurvatum. J. Bone Joint Surg., *29*:644, 1947.

524. Heyman, C. H.: Operative treatment of paralytic genu recurvatum. J. Bone Joint Surg., *44–A*:1246, 1962.

525. Hildebrandt, A.: Über eine neue Methode der Muskeltransplantation. Arch. Klin. Chir., *78*:75, 1906.

526. Hipps, H. E.: Clinical significance of certain microscopic changes in muscles of anterior poliomyelitis. J. Bone Joint Surg., *24*:68, 1942.

527. Hogshead, H. P., and Ponseti, I. V.: Fascia lata transfer to the erector spinae for the treatment of flexion-abduction contractures of the hip in patients with poliomyelitis and meningomyelocele. Evaluation of results. J. Bone Joint Surg., *46–A*:1389, 1964.

528. Hohmann, G.: Ersatz des gelähmten Biceps brachii durch den Pectoralis major. München. Med. Wschr., *65*:1240, 1918.

529. Hohmann, G.: Operative Verwertung erhaltener Muskeln bei Kinderlähmung. München. Med. Wschr., *92*:249, 1950.

530. Hoke, M.: An operation for stabilizing paralytic feet. Amer. J. Orthop. Surg., *3*:494, 1921.

531. Holmdahl, H. C.: Astragalectomy as a stabilizing operation for foot paralysis following poliomyelitis; results of a follow-up investigation of 153 cases. Acta Orthop. Scand., *25*:207, 1956.

532. Hovnanian, A. P.: Latissimus dorsi transplantation for loss of flexion or extension at the elbow. Ann. Surg., *143*:493, 1956.

533. Hunt, J. C., and Brooks, A. L.: Subtalar extra-articular arthrodesis for correction of paralytic valgus deformity of the foot. Evaluation of forty-four procedures with particular reference to associated tendon transference. J. Bone Joint Surg., *47–A*:1310, 1965.

534. Hunt, W. S., Jr., and Thompson, H. A.: Pantalar arthrodesis. A one-stage operation. J. Bone Joint Surg., *36–A*:349, 1954.

535. Inclan, A.: End results in physiological blocking of flail joints. J. Bone Joint Surg., *31–A*:748, 1949.

536. Ingersoll, R. E.: Transplantation of peroneus longus to anterior tibial insertion in poliomyelitis. Surg. Gynec. Obstet., *86*:717, 1948.

537. Ingram, A. J., and Hundley, J. M.: Posterior bone block of the ankle for paralytic equinus. An end-result study. J. Bone Joint Surg., *33–A*:679, 1951.

538. Irwin, C. E.: Transplants to the thumb to restore function of opposition: End results. Southern Med. J., *35*:257, 1942.

539. Irwin, C. E.: Genu recurvatum following poliomyelitis; controlled method of operative correction. J.A.M.A., *120*:277, 1942.

540. Irwin, C. E.: Subtrochanteric osteotomy in poliomyelitis. J.A.M.A., *133*:231, 1947.

541. Irwin, C. E.: The iliotibial band, its role in producing deformity in poliomyelitis. J. Bone Joint Surg., *31–A*: 141, 1949.

542. Irwin, C. E., and Eyler, D. L.: Surgical rehabilitation of the hand and forearm disabled by poliomyelitis. J. Bone Joint Surg., *33–A*:679, 1951.

543. Johnson, E. W., Jr.: Results of modern methods of treatment of poliomyelitis. J. Bone Joint Surg., *27*: 223, 1945.

544. Johnson, E. W., Jr.: Contractures of the iliotibial band. Surg. Gynec. Obstet., *96*:599, 1953.

545. Jones, G. B.: Paralytic dislocation of the hip. J. Bone Joint Surg., *36–B*:375, 1954.

546. Jones, G. B.: Paralytic dislocation of the hip. J. Bone Joint Surg., *44–B*:573, 1962.

547. Kettelkamp, D. B., and Larson, C. B.: Evaluation of the Steindler flexorplasty. J. Bone Joint Surg., *45–A*:513, 1963.

548. Key, J. A.: Arthrodesis of the shoulder by means of osteoperiosteal grafts. Surg. Gynec. Obstet., *50*:468, 1930.

549. King, B. B.: Ankle fusion for the correction of paralytic drop foot and calcaneus deformity. Arch. Surg., *40*:90, 1940.

550. Kleinberg, S.: The transplantation of the adductor longus in its entirety to supplement the quadriceps femoris. Bull. Hosp. Joint Dis., *18*:117, 1957.

551. Kreuscher, P. H.: The substitution of the erector spinae for paralyzed gluteal muscles. Surg. Gynec. Obstet., *40*:593, 1925.

552. Kuhlmann, R. F., and Bell, J. F.: A clinical evaluation of tendon transplantations for poliomyelitis affecting the lower extremities. J. Bone Joint Surg., *34–A*:915, 1952.

553. Lambrinudi, C.: New operation on drop-foot. Brit. J. Surg., *15*:193, 1927.

554. Lambrinudi, C.: A method of correcting equinus and calcaneus deformities at the sub-astragaloid joint. Proc. Roy. Soc. Med. (Section on Orthopaedics), *26*: 788, 1933.

555. Landsteiner, K., and Popper, E.: Übertragung der Poliomyelitis acuta auf Affen. Z. Immunitätsforsch. Exp. Ther. Orig., *2*:377, 1909.

556. Lange, F.: Die epidemische Kinderlähmung. München, J. F. Lehmann, 1930.

557. Leavitt, D. G.: Subastragaloid arthrodesis for the os calcis type of flat foot. Amer. J. Surg., *59*:501, 1943.

558. LeCoeur, P.: Procédés de restauration de la flexion du coude paralytique. Rev. Chir. Orthop., *39*:655, 1953.

559. Legg, A. T.: Transplantation of tensor fasciae femoris in cases of weakened gluteus medius. J.A.M.A., *80*: 242, 1923.

560. Legg, A. T.: Tensor fasciae femoris transplantation in cases of weakened gluteus medius. New Eng. J. Med., *209*:61, 1933.

561. Legg, A. T., and Merrill, J. T.: Physical Therapy in Infantile Paralysis. Hagerstown, Md., W. F. Prior Co., Inc., 1932.

562. Lewis, D. D.: Trapezius transplantation in the treatment of deltoid paralysis. J.A.M.A., *55*:2211, 1910.

563. Liebolt, F. L.: Pantalar arthrodesis in poliomyelitis. Surgery, *6*:31, 1939.

564. Lipscomb, P. R., and Sanchez, J. J.: Anterior transplantation of the posterior tibial tendon for persistent palsy of the common peroneal nerve. J. Bone Joint Surg., *43–A*:60, 1961.

565. Lorthioir, J.: Huit cas d'arthrodèse du pied avec extirpation temporaire de l'astragale. J. Chir. Ann. Soc. Belge Chir., *11*:184, 1911.

566. Lovett, R. W.: The Treatment of Infantile Paralysis. Philadelphia, P. Blakiston's Son & Co., 1916.

567. Lowman, C. L.: Abdominal Fascial Transplants. Los Angeles, privately printed, 1954.

568. Lowman, C. L.: Fascial transplants in paralysis of abdominal and shoulder girdle muscles. A.A.O.S. Instructional Course Lectures. Vol. 14. Ann Arbor, J. W. Edwards, 1957, p. 300.

569. Lowman, C. L.: Fascial transplants in relation to muscle function. J. Bone Joint Surg., 45–A:199, 1963.

570. MacAusland, W. R., and MacAusland, A. R.: Astragalectomy (the Whitman operation) in paralytic deformities of the foot. Ann. Surg., 80:861, 1924.

571. McFarland, B.: Paralytic instability of the foot (editorial). J. Bone Joint Surg., 33–B:493, 1951.

572. MacKenzie, I. G.: Lambrinudi's arthrodesis. J. Bone Joint Surg., 41–B:738, 1959.

573. Magoffin, R. L., Lennette, E. H., Hollister, A. C., Jr., and Schmidt, N. J.: An etiologic study of clinical paralytic poliomyelitis. J.A.M.A., 175:269, 1961.

574. Makin, M.: Tibiofibular relationship in paralyzed limbs. J. Bone Joint Surg., 47–B:500, 1965.

575. Makin, M., and Yossipovitch, Z.: Translocation of the peroneus longus in the treatment of paralytic pes calcaneus. A follow-up study of thirty-three cases. J. Bone Joint Surg., 48–A:1541, 1966.

576. Malvarez, O.: Arthrodesis subastragalina extraarticular en el pie valgo pronado pavalitico. Arthrodesis minima. Estudio de 87 casos. Rev. Ortop. Traum., Lat. Amer., 2:251, 1957.

577. Marek, F. M., and Schein, A. J.: Aseptic necrosis of the astragalus following arthrodesing procedures of the tarsus. J. Bone Joint Surg., 27:587, 1945.

578. Mayer, L.: The physiological method of tendon transplantation. I. Historical; anatomy and physiology of tendons. Surg. Gynec. Obstet., 22:182, 1916.

579. Mayer, L.: The physiological method of tendon transplantation. II. Operative technique. Surg. Gynec. Obstet., 22:298, 1916.

580. Mayer, L.: The physiological method of tendon transplantation. III. Experimental and clinical experiences. Surg. Gynec. Obstet., 22:472, 1916.

581. Mayer, L.: Transplantation of the trapezius for paralysis of the abductors of the arm. J. Bone Joint Surg., 9:412, 1927.

582. Mayer, L.: Fixed paralytic obliquity of the pelvis. J. Bone Joint Surg., 13:1, 1931.

583. Mayer, L.: Operative reconstruction of the paralyzed upper extremity. J. Bone Joint Surg., 21:377, 1939.

584. Mayer, L.: The significance of the iliocostal fascial graft in the treatment of paralytic deformities of the trunk. J. Bone Joint Surg., 26:257, 1944.

585. Mayer, L.: The physiologic method of tendon transplants. Reviewed after forty years. A.A.O.S. Instructional Course Lectures. Vol. 13. Ann Arbor, J. W. Edwards, 1956, p. 116.

586. Mayer, L., and Green, W.: Experiences with the Steindler flexorplasty at the elbow. J. Bone Joint Surg., 36–A:775, 1954.

587. Medin, O.: L'état aigu de la paralysie infantile. Arch. Méd. Enf., 1:257, 321, 1898.

588. Miller, O. L.: Paralytic knee fusions. Southern Med. J., 20:782, 1927.

589. Miller, O. L.: Surgical management of pes calcaneus. J. Bone Joint Surg., 18:169, 1936.

590. Mortens, J., and Pilcher, M. F.: Tendon transplantation in the prevention of foot deformities after poliomyelitis in children. J. Bone Joint Surg., 38–B:633, 1956.

591. Mortens, J., Gregersey, P., and Zachariae, L.: Tendon transplantation in the foot after poliomyelitis in children. Acta Orthop. Scand., 27:153, 1957–1958.

592. Mustard, W. T.: Iliopsoas transfer for weakness of the hip abductors; preliminary report. J. Bone Joint Surg., 34–A:647, 1952.

593. Mustard, W. T.: A follow-up study of iliopsoas transfer for hip instability. J. Bone Joint Surg., 41–B:289, 1959.

594. Nicoladoni, C.: Nachtrag zum Pes calcaneus und zur Transplantation der Peronealsehnen. Arch. Klin. Chir., 27:660, 1881.

595. Nieny, K.: Zur Behandlung der Fussdeformitaten bei ausgedehnten Lahmungen. Arch. Orthop. Unfallchir., 3:60, 1905.

596. Nyholm, K.: Elbow flexorplasty in tendon transposition (an analysis of the functional result in 26 patients). Acta Orthop. Scand., 33:30, 1963.

597. Ober, F. R.: An operation for relief of paralysis of the gluteus maximus muscle. J.A.M.A., 88:1063, 1927.

598. Ober, F. R.: Operative and postoperative treatment of infantile paralysis. New Eng. J. Med., 205:300, 1931.

599. Ober, F. R.: An operation to relieve paralysis of the deltoid muscle. J.A.M.A., 99:2182, 1932.

600. Ober, F. R.: Tendon transplantation in the lower extremity. New Eng. J. Med., 209:52, 1933.

601. Ober, F. R.: The role of the iliotibial band and fascia lata as a factor in the causation of low-back disabilities and sciatica. J. Bone Joint Surg., 18:105, 1936.

602. Ober, F. R.: Transplantation to improve the function of the shoulder joint and extensor function of the elbow joint. A.A.O.S. Lectures on Reconstructive Surgery. Vol. 2. Ann Arbor, J. W. Edwards, 1944, p. 274.

603. Ober, F. R., and Barr, J. S.: Brachioradialis muscle transposition for triceps weakness. Surg. Gynec. Obstet., 67:105, 1938.

604. Paluska, D. J., and Blount, W. P.: Ankle valgus after the Grice subtalar stabilization: the late evaluation of a personal series with a modified technic. Clin. Orthop., 59:137, 1968.

605. Parsons, D. W., and Seddon, H. J.: The results of operations for disorders of the hip caused by poliomyelitis. J. Bone Joint Surg., 50–B:266, 1968.

606. Patterson, R. L., Parrish, F. F., and Hathaway, E. N.: Stabilizing operations on the foot. A study of the indications, techniques used, and end results. J. Bone Joint Surg., 32–A:1, 1950.

607. Pauker, E.: Correction of the outwardly rotated leg from poliomyelitis. J. Bone Joint Surg., 41–B:70, 1959.

608. Peabody, C. W.: Tendon transposition; an end-result study. J. Bone Joint Surg., 20:193, 1938.

609. Peabody, C. W.: Tendon transposition in the paralytic foot. A.A.O.S. Instructional Course Lectures. Vol. 6. Ann Arbor, J. W. Edwards, 1949, p. 178.

610. Peabody, C. W., Draper, G., and Dochez, A. R.: A clinical study of acute poliomyelitis. Monograph No. 4, Rockefeller Inst. of Med. Research, New York, 1912.

611. Pollock, J. H., and Carrell, B.: Subtalar extra-articular arthrodesis in the treatment of paralytic valgus deformities. A review of 112 procedures in 100 patients. J. Bone Joint Surg., 46–A:533, 1964.

612. Pollock, L. J.: Accessory muscle movements in deltoid paralysis. J.A.M.A., 79:526, 1922.

613. Putti, V.: Rapporti statici fra piede e ginocchio nell' arto paralitico. Chir. Organi. Mov., 6:125, 1922.

614. Putti, V.: Due sindromi paralitiche del'arto superiore. Note di fisiopatologia della rotazione antibrachiale. Chir. Organi Mov., 26:215, 1940.

615. Pyka, R. A., Coventry, M. B., Moe, J. H.: Anterior subluxation of the talus following triple arthrodesis. J. Bone Joint Surg., 46–A:16, 1964.

616. Rapp, I. H.: Serratus anterior paralysis treated by transplantation of pectoralis minor. J. Bone Joint Surg., 36–A:852, 1954.

617. Reidy, J. A., Broderick, T. F., Jr., and Barr, J. S.: Tendon transplantations in the lower extremity. A review of end results in poliomyelitis. I. Tendon transplantations about the foot and ankle. J. Bone Joint Surg., 34–A:900, 1952.

618. Riedel, G.: Zur Frage der Muskeltransplantation bei Deltoides lähmung. Ergebn. Chir. Orthop., 21:489, 1928.

619. Riska, E. B.: Transposition of the tractus iliotibialis to the patella as a treatment of quadriceps paralysis and certain deformities of the lower extremity after poliomyelitis. Acta Orthop. Scand., 32:140, 1962.

620. Rissler, J.: Zur Kenntnis der Veranderungen des Nervensystems bei Poliomyelitis anterior acuta. Nord. Med. Ark., 11:22:1, 1888.

621. Rountree, C. R., and Rockwood, C. A., Jr.: Arthrodesis of the shoulder in children following infantile paralysis. Southern Med. J., 52:861, 1959.

622. Rugtveit, A.: Extra-articular arthrodesis according to Green-Grice, in flat feet. Acta Orthop. Scand., 34:367, 1964.

623. Ryerson, E. W.: Arthrodesing operations on the feet. J. Bone Joint Surg., 5:453, 1923.

624. Sabin, A. B.: Pathology and pathogenesis of human poliomyelitis. J.A.M.A., 120:506, 1942.

625. Sabin, A. B.: Oral poliovirus vaccine. History of its development and prospects. Eradication of poliomyelitis. J.A.M.A., 194:872, 1965.

626. Sabin, A. B., Michaels, R. H., Spigland, I., Pelon, W., Rhim, J. A., and Wahr, R. E.: Community-wide use of oral poliovirus vaccine. Amer. J. Dis. Child., 101:546, 1961.

627. Saha, A. K.: Theory of Shoulder Mechanism: Descriptive and Applied. Springfield, Ill., Charles C Thomas, 1961.

628. Saha, A. K.: Surgical rehabilitation of paralyzed shoulder following poliomyelitis in adults and children. J. Int. Coll. Surg., 42:198, 1964.

629. Saha, A. K.: Surgery of the paralyzed and flail shoulder. Acta Orthop. Scand., Suppl. 97, 1967.

630. Salk, J. E.: Studies in human subjects on active immunization against poliomyelitis. J.A.M.A., 151:1081, 1953.

631. Scheer, G. E., and Crego, C. H., Jr.: A two-stage stabilization procedure for correction of calcaneocavus. J. Bone Joint Surg., 38–A:1247, 1956.

632. Schnute, W. J., and Tachdjian, M. O.: Intermetacarpal bone block for thenar paralysis following poliomyelitis. J. Bone Joint Surg., 45–A:1663, 1963.

633. Schottsdaedt, E. R., Larsen, L. J., and Bost, F. C.: Complete muscle transposition. J. Bone Joint Surg., 37–A:897, 1955.

634. Schottstaedt, E. R., Larsen, L. J., and Bost, F. C.: The surgical reconstruction of the upper extremity paralyzed by poliomyelitis. J. Bone Joint Surg., 40-A:633, 1958.

635. Schwartz, R. P.: Arthrodesis of subtalus and midtarsal joints of the foot; historical review, preoperative determinations, and operative procedure. Surgery, 20:619, 1946.

636. Schwartzmann, J. R., and Crego, C. H., Jr.: Hamstring-tendon transplantation for the relief of quadriceps femoris paralysis in residual poliomyelitis. A follow-up study of 134 cases. J. Bone Joint Surg., 30–A:541, 1948.

637. Seddon, H. J.: Transplantation of pectoralis major for paralysis of the flexors of the elbow. Proc. Roy. Soc. Med., 42:837, 1949.

638. Segal, A., Seddon, H. J., and Brooks, D. M.: Treatment of paralysis of the flexors of the elbow. J. Bone Joint Surg., 41–B:44, 1959.

639. Seymour, N., and Evans, D. K.: A modification of the Grice subtalar arthrodesis. J. Bone Joint Surg., 50–B:372, 1968.

640. Sharp, N. N., Guhl, J. F., Sorensen, R. I., and Voshell, A. F.: Hip fusion in poliomyelitis in children. A preliminary report. J. Bone Joint Surg., 46–A:121, 1964.

641. Sharrard, W. J. W.: Muscle recovery in poliomyelitis. J. Bone Joint Surg., 37–B:63, 1955.

642. Siffert, R. S., Forster, R. I., and Nachamie, B.: "Beak" triple arthrodesis for correction of severe cavus deformity. *In* DePalma, A. F. (ed.): Clinical Orthopaedics and Related Research, Vol. 45. Philadelphia, J. B. Lippincott Co., 1966.

643. Smith, A. deF., and von Lackum, H. L.: Subastragaloid arthrodesis. Surg. Gynec. Obstet., 40:836, 1925.

644. Smith, E. T., Pevey, J. K., and Shindler, T. O.: The erector spinae transplant—a misnomer. Clin. Orthop., 30:144, 1963.

645. Smith, J.. B., and Westin, G.: Subtalar extra-articular arthrodesis. J. Bone Joint Surg., 50–A:1027, 1968.

646. Somerville, E. W.: Paralytic dislocation of the hip. J. Bone Joint Surg., 41–B:279, 1959.

647. Soule, R. E.: Further considerations of arthrodesis in the treatment of lateral deformity of the foot. Amer. J. Orthop. Surg., 12:422, 1915.

648. Soutter, R.: A new operation for hip contractures in poliomyelitis. Boston Med. Surg. J., 170:380, 1914.

649. Spira, E.: The treatment of dropped shoulder, a new operative technique. J. Bone Joint Surg., 30–A:229, 1948.

650. Spira, E.: Replacement of biceps brachii by pectoralis minor transplant. Report of a case. J. Bone Joint Surg., 39–B:126, 1957.

651. Staples, O. S.: Posterior arthrodesis of the ankle and subtalar joints. J. Bone Joint Surg., 38–A:50, 1956.

652. Staples, O. S., and Watkins, A. L.: Full active abduction in traumatic paralysis of deltoid. J. Bone Joint Surg., 25:85, 1943.

653. Steigman, A. J.: The control of poliomyelitis. J. Pediat., 59:163, 1961.

654. Steindler, A.: A muscle plasty for the relief of flail elbow in infantile paralysis. Interstate Med. J., 25:235, 1918.

655. Steindler, A.: Orthopedic reconstruction work on hand and forearm. N.Y. Med. J., 108:1117, 1918.

656. Steindler, A.: Operative treatment of paralytic conditions of the upper extremity. J. Orthop. Surg., 1:608, 1919.

657. Steindler, A.: The treatment of the flail ankle; panastragaloid arthrodesis. J. Bone Joint Surg., 5:284, 1923.

658. Steindler, A.: Reconstructive Surgery of the Upper Extremity. New York, D. Appleton & Co., 1923, p. 56.

659. Steindler, A.: Orthopedic Operations. Indications, Technique, and End Results. Springfield, Ill., Charles C Thomas, 1940, p. 129.

660. Steindler, A.: Muscle and tendon transplantation at the elbow. A.A.O.S. Instructional Course Lectures on Reconstruction Surgery. Ann Arbor, J. W. Edwards, 1944, p. 276.

661. Steindler, A.: Newer pathological and physiological concepts of anterior poliomyelitis and their clinical interpretation. J. Bone Joint Surg., 29:59, 1947.

662. Steindler, A.: Reconstruction of poliomyelitic upper extremity. Bull. Hosp. Joint. Dis., 15:21, 1954.

663. Storen, G.: Genu recurvatum. Treatment by wedge osteotomy of tibia with use of compression. Acta Chir. Scand., 114:40, 1957.

664. Straub, L. R., Harvey, J. P., Jr., and Fuerst, C. E.: A clinical evaluation of tendon transplantation in the paralytic foot. J. Bone Joint Surg., 39–A:1, 1957.

665. Sutherland, D. H., Bost, F. C., and Schottstaedt, E. R.: Electromyographic study of transplanted muscles about the knee in poliomyelitic patients. J. Bone Joint Surg., 42–A:919, 1960.

666. Thomas, C. I., Thompson, T. C., and Straub, C. R.: Transplantation of the external oblique muscle for abductor paralysis. J. Bone Joint Surg., 32–A:207, 1950.

667. Thompson, C. E.: Fusion of the metacarpals of the thumb and index finger to maintain functional position of the thumb. J. Bone Joint Surg., 24:907, 1942.

668. Thompson, T. C.: Astragalectomy and the treatment of calcaneovalgus. J. Bone Joint Surg., 21:627, 1939.

669. Thompson, T. C.: A modified operation for opponens paralysis. J. Bone Joint Surg., 24:632, 1942.

670. Toupet, R.: Technique d'enchevillement du tarse, réalisant l'arthrodèse de torsion et la limitation des movements d'extension du pied. J. Chir. (Paris), 16:268, 1920.

671. Towsend, W. R.: Treatment of the paralytic clubfoot by arthrodesis. Amer. J. Orthop. Surg., 3:378, 1905.

672. Tubby, A. H.: A case illustrating the operative treatment of paralysis of serratus magnus by muscle grafting. Brit. Med. J., 2:1159, 1904.

673. Underwood, M.: Treatise on Diseases of Children with General Directions of Infants from Birth. London, J. Churchill, 1789.

674. Von Baeyer, H.: Translokation von Sehnen. Z. Orthop. Chir., 56:552, 1932.

675. Von Heine, J.: Beobachtungen über Lähmungszustande der unteren Extremitäten und deren Behandlung. Stuttgart, Kohler, 1840.

676. Von Lesser, L.: Ueber operative Behandlung des Pes varus paralyticus. Zbl. Chir., 6:497, 1879.

677. Wagner, L. C.: Modified bone block (Campbell) of ankle for paralytic drop foot with report of twenty-seven cases. J. Bone Joint Surg., 13:142, 1931.

678. Wagner, L. C., and Rizzo, P. C.: Stabilization of the hip by transplantation of the anterior thigh muscles. J. Bone Joint Surg., 18:180, 1936.

679. Waterman, J. H.: Tendon transplantation. Its history, indications, and technic. Med. News, 81:54, 1902.

680. Watkins, M. B., Jones, J. B., Ryder, C. T., Jr., and Brown, T. H., Jr.: Transplantation of the posterior tibial tendon. J. Bone Joint Surg., 36-A:1181, 1954.

681. Watson-Jones, R.: Extra-articular arthrodesis of the shoulder. J. Bone Joint Surg., 15:862, 1933.

682. Waugh, T. R., Wagner, J., and Stinchfield, F. E.: An evaluation of pantalar arthrodesis. A follow-up study of one hundred and sixteen operations. J. Bone Joint Surg., 47–A:1315, 1965.

683. Weissman, S. L.: Capsular arthroplasty in paralytic dislocation of the hip. A preliminary report. J. Bone Joint Surg., 41–A:429, 1959.

684. Weissman, S. L., Torok, G., and Kharmosh, O.: L'arthrodèse extraarticulaire avec transplantation tendineuse concomitante dans le traitement du pied plat valgus paralytique du jeune enfant. Rev. Chir. Orthop., 43:79, 1957.

685. Westin, G. W.: Tendon transfers about the foot, ankle, and hip in the paralyzed lower extremity. (Instructional Course Lectures) J. Bone Joint Surg., 42–A:1430, 1965.

686. Whitman, A.: Astragalectomy and backward displacement of the foot. An investigation of its practical results. J. Bone Joint Surg., 4:266, 1922.

687. Whitman, R.: The operative treatment of paralytic talipes of the calcaneus type. Amer. J. Med. Sci.,122:593, 1901.

688. Wickman, O. I.: Studien über Poliomyelitis acuta. Arb. Path. Inst. Univ. Helsingfors. Berl., 1:109, 1905.

689. Willard, DeF. P.: Subastragalar arthrodesis in lateral deformities of paralytic feet. Amer. J. Orthop. Surg., 14:323, 1916.

690. Williamson, G. A., Moe, J. H., and Basom, W. C.: Results of the Lowman operation for paralysis of the abdominal muscles. Minn. Med., 25:117, 1942.

691. Wilson, F. C., Jr., Fay, G. F., Lamotte, P., and Williams, J. C.: Triple arthrodesis. A study of the factors affecting fusion after three hundred and one procedures. J. Bone Joint Surg., 11:40, 1929.

692. Wilson, P. D.: Posterior capsulotomy in certain flexion contractures of the knee. J. Bone Joint Surg., 11:40, 1929.

693. Yount, C. C.: The role of the tensor fasciae femoris in certain deformities of the lower extremities. J. Bone Joint Surg., 8:171, 1926.

694. Yount, C. C.: An operation to improve function in quadriceps paralysis. J. Bone Joint Surg., 20:314, 1938.

695. Zachariae, L.: The Grice operation for paralytic flat feet in children. Acta Orthop. Scand., 33:80, 1963.

696. Zancolli, E. A.: Paralytic supination contracture of the forearm. J. Bone Joint Surg., 49-A:1275, 1967.

697. Zaoussis, A. L.: Osteotomy of the proximal end of the radius for paralytic supination deformity in children. J. Bone Joint Surg., 45-B:523, 1963.

OBSTETRICAL BRACHIAL PLEXUS PALSY

698. Adler, J. B., and Patterson, R. L.: Erb's palsy. Long-term results of treatment in eighty-eight cases. J. Bone Joint Surg., 49-A:1052, 1967.

699. Aitken, J.: Deformity of the elbow joint as a sequel to Erb's obstetrical paralysis. J. Bone Joint Surg., 34-B:352, 1952.

700. Babbitt, D. P., and Cassidy, R. H.: Obstetrical paralysis and dislocation of the shoulder in infancy. J. Bone Joint Surg., 50-A:144, 1968.

701. Blount, W. P.: Osteoclasis for supination deformities in children. J. Bone Joint Surg., 22:300, 1940.

702. Bullard, W. N.: Obstetric paralysis. Amer. J. Med. Sci., 134:93, 1907.

703. Burman, M.: Paralytic supination contracture of the forearm. J. Bone Joint Surg., 38-A:303, 1956.

704. Clark, L. P., Taylor, A. S., and Prout, T. P.: A study of brachial birth palsy. Amer. J. Med. Sci., 130:670, 1905.

705. Duchenne, G. B. A.: De l'Éléctrisation Localisée et de Son Application à la Pathologie et à la Thérapeutique. 3rd Ed. Paris, Baillière, 1872, p. 357.

706. Erb, W. H.: Ueber eine Eigenthümliche Localisation von Lähmungen im Plexus Brachialis. Verhandl. Naturhist. Med. Heidelberg, N.F., 2:130, 1874.

707. Fairbank, H. A. T.: Birth palsy: Subluxation of shoulder joint in infants and young children. Lancet, 1:1217, 1913.

708. Gilmour, J.: Notes on the surgical treatment of brachial birth palsy. Lancet, 2:696, 1925.

709. Granberry, W. M., and Lipscomb, P. R.: Tendon transfers to the hand in brachial palsy. Amer. J. Surg., 108:840, 1964.

710. Green, W. T., and Tachdjian, M. O.: Correction of residual deformities of the shoulder in obstetrical palsy. J. Bone Joint Surg., 45-A:1544, 1963.

711. Klumpke, A.: Contribution à l'étude des paralysies radiculaires du plexus brachial. Paralysies radiculaires totales. Paralysies radiculaires inférieures. De la participation des filets sympathiques oculo-pupilaires dans ces paralysies. Rev. Méd. (Paris), 5:591, 1885.

712. L'Episcopo, J. B.: Tendon transplantation in obstetrical paralysis. Amer. J. Surg., 25:122, 1934.

713. L'Episcopo, J. B.: Restoration of muscle balance in the treatment of obstetrical paralysis. New York J. Med., 39:357, 1939.

714. Liebolt, F. L., and Furry, J. G.: Obstetrical paralysis with dislocation of the shoulder. J. Bone Joint Surg., 35-A:227, 1953.

715. Lovett, R.: The surgical aspect of the paralysis of newborn children. Boston Med. Surg. J., 127:8, 1892.

716. Mastandrea, G.: Il traplanto del muscolo tricitite brachiale sul bicipite negli esiti della paralisi obstetrica. Ortop. Traumatol., 23:953, 1953.

717. Moore, B. H.: A new operation for brachial birth palsy—Erb's paralysis. Surg. Gynec. Obstet., 61:832, 1935.

718. Moore, B. H.: Brachial birth palsy. Amer. J. Surg., 43:338, 1939.

719. Morison, J. E.: Peripheral brachial paralysis in infants and children. Arch. Dis. Child., 13:310, 1938.

720. Patterson, R. L., Jr.: Obstetrical paralysis. Physiother. Rev., 20:291, 1940.

721. Scaglietti, O.: The obstetrical shoulder trauma. Surg. Gynec. Obstet., 66:868, 1938.

722. Sever, J. W.: Obstetrical paralysis. Its etiology, pathology, clinical aspects, and treatment, with a report of 470 cases. Amer. J. Dis. Child., 12:541, 1916.

723. Sever, J. W.: The results of a new operation for obstetrical paralysis. Amer. J. Orthop. Surg., 16:248, 1918.

724. Sever, J. W.: Obstetrical paralysis. J.A.M.A., *85*:1862, 1925.
725. Sever, J. W.: Obstetrical paralysis. Surg. Gynec. Obstet., *44*:547, 1927.
726. Smellie, W.: Collection of Preternatural Cases and Observations in Midwifery, Compleating the Design of Illustrating His First Volume On That Subject. Vol. III. p. 504. London, Wilson and Durham, 1764.
727. Sulas, V.: La pasizione de deratazione esterna abbinate all abduzione dell'arto superiore nella cura della paralisi obstetrica nei primi mesi di vita. Rass. Ital. Chir. Med., *3*:53, 1954.
728. Taylor, A. S.: Results from the surgical treatment of brachial birth palsy. J.A.M.A., *48*:96, 1907.
729. Thomas, T. T.: The relation of posterior subluxation of the shoulder joint to obstetrical palsy of the upper extremity. Ann. Surg., *59*:197, 1914.
730. Wickstrom, J.: Birth injuries of the brachial plexus. J. Bone Joint Surg., *42-A*:1448, 1960.
731. Wickstrom, J.: Birth injuries of the brachial plexus. Treatment of defects in the shoulder. Clin. Orthop., *23*:187, 1962.
732. Wickstrom, J., Haslam, E. T., and Hutchinson, R. H.: The surgical management of residual deformities of the shoulder following birth injuries of the brachial plexus. J. Bone Joint Surg., *37-A*:27, 1955.
733. Wolman, B.: Erb's palsy. Arch. Dis. Child., *23*:129, 1948.
734. Zachary, R. B.: Transplantation of teres major and latissimus dorsi for loss of external rotation at the shoulder. Lancet, *2*:757, 1947.
735. Zancolli, E. A.: Paralytic supination contracture of the forearm. J. Bone Joint Surg., *49-A*:1275, 1967.
736. Zaoussis, A. L.: Osteotomy of the proximal end of the radius for paralytic supination deformity in children. J. Bone Joint Surg., *45-B*:523, 1963.

SCIATIC NERVE PALSY

737. Bates, C., and Page, A. P. M.: A new neonatal syndrome. Brit. Med. J., *2*:756, 1949.
738. Curtiss, P. H., Jr., and Tucker, H. J.: Sciatic palsy in premature infants—a report and follow-up study of 10 cases. J.A.M.A., *174*:586, 1960.
739. DiMargo, A.: On paralysis of the sciatic nerve caused by intragluteal injection of drugs. Clin. Pediat., *43*:230, 1961.
740. Fhrenfest, H.: Birth Injuries of the Child. 2nd Ed. New York and London, D. Appleton & Co., 1931.
741. Fahrini, W. H.: Neonatal sciatic palsy. J. Bone Joint Surg., *32-B*:42, 1950.
742. Gilles, F. H., and French, J. H.: Postinjection sciatic nerve palsies in infants and children. J. Pediat., *58*:195, 1961.
743. Hudson, F. P., McCandless, A., and O'Malley, A. G.: Sciatic paralysis in newborn infants. Brit. Med. J., *1*:223, 1950.
744. Johnson, E. W., Jr.: Sciatic nerve palsy following delivery. Postgrad. Med., *30*:495, 1961.
745. Meyer, M.: Paralysie obstetricale des membres inférieurs. Rev. Orthop. (Paris), *18*:767, 1931.
746. Mills, W. G.: A new neonatal syndrome. Brit. Med. J., *2*:464, 1949.
747. San Augustin, M., Nitowsky, H. M., and Borden, J. N.: Neonatal sciatic palsy after umbilical vessel injection. J. Pediat., *60*:408, 1962.
748. Shaw, N. E.: Neonatal sciatic palsy from injection into the umbilical cord. J. Bone Joint Surg., *42-B*:736, 1960.

PERONEAL MUSCULAR ATROPHY (CHARCOT-MARIE-TOOTH DISEASE)

749. Allan, W.: Relation of hereditary pattern to clinical severity as illustrated by peroneal atrophy. Arch. Intern. Med., *63*:1123, 1939.
750. Bourguignon, G.: Association of Friedreich's disease and atrophy of Charcot-Marie type. Rev. Neurol., *83*:284, 1950.
751. Brihaye, M., Nenquin-Klaassen, E., Berthdet, G.: Neurogenic muscular atrophy of Charcot-Marie-Tooth. Hoffman type combined with bilateral optic atrophy. Acta Neurol. Belg., *56*:302, 1956.
752. Brodal, A., Böyesen, S., Frövig, A. G.: Progressive neuropathic atrophy (Charcot-Marie-Tooth). A.M.A., Arch. Neurol. Psychiat., *70*:1, 1953.
753. Brody, L. A., and Wilkins, R. H.: Charcot-Marie-Tooth disease. Arch. Neurol., *17*:552, 1967.
754. Bulgarelli, R., and Leva, R.: Are Friedreich, Charcot-Marie-Tooth and Déjérine-Sottas diseases distinct nosologic entities? Minerva Pediat., *6*:497, 1954.
755. Charcot, J. M., and Marie, P.: Sur une forme particulière d'atrophie musculaire progressive, souvent familiale, débutant par les pieds et les jambes et atteignant plus tard les mains. Rev. Méd. (Paris), *6*:97, 1886.
756. Christiaens, L., Poingt, O., and Farriaux, J. P.: Charcot-Marie disease in a four-year-old. Lille Méd., *8*:513, 1963.
757. Christie, B. G.: Electrodiagnostic features of Charcot-Marie-Tooth disease. Proc. Roy. Soc. Med., *54*:321, 1961.
758. Crank, H. H., and Reider, N.: Genetic features in the Charcot-Marie-Tooth type of muscular atrophy. Bull. Menninger Clin., *3*:88, 1939.
759. Currie, R. A.: Case of the Charcot-Marie-Tooth type of muscular atrophy, with a note on the condition of the bones. Glasgow Med. J., *107*:28, 1927.
760. Dawson, C. W., and Roberts, J. B.: Charcot-Marie-Tooth disease. J.A.M.A., *188*:659, 1964.
761. Déjérine et Armand-Delille: Un cas d'atrophie musculaire, type Charcot-Marie, suivi d'autopsie. Rev. Neurol., *11*:1198, 1903.
762. Dyck, P. J., Lambert, E. H., and Mulder, D. W.: Charcot-Marie-Tooth disease. Nerve conduction and clinical studies of a large kinship. Neurology, *13*:1, 1963.
763. Dyck, P. J., Winkelmann, R. K., and Bolton, C. F.: Quantitation of Meissner's corpuscles in hereditary neurologic disorders. Charcot-Marie-Tooth disease. Roussy-Lévy syndrome, Déjérine-Sottas disease, hereditary sensory neuropathy, spinocerebellar degeneration and hereditary spastic paraplegia. Neurology, *16*:10, 1966.
764. Earl, W. C., and Johnson, E. W.: Motor nerve conduction velocity in Charcot-Marie-Tooth disease. Arch. Phys. Med., *44*:247, 1963.
765. Eisenbud, A., and Grossman, M.: Peroneal form of progressive muscular atrophy. A clinical report of two families. Arch. Neurol. Psychiat., *18*:766, 1927.
766. England, A. C., and Denny-Brown, D.: Severe sensory changes, and trophic disorder, in peroneal muscular atrophy (Charcot-Marie-Tooth type). Arch. Neurol. Psychiat., *67*:1, 1952.
767. Erwin, W. G.: A pedigree of sex-linked recessive peroneal atrophy. J. Hered., *35*:24, 1944.
768. Gilliatt, R. W., and Thomas, P. K.: Extreme slowing of nerve conduction in peroneal muscular atrophy. Ann. Phys. Med., *4*:104, 1957.
769. Haase, G. R., and Shy, G. M.: Pathological changes in muscle biopsies from patients with peroneal muscular atrophy. Brain, *83*:631, 1960.
770. Herringham, W. P.: Muscular atrophy of the peroneal type affecting many members of a family. Brain, *11*:230, 1889.
771. Hoffmann, J.: Ueber progressive neurotische Muskelatrophie. Arch. Psychiat. (Berlin), *20*:660, 1889.
772. Hoyt, W. F.: Charcot-Marie-Tooth disease with primary optic atrophy. A.M.A. Arch. Ophthal., *64*:925, 1960.
773. Jacobs, J. E., and Carr, C. R.: Progressive muscular atrophy of the peroneal type (Charcot-Marie-Tooth disease), orthopedic management and end-result study. J. Bone Joint Surg., *32-A*:27, 1950.

774. Karlholm, S. and Nilsonne, U.: Operative Treatment of the foot deformity in Charcot-Marie-Tooth disease. Acta Orthop. Scand., *39*:101, 1968.

775. LaPresle, J.: Contribution a l'étude de la dystasie aréflexique héréditaire. Etat actuel de quatre des sept cas princeps de Roussy et Mlle. Lévy, trente ans après la première publication de ces auteurs. Sem. Hôp. Paris, *32*:2473, 1956.

776. Lidge, R. T., and Chandler, F. A.: Charcot-Marie-Tooth disease. J. Pediat., *43*:152, 1953.

777. MacKlin, M. T., and Bowman, J. T.: Inheritance of peroneal atrophy. J.A.M.A., *86*:613, 1926.

778. Milhorat, A. T.: Progressive muscular atrophy of peroneal type associated with atrophy of the optic nerves. Arch. Neurol. Psychiat., *50*:279, 1943.

779. Ross, A. T.: Combination of Friedreich's ataxia and Charcot-Marie-Tooth atrophy in each of two brothers. J. Nerv. Ment. Dis., *95*:680, 1942.

780. Roussy, G., and Lévy, G.: Sept cas d'une maladie familiale particulaire: Troubles de la march, pieds, bots et aréfléxie tendineuse généralisée, avec accessoirement, légère maladresse des mains. Rev. Neurol. (Paris), *45*:427, 1926.

781. Roussy, G., and Lévy, G.: A propos de la dystasie aréflexique héréditaire. Rev. Neurol. (Paris), *62*:763, 1934.

782. Sachs, B.: The peroneal form or the leg-type of progressive muscular atrophy. Brain, *12*:447, 1890.

783. Schneider, D. E., and Bels, M. M.: Charcot-Marie-Tooth disease with primary optic atrophy. Report of two cases occurring in brothers. J. Nerv. Ment. Dis., *85*:541, 1937.

784. Schwartz, L. A.: Clinical histopathological and inheritance factors in peroneal muscular atrophy (Charcot-Marie-Tooth type). J. Mich. Med. Soc., *43*:219, 1944.

785. Spillane, J. D.: Familial pes cavus and absent tendon jerks: Its relationship with Friedreich's disease and peroneal muscular atrophy. Brain, *63*:275, 1940.

786. Stranak, V.: Charcot-Marie-Tooth-Hoffman syndrome. Beitr. Orthop. Trauma., *15*:564, 1968.

787. Symond, S. C. P., and Shaw, M. E.: Familial claw-foot with absent tendon-jerks. A "forme fruste" of the Charcot-Marie-Tooth disease. Brain, *49*:387, 1926.

788. Tooth, H. H.: The Peroneal Type of Progressive Muscular Atrophy. London, H. K. Lewis, 1886.

789. Van Bogaert, L., and Moreau, M.: Combinaison de l'amyotrophie de Charcot-Marie-Tooth et de la maladie de Friedreich, chez plusieurs membres d'une même famille. Encephale, *34*:312, 1939–1941.

790. Yudell, A., Dyck, P. J., and Lambert, E. H.: A kinship with the Roussy-Lévy syndrome. Arch. Neurol., *13*:432, 1965.

HYPERTROPHIC INTERSTITIAL NEURITIS

791. Austin, J. H.: Observations on the syndrome of hypertrophic neuritis (the hypertrophic interstitial radiculoneuropathies). Medicine, *35*:187, 1956.

792. Andermann, F., Lloyd-Smith, D. L., Mavor, H., and Mathieson, G.: Observations on hypertrophic neuropathy of Déjérine and Sottas. Neurology, *12*:712, 1962.

793. Bedford, P. D., and James, F. E.: A family with progressive hypertrophic polyneuritis of Déjérine and Sottas. J. Neurol. Neurosurg. Psychiat., *19*:46, 1956.

794. Byers, R. K., and Taft, L. T.: Chronic multiple peripheral neuropathy in childhood. Pediatrics, *20*:517, 1957.

795. Craft, P. B., and Wadia, N. H.: Familial hypertrophic polyneuritis. Review of a previously reported family. Neurology, *7*:356, 1957.

796. Déjérine, J., and Sottas, J.: Sur la névrite interstitielle, hypertrophique et progressive de l'enfance. C. R. Soc. Biol., *5*:63, 1893.

797. Gombault, A., and Mallet: Un cas de tabès ayant débuté dans l'enfance. Arch. Med. Exper., *1*:385, 1889.

798. Isaacs, H.: Familial chronic hypertrophic polyneuropathy with paralysis of the extremities in cold weather. S. Afr. Med. J., *34*:758, 1960.

799. Joiner, C. L., McArdle, B., and Thompson, R. H. S.: Blood pyruvate estimations in the diagnosis and treatment of polyneuritis. Brain, *73*:431, 1950.

800. Russell, W. R., and Garland, H. G.: Progressive hypertrophic polyneuritis, with case reports. Brain, *53*:376, 1930.

REFSUM'S DISEASE OR HEREDOPATHIA ATACTICA POLYNEURITIFORMIS

801. Ashenhurst, E. M., Millar, J. H. D., and Milliken, T. G.: Refsum's syndrome affecting a brother and two sisters. Brit. Med. J., *2*:415, 1958.

802. Eldjarn, L., Try, K., Stokke, O., Munthe-Kaas, A. W., Refsum, S., Steinberg, D., Avigan, J., and Mize, C.: Dietary effects on serum phytanic acid levels and on clinical manifestations in heredopathia atactica polyneuritiformis. Lancet, *1*:691, 1966.

803. Kahke, W., and Wagner, H.: Conversion of H3-phytol to phytanic acid and its incorporation into plasma lipid fractions in heredopathia atactica polyneuritiformis. Metabolism, *15*:687, 1966.

804. Refsum, S.: Heredopathia atactica polyneuritiformis: A familial syndrome not hitherto described. Acta Psychiat. Neurol., Suppl. 38, 1946.

805. Refsum, S.: Heredopathia atactica polyneuritiformis. J. Nerv. Ment. Dis., *116*:1046, 1952.

806. Refsum, S., Salmonsen, L., and Skatvedt, M.: Heredopathia atactica polyneuritiformis in children. J. Pediat., *35*:335, 1949.

807. Richterich, R., Van Mechelen, P., and Rossi, E.: Refsum's disease (heredopathia atactica polyneuritiformis). An inborn error of lipid metabolism with storage of 3,7,11,15-tetramethyl hexadecanic acid. Amer. J. Med., *39*:230, 1965.

808. Steinberg, D., Herndon, J. H., Jr., Uhlendorf, B. W., Mize, G. E., Avigan, J., and Milne, C. W. A.: Refsum's disease. Nature of the enzyme defect. Science, *156*:1740, 1967.

809. Steinberg, D., Vroom, F. Q., Engel, W. K., Cammermeyer, J., Mize, C. E., and Avigan, J.: Refsum's disease—a recently characterized lipidosis involving the nervous system. Ann. Intern. Med., *66*:365, 1967.

810. Steinberg, D., Mize, C. E., Avigan, J., Fales, H. M., Eldjarn, L., Try, K., Stokke, O., and Refsum, S.: Studies on the metabolic error in Refsum's disease. J. Clin. Invest., *46*:313, 1967.

CONGENITAL ANALGIA—CONGENITAL INDIFFERENCE TO PAIN, FAMILIAL DYSAUTONOMIA (RILEY-DAY SYNDROME), AND CONGENITAL SENSORY NEUROPATHY

811. Abell, J. M., Jr., and Hayes, J. T.: Charcot knee due to congenital insensitivity to pain. J. Bone Joint Surg., *46-A*:1287, 1964.

812. Arbuse, D. I., Cantor, M. B., and Barenberg, P. A.: Congenital indifference to pain. J. Pediat., *35*:221, 1949.

813. Baxter, D. W., and Olszewski, J.: Congenital universal insensitivity to pain. Brain, *83*:381, 1960.

814. Biemond, A.: Investigation of the brain in a case of congenital and familial analgesia. Excerpta Med. Neurol. Psychiat., *8*:885, 1955.

815. Boyd, D. A., Jr., and Nie, L. W.: Congenital universal indifference to pain. Arch. Neurol. Psychiat., *61*:402, 1949.

816. Critchley, M.: Some aspects of pain. Brit. Med. J., *4*:891, 1934.

817. Critchley, M.: Congenital indifference to pain. Ann. Intern. Med., *45*:737, 1956.

818. Dearborn, G. V.: A case of congenital pure analgesia. J. Nerv. Ment. Dis., *75*:612, 1932.

819. Denny-Brown, D.: Hereditary sensory radicular neuropathy. J. Neurol. Neurosurg. Psychiat., *14*:237, 1951.

820. Dimon, J. H., Funk, F. J., Jr., and Wells, R. E.: Congenital indifference to pain with associated orthopedic abnormalities. Southern Med. J., *58*:524, 1965.

821. Ervin, F. R., and Sternbach, R. A.: Hereditary insensitivity to pain. Trans. Amer. Neurol. Ass., *85*:70, 1960.

822. Fanconi, G., and Ferrazzini, F.: Kongenitale Analgie (Kongenitale generalisierte Schmerzindifferenz). Helv. Paediat. Acta *12*:79, 1957.

823. Farquhar, H. G., and Sutton, T.: Congenital indifference to pain. Lancet, *1*:827, 1951.

824. Feindel, W.: Note on the nerve endings in a subject with arthropathy and congenital absence of pain. J. Bone Joint Surg., *35-B*:402, 1953.

825. Ford, F. R., and Wilkins, L.: Congenital universal insensitiveness to pain. Bull. Johns Hopk. Hosp., *62*:448, 1938.

826. Gillespie, J. B., and Perucca, L. G.: Congenital generalized indifference to pain. Amer. J. Dis. Child., *100*:124, 1960.

827. Jewesbury, E. C. O.: Insensitivity to pain. Brain, *74*:336, 1951.

828. Johnson, J. T. H.: Neuropathic fractures and joint injuries. J. Bone Joint Surg., *49-A*:1, 1967.

829. Kroop, I. G.: The production of tears in familial dysautonomia. J. Pediat., *48*:328, 1956.

830. Kunkle, E. C., and Chapman, W. P.: Insensitivity to pain in man. Ass. Res. Nerv. Ment. Dis. Proc., *23*:100, 1943.

831. Lamy, J., Garcin, R., Jammet, M. L., and Aussannaire, M., et al.: L'analgésie généralisée congénitale. Arch. Franc. Pediat., *15*:433, 1958.

832. McMurray, G. A.: Experimental study of a case of insensitivity to pain with neuropathic arthropathy. Arthritis Rheum., *9*:820, 1966.

833. Madonick, M. J.: Congenital insensitiveness to pain. J. Nerv. Ment. Dis., *120*:87, 1954.

834. Mooney, V., and Mankin, H. J.: A case of congenital insensitivity to pain with neuropathic arthropathy. Arthritis Rheum., *9*:820, 1966.

835. Murray, R. O.: Congenital indifference to pain with special reference to skeletal changes. Brit. J. Radiol., *30*:2, 1957.

836. Odgen, T. E., Robert, F., and Carmichael, E. A.: Some sensory syndromes in children: Indifference to pain and sensory neuropathy. J. Neurol. Neurosurg. Psychiat., *22*:267, 1959.

837. Petrie, J. G.: A case of progressive joint disorders caused by insensitivity to pain. J. Bone Joint Surg., *35-B*:399, 1953.

838. Pinsky, L., and DiGeorge, A. M.: Congenital familial sensory neuropathy with anhidrosis. J. Pediat., *68*:1, 1966.

839. Riley, C. M., and Moore, R. H.: Familial dysautonomia differentiated from related disorders. Pediatrics, *37*:435, 1966.

840. Riley, C. M., Day, R. L., Greeley, D. M., and Langford, W. S.: Central autonomic dysfunction with defective lacrimation. Pediatrics, *3*:468, 1949.

841. Roe, W.: Congenital indifference to pain. Proc. Roy. Soc. Med., *43*:250, 1956.

842. Rose, G. K.: Arthropathy of the ankle in congenital indifference to pain. J. Bone Joint Surg., *35-B*:408, 1953.

843. Sandell, L. J.: Congenital indifference to pain. J. Fac. Radiol. (London), *9*:50, 1958.

844. Siegelman, S. S., Heimann, W. G., and Manin, M. C.: Congenital indifference to pain. Amer. J. Roentgen. *97*:242, 1966.

845. Silverman, F. N., and Gilden, J. J.: Congenital insensitivity to pain: A neurologic syndrome with bizarre skeletal lesions. Radiology, *72*:176, 1959.

846. Smith, A. A., and Dancis, J.: Response to intradermal histamine in familial dysautonomia: A diagnostic test. J. Pediat., *63*:889, 1963.

847. Swanson, A. G.: Congenital insensitivity to pain with anhydrosis. A unique syndrome in two male siblings. A.M.A. Arch. Neurol., *8*:299, 1963.

848. Westlake, E. K.: Congenital indifference to pain. Brit. Med. J., *1*:144, 1952.

849. Winkelmann, R. K., Lambert, E. H., and Hayles, A. B.: Congenital absence of pain. Arch. Derm. (Chicago), *85*:325, 1962.

ACUTE POLYRADICULONEURITIS (GUILLAIN-BARRÉ SYNDROME)

850. Arbesman, C. E., Hyman, I., Dauzier, G., and Kantor, S. Z.: Immunologic studies of a Guillain-Barré syndrome following tetanus antitoxin. New York J. Med., *58*:2647, 1958.

851. Aylett, P.: Five cases of acute infective polyneuritis in children. Arch. Dis. Child., *29*:531, 1954.

852. Bassoe, P.: Guillain-Barré syndrome and related conditions. Arch. Path., *26*:289, 1938.

853. Bendz, P.: Respiratory problems in acute Guillain-Barré syndrome. A.M.A. Arch. Neurol. Psychiat., *73*:22, 1955.

854. Berlacher, F. J., and Abington, R. B.: ACTH and cortisone in Guillain-Barré syndrome. Review of the literature and report of a tested case following primary atypical pneumonia. Ann. Intern. Med., *48*:1106, 1958.

855. Blood, A., Locke, W., and Carabasi, R.: Guillain-Barré syndrome tested with corticotropin. J.A.M.A., *152*:139, 1953.

856. Bradford, J. P., Bashford, E. F., and Wilson, J. A.: Acute infective polyneuritis. Quart. J. Med., *12*:88, 1918.

857. Casamajor, L., and Lapert, G. R.: Guillain-Barré syndrome in children. Amer. J. Dis. Child., *61*:99, 1941.

858. Clement, M., and Ketelbant: Syndrome de Guillain et Barré et varicelle chez un enfant. J. Belge Neurol. Psychiat., *38*:240, 1938.

859. Cohen: À propos de trois enfants présentant certain caractères du syndrome de Guillain-Barré. J. Belge Neurol. Psychiat., *38*:307, 1938.

860. Cook, S. D.: The Guillain-Barré syndrome. Relationship of circulating immunocytes. Its disease activity. Arch. Neurol., *22*:470, 1970.

861. Crozier, R. E., and Ainley, A. B.: Guillain-Barré syndrome. New Eng. J. Med., *252*:83, 1955.

862. Eden, A. N.: Guillain-Barré syndrome in a six-month-old infant. Amer. J. Dis. Child., *102*:224, 1961.

863. Gomirato, G., and Vignolo-Lutati, U.: Frequency and pathogenesis of Guillain-Barré-Strohl syndrome in children. Minerva Pediat., *2*:525, 1950.

864. Guillain, G.: Radiculoneuritis with acellular hyperalbuminosis of the cerebrospinal fluid. Arch. Neurol. Psychiat., *36*:975, 1936.

865. Guillain, G., Barré, J. A., and Strohl, A.: Sur un syndrome de radiculonévrite avec hyperalbuminose du liquide céphalo-rachidien sans réaction cellulaire. Bull. Soc. Méd. Hôp. Paris, *40*:1462, 1916.

866. Haymaker, W., and Kernohan, J. W.: The Landry-Guillain-Barré syndrome, a clinicopathologic report of 50 fatal cases and a critique of the literature. Medicine, *28*:59, 1949.

867. Hecht, M. S.: Acute infective polyneuritis. J. Pediat., *11*:743, 1937.

868. Heller, G. L., and DeJong, R. N.: Treatment of the Guillain-Barré syndrome. Arch. Neurol., *8*:179, 1963.

869. Jones, I.: Facial diplegia in Guillain-Barré syndrome. Brit. Med. J., *2*:84, 1954.

870. Marino, J. J., Motto, S., and Przypyzany, J. C.: Guillain-Barré syndrome in children. Illinois Med. J., *110*:73, 1956.

871. Marshall, J.: The Landry-Guillain-Barré syndrome. Brain, *86*:55, 1963.
872. Melnick, S. C.: Thirty-eight cases of the Guillain-Barré syndrome: An immunologic study. Brit. Med. J., *1*:368, 1963.
873. Moore, R. Y.: The Guillain-Barré syndrome. Develop. Med. Child. Neurol., *9*:639, 1967.
874. Osler, L. D., and Sidell, A. D.: The Guillain-Barré syndrome: The need for exact diagnostic criteria. New Eng. J. Med., *262*:964, 1960.
875. Parker, W., Wilt, J. C., Dawson, J. W., and Stackiu, W.: Landry-Guillain-Barré syndrome. The isolation of an ECHO virus type 6. Canad. Med. Ass. J., *82*:813, 1960.
876. Paulson, G. W.: The Landry-Guillain-Barré-Strohl syndrome in childhood. Develop. Med. Child. Neurol., *12*:604, 1970.
877. Peterman, A. F., Daly, D. D., Dion, F. R., and Keith, H. M.: Infectious neuronitis (Guillain-Barré syndrome) in children. Neurology, *9*:533, 1959.
878. Plangues, J., and Mas, R.: Relapse 24 years after the first attack of a case of Guillain-Barré syndrome. Toulouse Méd., *62*:115, 1961.
879. Posek, C. M., Fowler, C. W.: The nosologic situation of the Landry-Guillain-Barré syndrome. Acta Neurol. Scand., *39*:187, 1963.
880. Ravn, H.: The Landry-Guillain-Barré syndrome—a survey and a clinical report of 127 cases. Acta Neurol. Scand., *43*:1, 1967.
881. Reye, R. D. K.: Neuropathology of Landry-Guillain-Barré syndrome. Med. J. Aust., *2*:386, 1954.
882. Schuch, C. P., Farmer, T. W.: Physical therapy in acute infectious polyneuritis. Phys. Ther. Rev., *35*:238, 1955.
883. Singh, A., and Jolly, S. S.: Landry-Guillain-Barré syndrome. Report of 25 cases. Indian J. Med. Sci., *12*:347, 1958.
884. Stillman, J. S., and Ganony, W. F.: Case of Guillain-Barré syndrome healed with ACTH and cortisone. New Eng. J. Med., *246*:293, 1952.
885. Von Hagen, K. O., and Baker, R. N.: Infectious neuronitis, present concepts of etiology and treatment. J.A.M.A., *151*:1465, 1953.
886. Waksman, B. H., and Adams, R. D.: Experimental allergic neuritis produced in rabbits with nerve and adjuvants. Fed. Proc., *13*:516, 1954.
887. Wiederholt, W. C., Mulder, D. W., and Lambert, E. H.: The Landry-Guillain-Barré-Strohl syndrome or polyradiculoneuropathy: Historical review, report on 97 patients and present concepts. Mayo Clin. Proc., *39*:427, 1964.
888. Wolfenden, W. H., and McGuinness, A. E.: The Guillain Barré syndrome with special reference to respiratory paralysis and recurrence. Med. J. Aust., *15*:163, 1958.

HERPES ZOSTER

889. Abercrombie, R. G.: Herpes zoster with muscular paralysis and disturbance of sensation. Brit. Med. J., *1*:778, 1941.
890. Brain, R. T.: The relationship between the viruses of zoster and varicella as demonstrated by the complement-fixation reaction. Brit. J. Exp. Path., *14*:67, 1933.
891. Broadbent, W. H.: Case of herpetic eruption in the course of branches of the brachial plexus followed by partial paralysis in corresponding motor nerves. Brit. Med. J., *2*:460, 1866.
892. Carter, A. B., and Dunlop, J. B. W.: Paresis following herpes zoster. Brit. Med. J., *1*:934, 1941.
893. Cheatham, W. J.: The relation of heretofore unreported lesions to pathogenesis of herpes zoster. Amer. J. Path., *29*:401, 1953.
894. Denny-Brown, D., Adams, R. D., and Fitzgerald, P. J.:

Pathologic features of herpes zoster. Arch. Neurol. Psychiat., *51*:216, 1944.
895. Duncan, J.: On herpes zoster. Journal of Cutaneous Medicine, *2*:241, 1868–9.
896. Grant, B. D., and Rowe, C. R.: Motor paralysis of the extremities in herpes zoster. J. Bone Joint Surg., *43-A*:885, 1961.
897. Gupta, S. K., Helal, B. H., and Kiely, P.: The prognosis in zoster paralysis. J. Bone Joint Surg., *51-B*:593, 1969.
898. Halpern, S. L., and Covner, A. H.: Motor manifestations of herpes zoster. Report of a case of associated permanent paralysis of the phrenic nerve. Arch. Intern. Med., *84*:907, 1949.
899. Hamilton, J. G. M.: Herpes zoster. Practitioner, *159*:122, 1947.
900. Hardy, M.: Du zona. Gaz. Hôp., *49*:827, 1876.
901. Kendall, D.: Motor complications of herpes zoster. Brit. Med. J., *2*:616, 1957.
902. Lhermite, J., and Nicolas: Les Lésions spinales du zona. La myélite zosteriènne. Rev. Neurol. (Paris), *1*:361, 1924.
903. McIntyre, J. H.: Herpes zoster with involvement of anterior horn cells. Brit. Med. J., *2*:716, 1951.
904. Rake, G., Blank, H., Coriell, L. L., Magler, F. P. Q., and Scott, T. F. McN.: The relationship of varicella and herpes zoster: Electron microscopic studies. J. Bact., *56*:293, 1948.
905. Rubin, D., and Fusfeld, R. D.: Muscle paralysis in herpes zoster. Calif. Med., *103*:261, 1965.
906. Spiers, A. S. D.: Herpes zoster and its motor lesions, with a report of a case of phrenic nerve paralysis. Med. J. Aust., *1*:850, 1963.
907. Taterka, J. H., and O'Sullivan, M. E.: The motor complications of herpes zoster. J.A.M.A., *122*:737, 1943.
908. Thalhimer, W.: Herpes zoster. Central nervous system lesions similar to those of epidermic (lethargic) encephalitis. Report on a case. Arch. Neurol. Psychiat., *12*:73, 1924.
909. Waller, G.: Two cases of herpes with motor paralysis. Brit. Med. J., *2*:560, 1885.
910. Weller, T. H., and Witton, H. M.: The etiologic agents of varicella and herpes zoster. Serologic studies with the viruses as propagated in vitro. J. Exp. Med., *108*:869, 1958.
911. Weller, T. H., Witton, H. M., and Bell, E. J.: The etiologic aspects of varicella and herpes zoster. Isolation, propagation, and cultural characteristics in vitro. J. Exp. Med., *108*:813, 1958.
912. Weseley, M. S., and Barenfeld, P. A.: Motor involvement in herpes zoster. New York J. Med., *65*:913, 1965.

MISCELLANEOUS AFFECTIONS OF PERIPHERAL NERVES

913. Campbell, A. M. C.: Neurological complications associated with insecticides and fungicides. Brit. Med. J., *2*:415, 1952.
914. Collings, H.: Polyneuropathy associated with nitrofuran therapy. Arch. Neurol., *3*:656, 1960.
915. Dreyfus, P. M., Hakim, S., and Adams, R. D.: Diabetic ophthalmoplegia. Arch. Neurol. Psychiat., *77*:337, 1957.
916. Fischer, C. M., and Adams, R. D.: Diphtheritic polyneuritis, a pathological study. J. Neuropath. Exp. Neurol., *15*:243, 1956.
917. Goldberg, A.: Acute intermittent porphyria. Quart. J. Med., *28*:183, 1959.
918. Heyman, A., Pfeiffer, J. B., Willet, R. W., and Taylor, H. M.: Peripheral neuropathy caused by arsenical intoxication. New Eng. J. Med., *254*:401, 1956.
919. Lawrence, D. G., and Locke, S.: Neuropathy in children with diabetes mellitus. Brit. Med. J., *1*:784, 1963.
920. Miller, H. G., and Stanton, J. B.: Neurological sequelae of prophylactic inoculation. Quart. J. Med., *23*:1, 1954.

921. Rundles, R. W.: Diabetic neuropathy. Medicine, *24*:111, 1945.

CONGENITAL ABSENCE OF MUSCLES

922. Bing, R.: Ueber angeborene Muskeldefecte. Virchow. Arch. Path. Anat., *170*:175, 1902.
923. Brown, J. B., and McDowell, I.: Syndactylism with absence of the pectoralis major. Surgery, 7:599, 1940.
924. Christopher, F.: Congenital absence of the pectoral muscles. J. Bone Joint Surg., *10*:350, 1928.
925. Krabbe, K.: Les lésions embryonnaires à la lumière des défectuosités mammaire et pectorale de la syndactylie et de la microdactylie. Acta Psychiat. Neurol., *24*:539, 1949.
926. LeDouble, A. F.: Traité des Variations de Système Musculaire de l'Homme et Leur Signification au Point de Vue de l'Anthropologie Zoologique. Paris, Schleicher Frères, 1897.
927. Morley, E. B.: Congenital defect of the pectoral muscle. Lancet, *1*:1101, 1923.
928. Resnick, E.: Congenital unilateral absence of the pectoral muscles often associated with syndactylism. J. Bone Joint Surg., *24*:925, 1942.
929. Silverman, F. N., and Huang, N.: Congenital absence of the abdominal muscles associated with malformations of the genitourinary and alimentary tracts: Report of cases and review of literature. Amer. J. Dis. Child., *80*:91, 1950.

ACCESSORY MUSCLES

930. Cauldwell, E. W., Anson, B. J., and Wright, R. R.: The extensor indicis proprius muscle. A study of 263 consecutive specimens. Quart. Bull. Northwestern Univ. Med. School, *17*:267, 1943.
931. Dunn, A. W.: Anomalous muscles simulating soft tissue tumors in the lower extremities. Report of three cases. J. Bone Surg., *47–A*:1397, 1965.
932. Dunn, A. W., and Evarts, C. M.: The extensor digitorum brevis manus muscle: A case report. Clin. Orthop., *28*:210, 1963.
933. Gray, D. J.: Some anomalous hamstring muscles. Anat. Rec., *91*:33, 1945.
934. Humphrey, G. M.: Observations in Myology. London, MacMillan & Co., Ltd., 1872.
935. Jones, B. W.: An anomalous extensor indicis muscle. J. Bone Joint Surg., *41-B*:763, 1959.
936. King, T. S., and O'Rahilly, R.: Muscle palmaris accessorius and duplication of muscle palmaris longus. Acta Anat. (Basel), *10*:327, 1950.
937. LeDouble, A. F.: Traité de Variations du Système Musculaire de l'Homme et de leur Signification au Point de Vue de l'Anthropologie Zoologique. Paris, Schleicher Frères, 1897.
938. Lipscomb, P. R.: Duplication of hypothenar muscles simulating soft tissue of the hand. Report of a case. J. Bone Joint Surg., *42-A*:1058, 1960.
939. Thomas, C. G., Jr.: Clinical manifestation of an accessory palmaris muscle. J. Bone Joint Surg., *40-A*:929, 1958.

IDIOPATHIC FIBROSIS OF MUSCLES

940. Bhattacharyya, D.: Abduction contracture of the shoulder from contracture of the intermediate part of the deltoid. J. Bone Joint Surg., *48-B*:127, 1966.
941. Cellarius, T. L.: Die Abduktionskonkraktur im Schultergelenk. Chirurg, *19*:221, 1948.
942. Csink, L., and Imrie, J.: Isolated contracture of rectus femoris muscle. J. Bone Joint Surg., *45-B*:145, 1963.
943. Dufek, M.: Prispevek ke vzniku fibrozy m. vasti intermedii u deti. Acta Chir. Orthop. Traum. Cech., *29*:149, 1962.
944. Fairbank, T. J., and Barnett, A. M.: Vastus intermedius

945. Gammie, W. F. P., Taylor, J. H., and Ursch, H.: Contracture of the vastus intermedius in children. A report of two cases. J. Bone Joint Surg., *45-B*:370, 1963.
946. Goodfellow, J. W., and Nade, S.: Flexion contracture of the shoulder from fibrosis of the anterior part of the deltoid muscle. J. Bone Joint Surg., *51-B*:356, 1969.
947. Gunn, D. R.: Contracture of the quadriceps muscle. J. Bone Joint Surg., *46-B*:492, 1964.
948. Hagen, R.: Contracture of the quadriceps muscle in children. Acta Orthop. Scand., *39*:565, 1968.
949. Harrold, A. J.: Rigid valgus foot from fibrous contracture of the peronei. J. Bone Joint Surg., *47-B*:743, 1965.
950. Hněvkovský, O.: Progressive fibrosis of the vastus intermedius muscle in children. A cause of limited knee flexion and elevation of the patella. J. Bone Joint Surg., *43-B*:318, 1961.
951. Karlen, A.: Congenital fibrosis of the vastus intermedius muscle. J. Bone Joint Surg., *46-B*:488, 1964.
952. Lerch, H.: Die Abduktions Kontraktur im Schultergelenk. Chirurg, *20*:675, 1949.
953. Lloyd-Roberts, G. C., and Thomas, T. G.: The etiology of quadriceps contracture in children. J. Bone Joint Surg., *46-B*:498, 1964.
954. Sato, M., Honda, S., and Inoue, H.: Three cases of abduction contracture of the shoulder caused by fibrosis of the deltoid muscle. Orthop. Surg. (Tokyo), *16*:1052, 1965.
955. Saunders, F. P., Hoefnagel, D., and Staples, O. S.: Progressive fibrosis of the quadriceps muscle. J. Bone Joint Surg., *47-A*:380, 1965.
956. Williams, P. H.: Quadriceps contracture. J. Bone Joint Surg., *50-B*:278, 1968.

FIBRODYSPLASIA OSSIFICANS PROGRESSIVA, MYOSITIS OSSIFICANS PROGRESSIVA

957. Ackerman, L. V.: Extra-osseous non-neoplastic bone and cartilage formation (So-called myositis ossificans). J. Bone Joint Surg., *40-A*:279, 1958.
958. Burton-Fanning, F. W., and Vaughan, A. L.: A case of myositis ossificans. Lancet, 2:849, 1901.
959. Byers, W. M.: Almost complete ossification of the human body. New Orleans J. Med., *23*:122, 1870.
960. Cox, H. L.: Progressive myositis ossificans: Review of the literature and report of a case. N. Carolina Med. J., *18*:459, 1957.
961. Van Creveld, S., and Soeters, J. M.: Myositis ossificans progressiva. Amer. J. Dis. Child., *62*:1000, 1941.
962. Dixon, T. F., Mulligan, L., Nassim, R., and Stevenson, F. H.: Myositis ossificans progressiva. J. Bone Joint Surg., *36-B*:445, 1954.
963. Dobrzanieck, W.: The problem of myositis ossificans progressiva. Ann. Surg., *104*:987, 1936.
964. Eaton, W. L., Conkling, W. S., and Daeschner, C. W.: Early myositis ossificans progressiva occurring in homozygotic twins. J. Pediat., *50*:591, 1957.
965. Fairbank, H. A. T.: Myositis ossificans progressiva. J. Bone Joint Surg., *32-B*:108, 1950.
966. Frejka, B.: Heteropic ossification and myositis ossificans progressiva. J. Bone Joint Surg., *11*:157, 1929.
967. Gaster, D.: A case of myositis ossificans. W. Lond. Med. J., *10*:37, 1905.
968. Goto, S.: Pathologisch-anatomische und klinische Studien über die sogen. Myositis ossificans progressiva multiples. (Hyperplasia fascialis ossificans progressiva). Arch. Klin. Chir., *6*:730, 1912–1913.
969. Grewal, K. S., and Das, N.: Myositis ossificans progressiva. J. Bone Joint Surg., *35-B*:244, 1953.
970. Griffith, G.: Progressive myositis ossificans. Arch. Dis. Child., *24*:71, 1949.
971. Helferich, H.: Ein Fall von sogenannter Myositis ossi-

contracture in early childhood. Case report of identical twins. J. Bone Joint Surg., *43-B*:326, 1961.

ficans progressiva. Zerztliches Intelligenz-Blatt, *26*: 485, 1879.

972. Hutchinson, J.: Reports of hospital practice. Medical Times and Gazette, *1*:March 31, 1960.

973. Koontz, A. R.: Myositis ossificans progressiva. Amer. J. Med. Sci., *174*:406, 1927.

974. Lockhart, J. D., and Burke, F. G.: Myositis ossificans progressiva — report of a case treated with corticotropin (ACTH). A.M.A. Amer. J. Dis. Child., *87*:626, 1954.

975. Lutwak, L.: Myositis ossificans progressiva: mineral, metabolic, and radioactive calcium studies of the effects of hormones. Amer. J. Med., *37*:269, 1964.

976. McKusick, V. A.: Fibrodysplasia ossificans progressiva. *In* Heritable Disorders of Connective Tissue. 3rd Ed. St. Louis, The C. V. Mosby Co., 1966, p. 400.

977. Maini, P. S., and Singh, M.: Localized myositis ossificans progressiva. J. Bone Joint Surg., *49–A*:955, 1967.

978. Mair, W. F.: Myositis ossificans progressiva. Edinburgh Med. J., *39*:13, 69, 1932.

979. Mather, J. H.: Progressive myositis ossificans. Brit. J. Radiol., *4*:207, 1931.

980. Mandsley, R. H.: A case of myositis ossificans progressiva. Brit. Med. J., *1*:954, 1952.

981. Michelsohn, J.: Ein Fall von Myositis ossificans progressiva. Z. Orthop. Chir., *12*:424, 1904.

982. Nutt, J. J.: Report of a case of myositis ossificans progressiva with bibliography. J. Bone Joint Surg., 5: 344, 1923.

983. Patin, G.: Lettres choisies de feu Mr. Guy Patin. Cologne, Vol. 1:28, 1692.

984. Peck, G. T., and Braund, R. R.: The development of sarcoma in myositis ossificans. J.A.M.A., *119*:776, 1942.

985. Riley, H. D., and Christie, A.: Myositis ossificans progressiva. Pediatrics, 8:753, 1951.

986. Rolleston, H. D.: Progressive myositis ossificans with reference to other developmental diseases of the mesoblast. Clin. J., *17*:209, 1901.

987. Rosborough, D.: Ectopic bone formation associated with multiple congenital anomalies. J. Bone Joint Surg., *48-B*:499, 1966.

988. Rosenstirn, J.: A contribution to the study of myositis ossificans progressiva. Ann. Surg., *68*:485, 591, 1918.

989. Ryan, K. J.: Myositis ossificans progressiva: Review of the literature with report of a case. J. Pediat., 27: 348, 1945.

990. Singleton, E. B., and Holt, J. F.: Myositis ossificans progressiva. Radiology, *62*:47, 1954.

991. Smith, D. M., Zemam, W., Johnston, C. C., Jr., and Deiss, W. P., Jr.: Myositis ossificans progressiva. Metabolism, *15*:521, 1966.

992. Tunte, W., Becker, P. E., and Von Knorre, G.: Zur Genetik der Myositis ossificans progressiva. Humangenetik, *4*:320, 1967.

993. Tutunjian, K. H., and Kegerreis, R.: Myositis ossificans progressiva. J. Bone Joint Surg., *19*:503, 1937.

994. Uehlinger, E.: Myositis ossificans progressiva. Ergebn. Med Strahlenforsch., 7:175, 1936.

995. Vastine, J. H., Vastine, M. F., and Arango, O.: Myositis ossificans progressiva in homozygotic twins. Amer. J. Roentgen., *59*:204, 1948.

996. Wilkins, W. E., Regen, E. M., and Carpenter, G. K.: Phosphatase studies on biopsy tissue in progressive myositis ossificans. Amer. J. Dis. Child., *49*:1219, 1935.

PROGRESSIVE MUSCULAR DYSTROPHY

997. Adams, R. D., Denny-Brown, D., and Pearson, C. M.: Diseases of Muscle; A Study of Pathology. 2nd Ed. New York, Hoeber, 1962.

998. Allen, J. E., and Rodgin, D. W.: Mental retardation in association with progressive muscular dystrophy. Amer. J. Dis. Child., *100*:208, 1960.

999. Archibald, K. C., and Vignos, P. J., Jr.: A study of contractures in muscular dystrophy. Arch. Phys. Med., *40*:150, 1959.

1000. Batten, F. E.: The myopathies or muscular dystrophies; critical review. Quart. J. Med., *3*:313, 1909.

1001. Batten, F. E., and Gibb, H. P.: Myotonia atrophica. Brain, *32*:187, 1909.

1002. Berenbaum, A. A., and Horowitz, W.: Heart involvement in progressive muscular dystrophy. Report of a case with sudden death. Amer. Heart J., *51*:622, 1956.

1003. Carter, H. W.: A modified clamp for striated muscle biopsies. Amer. J. Clin. Path., *51*:516, 1969.

1004. Chung, C. S., Morton, N. E., and Peters, H. A.: Serum enzymes and genetic carriers in muscular dystrophy. Amer. J. Hum. Genet., *12*:52, 1960.

1005. Danowski, T. S., Wirth, P. M., Leinberger, M. H., Randall, L. A., and Peters, J. H.: Muscular dystrophy. III. Serum and blood solutes and other laboratory indices. Amer. J. Dis. Child., *91*:346, 1956.

1006. Dorando, C., and Newman, M. K.: Bracing for severe scoliosis of muscular dystrophy patients. Phys. Ther. Rev., *37*:230, 1957.

1007. Dreyfus, J. C., Schapira, G., and Schapira, F.: Biochemical study of muscle in progressive muscular dystrophy. J. Clin. Invest., *33*:794, 1954.

1008. Dreyfus, J. C., Schapira, G., and Schapira, F.: Serum enzymes in the pathophysiology of muscle. Ann. N. Y. Acad. Sci., *75*:235, 1958.

1009. Duchenne, G. B.: Recherches sur le paralysie musculaire pseudo-hypertrophique ou paralysie myosclérosique. Arch. Gén. Méd., *11*:5, 179, 305, 421, 552, 1868.

1010. Ebashi, S., Toyokura, Y., Momoi, H., and Sugita, H.: High creatine phosphokinase activity of sera of progressive muscular dystrophy patients. J. Biochem. (Tokyo), *46*:103, 1959.

1011. Erb, W. H.: Dystrophia Muscularis Progressive. Klinische und Pathologischanatomische Studien. Deutsch. Nervenheilk., *1*:13, 173, 1891.

1012. Eulenberg, A.: Über eine familiäre, durch 6 Generationen verfolgbare Form kongenitaler Paramyotonie. Zbl. Neurol., *5*:265, 1886.

1013. Fuchs, E.: Ueber isolieren doppelseitige Ptosia. Arch. Ophthal. (Chicago), *36*:234, 1890.

1014. Golarz, M. N., Bourne, G. H., and Richardson, H. D.: Histochemical studies on human muscular dystrophy. J. Histochem. Cytochem., *9*:132, 1961.

1015. Gowers, W. R.: Pseudohypertrophic Muscular Paralysis. London, Churchill, 1879.

1016. Gowers, W. R.: A lecture on myopathy of a distal form. Brit. Med. J., *2*:89, 1902.

1017. Gucker, T., III.: The orthopedic management of progressive muscular dystrophy. J. Amer. Phys. Ther. Ass., *44*:243, 1964.

1018. Hoffmann, J.: Ein Fall von Thomsen'scher Krankheit, complicert durch Neuritis multiplex. Deutsch. Z. Nervenheilk, *9*:272, 1897.

1019. Horvath, B., Berg, L., Cummings, D. J., and Shy, G. M.: Muscular dystrophy cation concentrations in residual muscle. J. Appl. Physiol., *8*:22, 1955.

1020. Hughes, B. P.: Studies on starch gel electrophoresis of some human muscle proteins. Clin. Chim. Acta, *6*: 794, 1961.

1021. Hutchinson, J.: An ophthalmoplegia externa or symmetrical immobility (partial) of the eye with ptosis. Trans. Med. Chir. Soc. Edinb., *62*:307, 1879.

1022. Kloepfer, H. W.: Genetic aspects of neuromuscular disease. *In* Walton, J. N. (ed.): Disorders of Voluntary Muscle. Boston, Little, Brown and Co., 1964.

1023. Landouzy, L., and Déjérine, J.: De la myopathie atrophique progressive (myopathie héréditaire), débutant, dans l'enfance, par la face, sans altération du système nerveux. C. R. Acad. Sci. (Paris), *98*:53, 1884.

1024. Levine, P. A., and Kristeller, L.: Factors regulating the creatinine output in man. Amer. J. Physiol., *24*:45, 1909.

1025. Leyden, E.: Klinik der Ruckenmarks-Krankheiten. Berlin, Hirschwald, 1876, Vol. 2, p. 531.

1026. Manning, G. W., and Cropp, G. J.: The electrocardiogram in progressive muscular dystrophy. Brit. Heart J., 20:416, 1958.

1027. Meryon, E.: On granular or fatty degeneration of the voluntary muscles. Trans. Med. Chir. Soc. Edinb., 35:72, 1852.

1028. Miller, J.: Management of muscular dystrophy. J. Bone Joint Surg., 49-A:1205, 1967.

1029. Möbius, P. J.: Ueber die hereditaren Nervenkrankheiten. Samml. Klin. Vortr., 171:1505, 1879.

1030. Oppenheimer, H., and Milhorat, A. T.: Serum proteins, lipoproteins, and glycoproteins in muscular dystrophy and related diseases. Ann. N.Y. Acad. Sci., 94:308, 1961.

1031. Pearce, J. M. S., Pennington, R. J. T., and Walton, J. N.: Serum enzyme studies in muscle disease. III. Serum creatine kinase activity in relatives of patients of the Duchenne type muscular dystrophy. J. Neurol. Neurosurg. Psychiat., 27:181, 1964.

1032. Pennington, R. J.: Some enzyme studies in muscular dystrophy. Proc. Ass. Clin. Biochem., 2:17, 1962.

1033. Rayport, M.: A disposable isometric muscle biopsy clamp. J.A.M.A., 210:1451, 1969.

1034. Rosenthal, M.: Handbuch der Diagnostik und Therapie der Nervenkrankheiten. Erlangen, F. Enke, 1870.

1035. Sibley, J. A., and Lehninger, A. L.: Aldolase in the serum and tissues of Tumour-bearing animals. J. Nat. Cancer Inst., 9:303, 1949.

1036. Spencer, G. E., Jr.: Orthopaedic care of progressive muscular dystrophy. J. Bone Joint Surg., 49-A: 1201, 1967.

1037. Spencer, G. E., Jr., and Vignos, P. J., Jr.: Bracing for ambulation in childhood progressive muscular dystrophy. J. Bone Joint Surg., 44-A:234, 1962.

1038. Staheli, L. T.: A clamp for isometric muscle biopsies. Surgery, 59:1154, 1966.

1039. Steinert, H.: Myopathologische Beitrage: I. Ueber das klinische und anatomische Bild des Muskelschwunds der Myotoniker. Deutsch. Z. Nervenheilk., 37:58, 1909.

1040. Swinyard, C. A., Deaver, G. G., and Greenspan, L.: Gradients of functional ability of importance in rehabilitation of patients with progressive muscular and neuromuscular diseases. Arch. Phys. Med., 38: 574, 1957.

1041. Thomasen, E.: Myotonia: Thomasen's Disease (Myotonia congenita), Paramyotonia and Dystrophia Myotonica: A Clinical and Heredobiologic Investigation. Aarhus, Denmark, Universitetsforlaget, 1948.

1042. Thomsen, J.: Tonische Krämpfe in willkürlich beweglichen muskeln in Folge von Ererbter psychischer Disposition (Ataxia muscularis?). Arch. Psychiat. Nervenkr., 6:706, 1876.

1043. Thomson, W. H., Leyburn, P., and Walton, J. N.: Serum enzyme activity in muscular dystrophy. Brit. Med. J., 5208:1276, 1960.

1044. Turner, J. W. A.: The relationship between amyotonia congenita and congenital myopathy. Brain, 63:163, 1940.

1045. Turner, J. W. A.: On amyotonia congenita. Brain, 72:25, 1949.

1046. Tyler, F. H., and Stephens, F. E.: Studies in disorders of muscle. IV. Clinical manifestations and inheritance of childhood progressive muscular dystrophy. Ann. Intern. Med., 35:169, 1951.

1047. Tyler, F. H., and Wintrobe, M. M.: Studies in disorders of muscle: I. The problem of progressive muscular dystrophy. Ann. Intern. Med., 32:72, 1950.

1048. Van Pilsum, J. F., and Wolin, E. A.: Guanidinium compounds in blood and urine of patients suffering from muscle disorders. J. Lab. Clin. Med., 51:219, 1958.

1049. Vignos, P. J., Jr.: Diagnosis of progressive muscular dystrophy. J. Bone Joint Surg., 49-A:1212, 1967.

1050. Vignos, P. J., Jr., and Archibald, K. C.: Maintenance of ambulation in childhood muscular dystrophy. J. Chron. Dis., 12:273, 1960.

1051. Vignos, P. J., Jr., and Lefkowitz, M.: A biochemical study of certain skeletal muscle constituents in human progressive muscular dystrophy. J. Clin. Invest., 38:873, 1959.

1052. Vignos, P. J., Jr., and Watkins, M. P.: The effect of exercise in muscular dystrophy. J.A.M.A., 197:843, 1966.

1053. Walton, J. N.: On the inheritance of muscular dystrophy. Ann. Hum. Genet., 20:1, 1955.

1054. Walton, J. N.: The inheritance of muscular dystrophy. Further observations. Ann. Hum. Genet., 21:40, 1956.

1055. Walton, J. N.: Clinical Aspects of Human Muscular Dystrophy. In, Bourne, G. H., and Golarz, N. (eds.): Muscular Dystrophy in Man and Animals. New York and Basle, Karger, S., 1962.

1056. Walton, J. N., (ed.): Disorders of Voluntary Muscle. Boston, Little, Brown, and Co., 1964.

1057. Walton, J. N., and Warrick, C. K.: Osseous changes in myopathy. Brit. J. Radiol., 27:1, 1954.

1058. Welander, L.: Myopathia distalis tarda hereditaria. Acta. Med. Scandinav., Suppl., 265:1, 1951.

1059. Whorton, C. M., Hudgins, P. C., and Connors, J. J.: Abnormal spectrophotometric absorption spectrums of myoglobin in two forms of progressive muscular dystrophy. New Eng. J. Med., 265:1242, 1961.

1060. Wohlfart, G.: Aktuelle Probleme der Muskelpathologie. Deutsch. Nervenheilk., 173:426, 1955.

1061. Worden, D. K., and Vignos, P. J., Jr.: Intellectual function in childhood progressive muscular dystrophy. Pediatrics, 29:968, 1962.

1062. Zatuchni, J., Aegerter, E. E., Molthan, L., and Shuman, C. R.: The heart in progressive muscular dystrophy. Circulation, 3:846, 1951.

MYOTONIA CONGENITA (THOMSEN'S DISEASE)

1063. Adams, R. D., Denny-Brown, D., and Pearson, C. M.: Diseases of Muscle. A Study in Pathology. 2nd Ed. New York, Harper and Bros., 1962, p. 650.

1064. Becker, P. E.: In Proceedings, Third International Congress Human Genetics, Chicago. Baltimore, Johns Hopkins Press, 1967.

1065. Birt, A.: A study of Thomsen's disease (congenital myotonia) by a sufferer from it. Montreal Med., 37: 771, 1908.

1066. Bourne, G. H.: The Structure and Function of Muscle, Vol. III. Pharmacology and Disease. New York, Academic Press, 1960.

1067. Celesia, G. G., Andermann, F., Wiglesworth, F. W., and Robb, J. P.: Monomelic myopathy—congenital hypertrophic myotonic myopathy limited to one extremity. Arch. Neurol., 17:69, 1967.

1068. Déjérine, J., and Sottas, J.: Sur un cas de maladie de Thomsen, suivi d'autopsie. Rev. Méd., 15:241, 1895.

1069. Denny-Brown, D., and Nevin, S.: The phenomenon of myotonia. Brain, 64:1, 1941.

1070. Erb: Ueber die Thomsen'sche Krankheit. Wien. Klin. Wschr., 2:931, 1889.

1071. Flora, G. C.: Differential diagnosis of myotonia. Postgrad. Med., 41:148, 1967.

1072. Floyd, W. F., Kent, P., and Page, F.: An electromyographic study of myotonia. Electroenceph. Clin. Neurophysiol., 7:621, 1955.

1073. Foix, C., and Nicolesco, I.: Note sur les altérations du système nerveux dans un cas de maladie de Thomsen. C. R. Soc. Biol. (Paris), 89:1095, 1923.

1074. Gerschwind, N., and Simpson, J. A.: Procaine amide in the treatment of myotonia. Brain, 78:81, 1955.

1075. Isaacs, H.: The treatment of myotonia congenita. S. Afr. Med. J., 33:984, 1959.

1076. Johnson, J.: Thomsen and myotonia congenita. Med. Hist., 12:190, 1968.

1077. Kuhn, E.: Liegt den Erbkrankheiten Myotonia congenita und Dystrophia myotonica eine biochemisch fassbare Störung zugrunde? Aerztl. Forsch., *15*:6, 1961.

1078. Liebenam, L.: Zwillingspathologische Beobachtung bei Myotonia congenita (Thomsen'sche Krankheit). Z. Mensch. Vererb. Konstitutionslehre, *24*:13, 1939.

1079. Maas, O., and Paterson, A. S.: The identity of myotonia congenita (Thomsen's disease), dystrophia myotonica (myotonia atrophica) and paramyotonia. Brain, *62*:198, 1939.

1080. Nissen, K.: Beiträge zur Kenntnis der Thomsenschen Krankheit (Myotonia congenita) mit besonderer Berucksichtigung des hereditären Momentes und seinen Beziehungen zu den Mendelschen Vererbungsregeln. Z. Klin. Med., *97*:58, 1923.

1081. Sanders, J.: Eine Familie mit Myotonia congenita. (Thomsen'sche Krankheit). Genetica, *17*:253, 1935.

1082. Thomasen, E.: Myotonia. Universitatis hafniensis, Copenhagen, Munksgaard, 1948.

1083. Thomsen, J.: Tonische Krämfe in willkürlich beweglichen Muskeln in Folge von ererbter psychischer Disposition, Arch. Psychiat. Nervenkr., *6*:706, 1876.

1084. Van Der Meulen, J. P., Gilbert, G. J., and Kane, C. A.: Familial hyperkalemic paralysis with myotonia. New Eng. J. Med., *264*:1, 1961.

1085. Winters, J. L., and McLaughlin, L. A.: Myotonia congenita. J. Bone Joint Surg., *52-A*:1345, 1970.

1086. Wohlfart, G.: Dystrophia myotonica and myotonia congenita. Histopathologic studies with special reference to changes in the muscles. J. Neuropath. Exp. Neurol., *10*:109, 1951.

TRAUMATIC MYOSITIS OSSIFICANS

1087. Ackerman, L. V.: Extra-osseus localized non-neoplastic bone and cartilage formation (so-called myositis ossificans). Clinical and pathological confusion with malignant neoplasms. J. Bone Joint Surg., *40-A*:279, 1958.

1088. Binnie, J. F.: On myositis ossificans traumatica. Ann. Surg., *38*:423, 1903.

1089. Coley, W. B.: Myositis ossificans traumatica. A report of three cases illustrating the difficulties of diagnosis from sarcoma. Ann. Surg., *57*:305, 1912.

1090. Constance, T. J.: Localized myositis ossificans. J. Path. Bact., *68*:381, 1954.

1091. Costello, F. V., and Brown, A.: Myositis ossificans complicating anterior poliomyelitis. J. Bone Joint Surg., *33-B*:594, 1951.

1092. Damanski, M.: Heteropic ossification in paraplegia. J. Bone Joint Surg., *13 B*:286, 1961.

1093. Fay, O. J.: Traumatic parosteal bone and callus formation. The so-called traumatic ossifying myositis. Surg. Gynec. Obstet., *19*:174, 1914.

1094. Fine, G., and Stout, A. P.: Osteogenic sarcoma of the extraskeletal soft tissue. Cancer, *9*:1027, 1956.

1095. Geschickter, C. F., and Mascritz, I. H.: Myositis ossificans. J. Bone Joint Surg., *20*:661, 1938.

1096. Hardy, A. G., and Dickson, J. W.: Pathological ossification in traumatic paraplegia. J. Bone Joint Surg., *45-B*:76, 1963.

1097. Hirsch, E. F., and Morgan, R. H.: Causal significance to traumatic ossification of the fibrocartilage in tendon insertions. Arch. Surg., *39*:824, 1939.

1098. Howard, C.: Traumatic ossifying myositis. U.S. Naval Med. Bull., *46*:724, 1946.

1099. Irving, J., and LeBrun, H.: Myositis ossificans in hemiplegia. J. Bone Joint Surg., *36-B*:440, 1954.

1100. Lewis, D.: Myositis ossificans. J.A.M.A., *80*:1281, 1923.

1101. Makins, G. H.: Traumatic myositis ossificans. Proc. Roy. Soc. Med., *4*:part 3 (Surg. Sec.): 133, 1911.

1102. Pack, G. T., and Braund, R. R.: The development of sarcoma in myositis ossificans. Report of three cases. J.A.M.A., *119*:776, 1942.

1103. Roberts, P. H.: Heteropic ossification complicating paralysis of intracranial origin. J. Bone Joint Surg., *50-B*:70, 1968.

1104. Thorndike, A.: Myositis ossificans traumatica. J. Bone Joint Surg., *22*:315, 1940.

POLYMYOSITIS, DERMATOMYOSITIS

1105. Adams, R. D., Denny-Brown, D., and Pearson, C. M.: Diseases of Muscle. 2nd Ed. New York, Harper & Row, 1962.

1106. Arundell, F. D., Wilkinson, R. D., and Haserick, J. R.: Dermatomyositis and malignant neoplasms in adults. Arch. Derm. Syph., *82*:772, 1960.

1107. Banker, B. Q., and Victor, M.: Dermatomyositis (systemic angiopathy) of childhood. Medicine, *45*:261, 1966.

1108. Bitnum, S., Daeschner, C. W., Travis, L. B., Dodge, W. F., and Hopps, H. C.: Dermatomyositis. J. Pediat., *64*:101, 1964.

1109. van Bogaert, L., Radermecker, M. A., Lowenthal, A., and Ketelaer, C. J.: VII. Les polymyosite chronique (essais avec la cortisone). Acta Neurol., Belg., *11*: 869, 1955.

1110. Carlisle, J. W., and Good, R. A.: Dermatomyositis in childhood: Report of studies on seven cases and a review of the literature. J. Lancet, *79*:266, 1959.

1111. Christianson, H. B., O'Leary, P. A., and Power, M. H.: Urinary excretion of creatine and creatinine in dermatomyositis. J. Invest. Derm., *27*:431, 1956.

1112. Dowling, G. B.: Scleroderma and dermatomyositis. Brit. J. Derm., *67*:275, 1955.

1113. Eaton, L. M.: The perspective of neurology in regard to polymyositis. Study of 41 cases. Neurology, *4*:245, 1954.

1114. Everett, M. M., and Curtis, A. C.: Dermatomyositis: A review of 19 cases in adolescents and children. Arch. Intern. Med., *100*:70, 1957.

1115. Garcin, R., LaPresle, J., Gruner, J., and Scherrer, J.: Les polymyosites. Rev. Neurol. (Paris), *92*:465, 1955.

1116. Lambert, E. H., Sayre, G. P., and Eaton, L. M.: Electrical activity of muscles in polymyositis. Trans. Amer. Neurol. Ass., *79*:64, 1954.

1117. Pearson, C. M.: Rheumatic manifestations of polymyositis and dermatomyositis. Arthritis Rheum., *2*,127, 1959.

1118. Pearson, C. M.: Polymyositis: Clinical forms, diagnosis, and therapy. Postgrad. Med., *31*:450, 1962.

1119. Pearson, C. M.: Patterns of polymyositis and their response to treatment. Ann. Intern. Med., *59*:827, 1963.

1120. Pearson, C. M.: Polymyositis and related disorders. *In* Walton, J. N., (ed.); Disorders of Voluntary Muscle. Boston, Little, Brown, and Co., 1964, p. 305.

1121. Roberts, H. M., and Brunsting, L. A.: Dermatomyositis in childhood: Summary of 40 cases. Postgrad. Med., *16*:396, 1954.

1122. Selander, P.: Dermatomyositis in early childhood. Acta Med. Scand., Suppl. 246, p. 187, 1950.

1123. Sheard, C.: Dermatomyositis. Arch. Intern. Med., *88*:640, 1951.

1124. Unverricht, H.: Polymyositis acuta progressiva. Z. Klin. Med., *12*:533, 1887.

1125. Wagner, E.: Fall einer seltnen Muskelkrankheit. Arch. Heilk., *4*:288, 1863.

1126. Walton, J. N., and Adams, R. D.: Polymyositis. Baltimore, Williams & Wilkins Co., 1958.

1127. Wedgwood, R. J. P., Cook, C. D., and Cohen, J.: Dermatomyositis: Report of 26 cases with a discussion of endocrine therapy in 13. Pediatrics, *12*:447, 1953.

1128. Williams, R. C.: Dermatomyositis and malignancy: a review of the literature. Ann. Intern. Med., *50*:1174, 1959.

PERIODIC PARALYSIS

1129. Allot, E. W., and McArdle, B.: Further observations on familial periodic paralysis. Clin. Sci., *3*:229, 1938.

1130. Buchthal, F., Engbaek, L., and Gamstorp, I.: Paresis

and hyperexcitability in adynamia episodica hereditaria. Neurology, 8:347, 1958.

1131. Creutzfeldt, O. D., Abbott, B. C., Fowler, W. M., and
Pearson, C. M.: Muscle membrane potentials in epi-
sodic adynamia. Electroenceph. Clin. Neurophysiol.,
15:508, 1963.

1132. Drager, G. A., Hammill, J. F., and Shy, G. M.: Paramyotonia Congenita. Arch. Neurol. Psychiat., 80:1, 1958.

1133. Egan, T. J., and Klein, R.: Hyperkalemic familial
periodic paralysis. Pediatrics, 24:761, 1959.

1134. Gammon, G. D., Austin, J. A., Blithe, M. D., and Reid,
G. G.: The relation of potassium to periodic family
paralysis. Amer. J. Med. Sci., 197:326, 1939.

1135. Gamstorp, I.: Adynamia episodica hereditaria. Acta
Paediat. Suppl. 108, 45:1, 1956.

1136. Gamstorp, I.: A Study of Transient Muscular Weakness.
Acta Neurol. Scand., 38:3, 1962.

1137. Grob, D., Liljestrand, A., and Johns, R. J.: Potassium
movement in patients with familial periodic paralysis.
Amer. J. Med., 23:356, 1957.

1138. Klein, R., Egan, T., and Usher, P.: Changes in sodium,
potassium, and water in hyperkalemic familial periodic paralysis. Metabolism, 9:1005, 1960.

1139. Liljestrand, A.: A case of adynamia episodica hereditaria. Opusc. Med., 2:183, 1957.

1140. McArdle, B.: Familial periodic paralysis. Brit. Med.
Bull., 12:226, 1956.

1141. McArdle, B.: Adynamia episodica hereditaria and its
treatment. Brain, 85:121, 1962.

1142. Morrison, J. B.: Electromyographic changes in hyperkalemic familial periodic paralysis. Ann. Phys. Med.,
5:153, 1960.

1143. Poskanzer, D. C., and Kerr, D. N. S.: Periodic paralysis
with response to spironolactone. Lancet, 2:511, 1916.

1144. Poskanzer, D. C., and Kerr, D. N. S.: A third type of
periodic paralysis with normokalemia and favorable
response to sodium chloride. Amer. J. Med., 31:328,
1961.

1145. Shy, G. M., Wanko, T., Rowley, P. T., and Engel, A. G.:
Studies in familial periodic paralysis. Exp. Neurol.,
3:53, 1961.

1146. Tyler, I. H., Stephens, F. E., Gunn, F. D., and Perkoff,
G. T.: Studies in disorders of muscle. VII. Clinical
manifestations and inheritance of a type of periodic
paralysis without hypopotassemia. J. Clin. Invest.,
30:492, 1951.

1147. Van der Muelen, J. P., Gilbert, G. J., and Kane, C. A.:
Familial hyperkalemic paralysis with myotonia. New
Eng. J. Med., 264:1, 1961.

1148. Zierler, K. L., and Andres, R.: Movement of potassium
into skeletal muscle during spontaneous attack in
family periodic paralysis. J. Clin. Invest., 36:730,
1957.

McARDLE'S SYNDROME

1149. Engel, W. K., Eyerman, E. L., and Williams, H. E.: Late-
onset type of skeletal-muscle phosphoyrlase deficiency: New familial variety with completely and
partially affected subjects. New Eng. J. Med., 268:135,
1963.

1150. McArdle, B.: Myopathy due to a defect in muscle glycogen breakdown. Clin. Sci., 10:13, 1951.

1151. Mellick, R. S., Mahler, R. E., and Hughes, B. P.: Mc
Ardle's syndrome: Phosphorlylase-deficient myopathy. Lancet, 1:1045, 1962.

1152. Mommaerts, W. F. H. M., Illingworth, B., Pearson,
C. M., Guillory, R. J., and Saraydarian, K.: A functional disorder of muscle associated with the absence
of phosphorylase. Proc. Nat. Acad. Sci., 46:791, 1959.

1153. Pearson, C. M., Rimer, D. G., and Mommaerts, W. F. H.
M.: A metabolic myopathy due to absence of muscle
phosphorylase. Amer. J. Med., 30:502, 1961.

1154. Porte, D., Jr., Crawford, D. W., Jennings, D. M., Aber,
O., and McIlroy, M. B.: Cardiovascular and metabolic responses to exercise in a patient with McArdle's
syndrome. New Eng. J. Med., 275:406, 1966.

1155. Schmid, R., and Hammaker, L.: Hereditary absence of
muscle phosphorylase (McArdle's syndrome). New
Eng. J. Med., 264:223, 1961.

1156. Schmid, R., and Mahler, R.: Chronic progressive myopathy with myoglobinuria: Demonstration of a glyco-
genolytic defect in the muscle. J. Clin. Invest., 38:
1044, 1959.

1157. Ratinov, G., Baker, W. P., and Swaiman, K. F.: Mc
Ardle's syndrome with previously unreported elec-
trocardiographic and serum enzyme abnormalities.
Ann. Intern. Med., 62:328, 1965.

IDIOPATHIC PAROXYSMAL MYOGLOBINURIA

1158. Berenbaum, M. C., Birch, C. A., and Moreland, J. D.:
Paroxysmal myoglobinuria. Lancet, 1:892, 1955.

1159. Bowden, D. H., Fraser, D., Jackson, S. H., and Walker,
N. F.: Acute recurrent rhabdomyolysis (paroxysmal
myohaemoglobinuria). Medicine, 35:335, 1956.

1160. Buchanan, D., and Steiner, P. R.: Myoglobinuria with
paralysis (Meyer-Betz disease). A.M.A. Arch Neurol.
Psychiat., 66:107, 1951.

1161. Kohler, H. J.: Die Myoglobinurien. Erglebn. Inn. Med.
Kinderheilk., 11:1, 1959.

1162. Korein, J., Coddon, D. R., and Mowrey, F. H.: The
clinical syndrome of paroxysmal paralytic myoglobinuria. Neurology, 9:767, 1959.

1163. Meyer-Betz, F.: Beobachtungen an einem eigenartigen
mit Muskellähmungen verbundenem Fall von Hämo-
globinurie. Deutsch. Arch. Klin. Med., 101:85, 1911.

1164. Pearson, C. M., Beck, W. S., and Blahd, W. H.: Idiopathic paroxysmal myoglobinuria. Detailed study of
a case including radioisotope and serum enzyme
evaluations. A.M.A. Arch Intern. Med., 99:376, 1957.

1165. Prankerd, T. A. J.: Electrophoretic properties of myoglobin and its character in sickle cell disease and
paroxysmal myoglobinuria. Brit. J. Haemat., 2:80,
1956.

1166. Reiner, L., Konikoff, N., Altschule, M. D., Dammin, G.,
and Merrill, J. P.: Idiopathic paroxysmal myoglobinuria. Report of two cases and evaluation of the
syndrome. A.M.A. Arch. Intern. Med., 97:537, 1956.

1167. Schaar, F. E., LaBree, J. W., and Gleason, D. F.: Paroxysmal myohemoglobinuria with fatal renal tubular
injury. Central Soc. Clin. Res. Proc., 22:71, 1949.

STIFF-MAN SYNDROME

1168. Asher, R.: A woman with the stiff-man syndrome. Brit.
Med. J., 1:265, 1958.

1169. Moersch, F. P., and Woltman, H. W.: Progressive fluc-
tuating muscular rigidity ("stiff-man syndrome").
Proc. Staff Meet. Mayo Clin., 31:421, 1956.

1170. Price, T. M. L., and Allott, E. M.: The stiff-man syndrome. Brit. Med. J., 2:682, 1958.

MYASTHENIA GRAVIS

1171. Bowman, J. R.: Myasthenia gravis in young children.
Pediatrics, 1:472, 1948.

1172. Eaton, L. M.: Diagnostic tests for myasthenia with
prostigmin and quinine. Proc. Staff Meet. Mayo Clin.,
18:230, 1943.

1173. Erb, W.: Zur Casuistik der bulbären Lähmungen. Ueber
einen neuen, wahrscheinlich bulbären Symptomencomplex. Arch. Psychiat., 9:336, 1879.

1174. Goldflam, S.: Ueber einen scheinbar heilbaren bul-
bärparalytischen Symptomencomplex mit Betheili-
gung der Extremitäten. Deutsch. Z. Nervenheilk.,
4:312, 1893.

1175. Guthrie, L. G.: Myasthenia gravis in the seventeenth
century. Lancet, 1:330, 1903.

1176. Harvey, A. M., and Johns, R. J.: Myasthenia gravis and
the thymus. Amer. J. Med., 32:1, 1962.

1177. Grob, D.: Course and management of myasthenia gravis. J.A.M.A., *153*:529, 1953.

1178. Jolly, F.: Ueber Myasthenia gravis pseudoparalytica. Berl. Klin. Wschr., *32*:1, 1895.

1179. Kibrick, S.: Myasthenia gravis in the newborn. Pediatrics, *14*:365, 1954.

1180. MacRae, D. D.: Myasthenia gravis in early childhood. Pediatrics, *13*:511, 1954.

1181. Millichap, J. G., and Dodge, P. R.: Diagnosis and treatment of myasthenia gravis in infancy, childhood, and adolescence. Neurology, *10*:1007, 1960.

1182. Osserman, K. E.: Myasthenia Gravis. New York, Grune & Stratton, 1958.

1183. Pritchard, E. A. B.: "Prostigmin" in the treatment of myasthenia gravis. Lancet, *1*:432, 1935.

1184. Rowland, L. P.: Fatalities in myasthenia gravis. J. Amer. Neurol. Ass., *78*:158, 1953.

1185. Rowland, L. P.: Prostigmin responsiveness in the diagnosis of myasthenia gravis. Neurology, *5*:612, 1955.

1186. Rowland, L. P., and Eskenzai, A. M.: Myasthenia gravis with features resembling muscular dystrophy. Neurology, *6*:667, 1956.

1187. Simpson, J. A.: Myasthenia gravis and myasthenic syndromes. *In* Walker, J. N. (ed.): Disorders of Voluntary Muscle. Boston, Little, Brown and Co., 1964, p. 336.

1188. Stortebecker, T. P.: Signs of myositis in myasthenia gravis and in myopathy clinically resembling progressive muscular dystrophy. Acta Med. Scand., *151*:451, 1955.

1189. Strickroot, F. L., Schaeffer, R. L., and Bergs, H. L.: Myasthenia gravis occurring in an infant born of a myasthenic mother. J.A.M.A., *120*:1207, 1942.

1190. Teng, P., and Osserman, K. E.: Studies in myasthenia gravis: Neonatal and juvenile types. A report of 21 and a review of 188 cases. J. Mount Sinai Hosp., *23*:711, 1956.

1191. Viets, H. R.: A historical review of myasthenia gravis from 1672 to 1900. J.A.M.A., *153*:1273, 1953.

1192. Viets, H. R., and Brown, M. R.: Medical progress: Diseases of muscles. New Eng. J. Med., *245*:647, 1951.

1193. Viets, H. R., and Schwab, R. S.: Prostigmin in the diagnosis of myasthenia gravis. New Eng. J. Med., *213*:1280, 1935.

1194. Walker, M. B.: Treatment of myasthenia gravis with prostigmin. Lancet, *1*:1200, 1934.

1195. Walker, M. B.: Case showing effect of prostigmin on myasthenia gravis. Proc. Roy. Soc. Med., *28*:759, 1935.

1196. Westerberg, M. R., and MaGee, K. R.: Treatment review: Myasthenia gravis. Neurology, *5*:728, 1955.

1197. Willis, T.: De anima brutorum. Oxford, Theatro Sheldoniano, 1672, pp. 404–406.

1198. Wilkes, S.: On cerebritis, hysteria, and bulbar paralysis, as illustrative of arrest of function of the cerebrospinal centers. Guy's Hosp. Rep., *22*:7, 1877.

1199. Wyllie, W. G., Bodian, M., and Burrows, N. F. E.: Myasthenia gravis in children. Arch. Dis. Child., *26*:457, 1951.

GENERAL REFERENCES

1200. Adams, R. D., Denny-Brown, D., and Pearson, C. M.: Diseases of Muscle. 2nd Ed. New York, Paul B. Hoeber, Inc., 1963.

1201. Bourne, G. H.: The Structure and Function of Muscle, Vol. III. Pharmacology and Disease. New York, Academic Press, 1960.

1202. Dreyfus, J. C., and Schapira, G.: Biochemistry of Hereditary Myopathies. Springfield, Ill., Charles C Thomas, 1962.

1203. Greenfield, J. G., Shy, G. M., Alvord, E. C., and Berg, L.: Atlas of Muscle Pathology in Neuromuscular Diseases. London, E. & S. Livingstone, 1957.

1204. Murphy, E. G.: The Chemistry and Therapy of Disorders of Voluntary Muscle. Springfield, Ill., Charles C Thomas, 1964.

1205. Stanbury, J. B., Wyngaarden, J. B., and Frederickson, D. S.: The Metabolic Basis of Inherited Disease. 2nd Ed. New York, McGraw-Hill Book Co., 1966.

1206. Walton, J. N.: Disorders of Voluntary Muscle. Boston, Little, Brown and Co., 1964.

6. *The Spine*

Posture and Postural Defects

Posture can be defined as the relationship of the parts of the body to the line of the center of gravity. The orthopedic surgeon is concerned with posture as a gauge of mechanical efficiency of the neuromusculoskeletal system in the erect position.

Development of Posture

In the uterus the fetus is almost invariably in a position of flexion, with the convex curve of the spine lying against the curve of the uterine wall. The head, arms, and legs of the fetus are flexed on the torso (Fig. 6–1). The entire fetus lives suspended in the amniotic fluid, which has a specific gravity similar to that of the fetus. Following birth the development of posture is affected by the constant forces exerted by gravity.

The newborn holds his shoulders, elbows, hips, and knees in flexion, with his limbs slightly bowed and rotated inward (Fig. 6–2 A). Fifteen to thirty degrees of flexion

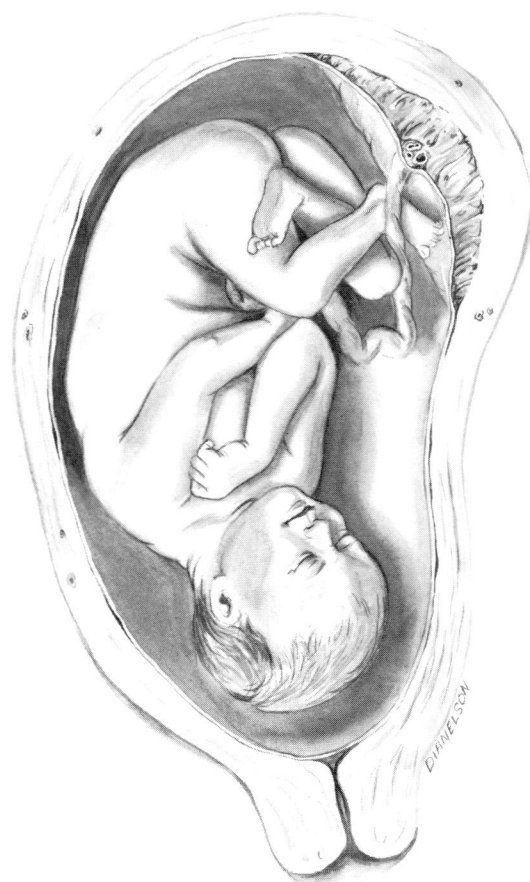

FIGURE 6–1. Posture of fetus in utero.

Note the position of flexion.

contracture of the knee is a normal physical finding. The infant lies in a nearly horizontal position, unable to support his head or trunk. In either the prone or the supine position, gravitational force is exerted on a horizontal plane and tends to unroll the "coiling" that was previously assumed within the uterus.

The rate of development of muscle strength varies in the different parts of the body. When the infant is in a horizontal position, the hip flexors, the anterior muscles of the neck, and the abdominal muscles are stretched and used minimally, whereas the extensors of the neck, back, and thigh are relaxed and are the first to increase their motor power. When the child is able to support his head and begins to sit up, the weight of the head, combined with the persistent flexion attitude of the hips and the associated flexion of the pelvis on the spine, produces a long convex curve of the entire spine. In the prestanding stage, this total convex curve of the back is normal (Fig. 6–2 B).

When the child begins to stand and walk, the extensor muscles of the back, neck, and hips are well developed and the spine is usually straight. In the upright position, the force of gravity is exerted in a vertical direction, causing an exaggerated lumbar lordosis and a protuberant abdomen (Fig. 6–2 C). With further growth and development, the child improves his stance and becomes more agile in walking and running. In studying posture, one should bear in mind the interdependence of various parts of the body. For example, mild pronation of the feet is normal and common in a child of preschool age. The gastrocnemius-soleus muscles are long enough to allow dorsiflexion of the feet 20 to 30 degrees beyond neutral. In stance, mild genu valgum is common. These physical findings are normal and not pathologic.

Normal Posture

The posture of each person has characteristics that are uniquely his. Various factors affecting posture are:

Bony contours. The shape of the vertebrae may be modified by diseases such as tuberculosis or Scheuermann's disease, which produce dorsal kyphosis.

Laxity of Ligamentous Structures. The degree of ligamentous laxity varies in different individuals, giving rise to looseness or tightness of the joints. The spine is composed of many joints, and is itself dependent upon the articulations inferior to it, such as those of the feet, knees, and hips.

Fascial and Musculotendinous Tightness. Tightness of soft tissue structures, especially the fascia lata, hamstrings, anterior hip capsule, and pectorals, affect posture.

Muscle Strength. Particularly important is the strength of the gluteus maximus, abdominal, erector spinae, and scapular adductor muscles.

Pelvic Inclination. The pelvis is the base upon which the vertebral column rests. Any change in its inclination will cause a corresponding change in the position of the fifth lumbar vertebra in relation to the sacrum, which in turn alters the posture of the entire spine. Inclination of the pelvis is ordinarily controlled by the muscles about the hip (Fig. 6–3). It is increased by contraction of the extensors of the hip, i.e., the glutei, hamstrings, and the posterior portion of the hip adductors, and it is decreased by contraction of the hip flexors, i.e., the iliopsoas, rectus femoris, pectineus, and the more anterior portion of the hip adductors. The spine is flexed by the iliopsoas and abdominal muscles, and is extended by the erector spinae. The abdominal muscles act synergetically with the glutei, the latter decreasing the pelvic inclination and the former reducing the lumbar lordosis. Motion of the vertebral column is greatest in the lumbar region; in the thoracic spine, however, rotation is of con-

siderable magnitude, but flexion and extension are limited. The muscles of respiration (the diaphragm and intercostals) produce a secondary effect on posture, as there is some extension of the dorsal spine with each inspiration.

In normal posture the body weight is carried forward on the balls of the feet, the legs are straight, the pelvic inclination is about 60 degrees to the vertical, the abdomen is retracted, the shoulders are level and flat, and the head is held erect. The line of the center of gravity of the body passes from the mastoid process to the cervicodorsal junction, crossing the bodies of the vertebrae at the dorsolumbar junction, and falling just anterior to the sacroiliac articulation and slightly posterior to the hip joint; it passes through the anterior

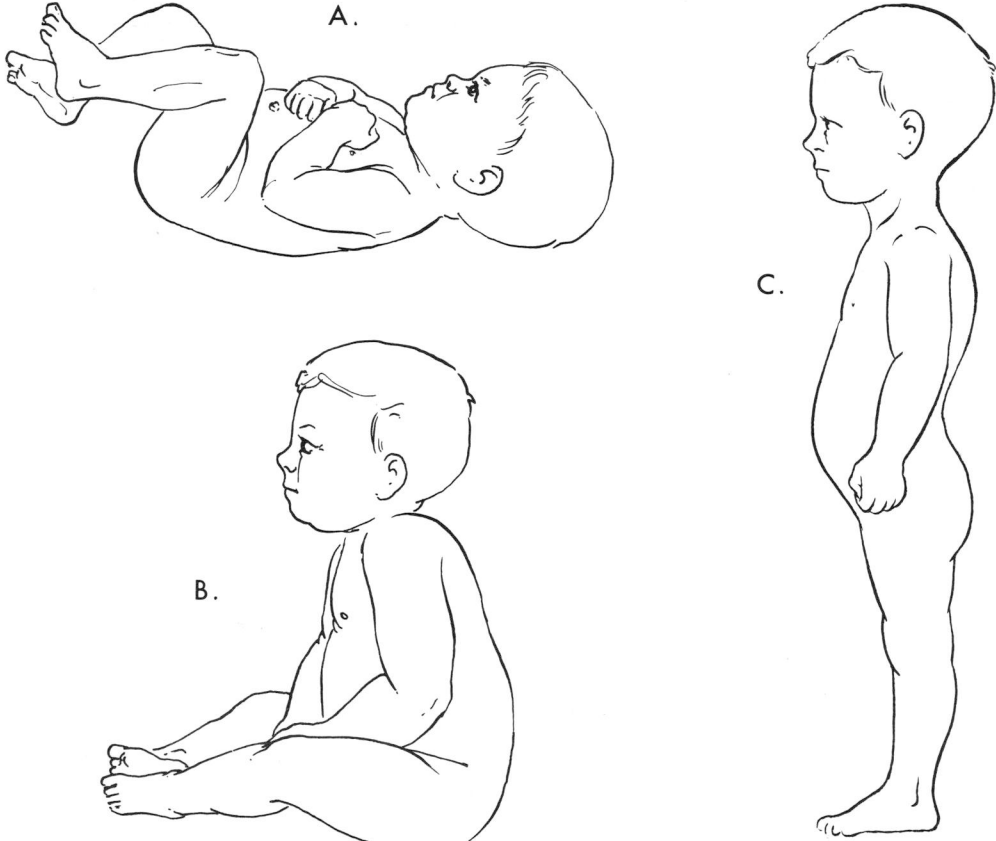

FIGURE 6–2.   Development of posture.

   A. In the newborn. Note the flexion attitude of the hips and knees. **B.** In the prestanding stage. Total convex curve of the spine is normal. **C.** In the 18-month-old child. A prominent abdomen and exaggerated lumbar lordosis are normal.

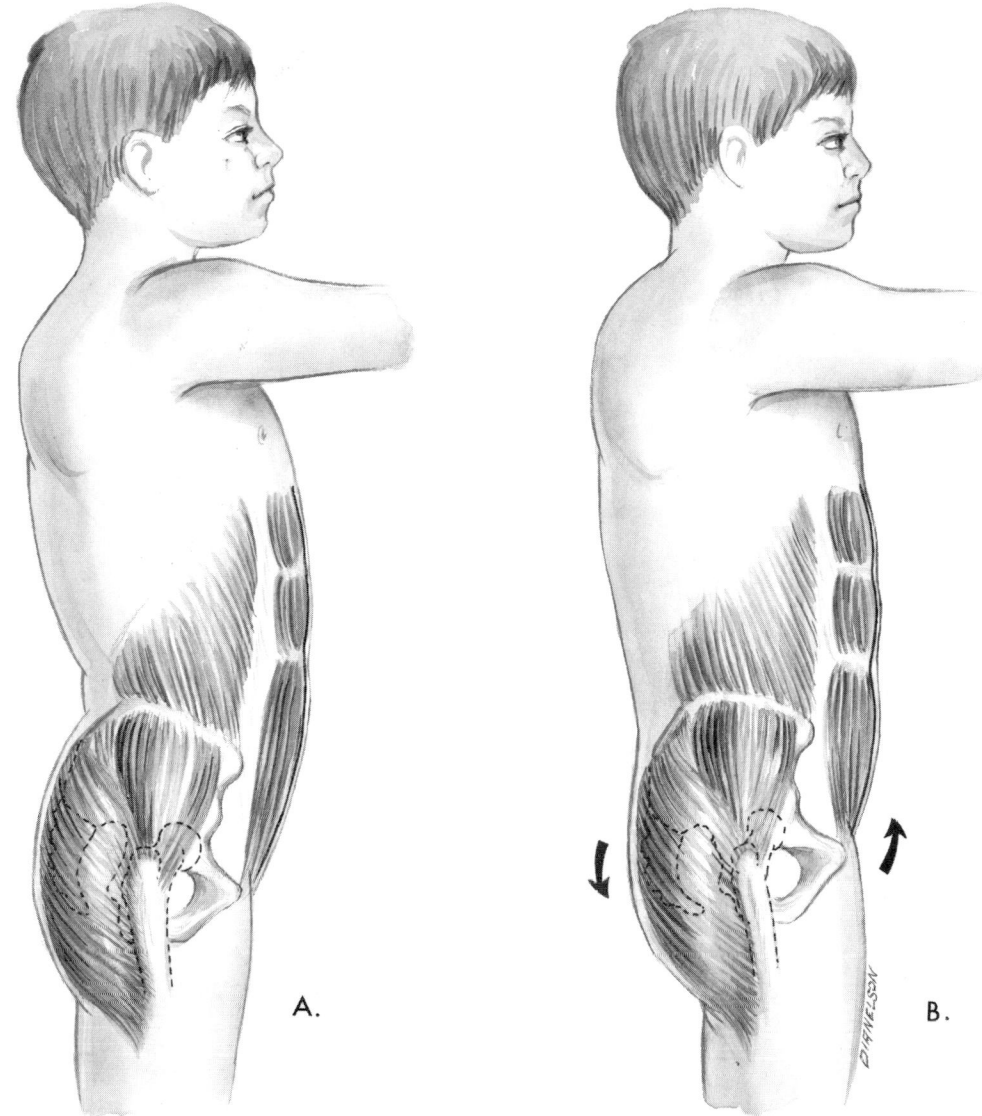

FIGURE 6–3. *Pelvic tilt.*

knee joint and terminates at the front of the talus in the ankle.

Gradation of Posture

Posture can be classified into four grades (Fig. 6–4 A to D):

A—*excellent* or almost perfect posture

B—*good*, but not ideal posture

C—*poor*, but not the worst possible posture

D—*bad* and very possibly symptom-producing posture

In excellent (*A*) posture, the head and shoulders are balanced over the pelvis, hips, and ankles, with the head erect and the chin held in. The sternum is the part of the body farthest forward, the abdomen is drawn in and flat, and the spinal curves are within normal limits. In bad (*D*) posture, the head is held forward to a marked degree, the chest is depressed, the abdomen is completely relaxed and protuberant, the spinal curves are exaggerated, and the shoulders are held behind the pelvis.

(*Text continued on page 1146.*)

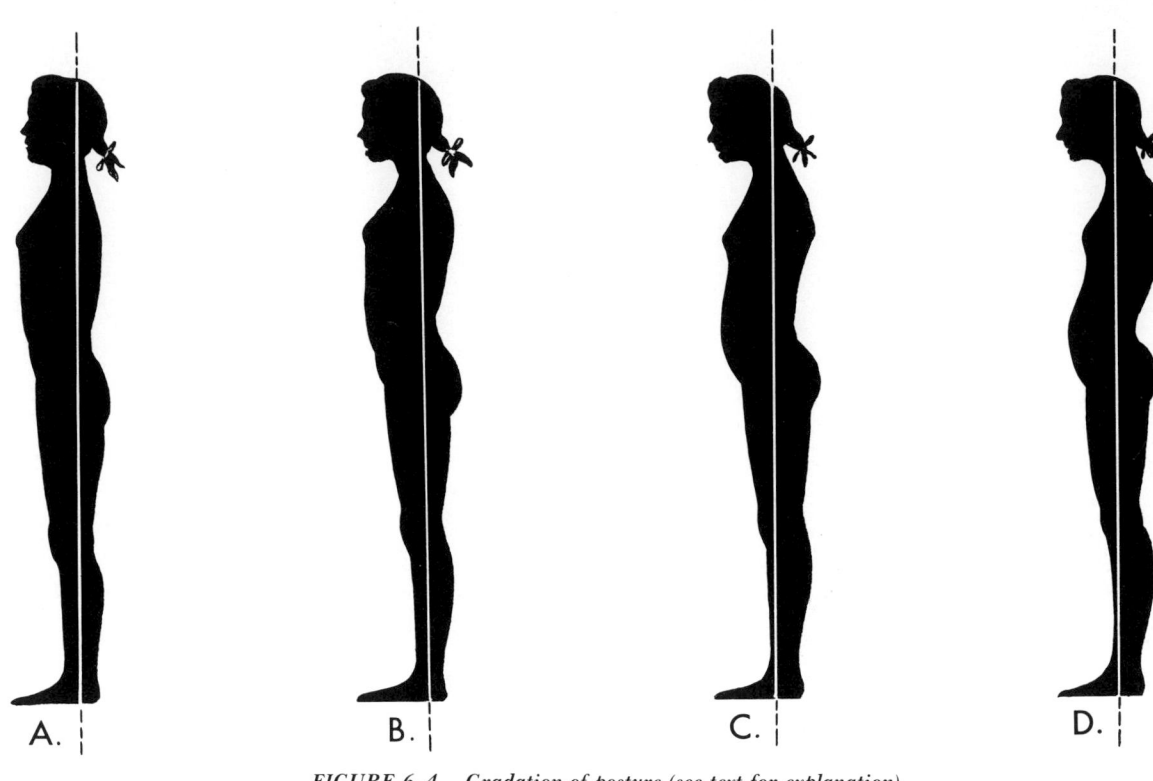

FIGURE 6–4. *Gradation of posture (see text for explanation).*

FIGURE 6–5. **Passive exercises for poor posture.**

Stretching of contracted anterior neck structures and pectorals. **A.** The child lies supine with a bolster just distal to the apex of kyphosis for 15 minutes once or twice a day. **B.** With the child sitting on a chair, parent passively stretches the contracted pectorals by pushing the forward drooped shoulders posteriorly. **C.** The child lies on his side, knees flexed on the chest, while an assistant places one hand at the apex of the kyphosis with same forearm steadying the lower spine, and with the other hand, pushes the upper spine above the kyphosis into hyperextension.

Stretching of contracted lumbosacral fascia. **D.** Knee-chest exercises. Lying supine, bring knees on chest, flattening the lumbar spine and passively stretching the contracture of the lumbosacral fascia; count to 10 and lower legs to starting position.

Passive stretching of contracture of anterior soft tissues of the neck. **E.** Head-neck traction in a Sayre sling.

Hamstring stretching. **F-1.** The child lies supine; an assistant steadies the pelvis with one hand and, with the other hand, holds the leg in extension, raises the leg to a right angle, or as close to it as possible, then lowers it to starting position. The knee should always be in complete extension and the pelvis steadied flat on the floor. **F-2.** Toe-touching. Stand erect with the feet flat on the floor and 6 inches apart and the arms extended over the head; keeping the knees extended, bend forward to touch the floor between the feet, count to 5, and return to starting position.

Gastrocnemius-soleus stretching. **G-1.** Stand 2 to 3 feet away from the wall. Keep the feet, especially the heels, flat on the floor; curl the toes; the feet should be in slight inversion with the big toes pointing medially. Steady the trunk by placing hands against the wall. A wooden block may be used under the forefeet for more effective stretching. **G-2.** Keeping knees and hips in extension and the heels on the floor, carry the buttocks and trunk toward the wall. Count to 5 and return to starting position.

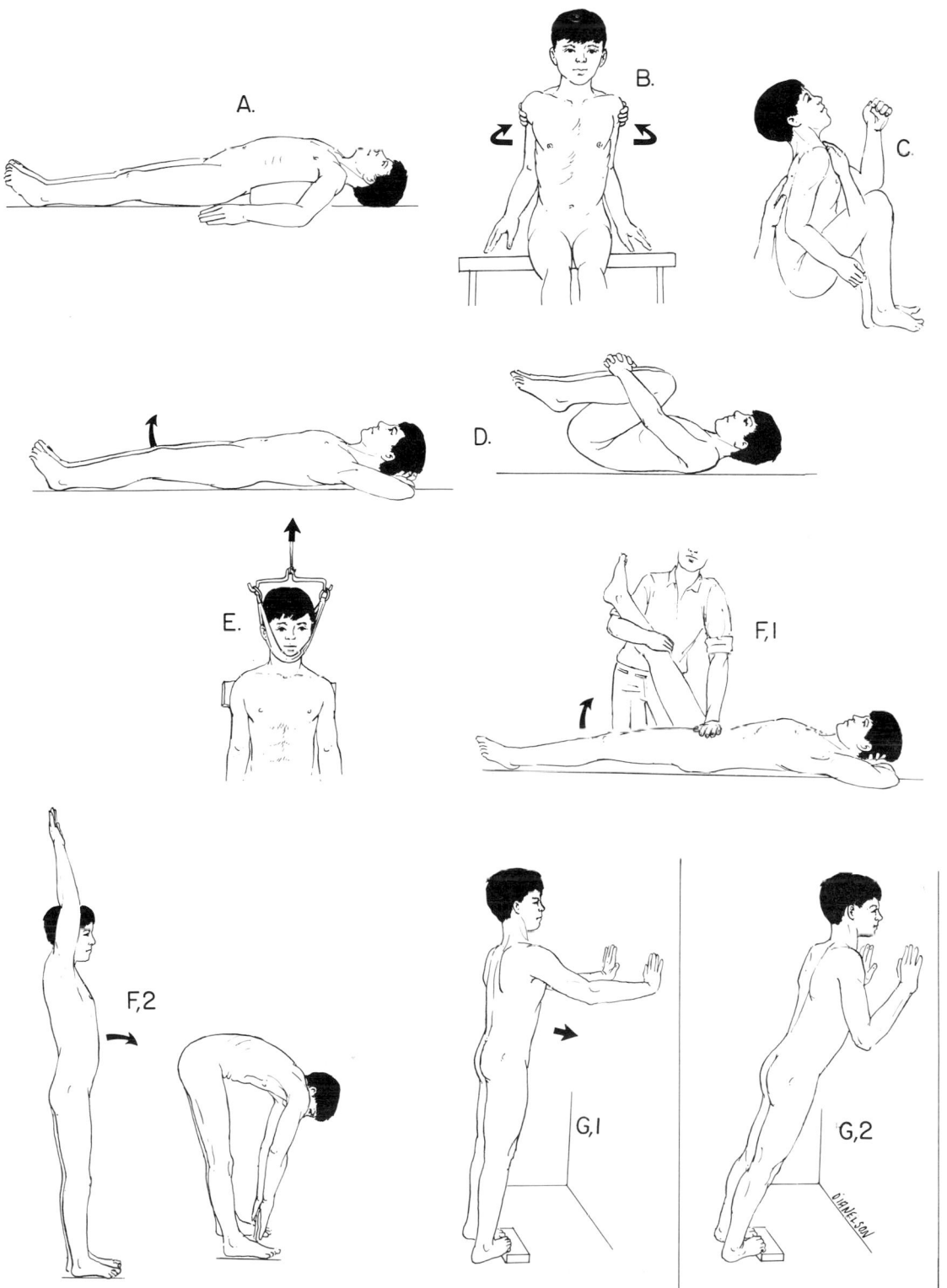

FIGURE 6–5. **Passive exercises for poor posture.** *See opposite page for legend.*

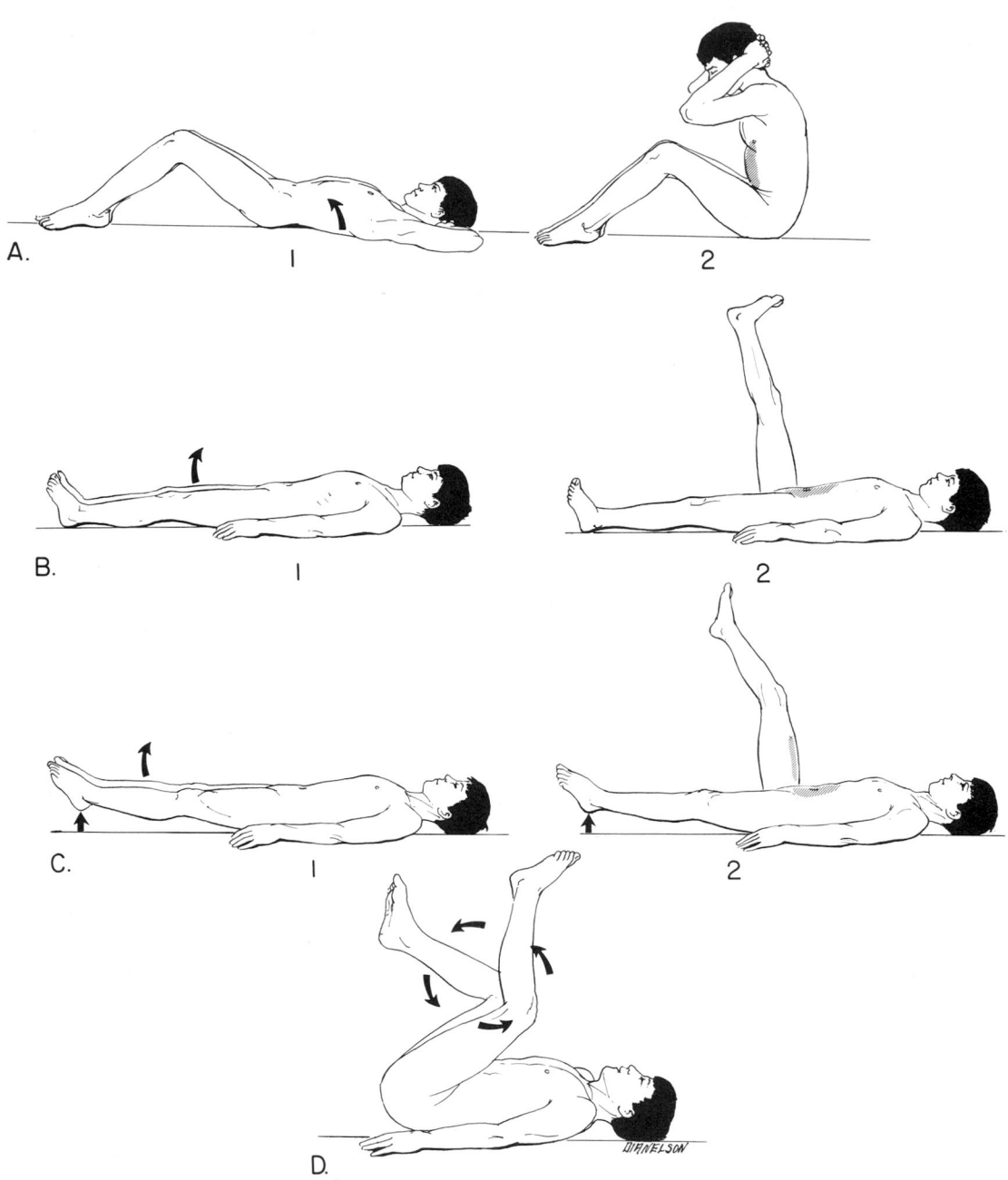

FIGURE 6–6.   *Active exercises for poor posture.*

Abdominal exercises. **A.** Sit-ups. **1.** Lie supine, hips and knees flexed 30 degrees and in neutral rotation, hands clasped behind head, keeping the feet on the floor (support may be used if necessary) and the back straight. **2.** Move to sitting position to the count of 5, then lower body to starting position. **B.** Leg raising. **1.** Lie supine, legs together, knees and hips in extension, arms at the side and lumbar spine flat. **2.** Raise right leg until it is at a right angle to the trunk, or as close to this position as possible, then slowly lower it. Repeat the same with left leg. Continue the exercise by alternating legs. **C.** Flutter-kick. **1.** Same position as in **B,** but keep the feet off the floor to a height of 2 or 3 inches. **2.** Slowly raise the right leg until it is perpendicular to the trunk, or as close to this position as possible, then slowly lower the leg to the starting position. Repeat the same with left lower extremity. Always keep feet and legs off the floor. **D.** Bicycling.

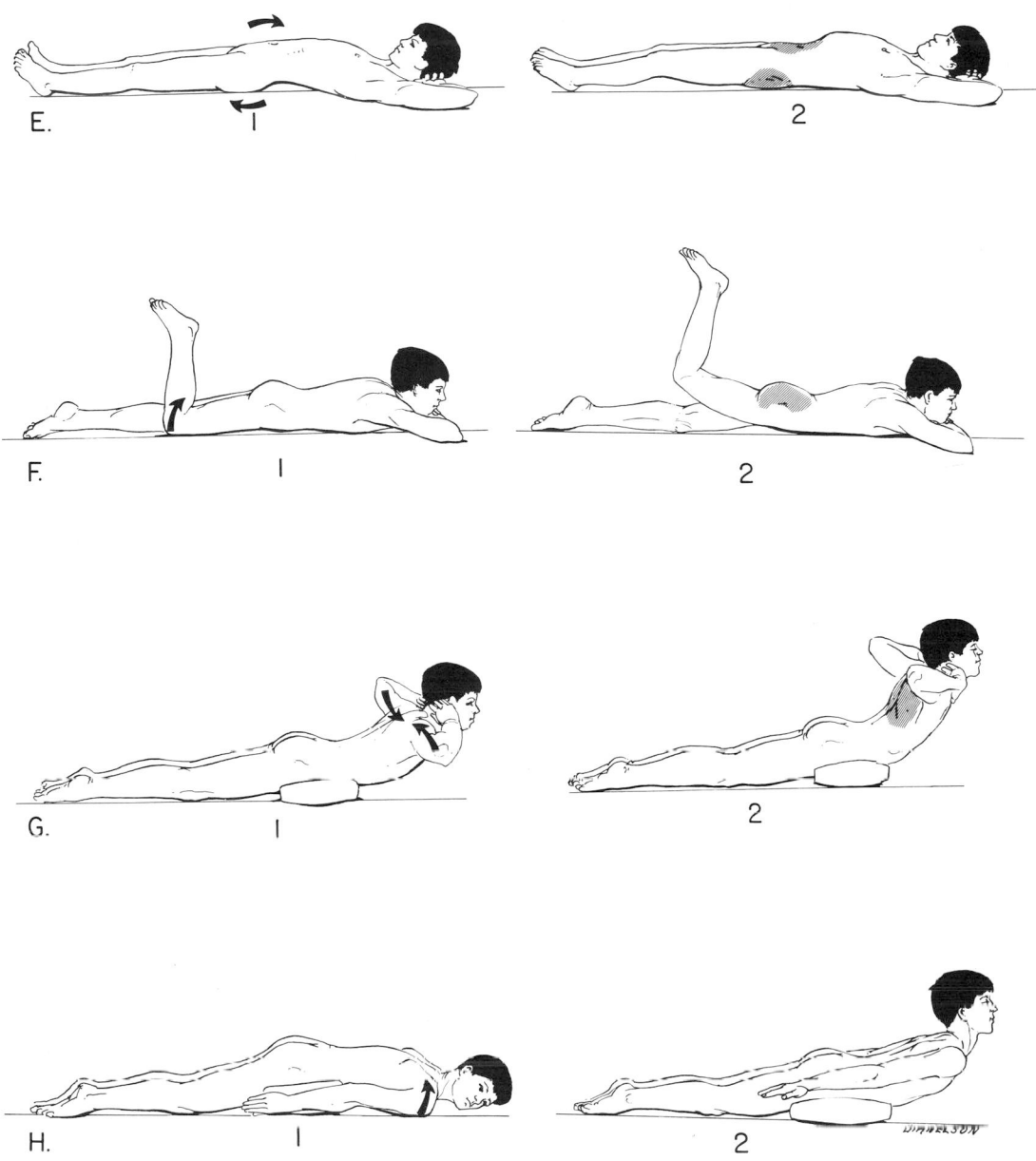

FIGURE 6–6 Continued. *Active exercises for poor posture.*

Pelvic tilt. **E–1.** Lying supine on the floor, pinch buttocks together and, without taking a deep breath, pull in abdominal muscles to flatten the lumbar spine. **E–2.** Graduate this exercise by performing the pelvic tilt exercise in stance while standing against the wall, and then in gait while walking away from the wall (Fig. 6–3).

Gluteus maximus exercises. **F–1.** Lie prone with knee flexed at right angle (to eliminate action of hamstrings) and arms under chin. **F–2.** Raise right thigh off floor as high as possible while keeping the knee flexed, count to 5, then lower it. Repeat the same with opposite side. Graduate this exercise to lifting both thighs off the floor at the same time.

Scapular adduction. **G–1.** Lying prone with one or two pillows under abdomen with shoulders abducted and hands clasped behind the neck, raise the head, neck, and upper trunk off the floor. **G–2.** Bring the shoulder blades together, count to 5, then return to starting position. The same exercise could be performed sitting on a chair with lower spine acutely flexed.

Dorsal hyperextension. **H–1.** Lie prone with the arms along the sides and the palms of the hands pressing against the thighs. **H–2.** Slowly raise the head, neck, and shoulders off the floor as high as possible, count to 5, then gradually return to starting position.

Treatment of Postural Defects

Poor posture in children should be noted, and corrective measures taken to increase the strength of the back so that it will be less susceptible in adult life to fatigue, back strain, and injury. Children rarely complain of backache from poor posture. In adults, however, poor body mechanics and posture are frequent causes of low back strain.

Treatment consists of passive and active exercises (Figs. 6–5 and 6–6). First, if there are any contracted soft tissues—such as triceps surae, hamstrings, anterior hip structures, lumbosacral fascia, pectorals, and neck flexors—they should be passively stretched. The tight anterior neck and shoulder structures may be stretched by lying down with a small bolster between the two scapulae for 15 minutes twice a day. The child is also instructed to perform exercises to increase the motor strength of the key muscles affecting posture; namely,

the abdominal muscles (sit-ups, flutter-kick, and bicycling), gluteus maximus (hip extension against gravity with knees in flexion), erector spinae (hyperextension of spine against gravity in prone position) and scapular adductors (bringing shoulder blades together in prone or sitting position).

The most important exercise is the pelvic tilt (Figs. 6–3 and 6–6 E). The patient is instructed to decrease the pelvic inclination by use of the abdominal and gluteus maximus muscles. Initially, he performs the pelvic tilt exercise in a supine position, then standing against the wall. By reduction of the pelvic tilt, all the exaggerated curves of the spine are decreased. The shoulders are brought over the pelvis with the head held erect and chin held in, thus correcting the poor posture. Postural exercises should be carried out until the individual is able to maintain the correct posture naturally. The patient should continue the exercises until they become part of his normal stance and gait.

Congenital and Developmental Anomalies

CONGENITAL SCOLIOSIS

Classification

There are various types of structural scoliosis due to congenital vertebral and rib anomalies. Winter, Moe, and Eilers have amended MacEwen's classification, which is based on the type and quantity of segmentation defects (Fig. 6–7).[13, 17] The six types are as follows:

I. Partial unilateral failure of formation of a vertebra producing a wedge and trapezoid shape of vertebra (Fig. 6–7 A). A small vestigial pedicle may be seen on the roentgenogram.

II. Complete unilateral failure of formation of a vertebra. A hemivertebra is produced, which may be unbalanced or balanced (Fig. 6–7 B to D).

III. Bilateral failure of segmentation in which there is absence of the disc space between adjacent vertebral bodies (Fig. 6–7 E).

IV. Unilateral failure of segmentation which produces an unsegmented bar (Fig. 6–7 F). Two or more vertebrae may be affected with involvement of either the vertebral bodies, the posterior elements, or both (Fig. 6–7 G to I). Unsegmented unilateral bars have the worst prognosis for progression and deformity (Fig. 6–7 J). Bilateral failure of segmentation may affect only the posterior elements, producing a fixed and progressive lordosis.

V. Fusion of ribs

A. The ribs may be fused into a bony mass close to and continuous with the vertebrae (usually associated with an unsegmented bar). These curves do progress, and correction cannot be obtained unless rib resection and osteotomy of the bar are performed.

B. The ribs may also be fused anteriorly at a distance from the vertebrae. This anomaly appears to have no significant relationship to curvature of the spine.

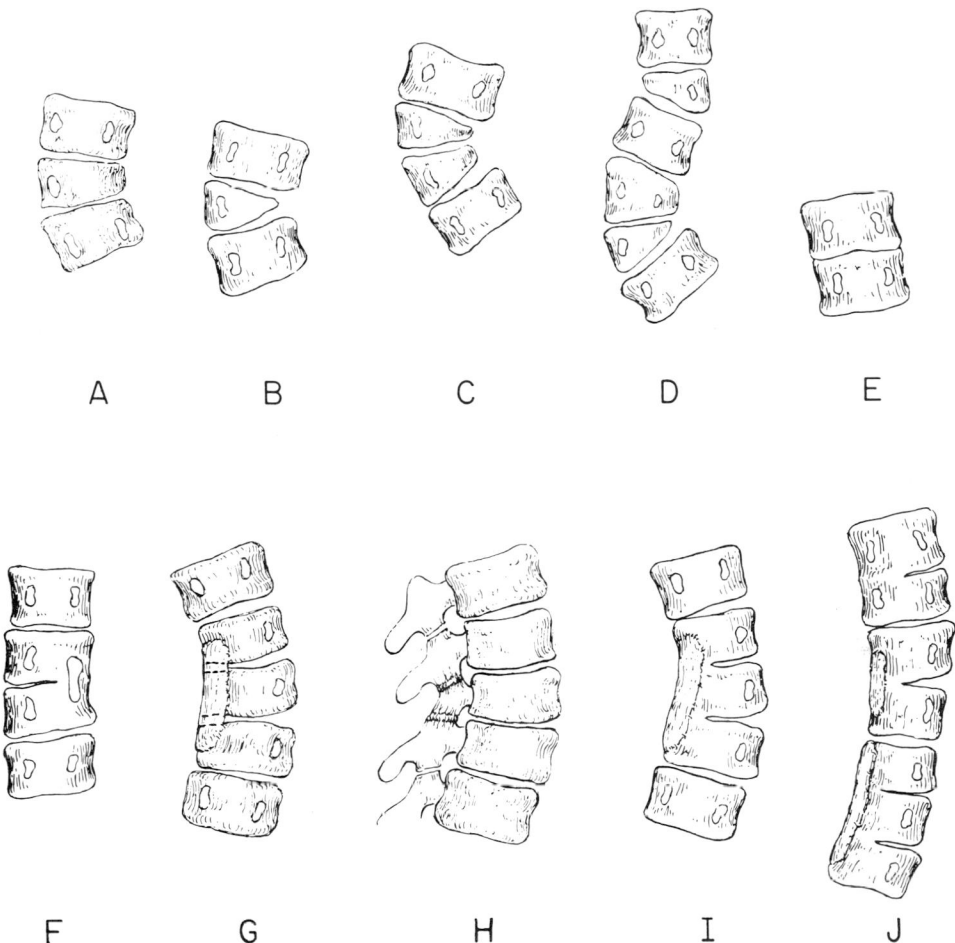

FIGURE 6–7. *Types of vertebral anomalies producing congenital scoliosis.*

A. Wedged vertebra due to partial unilateral failure of formation of a vertebra. **B.** Hemivertebra due to complete unilateral failure of formation of a vertebra. **C.** Double hemivertebra, unbalanced. **D.** Double hemivertebra, balanced. **E.** Bilateral symmetrical failure of segmentation. Note the absence of disc interspace and fusion of the adjacent vertebral bodies. **F.** Asymmetrical failure of segmentation (unsegmented bar). **G.** Asymmetrical failure of segmentation (unsegmented bar involving posterior elements only, anteroposterior view). **H.** Asymmetrical failure of segmentation, oblique view. Note the intact disc space and the confinement of lack of segmentation to the posterior elements only. **I.** Unsegmented bar involving both the disc area and posterior elements. **J.** Multiple unsegmented bars, unbalanced. (From Winter, R. B., Moe, J. H., and Eilers, V. E.: Congenital scoliosis: A study of 234 patients treated and untreated. J. Bone Joint Surg., *50–A*:3, 1968.)

VI. Unclassifiable. There are some types of segmentation defects that are not characterized by a single preponderant anomaly. Laminagrams are occasionally indicated to delineate the components of a jumbled mass of abnormal bones.

Associated congenital anomalies other than those of the vertebral column or ribs are not uncommon. Winter et al. found 115 associated anomalies in 73 of the 234 patients having congenital scoliosis. In their series, some of the common ones were as follows: congenital heart disease (16 patients), Sprengel's deformity (14 patients), cleft palate (9 patients), hypoplasia of one leg (9 patients), talipes equinovarus (6 patients), extra thumbs (4 patients), hypoplastic thumbs (4 patients), vertical talus (2 patients), pectus carinatum (2 patients), and cleft lip (2 patients).[17] In general, the curves in the cervicothoracic area tended to be associated with cardiac anomalies, Sprengel's deformity, and congenital anomalies of the upper limb, such as partial amelia or congenital absence of the radius; whereas, those in the lumbar area tended to be associated with anomalies of the genitourinary tract or the lower limbs.

A thorough neurologic examination should always be performed. Whenever there is evidence of neurologic deficit distal to an abnormal region of the spine, myelography is in order. Diastematomyelia was found in 14 patients in the series of Winter et al. When routine roentgenograms suggest diastematomyelia, myelography is indicated, even in the absence of a neurologic deficit, because the lesion should be resected before paresis develops.

Natural History

In the past, it has been an unfortunate tendency of many physicians to assume that congenital scoliosis does not progress and therefore treatment is not indicated. Kuhns and Hormell, in a study of 165 patients with congenital scoliosis, were able to obtain data on 85 children followed to maturity. They found that 13 showed no progression; 40, moderate progression (5 to 30 degrees); and 32, progression of more than 30 degrees.[12] Shands and Bundens noted sudden progression during adolescence.[14] Blount emphasized that unsegmented bars cause severe progression.[7] Winter, Moe, and Eilers, in the analysis of their 234 patients (of whom 110 had reached skeletal maturity), noted that congenital scoliosis is usually slowly but relentlessly progressive; an unacceptable deformity results if active treatment is not given.[17] One of the most common pitfalls is the failure to detect this

subtle but steady progression of the curvature. When one carefully measures serial standing roentgenograms and compares the most recent roentgenogram with the initial one, the slow and steady progression will become apparent. The following factors seem to affect the natural history of congenital scoliosis:

Specific Anomaly. Unilateral unsegmented bars, a common anomaly, are most often seen in the thoracic area and have the worst prognosis for progression and deformity (Fig. 6–8). With this exception, the specific anomaly present is of less prognostic value than the pattern of the curve and the area of the spine involved.

Area of the Spine Involved. In general, cervicothoracic and lumbar curves are less progressive than are curves in the thoracic region. One should be cognizant of the fact that a mild cervicothoracic curve may produce an unsightly appearance because of head and neck tilt and asymmetry and depression of one shoulder. Lumbar curves do not tend to cause much cosmetic deformity unless decompensation or pelvic obliquity occurs. Thoracic curves are likely to be more progressive than those primarily in other areas. Congenital scoliosis in the thoracolumbar area is largely due to hemivertebrae, which may be located laterally, posterolaterally, or sometimes directly posteriorly. The more posterior the hemivertebrae, the worse the kyphosis and the more ominous the prognosis.

Balance and Pattern of the Curve. In general, multiple balanced anomalies throughout the spine do not progress and there is a satisfactory cosmetic appearance (Fig. 6–9). The more unbalanced the

---

FIGURE 6–8. *The natural history of an unsegmented unilateral bar in the thoracic area.*

A. Clinical appearance of a girl three years old. **B.** Roentgenogram of the spine of the same patient at three years of age. Note the unsegmented unilateral bar on the left side from the third through the sixth thoracic vertebrae. The right thoracic curve is 38 degrees. The beginning of a left thoracolumbar compensatory curve is apparent. This patient was treated ineffectively with a leather and steel underarm Brace. **C.** Photograph of same patient at the age of 12 years, showing the severe clinical deformity. **D.** Roentgenogram of same patient at the age of 12 years. Note the progression of the major curve from 38 to 98 degrees and the development of severe structural secondary curve from the eighth thoracic vertebra to the second lumbar cuve. This child well demonstrates that unsegmented unilateral bars in the thoracic area have the worst prognosis for progression and deformity. (From Winter, R. B., Moe, J. H., and Eilers, V. E.: Congenital scoliosis. A study of 234 patients treated and untreated. J. Bone Joint Surg., *50–A*:12, 1968.)

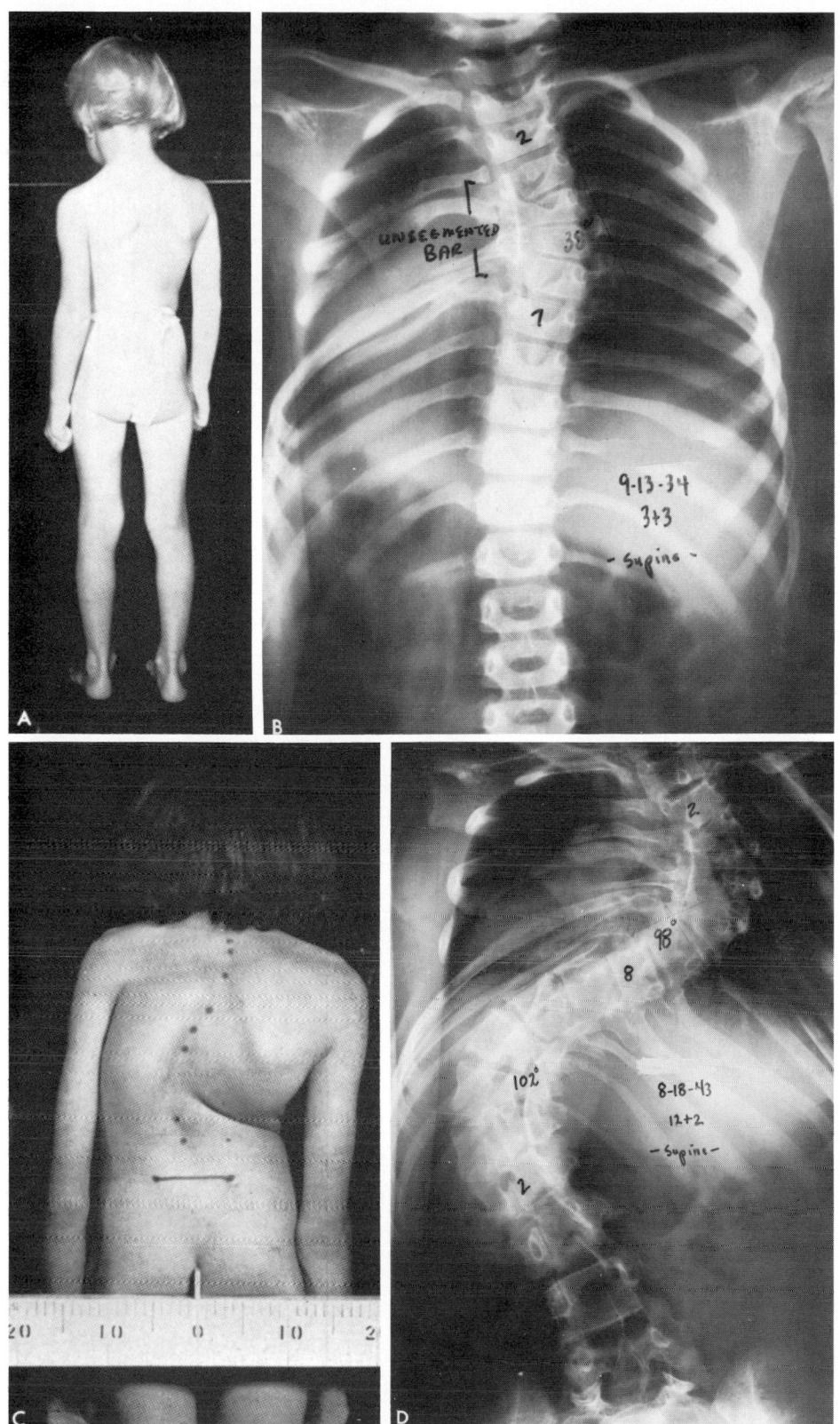

FIGURE 6–8. *The natural history of an unsegmented unilateral bar in the thoracic area.*
See opposite page for legend.

1149

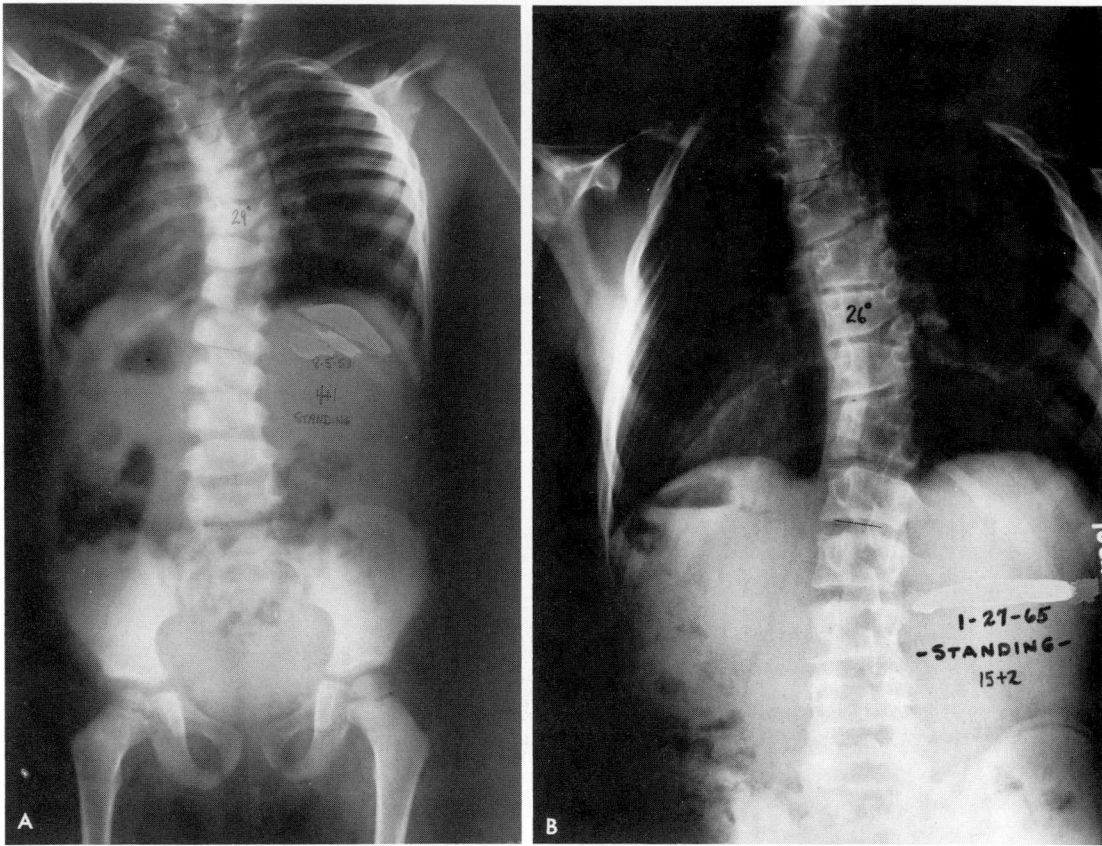

FIGURE 6–9. *The natural history of multiple balanced anomalies of the spine.*

A. Roentgenogram of the spine depicting multiple fairly well-balanced anomalies throughout the spine in a boy when he was four years old. Excellent clinical appearance. He received no treatment. **B.** Roentgenograms of the same boy at the age of 15 years. Note that the curve has not progressed. Cosmetic appearance and function of spine are excellent. (From Winter, R. B., Moe, J. H., and Eilers, V. E.: Congenital scoliosis. A study of 234 patients, treated and untreated. J. Bone Joint Surg., *50–A*:9, 1968.)

anomalies, the more likely is progression of the scoliosis (Fig. 6–10).

Age of the Patient and Prognosis. Congenital scoliosis, like idiopathic scoliosis, tends to progress most rapidly during the preadolescent growth spurt; however, it is common for most curves to progress slowly, even in infancy and throughout growth. Steady progression during the entire growth period is characteristic of curves due to unilateral unsegmented bars or to multiple unbalanced thoracic hemivertebrae. Once a curve begins to progress, it does so as long as there is growth.

Severity of the Curve. The severity of the curve and the rate of progression cannot be related, because some of the mild curves

progress more rapidly than the severe ones.

Progression patterns in congenital scoliosis are shown in Figure 6–11.

Treatment

CONSERVATIVE MANAGEMENT

In the neonatal period and early infancy, passive stretching exercises consisting primarily of lateral bending and head-neck traction are performed to keep the curve as flexible as possible. Moderately severe unbalanced curves are treated by placing the child in an infant scoliosis splint, which facilitates bathing, nursing, and diaper

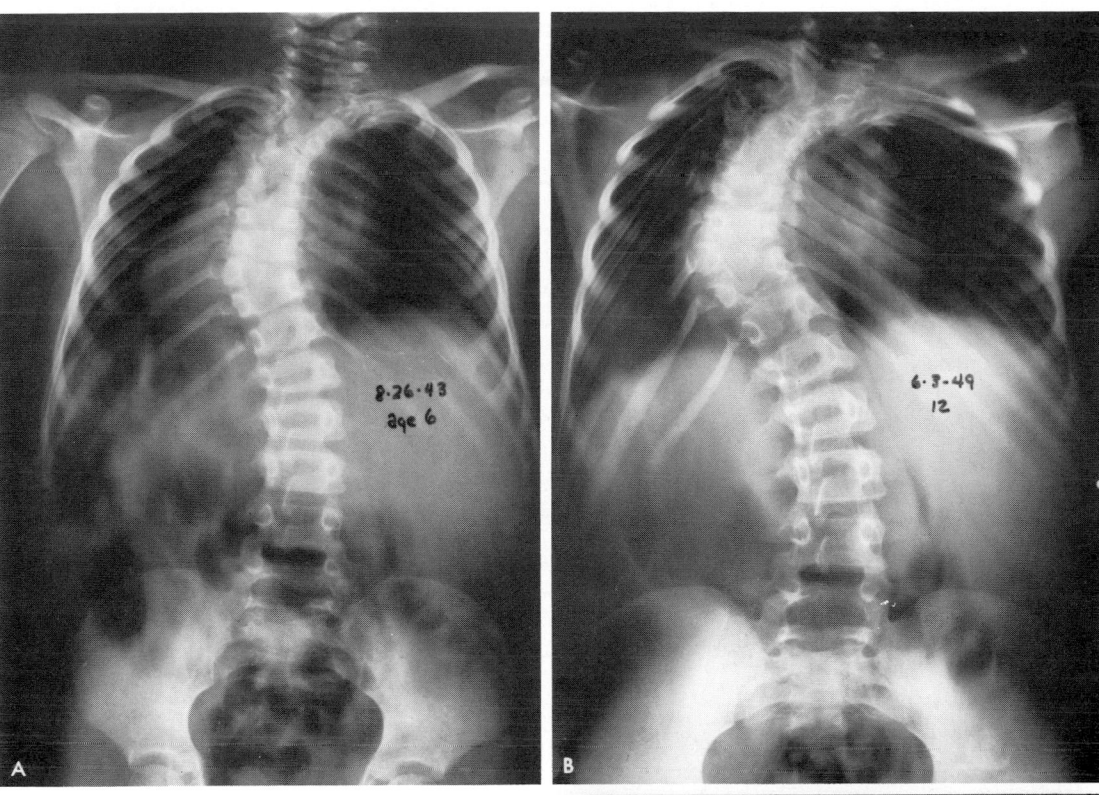

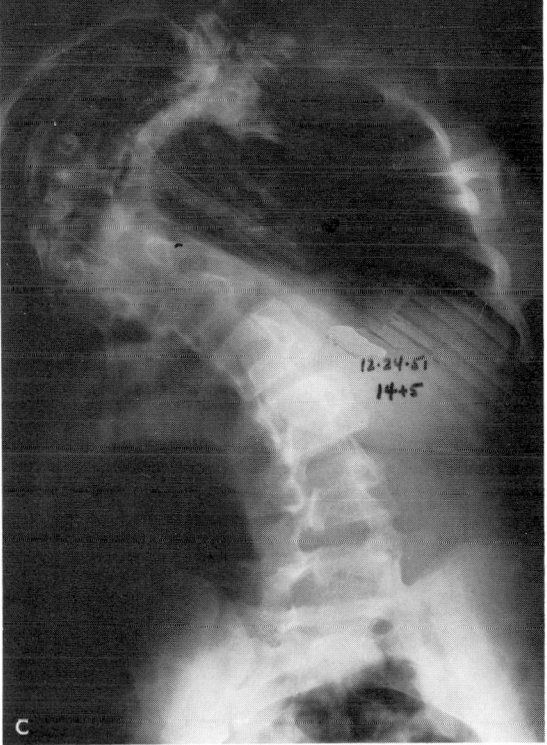

FIGURE 6–10.　*The natural history of unbalanced multiple congenital anomalies in the thoracic region.*

They usually increase to a marked degree and tend to progress more rapidly in adolescence. **A.** Patient was first seen at the age of six with a thoracic curve of 55 degrees and extending from the second thoracic to the eleventh thoracic vertebra with unbalanced multiple congenital deformities. The scoliosis was first noted at the age of five years. No active treatment was given. **B.** Roentgenograms of the spine of the same patient at the age of 12 years. The curve was 78 degrees. **C.** At the age of 14 years the curve was 120 degrees. Note the marked late progression. (From Winters, R. B., Moe, J. H., and Eilers, V. E.: Congenital scoliosis. A study of 234 patients treated and untreated. J. Bone Joint Surg., *50–A*:16–17, 1968.)

changing (Fig. 6–12). The splint is used for about 23 hours of the day.

When the infant begins to sit, crawl, or stand, a Risser localizer or turnbuckle cast is applied, permitting greater activity. The Risser cast is changed every two or three months. Under this aggressive, active regimen of therapy, the curve can be prevented from progressing and some degree of improvement can be expected.

The Risser cast is not desirable for long-term conservative care, as it cannot be removed for bathing and is often uncomfortably warm. The ambulatory Milwaukee brace is used as soon as it can be properly made and fitted to the young child. Usually this is done around two years of age. Use of the orthosis is continued as long as the spine is maintained in satisfactory correction. The cosmetic improvement is most dramatic when the Milwaukee brace is used in high thoracic or cervicothoracic curves with head tilt, asymmetrical neck line, and elevation of one shoulder.

OPERATIVE TREATMENT

When a curve is progressing despite the faithful use of Milwaukee brace or an unacceptable deformity is present that is not corrected by the use of the brace, maximal correction is obtained by application of a Risser localizer cast, and the involved vertebrae are fused. This is done regardless of the age of the child. Extension of scoliosis by growth of the vertebral column and addition of vertebrae to those involved in the initial curve can then be prevented by postoperative use of the Milwaukee brace; this obviates the need for more extensive fusions in young children. However, spinal fusion is hazardous in children with congenital heart disease and poor cardiorespiratory function. In such a case, the use of the Milwaukee brace should be continued.

Osteotomy of a unilateral unsegmented bar combined with resection of fused ribs on the concave side will significantly improve postoperative correction of severe

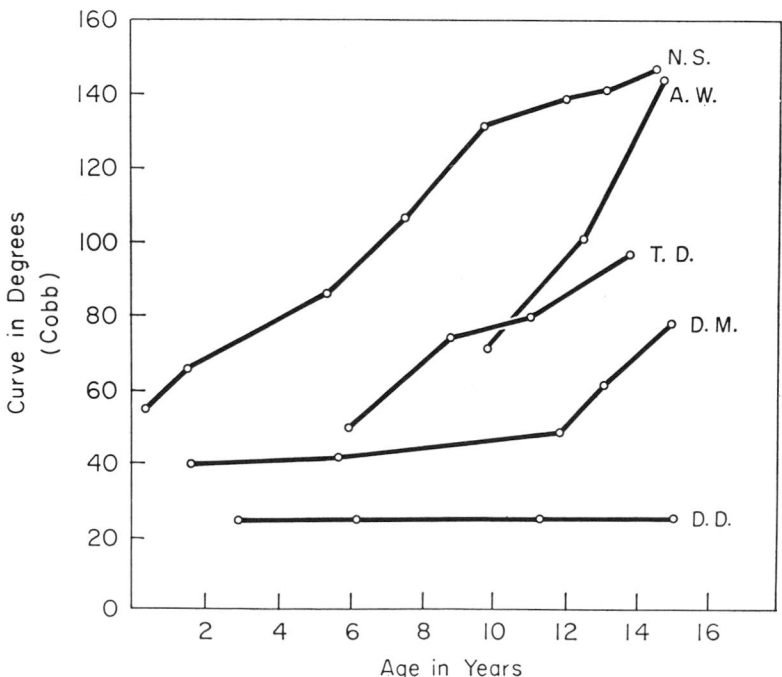

FIGURE 6–11. *Progression pattern in congenital scoliosis in untreated patients.*

N.S., a unilateral thoracic unsegmented bar; A.W., a single hemivertebra, third thoracic vertebra; T.D., multiple unbalanced thoracic anomalies; D.M., unbalanced anomalies, thoracolumbar junction; and D.D., multiple balanced anomalies of the entire spine. (From Winters, R. B., Moe, J. H., and Eilers, V. E.: Congenital scoliosis. A study of 234 patients treated and untreated. J. Bone Joint Surg., *50–A:8*, 1968.)

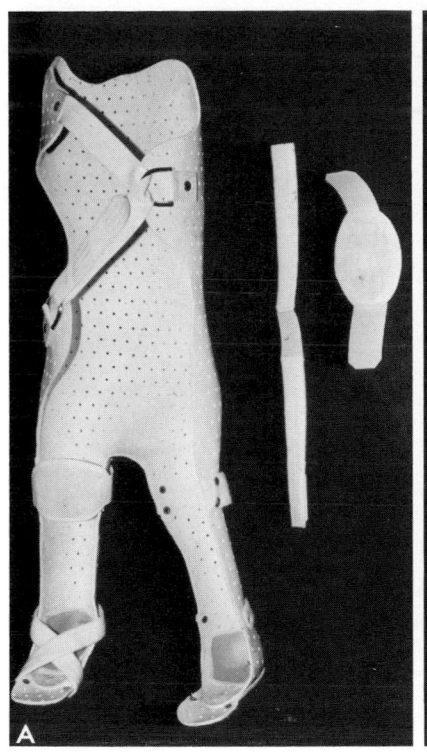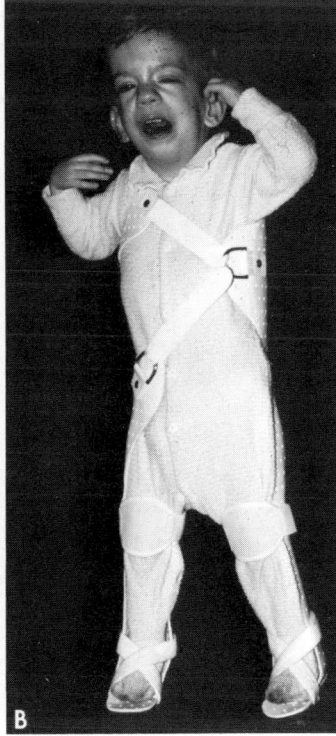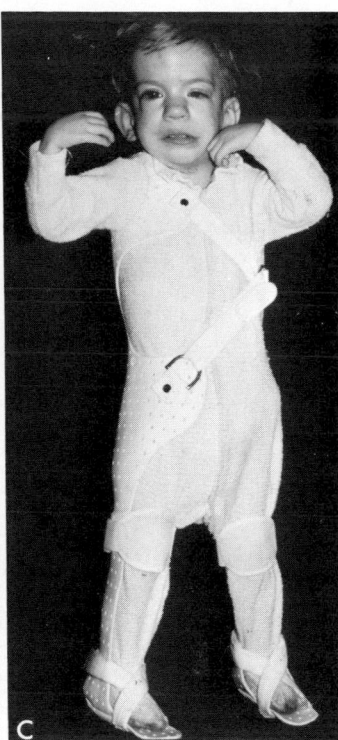

FIGURE 6–12.   Infant scoliosis splint.

curves. It is important that these procedures be performed by experienced surgeons, as neurologic complications are not uncommon. Halo-femoral (or halo-tibial or halo-pelvic) distraction with lateral sling pressure over the convexity of the curve is the most effective means of correction after the osteotomy.[10, 16] Fixed pelvic obliquity is best treated by fusing the lumbar spine to the sacrum in the compensated position.

Excision of hemivertebrae is rarely indicated, except in the case of a single lumbar hemivertebra that produces marked decompensation.[9, 14] Following excision, correction is maintained by external means, such as a Risser cast or a Milwaukee brace.

CONGENITAL KYPHOSIS

Congenital kyphosis is a rare condition that may be due to localized malformation of the spine, the rest of the skeleton being normal, or may be associated with a generalized disturbance of ossification, such as Morquio's disease, gargoylism, or cre-

tinism.[18–25] Only the first type is considered here.

Etiology

The cause is obscure. There is no definite familial incidence. It is more common in the female.

Clinical Picture

The deformity is usually noticed in infancy and becomes more pronounced as the child starts to stand and walk (Fig. 6–13). With further growth of the spine the kyphosis will usually increase. In children it is painless and there is no local tenderness or muscle spasm; however, in adult life, pain may be a symptom when degenerative arthritic changes develop. Ordinarily, the total height of the patient is somewhat below normal.

Compression of the spinal cord or *cauda equina* has been reported in one fourth of the published cases. A thorough neurologic evaluation is necessary, and myelography should be performed when indicated.

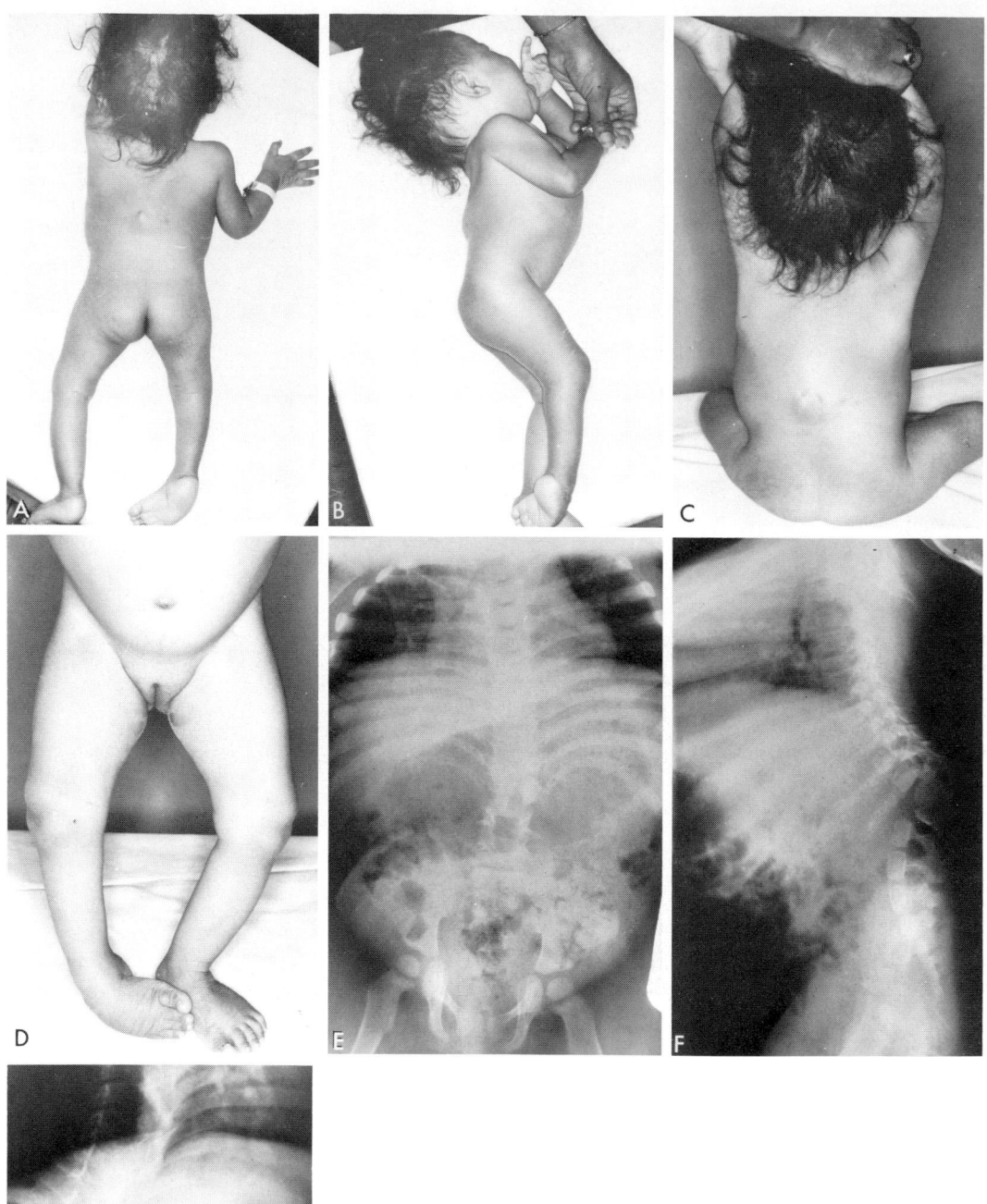

FIGURE 6-13. *Congenital kyphosis due to absence of the body of the second lumbar vertebra.*

A and **B.** Posterior and lateral views, recumbent, showing kyphosis. **C.** Sitting posterior view. **D.** Anterior view of lower limbs; note the talipes equinovarus deformity of right foot. **E** and **F.** Anteroposterior and lateral roentgenograms showing congenital absence of first lumbar vertebra. **G.** Oblique lateral view one year postoperatively following local spinal fusion.

Roentgenographic Features

The most common site of kyphosis is between the tenth thoracic and second lumbar vertebrae; however, it has been observed anywhere between the fourth thoracic and fourth lumbar segments.

Anatomically, the defect may be classified into the following seven types (Fig. 6–14):

1. Absence of the body of the vertebra
2. Absence of the body of the vertebra associated with microspondyly of a neighboring vertebra
3. Microspondyly of one vertebra
4. Microspondyly of two neighboring vertebrae
5. Incomplete segmentation of neighboring vertebrae
6. Absence of a corner of a vertebra
7. Wedging of a vertebra on the lateral

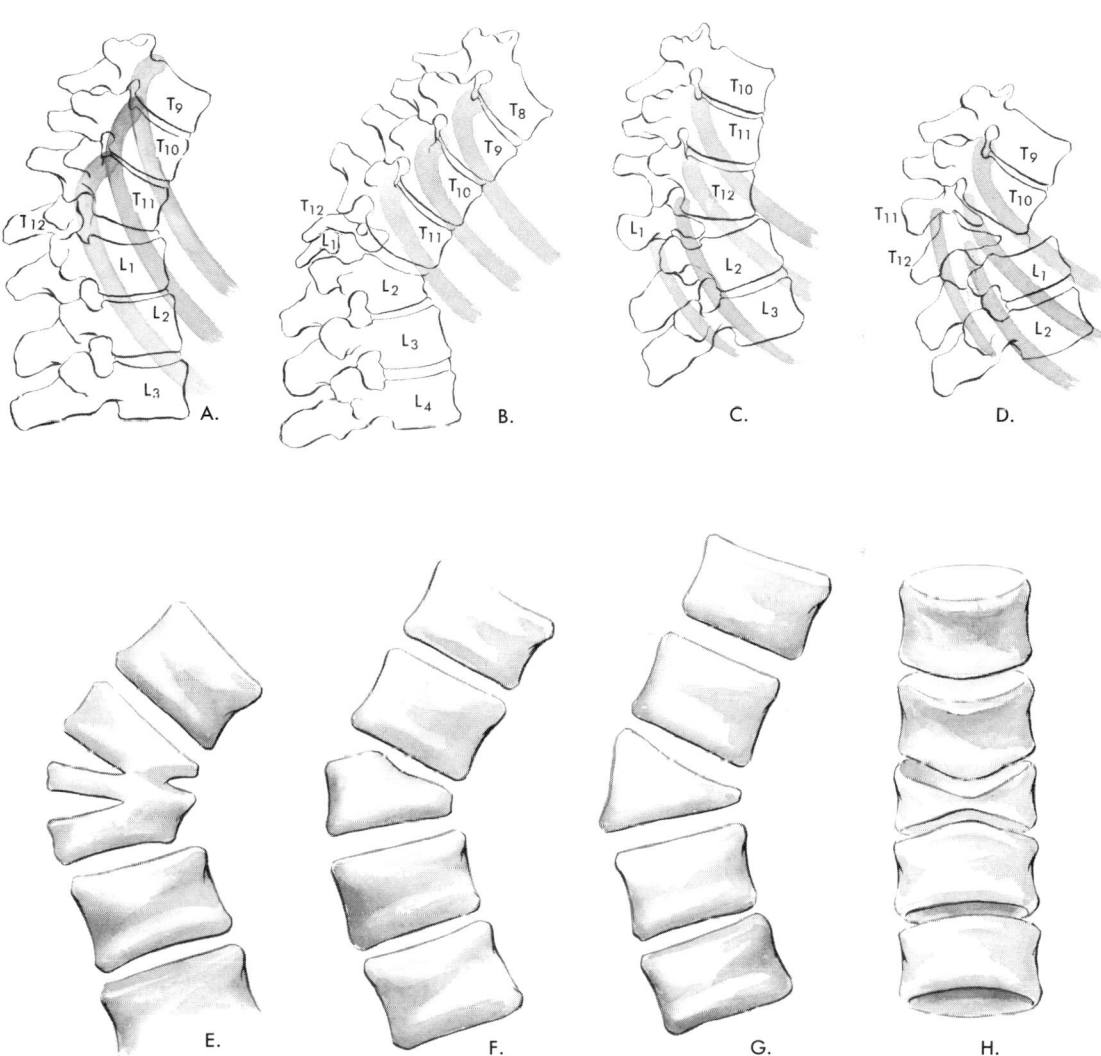

FIGURE 6–14. *Types of congenital kyphosis.*

A. Absence of the body of the vertebra (L1). **B.** Absence of the body of one vertebra (L1) and microspondyly of a neighboring vertebra (T12). Note the pedicles are present. **C.** Microspondyly of one vertebra (L1). **D.** Microspondyly of two neighboring vertebrae (T11, T12). **E.** Incomplete segmentation of neighboring vertebrae. **F.** Absence of a corner of the vertebra. **G.** Wedged vertebra, lateral view. **H.** Wedged vertebra, anteroposterior view. Note its butterfly appearance. (Redrawn after Bingold, A. C.: Congenital kyphosis. J. Bone Joint Surg., *35–B*:579, 1953.)

view, which gives a butterfly appearance to the same vertebra in the anteroposterior view[19]

The vertebra above the kyphosis may occasionally have a notch on its anterior border. In the differential diagnosis of congenital kyphosis one should always consider tuberculosis. Tuberculous spondylitis may be ruled out by a lack of systemic signs, a normal sedimentation rate, and negative tuberculin skin tests, and by the absence of bone or disc destruction, osteoporosis, or paravertebral abscess, which would normally produce a shadow in the roentgenograms. When indicated, roentgenograms and laminagrams of the kyphotic area of the spine should be taken for better visualization of bone and joint detail.

Treatment

Treatment is by local spinal fusion. In the presence of progressive neurologic deficit and spinal block, as shown by manometric and myelographic studies, laminectomy and decompression of the spinal cord are indicated. This should be done early and the spine should be stabilized by local arthrodesis.

When there are no neurologic symptoms, it is best to support the spine and wait until the child is one or two years of age before spinal fusion. The deformity cannot be corrected by conservative measures. The natural history of spinal cord or cauda equina compression is not known at present because of a lack of long-term follow-up studies of children with this condition. The author does not advise total excision of the posterior elements and posterior hemivertebrae prior to fusion.

SPONDYLOLISTHESIS

History and Terminology

The term *spondylolisthesis* is derived from the Greek word *spondylos*, meaning "spine," and *olisthanein*, meaning "to slip." The condition originally attracted the attention of obstetricians as a cause of obstruction in labor, although in 1741 André had already

described the cause of a "hollow back" as inward warping of the spine.[80] During the early part of the nineteenth century, it was described as a luxation of the lumbosacral joint. The term *spondylolisthesis* was coined in 1854 by Kilian, who pointed out that it represented a slow displacement of the last lumbar vertebra due to superimposed body weight.[87] Robert, in 1855, was the first to focus attention on a lesion of the neural arch. By careful dissection and freeing of the fifth lumbar vertebra of all soft tissues, he demonstrated that it was impossible for the vertebra with an intact neural arch to slip. However, if the neural arch was cut, the vertebra was free to slip.[125] The discontinuity in the pars interarticularis was demonstrated by Lambl in 1858.[92] Neugebauer studied anatomic specimens of vertebral columns and discovered in some a lesion of continuity in the pars interarticularis, with or without forward displacement of the vertebral body.[114]

When there is a defect in the pars interarticularis with no forward slipping, the term *spondylolysis* is applied (formed by combining *spondylo* with *lysis*, "to disintegrate." *Spondyloschisis*, *schisis* meaning "cleavage, crack, or fissure," is another term that has been used.

Junghanns used the term *pseudospondylolisthesis* to describe spondylolisthesis between the fourth and fifth lumbar vertebrae with an intact neural arch. He preferred to reserve the term *spondylolisthesis* for slipping caused by any lesion of the pars interarticularis.[86] However, the term *spondylolisthesis*, originally introduced by Kilian in 1854, referred to slipping of a vertebra, not to a lesion of continuity in the neural arch. This is significant when considering the true nature of spondylolisthesis and the different types that occur.

Spondylolisthesis was considered comparatively rare in the past, until the discovery of roentgen rays in 1895 made it a common diagnostic entity.

The term *neural arch defects* is a general one that can refer to several defects. "Pars defect," "interarticular defect," or "isthmal defect" all refer to a defect in that portion of the lamina located between the superior and inferior articular processes called the *pars interarticularis.* "Pedicle defect" refers to a bony discontinuity in that portion of the arch extending from the body of the vertebra to the lamina. Defects of the lamina may occur near the midline, thus involving the spinous process as well.

Types of Spondylolisthesis

Newman described five different types of spondylolisthesis encountered in a study of 319 patients.[116] In classifying these various groups, he considered the three main possible causes of spondylolisthesis; namely, defect of the facets, which may be congenital or acquired; defect of the neural arch or pedicle, congenital or acquired; and structural inadequacy of bone. The salient features of the five types are as follows (Fig. 6–15):

Type I — Congenital Spondylolisthesis. In this type, slipping at the lumbosacral junction is due to a congenital sacral defect, including the articular facets, with attenuation of the neural arch. A secondary break of the neural arch may result occasionally.

Type II — Spondylolytic Spondylolisthesis. In this true spondylolisthesis, slipping of the vertebra is due to elongation or, more

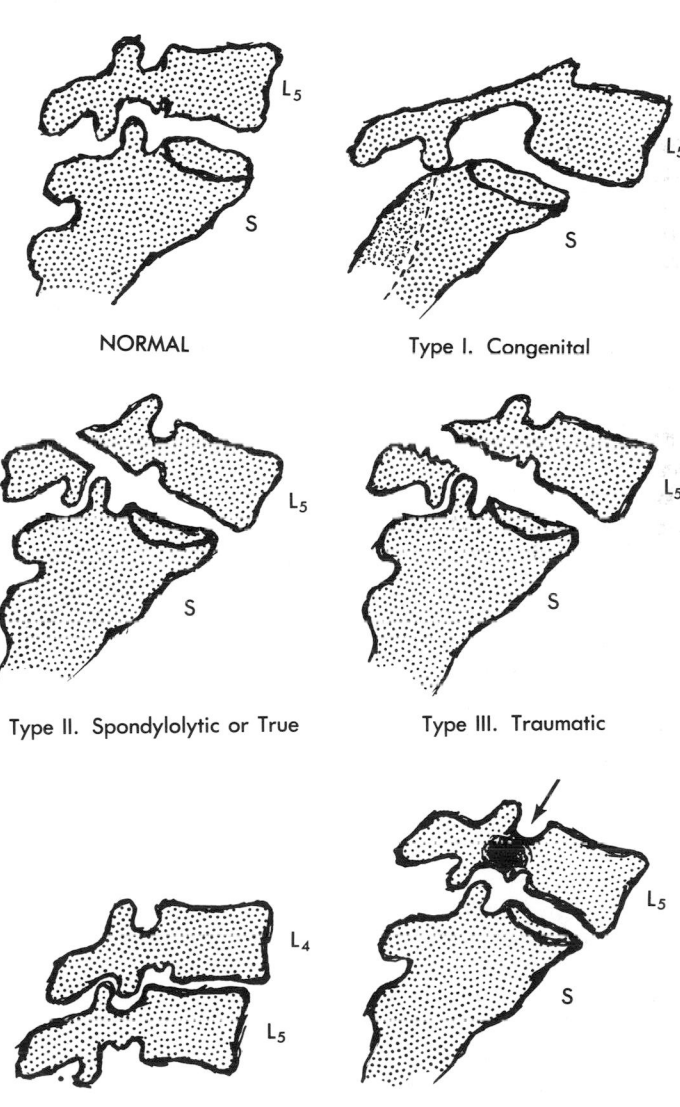

FIGURE 6–15. *Types of spondylolisthesis.*

Normal. Type I, congenital spondylolisthesis. Note the deficient development of the sacral neural arches with deficiency of the superior sacral facets. The pars interarticularis is attenuated and bent downward, but usually remains intact. Type II, spondylolytic spondylolisthesis (true spondylolisthesis). Note the break in the pars interarticularis. Type III, traumatic spondylolisthesis. Note the fracture of the neural arch. Type IV, degenerative spondylolisthesis. The slipping is due to degenerative joint changes causing facet deficiency. It is not seen in patients under 40 years. There is a high incidence of nerve root involvement, almost always at the fourth lumbar level. Type V, pathologic spondylolisthesis. Forward slipping is caused by insufficiency of bone structure from neoplasm or developmental defects such as osteogenesis imperfecta. (Redrawn from Newman, P. H.: The etiology of spondylolisthesis. J. Bone Joint Surg., 45–B:41, 1963.)

NORMAL

Type I. Congenital

Type II. Spondylolytic or True

Type III. Traumatic

Type IV. Degenerative

Type V. Pathologic

commonly, a break of the pars interarticularis, or a combination of both, with the facets remaining intact.

Type III—Traumatic Spondylolisthesis. Slipping is due to instability caused by an acute fracture of the neural arch.

Type IV—Degenerative Spondylolisthesis. This type is also known as pseudospondylolisthesis (Junghanns, 1931) and spondylolisthesis with intact neural arch (Macnab, 1950). Slipping is due to facet deficiency caused by degenerative joint changes. It almost always occurs at the fourth lumbar level. It is three times more common in women than in men, and has not been encountered in patients under 40 years of age. In this type there is high incidence of involvement of nerve tissue, such as the fifth lumbar root or the cauda equina.

Type V—Pathologic Spondylolisthesis. This is rare and is characterized by forward slipping of one or more vertebrae due to insufficiency of the bone structure. Bone weakness may stem from a developmental defect such as osteogenesis imperfecta, or from a local disease, such as tuberculosis or a neoplastic lesion.

Because degenerative spondylolisthesis is not seen in children, and because of the rarity of traumatic and pathologic spondylolisthesis, they are not discussed in this textbook.

SPONDYLOLYTIC SPONDYLOLISTHESIS (True Spondylolisthesis)

Incidence

This is the most common type of spondylolisthesis and apparently occurs only in man, who has a true upright stance, lumbar lordosis, and a bipedal gait.

The total incidence of spondylolytic spondylolisthesis varies in different races. Absolutely accurate studies are unavailable. The overall incidence in white Americans and Europeans is approximately 4 to 5 per cent. Roche and Rowe, in a study of 4,200 skeletons, found a total incidence of 4.2 per cent. On the basis of sex and ethnic groups, however, the incidence was found to be 6.4 per cent in the white male, and in the white female, 2.3 per cent; in the Negro male, it was 2.8 per cent, and in the Negro female, 1.1 per cent.[130] Willis, in 1923, in 1,520 unselected skeletons, found an incidence of 5.2 per cent.[165] Bailey, in 1947, reported the results of 2,080 roentgenographic examinations of army draftees in which he found neural arch defects in 4.4 per cent.[34] Runge, in 1954, noted an incidence of 3.09 per cent in 4,654 roentgenograms made in unselected pre-employment examinations, with an occurrence of actual spondylolisthesis of 2.08 per cent.[133]

In the Japanese, the incidence was reported to be 5.5 per cent in 125 skeletons studied by Hasebe in 1913.[78] Stewart, in 1953, described the Eskimos as having by far the highest incidence (24 per cent).[150] Even more striking were the differences recorded among three groups of Eskimos according to geographic location, indicating more penetrance of hereditary factors by inbreeding. South of the Yukon River, 18.8 per cent of the individuals examined had arch defects; 31.6 per cent of the Kodiak and Aleutian Islanders were affected; and north of the Yukon River, the incidence increased to 52.6 per cent.

Age Incidence

Spondylolytic spondylolisthesis is not present at birth and seldom before the age of four years. The youngest patient, an infant of 17 months, was reported by Kleinberg in 1934.[89] Defects in the pars interarticularis appear most frequently between the ages of five and one half and seven years. The incidence increases with age until adulthood, but not thereafter. In 1953, Stewart reported the following age incidence of neural arch defects in Alaskan natives: 5 per cent at the age of 6 years; 17 per cent at the age of 30 years; 34 per cent at 30 to 40 years of age, with no increase after the age of 40, a striking example of increasing age incidence.[150]

Slipping occurs before the age of 20 years. The period of most rapid olisthy is between the ages of 10 and 15 years. Unless there has been surgical intervention, slipping rarely, if ever, increases after the age of 20.

Etiology

The true etiology of spondylolysis has given rise to much controversy. Its pathogenesis is not yet established. Wiltse and Newman, in reviews of the etiology of spondylolisthesis, refuted several of the theories of etiology that had been advanced over the years.[116, 166, 167]

Abnormal Ossification. This theory was one of the first to be presented. It proposed that in patients with spondylolisthesis, each lateral mass, which normally ossifies from one center, instead ossified from two centers. The origin of the defect was thought to be a lack of fusion between two separate centers of ossification. Anatomic sections of over 700 fetuses have shown neither separate ossification nor any defect in the pars interarticularis.[37, 39, 51, 52, 63, 99, 117, 128, 137] Roentgenograms of newborn infants have not shown any evidence of spondylolisthesis nor any defect in the pars interarticularis.[35, 82]

Trauma. This has been eliminated as a causative factor, at birth or during postnatal life, by the failure of Rowe and Roche to produce a fracture of the pars interarticularis in experiments on stillborn infants.[132] Unquestionable fractures of the pars interarticularis reported in the literature have healed.[91, 129, 166] Studies by Stewart did not show the evidence of repair that one normally observes in fractures.[148, 150] In histologic sections of the defect there was neither evidence of callus formation nor anything that would seem to suggest a fracture.[128, 165]

Pinching-off of Pars Interarticularis by Impingement of Articular Process. In 1885, Lane suggested that the defect in the pars interarticularis of the fifth lumbar vertebra is produced by downward pressure of the inferior articular process of the fourth lumbar vertebra and upward pressure of the superior articular process of the sacrum eroding through the pars interarticularis (Fig. 6–16).[74] This theory has been supported by Capener in 1931 and 1960, by Meyer-Burgdorff in 1931, and by Nathan in 1959.[49, 50, 102, 111] However, the pinching-off process is not seen in roentgenograms of children and adolescents.

Following an extensive study of the etiology of spondylolisthesis, Wiltse formulated the theory that the defect in the pars interarticularis is caused by two factors: an inherited dysplasia or defect present in the cartilage model of the arch of the affected vertebra, and a strain on the weakened pars interarticularis from physical forces resulting from man's characteristic stance and lumbar lordosis. He believes that stress and strain on the pars interarticularis will not itself produce the defect unless the dysplasia or hereditary weakness is already present. Dysplasia is characterized by lack of normal ability of the bone to repair itself. The result is bone resorption rather than new bone formation, and the production of the characteristic defect.[167]

Instability in the lumbosacral region due to weakness of the supporting structures and a deficiency of the lumbosacral fascia, the posterior spinal ligaments, and the intervertebral disc were suggested by Newman as being contributory factors. He believed that the defect in the pars interarticularis is not the cause of spondylolisthesis, but rather, is a result of the instability, which produces so much stress on the once normal pars interarticularis that it undergoes a stress fracture.[115] Roberts advanced the idea that the defect is a stress fracture.[126] In the literature there are several reports of spondylolisthesis occurring immediately above the level of fusion in the lumbosacral area.[30, 58, 59, 77, 152, 161]

Spondylolisthesis has also been observed in association with a congenitally fused segment of the spine and as a sequel to a disc space infection.[58, 136]

Genetic Factors

There is definite evidence that defects in the pars interarticularis have a familial incidence.[35, 36, 63, 76, 95, 148, 150, 167]

Baker and McHolick studied the roentgenograms of 400 unselected six- to seven-year-old children (225 boys and 175 girls) and found defects in the pars interarticularis in 18 of them (12 males and 6 females). Roentgenograms of the parents of these children revealed a total parental incidence of defects of 28 per cent.[35] Wiltse studied 36 families in which one member had spondylolisthesis. He found a parental incidence of 26 per cent (26 of 101 individuals).[167]

The mode of inheritance that is consistent

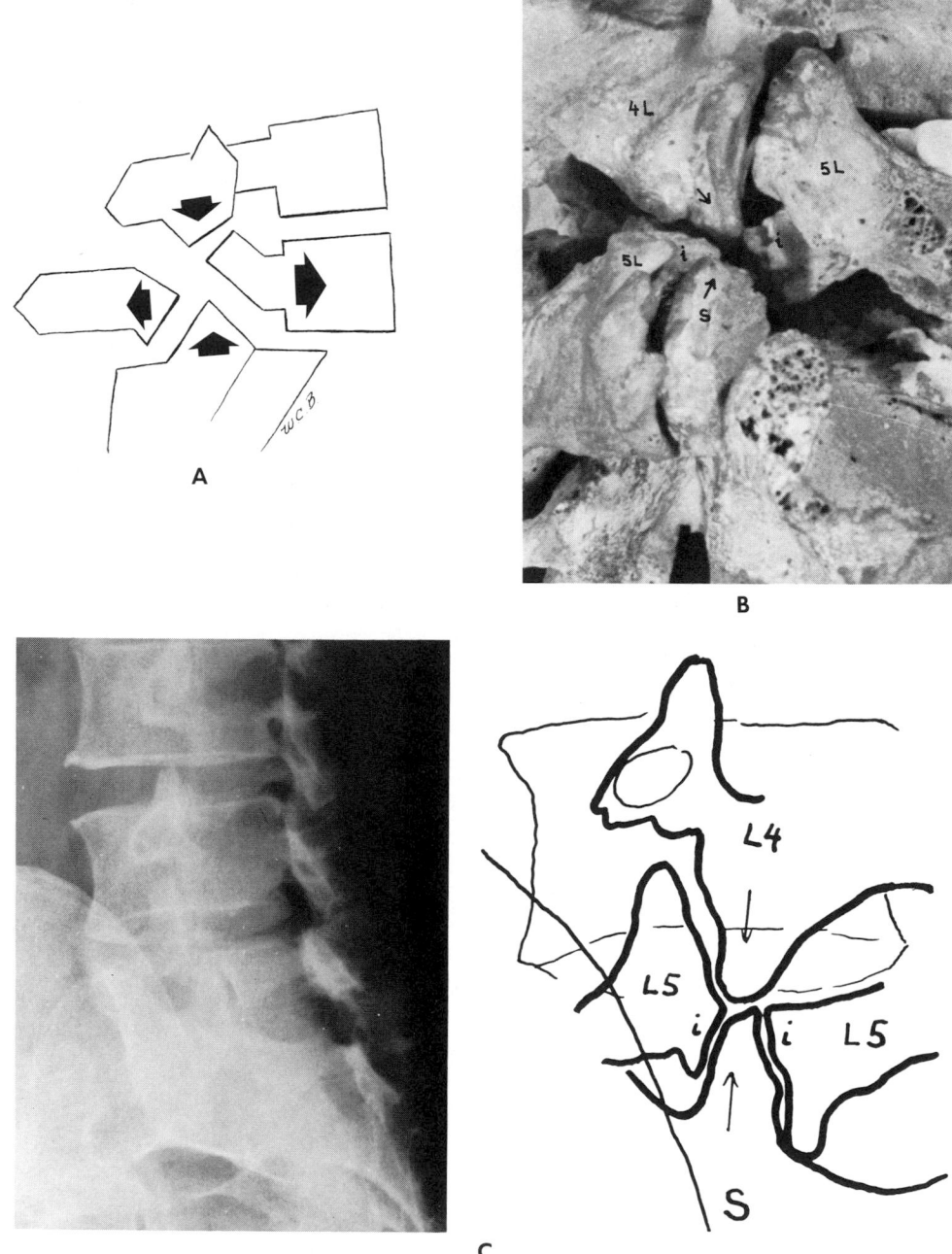

FIGURE 6–16. *Spondylolisthesis.*

A. Diagrammatic lateral view of the lower lumbosacral spine showing the wedgelike eroding forces on the defective pars interarticularis produced by downward pressure of the superior articular process of the first sacral vertebra. (Redrawn from Capener, N.: Spondylolisthesis. Brit. J. Surg., *19*:374, 1931.)
B. Gross specimen of typical spondylolisthesis of the fifth lumbar vertebra. Right lateral view of the articulated fourth lumbar vertebra, fifth lumbar vertebra, and sacrum. Note the cleft between the articular process of the fourth lumbar vertebra (*4L arrow*) and the articular process of the sacrum (*S arrow*). The cleft isthmus (*i., i.*) is thinner than normal. **C.** Left oblique roentgenogram and diagrammatic tracing of the roentgenogram of the lower spine with bilateral spondylolysis of the fifth lumbar vertebra. Note the articular process of the sacrum (*S arrow*) projects upward and penetrates deeply into the cleft, meeting the downward-projecting inferior articular process of the fourth lumbar vertebra (*L4 arrow*). (From Nathan, H.: Spondylolysis: Its anatomy and mechanisms of development. J. Bone Joint Surg., *41–A*:305, 310, 1959.)

with the data and that explains most of the pedigrees is that there is a single recessive gene with incomplete penetrance. There is the suggestion, however, that the involved gene sometimes shows incomplete dominance when neither parent is affected but four out of five siblings of the propositus are affected.

Pathology

The pathologic anatomy of the defect has been described by a number of observers.[41, 66, 123, 128, 165, 167] There was no evidence of callus formation in any of the studies, nor were there histologic findings to suggest fracture healing. However, the pathologic picture is not identical in every case. The tissue in the defect is more fibrous in nature when there is a wide gap. In some cases there may be a mass of fibrocartilage that appears to press on the nerve roots. When the gap is narrow, the bone ends tend to be smooth, blunt, and eburnated, or even to have some hyaline cartilage on the bone on each side of the defect. There is no periosteum over the bone ends. The transition from fibrous tissue to bone is usually abrupt. In some specimens the bone ends taper out at the defect.

The body of the fifth lumbar vertebra in the adult afflicted with spondylolisthesis is slightly trapezoid; its anterior border is longer than the posterior one (Fig. 6–17). The body of the fifth lumbar vertebra tends to become more trapezoid in shape as slipping takes place. To delineate this anatomic peculiarity, Vallois and Lozarthes described a lumbar index:[162]

Lumbar index =
$$\frac{\text{Height of posterior border of body in millimeters}}{\text{Height of anterior border of body in millimeters}} \times 100$$

An index of less than 100 means that the height of the posterior border of the body is less than the anterior. They found the average lumbar index to be 89 in 500 normal spines, 83 in 41 spines with spondylolysis, and 76 in 65 spines with spondylolisthesis.

In spines with severe slipping of the fifth lumbar vertebra, the top of the sacrum is dome-shaped.[109] The dome-shaped sacrum and severely trapezoid shape of the body of the fifth lumbar vertebra represent secondary changes that are not present in the very young child following the first appearance of the defect. These changes are of prognostic importance with regard to progression of slipping.

The 1962 study of Wiltse showed spina bifida to be 13 times as frequent in persons with a defect in the pars interarticularis as in those with normal spines. A severe degree of idiopathic structural scoliosis was noted to be four times as common.[167]

Level of Involvement

The fifth lumbar vertebra is most commonly involved (103 of 115 defects in the series of Bosworth et al., 1955); the next in frequency is the fourth (10 of 115 defects, Bosworth et al., 1955).[42] The third

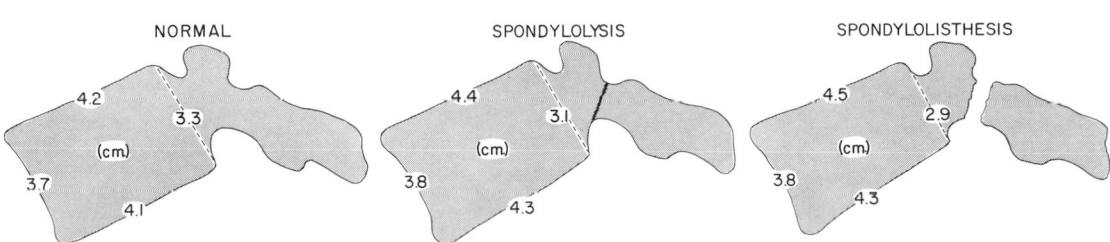

FIGURE 6–17. *Average dimensions of the adult fifth lumbar vertebra.*

Shown with no defects in the pars interarticularis, with spondylolysis, and with spondylolisthesis. Note the trapezoid shape of the fifth lumbar vertebra with spondylolisthesis. (Redrawn after Wiltse, L. L.: The etiology of spondylolisthesis. J. Bone Joint Surg., *44–A*:548, 1962.)

lumbar vertebra may be involved. Several vertebrae may be affected, usually two, involving the fourth and fifth lumbar segments. Spondylolisthesis may also occur in the cervical vertebrae.[60, 72, 120] The defect in the cervical spine is in the pedicle and not in the pars interarticularis.

Forward Slipping

The degree of severity of anterior displacement of spondylolisthesis is classified as Grade I, Grade II, Grade III, and Grade IV (Fig. 6–18).[103, 104] The superior border

of the anteroposterior diameter of the subjacent vertebra is divided into four equal parts; in Grade I, the displacement is 25 per cent or less, i.e., the posteroinferior angle of the anteriorly displaced vertebra lies within the first segment; in Grade II, between 25 and 50 per cent; in Grade III, between 50 and 75 per cent; and in Grade IV, greater than 75 per cent.

In the Meschan method of measuring the degree of spondylolisthesis on the lateral roentgenogram (Fig. 6–19), the first line extends between the posterior lip of the vertebral body superior to the one involved

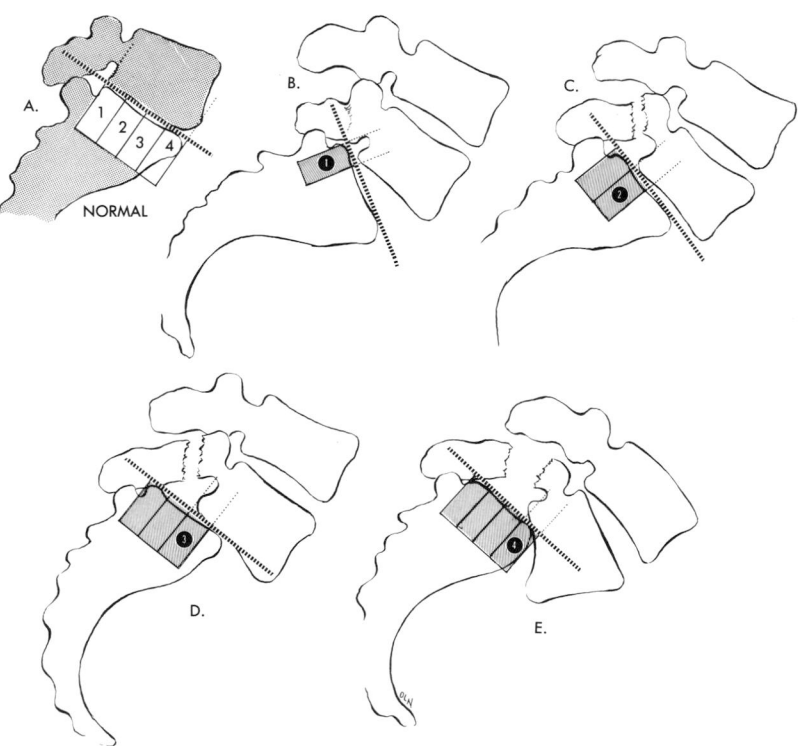

FIGURE 6–18. Gradation of degrees of spondylolisthesis.

A. Normal. The superior border of the anteroposterior diameter of the subjacent vertebra is divided into four equal parts. **B.** Grade I: The anterior displacement is 25 per cent or less, i.e., the posteroinferior angle of the displaced vertebra lies within the first segment. **C.** Grade II: The displacement is between 25 and 50 per cent. **D.** Grade III: The displacement is between 50 and 75 per cent. **E.** Grade IV: The displacement is greater than 75 per cent. (Redrawn after Meyerding, H. W.: Spondylolisthesis. Surg. Gynec. Obstet., 54:371, 1932.)

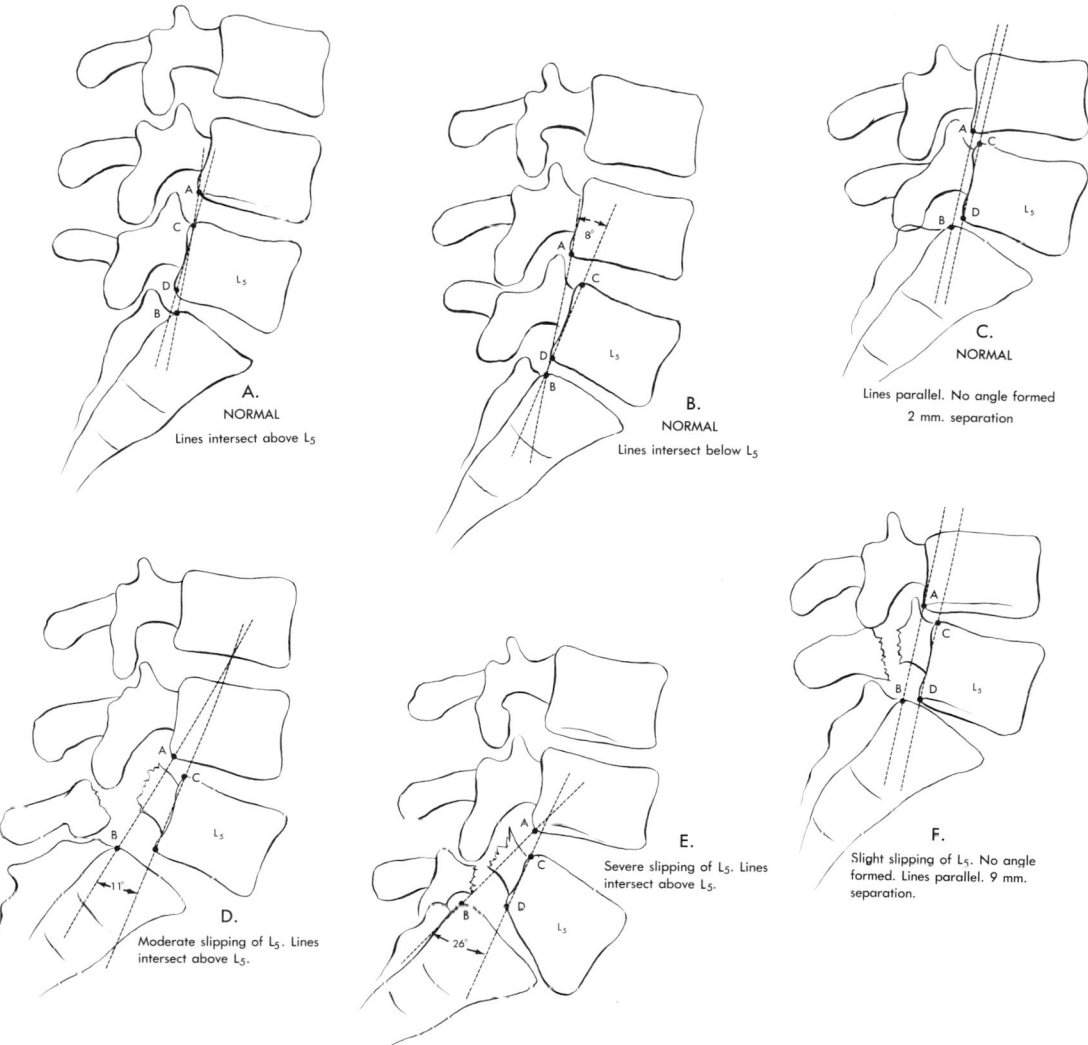

FIGURE 6–19. *The Meschan method of measuring the degree of spondylolisthesis.*

A to **C.** The three general types of normal lumbosacral spine. Note the position of the apex of the angles made by intersecting lines are at L5 in Figure 6–19 A or below L5 in Figure 6–19 B. **D** to **F.** Note the arrangement of the lines in cases of spondylolisthesis. See text for explanation. (Redrawn after Meschan, I.: Spondylolisthesis. Amer. J. Roentgen., 53:230–243, 1945.)

and the posterior lip of the vertebral body below (points A and B); the second line is drawn between the posterior upper and lower lips of the slipped vertebral body (points C and D). The lines are extended; if they are not parallel, they will meet and form an angle, which is measured with a protractor. If the lines are parallel (very occasionally this may occur in spondylolisthesis), the linear distance between the lines is measured. When the angle is as much as 10 degrees, the spondylolisthesis can be called slight; 11 to 20 degrees, mod-

erate; and greater than 20 degrees, severe. When the two lines are parallel, a distance of more than 3 mm. is abnormal. The degree of displacement should be reported accurately by stating, ". . . spondylolisthesis with a displacement through an angle of x degrees"; or, if the lines are parallel, ". . . a distance of x mm."

The degree of spondylolisthesis may also be measured by comparing the anteroposterior diameter of the slipped vertebra with the one above it (Fig. 6–20).[49] The Ullman's sign is demonstrated by drawing

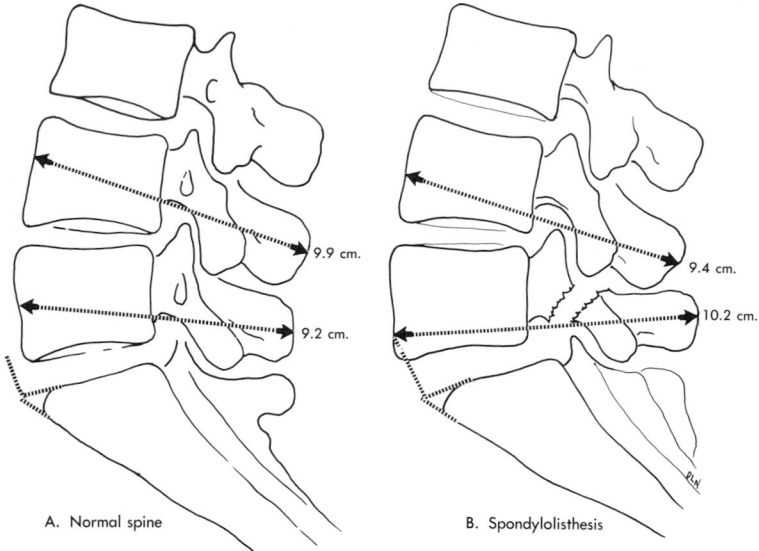

A. Normal spine   B. Spondylolisthesis

FIGURE 6–20.   Capener's method of determining the degree of spondylolisthesis.

Displacement is measured by comparison of anteroposterior diameters of the spondylolytic vertebra and the normal vertebra above it. Ullman's sign is demonstrated by drawing a line at right angles to the upper border of the sacrum at its anterior edge. Note in the normal spine **(A)** the fifth lumbar vertebra lies entirely behind this line, whereas, in spondylolisthesis, the perpendicular line is intersected by the slipped vertebral body. (Redrawn after Capener, N.: Spondylolisthesis. Brit. J. Surg., *19*:374, 1931.)

a line at a right angle to the upper border of the sacrum at its anterior edge; in the normal spine, the fifth lumbar vertebra lies entirely behind this line, whereas in spondylolisthesis the perpendicular line is intersected by the slipped vertebral body. In the method of Marique and Taillard the displacement is measured as a percentage of the anteroposterior diameter of the subjacent vertebral body (Fig. 6–21).[153]

Except in rare cases, spondylolisthesis does not usually appear until the age of four or five years. Progressive displacement of the vertebrae may occur during periods of rapid growth in childhood and adolescence, but once the age of 20 years is reached, further slipping usually does not take place unless there has been surgical intervention.

It is not known why only certain vertebrae are predisposed to slipping, nor why some types of slipping cease at a level of 25 per cent, some at 50 per cent, while a few others progress to complete olisthy. Severe slipping usually occurs at the level of the fifth lumbar vertebra. A severely wedge-shaped body of the fifth lumbar vertebra, a perpendicular sacrum with a dome-shaped top, and

more than 25 per cent slipping in a child, especially in one under ten years of age, are ominous, and the possibility of severe slipping or even complete olisthy is great.

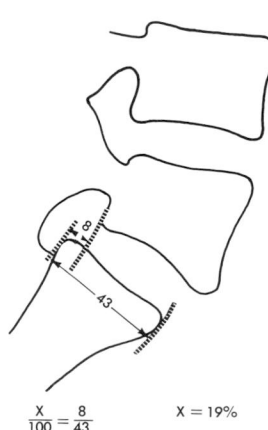

$$\frac{X}{100} = \frac{8}{43} \qquad X = 19\%$$

FIGURE 6–21.   The method of Marique and Taillard for measuring the degree of slipping.

The olisthy is measured as a percentage of the subjacent vertebral body. (Redrawn after Taillard, W.: Le spondylolisthesis chez l'enfant et l'adolescent: Étude de 50 cas. Acta Orthop. Scand., *24*:115, 1954.)

Clinical Features

In spondylolisthesis the defects are often discovered incidentally on roentgenograms taken for some other reason. Usually the condition is asymptomatic.

The clinical picture depends upon the age of the patient and upon the severity of the slipping. In children under ten years of age, it does not usually cause symptoms; poor posture and increasing lumbar lordosis may be the only presenting complaints.

Symptoms usually begin insidiously in the second or third decade of life, first as a dull low backache during standing or walking, which is usually relieved by rest. Later, pain may develop in the buttocks, radiating distally to one or both lower limbs along the course of the sciatic nerve, especially into the distribution of the fifth lumbar or first sacral dermatomes. Sciatica may be accompanied by sensory or motor disturbances and may be caused either by protrusion of an intervertebral disc (usually the one at the L 4–L 5 level) or by irritation of the nerve roots caused by the fibrocartilaginous mass at the defects in the pars interarticularis (Figs. 6–22 and 6–23). Complaints of weakness and stiffness of the lower back are common. Trauma, such as that from a fall or a twisting strain, may aggravate the symptoms of spondylolisthesis.

Physical findings depend upon the extent of slipping and on the presence or absence of nerve root irritation. In cases of severe spondylolisthesis, the torso is shortened and transverse skin creases are seen between the rib cage and the iliac crests. The distances between the xiphoid cartilage and the pubis and between the ribs and the crest of the ilium are diminished. The spine gives the appearance of having been telescoped into the pelvis. The sacrum is prominent and more vertical than normal. On palpation and inspection, the spinous process of the detached neural arch is prominent and there is a depression just above it. The bi-iliac diameter, which is normally less than the bitrochanteric diameter, becomes greater in spondylolisthesis. The pelvic inclination is increased and there is exaggeration of the normal lumbar lordosis. When displacement of the vertebra is severe, it produces angulation rather than curvature. There may be scoliosis due to unequal forward slipping of the vertebra and the consequent rotation. Anteroposterior motion of the spine in the affected area is restricted. There may be spasm of the erector spinae and hamstring muscles and tenderness over the spine of the involved vertebra. The body of the slipped lumbar vertebra may be palpable on abdominal or pelvic examination or both.

Neurologic findings depend upon the level and the degree of nerve root irritation or compression. When the condition is severe, the patient may have an awkward, waddling gait.

CONGENITAL SPONDYLOLISTHESIS

This type of spondylolisthesis was recognized and carefully described at postmortem examination by investigators prior to the discovery of roentgen rays.

It is more common in the female. The degree of slip is likely to be severe, and occasionally it is liable to cause obstruction during labor.

A sacral spina bifida is present, especially in the first vertebra, and development of the superior sacral facets is deficient. Because of the constant downward and forward thrust toward the lower lumbar vertebrae in erect posture, the lumbosacral facets give way, and the last lumbar vertebra gradually slips forward and downward over the top of the sacrum. The inferior facets of the last lumbar vertebra wear away the remnants of the superior sacral facets. The spinous process of the last lumbar vertebra is displaced forward and rests on the fibrous defect of the first sacral neural arch (Fig. 6–24). The pars interarticularis is attenuated and bent downward, but generally remains intact. Occasionally it may break under stress. The degree of slip is usually marked, and in very severe cases, the body of the last vertebra may become situated anterior to the sacrum.

In severe spondylolisthesis, the cauda equina and the first sacral nerve root, in particular, are liable to be stretched in an elongated S-bend between the neural arches of the last two lumbar vertebrae anteriorly and the protuberance of the back of the first sacral body posteriorly.

Ground between the vertebrae, the lum-

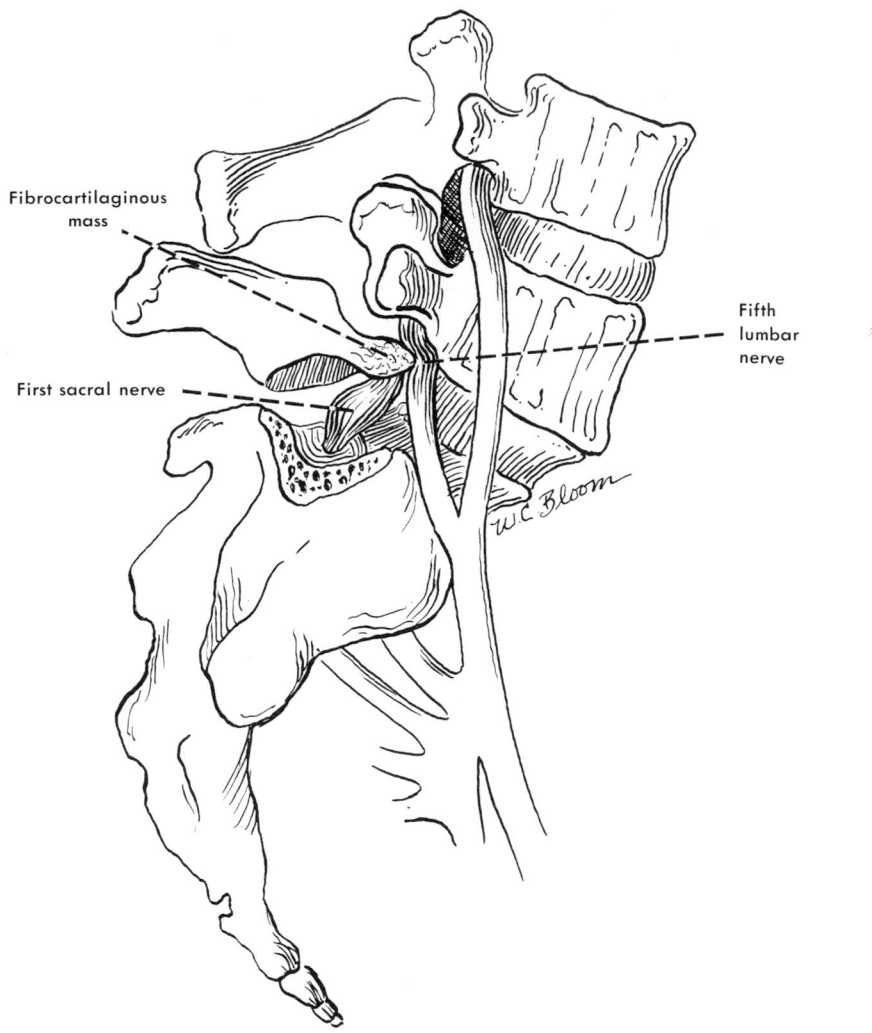

Fibrocartilaginous
mass

Fifth
lumbar
nerve

First sacral nerve

FIGURE 6–22.   Pathologic anatomy of spondylolisthesis at L5–S1 level.

Note the impingement upon the first sacral and fifth lumbar nerve roots by the fibrocartilaginous mass at the defect and the freely moveable fifth lumbar lamina. (Redrawn after Woolsey, R. D.: Mechanism of neurological symptoms and signs in spondylolisthesis at the fifth lumbar, first sacral level. J. Neurosurg., *11*:67, 1954.)

bosacral disc degenerates and is destroyed, and the cartilage of the apophyseal joints is worn. Occasionally, spontaneous bony fusion takes place during this period of instability—an attempt of nature to stabilize the process and prevent further slipping. Another such reaction is the formation of a buttress of bone from the anterior aspect of the first sacral vertebra (Fig. 6–25).

When there has been a sudden increase in the degree of slip, owing to trauma or a rapid spurt of growth, the presenting complaint may be acute low back pain. On examination, one will find a rigid lumbar

spine, spastic hamstrings, and often, scoliosis (Fig. 6–26). This has been described as the "clinical crisis" and "spondylolisthesis with tight hamstrings." It is due to stretching of nerve tissues.[116, 121]

Roentgenographic Findings

The diagnosis is confirmed by taking anteroposterior, lateral, right and left oblique (45-degree) views of the lumbosacral spine and a spot lateral view of the fifth lumbar and first sacral vertebrae.

Spondylolysis is best shown by a 25- to 45-

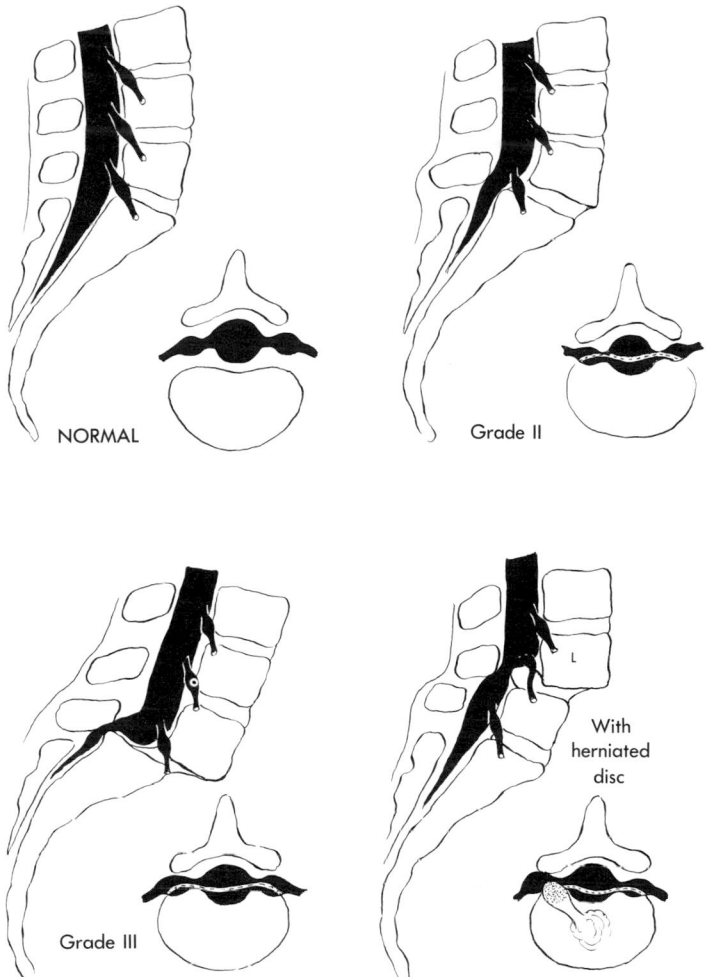

FIGURE 6-23. *Diagram demonstrating the effect on the spinal canal and nerve roots of varying degrees of spondylolisthesis and herniated disc.*

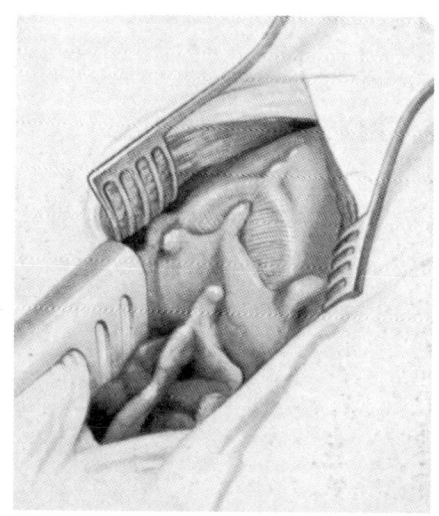

FIGURE 6-24. *Findings at operation in a case of congenital spondylolisthesis.*

Note the fibrous defect in the uppermost neural arches of the sacrum. The spinous process of the last lumbar vertebra lies on the fibrous defect. The lumbosacral apophyseal joints have given way. (From Newman, P. H., and Stone, K. H.: The etiology of spondylolisthesis. J. Bone Joint Surg., *45–B*:47, 1963.)

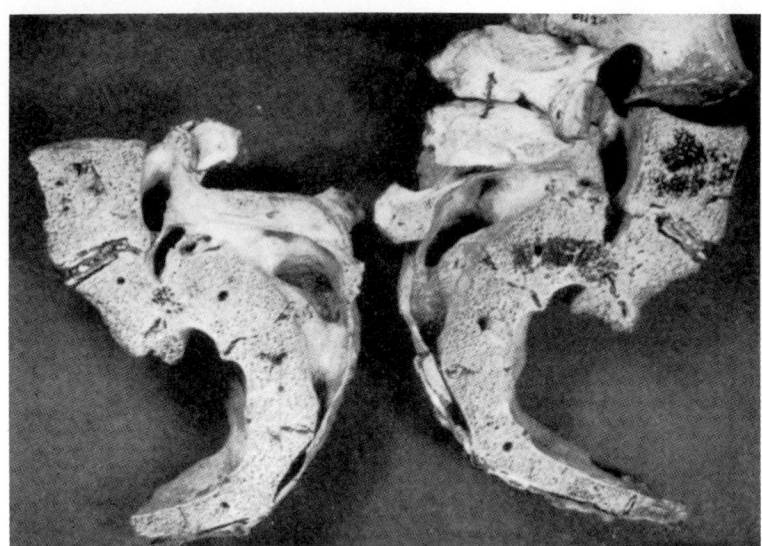

FIGURE 6–25. *Stabilization in spondylolisthesis by the formation of a buttress of bone from the anterior aspect of the first sacral vertebra.*

(From Newman, P. H., and Stone, K. H.: The etiology of spondylolisthesis. J. Bone Joint Surg., *45–B*:45, 1963.)

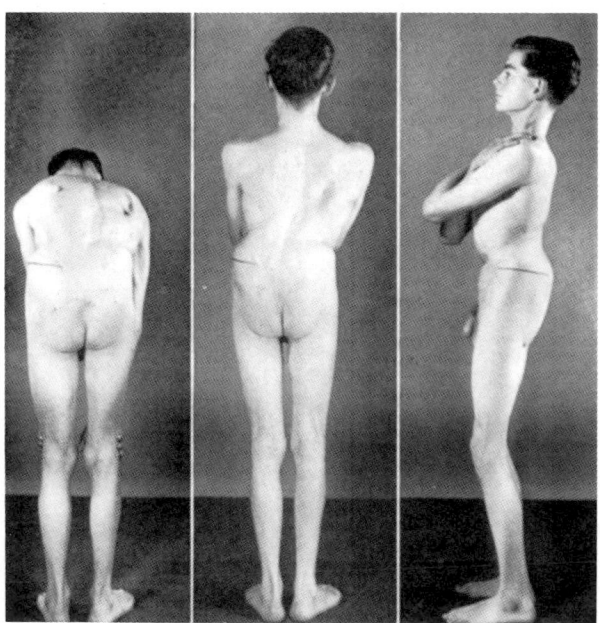

FIGURE 6–26. *"Clinical crisis" in sudden increase in degree of spondylolisthesis.*

Note the tightness of the hamstrings, the rigid lumbar spine, and the scoliosis. (From Newman, P. H., and Stone, K. H.: The etiology of spondylolisthesis. J. Bone Joint Surg., *45–B*:46, 1963.)

degree oblique view of the lumbosacral joint. In this view the lamina will flatten out and an outline resembling a Scotch terrier can be easily seen, the dog's "neck" being formed by the pars interarticularis. The defect in the pars interarticularis is shown as a break or a separation in the neck of the dog (Fig. 6–27) The defect in the pars interarticularis may also be seen in the lateral or the anteroposterior views.

Forward displacement of the vertebra is seen in the lateral radiograph. In the normal spine when a straight line is placed along the shadow of the anterior border of the body of the first sacral vertebra, it will project upward and forward well to the front of the shadow of the fifth lumbar body, whereas in spondylolisthesis the straight edge will transect the body of the fifth lumbar vertebra (Ullman's sign) (Fig. 6–20).

Brailsford has described the "bowline" appearance of the slipped fifth lumbar vertebra, which represents a converging of its inferior and lateral aspects with the inferior and lateral aspects of its transverse processes (Fig. 6–28).[13] It is seen clearly in advanced cases and is of value in diagnosis.

Treatment

CONSERVATIVE MANAGEMENT

When spondylolisthesis is discovered in a child or an adolescent, in whom there is a

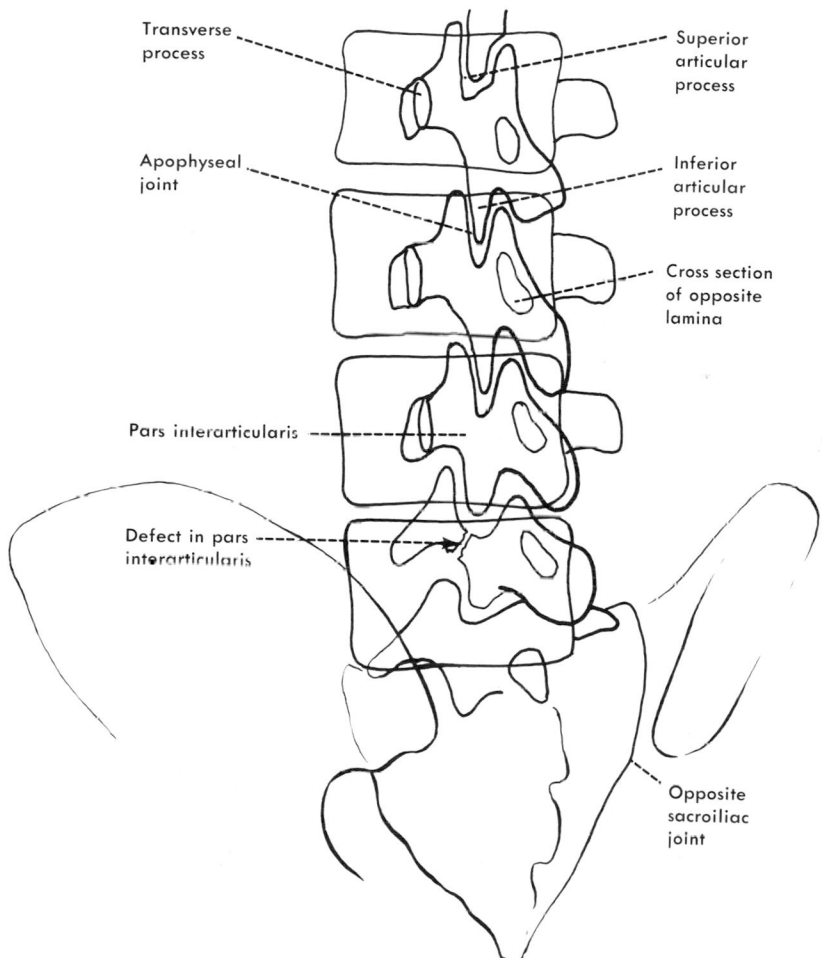

FIGURE 6–27. *Spondylolisthesis.*

Diagram of oblique view in roentgenogram shows the defect in the pars interarticularis.

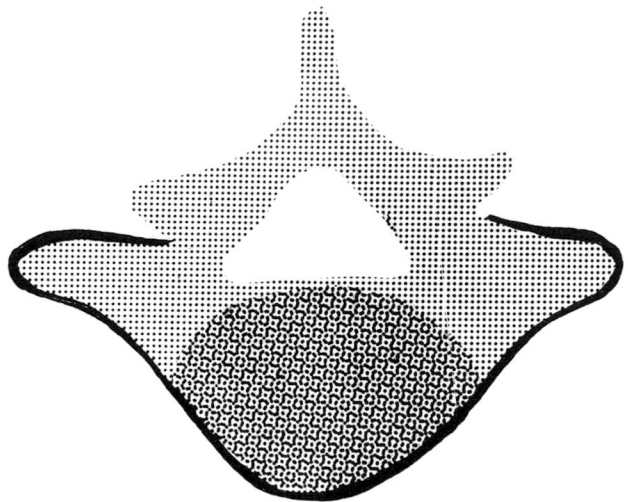

FIGURE 6–28.   The anteroposterior radiographic appearance of the spondylolisthetic vertebra.

The outline of the vertebra is that of a bow — the anterior convex outline of the body merges imperceptibly on each side by a gradual concavity into the outline of the lumbar transverse process. This outline is projected into the shadows of the first and second sacral vertebral bodies. (Redrawn after Brailsford, J.: Spondylolisthesis. Brit. J. Radiol., 6:666, 1933.)

greater tendency for further displacement, one should be more aggressive in treatment than one would be with an adult. If symptoms are minimal or absent and the displacement is slight, a trial of conservative management is usually indicated. It is important, however, to inform the parents of the possibility of further slipping and also to follow the child closely by periodic roentgenograms. Such patients are cautioned against overweight, overexertion in lifting, and participation in violent contact sports in which the risk of further displacement may be increased.

Most children and adolescents with spondylolisthesis have an exaggerated lumbar lordosis and an increase in pelvic tilt. In these patients postural exercises are in order. They consist of gluteus maximus, abdominal, and pelvic tilt exercises. Acute flexion of the trunk in abdominal exercises should be avoided. Pelvic tilt exercises are first done supine and then standing against the wall, rolling the buttocks under.

During periods of rapid growth or when symptoms are present, support to the spine in the form of a back brace is indicated.

OPERATIVE TREATMENT

When there is marked disability, persistent back pain, a moderate slip or progressive increase in the degree of slip, surgical intervention is indicated. The spine should be stabilized by arthrodesis of the olisthetic segment to the vertebrae above and below; i.e., in the case of fifth lumbar spondylolisthesis, the fusion should extend from the sacrum to the fourth lumbar vertebra.

When there is neurologic evidence of nerve root compression or irritation, removal of the loose neural arch, exploration of the nerve roots, and fusion are indicated. A preoperative myelogram is of great help.

In the recent literature several reports have appeared of treatment of spondylolisthesis with decompression alone by removal of the offending lamina and the fibrocartilaginous mass.[66, 84, 88, 170]

One should remember that not all sciatica is due to nerve root irritation alone. Sclerotome pain may closely simulate actual dermatome pain. Pseudosciatica may be the result of stretched ligaments in an unstable low back.

Decompression alone, without fusion, has no place in the treatment of spondylolisthesis in children or adolescents, as progression of forward slip occurs more frequently in individuals treated by this method. Even a defective neural arch provides some support to the slipped vertebrae. Further olisthy can and does occur after removal of the arch. In Bosworth's series of 64 patients who had the arch removed and subsequent fusion, 19 (30 per cent) had measurable progression of the olisthy. Pseudarthrosis was present in only 5 of these patients, while the remaining 14 suffered slipping during the four to five months required for solidification of the fusion.[42]

Many techniques for fusion of the lumbosacral spine have been devised; the one used varies with the surgeon. There is a relatively high rate of failure of fusion in attempted arthrodesis in spondylolisthesis as opposed to 17 per cent after laminectomy for protrusion of discs. Hammond et al. found an incidence of 60 per cent (36 of 73 fusions for spondylolisthesis).[74] Less than half of these 36 patients with pseudarthrosis, however, had sufficient symptoms to warrant exploration and repair. The relief of pain in the cases with pseudarthrosis is explained by the relative stability of the spine produced by the strong fibrous union of the vertebrae.

The author performs a modified Hibbs fusion supplemented by a large quantity of autogenous cancellous grafts and a stabilizing H-graft obtained from the ilium, as advocated by Bosworth and Barr.[38, 41] The large continuous iliac H-graft bridges the area between the fourth lumbar vertebra and the midsacrum, giving a relatively firm, immediate immobilization of the vertebrae to be fused (which is conducive to osteogenesis) and decreasing the danger of reparative reaction involving the roots. Postoperatively the spine is immobilized in a double hip spica cast for four to six months. The details of operative technique are illustrated in Plate 48. Preoperative and postoperative roentgenograms are shown in Figure 6–29.

Early ambulation after spinal fusion contributes to a higher rate of pseudarthrosis, and there is a greater chance of further slipping under the forces of body weight when the graft is still immature and not solid.

Anterior fusion or interbody arthrodesis has been advocated by several authors.[77, 92, 134] Posterior fusion is preferred because it is less hazardous and allows for exploration of nerve roots, defects, and intervertebral discs; it also provides an area for a larger mass of solid bone. The author has not yet encountered a case in which anterior or interbody fusion in children or adolescents was indicated.

Occasionally, reduction of the slipping has been attempted by various authors.[46, 61, 63, 68, 85, 153] Reduction is possible to achieve in children by means of skeletal traction through the long axis of the femur with the hips flexed and the trunk steadied with countertraction. Anterior skeletal traction through the innominate bones is applied in addition to femoral traction. The difficulty is to maintain the reduction with a local bone graft. Its only indication is in children with complete slipping, especially of the congenital type, who have so much deformity that it is difficult for them to walk because of the posterior projection of the pelvis, the shortening and forward displacement of the lumbar spine, and the severe compensatory lordosis (Fig. 6–30). To maintain the reduction, it is essential to keep the patient in traction for three to four months following spinal fusion and then immobilized in a double hip spica cast for another three months. As this requires a prolonged period of skeletal traction and hospitalization, one should preoperatively evaluate the patient's economic status as well as the psychologic effects of such confinement.

CONGENITAL ABSENCE OF THE SACRUM AND LUMBAR VERTEBRAE

Agenesis of the terminal segments of the vertebral column is rare. The failure of development ranges from mere absence of the lower coccygeal segment to complete aplasia of vertebrae below the twelfth thoracic segment. The lesser degrees of involvement, such as absence of the lower coccygeal segments, often go unnoticed and are usually recognized fortuitously during unrelated roentgenographic studies, whereas the more extreme degrees of involvement may be incompatible with life and have been described in reports on stillbirths.

The first case was described by Hohl in 1852, and since then several review articles and case reports have appeared in the literature.[171–193] Because of the wide range of possible vertebral anomalies, the recorded case presentations do not precisely depict the true incidence of the condition.

Total absence of the lumbosacral spine is a rare anomaly of severe axial skeletal

(Text continued on page 1180.)

Fusion for Spondylolisthesis with H (or Clothespin) Graft from Ilium

Under general endotracheal anesthesia the patient is placed in prone position with the table bent and flexed to flatten the lumbar spine and open the intervertebral spaces. Whole blood should be available for transfusion if it should be needed.

A. A midline incision about 4 inches long is made from the spinous process of the third lumbar vertebra to the midsacrum. Next, a separate incision is made over the iliac crest to obtain the bone graft. (An alternate skin incision is J-shaped, extending from the third lumbar spinous process to the posterior superior iliac spine of one side.

B. The supraspinous ligaments are incised from the fourth lumbar to the third sacral spinous process. Spina bifida of upper sacral and fifth lumbar vertebrae is often present in association with spondylolisthesis. Care should be taken not to open the dura.

C. Next, with a periosteal elevator the spinous processes, laminae, and facet joints are subperiosteally exposed. The muscles are held apart by self-retaining retractors. Hemostasis is secured by electrocautery or hot packs, or both. With a sharp curet, the laminae, the spinous processes, and the ligamenta flava are thoroughly denuded of all soft tissue.

D. With a bone clamp the looseness of the posterior neural arch is tested and demonstrated. If there is clinical and myelographic evidence of pressure on the nerve roots by the fibrocartilaginous mass at the partes interarticulares and anterior tilting of the proximal border of the loose neural arch, or both, one may have to excise both of them and free the nerve roots. For technical details the reader is referred to the description of Gill.[66] First, the middle parts of the loose neural arch are excised after freeing them from the tissues in the pars interarticularis and its articulation with the sacrum. Injury to the fifth lumbar and first sacral nerve roots should be avoided. The disc interspaces are examined for possible protrusion. If symptoms or signs of nerve root irritation are not present, the loose posterior neural arch should not be excised.

E. Next, the articular facets L4–L5 and L5–S1 are completely excised with osteotomes.

F. (1) With a curet all remaining articular cartilage is thoroughly removed from each facet joint. (2) Then a flap of bone is raised from the base of the transverse process and turned into the joint. (3) Multiple flaps of bone are raised from the laminae and sacrum. (4) They are crossed and their ends turned into appropriately placed trap doors in the bone. (5) The spinous process of the intervening vertebra (fifth lumbar) is excised.

Plate 48. Fusion for Spondylolisthesis with H (or Clothespin) Graft from Ilium

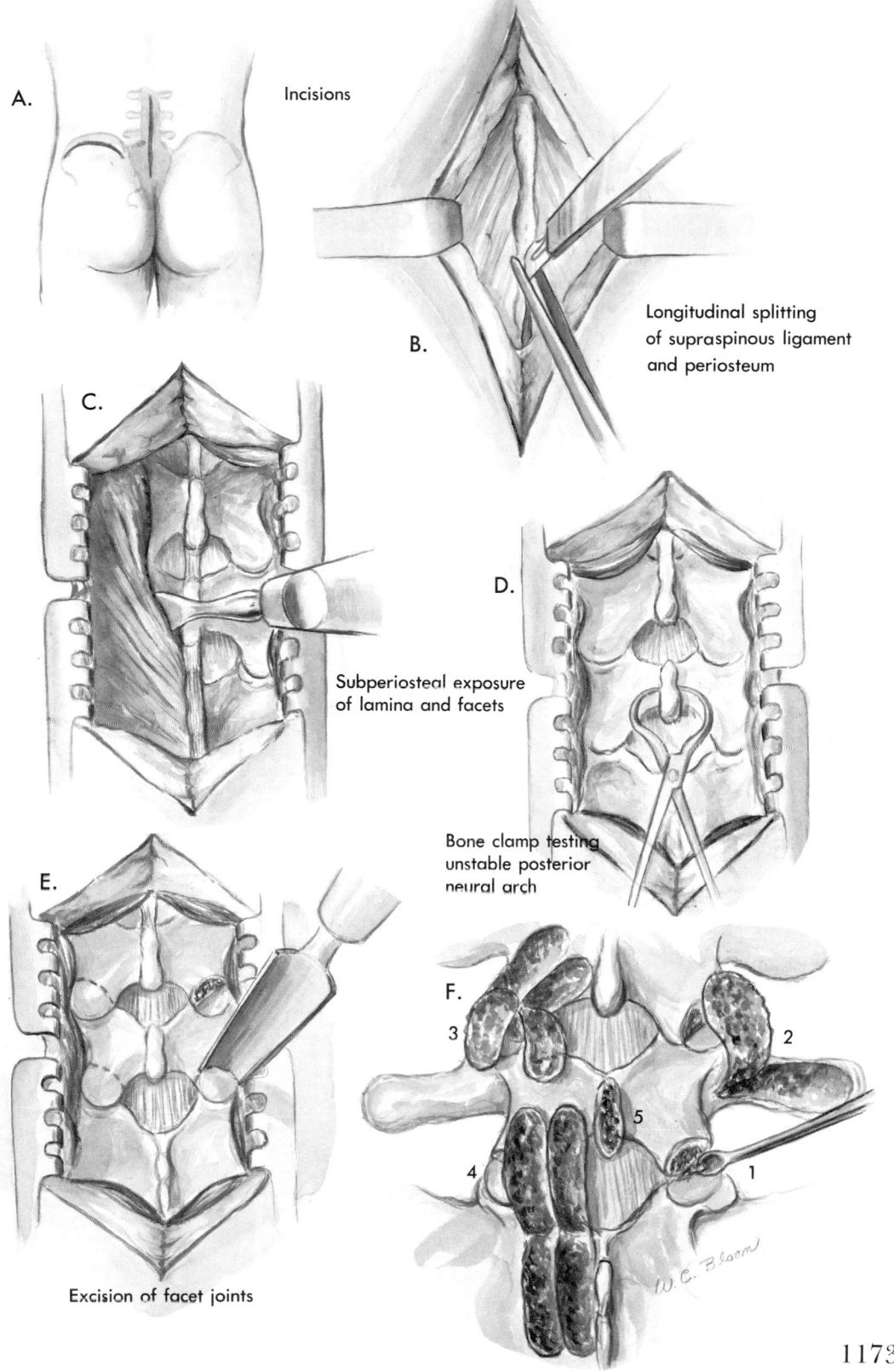

A. Incisions

B. Longitudinal splitting of supraspinous ligament and periosteum

C. Subperiosteal exposure of lamina and facets

D. Bone clamp testing unstable posterior neural arch

E. Excision of facet joints

F.

W. C. Bloom

Fusion for Spondylolisthesis with H (or Clothespin) Graft from Ilium (Continued)

G. The bone graft bed is prepared by decorticating all bone in the area. It is important that the fusion extend to the midsacrum.

H and **I.** Next, the posterolateral wall of the posterior two thirds of the ilium is exposed subperiosteally for taking of the autogenous bone graft. An incision is made along the subcutaneous border of the iliac crest at the point of contact of the periosteum with the origins of the gluteal and trunk muscles. The incision is carried down to bone, which is exposed subperiosteally to avoid hemorrhage. First, a large rectangular area on the outer table of the ilium is outlined with an osteotome. Then, a cortical graft from the outer table is removed with broad osteotomes. Next, an abundant amount of chips or sliver grafts of cancellous and cortical bone are removed with gouges and curved osteotomes. The periosteum and its muscular attachments are sutured together with interrupted sutures of silk or catgut. When bleeding from the ilium is profuse, Gelfoam and bone wax may be used to control it. One should always double-check to see that sponges are not left in the iliac wound.

J. Chip grafts of cortical and cancellous bone are packed laterally across the facet joints and transverse processes from the fourth lumbar vertebra to the sacrum. Lateral fusion is an integral part of lumbosacral fusion.

K. Then the ends of the clothespin graft are notched to receive the spinous process at each end of the fusion area. The spinous processes are separated by acutely flexing the spine. This can be done with a vertebral spreader or by bending the operating table, or both. The clothespin graft is inserted and held firmly in place by extension of the spine. As mentioned earlier, spina bifida of one or more of the sacral segments is not uncommon in spondylolisthesis. In such an instance, the lower end of the graft is fashioned as a double strut and is placed in grooves cut transversely in the region of the facet joints of the first sacral vertebra. If the spinous process of the first sacral vertebra is absent or underdeveloped, it is fitted to that of the second sacral vertebra. On occasion, one has simply to fit the lower end of the graft in the denuded posterior surface of the sacrum. Abundant cancellous bone is packed about the graft and across the laminae. The wound is closed in layers in the usual manner. A double long leg hip spica cast is applied for immobilization. Frequently a bivalved hip spica cast is made in which the patient is placed on completion of the operation.

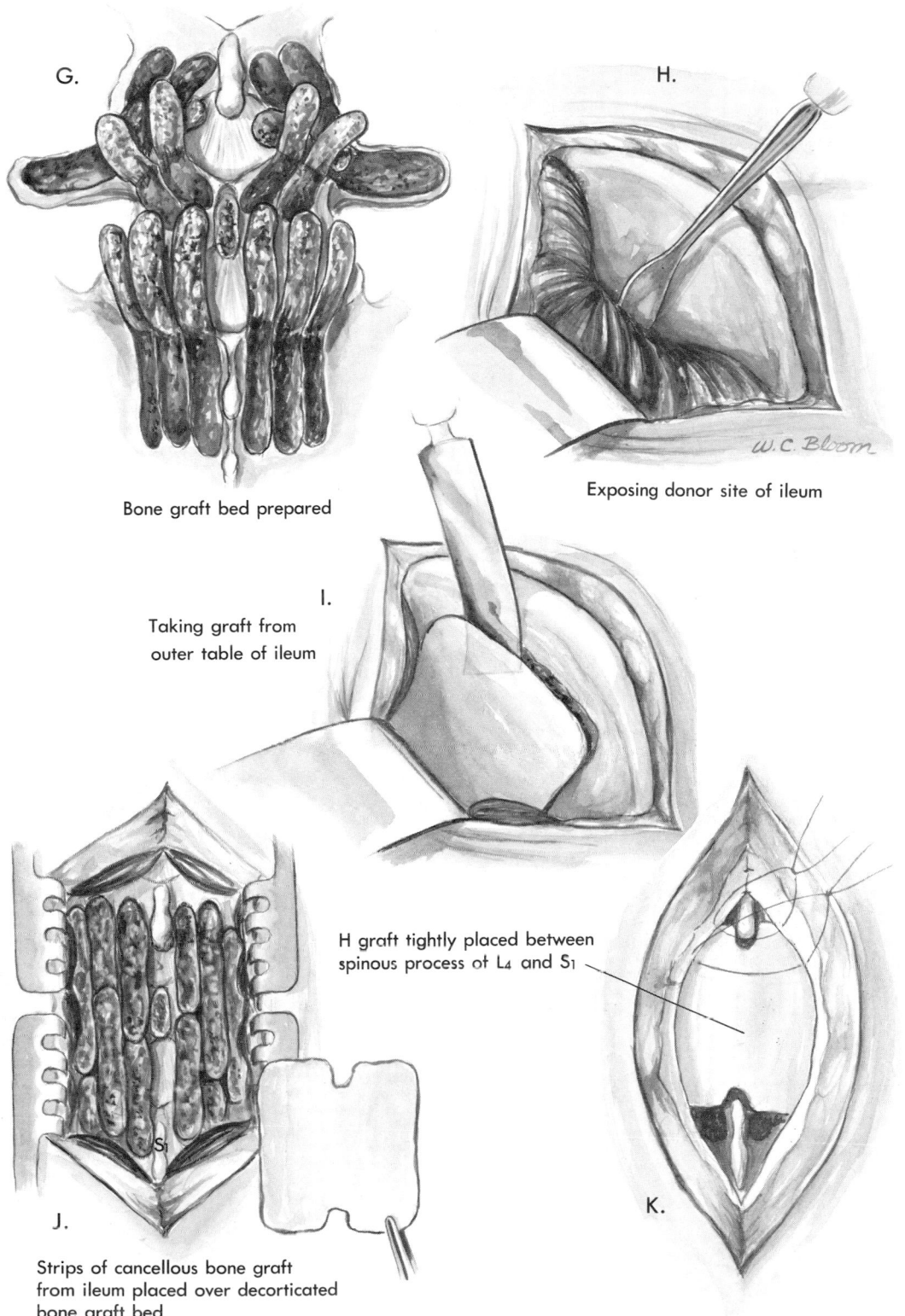

G.

Bone graft bed prepared

H.

Exposing donor site of ileum

W.C. Bloom

I.

Taking graft from outer table of ileum

H graft tightly placed between spinous process of L4 and S1

J.

Strips of cancellous bone graft from ileum placed over decorticated bone graft bed

K.

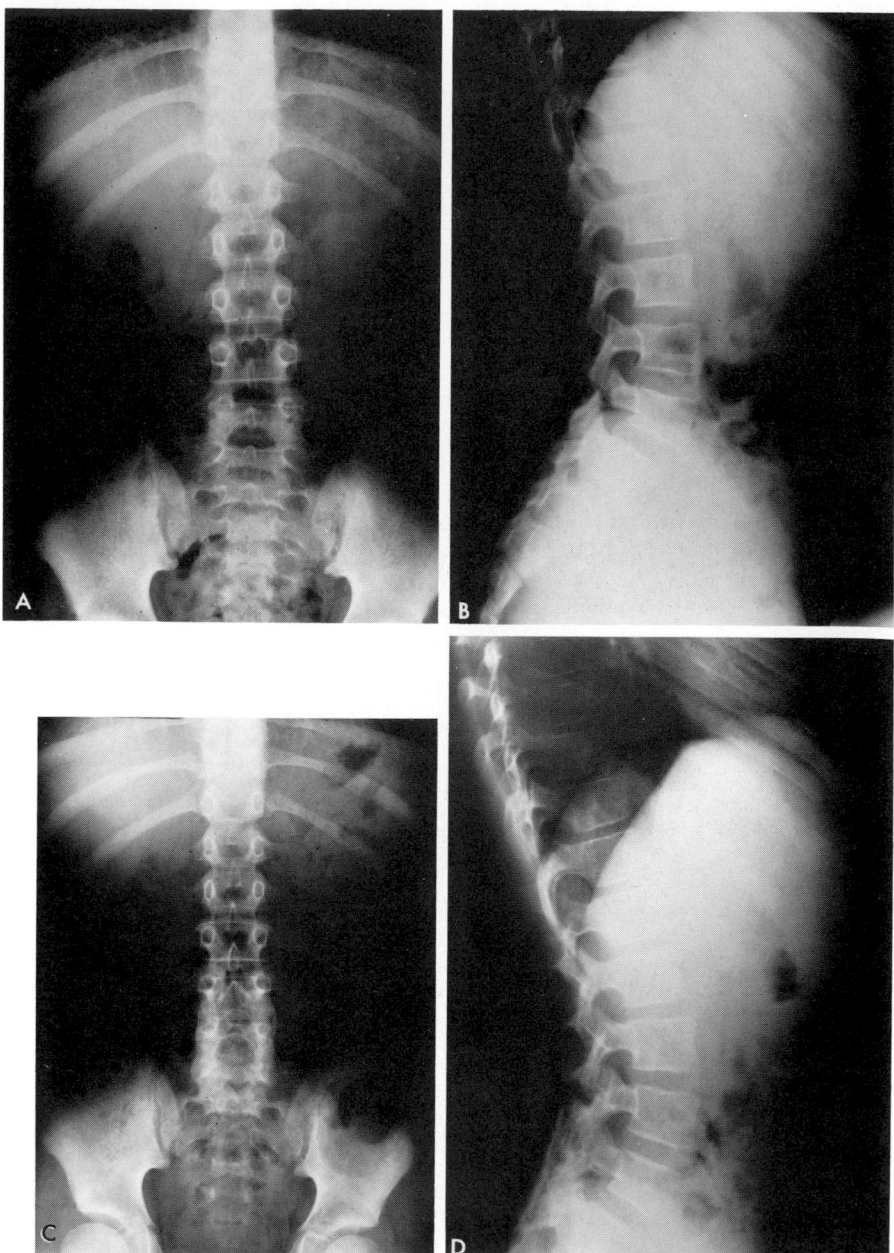

FIGURE 6–29. *Spondylolisthesis, first degree, between fifth lumbar and first sacral vertebra.*

A and **B.** Preoperative anteroposterior and lateral roentgenograms of lumbosacral spine. **C** and **D.** Postoperative roentgenograms one year after spinal fusion between fourth lumbar and mid-sacrum.

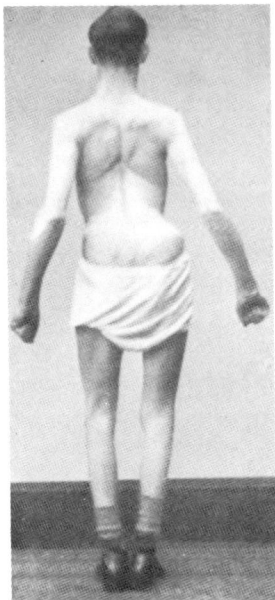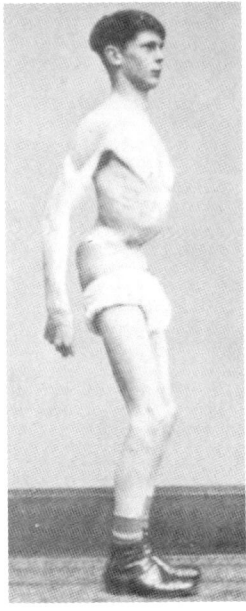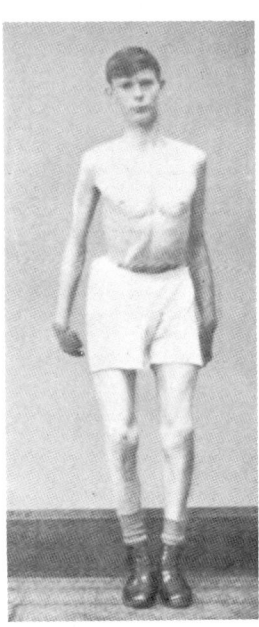

A

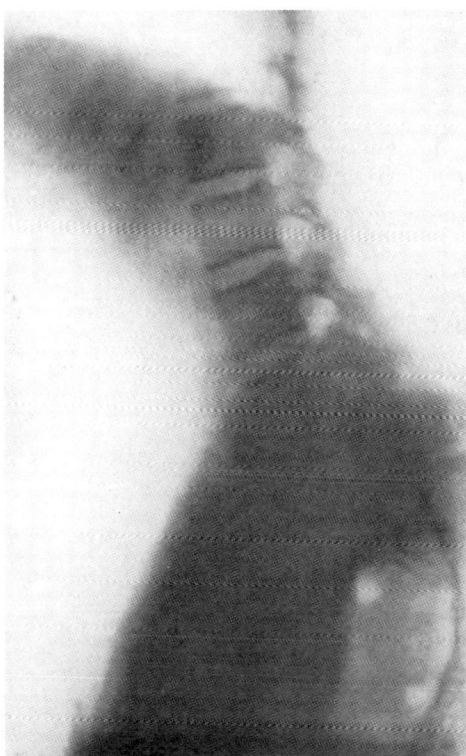

B

FIGURE 6–30. Severe spondylolisthesis with complete displacement of the fifth lumbar vertebra over the sacrum.

A. Clinical appearance of patient. Note severe compensatory lordosis. The posterior projection of the pelvis makes walking difficult. **B.** X-ray appearance. (From Jenkins, J. A.: Spondylolisthesis. Brit. J. Surg., *24*:80–85, 1936.)

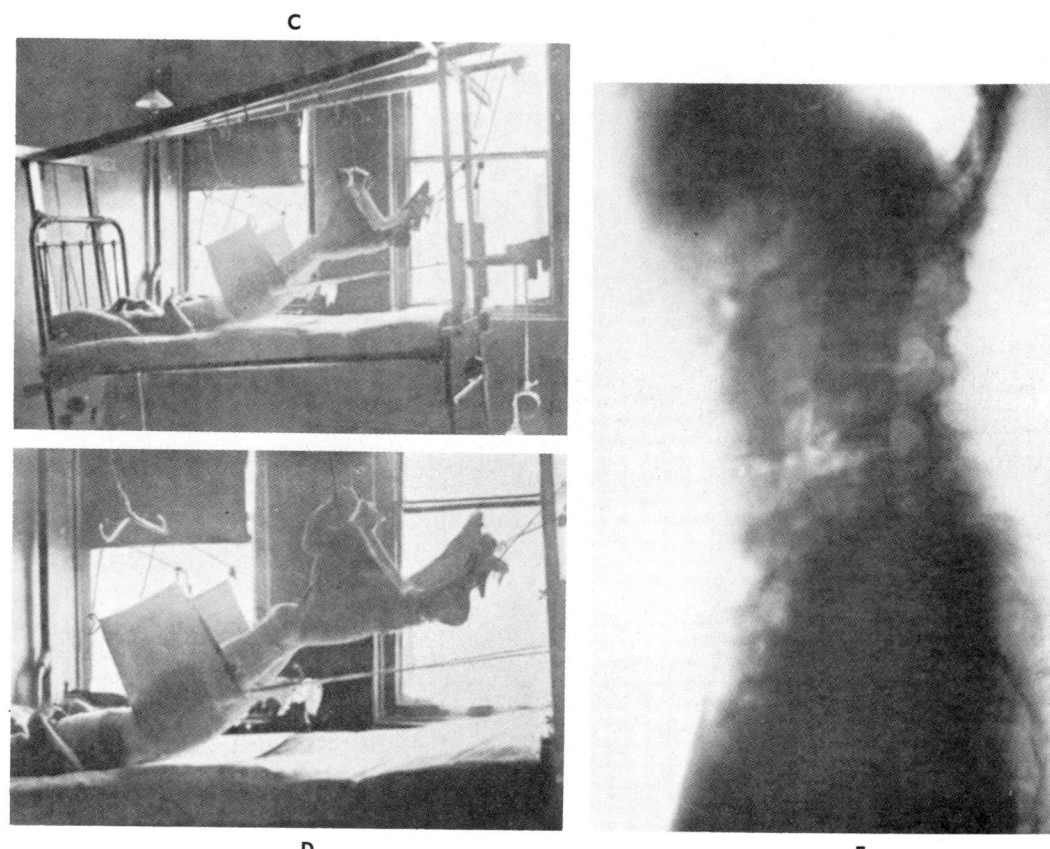

FIGURE 6–30 Continued. *Severe spondylolisthesis with complete displacement of the fifth lumbar vertebra over the sacrum.*

C and **D.** Method of reduction. (The author recommends direct skeletal traction with Steinmann pins through the distal femur and wires through both iliac wings.) **E.** Roentgenogram showing reduction. (From Jenkins, J. A.: Spondylolisthesis. Brit. J. Surg., *24*:80–85, 1936.)

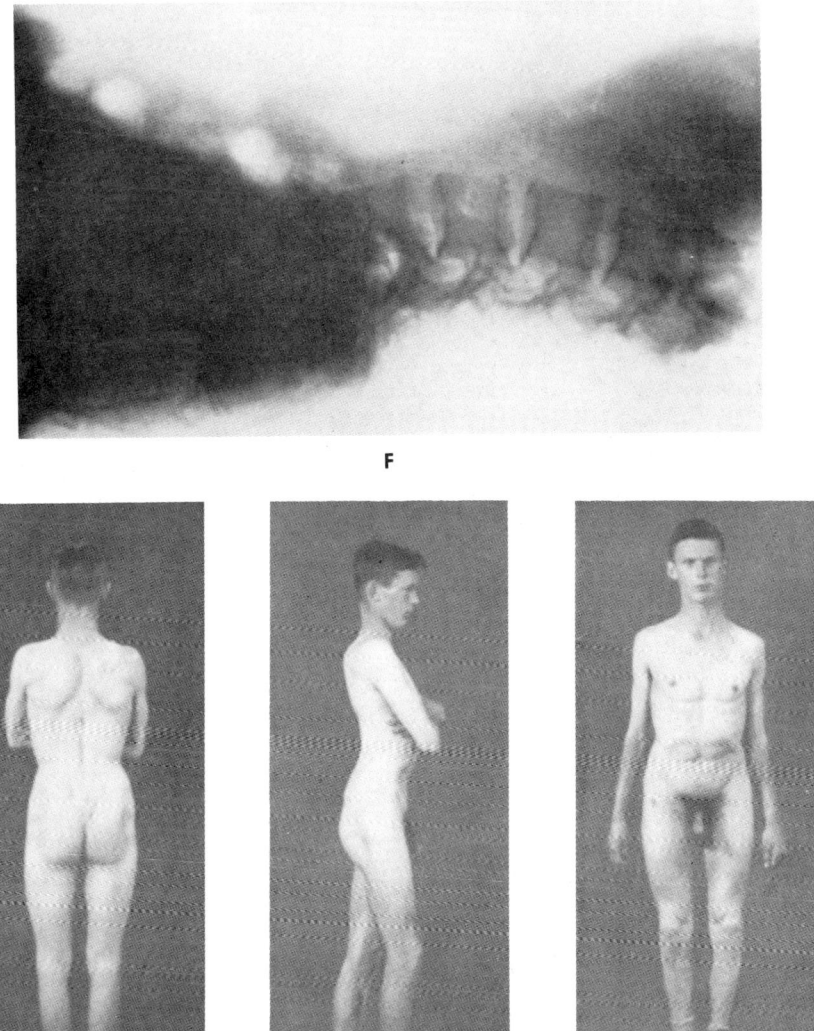

F

G

FIGURE 6–30 Continued.   Severe spondylolisthesis with complete displacement of the fifth lumbar vertebra over the sacrum.

F. Postoperative roentgenogram. **G.** Photographs a year after operation showing clinical improvement. (From Jenkins, J. A.: Spondylolisthesis. Brit. J. Surg., *24*:80–85, 1936.)

deficiency that results in a severely handicapped individual with contractural deformities and complete loss of function of
the lower limbs.[179, 181]

Etiology

In the human embryo, the stage of differentiation of the lumbar spine, sacrum,
and coccyx occurs between the fourth and
seventh postovulatory weeks. Duraiswami,
in his study of insulin-induced skeletal
abnormalities in developing chickens, found
that vertebral changes often resulted from
insulin injections made in the first two days
of incubation, whereas other skeletal aberrations resulted from later injections, indicating that the part most affected was
that which was in the most active stage of
development or differentiation.[177] The
noxious agent must exert its influence early
in embryonic development if it is to cause
congenital absence of the lumbosacral spine.

A higher than normal incidence of diabetes mellitus and spontaneous abortions
among women having offspring with congenital absence of the sacrum is reported
by Blumel and associates.[173]

Freedman suggested the theory of failure
of provocative mechanisms during early
embryonic differentiation.[180] Detwiler and
Holtzer presented evidence of inductive
and formative influence of the spinal cord
upon the vertebral column.[174] Animal experiments have shown that many defects
of the nervous system can result from a
failure of inductive interaction between
the presumptive notochord and neural
ectoderm during very early embryonic
stages.[182] One may attribute this failure to
a genetically determined exaggeration of
the pattern of ontogenic cellular death in
mesodermal and neural elements of the
posterior body regions.[90]

As to the importance of inheritable
genetic factors, a single instance of congenital absence of the sacrum occurring in
father and son has been reported by Pouzet,
in 1938.[189] Absence of the rump in the
fowl, closely resembling similar human
disorders, has been known for centuries.
In fowls, the anomaly occurs as a hereditary
anomaly as well as spontaneously as a
mutation.[175, 176]

Clinical Picture

The appearance of the patient depends
on the extent of spinal involvement and
on the degree of concomitant neurologic
deficit.

In complete absence of the lumbar spine
and sacrum, the patients are of short stature, having a characteristic cross-legged
Buddha-like attitude (Fig. 6–31). The
twelfth thoracic vertebra is dorsally prominent. There is marked disproportion between the thorax and the pelvis. The narrow, flat buttocks manifest a depressed
dimpling 2 or 3 inches lateral to the gluteal
cleft. The normal convexity of the sacrococcygeal region is lost. The anus is horizontal. The pelvis is very unstable under
the spine—on sitting unsupported, it tends
to roll up under the thorax and drops forward, seeming to rest anterior to the
thoracic spine as the patient tries to support
himself on his hands. The hips have flexion
and abduction contracture. The knees
show 60 to 90 degrees of flexion contracture
with large popliteal webs and heavily
callused knee pads. Fixed calcaneus deformities of the feet are present.

There is muscle paralysis and atrophy of
the lower limbs that is complete at and below the knees, with no voluntary or involuntary motor or reflex movement. Because of
marked muscle atrophy, a cone-shaped
appearance of the lower half of the body
develops. In the very extreme case, a
"mermaid" configuration is given, which
has merited the designation of "siren."

Sensation is usually normal down to the
knees. Distally, there may be spotty areas
of hypesthesia or anesthesia. Trophic
changes are absent. The patients have no
bladder or bowel control.

In total absence of the sacrum, the buttocks are flattened and the intergluteal
cleft is shortened with dimpling of each
buttock lateral to the cleft. There is loss
of the normal posterior convexity of the
sacrococcygeal region. On rectal examination the concavity of the sacrum and coccyx
is absent. The neurologic deficit varies
with the degree of involvement of the sacral
or lumbosacral plexus.

Many other unusual associated developmental anomalies have been recorded such
as: total absence of one lower limb, suppres-

(Text continued on page 1186.)

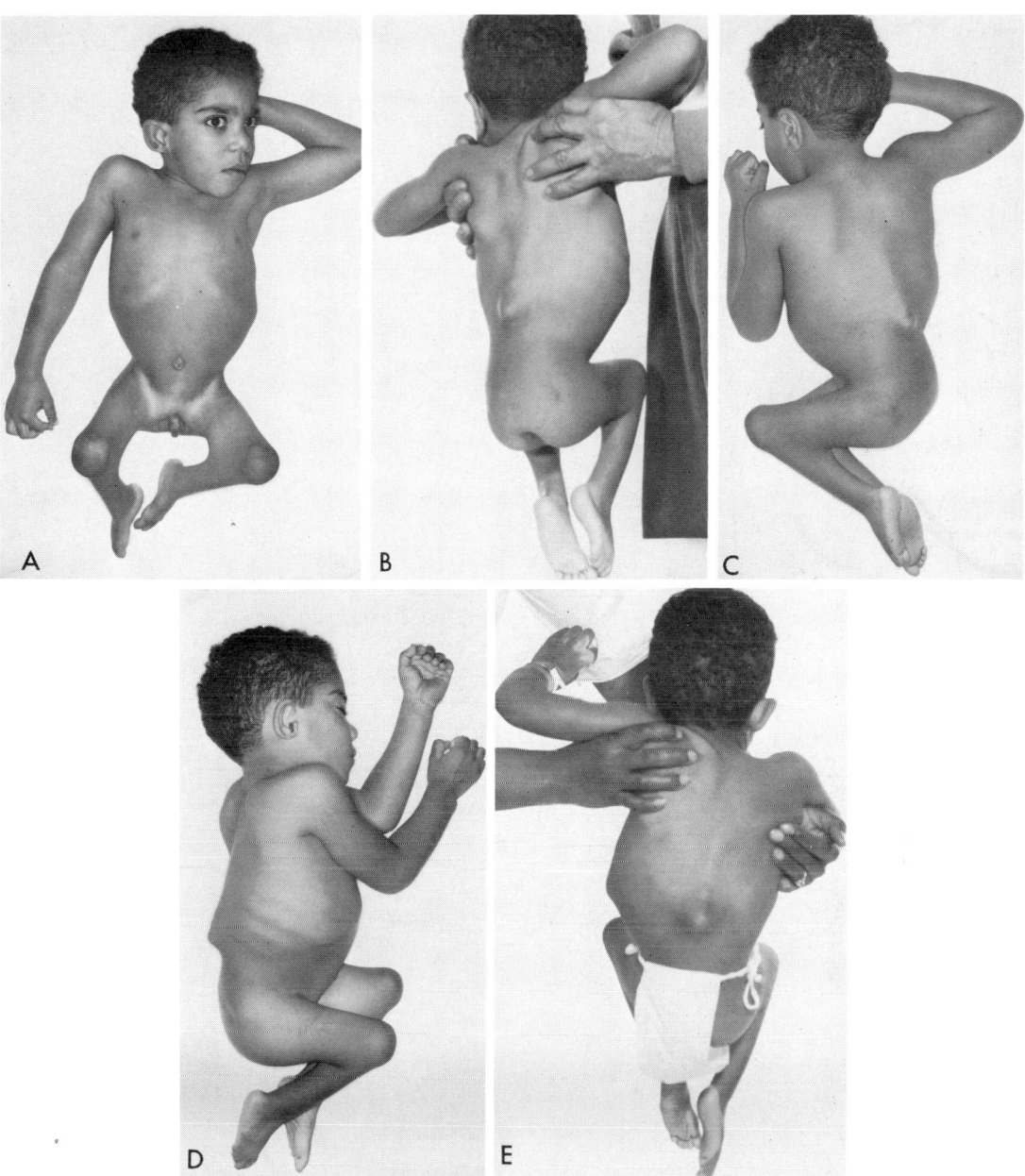

FIGURE 6–31. ***Congenital absence of the lumbosacral spine in a six-year-old child.***

A to **E.** Clinical appearance of patient in the front, right and left oblique, lateral, and back views.

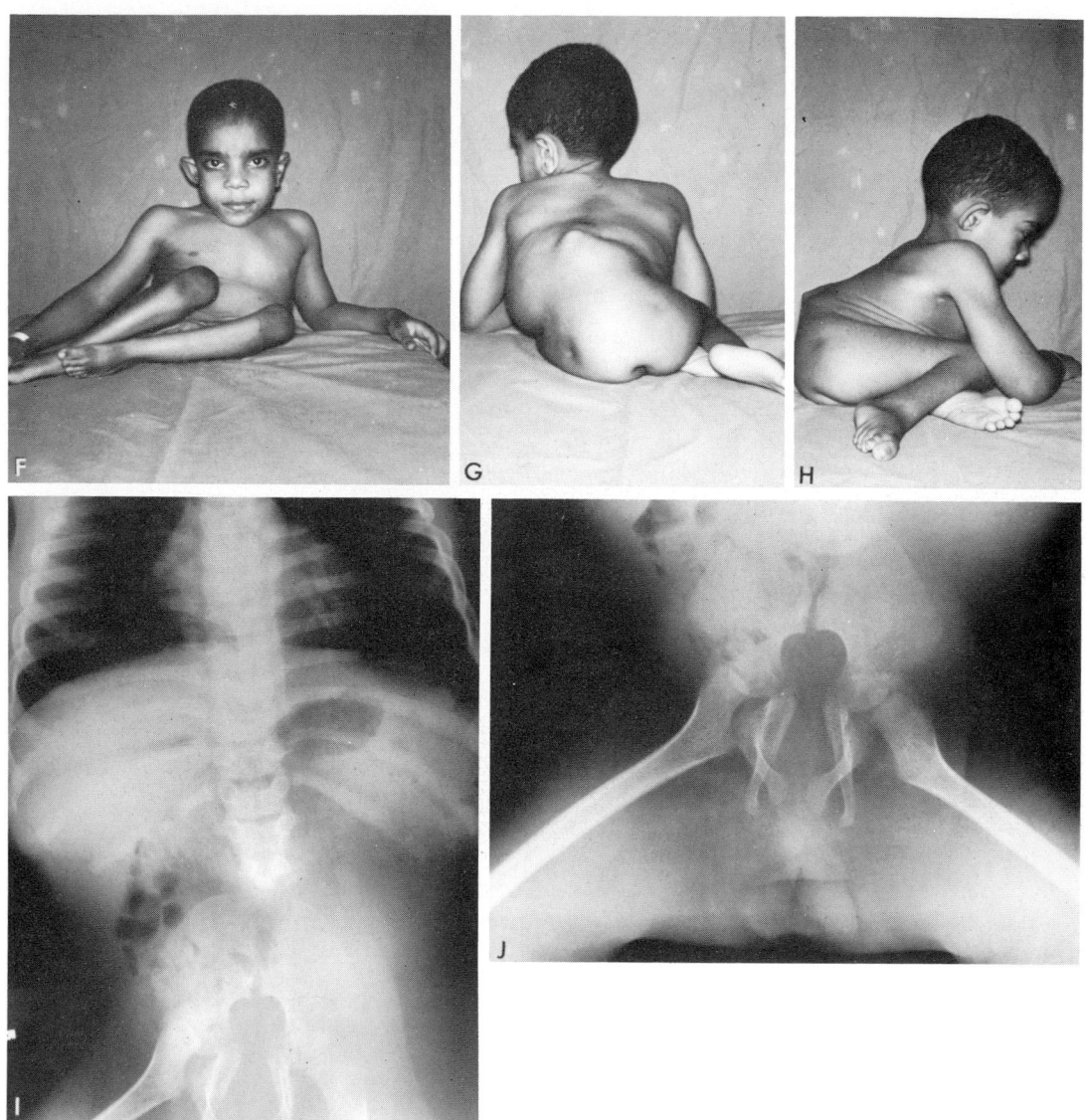

FIGURE 6–31 Continued.   Congenital absence of the lumbosacral spine in a six-year-old child.

F to H. Note the sitting posture. He has to support himself on his hands. The pelvis seems to roll up under the thorax. **I** and **J.** Anteroposterior roentgenogram of the spine (**I**) and pelvis (**J**). Note the absence of sacrum, coccyx, and distal three lumbar vertebrae. The second lumbar vertebra is the most distal segment present. The pelvis is narrow, with the ilia articulating amphiarthrodially. The hips are dislocated.

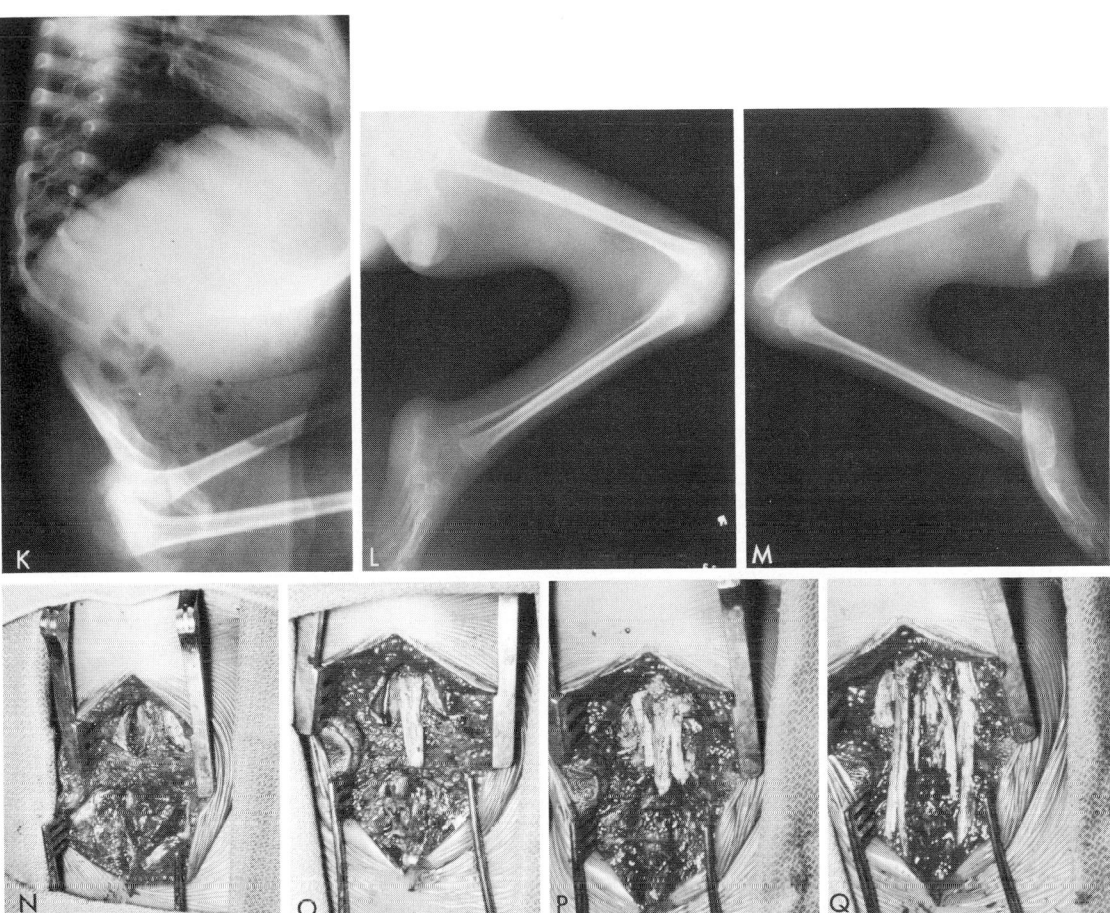

FIGURE 6–31 Continued. *Congenital absence of the lumbosacral spine in a six-year-old child.*

K. Lateral roentgenogram of the spine. **L** and **M.** Lateral roentgenograms of the lower extremities. Note the atrophy of the femora and tibiae. The knee joints are well formed but held in 120 degrees of flexion. **N.** Pathologic findings at operation. Note the absence of the spinal cord. There is no evidence of the lumbosacral plexus. **O.** The tibia of the patient's own amputated leg is used to stabilize the spine by grafting from the second lumbar vertebra to the pelvis. **P** and **Q.** Reinforcement of fusion by addition of large matchsticks of autogenous tibial graft.

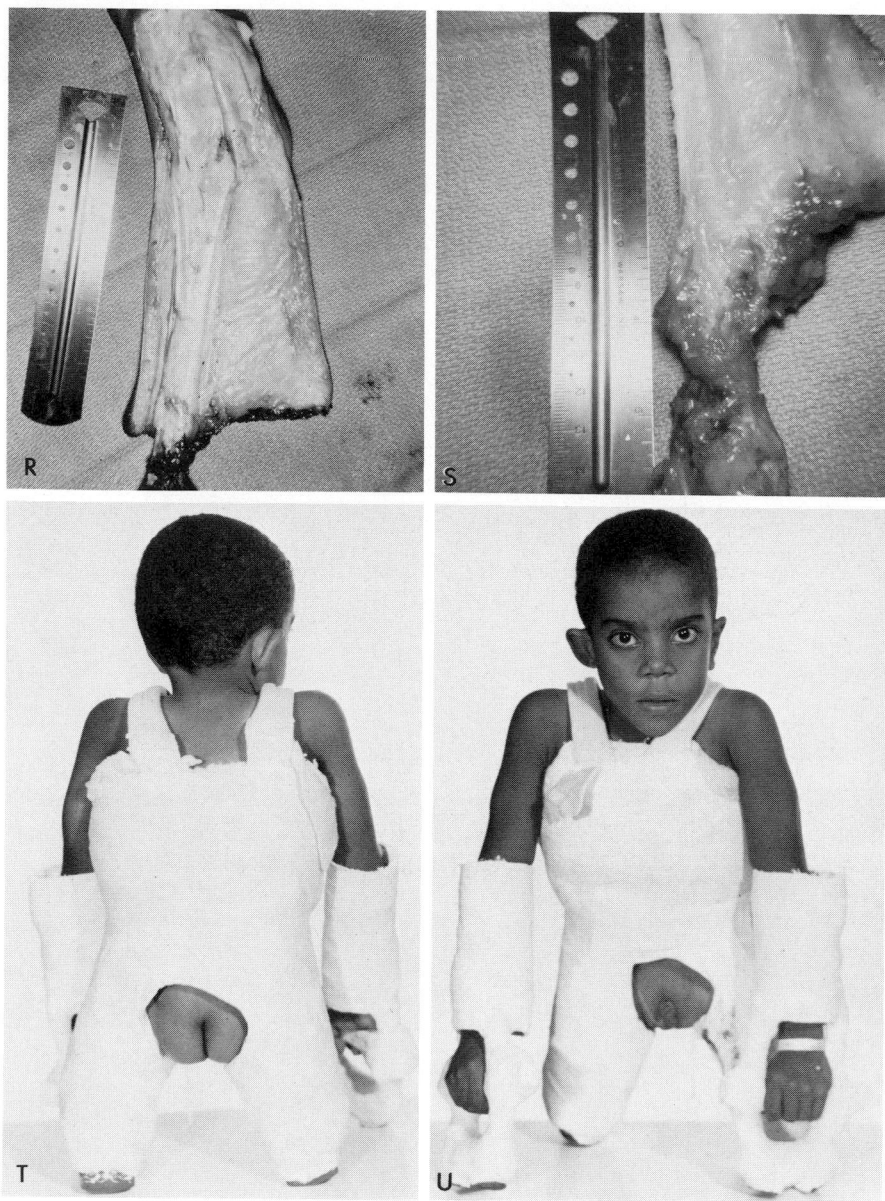

FIGURE 6–31 Continued.   Congenital absence of the lumbosacral spine in a six-year-old child.

R and **S.** Gross appearance of the amputated legs. Normal muscle tissue is replaced by large globules of soft deep yellow fat. Tendons are thin filaments, and the vessels very small. **T** and **U.** Hip-body spica cast with especially made short cast crutches used for ambulation in the immediate postoperative period.

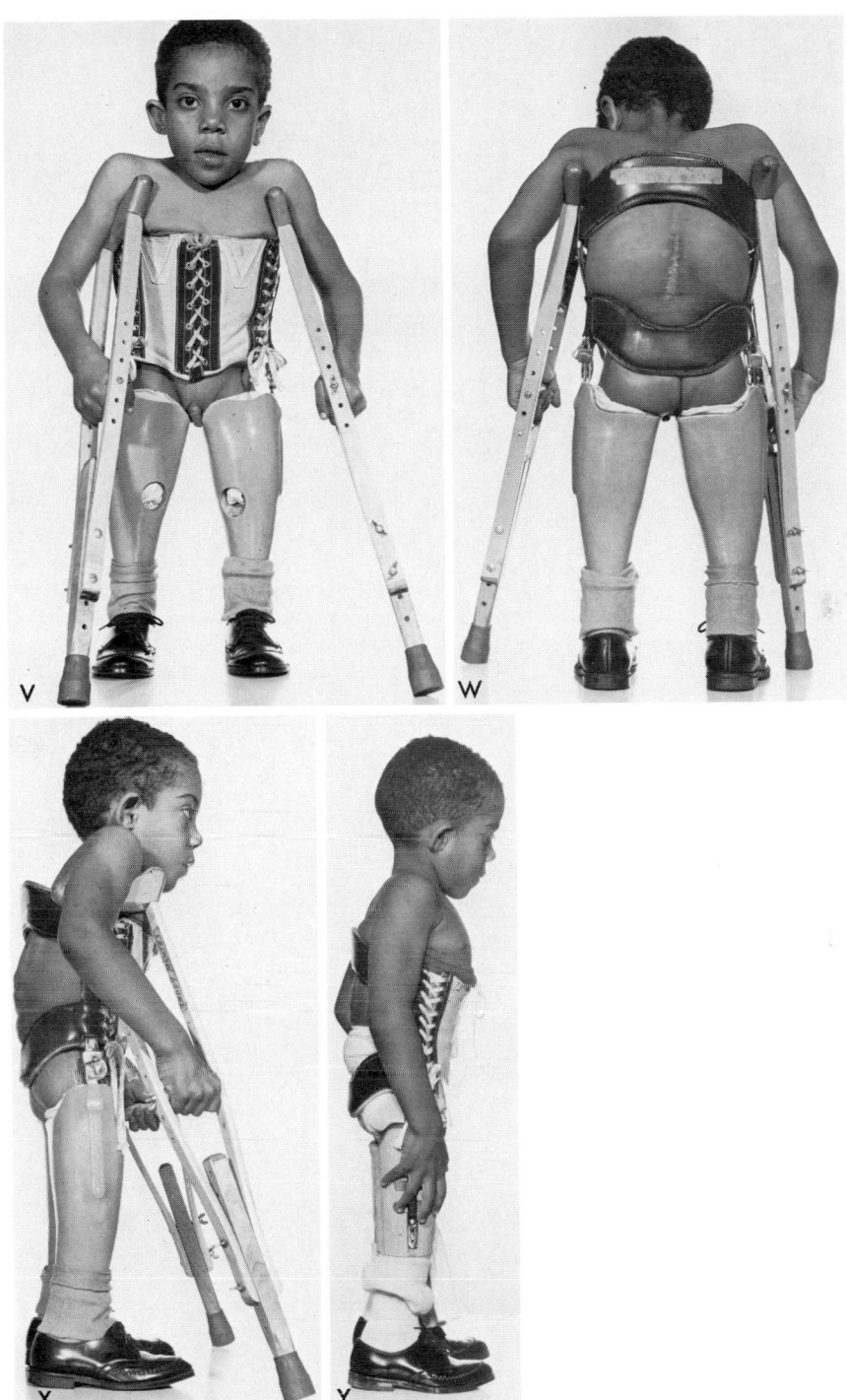

FIGURE 6–31 Continued.   *Congenital absence of the lumbosacral spine in a six-year-old child.*

V to **Y.** Patient is able to walk with his prosthetic limbs and spinal brace. He even can stand without support.

sion of neural elements, hemivertebrae, spina bifida, myelomeningocele, fusion of adjacent ribs, articulation of opposite ribs in the midline where corresponding vertebrae are absent, diminution in numbers of ribs, scoliosis, and anorectal abnormalities.

Roentgenographic Findings

The rib cage is normal. In total absence of the lumbosacral spine the twelfth thoracic vertebra is the most distal segment. The sacrum and coccyx are absent (Fig. 6–31 I to K). The pelvis is narrow with the ilia articulating amphiarthrodially. The femora and tibiae are atrophic, but normally formed. The femoral heads may be well seated in normal acetabuli, or the hip joints may be dislocated. The knee joints are well defined, but are held in 45 to 90 degrees of flexion (Fig. 6–31 L and M). The feet and ankles exhibit calcaneus deformity. Intravenous excretory pyelograms usually disclose normally functioning kidneys.

Pathologic Findings

The gross and histologic findings depend upon the level of the lesion. In total absence of the lumbosacral spine, normal muscle tissue is replaced by large globules of soft, deep, yellow fat. Femoral vessels are very small. Tendons are found as thin filaments, but have normal configuration. Femoral nerves are represented as gross fatty tissue adjacent to the small vessels. Afferent tracts are usually fairly well preserved, whereas efferent motor neuron pathways are impaired or missing.[191] The spinal cord does not disclose any lumbar enlargement or lumbosacral plexus and terminates at a higher level than usual, such as the seventh thoracic vertebra, when the spinal column ends at the second lumbar segment.

Treatment

Reconstruction of the lower limbs in total absence of the lumbosacral spine has not been successful because of the absence of muscle fibers and major motor nerves.[191]

Russell and Aitken and Frantz and Aitken have reported the results of treatment with bilateral subtrochanteric amputation and fitting with a pelvic-thoracic bucket and Canadian hip disarticulation prosthesis. These patients were able to be partially self-sufficient and to walk with the swing-to or swing-through gait, as performed by paraplegics.[179, 191]

The one major problem that has not been dealt with in this procedure is that of spinopelvic instability. As long as this defect remains uncorrected, the patient is able neither to sit unsupported nor to ambulate without the aid of a cumbersome pelvic-thoracic bucket.

Upon the suggestion of Dr. Robert L. Salter, bilateral knee disarticulation was performed and the tibiae were used to stabilize the spine by performing a fusion from T 11 or T 12 to the pelvis. These patients were able to sit up unsupported and were able to ambulate. Operative findings and preoperative and postoperative photographs are shown in Figure 6–31.

The neuromuscular deficit is less in congenital absence of the sacrum and coccyx. Patients are able to sit and walk with assistance. Treatment varies according to the degree of paralysis and the associated skeletal deformities. A patient with sacrococcygeal absence is illustrated in Figure 6–32.

Scoliosis

SCOLIOSIS

The word *scoliosis* is derived from the Greek word meaning "crooked." It is one of the most common deformities of the spine and presents a very difficult orthopedic problem. Despite great strides in methods of treatment, scoliosis can still be called the *crux orthopaedica*. André probably had that idea in mind when he devised his symbol for orthopedics.

The human spine is held erect by active

(Text continued on page 1190.)

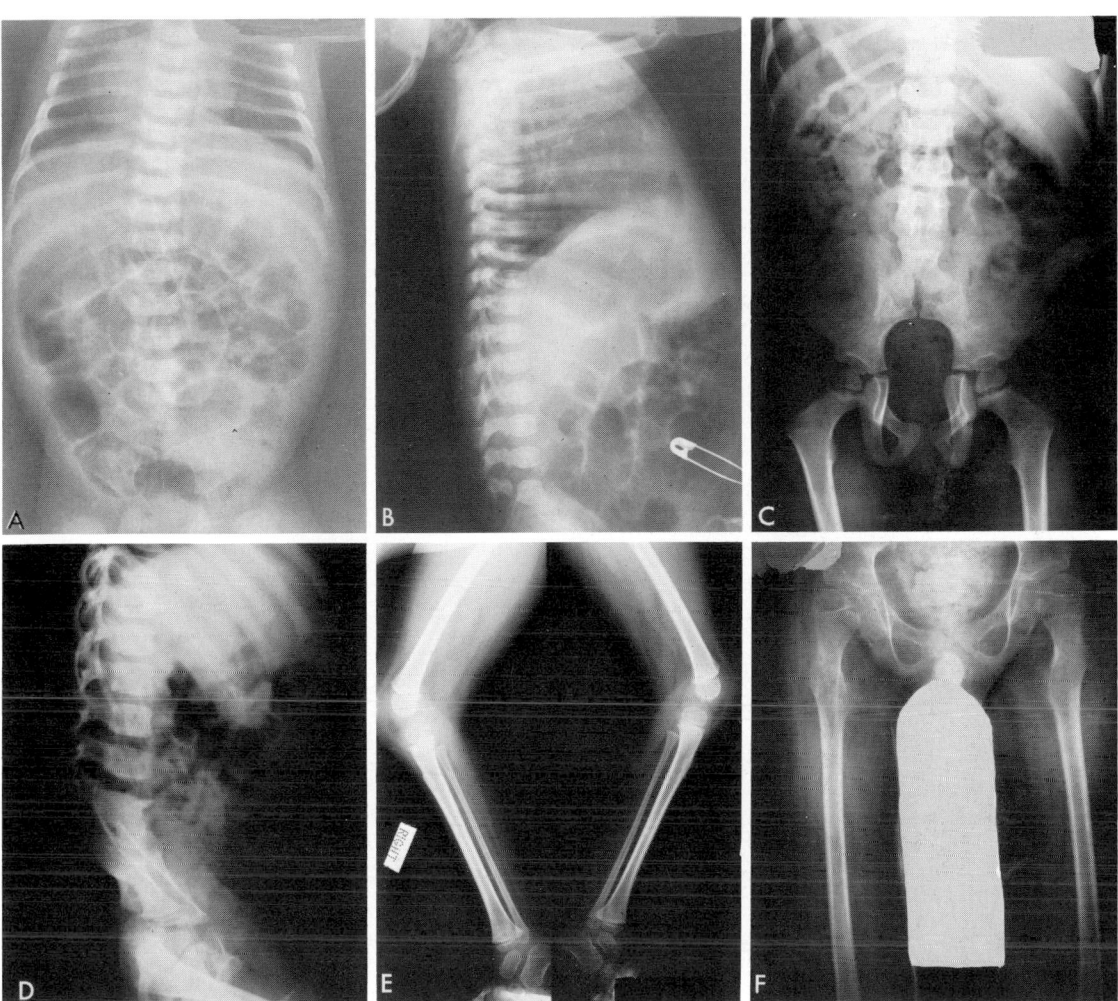

FIGURE 6-32. *Congenital absence of sacrum and coccyx.*

A and B. Anteroposterior and lateral roentgenograms of the spine at birth. Note the absence of the sacrum and coccyx. C and D. Anteroposterior and lateral roentgenograms of the spine at three years of age. E. Lateral roentgenograms of the lower limbs, showing normally developed bones. There is 35 degrees of flexion deformity of the knees. F. Anteroposterior roentgenogram of the hips and femora at seven years of age. Note the severe coxa valga and subluxation of the hips. At this time bilateral varization osteotomy of the proximal femora was performed to correct the coxa valga deformity.

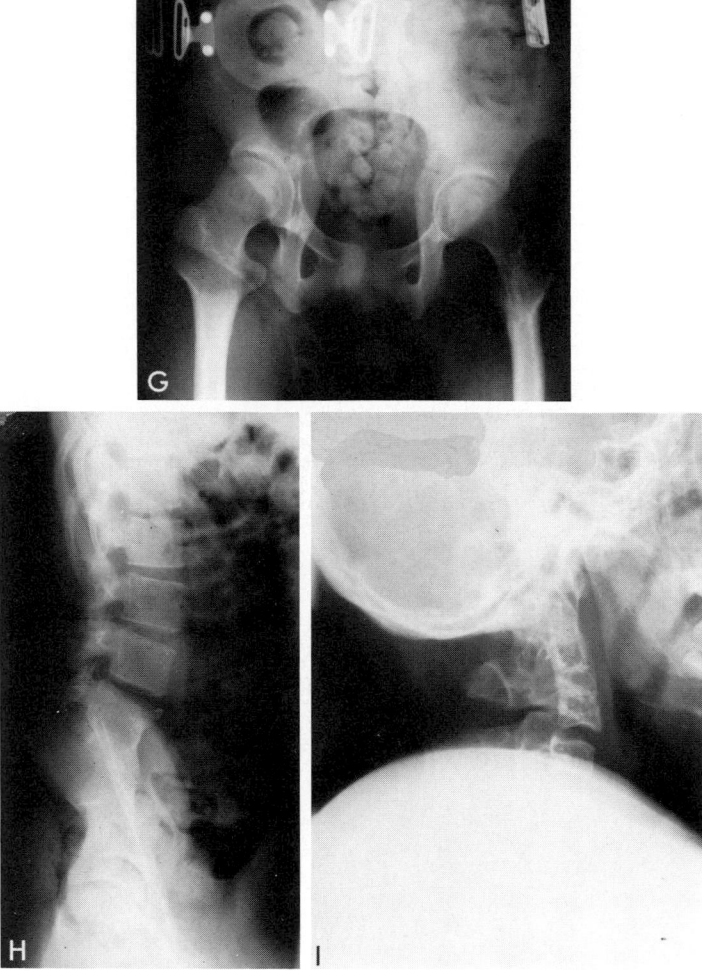

FIGURE 6–32 Continued.   Congenital absence of sacrum and coccyx.

G. Postoperative roentgenograms of the hips. The femoral heads are well seated in the acetabuli and the coxa valga deformity is corrected. **H.** Lateral roentgenogram of the lumbosacral spine at age 17 years. Note the spur at the superior-anterior margin on the fifth lumbar vertebra. **I.** Lateral roentgenogram of cervical spine, showing congenital fusion of upper five cervical vertebrae (Klippel-Feil).

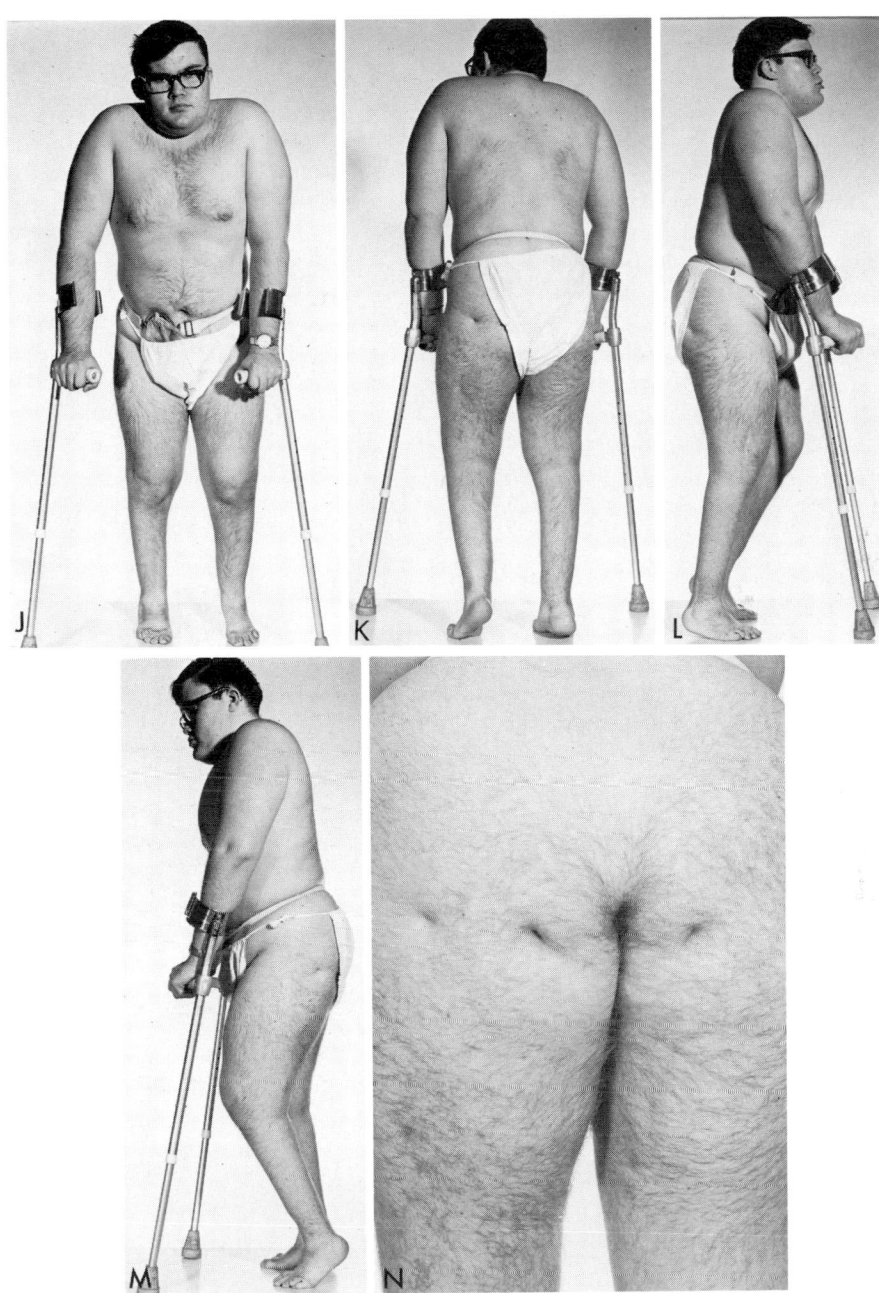

FIGURE 6–32 Continued.   Congenital absence of sacrum and coccyx.

J to **M.** Clinical appearance of patient. He is able to walk with crutches. **N.** Close view of buttocks showing the gluteal dimples.

muscular support and by the sense of balance. There is a definite tendency for the normal spine to grow straight. There are normally physiologic curves in the sagittal plane, but the spine is straight when viewed in the frontal plane, i.e., some degree of lumbar lordosis or dorsal kyphosis is normal, but there is no lateral curvature of the normal spine.

Scoliosis may be defined as lateral deviation and rotation of a series of vertebrae from the midline anatomic position of the normal spinal axis. The deformity occurs in two planes—lateral and rotatory. When the deviation cannot be corrected or the correction maintained, the scoliosis is considered pathologic. With progression of the curve, structural changes in the vertebrae will occur, and deformity of the rib cage will result from the rotation of the thoracic vertebral bodies. Associated pelvic deformity may take place. Relationships of intrathoracic and abdominal organs will be distorted.

Scoliosis is a deformity that has its genesis in childhood and adolescence, although the residual deformity persists throughout adult life.

Classification

There are two fundamental types of scoliosis—*functional* (or postural) and *structural*. The following simple and practical classification serves as a workable outline:
Functional or postural scoliosis
Structural scoliosis
  Congenital
  Acquired
    Idiopathic—unknown origin
      Lumbar
      Dorsolumbar
      Dorsal—infantile, juvenile, adolescent
      Combined dorsal and lumbar
      Cervicodorsal
    Known origin
      Neuromuscular
        Poliomyelitis
        Neurofibromatosis
        Intraspinal tumors
        Friedreich's ataxia
        Syringomyelia
        Spastic paralysis—cerebral palsy

        Muscular dystrophies and other myopathies
        Arthrogryposis multiplex congenita
      Postirradiation scoliosis
      Thoracogenic (postempyema, postthoracoplasty)
      Scoliosis in children with congenital heart disease
      Scoliosis due to affections of the vertebral column
        Osteochondrodystrophy
        Osteogenesis imperfecta
        Fracture-dislocation
        Tumors such as osteoid osteoma
        Inflammatory conditions such as rheumatoid, pyogenic, or tuberculous spondylitis

The importance of determining the etiologic diagnosis cannot be overemphasized. Structural scoliosis may be due to bone, nerve, or muscle lesions, or it may be of unknown etiology. Cobb suggested the following etiologic classification of structural scoliosis:[215]

Osteopathic
  Congenital
  Thoracogenic
  Other osteopathic
Neuropathic
  Congenital
  Postpolio
  Other neuropathic
Myopathic
  Congenital
  Muscular dystrophy
  Other myopathic
Idiopathic

The so-called sciatic and hysterical scolioses are not true scolioses, as the deformity is in only one plane.

Incidence

Scoliosis is usually recognizable before the age of 14 years. In a survey taken in 1955 of 50,000 chest roentgenograms in a population over 14 years of age in Delaware, Shands and Eisberg found the incidence of scoliosis to be 1.9 per cent. The etiology of the 230 curvatures that appeared in the first 15,000 films examined was as follows: approximately two thirds, the postural or functional type; one fourth, idiopathic; and the remaining 10 per cent, almost equally divided among congenital, paralytic, and post-thoracoplasty.[322] In the United States, the relative incidence of various types of scoliosis is changing, as poliomyelitis and tuberculosis are becoming more and more rare and a greater number of children with congenital heart disease survive. No statistically significant difference between the Caucasian and Negro races is found. During adolescence, the incidence of idiopathic scoliosis is five times greater in girls than in boys.

General population incidence was studied by Wynne-Davies in Edinburgh, Scotland. Her survey included children from two weeks to 18 years of age. The results are shown in Table 6–1. The total incidence of late-onset scoliosis was 1.8 per cent, and of early-onset, 1.3 per cent.[337]

FUNCTIONAL OR POSTURAL SCOLIOSIS

In functional scoliosis the curve is a single long thoracolumbar curve, and most often convex to the left (Fig. 6–33). Compensatory curves do not exist. It shows little rotation of the vertebrae, and as the spine is bent forward the rotation is toward the *concave* side of the curve, as opposed to structural scoliosis, in which rotation is to the convexity of the curve (Fig. 6–33 B). In recumbency and on suspension the curve disappears, and the spine bends equally well to both sides on lateral flexion of the trunk. There is no fixed rotation or lateral

angulation. The patient can voluntarily correct the lateral deviation of the spine and assume an erect posture. In roentgenograms of the spine, there is no evidence of wedging or other structural change in the vertebrae.

Functional scoliosis is seen in a variety of conditions. A short lower limb causes a compensatory functional scoliosis convex to the side of the depression of the pelvis, i.e., to the short side. Correcting the leg length discrepancy with a lift under the foot levels the pelvis, and the scoliosis disappears (Fig. 6–33 C and D). Functional scoliosis may also represent a compensatory adjustment to a pelvic tilt secondary to abduction or adduction contracture of the hip (Fig. 6-34). The lateral curvature starts at the lumbosacral junction.

Some degree of functional scoliosis is a common occurrence with poor posture. It is of little clinical importance, and ordinarily no treatment is indicated. However, if it is marked, general postural exercises are in order. Correction of contractural hip deformities and leg length equalization are indicated in some cases.

Functional scoliosis has never been known to become structural. A short leg will not of itself cause a structural curve. Parents should be reassured of this to relieve them of many years of anxiety.

IDIOPATHIC STRUCTURAL SCOLIOSIS

The term *idiopathic scoliosis* refers to a structural scoliosis whose etiology is unknown. This occurs in 80 per cent of the patients with structural scoliosis. One should remember, however, that scoliosis is a physical sign and *not* a diagnosis. Ordinarily when one has ruled out neurologic and paralytic causes by a thorough physical examination, and congenital anomalies by a negative roentgenogram, the diagnosis of idiopathic scoliosis is made. Idiopathic structural scoliosis may have its onset at any age during growth, but usually it has three fairly well-defined peak periods: in the first year of life, at five to six years of age, and from after the eleventh year to the end of growth. Therefore, it is subdivided into three chronological age groups: *infan-*

Table 6–1. *Incidence of Idiopathic Scoliosis: Survey of 11,087 Edinburgh Children*

Number of Children	Population Incidence per 1,000		
	Male	*Female*	*Total*
Early onset (3,193)	1.2 (2 of 1,653)	1.3 (1 and 1 resolving of 1,540)	1.3
Late onset (7,894)	0.3 (1 of 3,789)	3.9 (16 of 4,105)	1.8

*From Wynne-Davies, R.: J. Bone Joint Surg., 50–B:24, 1968.

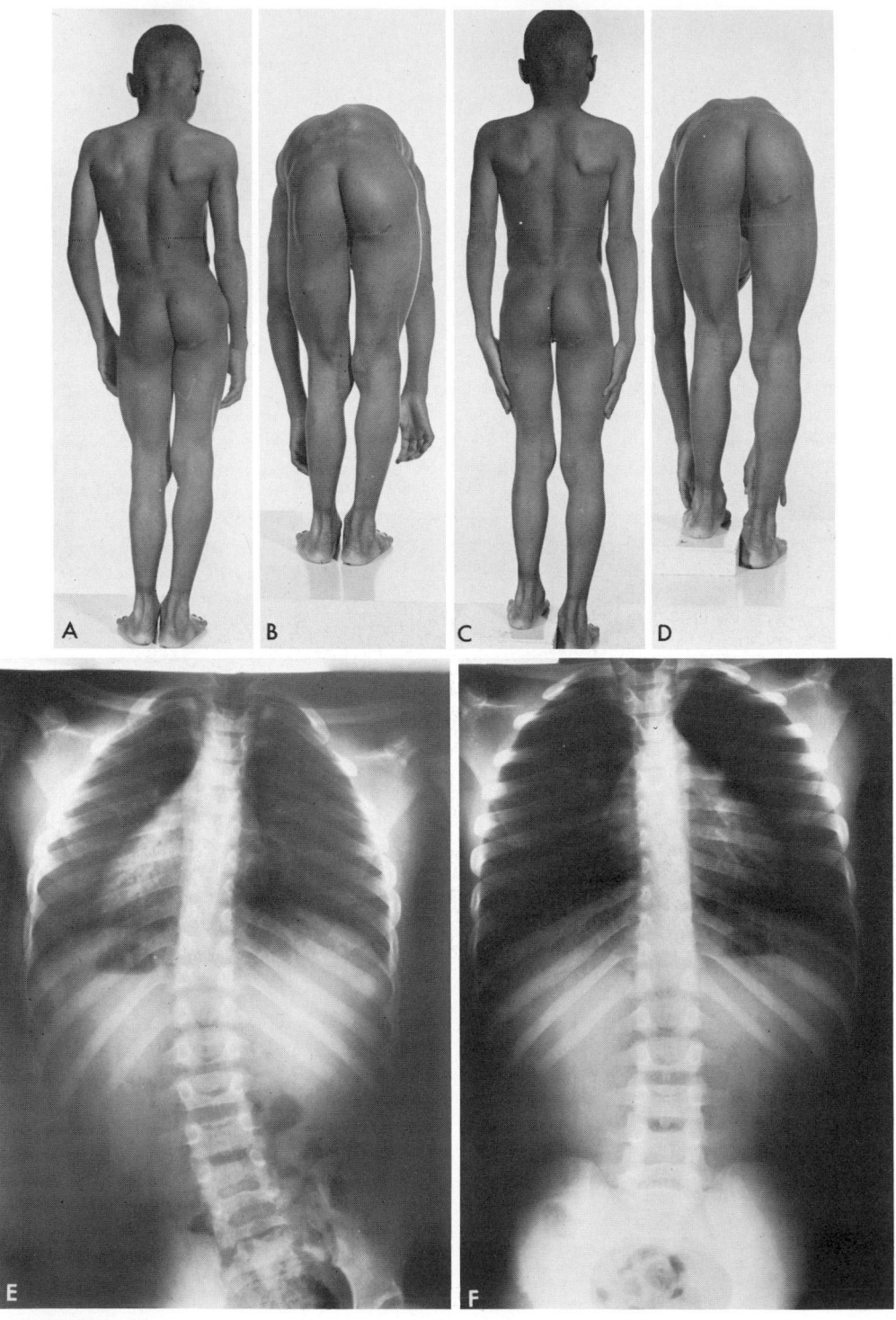

FIGURE 6–33. *The spine of a ten-year-old boy with functional scoliosis due to short left lower extremity.*

A. Note the single long thoracolumbar scoliosis without compensatory curves. It is convex to the left. **B.** The rotation of the vertebrae is toward the concave side of the curve as the patient bends forward. **C.** Note the disappearance of the scoliosis when the pelvis is leveled by correction of the leg length shortening with a lift under the foot. **D.** With the pelvis level, note correction of rotation of vertebrae. **E.** Roentgenogram of the spine. The lateral curvature starts at the lumbosacral junction. There is no evidence of wedging or other structural changes in the vertebrae. **F.** Roentgenogram of the spine demonstrating the disappearance of scoliosis by correction of the leg length discrepancy with a lift under the left foot and leveling of the pelvis.

1192

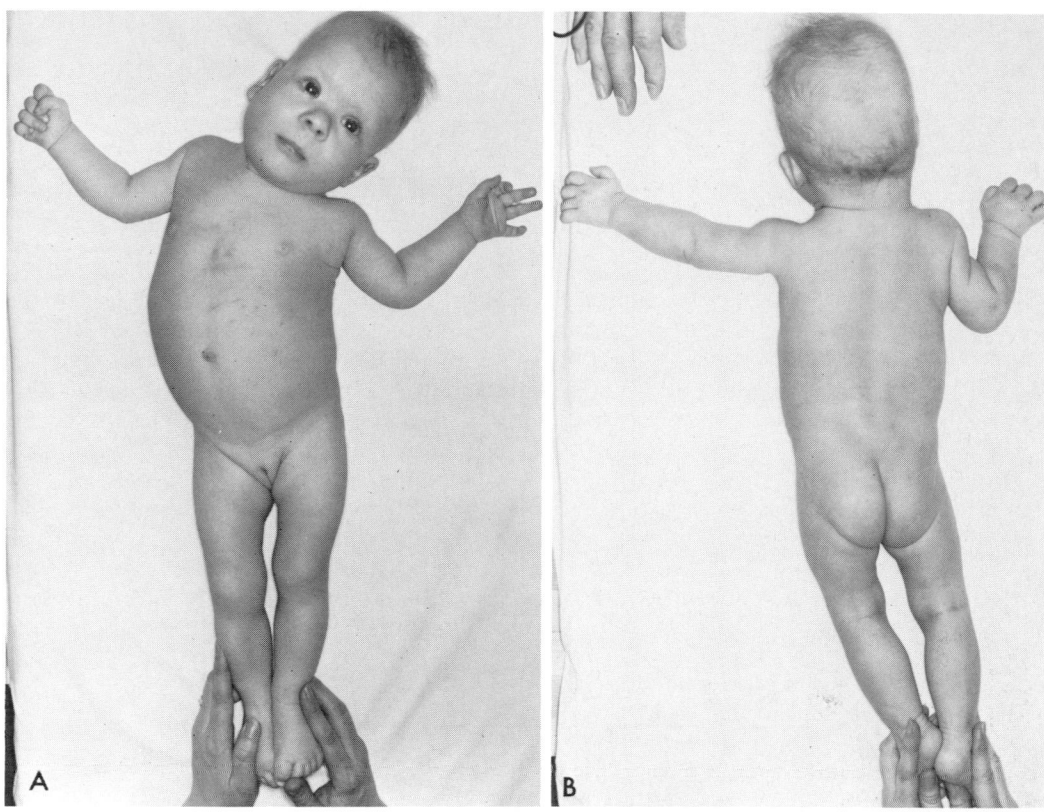

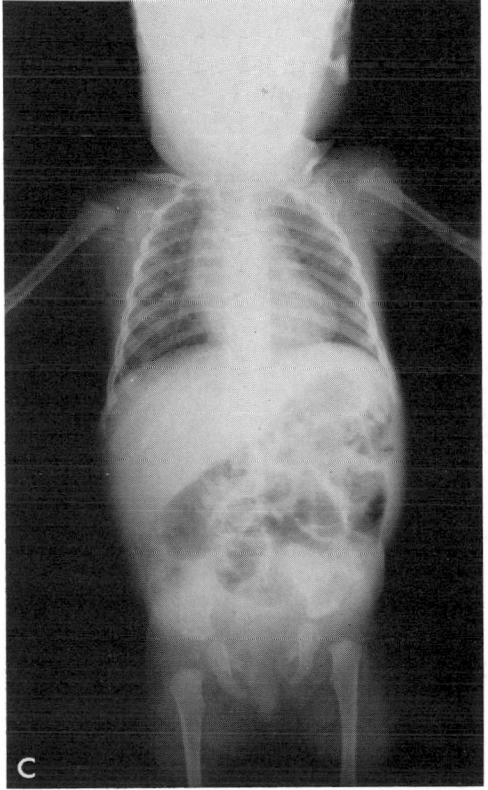

FIGURE 6–34. Functional scoliosis due to congenital abduction contracture of the right hip.

A and **B.** Clinical appearance of patient. **C.** Antero-posterior roentgenogram of the spine.

tile (from birth to three years of age); *juvenile* (from four years of age until the end of the ninth year): and *adolescent* (from the age of ten years to the end of skeletal growth).

Etiology

Several theories have been advanced to explain idiopathic scoliosis. It has been said that idiopathic scoliosis represents the effect of unrecognized poliomyelitis. With the development of prophylactic vaccine, the incidence of poliomyelitis has been greatly reduced; however, there has been no concomitant decrease in the incidence of idiopathic scoliosis.

The sex incidence, the stability of the spine, the type of curve, and the natural history of idiopathic and postpolio paralytic scoliosis are all different.

Nutritional deficiency has been incriminated as a causative factor, but this has never been proved. Neither have endocrine abnormalities been demonstrated. Weakness of the musculature or ligaments or insufficiency of the central nervous system may be underlying factors in the inability of the spine to withstand the stress and strain of body weight.

A normal spine tends to grow straight. Irrespective of its pathogenesis, idiopathic scoliosis represents a progressive structural deformity that is a product of abnormal growth. It does not occur, however, in the absence of active growth and it becomes static on completion of vertebral growth. Idiopathic structural scoliosis is a growth disturbance of the spine, most probably due to asymmetrical growth of the epiphyseal plates of the vertebrae.

Genetic Aspects

Idiopathic structural scoliosis is a familial condition. Wynne-Davies studied the family incidence of scoliosis in 114 patients by visiting and examining for scoliosis all their available relatives (well over 2,000 individuals), and compared these observations with the incidence of scoliosis in the general population (by examining a total of more than 10,000 children).[337] For purposes of

convenience in her genetic survey, Wynne-Davies divided scoliosis into two main groups: early-onset scoliosis (under eight years of age) and late-onset scoliosis (eight years of age and over). In the infant the side on which the great majority of curves was found was the left thoracic (90 per cent). Late-onset scoliosis was more frequent in girls (seven girls to one boy). Early-onset type is slightly more common in boys (five boys to four girls), and the curve may be "resolving" or "progressive." In the late-onset type, structural scoliosis does not disappear spontaneously.

Comparison of the incidence of scoliosis in the general population and among the relatives of scoliotic patients is shown in Figure 6–35. There is undoubtedly an increased incidence of scoliosis among families of the patients when compared with the general population. There is a marked rise in incidence of scoliosis 20 times more

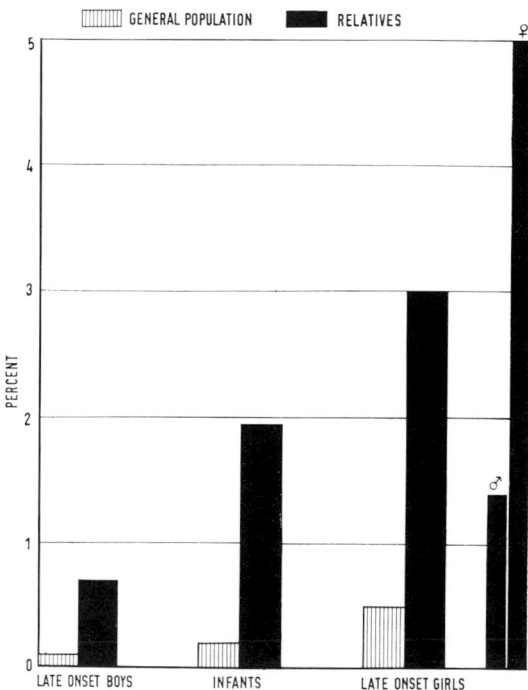

FIGURE 6–35. Comparison of incidence of scoliosis in the general population and among the relatives of scoliotic patients.

(From, Wynne-Davies, R.: Familial (idiopathic) scoliosis. A family survey. J. Bone Joint Surg., *50–B*: 24–30, 1968.)

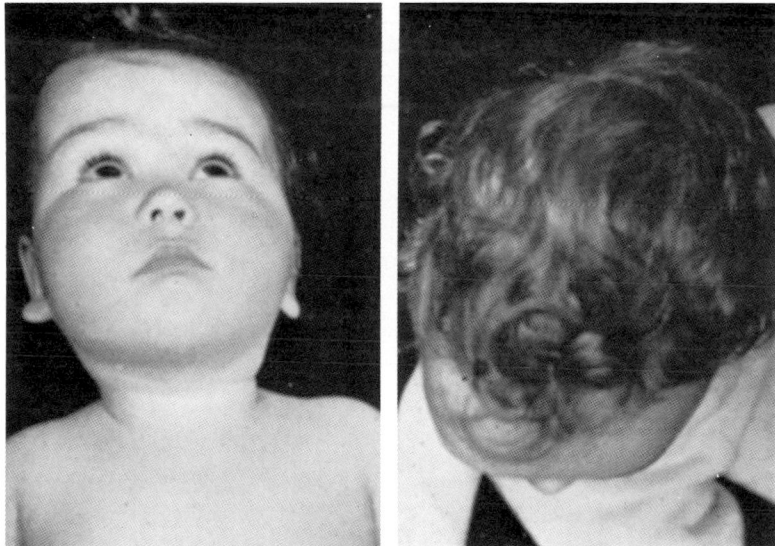

FIGURE 6–36. *Left-sided plagiocephaly associated with left thoracic scoliosis in infants.*

(From Wynne-Davies, R.: Familial (idiopathic) scoliosis. A family survey. J. Bone Joint Surg., *50–B*:24–30, 1968.)

common than in the general population) in the families of those girls with late-onset scoliosis. This strong evidence for a genetic factor suggests some of the characteristics of dominant inheritance. However, a larger series of patients must be studied to draw a firm conclusion regarding dominant or multiple gene inheritance.

The survey indicates that, despite certain clinical differences, the infantile and adolescent types of scoliosis probably share the same basic etiology, as the families studied contain instances of each. The finding of plagiocephaly in all infants with scoliosis under one year of age suggests the action of an environmental factor in the infantile group (Fig. 6–36). Infants with resolving-type scoliosis had affected relatives in the same proportion as children with infantile progressive scoliosis, suggesting that this may be a mild form of the same disorder. The most common defects associated with scoliosis were mental deficiency and epilepsy. Another finding of the survey was that the number of patients with onset of scoliosis in adolescence who were the offspring of older mothers was significantly greater than the expected figure for the normal population. Fisher and DeGeorge found a similar rise in the age of the mother.[233]

Experimental Scoliosis

As studies of scoliosis in man have not elucidated the pathogenesis of scoliosis, many authors have investigated the problem by animal experiments in an attempt to understand the normal processes of vertebral growth and the factors that may interfere with them. Scoliosis has been produced in animals by several means: (1) excision or denervation of muscles,[285, 318] (2) resection of ribs,[202] (3) division of posterior costotransverse ligaments,[267, 268] (4) fixation of vertebrae or ribs to each other,[336] (5) operations on growth zones of vertebrae,[203, 244, 284, 288, 289, 294] (6) radiation,[199, 227] and (7) feeding of *Lathyrus odoratus* seeds to produce lathyrism.[297–299, 301]

The experimental work of Ponseti and his co-workers is important, as it is the first example of scoliosis induced by metabolic changes. The basic substance in sweet pea seeds is an amino nitrite—glutamyl-amino propionitrite, a metabolic poison interfering with chondroitin sulfate. In the rat, feeding of *Lathyrus odoratus* causes slipping of epiphyses, ligamentous detachment, scoliosis, and aneurysm of the aorta. A biochemical cause of scoliosis may be conjectured, as metabolic abnormalities are commonly inherited and idiopathic scoliosis is familial.

The results of Langenskiöld and Mich-elsson correspond well with the general anatomic findings in human scoliosis. They found that excision of the posterior costotransverse ligaments produced a scoliosis with the convexity toward the side of the operation. They proposed that the costotransverse ligament transfers the forces of the spinal muscles from the ribs to the vertebrae, and the insufficiency of function of this ligament allows the spinal muscles on the opposite side to be overactive, producing rotation and lateral flexion deformity. Michelsson induced scoliosis in pigs by resection of the ribs and found that the neurocentral junction on the concave side remains open and grows, this being contrary to expectation based on human scoliosis.[277]

Mechanics of Scoliosis

The mechanics of scoliosis are still not entirely understood, but the following are important factors:[314, 327, 328]

The Law of Balance. Normally there is no lateral curvature of the human spine. Because of a natural sense of balance and equilibrium, the muscles controlling the vertebral column tend to hold the spine straight with the head erect over the mid-pelvis and the body in balance. When a curvature is initiated, compensatory curves promptly develop in an instinctive effort to maintain erect posture.

Structure of the Spine. The human spine is not a straight rod, but consists of a series of jointed segments that are arranged in an anteroposterior curve in the sagittal plane. It is a physical necessity that, if a lateral curve (frontal plane) is imposed upon a rod already bent in an anteroposterior direction (sagittal plane), a rotation in the third direction (transverse plane) must take place. Thus, any lateral motion in the spine is accompanied by rotation of the vertebrae and their attached appendages, the ribs. Conversely, rotary displacement of the vertebrae is accompanied by lateral inclination.

Intrinsic Equilibrium. In the normal spinal column there is an intrinsic equilibrium produced by the elasticity of the longitudinal ligaments on one side, which press the vertebrae together, and the expansile force of the discs on the other, which tends to separate the vertebrae. These elastic forces acting on the vertebral segments provide such a degree of stability that only a minimal amount of muscular force is necessary to maintain the spine in the erect position.

Inclinatory and Translatory Factors. The forces that produce scoliosis operate both in the inclinatory and translatory sense. It is important to make a distinction between the two, as they vary in importance and sequence in different types of scoliosis. The inclinatory factor is resisted normally by the muscle equilibrium; it is *intersegmental*, producing a contractural deformity between sections of the spine; it is characterized by a long-arc curve. The inclinatory factor is in the foreground and is the only one present in the earliest stages of paralytic scoliosis. The translatory factor is resisted normally by the intrinsic equilibrium of the spine; it is *intrasegmental*, producing a collapse between vertebrae; it is characterized by a short-arc curve. In idiopathic structural scoliosis the translatory factor is effective earlier than the inclinatory factor.[327, 328]

Pathology

The extent of structural changes varies with the degree of scoliosis.[228, 262, 266, 314] They are greatest at the apex of the curve, diminishing toward either end of the curve. In structural scoliosis, rotation of the vertebrae is to the convex side of the lateral curvature so that the spinous processes of the vertebrae are rotated toward the concavity of the curve.

Compressional and distractional forces act on the growing spine and produce changes in the vertebrae, which become wedge-shaped with the height of the vertebra higher on the convex side and lower on the concave side (Fig. 6–37). The vertebral body becomes condensed on the concave side as a result of the greater pressure, and it is expanded and thinned on the convex side. The vertebrae always rotate toward the convexity of the curve in structural scoliosis.

There are associated changes in the neural

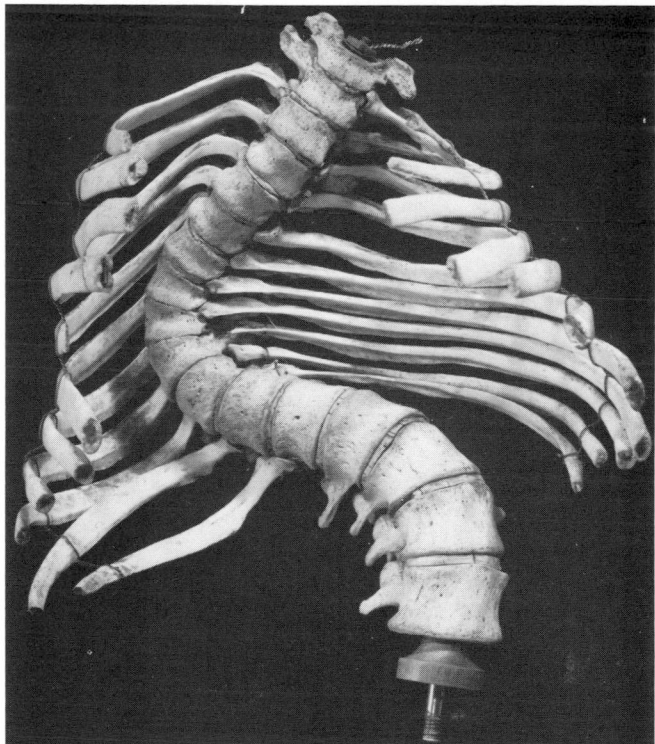

***FIGURE 6–37. Gross anatomic
specimen of the spine demonstrating
structural changes of right thoracic
scoliosis.***

Note the wedging of the vertebrae on the
concave side and rotation of the vertebral
bodies to the convexity of the curve. The
ribs on the concave side are rotated forward and on the convex side are thrust
backward. (From James, J. I. P.: Scoliosis.
Baltimore, Williams & Wilkins Co., 1967,
p. 13.)

canal and posterior arch. The laminae on
the convex side are broad and widely
separated, and those on the concave side
are narrow and close together (Fig. 6–38).
The pedicles are shorter and stubbier on
the concave side (Fig. 6–39). The transverse
processes more closely approach the sagittal plane on the convex side and are more
in the frontal plane on the concave side.
The intraspinal canal becomes distorted in
shape because of the misshapen pedicles
and articular processes (Fig. 6–39).

The intervertebral discs on the concave
side, as a result of pressure, are compressed
and show degenerative changes. The adjoining portion of the vertebra reacts with
sclerosis and marginal lipping. Later in
life degenerative arthritic changes take
place, especially in the lumbar area.

Significant adaptive changes take place
in the soft tissues. The muscles and ligaments are thickened and contracted on the
concave side, constituting a foremost obstacle to correction, and they become thin
and atrophied on the convex side. Later,
in severe curves, calcification of the liga-

mentary apparatus and synostosis between
the arches and intervertebral articulations
may take place.

The thoracic cage is also affected by
deformity. Because of rotation and translatory shift of the dorsal vertebrae, the ribs
on the convex side are thrust backward,
producing a posterior rib hump that is
aptly described as a "razor back" in severe
cases. On the concave side, the ribs are
rotated forward, producing prominence
of the anterior chest wall and the breast.
The sternum rotates on a vertical axis in
response to the change of position of the
ribs; thus, in a right dorsal curve, the left
border is in front of the right border. Also,
the sternum may be laterally displaced from
the median line.

With the translatory shift of the spine
sideward, the thorax is divided into two
asymmetrical halves. Its capacity is diminished on the convex side and increased on
the concave side. In severe cases, with
marked angulation of the ribs posteriorly,
the aeration of lung tissue is reduced on the
convex side. The abnormal pressure and

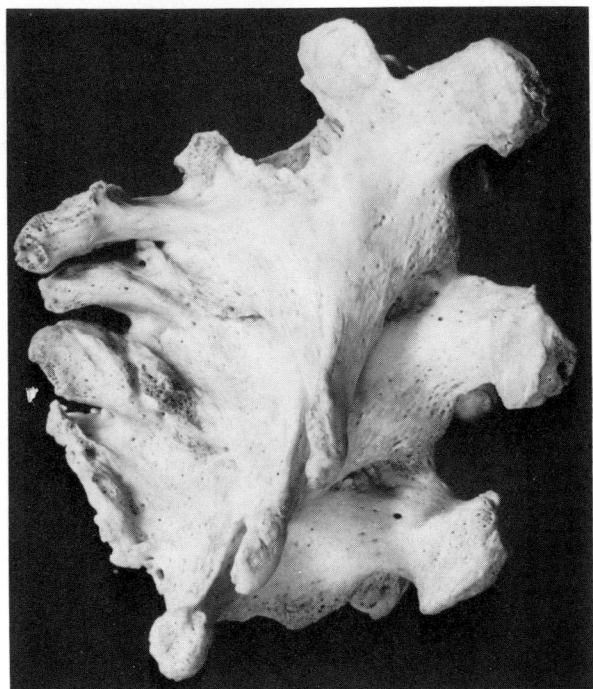

FIGURE 6–38. *Posterior view of the neural arch, showing the narrow laminae close together on the concave side.*

(From James, J. I. P.: Scoliosis. Baltimore, Williams & Wilkins Co., 1967, p. 15.)

FIGURE 6–39. *Superior view of a vertebra with structural scoliosis.*

Note that on the concave side the pedicle is short and stubby and the intraspinal canal is narrowed. (From James, J. I. P.: Scoliosis. Baltimore, Williams & Wilkins Co., 1967, p. 15.)

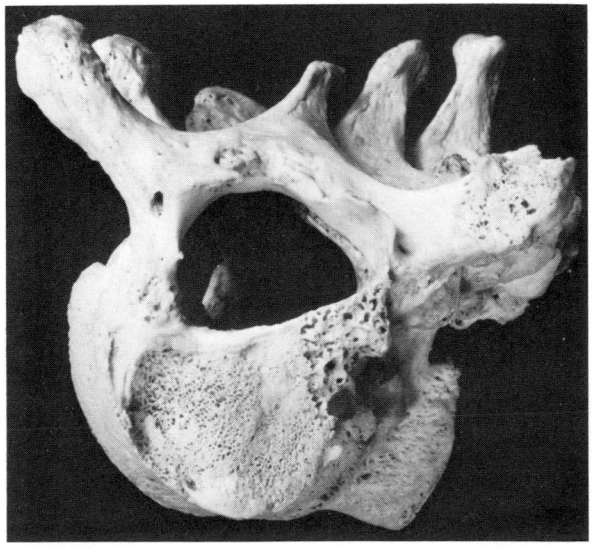

stresses exerted upon the heart may disturb cardiac function.*

In severe scoliosis with distortion of the shape of the intraspinal canal the spinal cord will be angulated and stretched; however, any interference with its function is very rare. Cord compression is due to an unusually tight dura mater and occurs only in severe deformities, especially in cases of marked dorsal kyphosis.[250]

Clinical Features

Patients with scoliosis usually seek medical attention with presenting complaints of a high shoulder, prominent shoulder blade or breast, high or prominent hip, asymmetry of flank creases and trunk, poor posture, and curvature. It is very seldom that a child with scoliosis will complain of backache and fatigue. A chest roentgenogram or intravenous pyelogram may reveal a previously undetected scoliosis. The deformity of scoliosis is the symptom in children.

In adults, particularly with lumbar scoliosis, backache is not uncommon and is due to degenerative arthritis in the posterior articulations; root pain may complicate local back pain. In very severe scoliosis, pressure of the ribs against the iliac crests may cause pain. Cardiorespiratory symptoms such as shortness of breath may occur in the severely scoliotic. Spinal cord compression is rarely encountered; it occurs during rapid growth periods of adolescence and is due to inability of the spinal cord to accommodate itself to structural changes in the intraspinal canal.

There are certain terms used to describe features of scoliosis. "Right" and "left" are used to indicate the direction of lateral angulation. "Cervicodorsal," "thoracic," "thoracolumbar," "lumbar," and "lumbosacral" relate to the segment of the spine affected. Usually the primary curves are mentioned first. "Combined dorsal and lumbar" curves indicate two primary curves with compensatory curves above and below. The degree of curvature might be

*See References 201, 213, 238, 243, 275, 276, 323, 324, 326, 334, 340.

designated as "mild," "moderate," or "severe."

The examination of the child with scoliosis should follow a definite order. First, the patient is observed standing while clothed, and next, without clothing and properly draped. The general posture and alignment of the spine are inspected from the front, side, and back (Fig. 6-40). The deformity of lateral angulation is best seen from directly behind with the child standing. The level of the shoulders and the position of the scapulae are noted. Are the head, neck, and shoulders balanced over the pelvis? When a plumb line is held over the spinous process of the seventh cervical vertebra, it should pass through the intergluteal cleft. Deviation of any number of spinous processes from this median line indicates a lateral curvature. The level and extent of lateral deviation should be recorded. The degree and direction of associated rotation of the vertebrae are best seen by observing the child from the back as he bends forward. In structural scoliosis, the rotation is to the convex side. The degree of rotation can be graded as "1," "2," "3," or "4 plus," depending on its severity; 1 plus is the mildest and 4 plus is the sharp "razor back." The patient is examined for asymmetry of the breasts, the rib cage, and the flank creases, prominence of the scapula and hip, and a low or high shoulder.

The amount of list of the trunk is noted. The height of the lift needed under the foot to correct the list (C 7 or occiput to intergluteal cleft) is recorded.

Next, the mobility of each curve is studied —on right and left lateral bends, head traction, and sitting or standing pelvic tilts. The extent, degree, and rigidity of each curve is again determined in the prone position. Is there any paravertebral muscle spasm or local tenderness?

Actual and apparent leg lengths are recorded. Is there any pelvic obliquity? If present, is it flexible or fixed? Are there any contractures about the hips on the Thomas and Ober tests? How tight are the hamstrings? What is the degree of chest expansion and the anteroposterior diameter of the thoracic cage? Muscle power should be examined, especially of the anterior and lateral abdominals, erector spinae, quadratus lumborum, and thoracic groups. Is

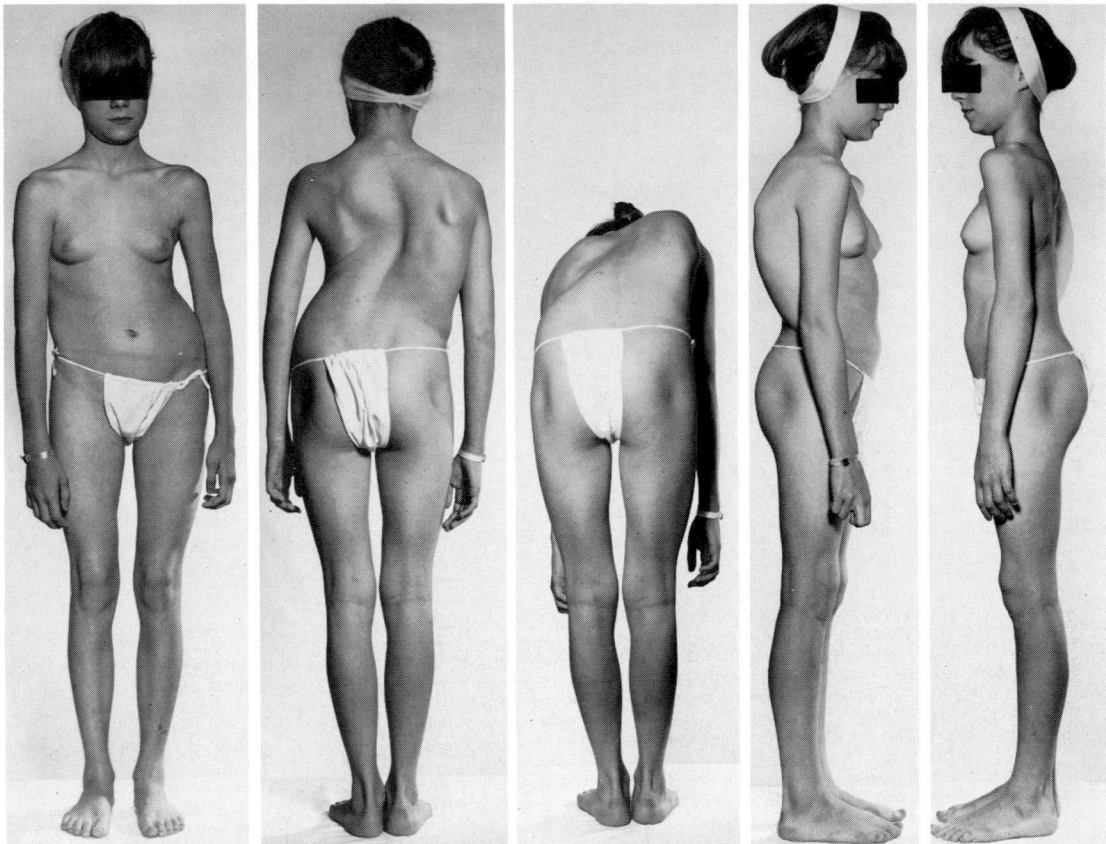

FIGURE 6–40.   *Idiopathic structural right thoracic scoliosis.*

there any other muscle weakness? Are there any café-au-lait spots or subcutaneous or pedunculated tumors to suggest neurofibromatosis? The presence or absence of various skin lesions associated with congenital anomalies of the spine is significant—e.g., a hairy patch, a skin dimple, a hemangioma, a lipoma, or a myelomeningocele. Are there any deformities of the foot? A pes cavus might suggest Friedreich's ataxia.

A thorough neurologic evaluation must always be a part of the examination for scoliosis. Occasionally an intraspinal tumor or other neurologic disease may be the cause of scoliosis. Also, all patients should have a complete physical examination, giving particular attention to the cardiovascular and pulmonary systems. Any abnormalities of the mandible and teeth should be recorded.

Standing and sitting heights should be measured in following the scoliotic patient,

for they have prognostic importance. It is encouraging to know that, during a period when a child has had a spurt of growth with increase in the height of the trunk, there has been no increase in the degree of scoliosis.

Routine photographs should be made to provide an objective record of the deformity and body posture, and to note any cosmetic improvement afforded by treatment. Photographic views should include front, back, and right and left standing views, and a back view with the patient bending forward (Fig. 6–41).

Roentgenographic Study

At the initial examination of a patient with more than minimal scoliosis, roentgen examination includes anteroposterior views of the spine from the iliac crests as high as possible, on a 14- by 17-inch film, standing and recumbent; right and left lateral bends in recumbency; and pelvic tilt films in the sitting or standing position, in which one side of the pelvis and then the other is elevated on a block to determine the effect of the tilt on the spine (Fig. 6–42 A to F). In paralytic scoliosis with collapsing spine, head traction views are indicated. A lateral view of the entire spine is taken to rule out epiphysitis, segmental deformities, spondylolisthesis, neoplastic or infectious lesions, or other disease, and to determine the degree of kyphosis or lordosis and the width of the sagittal diameter of the intraspinal canal (Fig. 6–42 G). Anteroposterior views of the hands and wrists are taken to determine skeletal maturity (Fig. 6–42 H).

In following the scoliotic child, it has been advocated frequently in the past that standing and supine roentgenograms of the spine be taken every three months until

maturity. With greater awareness of the dangers of irradiation, the author believes the patient should always be evaluated clinically before the x-rays are ordered; and unless the scoliosis is increasing or there is a change in the treatment, one standing roentgenogram of the spine no more frequently than every six months is adequate.

The angle of the curve is measured by Ferguson's or Cobb's method, or both. (Figs. 6–43 and 6–44). The end vertebrae of a given curve are the ones at each end of the curve nearest to the center and least rotated. The top vertebra of the curve is the highest one whose superior surface tilts to the side of the concavity of the curve to be measured. The superior surface of the vertebra above it usually tilts in the opposite direction to the side of the convexity, but it may be horizontal. The intervertebral space on the concave side is

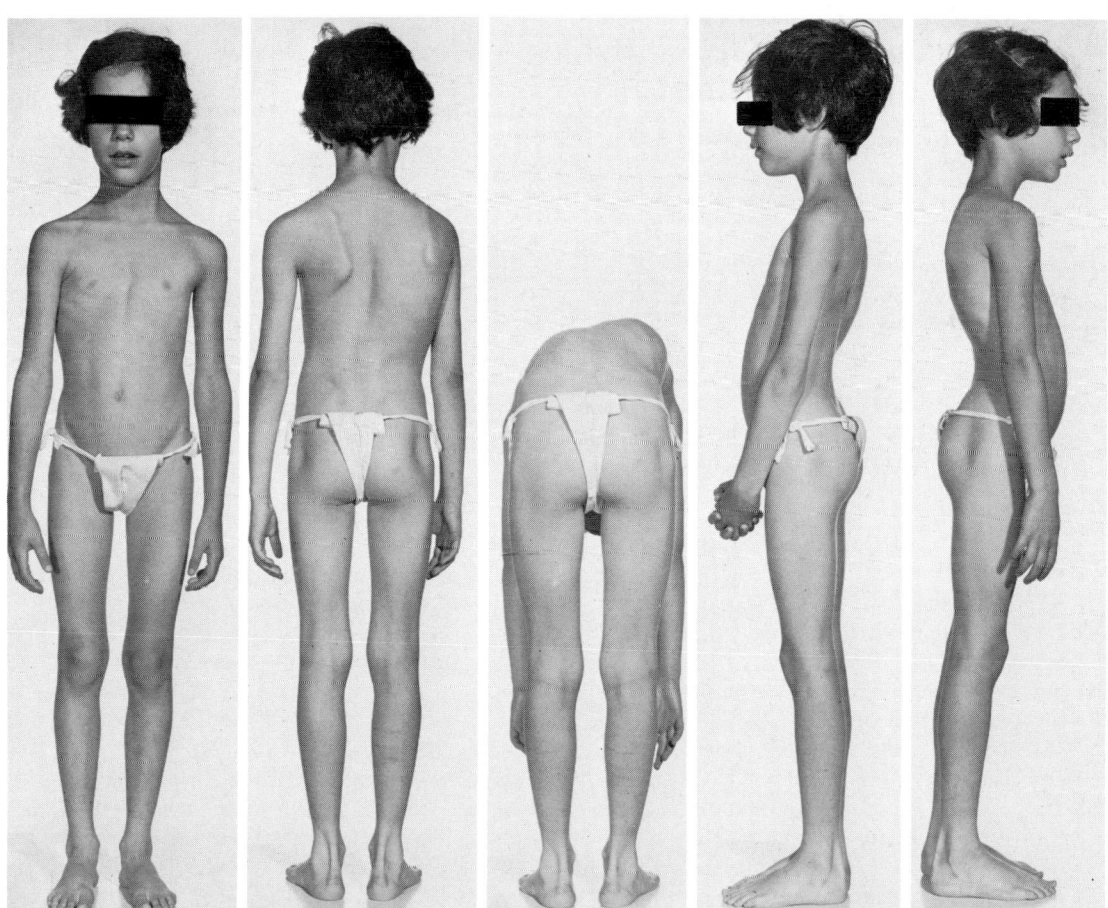

FIGURE 6–41. Routine photographic views of a patient with scoliosis.

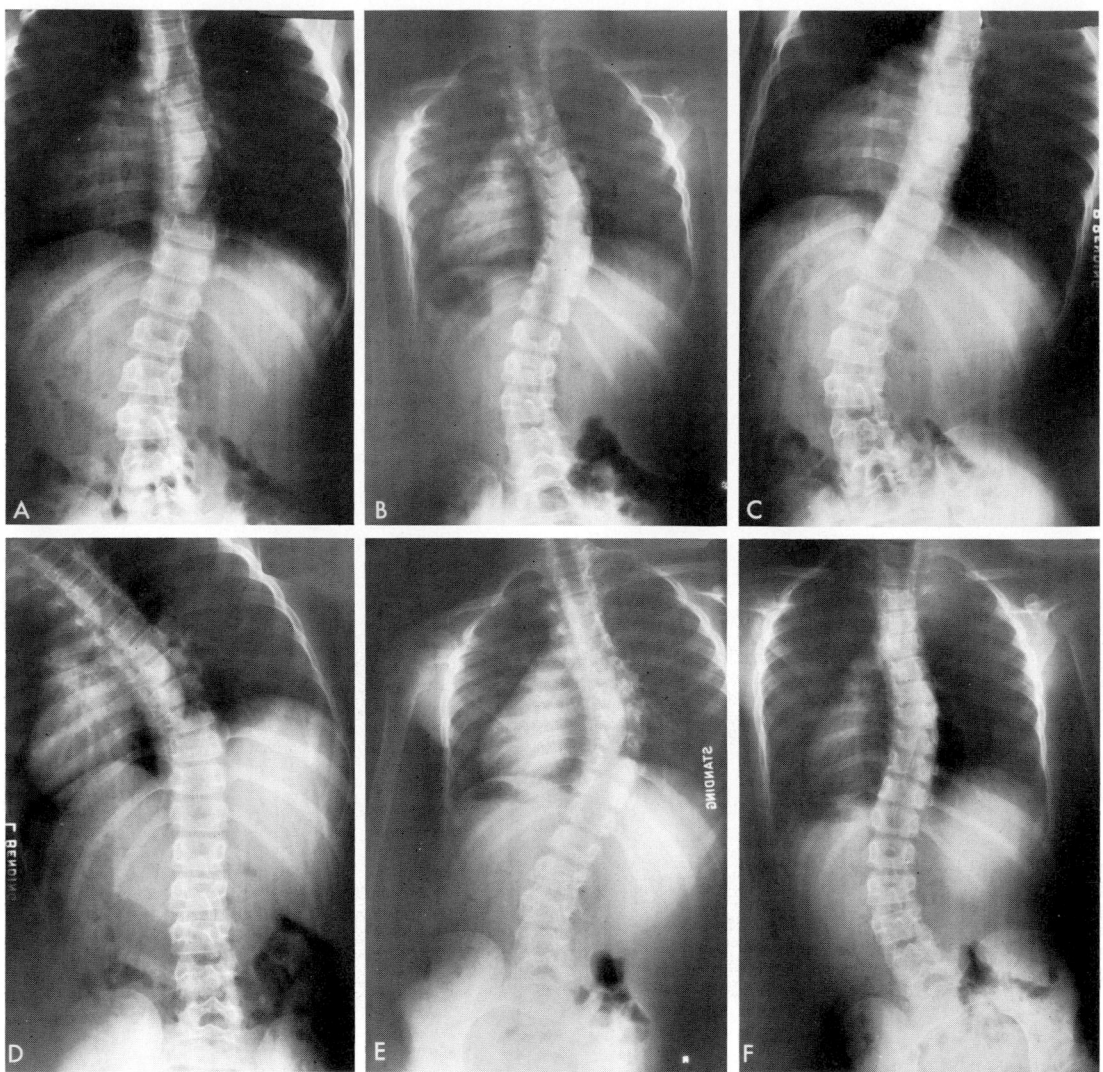

FIGURE 6–42.   *Routine roentgenographic views for structural scoliosis.*

These are roentgenograms of patient shown in Figure 6–41. **A.** Recumbent. **B.** Standing. **C.** Right bend. **D.** Left bend. **E.** Left pelvic tilt. **F.** Right pelvic tilt.

usually wider above the top vertebra and narrower below it, but if there is vertebral wedging, the width of this intervertebral space may vary. The same applies to the inferior surface of the bottom vertebra. Cobb draws intersecting perpendicular lines from the superior surface of the top and the inferior surface of the bottom vertebrae of the curve. The angle formed by these perpendicular lines is the "angle of the curve" (Fig. 6–43).[215] Ferguson marks a dot in the center of the shadow of the body in each of the three vertebrae—the two end

and the apical. (The apical vertebra is the one that is most rotated at the crest of the curve). Lines are drawn from the apex to each end. The angle of the curve is the divergence of these two lines from 180 degrees (Fig. 6–44).[230–232]

Identification of the Major Curve. Any angular deviation of the spine in one direction causes an opposite angular deviation when the erect position is assumed, so that the head is balanced above the pelvis. This secondary deviation is compensatory. Structural changes, such as wedging and rotation,

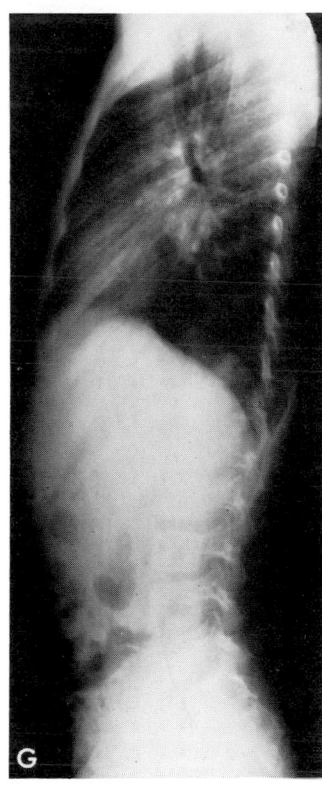
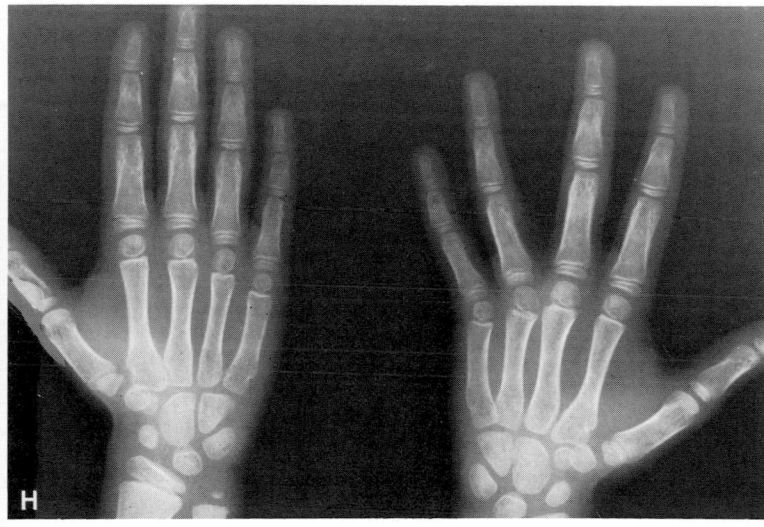

FIGURE 6–42 Continued. Routine roentgenographic views for structural scoliosis.

G. Lateral of dorsolumbar spine. **H.** Anteroposterior view of hands and wrists for skeletal age.

tend to develop in these secondary compensatory curves, which may make them difficult to distinguish from major curves. The following criteria are helpful in locating the major curve:

1. The curve with the least flexibility and corrigibility is the major one; this is determined by the lateral bend and by the pelvic tilt test roentgenograms. In the pelvic tilt test, anteroposterior roentgenograms are made with the patient sitting with an elevation beneath the buttock on the side of the convexity of the lumbar or dorsolumbar curve. The elevation should be 4 inches or as great as the patient can tolerate, but one with which he still retains spontaneous balance without external support. The patient should have no support, and the arms should be relaxed, with hands in the lap or outstretched. The pelvic tilt test film demonstrates the maximal possible voluntary correction of the lumbar curve. If there is little or no correction by the muscles at the convex aspect of the lumbar curve, it is a major curve.

2. The greater curve, or that toward which the trunk is shifted, is the major curve.

3. In the case of three curves ("triple curve"), the middle one is always the major one; whereas, in the case of four curves ("quadruple curve"), the two middle curves are usually major.

4. A major curve will deform and become fixed simultaneously, and show no tendency to reverse itself or to retain any correction that has been mechanically secured. Compensatory curves, on the other hand, only gradually become structural and tend to retain the power of spontaneous reversibility much longer. They are able to hold the reversed position after the primary correction.

Cardiopulmonary Function in Scoliosis*

An understanding of the cardiopulmonary problems of patients with scoliosis is essential for total care. This is especially true in children with congenital heart dis-

---

*See References 201, 213, 238, 243, 275, 276, 323, 324, 326, 334, 340.

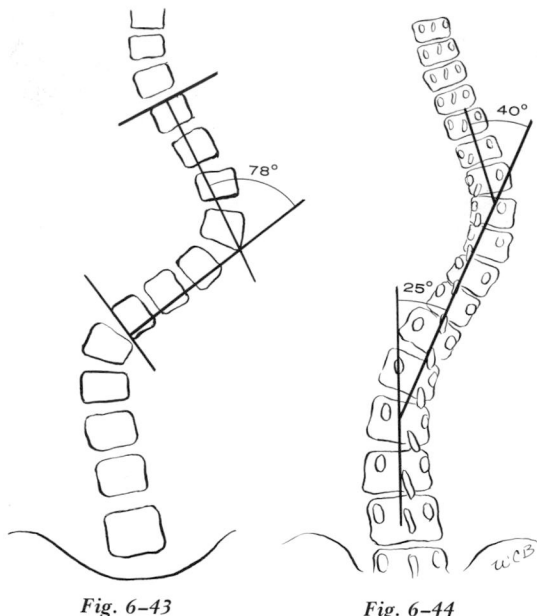

Fig. 6–43   *Fig. 6–44*

FIGURE 6–43.   *Cobb's method of measuring of the angle of the curve in scoliosis (see text for explanation).*

FIGURE 6–44.   *Ferguson's method of measuring of the angle of the scoliotic curve (see text for explanation).*

ease and with severe structural scoliosis. When the angle of a thoracic curve is 50 degrees or more, the vital capacity and the total lung capacity and peak flow rate are diminished. When the curve is 100 degrees or more, the patient may become symptomatic and have a respiratory pattern consisting of rapid frequent breathing. Hypoxia can occur. Pulmonary hypertension and cor pulmonale are grave complications.

Natural History and Curve Patterns of Idiopathic Scoliosis

It is important to know the natural history of scoliosis as it is a guide to prognosis and treatment. Scoliosis is likely to be progressive as long as there is potential for growth. Well over 140 years ago, in 1824, Bampfield observed that increasing scoliosis appeared only during growth of the body, and he thought it was due to increased growth on one side of the vertebral bodies with progressive absorption from pressure on the other side.[200] Bradford, in 1890, described scoliosis as having three

stages: initial, developmental, and stage of arrest. He stated that the stage of arrest occurred when all possible alteration in the shape of the bone had taken place with completion of ossification and when the vertebrae were sufficiently strong to sustain permanent weight without yielding laterally in the direction of torsion.[209]

The direct relationship between vertebral growth and increasing scoliotic deformity is well documented by the study of Risser and Ferguson.[310] The spine grows slowly in children from about seven to ten years of age, as indicated by comparison of vertical standing and sitting heights of the patients. In this age period the increase in scoliosis ranged from 3 to 5 degrees a year. In the preadolescent age of from 10 to 15 years, there was rapid growth of the spine and the scoliosis increased about 1 degree a month. It became essentially static after completion of vertebral growth, as shown by cessation of increase in sitting height. The spine stopped growing at an average age of 14½ years in girls and 16⅓ years in boys, the extremes being 13 to 16 years and 14½ to 17 years, respectively. However, the chrono-

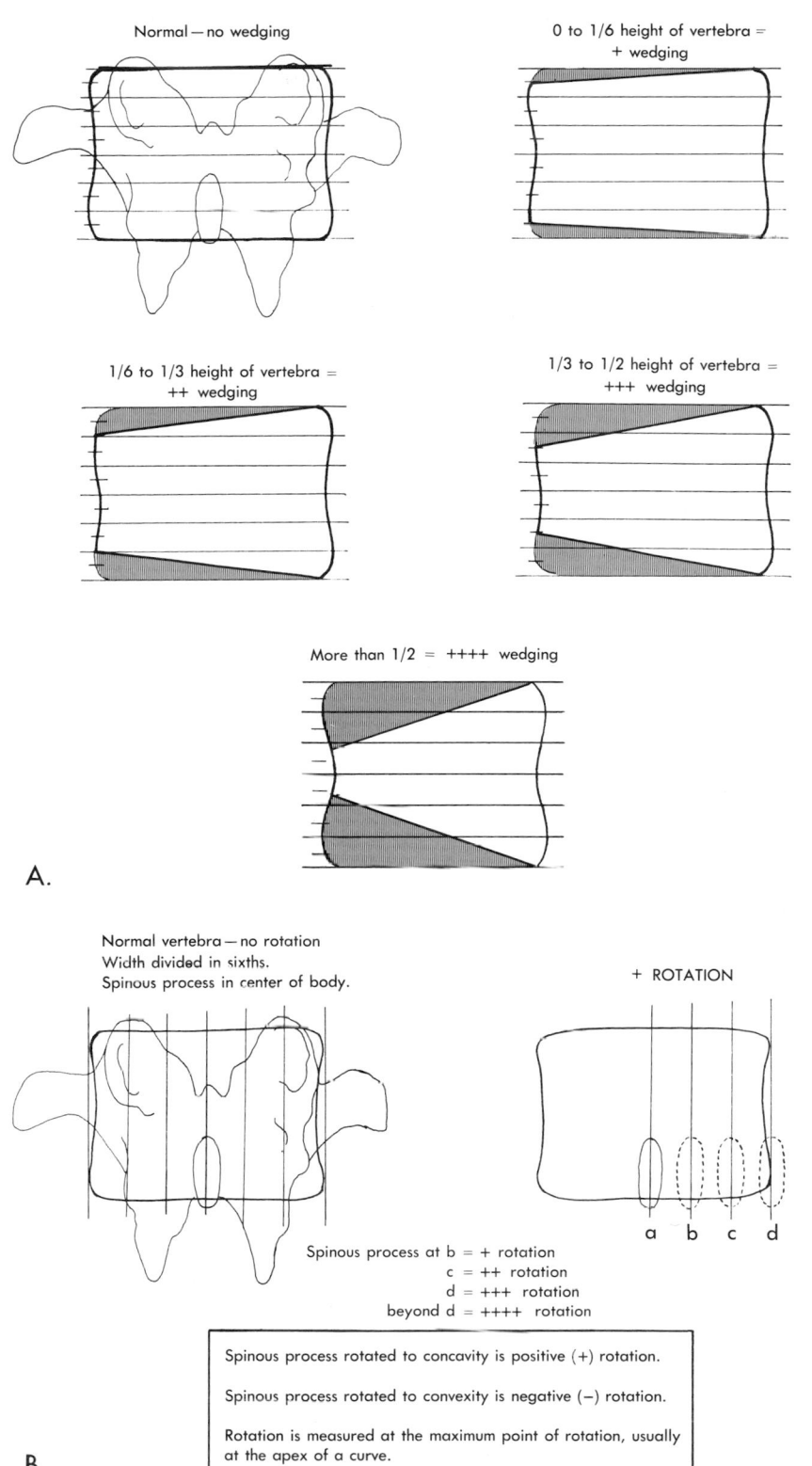

FIGURE 6–45. *Method of determination of degree of wedging (A) and rotation (B) of vertebrae in scoliosis.*

(Redrawn from Cobb, J. R.: A. A.O.S. Instructional Course Lectures, 5:261, 1948.)

logical age is not an accurate guideline for completion of vertebral growth. Risser observed that the completion of excursion of ossification of the iliac apophysis occurred simultaneously with completion of vertebral growth, and with it the scoliosis became static.[306, 307] The average ages at which the iliac apophyses completed their excursion of ossification across the iliac crests were 14 years in girls and 15½ years in boys. The average period of ossification excursion was one year from the first appearance of capping on the outer anterior border of the iliac crests to final completion, when the apophysis dipped down to come in contact with the ilium near the sacroiliac junction. The shortest period was seven months and the longest, more than two years. Occasionally, fragmentary development of the iliac apophysis occurs. Asymmetrical development of the two sides of the pelvis is seen in a number of cases.

Zaoussis and James, in a statistical study of patients with mature curves, confirmed that the cessation of spinal growth and curve progression coincides with the completion of growth in the iliac apophyses.[339] Their findings are shown in Figure 6–46. They also observed that menarche and growth of epiphyses of the vertebral bodies are early signs of maturation, almost always occurring in advance of ossification of the iliac apophyses and not reliable in the prognosis of curve progression.

In adults, the scoliotic deformity may increase up to 15 degrees as a result of degeneration and thinning of the intervertebral discs and osteoporosis of the spine.

In idiopathic scoliosis, the two chief factors that influence the prognosis seem to be the age of onset, and more important, the pattern of the curve. Ponseti and Friedman, from the University of Iowa Clinics, directed for many years by Dr. Arthur Steindler, reviewed 394 cases of idiopathic scoliosis in which surgical procedures had

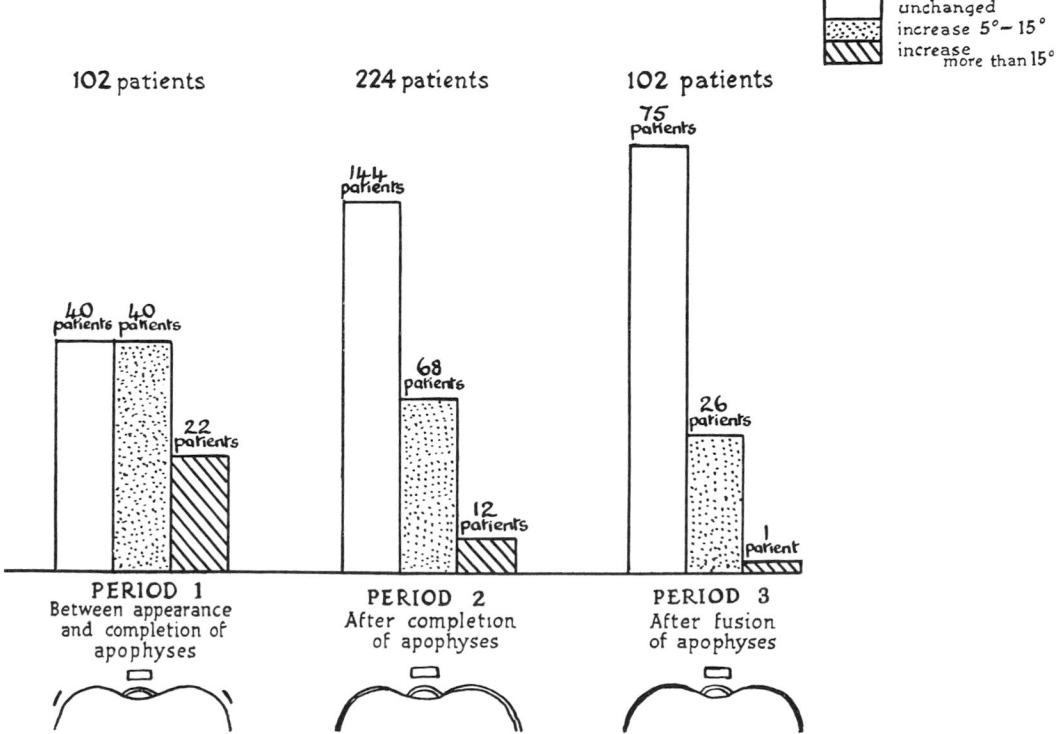

FIGURE 6–46.   *The evolution of curves during the three periods of growth of the iliac apophyses.*

(From Zaoussis, A. L., and James, J. I. P.: The iliac apophysis and the evolution of curves in scoliosis. J. Bone Joint Surg., *40–B*:442, 1958.)

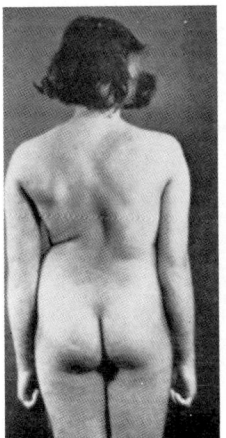 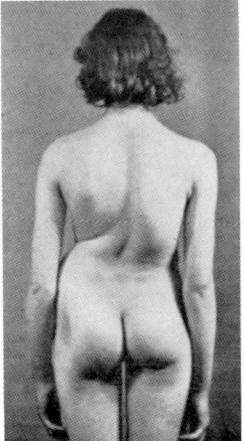 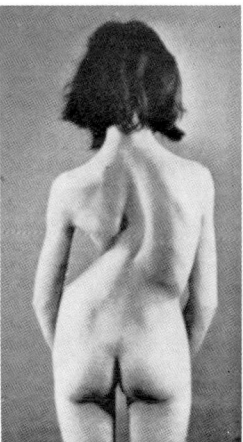 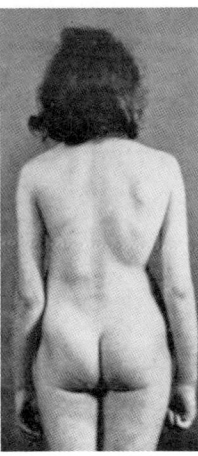

FIGURE 6–47. *Posterior view of four girls, each with 70 degrees of curvature.*

From left to right lumbar, thoracolumbar, thoracic, and double major cuvers. It clearly shows that the thoracic curve is the most decompensated and deformed with the low shoulder, the severe razor-back deformity, and the asymmetrical flank creases. Thoracic scoliosis has the worst prognosis for the expected severity of the degree of curvature. Note the girl with the double major curve is well balanced and least deformed. These photographs well illustrate that the deformity and prognosis in idiopathic scoliosis vary with the curve pattern. (From James, J. I. P.: Scoliosis. Baltimore, Williams & Wilkins Co., 1967, p. 53.)

not been performed; of these, 335 were observed to maturity.[300] James, in an intensive study of idiopathic scoliosis, came to essentially the same conclusions as did Ponseti and Friedman. In idiopathic scoliosis, most of the characteristics of the curve or curves are present at the onset of the deformity and rarely change. The curvature may progress considerably, and during the later stages, one or two vertebrae may be added to the original extent of the curve; however, the apex, direction of rotation, and location of the curve do not change. Only in very exceptional cases does a change in pattern occur during the development of scoliosis.

Idiopathic scoliosis may be classified into five main curve patterns; namely, major lumbar, thoracolumbar, combined thoracic and lumbar (double major), major thoracic, and cervicothoracic. The course and prognosis in idiopathic scoliosis vary with the curve patterns (Fig. 6–47). The age of the patient at onset of scoliosis is also important since the most deforming curves originate at an early age, and conversely, the curves with late onset that are detected near completion of growth increase only slightly or not at all. In a high percentage of cases, the final angular value of a curve can be corrrelated with the age at which scoliosis began. Each group is considered in detail in Table 6–2.

Moe and Kettleson studied 228 major idiopathic curves in 169 patients. They defined a *major curve* as one that produces a cosmetic deformity, has major structural changes, and requires correction in order to regain compensation and a satisfactory appearance. Thus, a patient may have a single major curve, or he may have double or even triple major curve patterns. The major curves were divided by Moe and Kettleson into three distinct groups: (1) *high thoracic* —extending from the seventh cervical to the seventh thoracic vertebra; (2) *thoracic* —extending from the third thoracic to the third lumbar; and (3) *lumbar* —extending from the tenth thoracic to the fifth lumbar. The incidence of the major curves in the 169 patients was as follows: 17 per cent, high thoracic; 84 per cent, thoracic; and 33 per cent, lumbar. (The sum of these percentages is over 100 because of the occurrence of double and triple major curve patterns in a single spine.) A single major curve was found in 56.8 per cent of the patients; a double major curve pattern in 41.4 per cent, and a triple major curve pattern in 1.8 per cent. The right thoracic pat-

Table 6–2. *Curve Patterns and Prognosis in Idiopathic Scoliosis**

	Curve Pattern				
	Primary Lumbar	Thoracolumbar	Combined Thoracic and Lumbar	Primary Thoracic	Cervicothoracic
Incidence (%)	23.6	16	37	22.1	1.3
Average age curve noted (yr.)	13.25	14	12.3	11.1	15
Average age curve stabilized (yr.)	14.5	16	15.5	16.1	16
Extent of curve	D 11–L 3 (5 vertebrae)	D 6 or D 7–L 1 or L 2 (6 to 8 vertebrae)	Dorsal, D 6–D 10 (5 segments) Lumbar, D 11–L 4 (5 segments)	D 6–D 11 (6 segments)	C 7 or D 1–D 4 or D 5 (4 to 6 vertebrae)
Apex of curve	L 1 or L 2	D 11 or D 12	Dorsal, D 7 or D 8 Lumbar, L 2	D 8 or D 9 (rotation extreme, convexity usually to right)	D 3
Average angular value at maturity (degrees)					
Standing	36.8	42.7	Dorsal, 51.9 Lumbar, 41.4	81.4	34.6
Supine	29.1	35	Dorsal, 41.4 Lumbar, 37,7	73.8	32.2
Prognosis	Most benign and least deforming of all idiopathic curves	Not severely deforming Intermediate between dorsal and lumbar curves	Good Body usually well aligned, curves even if severe tend to compensate each other High % of very severe scoliosis if onset before age of 10 yr.	Worst Progresses more rapidly, becomes more severe and produces greater clinical deformity than any other pattern Five years of active growth during which could increase	Deformity unsightly Poorly disguised because of high shoulder, elevated scapula, and deformed thoracic cage

*Adapted from Ponseti, I. V., and Friedman, B.: J. Bone Joint Surg., *32–A*:381–395, 1950.

tern was most common (43.2 per cent), followed in descending order of frequency by the double major right thoracic curve – left lumbar (26 per cent), double major left high thoracic, right thoracic (14.2 per cent), and left lumbar, 7.1 per cent. The double thoracic major curve pattern was first described by Moe and Kettleson.[282]

Treatment

Uncertainty as to the future course of scoliosis necessitates its early and efficient treatment. In some cases, the curvature may arrest itself spontaneously and early; in others, the deformity may progress rapidly and become so extreme as to impair the general health of the patient. Treatment should be directed to correct the deformity and to maintain the correction.

In 1941, after an end-result study of 425 cases of idiopathic scoliosis, the Research Committee of the American Orthopedic Association came to the following conclusions: (1) In approximately 60 per cent of the patients who were treated by exercises, the deformity increased; and in about 40 per cent, it remained unchanged. (2) In the majority of patients, correction without fusion was followed by complete loss of correction after support was discontinued. (3) Correction and subsequent fusion yielded better results than other forms of treatment.[198]

Cobb has estimated that surgery is required in about 5 per cent of the idiopathic cases, in 50 per cent of the postpoliomyelitic cases, in nearly all cases associated with neurofibromatosis, in 30 to 40 per cent of the congenital cases, and in only a few of the children with thoracogenic scoliosis, osteochondrodystrophies, and neurologic conditions.[215]

NONOPERATIVE MANAGEMENT

In general, a mild curve with good compensation and slight deformity is best treated conservatively. These patients should be closely observed with periodic roentgenograms of the spine to determine the rate of progression of the disease.

Exercises. The purposes of exercises are to improve posture and to maintain maximal spinal flexibility. They do not prevent progression to deformity.

Exercises consist of: *general postural*—abdominal, gluteus maximus, pelvic tilt, hyperextension, and bicycling; *asymmetrical exercises*—lateral bending toward the convexity of the greater curve, and trapeze-hanging (holding on with the upper limb on the concave side of the curve); *stretching exercises*, consisting of head and neck longitudinal traction applied by the parents; and if patient has a list to one side, *trunk shift* to balance head and neck above the pelvis and *respiratory exercises*, such as blowing balloons, to increase chest expansion and maximum breathing capacity.

The Milwaukee Brace

Of the many different types of orthoses devised for the treatment of scoliosis, the most effective is the Milwaukee brace, originated by Blount, Schmidt, and Bidwell, who presented a prototype of the orthosis in 1946 at the meeting of the American Academy of Orthopedic Surgeons in Chicago.[204–207] Since then, numerous changes have been made in the design of the brace.

The Milwaukee brace is designed to provide dynamic corrective action that incorporates distraction force between the head and pelvis by adjustable uprights as well as lateral corrective force directed toward the convex side of the major curve. Its efficient use has opened a new era in the conservative management of structural scoliosis. It has been substituted for the intermittent use of turnbuckle or localizer casts. With the Milwaukee brace, the patient is more comfortable; he can lie down, sit, stand, and walk; physiology is disturbed less, and better hygienic care can be given. It is the only orthosis that can effectively stretch the child, deflect the force of gravity away from the decompensating spine, relieve pressure on the vertebral epiphyses

on the concave side, and allow more normal vertebral growth.

The redesigned Milwaukee brace, shown in Fig 6–48, consists of the following components. (1) *A pelvic girdle* made of a thermoplastic material called Orthoplast. It is self-hinging, perforated for ventilation, waterproof, and can be remolded to relieve areas of skin pressure and to adjust for growth of the pelvis. In order to prevent early deterioration, the Orthoplast girdle is washed daily with soap and water. Ordinarily, the plastic pelvic girdle will last for a year and is much better tolerated than the older leather reinforced pelvic girdle, as it provides total contact. (2) Extensible anterior and posterior *upright bars.* The anterior vertical bar is made of an aluminum alloy and is radiolucent, whereas the two widely separated posterior bars are made of stainless steel. The metal uprights closely fit the upper torso but still leave room for deep breathing, lateral shifting pelvic tilt, and abdominal exercises. (3) *A cervical ring* connected with an occipital rest and "throat mold." The occipital rest fits snugly to the lower occiput. The throat mold has an advantage over the former chinpiece in that it relieves pressure against the mandible. (4) *Lateral pads* to apply pressure on the apical vertebrae. Additional parts that are sometimes used include a chin stop to prevent turning of the head, an axillary sling to provide balancing forces against a double major thoracic curve pattern, and a padded plastic shoulder-clavicular mold, which exerts a comfortable downward and posterior pull against a high thoracic curve that deforms the neckline.

Before undertaking treatment of a patient with a Milwaukee brace, the reader should carefully study the thorough monograph on the subject by Blount and Moe.[206]

There are several prerequisites for its effective use: first, access to a knowledgeable and cooperative orthotist who can supply and service a Milwaukee brace; second, an orthopedic surgeon trained and interested in the orthotic treatment of scoliosis (if his knowledge is cursory, he should refer the patient to a center where adequate therapy can be given); and third, a patient who will accept the orthosis and wear it full time until stability of correction has been demonstrated.

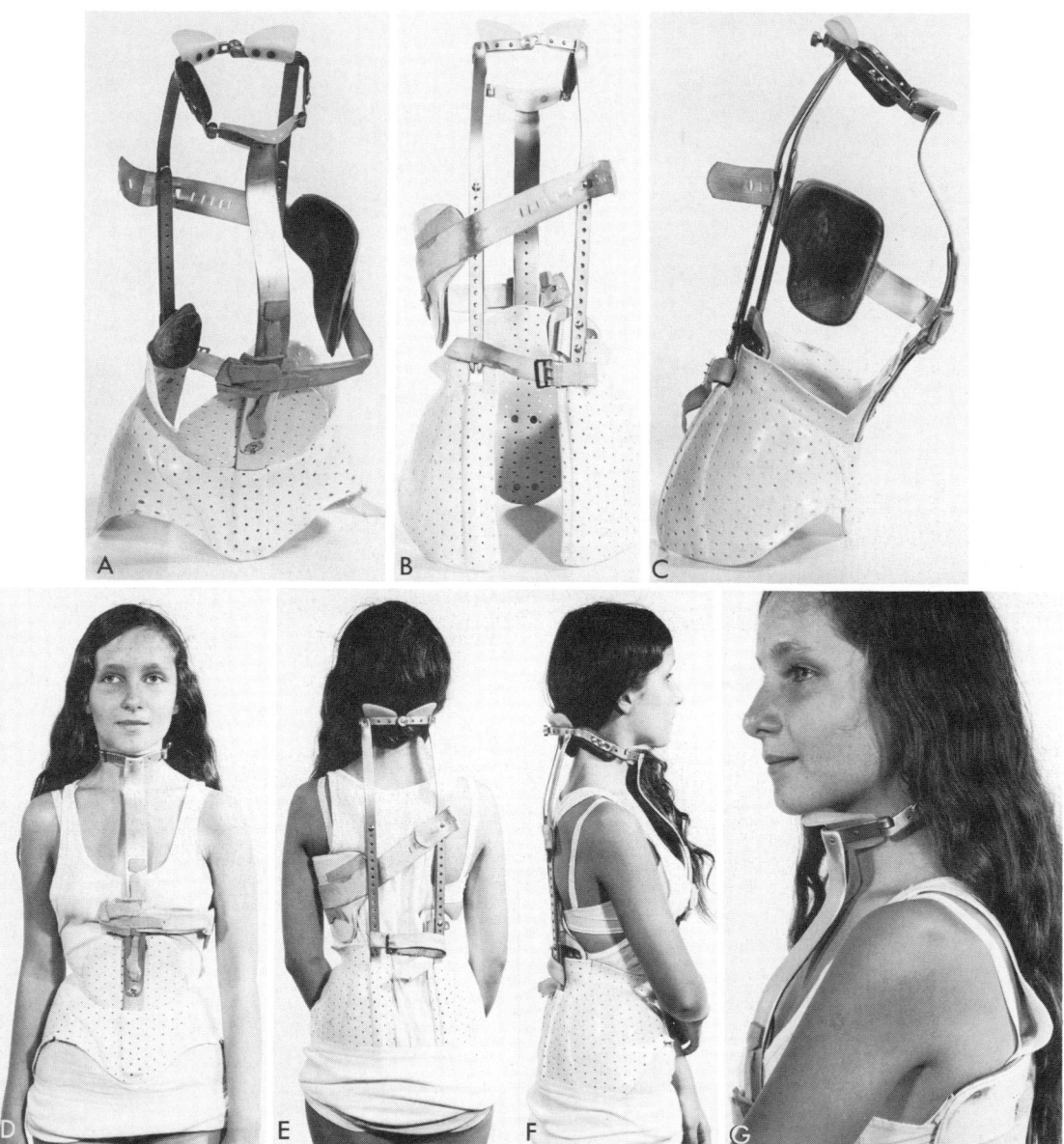

FIGURE 6–48.   *The Milwaukee brace—the modern design.*

A to **C.** Anterior, posterior, and lateral views of the orthosis (see text for explanation). **D** to **G.** An adolescent girl wearing the Milwaukee brace. Note the following: (1) the *pelvic girdle* made of a thermoplastic material called Orthoplast. It is self-hinging, perforated for ventilation, light, and waterproof. It can be remolded by using a heat gun to relieve areas of skin pressure and accommodate the increasing size of the pelvis. Deterioration of the Orthoplast pelvic girdle is prevented by daily washing with soap and water. (2) The "throat mold" is snugly approximated and there is complete lack of pressure against the mandible. (3) The occipital pad fits the lower occiput accurately, following its contour. (4) The uprights fit closely to the torso, allowing room for deep breathing, lateral shift, pelvic tilt, and abdominal exercises.

Orthopedic Evaluation of the Milwaukee Brace. This checklist, as outlined by Blount and Moe, is as follows:

PELVIC GIRDLE. This is the most important component in the successful fitting of the Milwaukee brace. It should be sufficiently long in the back, extending to about 1 inch above the seat of a hard chair when the patient is sitting; and in the front, the lower end of the pelvic girdle should extend to the pubis and should allow no lower abdominal protrusion. If the pelvic girdle is properly made, it is much lower posteriorly than anteriorly—the brace will not balance in an upright position on a flat surface. The pelvic girdle should be comfortably long in the groin and should be tight to a comfortable degree. The waistline should be at the proper level, not riding high on the ribs or low against the lateral margin of the iliac crests. The tightness of the pelvic girdle and the length of the uprights control the degree of constriction at the waist.

The tilt of the pelvic girdle and the posture of the lumbosacral spine are checked. A correctly fitted brace will hold the pelvis in a tilted position and flatten the lumbar spine. A common error is completion of the brace with a built-in lordosis. During preparation of the negative plaster model, the patient should tilt his pelvis and improve his posture. The lumbosacral lordosis can also be reduced by skiving the plaster mold in the abdominal and gluteal regions. During fitting of the brace, one can increase the tilt of the pelvic girdle and reduce the swayback by bending the vertical bars and adjusting their length.

CERVICAL RING, OCCIPITAL REST AND THROAT MOLD (Fig. 6–49). The occipital pads should fit snugly against the base of the occiput and closely follow the contour of the skull when the head is held in normal erect position. The occipital pad should not ride high on the back of the skull, as it will push the head forward, distraction force on the occiput will be lost, and excessive pressure will be exerted on the throat. The "throat mold" should be at a lower level than the occipital rest, the average angle being 30 degrees. In a properly fitted brace, the chin can be easily raised 3 cm. from the throat mold while the occiput pads remain closely fitted to the lower occiput. When this is being checked, the pelvic girdle should be tight and accurately placed. One pitfall is to lengthen the anterior vertical bar without simultaneously lengthening the posterior bars. The head should be held in neutral comfortable position. The length of the cervical ring should be correct: if it is too short, it will choke, and

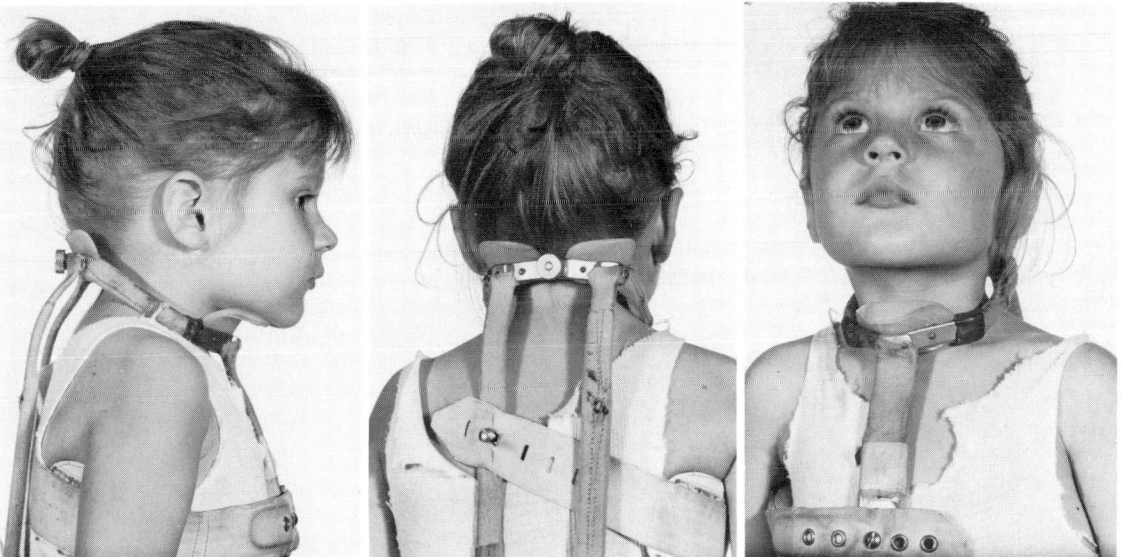

FIGURE 6–49. *The cervical ring, occipital rest, and throat mold (see text for explanation).*

if too long, pressure will be exerted on the mandible. Having the neck ring hinged anteriorly facilitates easy removal and reapplication of the brace. In infants, the neck ring is circularly padded and a throat mold is not used.

PLACEMENT OF LATERAL PADS.   With distraction alone, i.e., without the help of lateral pads, flexible curves will straighten. James does not use lateral pads.[262] Blount and Moe, however, strongly believe that the thoracic and lumbar lateral pads help to stretch the spine and also press upon the rotated areas, playing an important role in the effective use of the brace. The lateral pads are placed at sites where they will exert maximal corrective force on the apex of the deformity.[204-206, 280] This is checked on the roentgenograms made with the brace on. Pads are selected according to curve pattern. With longitudinal growth and correction of the curve, it is necessary to change the sites of the pads. For a detailed discussion of this the reader is advised to consult the monograph of Blount and Moe.[206]

THE FIT OF THE UPRIGHTS.   The vertical uprights should fit the torso closely, leaving adequate room for deep breathing, lateral shift, pelvic tilt, and abdominal exercises. There should be no restriction of deep inspiration and no pressure by the upright against the chest wall. The exact position of the bars depends upon the contours of the body. Leg length inequality, if present, should be corrected by appropriate lifts to correct listing of the uprights.

Orthopedic Follow-up of the Milwaukee Brace Patient.   The patient should be approached optimistically and reassured that soon he will be relieved of his feeling of claustrophobia and that, in a few weeks, he will hardly be aware that he is wearing the brace. It is also advisable and psychologically comforting for the patient to talk to another patient who has worn the brace for a period of time.

A patient who presents difficult fitting problems or one who is emotionally distressed is best hospitalized for rest and frequent observation during the first week. If he is comfortable while ambulatory, he is discharged and checked regularly on an outpatient basis.

After checking the fit of the brace on the second or third day, a standing anteropos-terior roentgenogram of the entire spine with the brace on is made. This permits visualization of the accurate placement of the pads and response to their holding force.

In the patient's early office visits, it should be emphasized that a tight pelvic girdle is more comfortable than a loose one, as the former presses into the soft tissues at the waist and causes fewer skin pressure problems than the latter, which rests on the sharp bony edges of the pelvis. The pelvic girdle is tightened as much as is comfortable for the patient and the strap is marked. Initially, the pelvic girdle may be loosened for short periods, but it should be re-tightened to maximal tolerance.

As correction of scoliosis occurs, the vertebral column lengthens, making the brace relatively shorter. The patient should be able to lift the chin at least one, but not more than three, fingerbreadths without pulling down on the ring. The brace is elongated both anteriorly and posteriorly and only one hole at a time. The neck ring may have to be shortened to bring the throat mold as close to the neck as can be tolerated without the feeling of choking. Again, a standing roentgenogram in the brace is taken to check the position of the pads and the general progress.

On subsequent office visits the orthopedic surgeon follows the same routine, checking tightness of the pelvic girdle, throat mold–occiput fit, length of the brace, presence or absence of any pain or pressure areas, location and proper holding force of the pads; reviewing the exercises to be performed in and out of the brace; and checking progress in straightening of the scoliosis. The spine should be carefully examined. Is the scoliosis compensating? Where does the plumb line fall when dropped from the vertebra prominens or the midocciput? Is there any overcorrection? Are the shoulders level? Is the scapula prominent? Is it necessary to add an axillary sling or shoulder pad, or both?

Roentgenograms of the spine are made as indicated, usually a standing film out of the brace, at intervals of three months. Superfluous x-rays should be avoided.

EXERCISES.   Physical activities of the patient should remain as near normal as possible. The only games that are forbidden are body contact sports because of the danger to other players. There is no need for the patient to be excused from physical education at school; he should be allowed to participate in sports such as tennis, volley ball, or bicycling. Swimming is an excellent sport for the scoliotic patient and should be encouraged, the patient being permitted to remove the brace and swim for an hour each day. When not in the water, he must be recumbent and must not sit around the pool without wearing the brace.

The child should be taught general good posture by a physical therapist during the first week and at regular intervals thereafter. Exercises are necessary to maintain muscle tone and proper body mechanics. Out of the brace the patient performs abdominal, dorsal hyperextension, gluteus maximus, lateral bend, and pelvic tilt exercises, the last-named exercise being the most important. It is done first with knees bent, later with knees straight and standing with back against the wall, and last in stance and in gait. Contractural deformities such as tight hamstrings and hip flexion, if present, should be stretched by passive exercises.

Active corrective exercises for the scoliotic deformities are performed in the brace and consist of the following: *active distraction*—the patient pushes down on the anterior bar and then stretches up out of the brace as far as possible; *deep breathing*—the child inhales deeply and then exhales and arches his back like a cat against the major pad; *thoracic retraction*—while holding the position of pelvic tilt, the patient pulls away from the lateral pads and corrects the thoracic curve.

Complications with the Milwaukee Brace

EFFECT ON TOOTH POSITION AND MAXILLO-FACIAL VERTICAL GROWTH. Growing bone reacts to external pressure. The old Milwaukee brace exerted upward force on the mandible and occiput. Logan measured the force applied to the mandible by the Milwaukee brace by inserting a hydrostatic bag between the jaw and the brace and noted that an average intermittent pressure of 4 lb. was produced.[271] The greatest pressure occurred at night when the children were asleep and relaxed, when they "fell into" the brace.

The first documented case of alteration of growth pattern and potential configuration of teeth and mandible by external pressure was reported by Howard in 1926.[255]

He described the case of a patient wearing a plaster body cast who developed malocclusion of the incisor teeth three weeks after the cast was applied. Within six months there was shortening of the lower part of the face. Later, in 1929, he reported these patients as showing only a slight tendency to regain their former normal state at the end of 12 months following removal of orthopedic casts.[256] Recent work in this field was published by Bunch, in 1961, and Alexander, in 1966.[197, 210] The detrimental effects of the old Milwaukee brace on the dentition and surrounding maxillofacial complex are well documented (Fig. 6–50). Alexander obtained beginning and progress study models, cephalograms, and photographs of 14 patients who were being treated for scoliosis with the Milwaukee brace. Seven patients (the control group) did not wear any auxiliary appliance to stabilize the dentition; the other seven wore a positioner-type appliance for stabilization. He showed that the Milwaukee brace affects the dentition by extruding the incisors and depressing the molars. The effect is more pronounced in the lower molars. A shortening of the vertical dimension of the lower anterior face was found in all patients. Vertical growth seemed to be affected in the lower border of the body of the mandible.

Since 1969, the chinpiece has been eliminated and a throat mold has been substituted that serves to hold the head erect and the lower occiput over the occipital pads. In this way, distraction forces are exerted on the occiput and pressure against the mandible is completely avoided, thus preventing deformities of the mandible and disturbances of bite; also, it is less disturbing cosmetically than is the chin rest.

An orthodontic examination prior to initiation of treatment with the Milwaukee brace is desirable; such an evaluation is particularly important if there is pre-existing malocclusion.

EMOTIONAL HYPERREACTION. This can occur and is best controlled by association with other patients in braces. It takes a few weeks for children suffering from this complication to adjust to the brace. The author allows the child to go to school without the brace during the first two weeks, breaking him in gradually. Like a new shoe, the brace must be worn for several weeks

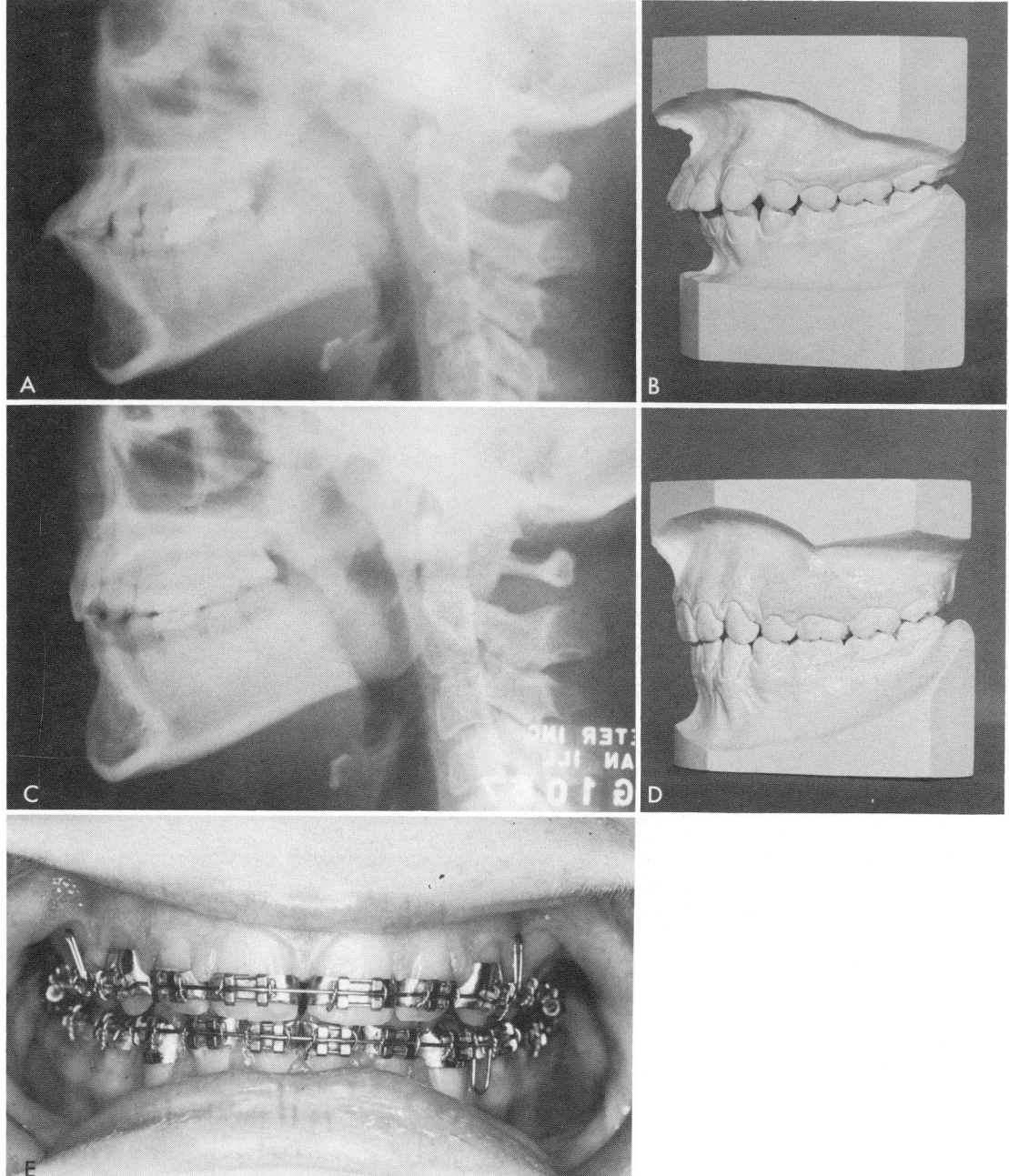

FIGURE 6–50. *Detrimental effect of the old Milwaukee brace upon dentition and maxillofacial complex.*

In the *new* Milwaukee brace, the chin rest is discontinued and the throat mold is substituted. Distraction force is exerted on the lower occiput and not on the mandible; thus deformities of the lower face and disturbance of bite are eliminated. **A** and **B**. Roentgenogram and mold demonstrating the extrusion of the incisors and the depression of the molars. Vertical growth of the body of the mandible is retarded. **C** to **E**. Views showing correction of deformity by orthodontic treatment with braces.

before it is comfortable. After a month almost invariably the patients start wearing the brace day and night by themselves. In some children it is best to initiate corrective treatment for a month or two by application of a Risser localizer cast. The child becomes accustomed to a corrective device and the transition from Risser localizer cast to

Milwaukee brace is then smoothly accomplished with good cooperation from the patient.

PRESSURE SORES. These should not occur under a properly made and fitted brace. If they are encountered, the brace is adjusted to relieve the pressure and daily skin care is given.

WEANING. In nonoperative treatment of scoliosis, the Milwaukee brace is worn continually until maximal correction is obtained. After the corrected spine is stable, gradual weaning from the brace may be started. The periods that the patient is permitted out of the brace depend upon the patient's ability to maintain correction, as demonstrated by roentgenograms made after the patient has been out of the brace for a specific period.

First, a standing roentgenogram of the spine is taken after the patient has been out of the brace for three hours. If there is no loss of correction the patient is allowed gradually to remove the brace for three hours daily. These periods out of the brace should be increased gradually to four, then to six and eight hours daily. When the child is able to be out of the brace for eight hours without loss of correction, as shown by standing roentgenograms, he is gradually allowed to go to school without it. The brace is worn during the night for the last six months. Too sudden weaning can cause substantial loss of correction.

Moe and Kettleson published a retrospective study of 228 major idiopathic curves in 169 patients who had either completed Milwaukee brace treatment (132 patients) or were then wearing the brace at night only during the weaning process (37 patients). The median total brace wearing time was 34.4 months; included in this are the three treatment phases: (1) *full time*—that period when the patient wore the brace during all but one or two hours per day (median 18.7 months); (2) *part-time* (four to eight hours out) or that period during which the patient's wearing time was gradually being reduced from full time to nights only (median 9.5 months); and (3) *nights only*—the final period, when the brace was worn only while the patient was in bed at night (median 11.7 months).

This study, despite the obvious lack of important data of skeletal age and spinal maturity, demonstrated that the Milwaukee brace is effective in controlling and correcting a high percentage of moderate and mild idiopathic spinal curves. The best results are obtained when: (1) treatment is begun before the iliac apophyses have become capped, with great potential of vertebral growth still remaining; (2) there is full cooperation by the patient; (3) the curve is long; and (4) the degree of curvature is not severe—only one curve of less than 40 degrees at the start of brace treatment required correction and fusion (the patient was completely uncooperative). The best response to orthotic treatment was obtained in the thoracic and lumbar curves. The high thoracic curves gave the poorest response. The maximal degree of correction is achieved in the first two years in 97 per cent, and within two and one half years in all patients. The median loss of correction after removal of the brace was 1 per cent in thoracic curves, and 5 per cent in lumbar curves. Despite the fact that in some of the larger (45 to 50 degrees) double major curves of the right thoracic left lumbar pattern there was no roentgenographic improvement, substantial cosmetic improvement with better balance and lessening of the rib prominence was achieved. With adequate Milwaukee brace treatment, severe deformities in *some* young children can be prevented from progressing or even improved so that the necessary surgery can be safely delayed until a more desirable age for surgery is reached.[282]

It is imperative to detect and treat scoliosis in its incipient stage. All idiopathic curves have their genesis in spines that at one time were straight. Early diagnosis and immediate treatment with the Milwaukee brace, even part-time, will provide a check-rein on these minimal curves, preventing them from progressing and becoming fixed severe deformities. The pediatrician and general practitioner should be educated to inspect the unclothed spine of every child who is in his office for routine general examination.

The Milwaukee brace should be used when a *minimal curve* shows structural rigidity of the soft tissues on its concave side, i.e., the curve is not completely flexible and cannot be overcorrected on side-bending, as shown by roentgenograms. The brace can be withheld when a 10- or 15-degree curve is fully flexible; however, on the slightest evidence of progression, treatment with the Milwaukee brace should be started. These slight curves with minimal structural changes can be readily corrected by early orthotic treatment. When confronted with a *moderate* idiopathic curve, the age of the child and skeletal maturity of his spine are important factors to consider in deciding which method of treatment, surgery or Milwaukee brace, is preferred. The following guidelines are based upon the recommendations of Moe:

1. Use the Milwaukee brace in a structural curve that measures 40 degrees or less (by the Cobb method) in a spine that is skeletally immature and has substantial growth remaining. Adequate permanent correction may be achieved in such cases. Sometimes in the younger juvenile patient, satisfactory response may be obtained in single thoracic curves of 50 or even 60 degrees. The brace can be tried in such cases.

2. Surgery (correction in cast and fusion with or without Harrington instrumentation) is the treatment of choice in single major curves of 60 or more degrees in the older adolescent whose growth is nearing completion.

3. Surgical treatment should also be carried out in the early adolescent or juvenile patient with an 80- or 90-degree curve—such severe curvatures should *not* be treated conservatively with the Milwaukee brace.

4. Infantile structural scoliosis responds well to Milwaukee brace treatment. It is possible (with the new plastic girdle) to fit the Milwaukee brace satisfactorily to a six-month-old infant.

5. In congenital scoliosis with unsegmented bars, hemivertebrae, and other major curve-producing anomalies, *solid fusion* in early life is required, followed by support in the Milwaukee brace.

6. In some cases, the spine of a child with paralytic scoliosis can be supported and progression of the curve inhibited until the patient has regained motor power; such a patient can be weaned away from the Milwaukee brace before puberty without resorting to a surgical procedure. In other cases, operative treatment can be postponed until the child has grown to a reasonable height, when fusion of a collapsing spine can be accomplished without stunting growth. When paralytic scoliosis is associated with severe pelvic obliquity, it is difficult to use the Milwaukee brace effectively. It is best to release all contractural deformities and to fuse the curve to include the sacrum whenever pelvic obliquity is present. In myelomeningocele children with sensory loss about the pelvis, it is very difficult to use the Milwaukee brace; however, with intelligent parents and a cooperative patient, its use may be feasible in these children.

7. In the postoperative management of a fused spine, the brace will prevent worsening of compensatory curves.[280]

OPERATIVE TREATMENT

The indications for correction of the curve and spinal fusion are: (1) a cosmetically objectionable deformity with decompensation of the spine and asymmetry of the trunk in an adolescent or postadolescent patient, regardless of whether growth of the spine has ceased (Fig. 6–51); (2) a proved progressive curve in a young and growing child in whom conservative measures have failed (Fig. 6–52), and (3) persistent backache that cannot be controlled by conservative means (seen especially in the older patient with lumbar scoliosis).

The traditional operation that has been universally used for many years is extensive posterior spinal fusion. This is performed after as much correction as possible has been obtained by conservative means.

Methods of Forcible Correction of Curves

Of the various methods that have been developed for correction of scoliosis prior to fusion, the turnbuckle cast, the Risser localizer cast, the transection shift jacket of Von Lackum, and the Harrington method of spinal instrumentation have proved to be effective.[204–208, 246–248, 312, 330–332] Whichever method is used, it is essential to remember that the primary purpose of scoliosis treatment is to restore compensation of the spine with a symmetrical trunk and with head, neck, and shoulders centered over the pelvis.

The Turnbuckle Cast. Use of a turnbuckle cast is based on the principle that bending is more effective than straight traction in straightening a curved rod. The principle had been previously employed by Abbott, in 1912, and by Lovett and Brewster, in 1924.[196, 272] The turnbuckle cast technique used now is the one devised by Risser.[306, 312] Prior to application of the

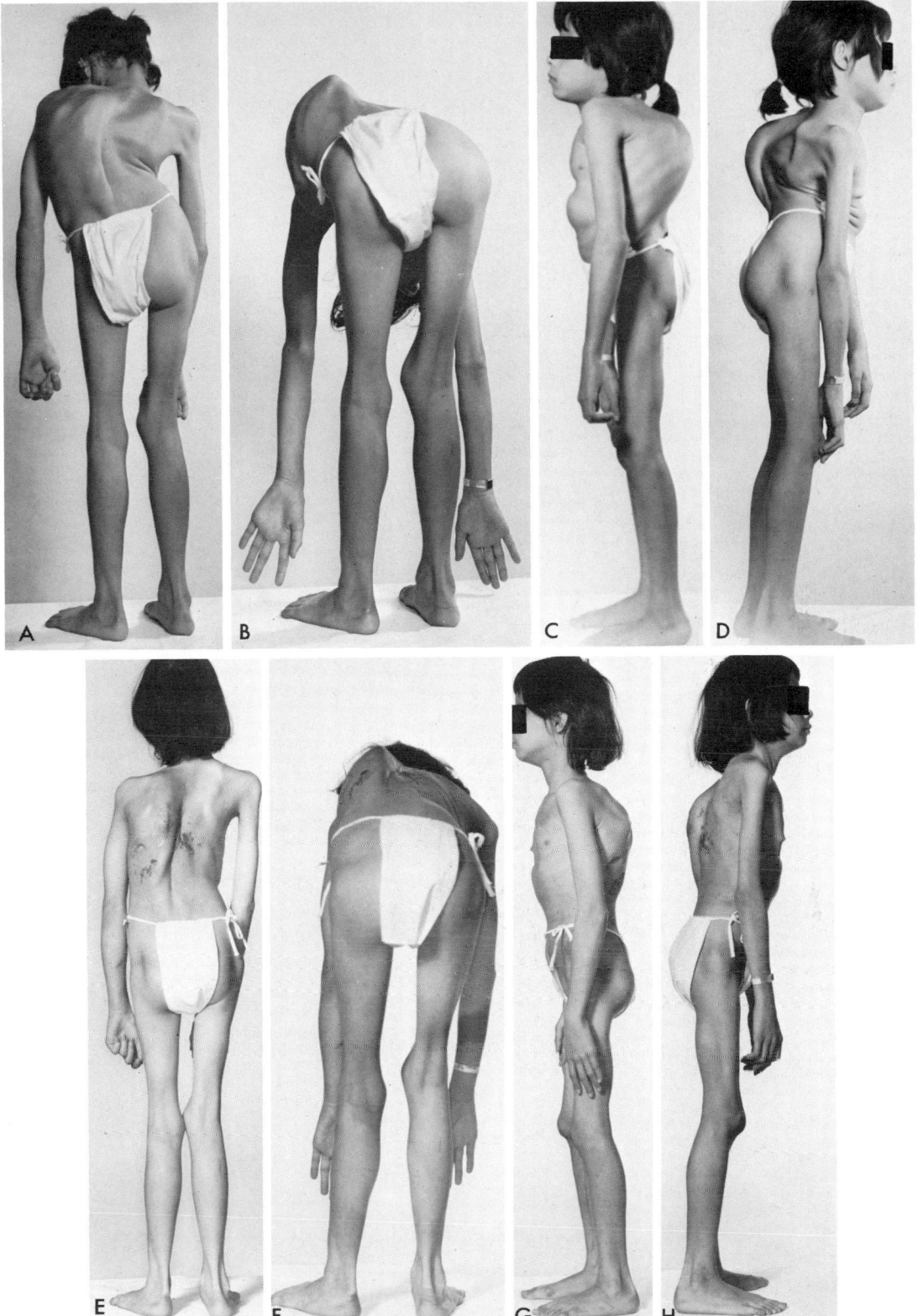

FIGURE 6–51. Severe structural scoliosis.

A to **D.** Preoperative views. The spine is decompensated and the deformity is very severe. **E** to **H.** Postoperative views showing improvement of deformity.

1217

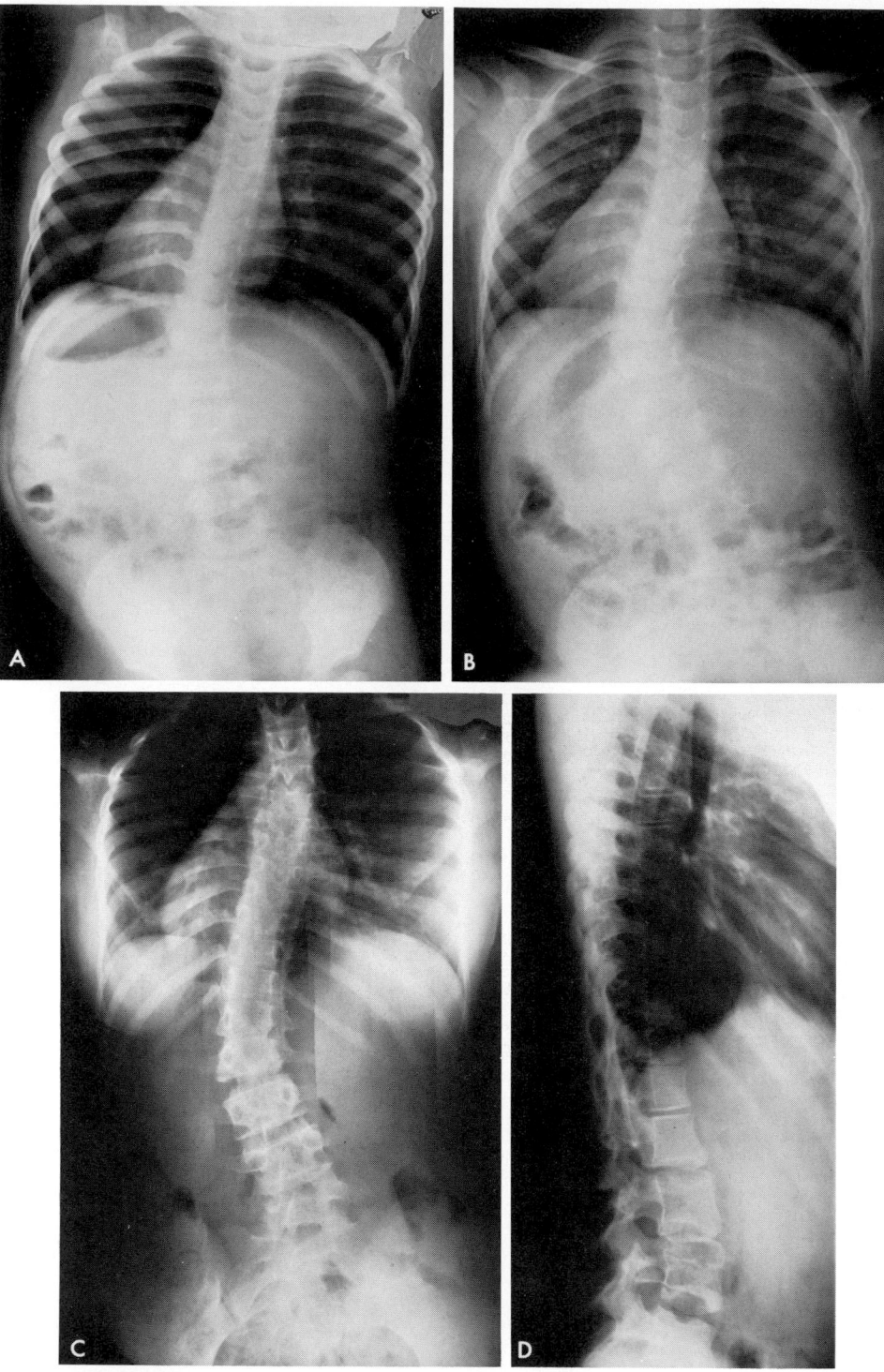

FIGURE 6–52. *Infantile structural idiopathic left thoracolumbar scoliosis.*

A. Anteroposterior standing roentgenogram of the spine at one and a half years. **B.** At three years of age. Note progression of the curve. Treatment consisted of intermittent use of a Risser localizer cast, which did not prevent progression of the scoliosis. Spinal fusion of the fifth dorsal to the second lumbar vertebrae, inclusive, was performed to stabilize the spine. **C** and **D.** Anteroposterior and lateral roentgenograms of the spine 11 years postoperatively at age 14 years. Stability and correction of the spine have been maintained, but note the retarded growth of the fused vertebrae.

turnbuckle cast, it is essential to study the flexibility of the secondary curves by pelvic tilt and bending tests. As the primary curve is straightened, the secondary curves are increased and the trunk is thrown out of balance. The possible spontaneous correction in the compensatory lumbar curve with the common right dorsal primary curve is determined by a left pelvic tilt test. The possibility of correction of the upper compensatory curve is determined by side-bending films. The sum of the residual angles of the secondary curves is the total residual curve of the spine in one direction caused by the primary curve. For the spine to be completely compensated, there must be an equally restored curvature in the opposite direction.

At the Children's Hospital Medical Center in Boston, Massachusetts, the turnbuckle cast was used almost exclusively, and difficulty of restoration of compensation has not been a problem.[242]

In application of the cast it is essential to pay careful attention to details. (1) Exposure of the patient to other children who are presently wearing a cast or to those who have worn one is of great psychologic help. One should take time to explain to the patient the steps in the application of the cast. (2) The patient should have an empty stomach and be adequately sedated. (3) Lower limbs, trunk, head, and neck are put into a body stockinette with holes over the nostrils for breathing. (4) A large piece of white felt, two and one half times the width of the patient and long enough to extend from below the knees to above the head, is cut, carefully trimmed, and sewed while on the patient. It should include the arm on the concave side and the thigh on the convex side of the primary curve. Suture lines on the felt should be strategically placed to avoid pressure sores. A rectangular piece of felt is loosely sutured over the axilla of the included arm. Two or three layers of removable felt are placed under the proposed location of the anterior and posterior hinges; these "hinge pads" are removed later to allow space for correction of the chest deformity. (5) The patient is placed supine on a scoliosis frame. Various types of frames can be used. The author uses the Risser cast table; the Albee-Comper fracture table with Cobb attachments, or a modified Goldthwait frame can be used. (6) The

patient holds a pole with the arm that will be in the cast. The included shoulder should be in 30 to 40 degrees of forward flexion to avoid traction on the brachial plexus. The patient's trunk and head are somewhat bent to the concavity of the primary curve to partially straighten the compensatory curves and allow maximal correction of the primary curve with minimal increase of the compensatory countercurves. The position of the included hip should be 40 to 50 degrees of flexion. The head and neck are included in the jacket if the apex of the primary curve is at T 9 or higher. (7) Next, the body cast is applied. It should be well molded over the occiput, chin, and iliac crests. (8) Thumb-tack localizer roentgenograms are taken for accurate placement of the hinges. The hinges are positioned on the anterior and posterior aspects of the cast, with the joint placed lateral and slightly distal to the apex of the primary curve, so that a distracting as well as a lateral bending force is exerted as the turnbuckle bends the spine laterally. The more severe the deformity, the more eccentrically the hinges should be placed. The eccentricity of the hinges can be changed by shifting the holes. (9) The cast is allowed to dry for three to four days, and then is cut transversely at the level of the hinges on the concave side. The cut is extended anteriorly and posteriorly to the hinges. From the opposite side of the cast, a large elliptical window between the hinges is opened to allow lateral bending in that direction. All cast debris on the patient should be removed. The turnbuckle lugs are secured firmly with plaster of Paris to the superior part of the lower cast and the inferior surface of the arm cast. The felt and stockinette are cut and anchored to plaster edges with adhesive tape. A turnbuckle is attached to the lugs. (10) The turnbuckle is turned each morning, and the distance between the two lugs and the date are recorded on the cast. The correction must be slow, gradual, and painless. (11) Any pressure points at the window edges and deep at the hinges are eliminated with appropriate padding. Brachial plexus nerve function is checked every day. If necessary, the superior half of the arm cast can be bivalved for better evaluation of neuromuscular function. (12) At various time intervals, roentgenograms are made to determine the degree of correction. The

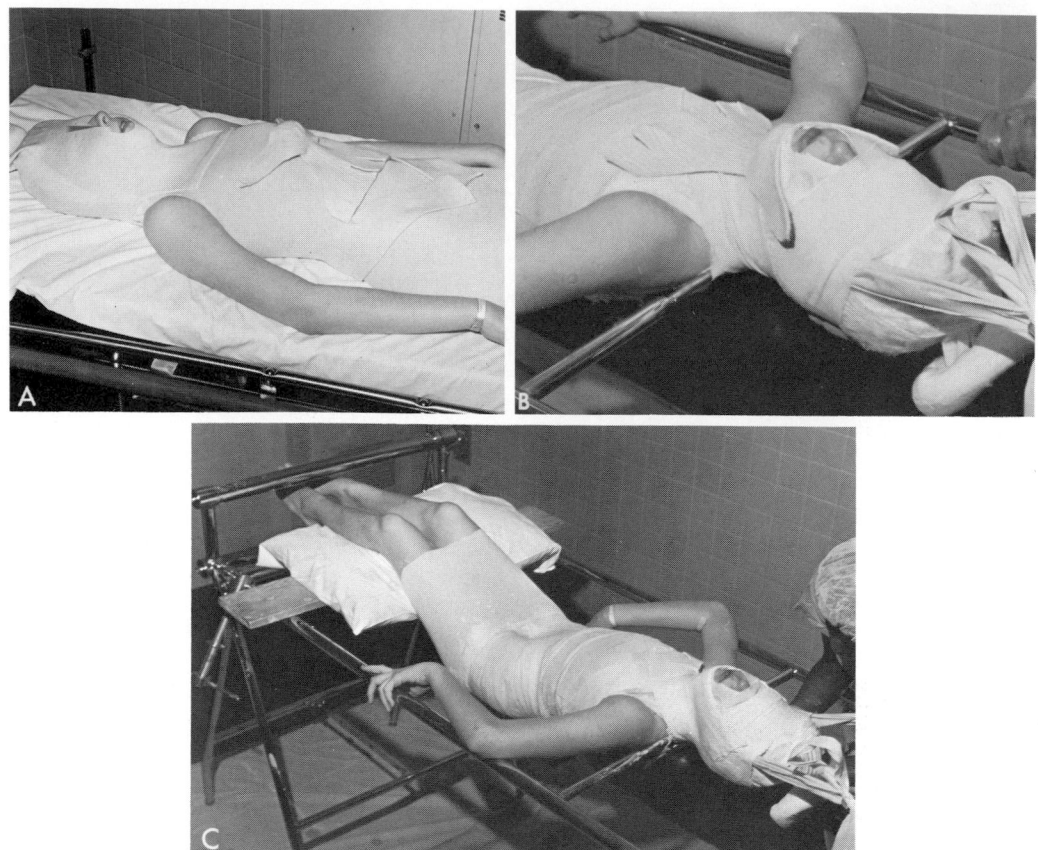

FIGURE 6–53.   *Risser localizer cast.*

A and **B.** Photograph showing stockinette stretched over patient and felt padding over her lower chest and trunk and pelvis. **C.** Patient on the Risser localizer table with cast completed.

maximal amount of correction that is permissible or obtainable usually requires two to four weeks.

Localizer Cast Correction (Risser).   In the Risser localizer cast, correction is obtained by the application of localized pressure from a posterolateral direction over the rib deformity at a point level with the apex of the curve, while traction is exerted on the head and pelvis. The apex of the curve is forced between the ends of the curve, which are fixed by traction.[306, 312]

Supposedly the localizer cast gives greater correction of rotation and rib prominence than that afforded by the turnbuckle cast. The patient may walk in a localizer cast. In many centers, the localizer cast is used almost exclusively. Its disadvantage is the rapidity and suddenness of correction with its inherent dangers of more skin trouble and decreased tolerance by the patient. In severe fixed curves one can obtain more cor-

rection of angulation with the turnbuckle cast, which can be used initially to make the curve more flexible, and a localizer Risser cast may be applied later for better balancing.

The patient is placed supine on the Risser localizer table, upon the canvas strap, with stockinette stretched over him from the head to the knees. Next, circular felt strips of padding are smoothly applied to the trunk, back of the head, neck, chin, and pelvic girdle (Fig. 6–53). A heavy piece of felt is covered with a previously made contoured square of plaster to distribute the localizer pressure. In a double primary curve, another such felt-plaster piece is made for the second curve.

The plaster cast is applied in sections. First, the pelvic girdle portion is applied, and the plaster molded snugly and carefully around the iliac crests, the sacrum, and the symphysis pubis. The hips should be in

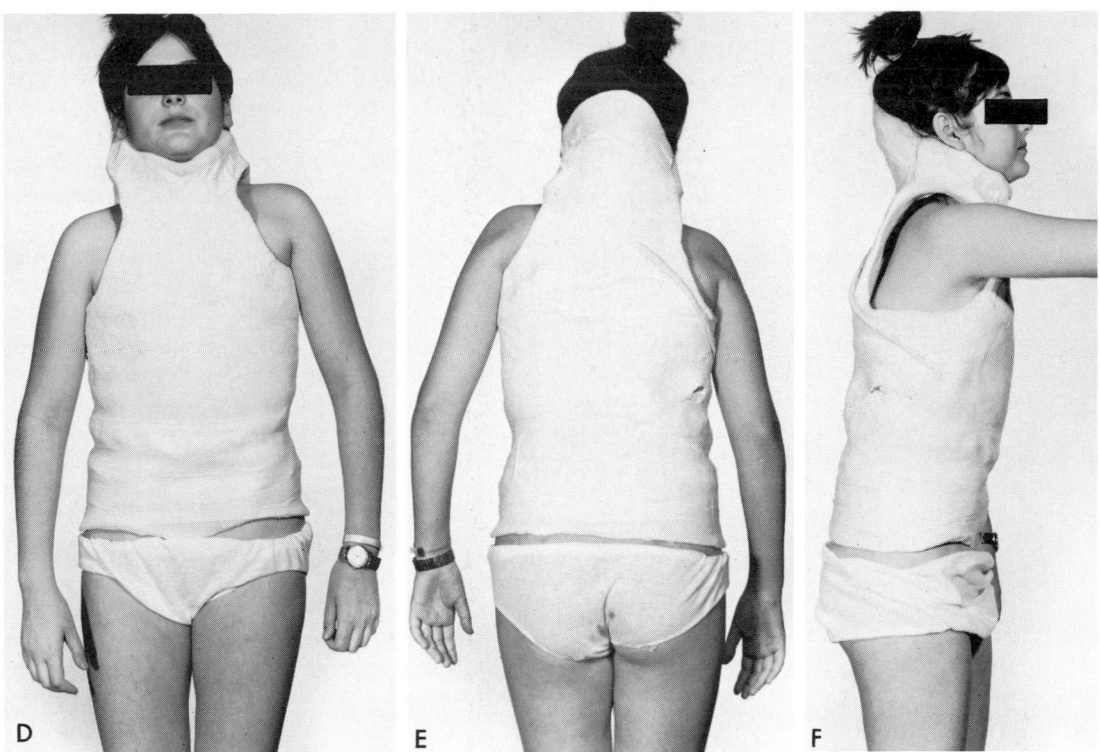

FIGURE 6–53 Continued.   Risser localizer cast.

D to **F.** Views of patient standing with cast on.

flexion to reduce excessive lumbar lordosis. Next, gentle traction is applied to the head with a halter, and then a well-molded cast is applied over the neck, chin, occiput, and shoulders. Traction is applied to the pelvis with a pelvic belt anchored over the plaster girdle. Gradually and simultaneously, traction forces are increased on both the pelvis and the head. The localizer pusher is then gradually turned to increase the pressure over the posterolateral aspect of the thoracic deformity for correction of the dorsal curve. Next the entire trunk is incorporated in the cast, connecting the head and pelvic portions. The alignment of the spine should be carefully watched. A V-shaped notch is cut in the cast under the chin to relieve any undue pressure.

Transection Shift Jacket (Von Lackum).[330–332] This is a body cast that includes both thighs and the chin and occiput. It is applied in sections, the dividing line being opposite the apex of a single deforming curve or at the juncture of two primary curves. It is well padded throughout, but particularly so on the lateral margins, where there is pressure during the lateral shift. No hinges or turnbuckles are employed. Correction can be made within an hour after the jacket is applied. The single transection jacket is indicated for the flexible double primary curve, whereas the double transection type is indicated for flexible single primary ("triple curve") patterns of scoliosis, excluding cervicodorsal and high dorsal areas. Correction is accomplished by the manual shift of one section against the other or by shifting the center section against the end sections.

Spinal Fusion

Two or three days prior to operation, the cast is removed, and the patient is allowed to be ambulatory in order to allow the vasomotor system to return to normal. The trunk and lower limbs are prepared with pHisoHex or some other surgical soap several times a day.

The surgeon and his assistants should familiarize themselves with the anatomic landmarks of the spine prior to operation. The spinous processes are palpated and studied as to their size, shape, and direction, and correlated with superficial skin marks. Films are taken with a paper clip placed over the spinous processes of the seventh cervical, apical, and end vertebrae to verify their respective levels. The quality of a regular roentgenogram is always better than that of a film taken with portable equipment in the operating room.

Another method frequently used by others is to make a marker film after injecting a small amount of sterile methylene blue into the periosteum and bone of the spinous process of one of the vertebrae within the fusion area. The findings should be recorded on the patient's chart. At the time of operation, if there is any doubt, roentgenograms are made in the operating room. If these precautions are not taken, the fusion may include an area lower or higher than planned, thus adversely affecting the outcome.

Some surgeons prefer to perform spinal fusion through a window in the cast. Despite endotracheal anesthesia and modern improved techniques, cardiac arrest and respiratory difficulties are always a potential danger. When the patient is in a cast during an operation, an adequate window should be cut out over the precordium, and a cast cutter and other instruments for removing the body cast immediately must be available in the operating room. If Harrington instrumentation is planned with the fusion, the operation is performed through a window in the cast.

Selection of Fusion Area. The primary or major curve, which is also the most deforming, is obviously the part of the spine to be fused. This is clinically determined on the basis of the original roentgenograms of the spine made with the patient standing, the position in which the deformity is most severe, and after study of lateral bend and pelvic tilt roentgenograms. The major curve is usually the longer and least flexible one, and it has the greatest structural changes. The dorsal curve is more rigid, as wedging of the vertebral bodies occurs earlier in the thoracic than in the lumbar curves. Also the thoracic curve, because of the associated rib rotation and "razor back," causes the greatest deformity. With double curves the dorsal region is usually fused, as it is most deforming. When there is severe deformity and rigidity in both lumbar and dorsal curves, both are corrected and fused.

As a general rule, the minimum fusion area should extend from end vertebra to end vertebra of the primary curve. The end vertebrae are determined in the original standing films by the maximal vertebral tilting and paralleling or reversal of the intervertebral space wedging. On glancing at the roentgenograms one can easily locate the maximally tilted end vertebrae; the inexperienced may need to draw lines along the vertebral body margins in order to determine when these lines converge into the concavity of a curve and when they begin to diverge on the convex side of the adjacent curve. The intervertebral spaces within a curve will be wedge-shaped, with the lesser thickness of the wedge pointing into the concavity of a curve; the wedge will point in the opposite direction in the opposing curve.

The end vertebrae and their rotation are readily recognized when the patient is lying prone on the operating table out of the cast, and when all posterior neural arches of the primary curve are exposed in a one-stage operation.

Another important factor in determining the fusion area is the extent of rotation of the vertebral bodies toward the convexity of the curve.[281] The maximally tilted vertebra is still rotated to the convexity of the major curve, and such rotation may continue one or two vertebrae beyond the maximally tilted vertebra. In this event, it is essential to extend the fusion area beyond the major curve and to fuse all the vertebrae that are rotated toward the convexity of the major curve, including the neutrally rotated vertebrae above and below. Rotation should be studied by the position of the pedicles and spinous processes in the roentgenograms before and after correction and also when the patient is prone on the operating table. In scoliosis with maximally tilted vertebra in the lower lumbar area and a short compensatory curve below, one should disregard rotation persisting below the maximally tilted vertebra.

The age of the patient should be considered when determining the extent of the fusion. Errors in the young have arisen through failure to fuse a long enough portion of the spine. With growth of the spine, the original curve lengthens and the correction may be lost. Addition of one or two vertebrae will provide security in the young.

Fusion should not extend into compensatory curves if they are rigid and the vertebrae are structurally deformed. It is essential for the spine in the upright position to be symmetrical and in normal balance and equilibrium. The hazard of imbalance is greater in the turnbuckle correction and minimal, but still present, in the localizer correction.

The use of Harrington instrumentation should be individualized. The procedure delays the time of operation, increases the risk of infection, and there is always the possible complication of paralysis. At present, the author considers the use of Harrington instrumentation (only the distraction component) in patients who have a sensitive and allergic skin that cannot tolerate local pressure from the cast, in cases in which there are definite reasons for early ambulation, in flexible but severe paralytic curves, and in curves that extend to the lumbar spine, where the likelihood of pseudarthrosis is great (Fig. 6–54).

Technique of Spinal Fusion for Scoliosis.
The subsequent discussion of the operative treatment of scoliosis is based on the works of Hibbs, Risser, A. DeF. Smith, Von Lackum, Cobb, Blount, Schmidt, Moe, and Goldstein.*

Hibbs, in 1911, reported the first spinal fusion procedure, which consisted of partially shearing off the base of the spinous processes, then breaking them down to bridge the interlaminar spaces.[251] The spinal fusion was performed on three patients with Pott's disease. In this paper, Hibbs suggested that the procedure might well be used in scoliosis, which was first done in 1914. In 1924 Hibbs reported a series of 59 patients with scoliosis treated by fusion, in some of whom there was correction and in some, not.[252] Howorth has reviewed the history of the evolution of spinal fusion.[257]

_____

*See References 208, 214–219, 239–241, 251–253, 281, 282, 306–312, 317, 325, 330–332.

The exact techniques of fusion vary with different surgeons. Any method in which fragments or leaves of bone are elevated from the laminae and spinous processes and are turned up and down so that they overlap is a modification of the Hibbs technique. Because it is used by every surgeon, a review of the Hibbs method of fusion, as described by him in 1924, is appropriate.

An incision is made through the skin and subcutaneous tissue, from above downward, exposing the tips of the spinous processes of the vertebrae to be fused. The periosteum over the tips of these processes is split longitudinally, and, with a periosteal elevator, pushed to either side, leaving them bare. The periosteum and interspinous ligaments in turn are still farther split and pushed forward a short distance from each spinous process as two lateral halves, gauze packs being inserted to prevent oozing. The dissection is carried farther and farther forward upon each vertebra in turn, until the spinous processes, the posterior surfaces of the laminae, and the base of the transverse processes are bared, thereby exposing the ligamentum subflavum attached to the margins of the laminae and the articulations of the lateral processes.

The ligament is removed from the laminae with a curette, and the articulation of the lateral processes is destroyed in order to establish bone contact at this point. With a bone gouge, a substantial piece of bone is elevated from the adjacent edges of each lamina, of half its thickness and of half its width. The free end of the piece from above is turned down to make contact with the lamina below, and the free end of the piece from the lamina below is turned up to make contact with the lamina above. In transposing these pieces of bone from the laminae, it is better to avoid severing their continuity.

Each spinous process is then partially divided with bone forceps and broken down, forcing the tip to come into contact with the bare bone of the vertebra below. The spinous process of the last vertebra below should be turned up to bring about contact with the next above. As the spinous processes of the lumbar region are wide, it is sometimes practicable to split them, turning one half up and the other half down. Thus is established contact of abundant cancellous bone at the articulations of the lateral processes, laminae, and spinous processes. The periosteum and ligament, which together have been pushed to either side and lie practically as an unbroken sheet, are brought together in the middle with interrupted sutures of ten-day chromic catgut.[252]

Details of the technique of spinal fusion

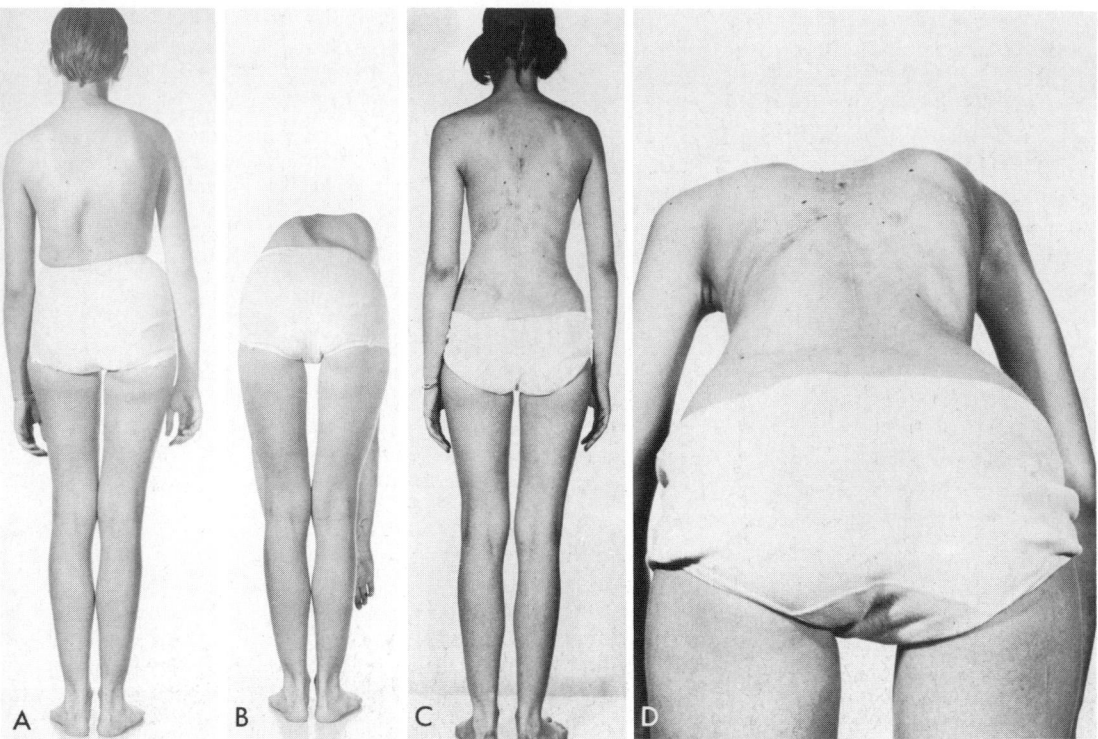

FIGURE 6–54.   *Idiopathic scoliosis—double major (left lumbar right thoracic) curve pattern in an adolescent girl.*

A and **B.** Preoperative photographs. **C** and **D.** Following correction in the cast, spinal fusion, and Harrington instrumentation, showing improvement in deformity.

as performed by the author are illustrated in Plate 49.

Postoperative Management.   Ten to fourteen days postoperatively, after removal of sutures, a corrective cast is reapplied and roentgenograms are made through the cast to check the degree of correction. If the desired correction has been obtained and the cast is comfortable, the patient is discharged from the hospital after thorough instructions have been given to the parents concerning care of the patient and of the cast. Arrangements are made to procure a hospital bed; this greatly facilitates home care. Home tutoring should be arranged. The patient is to remain recumbent for a period of six months following the operation. He may turn, move around in bed, and elevate the torso to a 45-degree angle from the horizontal without harm.

Breathing, pelvic tilt, and active longitudinal stretching exercises are outlined. A low-calcium diet during the period of re-

cumbency will help to prevent formation of calculi in the urinary tract.

In the average case, after six months following surgery, the patient is readmitted to the hospital. The cast is removed and roentgenograms are made in both antero-posterior and oblique lateral views. The x-ray requisition for oblique lateral views should read "Center on the scar and to show the graft." At times, more than one oblique lateral view is taken to visualize the graft. These roentgenograms are carefully studied as to the extent and maturity of the fusion mass. Is there any evidence of pseudarthrosis? The degree of curvature should be measured and compared with the correction obtained in the immediate postoperative cast. Has there been any loss of correction while in the cast?

The patient is allowed to turn and move around in bed. He should not be allowed to sit, as this would put stress on the graft. Skin care is given. If a turnbuckle Risser

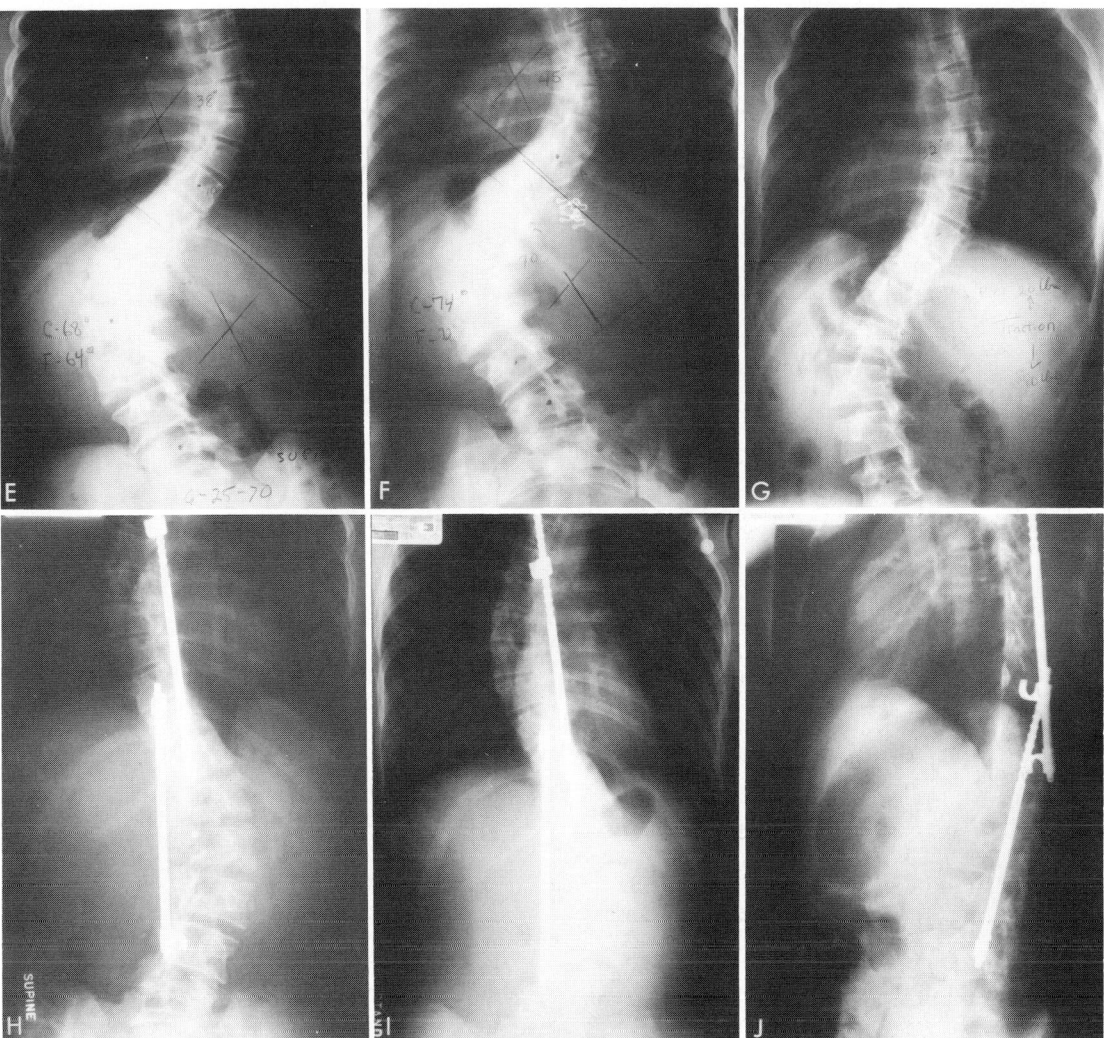

FIGURE 6-54 Continued.   Idiopathic scoliosis — double major (left lumbar right thoracic) curve pattern in an adolescent girl.

E to **G.** Preoperative roentgenograms, supine, standing, and in traction. **H** to **J.** Postoperative roentgenograms showing degree of correction.

cast is used for correction, it is essential to obtain flexibility of compensatory curves and balance the head and neck above the pelvis, which might take one or two weeks. Then a new localizer cast is applied, and the patient is allowed to ambulate with the support of crutches until balance and general strength are regained. Roentgenograms of the spine are made through the cast with the patient standing, and the degree of curvature is compared with that shown in recumbent films. He is then allowed to return gradually to relatively full activity.

The localizer cast is worn for two additional months, after which it is again removed and roentgenograms of the spine are made. If the fusion appears solid and there is no loss of correction, external support is discontinued and the patient is allowed to be increasingly active. If there is any doubt, it is best to apply another snug, well-molded body cast, which is worn for two more months. General postural and gradual muscle-strengthening exercises are performed to rehabilitate the spine and the patient in general. Areas suspected of possible pseudarthrosis, if present, are

(Text continued on page 1234.)

Spinal Fusion for Scoliosis

Under general endotracheal anesthesia, using a nonexplosive agent, the patient is turned in the prone position. In order to replace blood throughout the procedure two large-gauge intravenous needles, usually of the plastic type, are mandatory. The availability of whole blood should be double-checked before starting the operation. The surgeon himself should supervise the positioning of the patient.

The author prefers to take the osteoperiosteal graft from the tibia. In the growing child, the donor leg is the one toward which his spine lists. As always, roentgenograms of the tibia are essential and should be studied prior to taking of the graft. A pneumatic tourniquet is placed on the proximal thigh, which, with a large sandbag, is elevated to facilitate its preparation. The whole back is prepared and draped. The use of a large self-adhering drape is of great help in ensuring asepsis. The spinous process of the seventh cervical vertebra and the ilium on both sides should be in the sterile field. The donor leg for the osteoperiosteal graft is acutely flexed at the knee and is firmly attached to the operating table.

A. The incision is made from above downward, through skin and subcutaneous tissue from a level one vertebra superior to the proposed fusion area to a level one vertebra inferior to it. The direction of skin incision is planned so that when the curve is recorrected in the cast, the operative scar will be straight. This improves the appearance of the back and draws less attention to any residual curve.

B. The superficial and deep fasciae are divided in a straight line over the spinous processes to be fused. Three or four Wheatlander retractors are placed to spread the wound under tension.

C. The median raphe is incised, exposing the tips of the spinous processes. Starting at the proximal end, the assistant presses down over the spinous process with a Kelly clamp, and the surgeon, with a scalpel, splits the cartilaginous tip of the spinous process longitudinally in the *midline* down to bone.

Plate 49. *Spinal Fusion for Scoliosis*

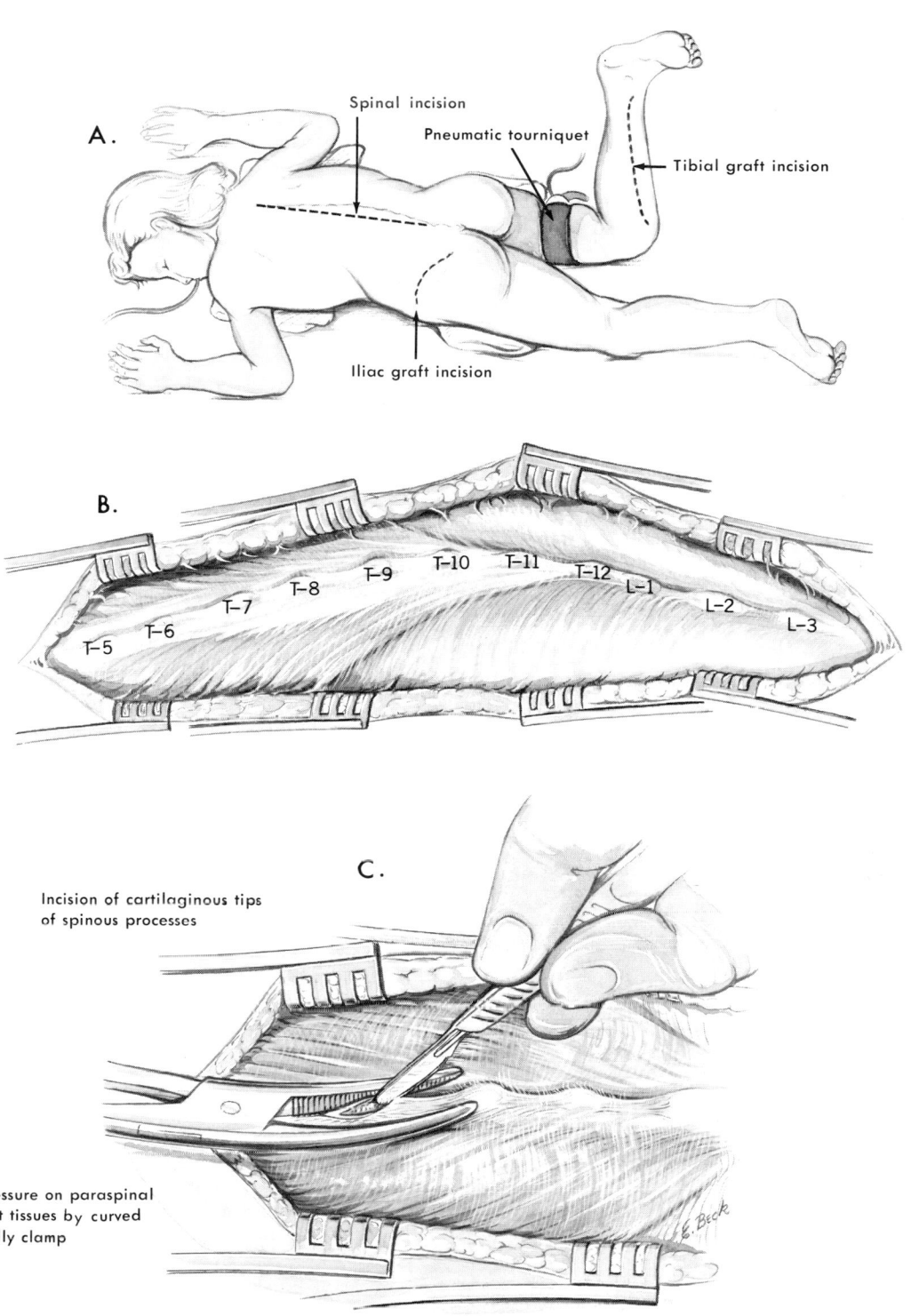

A.

Spinal incision

Pneumatic tourniquet

Tibial graft incision

Iliac graft incision

B.

T-5 T-6 T-7 T-8 T-9 T-10 T-11 T-12 L-1 L-2 L-3

C.

Incision of cartilaginous tips
of spinous processes

Pressure on paraspinal
soft tissues by curved
Kelly clamp

E. Beck

Spinal Fusion for Scoliosis *(Continued)*

D. Next, with Cobb periosteal elevators the spine is subperiosteally exposed as far laterally as the transverse process in the dorsal area and beyond the articular facets in the lumbar area. Subperiosteal stripping of muscle and soft tissues from the spinous process, lamina, and transverse process should be very meticulous. As the subperiosteal dissection is carried out, each level is packed firmly with gauze to minimize bleeding. When this is completed, the packing is removed and Wheat-lander retractors or laminectomy spreader retractors, or both, are placed deeply to spread the soft tissues out of the field. Next, with the scalpel, rongeurs, and curets, the interspinous ligaments and all remaining soft tissue tags are removed from the spinous processes, laminae, facet joints, and the transverse processes. The soft-tissue clean-up should be very thorough. Any bleeding, which may be vigorous in the intertransverse process spaces, is controlled with electrocautery.

E. Intra-articular fusion in the dorsal area is performed as follows: First, the posterior half of the facet joint is removed with a Hibbs or Cobb gouge.

F. Then, with a curet, all of its articular cartilage is removed.

G. Next, flaps of bone from the base of the transverse process are elevated and turned into the joint.

Plate 49. *Spinal Fusion for Scoliosis*

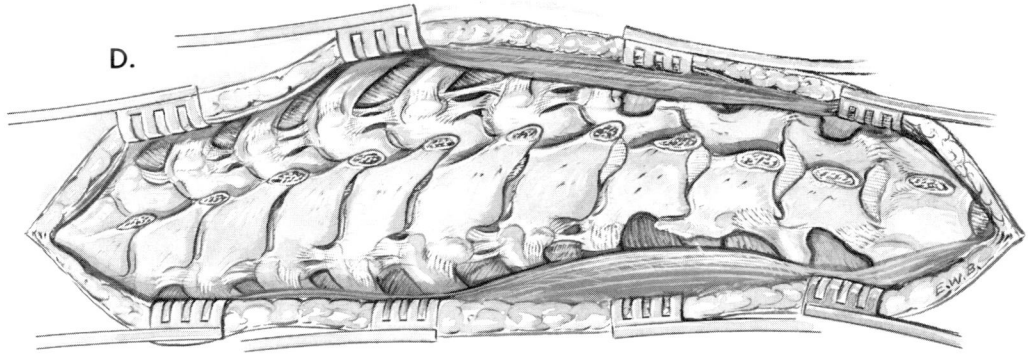

D.

Exposure of spinous processes, laminae, and transverse
processes of vertebrae to be fused

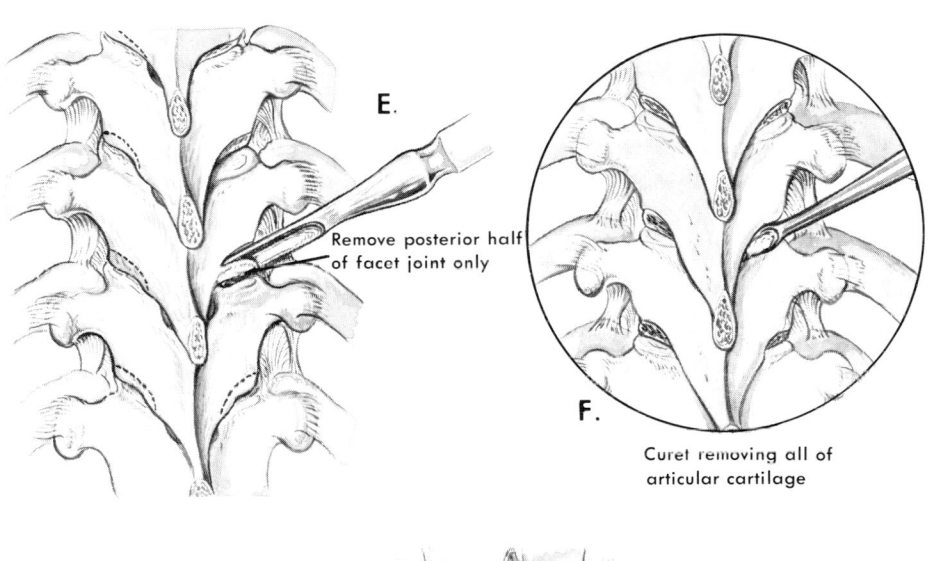

E.

Remove posterior half
of facet joint only

F.

Curet removing all of
articular cartilage

Facet joint fusion

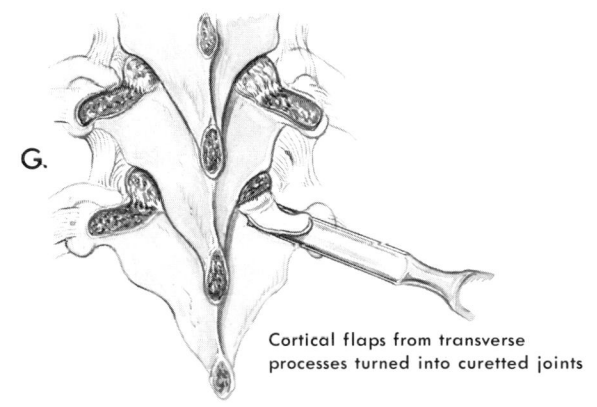

G.

Cortical flaps from transverse
processes turned into curetted joints

Spinal Fusion for Scoliosis *(Continued)*

H. In the lumbar area the articular facet is completely excised with osteotomes.

I. The articular cartilage is curetted out, and into each joint a block of bone (obtained from the spinous processes or ilium) is inserted and countersunk.

J. Next, with sharp Hibbs or Cobb gouges, multiple flaps of bone, half of its thickness and half of its width, are elevated from the base of the spinous processes and laminae. The assistant, with a suction tip, keeps the edge of the bone gouge free of blood and clearly visible to the surgeon. It is easy to keep the flaps attached at their base by rotating the edge of the sharp gouge. The free end of the flap from the lamina below is turned up and locked under the laterally bent flap of the lamina above. The superior half of the spinous process of the most cephalad vertebra of the fusion area and the most inferior one are left intact. The facet joints at the extremes of the fusion area (i.e., between the superior vertebra and the one above, and the inferior vertebra and the one below) are not disturbed. Then the remaining portion of each spinous process is partially divided with a Hibbs bone cutter, broken down, and turned up to bring it in contact with the next above. Thus, when decortication is completed, there is contact of abundant cancellous bone at the laminae, spinous processes, and at the facet joints.

Plate 49.   Spinal Fusion for Scoliosis

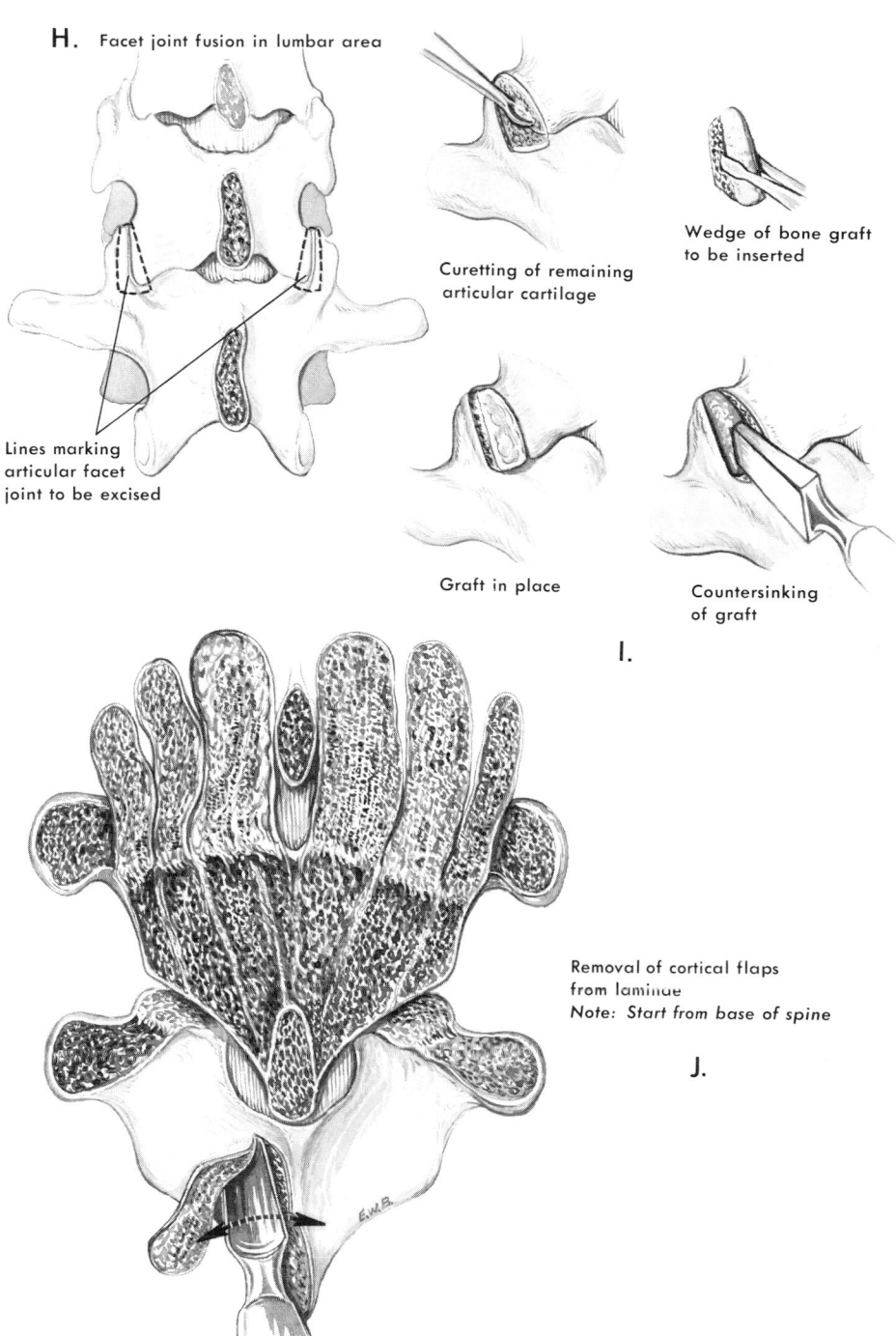

H. Facet joint fusion in lumbar area

Lines marking
articular facet
joint to be excised

Curetting of remaining
articular cartilage

Wedge of bone graft
to be inserted

Graft in place

Countersinking
of graft

I.

Removal of cortical flaps
from laminae
Note: Start from base of spine

J.

Spinal Fusion for Scoliosis *(Continued)*

K. The wound is irrigated. The osteoperiosteal bone graft taken from the tibia is divided into two unequal pieces. The longer piece should reach the end vertebrae of the fusion area. It is sutured to the base of the intact half of the spinous process of the inferior vertebra and placed snugly on the convex side of the curve. The shorter piece is sutured to the base of the intact half of the spinous process of the superior vertebra and also fitted on the convex side of the curve. There should be adequate overlap of the two fragments because the vertebral column will elongate as the scoliosis is corrected.

L. Fragments of autogenous bone from the tibia are laid down over the facet joint in the intertransverse process spaces and overlapping the laminae. Often surgeons dislike removing grafts from the patient's tibia and obtaining autogenous iliac grafts through a separate curved incision made just distal to the posterior half of the iliac crest. They place the cancellous and cortical bone grafts over the facet joints and overlapping the laminae.

M. The retractors are removed and the muscles are allowed to fall into place. The periosteum, with the deep layers of the muscle, is closed with interrupted sutures. The remaining wound is closed in layers in the usual manner.

Plate 49. Spinal Fusion for Scoliosis

K.

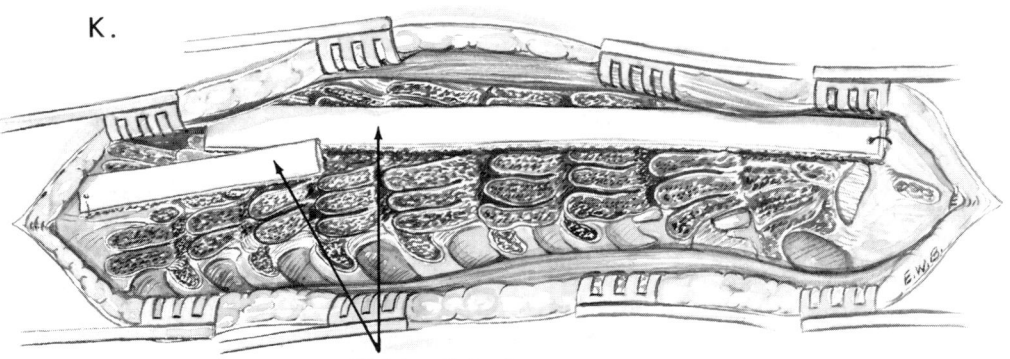

Tibial grafts in place.
Note: Long piece reaches the end
vertebrae of fusion area on convex side

L.

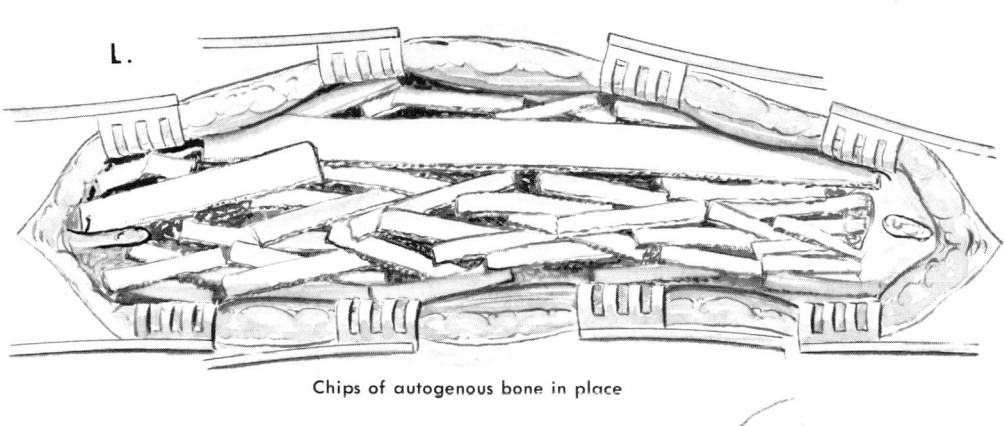

Chips of autogenous bone in place

M.

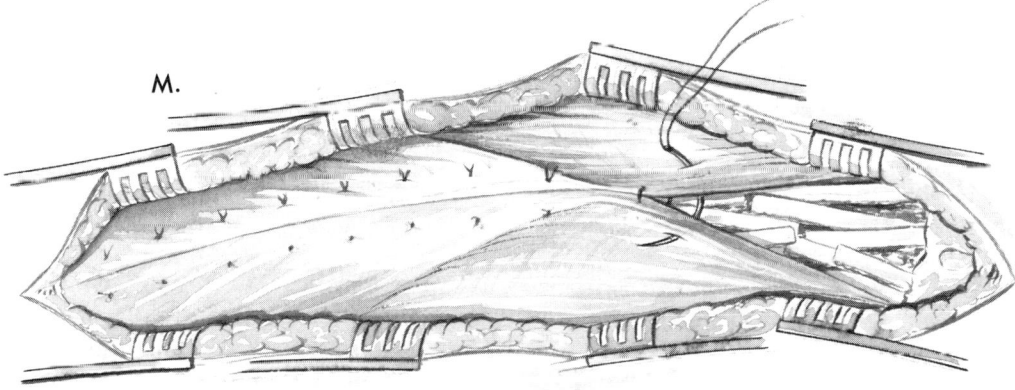

Deep closure

watched for an additional two months, during which walking is not permitted.

If the six-months-postoperative roentgenograms disclose an obvious pseudarthrosis, it is explored and fused without delay, and immobilization in the full localizer cast is continued for an additional three months.

Complications. Treatment of scoliosis by means of forcible correction and fusion may be beset with many complications. During correction of the curves by the cast, pressure sores may develop from friction of the cast against the skin in regions of inadequately padded bony prominences. The chin, occiput, scapula, iliac crests, sacrum, and ribs must be carefully padded before the cast is applied, and the cast should be well molded over or trimmed about them. It is best to make a V-shaped cut in the cast under the chin. Any complaints of pain, especially persistent burning pain, must be investigated. Brachial plexus palsy may develop as a result of traction on the cervical nerve roots or from direct pressure of the neckpiece or armpiece. It is usually encountered in patients in a turnbuckle Risser cast and can be avoided by bending the head toward the concavity of the curve and by forward flexion of 35 to 45 degrees of the shoulder with the armpiece while the cast is being applied. The author usually bivalves the superior half of the cast incorporating the arm. When the serious complication of brachial plexus palsy develops, correction of the curvature must be interrupted and resumed with extreme care only after the signs of palsy have disappeared.

Shock, respiratory or cardiac arrest, postoperative atelectasis, pneumonia, and wound infection are complications that may develop during the operation or in the immediate postoperative period. Generally, however, spinal fusion is a safe operation and the foregoing complications can be prevented when the necessary precautions are taken and the patient is carefully prepared for the procedure.

Loss of initial correction and recurrence of scoliotic deformity may be due to various causes. An inefficient cast may not hold the correction after spinal fusion. This is termed *holding loss*, and it is encountered more commonly with the use of turnbuckle jackets than with localizer casts. Early ambulation after surgery, delayed fusion, and pseudarthrosis are other factors to consider in determining the reason for loss of initial correction while the patient is in the cast.

Pseudarthrosis is the chief cause of recurrence of scoliosis. The reported incidence of pseudarthrosis varies in different centers. The relatively immobile thoracic spine fuses solidly in a much greater percentage of patients than do the more mobile thoracolumbar and lumbar spines. The longer the fusion area or the more severe the deformity, the higher is the incidence of pseudarthrosis. These factors are variables that influence the stress on the graft. The incidence of pseudarthrosis is greatest in paralytic scoliosis and in neurofibromatosis. The rate of pseudarthrosis can be diminished by excellent surgical technique, use of abundant autogenous bone in the fusion area, and an adequate period of effective immobilization of the spine to permit the fusion mass to mature.

Pseudarthrosis may be single or multiple. It may be easily seen on roentgenograms as a wide transverse radiolucent defect in the fusion area, or it may be a narrow transverse defect that may not be visible on roentgenograms and may be detected only because correction has been lost. Clinically, in addition to loss of correction, local tenderness over the fusion area should make one suspicious of the presence of pseudarthrosis. The roentgenograms, especially the oblique views, should be studied carefully. The danger of pseudarthrosis lies in the failure to diagnose and treat it.

Routine exploration of the fusion mass for pseudarthrosis is not justified, for this would result in about four out of five patients being subjected to an unnecessary surgical procedure. At the end of six months, when roentgenograms disclose suspicious defects, immobilization is continued for another two to three months, during which time ambulation is not allowed. Obviously defective grafts are explored and re-fused without further delay and the spine immobilized in recumbency in a full localizer corrective cast. When a single defect in the graft is demonstrated by the roentgenogram, it is best to explore the entire fusion area, as there may be others that cannot be visualized. On testing on the operating table, motion can be demonstrated between the two fragments. At exploration there will be a heavy solid graft covered by periosteum that strips readily up to the area of pseudarthrosis, where there is fibrous tissue tightly adherent to it.

Occasionally, a sinuous narrow defect may be hidden under an incomplete shell of apparently viable bone. If there is no motion between the fragments, one should leave its center third undisturbed for stability. Only the lateral thirds are cleared of all fibrous tissue down to raw bleeding bone with curet and rongeurs. The edges of the graft are undercut and packed with cancellous bone and slivers of cortical bone. When the pseudarthrosis is wide and there is motion between the fragments, the fibrous tissue should be removed with any sclerotic bone down to raw bleeding bone, and again the defect should be packed with cancellous bone. Flaps of bone should be raised up and down from the neighboring fusion mass to straddle the pseudarthrosis site along its full width, and long pieces of bone graft should be placed lengthwise across the defect.

The period of immobilization recumbency after repair of pseudarthrosis is usually shorter than that for primary correction of curves and fusion.

Errors in the selection of fusion area and inadequacy of fusion length are common causes of recurrence of scoliosis. When correction and fusion are done early in life, one or more adjacent vertebrae may become included in the major curve with further vertebral growth; this is another cause of recurrence of the deformity in the newly annexed section of the major curve. A short fusion has the same effect. The loss of correction will be progressive until vertebral growth is complete. Early recognition of the error and extension of the short fusion area will prevent loss of correction.

Fusion of just one of the double major curves or selection of the wrong curve for fusion are other causes of recurrence of scoliotic deformity. In such instances, the total balance of the patient and his spine should be evaluated with a thorough study of the roentgenograms of the spine, in-

cluding bending and pelvic tilt films, to determine which additional area or areas of the vertebral column should be corrected and fused. Sometimes the previous fusion mass should be osteotomized at the apex of the curve and the deformity corrected by application of a cast, the primary objective being compensation of the curves and balance of the spine.

COSMETIC SURGERY FOR SCOLIOSIS

Rotational and angular deformities of the spine may be so fixed that it may be impossible to effect any correction. Under these circumstances, operations to improve external appearance may be indicated. The two available surgical procedures are resection of the prominent rib hump and subtotal scapulectomy. These two procedures may be combined.

Resection of Prominent Rib Hump. Preoperative studies should be undertaken to determine the cause of the razor-back deformity. Where is the site of angulation of the ribs? Careful clinical palpation and tangential roentgenographic views of the spine in the forward-bend position are of some help. If the prominence of the ribs is a few inches away from the transverse processes, a pleasing cosmetic improvement will be obtained by resection of the posterior inner third and ends of the ribs in which the transverse processes are prominent (Fig. 6–55); whereas, if the main causes of razor-back deformity are rotated transverse processes and vertebral bodies with the rib angulation very close to the transverse process, improvement will be slight (Fig. 6–56). Pulmonary function studies are in order before advising such an operation.

The surgical approach is through the old midline spinal fusion incision with transverse lateral extensions for 3 to 4 inches along the lowest and highest rib to be resected. Resection of the supraspinous portion of the scapula is of great help in obtaining adequate access to the upper ribs. The skin, subcutaneous tissues, and deep fascia are divided in the line of incision. From the lateral border of the erector spinae muscles, parallel incisions are made along the center of each rib with a diathermy knife, the periosteum is stripped

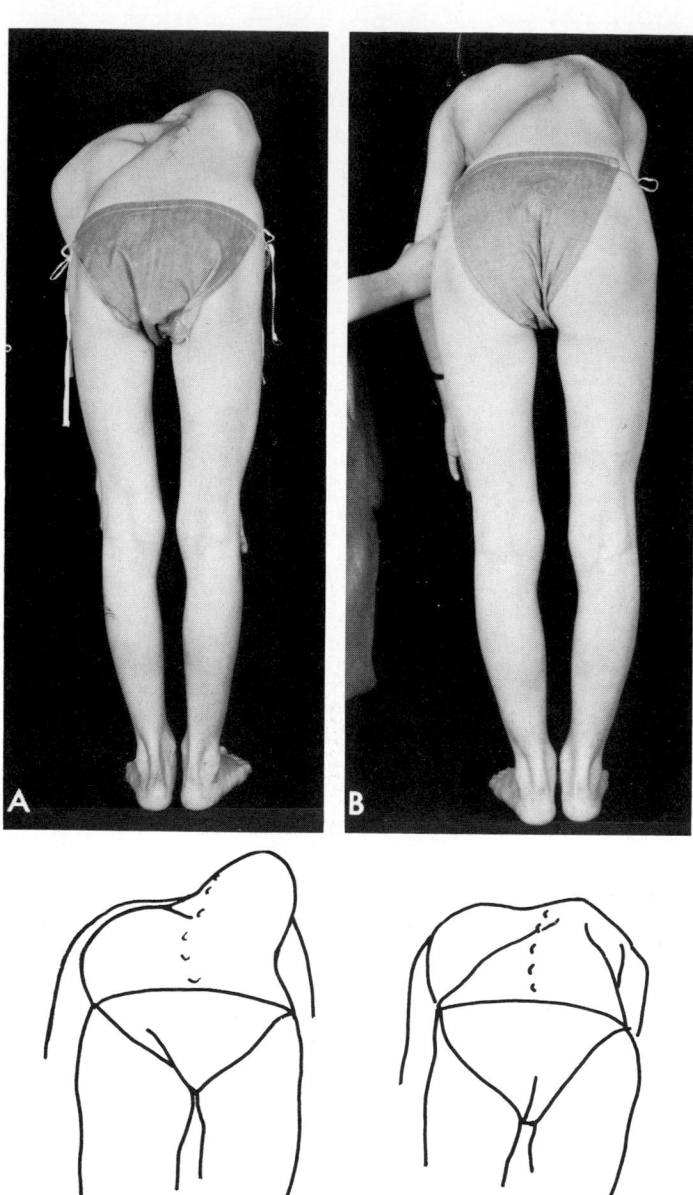

FIGURE 6–55.   *Forward bend photographs and sketches of patient before and after rib resection.*

Note the marked improvement in razor-back deformity in severe structural scoliosis. (From Roaf, R.: Scoliosis. Baltimore, Williams & Wilkins Co., 1966.)

off the ribs, and the posterior inner 4 or 5 inches of each rib is resected, including the transverse processes up to their base and the necks of the ribs up to the heads. The pleura should not be opened. Roaf recommends stabilization of the chest wall with No. 1 Mersaline sutures inserted through a hole (made with a rib punch) in each of the free ends of the resected ribs and secured to the corresponding interspinous ligaments.[314] It is desirable to drain

the extrapleural space with closed suction Hemovac drainage for a period of 24 to 48 hours. If the pleura is inadvertently opened, a separate intrapleural underwater drain is inserted, which is removed as soon as lung expansion is demonstrated in the postoperative roentgenograms.

Cosmetic improvement is usually satisfactory in the carefully chosen patient.

Subtotal Scapulectomy.   This is indicated when there is marked protrusion of the

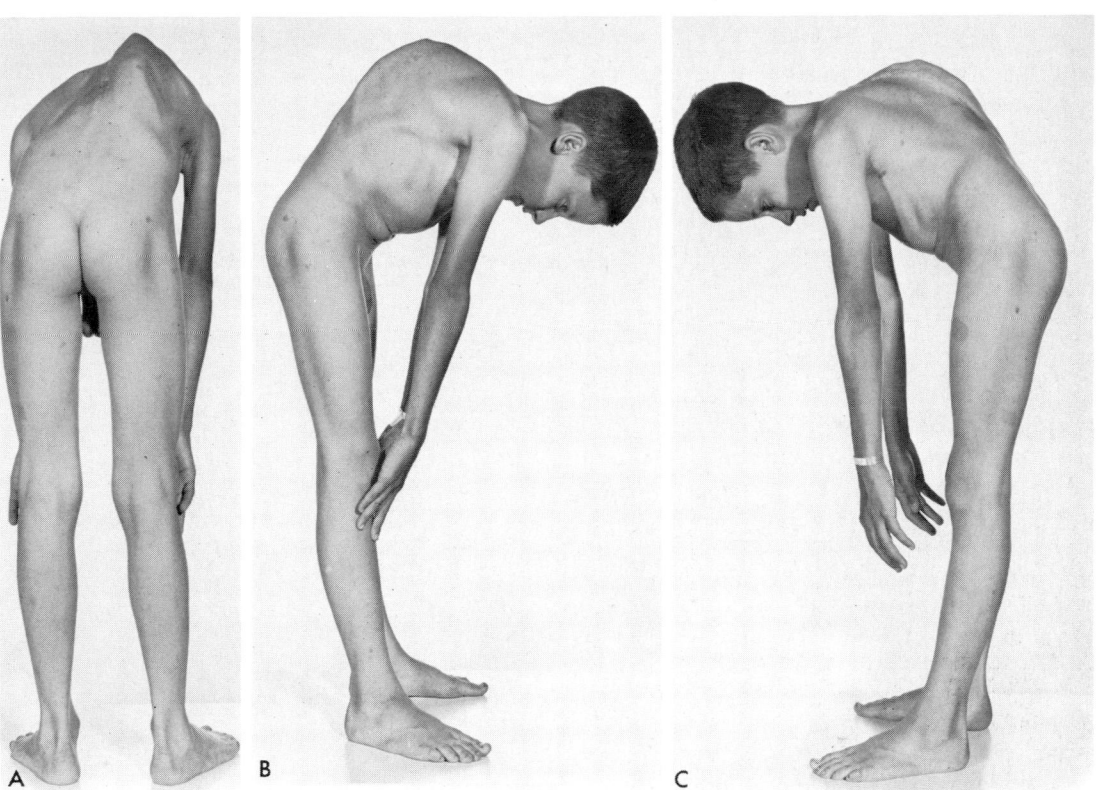

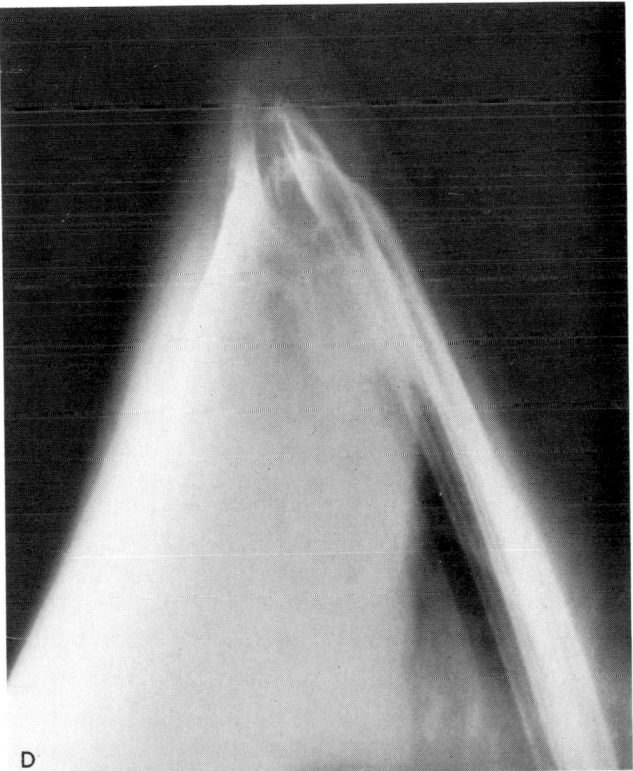

FIGURE 6–56.   Razor-back deformity in a ten-year-old boy with multiple neurofibromatosis and severe structural scoliosis.

Note the café-au-lait spots. Spinal fusion was performed at four years of age. **A** to **C.** Forward bend and side views showing the severe razor-back deformity. **D.** Tangential roentgenogram of the spine in forward bend position. Note the principal cause of razor-back deformity is the rotated transverse processes and the vertebral bodies with the rib angulation very close to the transverse processes. Improvement following rib and transverse process resection will be slight.

vertebral border and prominence of the scapula. It is advisable to excise most of the blade of the scapula, because, with limited excisions, one often finds that part of the stump now appears to protrude and a further procedure is necessary.

Equalization of Apparent Leg Length Inequality. If there is fixed lumbosacral scoliosis with marked tilting of the pelvis, the patient will have a noticeable list to one side. To compensate for the imbalance of the spine, the patient may stand with the knee flexed on the convex side and the ankle in equinus position on the concave side. The apparent leg length discrepancy may be corrected by a suitably built-up shoe, but many girls will not accept a raised shoe permanently. On such occasions, equalization of the inequality in leg length can be achieved by epiphysiodesis at the appropriate age in a young child or by shortening of the femur over an intramedullary rod on the long side. The femur can also be shortened in the subtrochanteric region and internally fixed with a large blade plate. Lengthening of the tibia on the short side in a mature person is a formidable procedure. It should not be undertaken unless the patient fully understands the problem and the possible risks.

INFANTILE STRUCTURAL IDIOPATHIC SCOLIOSIS

In this condition, scoliosis develops in infants and children before the age of three years. It is differentiated from congenital scoliosis by the absence of anomalies of the vertebrae or of the ribs at birth. It has been described by James, Scott, Morgan, and Lloyd-Roberts and Pilcher.[261, 270, 283, 320]

There are two forms of infantile structural scoliosis, the benign resolving type and the progressive type.

The *progressive type* always causes severe scoliotic deformity by the time of maturity. Progression is usually rapid and early, as much as 60 to 80 degrees within two years. As a general rule, if a curve exceeds 30 degrees at the age of one year, it will worsen. The progressive type is more common in boys and is most often located in the thoracic region. Eighty per cent of the curves are on the left. This type of deformity is always accompanied by compensatory curves. It is rare in the United States.

The *resolving type* is also common in boys and is often left-sided, but the curve does not exceed 37 to 40 degrees. Compensatory curves do not accompany the primary curve, and regardless of treatment, it resolves spontaneously within a few years.

Treatment should be aggressive in the progressive type. In the infant up to two years of age, a localizer Risser cast will correct and prevent progression of the curve. After two to three years, the child can wear the Milwaukee brace with good results. If conservative measures fail to check progression of the scoliosis, correction and fusion are indicated. In the young child, one should make sure the fusion is long enough because of the possible involvement of more vertebrae above and below the fused primary curve as growth proceeds.

PARALYTIC SCOLIOSIS

In this condition the primary cause of scoliosis is paralysis of one or more of the groups of trunk and abdominal muscles, commonly following an onset of poliomyelitis. The scoliosis generally presents a long "C" curve and is more flexible than other types of structural scoliosis. The degree and severity of collapse of the spine is dependent upon the extent of paralysis. Rapid progression of the curve can occur during a growth spurt.[221, 236, 237, 260, 280, 295, 313]

Stabilization of the spine is an important consideration in the treatment of paralytic scoliosis. When there is marked muscle weakness and respiratory difficulty, it is best to fuse the entire dorsal spine and most of the lumbar spine. High cervicodorsal curves should be fused early. The Harrington instrumentation procedure is used if the paralytic curve is severe but flexible; however, it should be performed only by the experienced who have mastered the technique. It should never be used without performing a meticulous spinal fusion at the same time. The bones should be large and strong enough to hold the metal device; consequently, use of the Harrington instrumentation is seldom indicated in patients under the age of ten years.

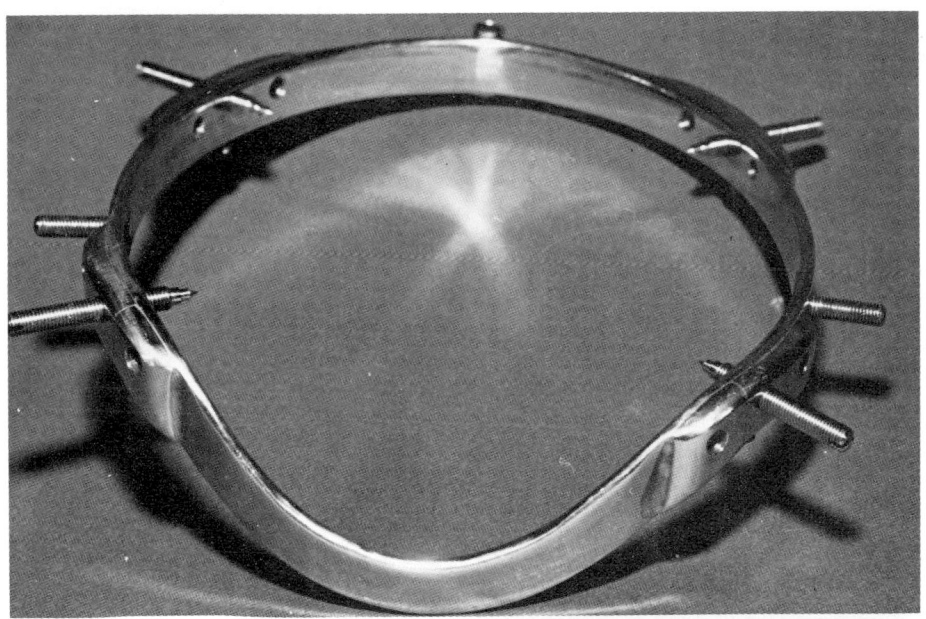

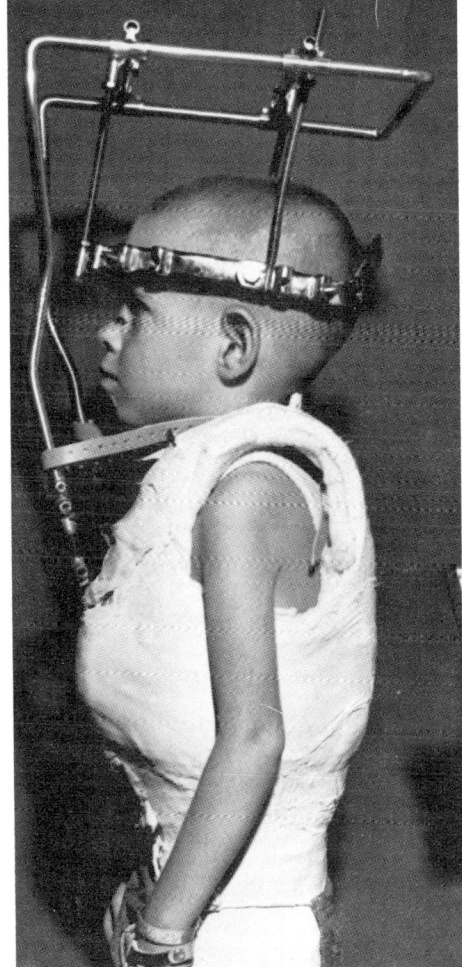

FIGURE 6–57. *Halo distraction apparatus.*

Top. Anterior view of the halo. **Bottom.** The halo distraction apparatus attached to patient and cast. (From Garrett, A. L., Perry, J., and Nickel, V. L.: Stabilization of the collapsing spine. J. Bone Joint Surg., 43–A:476, 1961.)

The halo distraction apparatus, attached to the patient and to the body cast, provides a method for correction and stabilization of curves involving the cervical and upper thoracic spine without external pressure upon the thoracic cage, a definite advantage when respiratory function is impaired (Fig. 6–57).[236, 237] Occasionally, one has to combine with the halo the use of bilateral femoral or tibial Steinmann pins or a pin through the pelvis to obtain skeletal distraction.[226] The use of fascial transplants may be indicated to support the paralyzed abdominal and trunk muscles.

SCOLIOSIS IN NEUROFIBROMATOSIS

The usual type of scoliosis associated with neurofibromatosis is characterized by a sharply localized short curve caused by a circumscribed area of neurofibromatosis adjacent to or in the vertebral column. The curve is often rapidly progressive and produces severe deformity. If it cannot be controlled by Milwaukee brace stabilization, early correction and fusion should be performed. Care should be taken to include enough of the spine on each side of the sharp curve to prevent recurrence of the scoliosis due to the involvement of additional vertebrae above and below the fused primary curve as the patient grows.

Occasionally, the scoliosis of neurofibromatosis is a long, gentle curve produced by conditions outside the vertebral column, such as the presence of marked leg length discrepancy or a heavy hypertrophied arm. Management of these curves is conservative, and correction and spinal fusion are rarely indicated.

POSTIRRADIATION SCOLIOSIS

Radiation of the area of the spine for conditions such as Wilms' tumor or neuroblastoma may affect growth of the vertebral column asymmetrically, producing scoliosis.[199, 264, 335] In the young child, if the curve is flexible, the use of the Milwaukee brace is indicated; however, if progression cannot be controlled by conservative measures, early surgical fusion is required.

SCOLIOSIS IN ARTHROGRYPOSIS MULTIPLEX CONGENITA

Some patients with arthrogryposis multiplex congenita develop scoliosis when they begin to sit and walk. Usually it is characterized by a long "C" curve caused by asymmetrical contracture of the muscles and ligaments of the trunk rather than by any abnormality of the vertebrae. Treatment is often conservative, consisting of passive stretching exercises and the use of the Milwaukee brace. Usually the severely afflicted child with marked involvement of the spinal musculature has decreased anteroposterior diameter of the chest and poor respiratory function (Fig. 6–58). Such children usually succumb to pulmonary infections, and operative procedures on the spine should be undertaken with great caution.

SCHEUERMANN'S JUVENILE KYPHOSIS

Definition

Scheuermann's juvenile kyphosis is an arcuate and fixed kyphosis developing around the time of puberty. It is caused by a wedge-shaped deformity of one or more vertebrae that show certain roentgenographic changes. This characteristic wedging of the vertebral bodies with diminished anterior height was first described in 1920 by Scheuermann, who emphasized that a definite diagnosis is possible only by means of roentgenographic study.[359] In his original description, Scheuermann nearly always found three abnormal wedge-shaped vertebrae in each case, but he reported in 1936 that the number might vary from one to five.[360] The presence of wedge-shaped vertebrae is an important sign, and according to measurements of vertebral wedging, the limit between abnormal and normal appears to be in the vicinity of a wedging of 5 degrees.[347, 349] The roentgenographic definition of Scheuermann's juvenile kyphosis is a kyphosis including at least three adjacent vertebrae with wedging of 5 degrees or more.[362]

Incidence

The absolute incidence of Scheuermann's kyphosis in the general population is not known. The reported incidence is 6 per cent in soldiers and 8 per cent in men working in industry.[362] Reports regarding the incidence in adult females are not available.

Etiology and Pathogenesis

Its cause is still unknown. Many theories have been advanced, however. Initially, Scheuermann, in 1920, considered the changes to be caused by aseptic necrosis of bone of the same nature as that of Legg-Perthes disease.[359] The wedging of the vertebra was explained as the result of aseptic necrosis in the limbus primordium, which disturbed the growth of the height of the vertebral body anteriorly, it being assumed that this growth took place from the limbus. In the beginning this theory was widely accepted, but later Scheuermann emphasized that the changes must be caused by an unknown basic factor.[360]

Some authors proposed damage to the limbus primordium by inflammation or mild infection (epiphysitis). The theory that proposed epiphysitis to be the etiologic factor could not be accepted by others because inflammatory changes could not be demonstrated.[350–352]

Pathologic studies on patients with Scheuermann's juvenile kyphosis disclosed limbi that were grossly as well as microscopically normal.[356, 361] Wedging in patients as young as nine years, even before onset of ossification of the limbus, was found by Scheuermann in roentgenographic studies.[360] These findings tend to refute the theory of aseptic necrosis of the limbus.

Schmorl performed autopsies on six patients with Scheuermann's kyphosis aged 16 to 24 years. He advanced the theory that juvenile kyphosis was due to changes of the discs in the middle and lower thoracic spine. The bulged discs would rupture into the spongiosa through preformed or traumatic tears in the end-plates, with the resultant diminution in mass and deformity of the discs. At the site of the perforation of the cartilage plates, enchondral skeletal growth was inhibited. Growth would also be delayed in the anterior part of the vertebral bodies, which were exposed to relatively great pressure because of the kyphosis. He claimed that these changes were not present in other types of kyphosis than the juvenile one.[361]

Schmorl's theory, however, was challenged by the finding of such changes in the vertebrae outside the area of kyphosis in patients with Scheuermann's kyphosis, and even in persons who did not have Scheuermann's disease.[360, 364]

Mechanical and static forces have been considered to be of etiologic importance. Ferguson implicated the anterior groove as a causative factor. He reviewed unselected normal lateral chest films in the age group from 6 to 11 years and observed the anterior vascular groove to close with anterior wedging and the development of a round back in preadolescents.[348] On dissection, it was found that the indentation in the anterior border of the vertebra, as seen on the roentgenogram was occupied by a large endothelium-lined vascular lake formed by the confluence of veins at this point. The stresses of upright posture and reduction of the spring action of the spine was implicated by Lambrinudi as a cause of wedging of the vertebrae.[351]

Injuries prior to clinical onset of Scheuermann's kyphosis have only been described in 5 per cent to 12 per cent of the cases.[351, 360]

The theory of mechanical factors as a cause of Scheuermann's kyphosis does not have an experimental basis. Investigators inserted steel wires subcutaneously into the tails of castrated and noncastrated male rats, fixing the steel wires to subcutaneous tissues and bending them to create a fixed kyphotic position that was maintained for a period of three to six months. Even at the end of six months, histologic studies did not reveal any pressure necrosis or areas of degeneration in the cartilage or bone. Roentgenograms did not disclose wedging of the vertebral bodies in any case.[353]

The studies of Sørensen showed a very high familial occurrence of Scheuermann's kyphosis, but could not demonstrate any mode of inheritance.[362]

Accumulated data of pathologic findings in the early stages of the disease are very

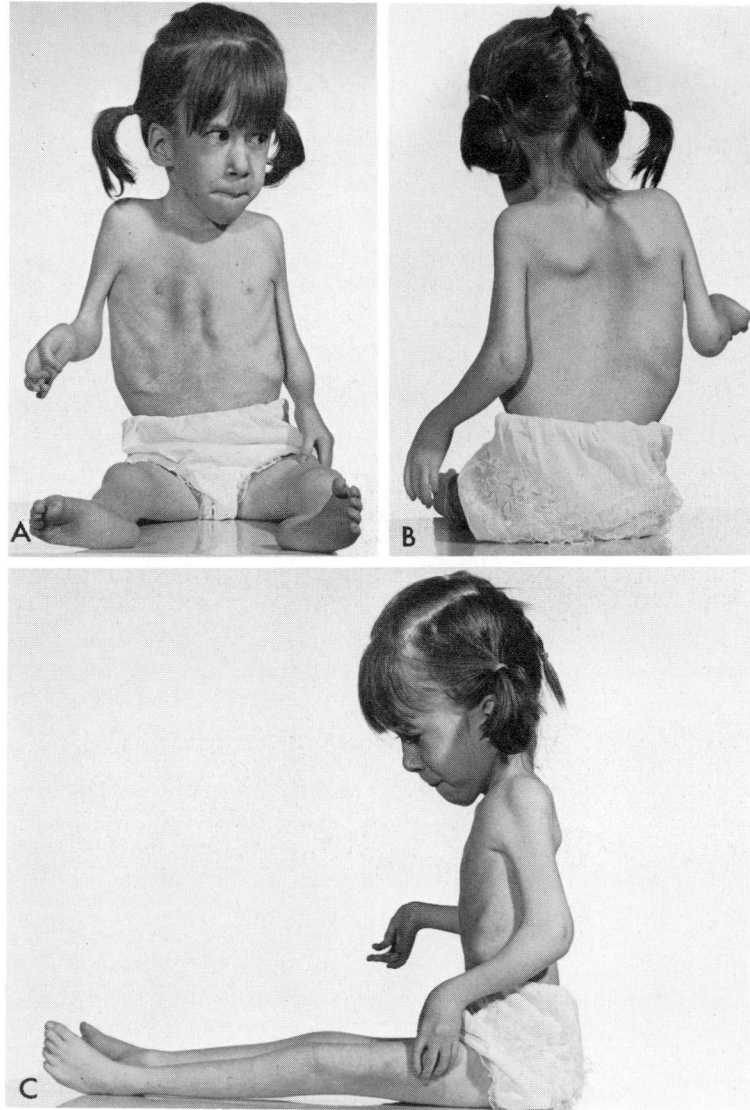

FIGURE 6–58.   Scoliosis in arthrogryposis multiplex congenita.

A to **C.** Anterior, posterior, and lateral views of a three-year-old child with severe arthrogryposis multiplex congenita. Note the severe contractural deformities, hydrocephalus, and right thoracolumbar scoliosis. There is marked dorsal lordosis and decrease of anteroposterior diameter of the chest.

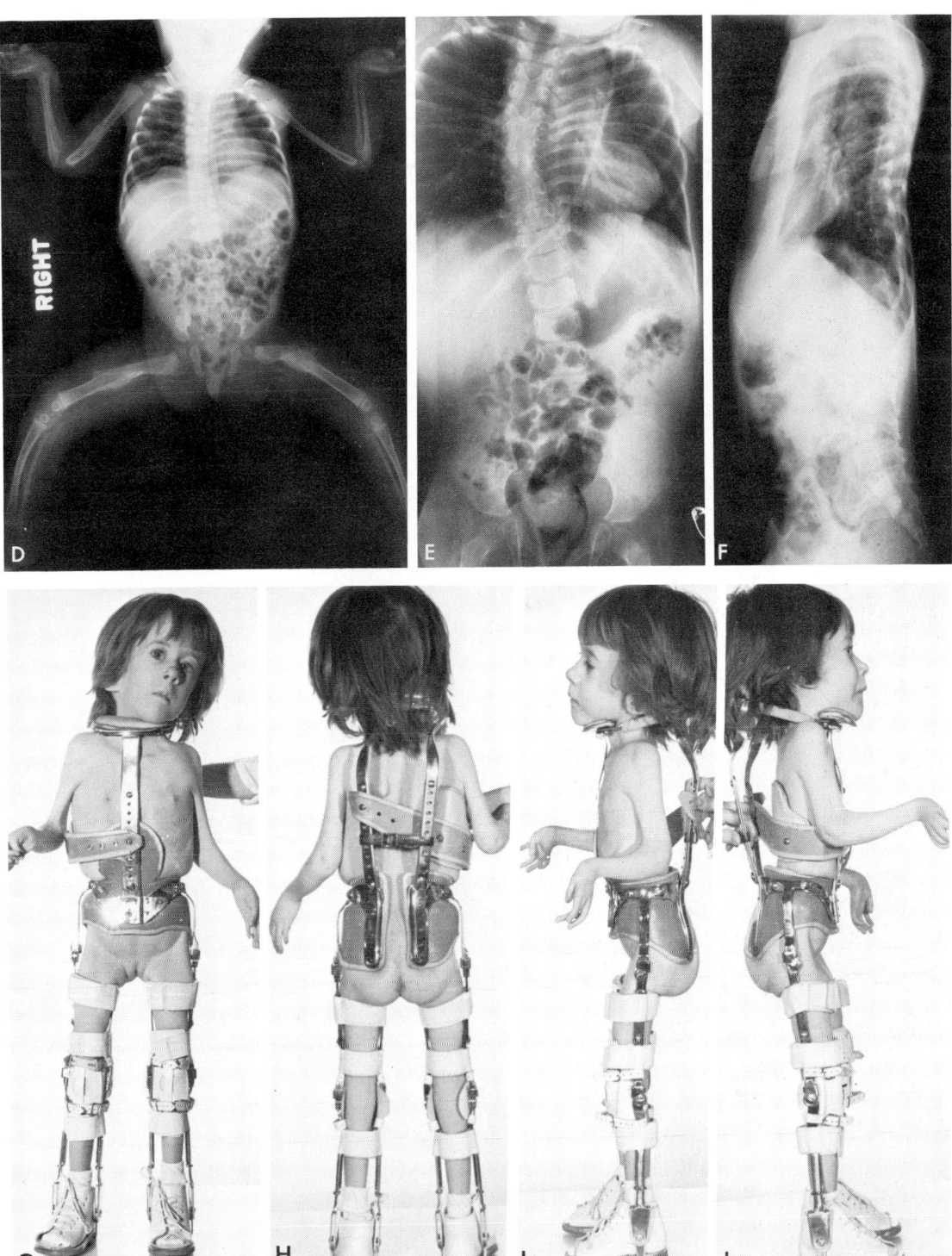

FIGURE 6–58 Continued. *Scoliosis in arthrogyposis multiplex congenita.*

D. Roentgenograms of spine, depicting the scoliosis at three months of age. **E** and **F.** Roentgenograms of spine, anteroposterior and lateral, at 18 months of age showing the increased scoliosis and the severe dorsal lordosis. **G** to **J.** Views of child in Milwaukee brace (old type). A chin guard was added to control rotation of neck. Long leg orthoses are used for ambulation.

meager because of the rarity of the opportunity to perform postmortem studies.

Clinical Features

The disease is equally common in both sexes. The age of clinical manifestation is from 13 to 17 years, i.e., around puberty, occurring somewhat earlier in girls than in boys. In a few cases, it has been observed as early as nine years of age.

The patient is usually presented with the complaint of poor posture. He may complain of fatigue or pain in the region of the kyphosis. The aching sensation is aggravated after standing in the same position for a long time and is relieved by a change in position, particularly by lying down.

The physical findings depend upon the location of the apex of kyphosis. Its site is purely thoracic in about three fourths, thoracolumbar in nearly one fourth, and lumbar in only a few of the patients. If the summit is in the thoracic area, there is marked accentuation of the normal dorsal kyphosis, increased lumbar lordosis, and a protuberant abdomen. The upper trunk and drooping shoulders are held backward with the center of gravity falling behind the sacrum, and the normal pelvic tilt is exaggerated. As a rule, the cervical lordosis also becomes increased. The exaggerated cervical and lumbar lordosis is a compensatory phenomenon.

If the apex is at the thoracolumbar level, the result is a long kyphosis and a short, low lumbar lordosis. If the lesion is purely lumbar, the postural defect is that of a straight back with a flat thoracic spine and an angular transition between the kyphosis and the sacrum.

In the beginning stages, the postural defect may be corrected both actively and passively, but gradually, within a period of six to nine months, the kyphosis becomes fixed.

A minimal structural scoliosis in the area of kyphosis is present in about 30 to 40 per cent of patients.

Local tenderness on direct manual pressure or light percussion may be present. Muscle and neurologic examination is usually within normal limits. The hamstrings are commonly shortened, as shown by limitation of straight leg raising and inability to touch the floor on forward flexion of the spine.

Roentgenographic Findings

A positive diagnosis of Scheuermann's juvenile kyphosis is only possible by means of radiography. In the lateral view the constant finding is the wedge shape of the affected vertebrae (Fig. 6–59). The wedging is most marked in the central area of the kyphosis and diminished cephalad and caudad. Measurement of the vertebral wedging (vw) is carried out on the lateral roentgenogram by drawing lines through the levels of the two end-plates and determining the angle between the two lines with an ordinary goniometer (Fig. 6–60). The limit between abnormal and normal vertebral wedging appears to be 5 degrees. The *kyphotic angle* (kw) is the angle between the upper end-plate of the cranial vertebra in the kyphosis and the lower end-plate of the caudal vertebra in the kyphosis.

Disc protrusions into the spongiosa of the vertebra described by Schmorl, and known as Schmorl's nodules, are frequently found on x-rays in the lateral views.[361] The Schmorl's nodules may be single or paired in the two vertebrae on either side of the disc and are delimited from the spongiosa by a narrow, more or less dense osseous zone.

Irregularity of the end-plates, which may be "moth-eaten," frayed, or indented, is often seen. These changes are frequently observed in the vertebrae that are deformed by Schmorl's nodules. The intervertebral discs are normal in the early stage of the disease, maintaining their height between the wedged vertebrae; later, they narrow, particularly in the central area of kyphosis. The anteroposterior diameter of wedged vertebrae may be increased.

The vascular groove from the anterior border into the body has been reported by Ferguson to be visibly longer than normal; however, this finding has not been confirmed by others.[348, 362]

Toward the end of the growth period the anterior corners of the kyphotic vertebrae may be sharpened. Later in adult life osteo-

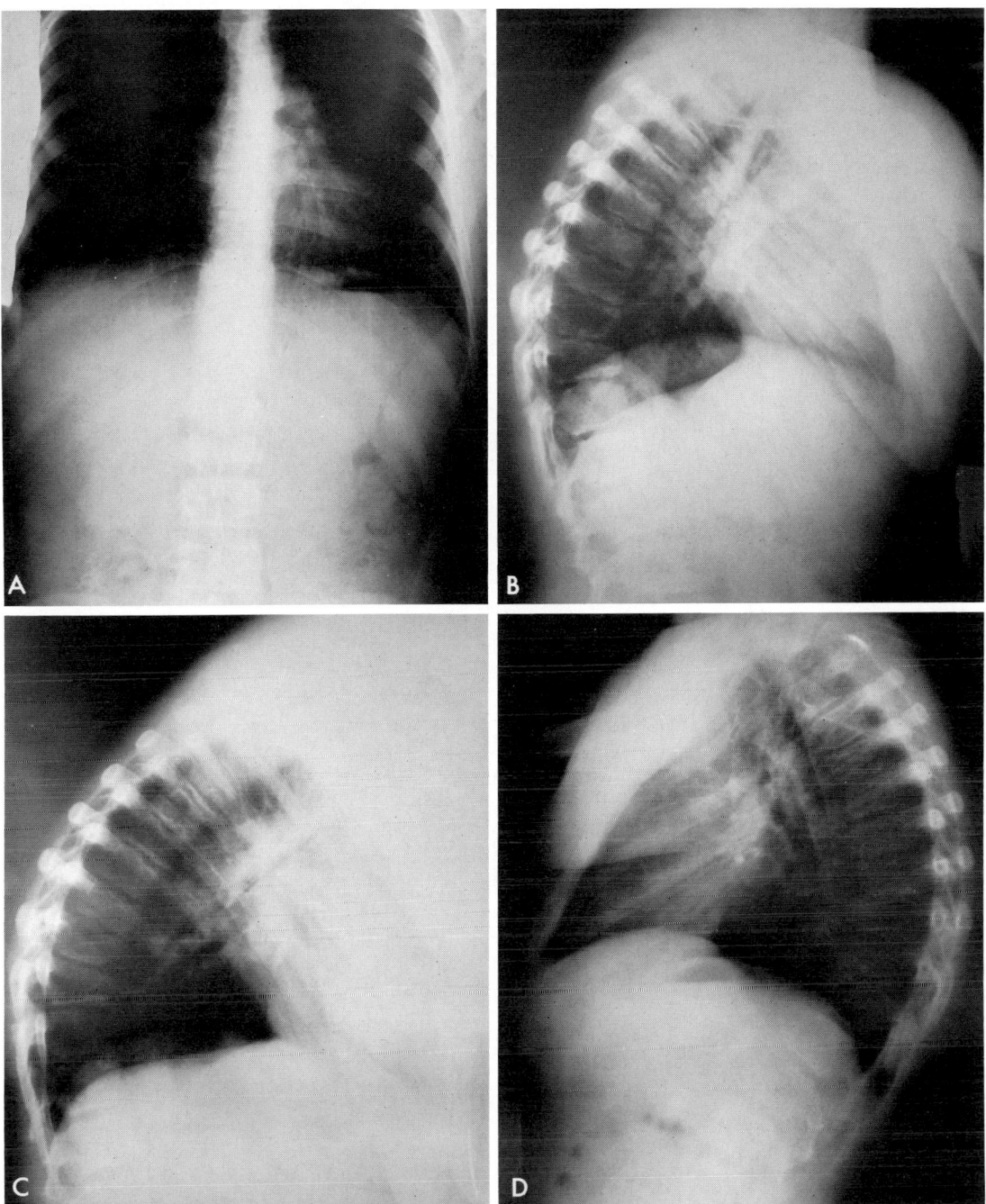

FIGURE 6–59. *Scheuermann's juvenile kyphosis involving the eighth, ninth, and tenth thoracic vertebrae.*

A and **B.** Anteroposterior and lateral views of dorsal spine. **C** and **D.** Flexion and extension views.

phytes may develop at the anterior border of the deformed vertebral bodies.

Natural History, Course, and Prognosis

From the onset of the disease until the cessation of growth the roentgenographic changes have been divided into several stages. Mau, in 1925, grouped them as follows:

  I. Stage of irritation (limbus changes)
  II. Stage of deformation development of wedging)
  III. Stage of repair (epiphyseal synostosis at cessation of growth)
  IV. Stage of proliferation (development of exostosis)[352]

Nathan and Kuhns classified the course into the *early* stage, the *healing* stage, and the *healed* stage, corresponding approximately to the classification of Mau. They noted that during the healing stage there was no progression of the wedge deformity and the structural changes present in the healed stage remained constant throughout life.[355]

A combined clinical-roentgenographic course of the disease was subdivided into the following stages by Brocher:

  I. *Functional phase*, characterized clinically by poor posture from the age of nine or ten years. There may be some exaggeration of dorsal kyphosis, but there is no pain or other clinical symptom. It is rare, however, that one diagnoses Scheuermann's kyphosis in this stage. It is usually found accidentally while studying roentgenograms of the chest or spine that were taken for other reasons, or by examining the younger siblings of patients with known Scheuermann's kyphosis. In the roentgenogram, this phase is characterized by regular but abnormal wedging of several vertebrae.

  II. *Florid stage*, which represents the typical clinical picture in the age range of 12 to 18 years. There is fixation of the kyphosis and possible minimal scoliosis in the area. Pain and fatigue in the back are usual complaints. Radiologically, this phase is characterized by abnormal wedging of the vertebrae with irregular end-plates, and not infrequently by Schmorl's nodules.

  III. *Late stage*, seen in adult life. There is wedge deformity of the vertebrae with more regular end-plates, narrowing of the discs, and development of osteophytes. Local back pain is common. The muscles at the site of the kyphosis are poorly developed and may be the site of fibrositis.[344, 345]

Sørensen, in his long-term study, came to the following conclusions: (1) Back pain and fatigue are less common after the completion of growth than before its completion, having no effect on the working capacity of the patient. (2) One half of the patients develop low back pain later in life, and about one quarter of the patients develop low lumbar disc degeneration. In general, the extent and severity of kyphosis could not be correlated with low back pain, low lumbar disc degeneration, or strenuosity of the patient's work. (3) When the site of kyphosis was low or when it was long, involving the second lumbar vertebra cau-

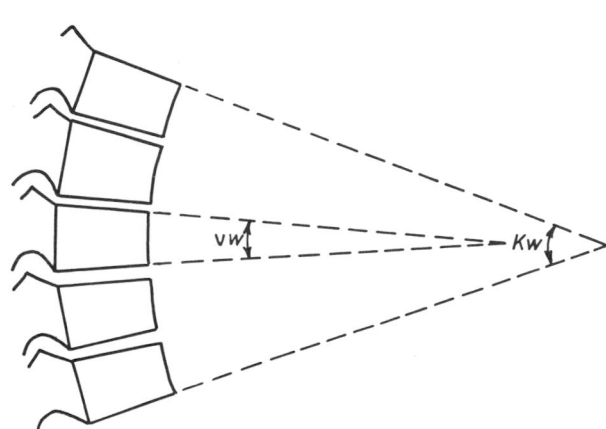

FIGURE 6–60. *The method of measuring the degree of vertebral wedging (vw) and of kyphosis (kw). See text for explanation.*

(From Sørensen, H. K.: Scheuermann's Juvenile Kyphosis. Copenhagen, Munksgaard, 1964.)

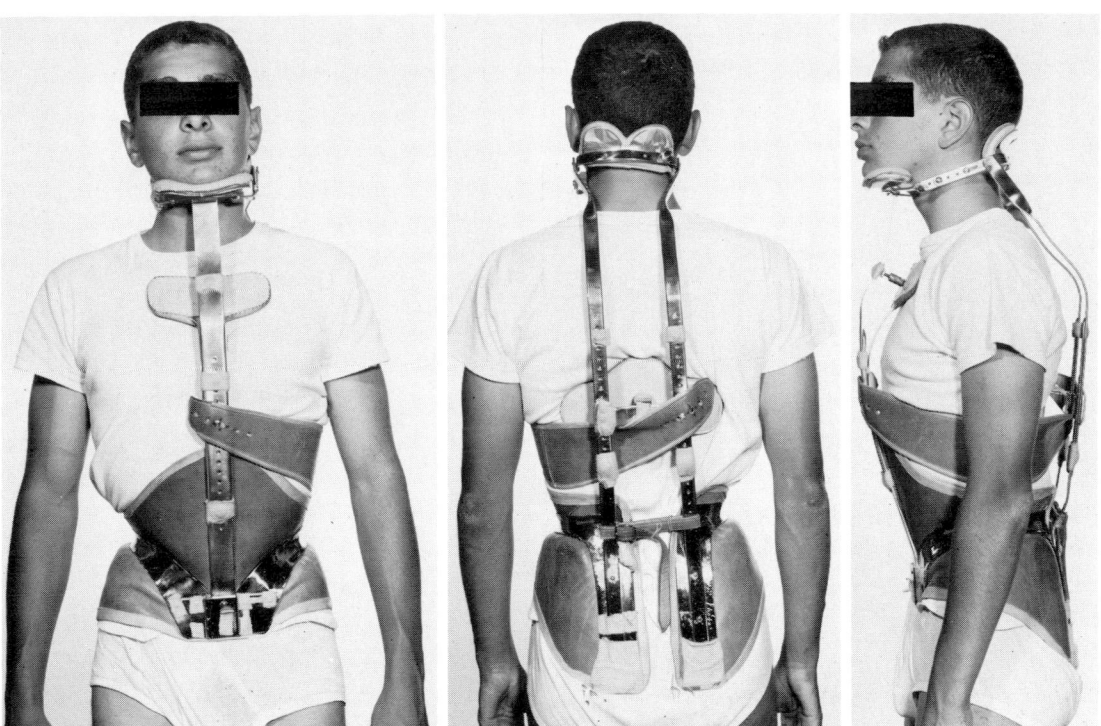

FIGURE 6–61. *Milwaukee brace used for Scheuermann's disease.*

Note the sternal pad and the kyphos pad located posteriorly just below the apex of the kyphosis. With the new throat mold and close fit of the uprights these pads are usually unnecessary.

dally, the incidence of low lumbar disc degeneration causing pain was very high. (4) Roentgenologically, there will be a slow progression of the kyphosis due to very slight increase in vertebral wedging and to narrowing of the discs. (5) The prognosis appears to be most unfavorable for patients with low kyphosis if the lordosis below is entirely abolished, whereas it is extremely favorable in the classic type of Scheuermann's kyphosis confined to the thoracic spine.[362]

Treatment

The most effective method of treatment is the Milwaukee brace. In the past, a sternal pad and a kyphos pad were used (Fig. 6–61). With the new throat mold and close fit of the uprights, these pads are usually not necessary, as the dorsal kyphosis can be effectively corrected by the distraction forces and by increasing the pelvic tilt and decreasing the exaggerated lumbar lordosis. Results of treatment of Scheuermann's disease with the Milwaukee brace have been excellent according to the experience of the author. The brace is worn continuously for at least 12 months until there is radiologic evidence of healing; then the brace is used only at night for another 12 months.

General postural exercises are performed out of the brace and are continued for a considerable period of time after use of the brace has been discontinued.

Disorders of Intervertebral Discs in Children

INTERVERTEBRAL DISC CALCIFICATION

Calcification of intervertebral discs was first described by Calvé and Galland in 1922.[369] It is common after the fifth decade of life, when, in most cases, it is an accidental roentgenographic finding, usually occurring in the thoracic or thoracolumbar region. In adults, it is thought to be a degenerative process.

In children, intervertebral disc calcification is rare, but in recent years has been recognized more frequently. It is commonly located in the cervical spine, but does occur in the thoracic or lumbar disc spaces. The comprehensive papers of Eyring et al, Newton, Silverman and Weens have reviewed most of the cases.[376, 386, 394, 398]

Etiology

Despite many theories, the cause of this disease is uncertain. It has been suggested that disc calcification is the result of a metastatic infective process.[382] The normal adult disc is avascular, but in children the intervertebral disc is supplied by a number of blood vessels that penetrate the cartilage plate, connecting it with the general circulation. These vascular channels in the discs undergo degeneration early in life, gradually disappearing by the age of 20 or 30 years. Thus, the discs in children may be exposed to infectious agents carried in the blood stream. However, strong evidence against infection is the fact that in the majority of cases there is no sign of pyogenic infection and the course of the disease is not the same as in infectious discitis. Calcification of discs in children may represent a nonspecific inflammatory reaction.

Trauma has often been implied as a predisposing factor, but in many children with disc calcification, a definite history of preceding injury cannot be obtained. In children, it seems unlikely that degenerative and vascular disease processes are etiologic agents. Generalized metabolic diseases such as alkaptonuric ochronosis have been ruled out by the negative urinary studies for ochronosis. The multiple disc calcifications in ochronosis do not develop until middle age.

Clinical Picture

Intervertebral disc calcification in childhood presents a distinct clinical syndrome. It is more frequent in the male, approximately in the ratio of two to one. The average age at the time of initial symptoms and diagnosis is seven years. When calcification occurs in the cervical spine, almost all patients have complaints and positive findings consisting of (1) neck pain, local or referred; (2) limitation of neck motion associated frequently with varying degrees of torticollis; (3) local tenderness; and (4) evidence of inflammation, as shown by elevation of temperature, or erythrocyte sedimentation rate, and of white blood count. Most patients are symptom-free within 14 days; however, a few will continue to have occasional neck pain for one or two years.

Calcified thoracic and lumbar discs, often an incidental roentgenographic finding, are generally multiple, asymptomatic, and persistent (Fig. 6–62). A definite association of this condition with congenital heart disease has been reported.

Roentgenographic Findings

In the cervical spine, the highest incidence of calcification is in the lower cervical region, but it does occur in all interspaces from the second to the seventh cervical vertebrae. More than one disc may be calcified. The site of calcification is usually central in the disc, presumably in the nucleus pulposus. Usually radiographic appearance of calcium is seen from several days to three weeks after the onset of symptoms. However, there are reported cases in which intervertebral disc calcification was noted long prior to the onset of symptoms, as

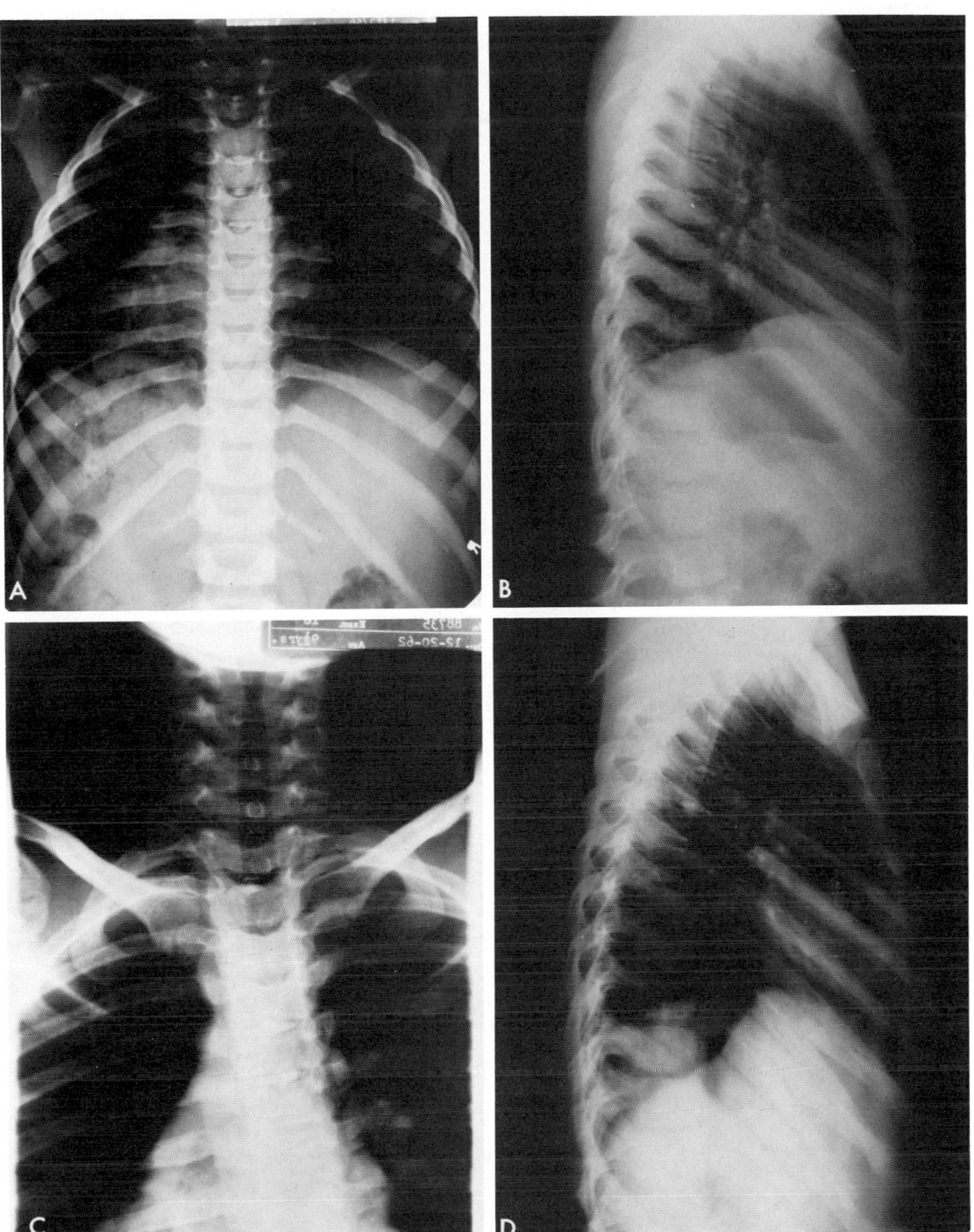

FIGURE 6–62. *Intervertebral disc calcification in upper dorsal vertebrae.*

A and **B.** Anteroposterior and lateral roentgenograms of dorsal spine. Note the calcified intervertebral discs between T3, T4, and T5 vertebrae. **C** and **D.** Anteroposterior and lateral roentgenograms of dorsal spine of same patient six years later. Note the persistence of calcification.

if they were lying dormant. Usually there is subsequent regression and disappearance of calcification following the onset of neck symptoms. Resolution of these calcifications supports the presence of the previously described blood vessels supplying the discs.

In long-term follow-up of some patients there has been persistence of residual calcification of the disc interspace, flattening of the vertebral bodies, and osteophytes.[376]

Treatment

Simple conservative measures such as neck traction, cervical collar, and analgesics are effective in controlling symptoms. The prognosis is good. The use of roentgen therapy, chelating agents, and antibiotics is not justifiable. Occasionally, the involved disc may prolapse posteriorly or laterally.[389, 396] In such cases, appropriate treatment such as decompression and disc excision is carried out if persistence and severity of neurologic deficit and symptoms warrant it.

DISCITIS

Discitis is an infectious or inflammatory lesion affecting the intervertebral disc in children. In the embryo and the young child the intervertebral discs receive their blood supply from the surfaces of the adjacent vertebral bodies.[399, 403, 422] The blood supply to the intervertebral disc in childhood makes it possible for bacteria to gain entrance into the disc through the hematogenous route, which is not possible in the adult. The vascular supply to the intervertebral discs is greater in early life, and it gradually decreases with advancing age. Böhmig states that infectious blood diseases could affect the disc up to the twentieth year of age.[399] Another source of infection of the intervertebral disc is by direct inoculation of the bacteria, as in lumbar puncture or myelography.

Narrowing of the intervertebral disc due to infection or inflammation has been described under various names in the literature.[399–424] A. DeF. Smith, in 1933, described it under the title "A Benign Form of Osteomyelitis of the Spine."[421] Harbin and Epton

observed that, in some patients with osteomyelitis of the spine, the infection involved only the intervertebral disc, without osseous involvement.[409] Ghormley et al., in 1940, described 20 adult patients with narrowing of an intervertebral disc in a "Study of Acute Infectious Lesions of Intervertebral Discs," proposed that, if osseous involvement of the vertebrae was extensive, a diagnosis of osteomyelitis should be made; if absent or minimal, it was assumed that the lesion represented an infection of the disc and not osteomyelitis.[407] In describing the clinical entity the term "acute osteitis of the spine" was used by Bremner and Neligan, and "spondylarthritis" by Saenger.[400, 419] Mathews et al. reported on nine children, calling the condition a "destructive lesion involving the intervertebral disc in children," and proposed that the disorder is a primary disease of the intervertebral disc that is self-limited and has a good prognosis.[416] Doyle reported 16 children with this condition under the title "Narrowing of the Intervertebral Disc Space in Children. Presumably an Infectious Lesion of the Disc."[404] DuPont and Anderson and Jamison et al. called it nonspecific spondylitis; Menelaus reported on 35 children and gave credit to Price for coining the word *discitis* to describe the disorder as essentially an inflammation affecting a disc with little or no evidence of primary bone involvement.[405, 410, 417] In the series of 35 children reported on by Menelaus, the lumbar spine was involved in 74 per cent, the thoracic spine, in 24 per cent, and in one child, the cervical spine was affected. More than one intervertebral disc may be involved.

Clinical Findings

The typical patient is a young child between two and seven years of age who is brought to the physician with a complaint of pain in the back of one or two weeks' duration. The backache is localized around the involved vertebral area, although it may radiate as vague pains in the buttock, thigh, knee, or abdomen. However, it lacks any true radicular nature. Parents usually state that the child has a limp or refuses to sit, stand, or walk. An upper respiratory infection or an episode of diarrhea may precede the onset of the illness.

On physical examination the child does not appear to be acutely ill, but is irritable and prefers the recumbent position. The temperature may be elevated, but generally not above 100° or 101° F. Paravertebral muscle spasm is the principal physical finding (Fig. 6–63). The normal lumbar lordosis may be lost. Hamstring muscle spasm, if present, will limit straight leg raising. Koenig's sign may be positive, with pain in the back on flexion of the neck. On careful examination, in a cooperative child, tenderness at the site of the lesion may be noted. There is no neurologic deficit; sensation, reflexes, and motor strength are normal. At first, the erythrocyte sedimentation rate and white blood count are usually elevated, but they return to normal in four to six weeks. Initially, the possibility of tuberculosis should be considered, but in discitis, the tuberculin skin test is negative and the natural course of the condition is quite unlike that of tuberculosis of the spine. If, because of certain radiologic features, there is a possibility of brucellosis or typhoid fever, routine agglutination tests should be performed.

Attempts to obtain the bacterial organism and determine its sensitivity are made. In addition to blood and throat culture, a needle aspiration of the affected intervertebral space is performed under image intensifier control (Fig. 6–64). If no pus or sanguinous fluid is obtained, 1 ml. of normal saline solution is instilled and then reaspirated. Often these children have been given antibiotics for some reason before the diagnosis is made, and the condition is modified. In some cases, staphylococci or *Escherichia coli* has been cultured.

Treatment

The principle of treatment is to rest the spine in recumbency in a plaster of Paris jacket, which includes the hips and thighs when the lumbar spine is affected, or the head and neck (Minerva jacket) when the thoracic or cervical spine is involved. This treatment is continued until back pain, muscle spasm, or local tenderness have subsided and until the blood sedimentation rate, temperature, and white blood count are normal and the roentgenograms indicate that bony erosion is not progressing. With healing, some sclerosis of the adjacent bony surfaces is usually seen (Fig. 6–65). This usually takes place in two to three months. These children are then gradually per-

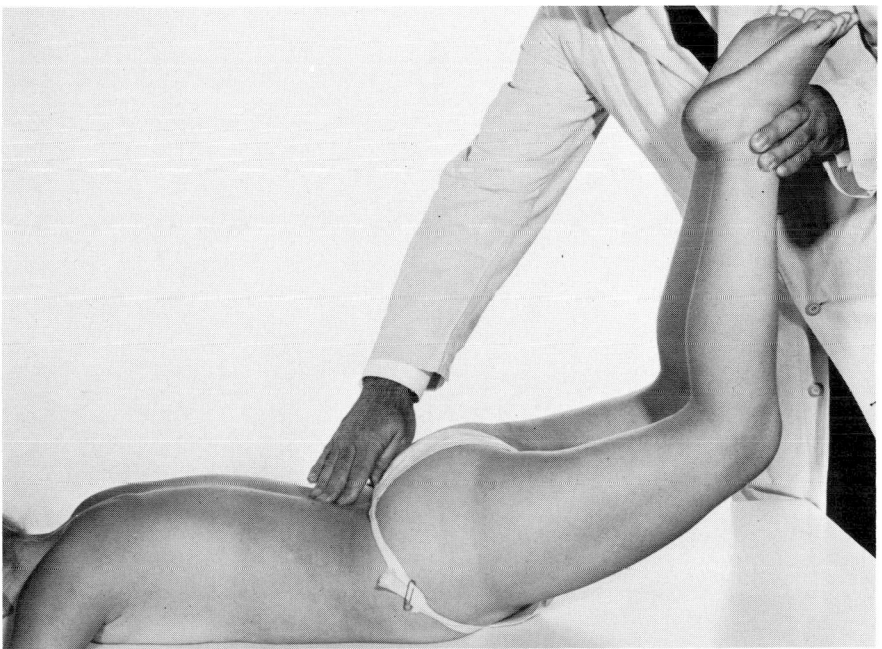

FIGURE 6–63. *Method of demonstrating paravertebral muscle spasm in the lumbar spine in a child.*

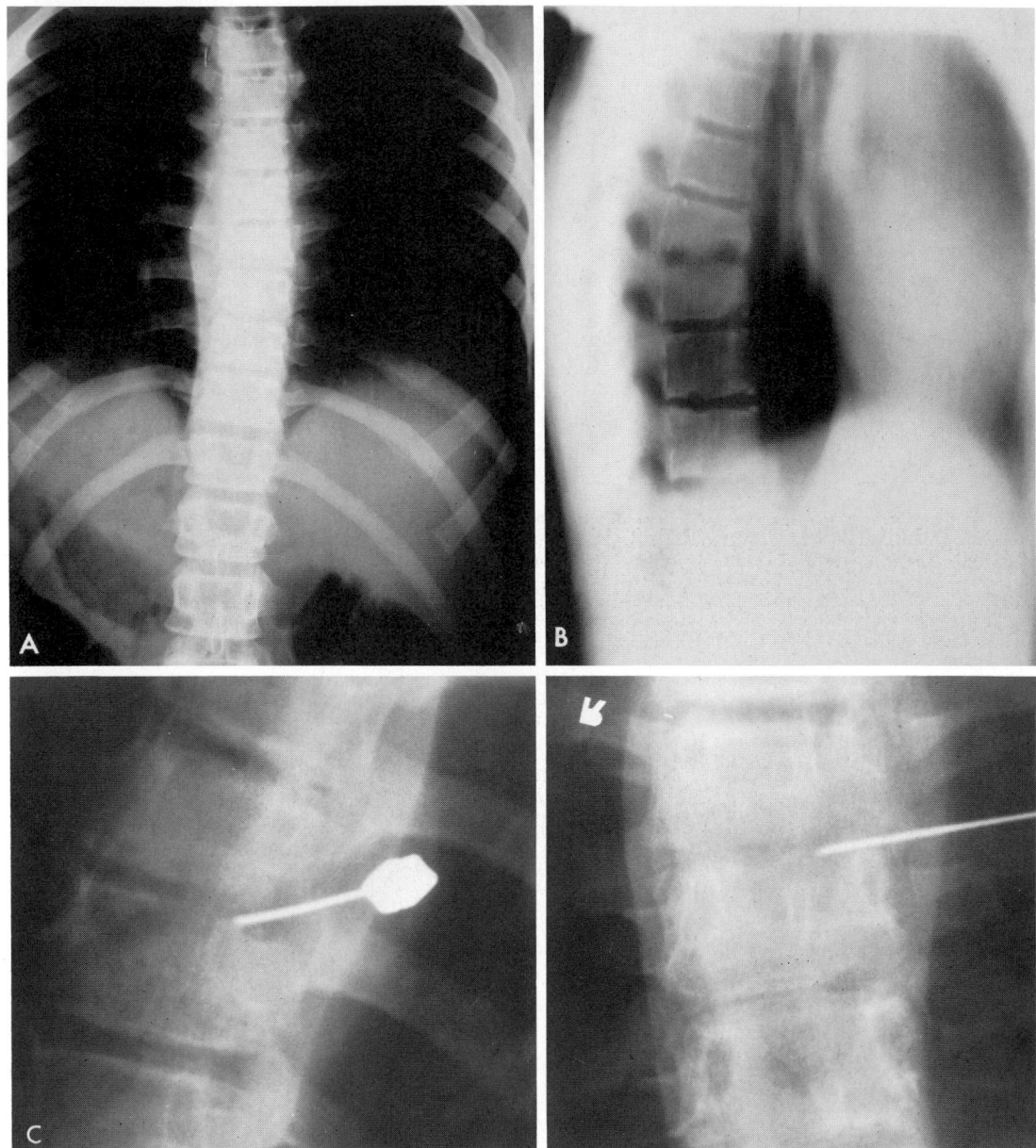

FIGURE 6-64. *Discitis — an infectious disease affecting the intervertebral disc between the eighth and ninth dorsal vertebrae.*

A and **B.** Anteroposterior and lateral (laminogram) roentgenograms of the dorsal spine. Note the erosion and partial wedging of the inferior surface of the eighth thoracic vertebra. **C.** Aspiration of the disc interspace between T8 and T9 under image intensifier radiographic control. The organism cultured was *Staphylococcus aureus*.

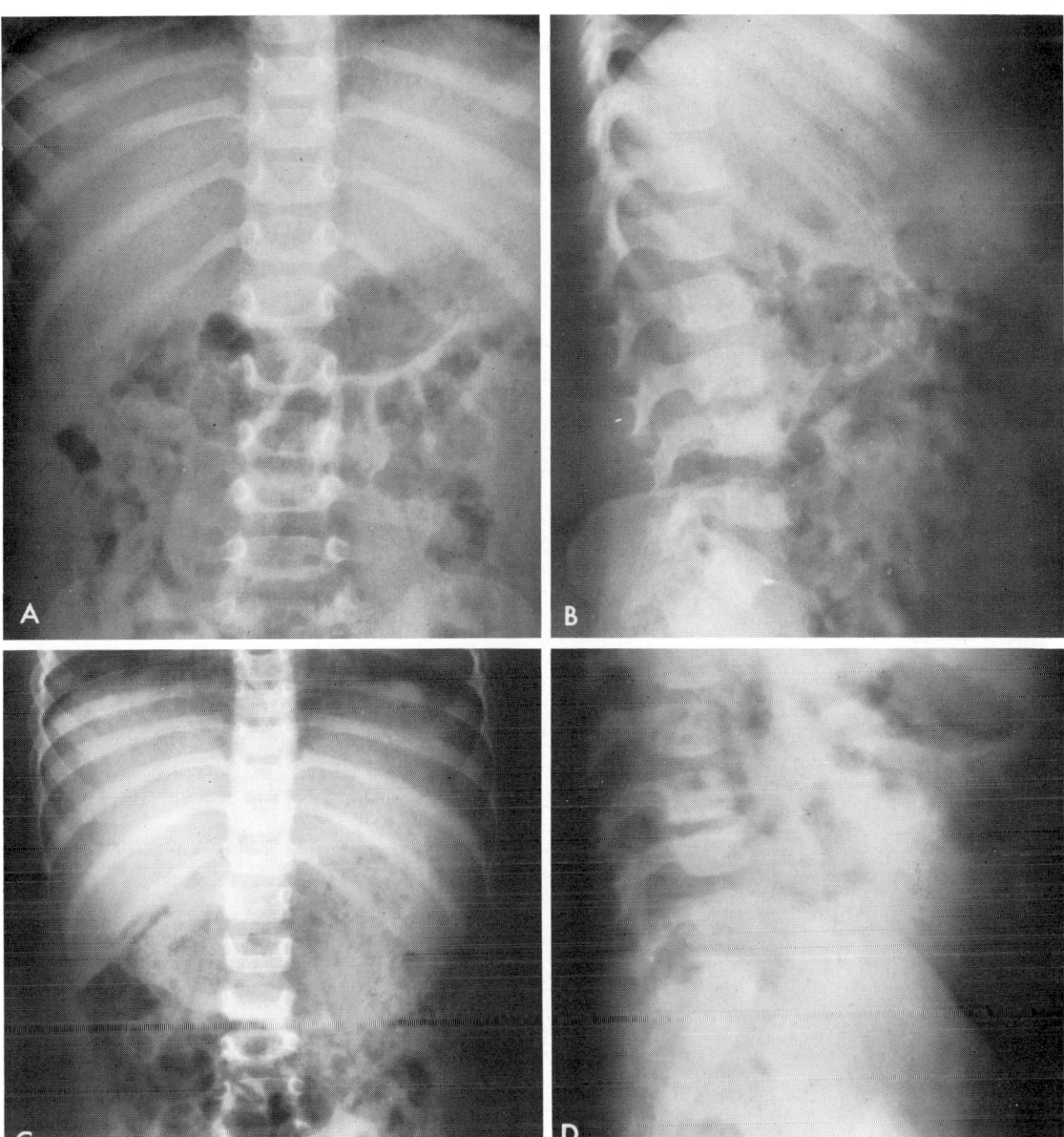

FIGURE 6–65. *Discitis affecting the disc between third and fourth lumbar vertebrae.*

A and **B.** Anteroposterior and lateral roentgenograms. Note the erosion of adjacent bony surfaces between L3 and L4. Bacterial organism cultured was *Staphylococcus aureus.* Treatment consisted of immobilization in a plaster of Paris body jacket for three months and penicillin for four weeks. **C** and **D.** Anteroposterior and lateral roentgenograms of the spine six months later. Note the healing and sclerosis of adjacent bony surfaces.

mitted to walk. A spinal hyperextension brace is used for another one or two months if moderate narrowing is still present in the disc interspace.

Antibiotics are administered for a period of four to six weeks, especially in cases of pyrexia and when a bacterial organism has been cultured. Suppuration as a complication of discitis has been reported.[417] When a paravertebral abscess forms, it is surgically explored and drained by a closed suction-irrigation system.

HERNIATED INTERVERTEBRAL DISC

Protruded intervertebral discs are rarely seen in children.[427, 428, 430, 432, 433] However, they should be considered in the differential diagnosis of low backache and sciatica in a child. The history and findings on neurologic examination do not differ from those in adults. They usually are encountered in the second decade and are equally common in boys and girls.

Trauma plays a conspicuous role in the onset of complaints. If an adequate trial of conservative therapy fails to provide relief of symptoms, surgery is indicated. A preoperative myelogram should be performed for localization of the lesion.

References

POSTURE AND POSTURAL DEFECTS

1. Hellebrandt, F. A., and Franseen, E. B.: Physiological study of the vertebral stance of man. Physiol. Rev., 23:220, 1943.
2. Howorth, B.: Dynamic posture. J.A.M.A., 131:1398, 1946.
3. Keith, A.: Man's posture: Its evolution and disorders. Brit. Med. J., 1:451, 1923.
4. Klein, A.: Posture Clinics: Organization and Exercises. Washington, D.C., U.S. Department of Labor, Children's Bureau, 1931, Publication Number, 164.
5. Lowman, C. L., and Young, C. H.: Postural Fitness: Significance and Variances. Philadelphia, Lea and Febiger, 1960.
6. Phelps, W. M., Kiphuth, R. J. H., and Goff, C. W.: The Diagnosis and Treatment of Postural Defects. 2nd Ed. Springfield, Ill., Charles C Thomas, 1956.

CONGENITAL SCOLIOSIS

7. Blount, W. P.: Congenital Scoliosis. In Huitième Congrès de la Société International de Chirurgie Orthopedique et de Traumatologie, New York, 4–9 Septembre 1960. Bruxelles, Imprimerie des Sciences, 1961, p. 748.
8. Browne, D.: Congenital postural scoliosis. Proc. Roy. Soc. Med., 49:395, 1956.

9. Compere, E. L.: Excision of hemivertebrae for correction of congenital scoliosis. Report of Two Cases. J. Bone Joint Surg., 14:555, 1932.
10. Garrett, A. L., Perry, J., and Nickel, V. L.: Stabilization of the collapsing spine. J. Bone Joint Surg., 43–A:474, 1961.
11. Harrington, P. R.: Treatment of scoliosis. Correction and internal fixation by spine instrumentation. J. Bone Joint Surg., 44–A:591, 1962.
12. Kuhns, J. G., and Hormell, R. S.: Management of congenital scoliosis. Review of one hundred and seventy cases. Arch. Surg., 65:250, 1952.
13. MacEwen, G. D.: Congenital scoliosis with a unilateral bar. Radiology, 90:711, 1968.
14. Shands, A. R., Jr., and Bundens, W. D.: Congenital deformities of the spine. An analysis of the roentgenograms of 700 children. Bull. Hosp. Joint Dis., 17:110, 1956.
15. Von Lackum, H. L., and Smith, A. DeF.: Removal of the vertebral bodies in the treatment of scoliosis. Surg. Gynec. Obstet., 57:250, 1933.
16. Wiles, P.: Resection of dorsal vertebrae in congenital scoliosis. J. Bone Joint Surg., 33–A:151, 1951.
17. Winter, R. B., Moe, J. H., and Eilers, V. E.: Congenital scoliosis. A study of 234 patients treated and untreated. J. Bone Joint Surg., 50–A:1, 1968.

CONGENITAL KYPHOSIS

18. Bauer, H.: Über Angeborene Wirbelsäulenmissbildungen, insbesondere angeborene Kyphosen. Z. Orthop. Chir., 58:354, 1933.
19. Bingold, A. C.: Congenital kyphosis. J. Bone Joint Surg., 35–B:579, 1953.
20. Lindemann, K.: Zur Kasuistik der angeboren Kyphosen. Arch. Orthop. Unfallchir., 30:27, 1931.
21. Lombard, P., and Le Génissel: Cyphoses congénitales. Rev. Orthop., 25:532, 1938.
22. Müller, W.: Die angeborene Gibbusbildung mit Wirbelkörperspaltung an der unteren Brustwirbelsäule. Arch. Orthop. Unfallchir., 30:319, 1931.
23. Saidman, J.: Diagnostic et Traitement des Maladies de la Colonne Vertébrale. Paris, G. Doin and Cie, 1948.
24. Schapira, C.: Su alcune forme rare di malformazioni congenite del rachide (sinostosi vertebrali-cifosi congenite). Chir. Organi Mov., 22:39, 1936.
25. Van Assen, J.: Angeborene Kyphose. Acta Chir. Scand., 67:14, 1930.

SPONDYLOLISTHESIS

26. Adkins, E. W. O.: Spondylolisthesis. J. Bone Joint Surg., 37–B:48, 1955.
27. Allen, M. L., and Lindem, M. C.: Significant roentgen findings in routine pre-employment examination of the lumbosacral spine: A preliminary report. Amer. J. Surg., 80:762, 1950.
28. Amuso, S. J., and Mankin, H. J.: Hereditary spondylolisthesis and spina bifida. Report of a family in which the lesion is transmitted as an autosomal dominant through three generations. J. Bone Joint Surg., 49:507, 1967.
29. Amuso, S. J., Neff, R. S., and Coulson, D. B.: The surgical treatment of spondylolisthesis by posterior element resection. A long-term follow-up study. J. Bone Joint Surg., 52:529, 1970.
30. Anderson, C. E.: Spondylolisthesis following spine fusion. J. Bone Joint Surg., 38–A:1142, 1956.
31. André, N.: L'orthopédie ou l'art de prévenir et de corriger dans les enfants les déformités du corps. Paris, La Veuve Alix, 1741; English Edition, London, Printed for A. Millar, 1743; Philadelphia, reproduced by J. B. Lippincott Co., 1961.
32. Arden, G. P.: Spondylolisthesis with bilateral drop foot. Proc. Roy. Soc. Med., 42:601, 1949.
33. Bailey, W.: Persistent vertebral process epiphysis. Amer. J. Roentgen., 42:85, 1939.

34. Bailey, W.: Observations on the etiology and frequency of spondylolisthesis and its precursors. Radiology, 48:107, 1947.

35. Baker, D. R., and McHolick, W.: Spondyloschisis and spondylolisthesis in children. In Proceedings of the American Academy of Orthopedic Surgeons. J. Bone Joint Surg., 38–A:933, 1956.

36. Bakke, S. N.: Roentgenologische Beobachtungen über die Bewegungen der Wirbelsäule. Acta. Radiol., 13:Suppl., 1931.

37. Bardine, C. R.: Numerical Vertebral Variations in the Human Adult and Embryo. Anat. Anz., 25:497, 1904.

38. Barr, J. S.: Spondylolisthesis. J. Bone Joint Surg., 37–A: 878, 1955.

39. Batts, M., Jr.: The etiology of spondylolisthesis. J. Bone Joint Surg., 21:879, 1939.

40. Beeler, J. W.: Further evidence on the acquired nature of spondylolysis and spondylolisthesis. Amer. J. Roentgen., 108:796, 1970.

41. Bosworth, D. M.: Technique of spinal fusion in the lumbosacral region by the double clothespin graft (distraction graft, "H" graft) and results. A.A.O.S. Instructional Course Lectures, 9:44, 1952.

42. Bosworth, D. M., Fielding, J. W., Demarest, L., and Bonoquist, M. I.: Spondylolisthesis. A critical review of the consecutive series treated by arthrodesis. J. Bone Joint Surg., 37–A:767, 1955.

43. Brailsford, J.: Spondylolisthesis. Brit. J. Radiol., 6:666, 1933.

44. Briggs, H., and Keats, S.: Laminectomy and foraminotomy with chip fusion; operative treatment for relief of low-back pain and sciatic pain associated with spondylolisthesis. J. Bone Joint Surg., 29:328, 1947.

45. Brocher, J. E. W.: L'étiologie du spondylolisthésis. Schweiz. Med. Wschr., 83:788, 1953.

46. Burckhardt, E.: Spondylolisthesis. Schweiz. Med. Wschr., 70:1093, 1940.

47. Burns, B. H.: Two cases of spondylolisthesis. Proc. Roy. Soc. Med., 25:571, 1932.

48. Burns, B. H.: Operation for spondylolisthesis. Lancet, 1:1233, 1933.

49. Capener, N.: Spondylolisthesis. Brit. J. Surg., 19:374, 1931.

50. Capener, N.: The origins of spondylolisthesis. Bull. Hosp. Joint Dis., 21:111, 1960.

51. Chandler, F. A.: Lesions of the "isthmus" (pars interarticularis) of the laminae of the lower lumbar vertebrae and their relation to spondylolisthesis. Surg. Gynec. Obstet., 53:273, 1931.

52. Ciccone, R., and Richman, R. M.: Mechanism of injury and distribution of 3,000 fractures and dislocations caused by parachute jumping. J. Bone Joint Surg., 30–A:77, 1948.

53. Cleveland, M., Bosworth, D. M., and Thompson, F. R.: Pseudoarthrosis in lumbosacral spine. J. Bone Joint Surg., 30–A:302, 1948.

54. Colcher, A. E., and Hursh, A. M. W.: Pre-employment low-back x-ray survey; review of 1500 cases. Industr. Med. Surg., 21:319, 1952.

55. Colonna, P. C.: Spondylolisthesis; analysis of 201 cases. J.A.M.A., 154:398, 1954.

56. Congdon, R. T.: Spondylolisthesis and vertebral anomalies in skeletons of american aborigines. With clinical notes on spondylolisthesis. J. Bone Joint Surg., 14:511, 1932.

57. Cornish, B. L.: Traumatic spondylolisthesis of the axis. J. Bone Joint Surg., 50:31, 1968.

58. Cozen, L.: The development of the origins of spondylolisthesis. J. Bone Joint Surg., 43–A:180, 1961.

59. DePalma, A. F., and Marone, P. J.: Spondylolysis following spinal fusion. Clin. Orthop., 15:208, 1959.

60. Durbin, F. C.: Spondylolisthesis of the cervical spine. J. Bone Joint Surg., 38–B:734, 1956.

61. Faugeron, P.: Spondyloptosis lombo-sacré. Rev. Chir. Orthop., 37:504, 1951.

62. Freebody, D.: Lumbosacral fusion by the transperitoneal approach. In Proceedings and reports of universities, colleges, councils and associations. J. Bone Joint Surg., 44–B:217, 1962.

63. Friberg, S.: Studies on spondylolisthesis. Acta Chir. Scand., 82:Suppl. 55, 1, 1939.

64. Galluccio, A. C.: Spondylolisthesis; general considerations with emphasis on radiologic aspects. Radiology, 42:143, 1944.

65. George, E. M.: Spondylolisthesis. Surg. Gynec. Obstet., 68:774, 1939.

66. Gill, G. G., Manning, J. G., and White, H. L.: Surgical treatment of spondylolisthesis without spinal fusion. J. Bone Joint Surg., 37–A:493, 1955.

67. Glorieux, P., and Roederer, C.: La Spondylolyse et Ses Conséquences: Spondylolisthésis — Scoliose Listhésique. Étude Radiologique — Clinique — Médicolégale. Paris, Masson et Cie., 1937.

68. Green, W. T., and Griffin, P. T.: Personal communication.

69. Hadley, L. A.: Congenital absence of pedicle from the cervical vertebra; report of three cases. Amer. J. Roentgen., 55:193, 1946.

70. Hadley, L. A.: Bony masses projecting into the spinal canal opposite a break in the neural arch of the fifth lumbar vertebra. J. Bone Joint Surg., 37–A:787, 1955.

71. Hadley, L. A.: The Spine. Anatomico-Radiographic Studies. Development and the Cervical Region. Springfield, Ill., Charles C Thomas, 1956.

72. Hadley, L. A.: Secondary ossification centers and the intraarticular Ossicle. Amer. J. Roentgen., 76:1095, 1956.

73. Hallgrimsson, S.: Case of pseudospondylolisthesis with affection of spinal roots. Acta Orthop. Scand., 12:309, 1941.

74. Hammond, G., Wise, R. E., and Haggart, G. E.: Review of seventy-three cases of spondylolisthesis treated by arthrodesis. J.A.M.A., 163:175, 1957.

75. Harnach, Z. G., Gotfryd, O., and Baudysova, J.: Spondylolisthesis with hamstring spasticity. A case report. J. Bone Joint Surg., 48:878, 1966.

76. Harris, R. I.: Spondylolisthesis. Hunterian lecture. Ann. Roy. Coll. Surg. Eng., 8:259, 1951.

77. Harris, R. I., and Wiley, J. J.: Acquired spondylolysis as a sequel to spine fusion. J. Bone Joint Surg., 45–A: 1159, 1963.

78. Hasebe, K.: Die Wirbelsäule der Japaner. Z. Morph. Anthrop., 15:259, 1912–13.

79. Henderson, E. D.: Results of the surgical treatment of spondylolisthesis. J. Bone Joint Surg., 48:619, 1966.

80. Herbiniaux, G.: Traité sur Divers Accouchements Laborieux, et sur les Polypes de la Matrice. Bruxelles, J. L. DeBoubers, 1782.

81. Hirsch, C.: Anterior grafting in extensive spondylolisthesis. Arch. Orthop. Unfallchir., 60:46, 1966.

82. Hitchcock, H. H.: Spondylolisthesis: Observations on its development, progression, and genesis. J. Bone Joint Surg., 22:1, 1940.

83. Hulbert, N. G.: Spondylolisthesis with cauda equina lesion. Proc. Roy. Soc. Med., 41:97, 1948.

84. James, A., and Nisbet, N. W.: Posterior intervertebral fusion of lumbar spine: Preliminary report of new operation. J. Bone Joint Surg., 35–B:181, 1953.

85. Jenkins, J. A.: Spondylolisthesis. Brit. J. Surg., 24:80, 1936.

86. Junghanns, H.: Spondylolisthesen ohne Spalt im Zwischengelenkstück. ("Pseudospondylolisthesen"). Arch. Orthop. Unfallchir., 29:118, 1931.

87. Kilian, H. F.: De Spondylolisthesis gravissmae Pelvangustiae caussa Nuper Detecta. Commentatio anatomico-obstetrica. Bonn, Lit. C. Georgii, 1854.

88. King, A., Baker, D. R., and McHolick, W. J.: Another approach to the treatment of spondylolisthesis and spondyloschisis. Clin. Orthop., 10:257, 1957.

89. Kleinberg, S.: Spondylolisthesis in an infant. J. Bone Joint Surg., 16:441, 1934.

90. Klenerman, L.: Posterior spinal fusion in spondylolisthesis. J. Bone Joint Surg., 44–B:637, 1962.

91. Lambert, R. G., and Billings, E. L.: Traumatic spondylolisthesis. Read at the Annual Meeting of the Western Orthopedic Association. Coronado, California, 1960.

92. Lambl: Cited by Chandler. Sec Ref. 47.

93. Lance, E. M.: Treatment of severe spondylolisthesis with neural involvement. A report of two cases. J. Bone Joint Surg., 48:883, 1966.

94. Lane, W. A.: Some of the changes which are produced by pressure in the lower part of the spinal column, spondylolisthesis, displacement backwards of the fifth lumbar vertebra, torticollis, etc. Trans. Path. Soc., 36:364, 1885.

95. Laurent, L. E.: Spondylolisthesis. Acta Orthop. Scand. Suppl., 35:7, 1958.

96. Laurent, L. E., and Einola, S.: Spondylolisthesis in children and adolescents. Acta Orthop. Scand., 31:45, 1961.

97. Lerner, H. H., and Gazin, A. L.: Interarticular isthmus hiatus (spondylolysis). Radiology, 46:573, 1946.

98. Macnab, I.: Spondylolisthesis with an intact neural arch—the so-called pseudo-spondylolisthesis. J. Bone Joint Surg., 32–B:325, 1950.

99. Mall, F. P.: On ossification centers in the human embryos less than one hundred days old. Amer. J. Anat., 5:433, 1906.

100. Mercer, W.: Orthopaedic Surgery. Baltimore, William Wood & Co., 1936.

101. Meschan, I.: Spondylolisthesis; Commentary on etiology and improved method of roentgenographic mensuration and detection of instability. Amer. J. Roentgen., 53:230, 1945.

102. Meyer-Burgdorff, H.: Untersuchungen über das Wirbelgleiten. Leipzig, George Thieme, 1931.

103. Meyerding, H. W.: Spondylolisthesis. J. Bone Joint Surg., 13:39, 1931.

104. Meyerding, H. W.: Spondylolisthesis. Surg., Gynec. Obstet., 54:371, 1932.

105. Meyerding, H. W.: Spondylolisthesis as an etiologic factor in backache. J.A.M.A., 111:1971, 1938.

106. Meyerding, H. W.: Low backache and sciatic pain associated with spondylolisthesis and protruded intervertebral disc: Incidence, significance and treatment. J. Bone Joint Surg., 23:461, 1941.

107. Meyerding, H. W.: Spondylolisthesis: Surgical treatment and results. J. Bone Joint Surg., 25:65, 1943.

108. Mosimann, P.: Die Histologie der Spondylolyse. Arch. Orthop. Unfallchir., 53:264, 1961.

109. Mouchet, A., and Roederer, C.: Le spondylolisthesis. Presse Méd., 39:569, 1931.

110. Mutch, J., and Walmsley, R.: The aetiology of cleft vertebral arch in spondylolisthesis. Lancet, 270:74, 1956.

111. Nathan, H.: Spondylolysis: Its anatomy and mechanism of development. J. Bone Joint Surg., 41–A:303, 1959.

112. Neugebauer, F. L.: Die Entstehyng der Spondylolisthesis. Zbl. Gynäk., 5:260, 1881.

113. Neugebauer, F. L.: Zur Entwicklungsgeschichte des Spondylolisthetischen Beckens und Seiner Diagnose (mit Berücksichtigung von Körperhaltung und Gangspur). Casuistisch-Kritische Monographie. Halle, Max Niemeyer, 1882.

114. Neugebauer, F. L.: A New Contribution to the History and Etiology of Spondylolisthesis. The New Sydenham Society. Selected Monographs. London, The New Sydenham Society, 1888.

115. Newman, P. H.: Spondylolisthesis, its cause and effect. Ann. Roy. Coll. Surg. Eng., 16:305, 1954–55.

116. Newman, P. H., and Stone, K. H.: The etiology of spondylolisthesis. J. Bone Joint Surg., 45–B:39, 1963.

117. Noback, C. R.: The developmental anatomy of the human osseous skeleton during the embryonic, fetal, and circumnatal periods. Anat. Rec., 88:91, 1944.

118. Orth, J. O., Penning, A., and Kluft, O.: Unilateral spondylolysis of the sixth cervical vertebra. J. Bone Joint Surg., 51:1379, 1969.

119. Pease, C. N., and Nagat, H.: Spondylolisthesis in children. Special reference to the lumbosacral joint and treatment by fusion. Clin. Orthop., 52:187, 1967.

120. Perlman, R., and Hawes, L. E.: Cervical spondylolisthesis. J. Bone Joint Surg., 33–A:1012, 1951.

121. Phalen, G. S., and Dickson, J. A.: Spondylolisthesis and Tight Hamstrings. J. Bone Joint Surg., 43–A:505, 1961.

122. Potter, R. M., and Norcross, J. R.: Spondylolisthesis without isthmus defect. Radiology, 63:678, 1954.

123. Raney, R. B.: Isthmus defects of the fifth lumbar vertebra. Southern Med. J., 38:166, 1945.

124. Rhodes, M. P., and Colangelo, C.: Spondylolysis and its relations to spondylolisthesis. Amer. J. Surg., 72:20, 1946.

125. Robert (zu Coblenz): Eine eigenthümliche angeborene Lordose, wahrscheinlich bedingt durch eine Verschiebung des Korpers des letzten Lendenwirbels auf die vordere Fläche des ersten Kruezbeinwirbels (spondylolisthesis Kilian, bebst Bemerkungen über die Mechanik dieser Beckenformation. Mschr. Geburtskunde Frauenk., 5:81, 1855.

126. Roberts, R. A.: Chronic Structural Low Back Ache due to Low Back Structural Derangements. London, H. K. Lewis, 1947.

127. Roche, M. B.: Bilateral fracture of the pars interarticularis of a lumbar neural arch. J. Bone Joint Surg., 30–A:1005, 1948.

128. Roche, M. B.: The pathology of the neural arch defects; a dissection study. J. Bone Joint Surg., 31–A:529, 1949.

129. Roche, M. B.: Healing of bilateral fracture of the pars interarticularis of the lumbar neural arch. J. Bone Joint Surg., 32–A:428, 1950.

130. Roche, M. B., and Rowe, G. G.: Incidence of separate neural arch and coincident bone variation; Survey of 4,200 skeletons. Anat. Rec., 109:233, 1951.

131. Rombold, C.: Treatment of spondylolisthesis by posterolateral fusion, resection of the pars interarticularis and prompt mobilization of the patient. An end-result study of seventy-three patients. J. Bone Joint Surg., 48:1282, 1966.

132. Rowe, G. G., and Roche, M. B.: The etiology of separate neural arch. J. Bone Joint Surg., 35–A:102, 1953.

133. Runge, C. F.: Roentgenographic examination of the lumbosacral spine in routine pre-employment examinations. J. Bone Joint Surg., 36–A:75, 1954.

134. Schmorl, G.: Beitrag zur kenntnis der Spondylolisthese. Deutsche. Z. Chir., 237:422, 1932.

135. Schmorl, G., and Junghanns, H.: Die Gesunde und Kranke Wirbelsäule. Leipzig, George Thieme, 1932.

136. Schneider, C. C., and Melamed, A.: Spondylolysis and spondylolisthesis: Case report clarifying the etiology of spondylolysis. Radiology, 69:863, 1957.

137. Sensing, E. G.: The Early Development of the Human Vertebral Column. Contrib. to Embryology, Vol. 33:21, Washington Carnegie Institute, 1949.

138. Serre, H.: Spondylolyse traumatique vraie: Fracture isolée des isthumus de L5 anterieurement normaux. Rev. Rhum., 23:44, 1956.

139. Shahriaree, H., and Harkess, J. W.: A family with spondylolisthesis. Radiology, 94:631, 1970.

140. Shands, A. R., Jr., and Bundens, W. D.: Congenital deformities of the spine. An analysis of the roentgenograms of 700 children. Bull. Hosp. Joint Dis., 17:110, 1956.

141. Shore, L. R.: A report of a specimen of spondylolisthesis found in a skeleton of a Bantu native of South Africa; with further specimens illustrating an anomalous mode of development of the lower lumbar vertebrae. Brit. J. Surg., 16:431, 1929.

142. Shore, L. R.: Abnormalities of the vertebral column in a series of skeletons of Bantu natives of South Africa. J. Anat., 64:206, 1930.

143. Sicard, A., and Leca, A.: Les spondylolisthesis traumatiques. Presse Méd., 60:914, 1952.

144. Siehl, D.: Heredity in spondylolisthesis and spondylolysis. J. Amer. Osteopath Ass., 53:154, 1953.

145. Southworth, J. D., and Bersack, S. R.: Anomalies of the lumbosacral vertebrae in five hundred and fifty individuals without symptoms referable to the low back. Amer. J. Roentgen., *64:*624, 1950.

146. Speed, K.: Spondylolisthesis: Treatment of anterior bone graft. Arch. Surg., *37:*175, 1938.

147. Steiner, G.: Isolated fractures of the vertebral arch. Amer. J. Roentgen., *39:*43, 1938.

148. Stewart, T. D.: Incidence of separate neural arch in the lumbar vertebrae of Eskimos. Amer. J. Phys. Anthrop., *16:*51, 1931.

149. Stewart, T. D.: Spondylolisthesis without separate neural arch (pseudo-spondylolisthesis of Junghanns). J. Bone Joint Surg., *17:*640, 1935.

150. Stewart, T. D.: The age incidence of Neural-arch defects in Alaskan natives considered from the standpoint of etiology. J. Bone Joint Surg., *35–A:*937, 1953.

151. Stewart, T. D.: Examination of the possibility that certain skeletal characters predispose to defects in the lumbar neural arches. Clin. Orthop., *8:*44, 1956.

152. Sullivan, C. R., and Bickel, W. H.: The problem of traumatic spondylolysis; a report of three cases. Amer. J. Surg., *100:*698, 1960.

153. Taillard, W.: Le spondylolisthesis chez l'enfant et l'adolescent: étude de 50 cas. Acta Orthop. Scand., *24:*115, 1954.

154. Thieme, F. P.: Lumbar breakdown caused by erect posture in man; with emphasis on spondylolisthesis and herniated intervertebral disc. Anthrop. Papers, Museum of Anthrop., University of Michigan, Paper No. 4, 1950.

155. Todd, T. W.: Age changes in the pubic bone. Amer. J. Phys. Anthrop., *3:*285, 1920.

156. Toland, J. J.: Spondylolisthesis in identical twins. Clin. Orthop., *5:*194, 1955.

157. Turner, H., and Markeloff, N.: Die Röntgenidagnostik der Spondylolysis im Lichte Experimenteller Forschung am Kadaver. Acta Chir. Scand., *67:*914, 1930.

158. Turner, H., and Tchirkin, N.: Spondylolisthesis. J. Bone Joint Surg., *7:*763, 1925.

159. Turney, J. P.: Cauda equina lesion due to spondylolisthesis. Brit. Med. J., *2:*1028, 1952.

160. Ullman, H. J.: Diagnostic line for determining subluxation of fifth lumbar vertebra. Radiology, *2:*305, 1924.

161. Unander-Scharin, L.: A case of spondylolisthesis lumbalis acquista. Acta Orthop. Scand., *19:*536. 1950.

162. Vallois, H. V., and Lozarthes, G.: Indices lombares et indice lombaire totale. Bull. Soc. Anthrop., *3:*117, 1942.

163. Weitzman, G.: Dilatation of the common iliac vein and the inferior vena cava in spondylolisthesis. Report of a case with reference to three other cases. Clin. Orthop., *42:*157, 1965.

164. Willis, T. A.: The lumbo-sacral vertebral column in man: Its stability of form and function. Amer. J. Anat., *32.*95, 1923.

165. Willis, T. A.: The separate neural arch. J. Bone Joint Surg., *13:*709, 1931.

166. Wiltse, L. L.: Etiology of spondylolisthesis. Clin. Orthop., *10:*48, 1957.

167. Wiltse, L. L.: The etiology of spondylolisthesis. J. Bone Joint Surg., *44–A:*539, 1962.

168. Wiltse, L. L., and Hutchinson, R. H.: Surgical treatment of spondylolisthesis. Clin. Orthop., *35:*116, 1964.

169. Woolsey, R. D.: Mechanism of neurological symptoms and signs in spondylolisthesis at the fifth lumbar, first sacral level. J. Neurosurg., *11:*67, 1954.

170. Woolsey, R. D.: Simple laminectomy for spondylolisthesis without spinal fusion. J. Int. Coll. Surg., *29:*101, 1958.

CONGENITAL ABSENCE OF THE SACRUM AND LUMBAR VERTEBRAE

171. Aitken, G. T., and Frantz, C. H.: Management of the child amputee. A.A.O.S. Instructional Course Lectures, *17:*246, 1960.

172. Araujo, A. De.: Distrofia cruro-vesico-glutea por agenesia total do sacro-coccyx. Arq. Brasil. Cir. Ortop., *4:*43, 1936.

173. Blumel, J., Evans, E. B., and Eggers, G. W. N.: Partial and complete agenesis or malformation of the sacrum with associated anomalies. J. Bone Joint Surg., *41–A:* 497, 1959.

174. Detwiler, S. R., and Holtzer, H.: The inductive and formative influence of the spinal cord upon the vertebral column. Bull. Hosp. Joint Dis., *15:*114, 1954.

175. Dunn, L. C.: The inheritance of rumplessness in the domestic fowl. J. Hered., *16:*127, 1925.

176. Dunn, L. C., and Landauer, W.: The genetics of the rumpless fowl with evidence of a case of changing dominance. J. Genet., *29:*217, 1934.

177. Duraiswami, P. K.: Insulin-induced skeletal abnormalities in developing chickens. Brit. Med. J., *2:*384, 1950.

178. Feller, A., and Sternberg, H.: Zur Kenntnis der Fehlbildungen der Wirbesäule. III Mitteilung. Über den vollständigen Mangel der unteren Wirbelsäulenabschnitte und seine Bedeutung für die formale genese der Defektbildungen des hinteren Körperendes. Virchow. Arch. Path. Anat., *280:*649, 1931.

179. Frantz, C. H., and Aitken, G. T.: Complete absence of the lumbar spine and sacrum. J. Bone Joint Surg., *49–A:*1531, 1967.

180. Freedman, B.: Congenital absence of the sacrum and coccyx. Report of a case and review of the literature. Brit. J. Surg., *37:*299, 1950.

181. Friedel, G.: Defekt der Wirbelsäule vom 10. Brustwirbel an abwärts bei einem Neugeborenen. Arch. Klin. Chir., *93:*944, 1910.

182. Grüneberg, H.: The Pathology of Development. Oxford, Blackwell, 1963.

183. Hilgenreiner, H.: Ein Fall von Anchypodie. Beitrag zum vollständigen Kreuzbein defekt. Z. Orthop., *66:*224, 1937.

184. Hohl, A. F.: Zur Pathologie des Beckens. I. Das schägovale Becken. Leipzig, Wilhelm Englemann, 1852, p. 61.

185. Katz, J. F.: Congenital absence of the sacrum and coccyx. J. Bone Joint Surg., *35–A:*398, 1953.

186. Lichtor, A.: Sacral agenesis. Report of a case. Arch. Surg., *54:*430, 1947.

187. Pearlman, C. K., and Bors, E.: Congenital absence of the lumbosacral spine. J. Urol., *101:*374, 1969.

188. Perry, J., Bonnett, C. A., and Hoffer, M. M.: Vertebral pelvic fusions in the rehabilitation of patients with sacral agenesis. J. Bone Joint Surg., *52:*288, 1970.

189. Pouzet, F.: Les anomalies du développement du sacrum. Lyon Chir., *35:*371, 1938.

190. Rosenthal, R. K.: Congenital absence of the coccyx. sacrum, lumbar vertebrae and the lower thoracic vertebrae. Report of a case. Bull. Hosp. Joint Dis., *29:*287, 1968.

191. Russell, H. E., and Aitken, G. T.: Congenital absence of the sacrum and lumbar vertebrae with prosthetic management. J. Bone Joint Surg., *45–A:*501, 1963.

192. Salter, R. L.: Personal communication.

193. Saunders, J. W., Jr.: Death in embryonic systems. Science, *154:*604, 1966.

194. Sinclair, J. G., Duren, N. and Rude, J. C.: Congenital lumbosacral defect. Arch. Surg., *43:*474, 1941.

195. Zeligs, I. M.: Congenital absence of the sacrum. Arch. Surg., *41:*1220, 1940.

SCOLIOSIS

196. Abbott, E. G.: Correction of lateral curvature of the spine. N.Y. Med. J., *95.*833, 1912.

197. Alexander, R. G.: The Effects of Tooth Position and Maxillofacial vertical growth during treatment of scoliosis with the Milwaukee brace. Amer. J. Orthodont., *52:*161, 1966.

198. American Orthopedics Association Research Committee Report: End-result study of the treatment of idiopathic scoliosis. J. Bone Joint Surg., *23:*963, 1941.

199. Arkin, A. M., and Simon, N.: Radiation scoliosis—an

experimental study, J. Bone Joint Surg., *32A*:396, 1950.

200. Bampfield, R. W.: "An Essay on Curvature and Diseases of the Spine, Including all the Forms of Spinal Distortion." London, Longman, Hurst, Rees, Orme, Brown & Green, 1824.

201. Bergofsky, E. H., and Turino, F.: Cardiorespiratory failure in kyphoscoliosis. Medicine, *38*:263, 1959.

202. Bisgard, J. D.: Experimental thoracogenic scoliosis. J. Thorac. Surg., *4*:435, 1935.

203. Bisgard, J. D., and Musselman, M. M.: Scoliosis. Its experimental production and growth correction; growth and fusion of vertebral bodies. Surg. Gynec. Obstet., *70*:1029, 1940.

204. Blount, W. P.: Scoliosis and the Milwaukee brace. Bull. Hosp. Joint Dis., *19*:152, 1958.

205. Blount, W. P., and Bolinske, J.: Physical therapy in the nonoperative treatment of scoliosis. Phys. Ther., *47*:919, 1967.

206. Blount, W. P., and Moe, J. H.: The Milwaukee Brace. Baltimore, Williams & Wilkins Co., 1972. In press.

207. Blount, W. P., Schmidt, A. C., and Bidwell, R. G.: Making of the Milwaukee brace in the operative treatment of scoliosis. J. Bone Joint Surg., *40–A*:526, 1958.

208. Blount, W. P., Schmidt, A. C., Keever, B. D., and Leonard, E. T.: The Milwaukee brace in the operative treatment of scoliosis. J. Bone Joint Surg., *40–A*:511, 1958.

209. Bradford, E. H.: Trans. Amer. Orthop. Ass., *3*:125, 1890.

210. Bruderman, I., and Stein, M.: Physiologic evaluation and treatment of kyphoscoliosis patients. Ann. Intern. Med., *55*:94, 1961.

211. Bunch, W. B.: Orthodontic positioner treatment during orthopedic treatment of scoliosis. Amer. J. Orthodont., *47*:174, 1961.

212. Butterworth, T. R., Jr., and James C.: Electromyographic studies in idiopathic scoliosis. Southern Med. J. *62*:1008, 1969.

213. Caro, C., and Dubois, A.: Pulmonary function in kyphoscoliosis. Thorax, *16*:282, 1961.

214. Cobb, J. R.: The treatment of scoliosis. Conn. Med. J., *7*:467, 1943.

215. Cobb, J. R.: Outline for the study of scoliosis. A.A.O.S. Instructional Course Lecures, *5*:261, 1948.

216. Cobb, J. R.: Correction of scoliosis. *In* Poliomyelitis, Second International Poliomyelitis Congress. Philadelphia, J. B. Lippincott Co., 1953.

217. Cobb, J. R.: Technique, after-treatment, and results of spine fusion for scoliosis. A.A.O.S. Instructional Course Lectures, *9*:65, 1952.

218. Cobb, J. R.: Spine arthrodesis in the treatment of scoliosis. Bull. Hosp. Joint Dis., *19*:187, 1958.

219. Cobb, J. R.: The problem of the primary curve. J. Bone Joint Surg., *42–A*:1413, 1960.

220. Collis, D. K., and Ponseti, I. V.: Long-term follow-up of patients with idiopathic scoliosis not treated surgically. J. Bone Joint Surg., *51*:425, 1969.

221. Colonna, P. C., and Vom Saal, F.: A study of paralytic scoliosis based on 500 cases of poliomyelitis. J. Bone Joint Surg., *23*:335, 1941.

222. Conner, A. N.: Developmental anomalies and prognosis in infantile idiopathic scoliosis. J. Bone Joint Surg., *51*:711, 1969.

223. Cook, C. D., Barrie, H., Deforest, S. A., and Heliesen, P. J.: Pulmonary physiology in children. Pediatrics, *25*:766, 1960.

224. DeGeorge, F. V., and Fisher, R. L.: Idiopathic scoliosis: Genetic and environmental aspects. J. Med. Genet., *4*:251, 1967.

225. Del Norto, U.: Rib resection with Marino-Zerco-Harrington instrumentation. Clin. Orthop., *65*:191, 1969.

226. Dewald, P. L., and Ray, R. D.: Skeletal traction for the treatment of severe scoliosis. The University of Illinois Dalo loop apparatus. J. Bone Joint Surg., *52*:233, 1970.

227. Engel, D., and Richter, A.: Experiments on the produc-

tion of spinal deformities by radium. Amer. J. Roentgen., *42*:217, 1939.

228. Enneking, W. F., and Harrington, P.: Pathological changes in scoliosis. J. Bone Joint Surg., *51*:165, 1969.

229. Farkas, A.: Basic factors in the development of scoliosis. Bull. Hosp. Joint. Dis., *28*:131, 1967.

230. Ferguson, A. B.: The study and treatment of scoliosis. Southern Med. J., *23*:116, 1930.

231. Ferguson, A. B.: Roentgen diagnosis of the extremities and spine. New Yorker, Hoeber, 1945.

232. Ferguson, A. B.: Roentgen interpretations and decisions in scoliosis. A.A.O.S. Instructional Course Lecures, Vol. 7. 1950, p. 160.

233. Ficher, R. L., and DeGeorge, F. V.; Idiopathic scoliosis: An investigation of genetic and environmental factors. J. Bone Joint Surg., *49–A*:1005, 1967.

234. Flinchum, D.: Rib resection in the treatment of scoliosis. Southern Med. J., *56*:1378, 1963.

235. Galante, J., Schultz, A., and Dewald, R. L.: Forces acting in the Milwaukee brace on patients undergoing treatment for idiopathic scoliosis. J. Bone Joint Surg., *52*:498, 1970.

236. Garrett, A. L., Perry, J., and Nickel, V. L.: Stabilization of the collapsing spine. J. Bone Joint Surg., *43–A*:474, 1961.

237. Garrett, A. L., Perry, J., and Nickel, V. L.: Paralytic scoliosis. Clin. Orthop., *21*:117, 1961.

238. Gazioglee, K., Goldstein, L. A., and Femi-Pearse, D.: Pulmonary function in idiopathic scoliosis. Comparative evaluation before and after orthopaedic correction. J. Bone Joint Surg., *50*:1391, 1968.

239. Goldstein, L. A.: Results in the treatment of scoliosis with turnbuckle plaster cast correction and fusion. J. Bone Joint Surg., *41–A*:321, 1959.

240. Goldstein, L. A.: The surgical management of scoliosis. Clin. Orthop., *35*:95, 1964.

241. Goldstein, L. A.: Treatment of idiopathic scoliosis by Harrington instrumentation and fusion with fresh autogenous iliac bone grafts. J. Bone Joint Surg., *51*:209, 1969.

242. Griffin, P. P.: Personal communication.

243. Gucker T., III: Changes in vital capacity in scoliosis: Preliminary report on effects of treatment. J. Bone Joint Surg., *44–A*:469, 1962.

244. Haas, S. L.: Experimental production of scoliosis. J. Bone Joint Surg., *21*:963, 1939.

245. Hamilton, F., Thomas, M. P., and Peralta, M. M., Jr.: Ventilation effects on the Harrington procedure for the treatment of scoliosis. Surg. Gynec. Obstet., *130*:1067, 1970.

246. Harrington, P. R.: Treatment of scoliosis. Correction and internal fixation by spine instrumentation. J. Bone Joint Surg., *44–A*:591, 1962.

247. Harrington, P. R.: Scoliosis in the growing spine. Pediat. Clin. N. Amer., *10*:225, 1963.

248. Harrington, P. R.: The management of scoliosis by spine instrumentation. An evaluation of more than 200 cases. Southern Med. J., *56*:1367, 1963.

249. Harrington, P. R.: Nonoperative treatment of scoliosis. Texas Med., *64*:54, 1968.

250. Heyman, C. H.: Spinal-cord compression associated with scoliosis. J. Bone Joint Surg., *19*:1081, 1937.

251. Hibbs, R. A.: An operation for progressive spinal deformities. A preliminary report of three cases from the service of the Orthopaedic Hospital. N.Y. Med. J., *93*:1013, 1911.

252. Hibbs, R. A.: A report of fifty-nine cases of scoliosis treated by the fusion operation. J. Bone Joint Surg., *6*:3, 1924.

253. Hibbs, R. A., Risser, J. C., and Ferguson, A. B.: Scoliosis treated by the fusion operation. J. Bone Joint Surg., *13*:91, 1931.

254. Hirsch, C., and Waugh, T.: The introduction of force measurements guiding instrumental correction of scoliosis. Acta Orthop. Scand. *39*:136, 1968.

255. Howard, C. C.: A preliminary report infraocclusion of the molars and premolars produced by orthopedic treatment of scoliosis. Int. J. Orthodont., *12*:434, 1926.

256. Howard, C. C.: A second report of infraocclusion of the molars and premolars produced by orthopedic treatment of scoliosis. Int. J. Orthodont., *15*:329, 1929.

257. Howorth, M. B.: Evolution of spinal fusion. Ann. Surg., *117*:278, 1943.

258. Huebert, H., and Mackinnon, W. B.: Syringomyelia and scoliosis. J. Bone Joint Surg., *51*:338, 1969.

259. James, J. I. P.: Idiopathic scoliosis. The prognosis, diagnosis and operative indications related to curved patterns and the age at onset. J. Bone Joint Surg., *36-B*:36, 1954.

260. James, J. I. P.: Paralytic scoliosis. J. Bone Joint Surg., *38-B*:660, 1956.

261. James, J. I. P.: Infantile idiopathic scoliosis. Clin. Orthop., *21*:106, 1961.

262. James, J. I. P.: Scoliosis. Baltimore, Williams & Wilkins Co., 1967.

263. James, J. I. P., Lloyd-Roberts, G. C., and Pilcher, M. F.: Infantile structural scoliosis. J. Bone Joint Surg., *41-B*: 719, 1959.

264. Katzman, H., Waugh, T., and Berdon, W.: Skeletal changes following irradiation of childhood tumors. J. Bone Joint Surg., *51-A*:825, 1969.

265. Kittleson, A. C., and Lim, L. W.: Measurement of scoliosis. Amer. J. Roentgen., *108*:775, 1970.

266. Kleinberg, S.: Scoliosis: Pathology, Etiology and Treatment. Baltimore, Williams & Wilkins Co., 1951.

267. Langenskiöld, A., and Michelsson, J. E.: Experimental progressive scoliosis in the rabbit. J. Bone Joint Surg., *43-B*:116, 1961.

268. Langenskiöld, A., and Michelsson, J. E.: The pathogenesis of experimental progressive scoliosis. Acta Orthop. Scand. Suppl., *59*:1, 1962.

269. Lindahl, O., and Movin, A.: Measurement of the deformity in scoliosis. Acta Orthop. Scand., *39*:291, 1968.

270. Lloyd-Roberts, G. C., and Pilcher, M. F.: Structural idiopathic scoliosis in infancy. A study of the natural history of 100 patients. J. Bone Joint Surg., *47-B*:520, 1965.

271. Logan, W. R.: The effect of the Milwaukee brace on the developing dentition. Dent. Pract., *12*:447, 1962.

272. Lovett, R. W., and Brewster, A. H.: Correction of the structural lateral curvature of spine. J.A.M.A., *82*: 1115, 1924.

273. Luke, M. J., and McDonnell, E. J.: Congenital heart disease and scoliosis. J. Pediat., *73*:725, 1968.

274. Macewen, G. D., and Shands, A. R., Jr.: Scoliosis — a deforming childhood problem. Clin. Pediat., *6*:210, 1967.

275. Makley, J. T., Herndon, C. H., and Inkley, S.: Pulmonary function in paralytic and non-paralytic scoliosis before and after treatment. A study of sixty-three cases. J. Bone Joint Surg., *50*:1379, 1968.

276. Mankin, J. J., Graham, J. J., and Schack, J.: Cardiopulmonary function in mild and moderate idiopathic scoliosis. J. Bone Joint Surg., *46-A*:53, 1964.

277. Michelsson, J. E.: The development of spinal deformity in experimental scoliosis. Acta Orthop. Scand., Suppl. *81*:1965.

278. Miles, M.: Vertebral changes following experimentally produced muscle imbalance. Arch. Phys. Med., *28*:284, 1947.

279. Moe, J. H.: A critical analysis of methods of fusion for scoliosis; an evaluation in 276 patients. J. Bone Joint Surg., *40-A*:529, 1958.

280. Moe, J. H.: The Milwaukee brace in the treatment of scoliosis. Clin. Orthop., *77*:18, 1971.

281. Moe, J. H., and Gustillo, R. B.: Treatment of scoliosis; Results in 196 patients treated by cast correction and fusion. J. Bone Joint Surg., *46-A*:293, 1964.

282. Moe, J. H., and Kettleson, D.: Idiopathic scoliosis, analysis of curve patterns and preliminary results of Milwaukee brace treatment in 169 patients. J. Bone Joint Surg., *52-A*:1509, 1970.

283. Morgan, T. H., and Scott, J. C.: Treatment of infantile idiopathic scoliosis. J. Bone Joint Surg., *38-B*:450, 1956.

284. Moser, H.: Experimentelle Untersuchungen zur Frage der Entwicklung und Beeinflussung der Angeborenen Skoliose. Wien. Klin. Wschr., *68*:230, 1956.

285. Müller, W.: Skoliosen im Tierversuch. Beit. Klin. Chir., *142*:343, 1928.

286. Nachenson, A.: A long-term follow-up study of non-treated scoliosis. Acta Orthop. Scand., *39*:466, 1968.

287. Nachenson, A., and Elfstrom, G.: A force-indicating Distractor for the Harrington-rod procedure. J. Bone Joint Surg., *51*:1660, 1969.

288. Nachlas, I. W., and Borden, J. N.: Experimental scoliosis — the role of the epiphysis. Surg. Gynec. Obstet., *90*:672, 1950.

289. Nachlas, I. W., and Borden, J. N.: The cure of experimental scoliosis by directed growth control. J. Bone Joint Surg., *33-A*:24, 1951.

290. Naeye, R. L.: Kyphoscoliosis and cor pulmonale. Amer. J. Path., *38*:561, 1961.

291. Nash, C. L., Jr., and Moe, J. H.: A study of vertebral rotation. J. Bone Joint Surg., *51*:223, 1969.

292. Neuhauser, E. B. D., Wittenborg, M. H., Berman, C. Z. and Cohen, J.: Irradiation effects of roentgen therapy on the growing spine. Radiology, *59*:637, 1952.

293. Nilsonne, U.: Long-term prognosis in idiopathic scoliosis. Acta Orthop. Scand., *39*:456, 1968.

294. Pacher, W.: Operative Erzeugung einer Skoliose im Tierversuch. Z. Orthop., *69*:140, 1939.

295. Perry, J., and Nickel, V. L.: Total cervical spine fusion for neck paralysis. J. Bone Joint Surg., *41-A*:37, 1959.

296. Peterson, H. A., and Peterson, L. F.: Hemivertebrae in identical twins with dissimilar spinal columns. J. Bone Joint Surg., *49*:938, 1967.

297. Ponseti, I. V.: Prevention of amononitrile lesions in rats with L-triiodothyronine. Proc. Soc. Exp. Biol. Med., *96*:14, 1957.

298. Ponseti, I. V.: Experimental scoliosis. Bull. Hosp. Joint Dis., *19-20*:216, 1958-59.

299. Ponseti, I. V., and Baird, W. A.: Scoliosis and dissecting aneurysm of the aorta in rats fed with Lathyrus odoratus seeds. Amer. J. Path., *28*:1059, 1952.

300. Ponseti, I. V., and Friedman, B.: Changes in scoliotic spine after fusion. J. Bone Joint Surg., *32-A*:381, 1950.

301. Ponseti, I. V., and Shepard, R. S.: Lesions of the skeleton and other mesodermal tissues in rats fed with sweet-pea (Lathyrus odoratus) seeds. J. Bone Joint Surg., *36-A*: 1031, 1954.

302. Redford, J. B., Butterworth, T. R., and Clements, E. L., Jr.: Use of electromyography as a prognostic aid in the management of idiopathic scoliosis. Arch. Phys. Med., *50*:433, 1969.

303. Relton, J. E., and Hall, J. E.: An operation frame for spinal fusion. A new apparatus designed to reduce haemorrhage during operation. J. Bone Joint Surg., *49*:327, 1967.

304. Riseborough, E. J.: Treatment of scoliosis. New Eng. J. Med., *276*:1429, 1967.

305. Riska, E. B.: End results in the treatment of scoliosis. A survey of 57 cases. Acta Orthop. Scand. Suppl., *102*:7, 1967.

306. Risser, J. C.: Important practical facts in the treatment of scoliosis. A.A.O.S. Instructional Course Lecures, *5*:248, 1948.

307. Risser, J. C.: Modern trends in scoliosis. Bull. Hosp. Joint Dis., *19*:166, 1958.

308. Risser, J. C.: The iliac apophysis: An invaluable sign in the management of scoliosis. Clin. Orthop., *2*:111, 1958.

309. Risser, J. C.: Scoliosis: Past and present. J. Bone Joint Surg., *46-A*:167, 1964.

310. Risser, J. C., and Ferguson, A. B.: Scoliosis: Its prognosis. J. Bone Joint Surg., *18*:667, 1936.

311. Risser, J. C., and Norquist, D. M.: A follow-up study of the treatment of scoliosis. J. Bone Joint Surg., *40-A*: 555, 1958.

312. Risser, J. C., Lauder, C. H., Norquist, D. M., and Craig, W. A.: Three types of body casts. A.A.O.S. Instructional Course Lectures, *10:*131, 1953.

313. Roaf, R.: Paralytic scoliosis. J. Bone Joint Surg., *38–B:*640, 1956.

314. Roaf, R.: Scoliosis. Baltimore, Williams & Wilkins Co., 1966.

315. Roaf, R.: The basis anatomy of scoliosis. J. Bone Joint Surg., *48:*786, 1966.

316. Robson, P.: The prevalence of scoliosis in adolescents and young adults with cerebral palsy. Develop. Med. Child Neurol., *10:*447, 1968.

317. Schmidt, A. C.: Fundamental principles and treatment of scoliosis. A.A.O.S. Instructional Course Lectures, *16:*184, 1959.

318. Schwartzmann, J. R., and Miles, M.: Experimental production of scoliosis in rats and mice. J. Bone Joint Surg., *27:*59, 1945.

319. Scott, J. C.: Scoliosis and neurofibromatosis. J. Bone Joint Surg., *47–B:*240, 1965.

320. Scot, J. C., and Morgan, T. H.: The natural history and prognosis of infantile idiopathic scoliosis. J. Bone Joint Surg., *37–B:*400, 1955.

321. Sevastikoglou, J. A., and Bergquist, E.: Evaluation of the reliability of radiological methods for registration of scoliosis. Acta Orthop. Scand., *40:*608, 1969.

322. Shands, A. R., Jr., and Eisberg, H. B.: The incidence of scoliosis in the state of Delaware, a study of 50,000 minifilms of the chest made during a survey for tuberculosis. J. Bone Joint Surg., *37–A:*1243, 1955.

323. Shannon, D. C., Riseborough, E. J., and Valenca, L. M.: The distribution of abnormal lung function in kyphoscoliosis. J. Bone Joint Surg., *52:*131, 1970.

324. Shaw, B., and Read, J.: Hypoxia and thoracic scoliosis. Brit. Med. J., *2:*1486, 1960.

325. Smith, A. DeF., Butte, F. L., and Ferguson, A. B.: Treatment of scoliosis by the wedging jacket and spine fusion; a review of 265 cases. J. Bone Joint Surg., *20:*825, 1938.

326. Steinberg, I.: Cor pulmonale in kyphoscoliosis. Angiocardiographic features of a case. Amer. J. Roentgen., *97:*658, 1966.

327. Steindler, A.: Nature and course of idiopathic scoliosis. A.A.O.S. Instructional Course Lectures, *7:*150, 1950.

328. Steindler, A.: Kinesiology of the Human Body. Springfield, Ill., Charles C Thomas, 1955.

329. Tambornino, J. M., Armbrust, E. N., and Moe, J.: Harrington instrumentation in correction of scoliosis; a comparison with cast correction. J. Bone Joint Surg., *46–A:*313, 1964.

330. Von Lackum, W. H.: The Surgical Treatment of Scoliosis. A.A.O.S. Instructional Course Lectures, *5:*236, 1948.

331. Von Lackum, W. H.: The surgical treatment of scoliosis. *In* Bancroft, F. W., and Marble, H. C. (eds.): Surgical Treatment of the Motor-Skeletal System. 2nd. Ed. Philadelphia, J. B. Lippincott, Co., 1951.

332. Von Lackum, W. H., and Miller, J. P.: Critical observations of the results of the operative treatment of scoliosis. J. Bone Joint Surg., *31–A:*102, 1949.

333. Waugh, T. R.: Intravital measurements during instrumental correction of idiopathic scoliosis. Acta Orthop. Scand, Suppl., *93:*1, 1966.

334. Westgate, H. D., Fisch, R. O., and Langer, L. O., Jr.: Pulmonary function in kyphoscoliosis before and after correction by the Harrington instrumentation method. J. Bone Joint Surg., *51:*935, 1969.

335. Whitehouse, W. M., and Lampe, I.: Osseous damage in irradiation of renal tumors in infancy and childhood. Amer. J. Roentgen., *70:*721, 1953.

336. Wullstein, L.: Die Skoliose in ihrer Behandlung und Entstehung nach klinischen und experimentellen Studien. Z. Orthop. Chir., *10:*177, 1902.

337. Wynne-Davies, R.: Familial (idiopathic) scoliosis. A family survey. J. Bone Joint Surg., *50–B:*24, 1968.

338. Young, L. W., Oestreich, A. E., and Goldstein, L. A.: Roentgenology in scoliosis: Contribution to evaluation and management. Amer. J. Roentgen., *108:*778, 1970.

339. Zaoussis, A. L., and James, J. I. P.: The iliac apophysis and the evolution of curves in scoliosis. J. Bone Joint Surg., *40–B:*442, 1958.

340. Zorab, P.: The lungs in kyphoscoliosis. Develop. Med. Child Neurol., *4:*339, 1962.

SCHEUERMANN'S DISEASE

341. Axhausen, G.: Über den Abgrenzungvorgang am epiphysären Knochen (Osteochondritis dissecans König). Virchow. Arch., *252:*458, 1924.

342. Bradford, D. S., and Garcia, A.: Neurological complications in Scheuermann's disease. A case report and review of the literature. J. Bone Joint Surg., *51:*567, 1969.

343. Brocher, J. E. W.: Die Scheuermannsche Krankheit und ihre Differentialdiagnose. Basel, B. Schwade & Co., 1946.

344. Brocher, J. E. W.: Die Wirbelsäulentuberkulose und ihre Differentialdiagnose. Stuttgart, G. Thieme, 1953.

345. Brocher, J. E. W.: Die Prognose der Wirbelsäulenleiden. Stuttgart, G. Thieme, 1957.

346. Buchman, J.: Vertebral epiphysitis; cause of spinal deformity. J. Bone Joint Surg., *7:*814, 1925.

347. Burdzik, G., and Wuensch, K.: Beitrag zum Röntgenbild der Brustkyphose und seiner Deutung. Z. Orthop., *84:*591, 1954.

348. Ferguson, A. B., Jr.: The etiology of preadolescent kyphosis. J. Bone Joint Surg., *38–A:*149, 1956.

349. Fletcher, G. H.: Anterior vertebral wedging—frequency and significance. Amer. J. Roentgen., *57:*232, 1947.

350. Lachapèle, A. P., and Lagarde, C.: De la maladie de Scheuermann (dite épiphysite vertébrale). J. Radiol. Electr., *28:*10, 1947.

351. Lambrinudi, C.: Adolescent and senile kyphosis. Brit. Med. J., *2:*800, 1934.

352. Mau, C.: Die Kyphosis dorsalis adolescentium im Rahmen er Epiphysen und Epiphysentinienerkrankungen des Wachstumsalters. Z. Orthop. Chir., *46:*145, 1925.

353. Mau, C.: Tierexperimentelle Studien zur Frage der pathologischen Anatomie der Adoleszentenkyphose. Z. Orthop. Chir., *51:*106, 1929.

354. Mooney, A. C.: Disc lesions in relation to pain. Brit. J. Radiol., *18:*153, 1945.

355. Nathan, L., and Kuhns, J. G.: Epiphysitis of spine. J. Bone Joint Surg., *22:*55, 1940.

356. Niedner, F.: Zur Kenntnis der normalen und pathologischen Anatomie der Wirbelkörperrandleiste. Fortschr. Röntgenstr., *46:*628, 1932.

357. Ober, F. R.: The clinical diagnosis, treatment and prognosis of epiphyseal disturbances in childhood. J.A.M.A., *127:*320, 1945.

358. Roaf, R.: Vertebral growth and its mechanical control. J. Bone Joint Surg., *42–B:*40, 1960.

359. Scheuermann, H. W.: Deforming osteochondritis of spine. Ugesk. Laeg., *82:*385, 1920.

360. Scheuermann, H. W.: Kyphosis juvenilis (Scheuermann's Krankheit). Fortschr. Röntgenstr., *53:*1, 1936.

361. Schmorl, G.: Beiträge zur pathologischen Anatomie der Wirbelbandscheiben und ihre Beziehungen zur den Wirbelkörpern. Arch. Orthop. Unfallchir., *29:*389, 1931.

362. Sørensen, H. K.: Scheuermann's Juvenile Kyphosis. Copenhagen, Munksgaard, 1964.

363. Stagnara, P., Du Peloux, J., and Fauchet, R.: Traitement orthopédique ambulatoire de la maladie de Scheuermann en periode d'évolution. Rev. Chir. Orthop., *52:*585, 1966.

364. Wissing, O.: Prolaps af Nucleus Pulposus. Nord. Med., *2:*1384, 1939.

INTERVERTEBRAL DISK CALCIFICATION

365. Asadi, A.: Calcification of intervertebral discs in children. Amer. J. Dis. Child., *97:*282, 1959.

366. Baron, A.: Über eine neue Erkrankung der Wirbelsäule. Jb. Kinderheilk, *104:*357, 1924.
367. Bjelkhagen, I., and Gladnikoff, H.: Calcified disc protrusion in children. Acta Radiol., *48:*151, 1957.
368. Böhmig, R.: Die Blutgefässversorgung der Wirbelbandscheiben, das Verhalten des intervertebralen Chordasegments und die Bedeutung beider für die Bandscheibendegeneration; Zugleich ein Beitrag zur enchondralen Ossification der Wirbelkoerper. Arch. Klin. Chir., *158:*374, 1930.
369. Calvé, J., and Galland, M.: Sur une affection particulière de la colonne vertébrale simulant le mal de Pott. J. Radiol. Electr., *6:*21, 1922.
370. Cohen, R., Burhip, R., and Wagner, E.: Calcification of the intervertebral disc in a child; report of a case. Ann. Western Med. Surg., *3:*202, 1949.
371. Connell, M. C.: Calcification of intervertebral discs in children. Clin. Radiol., *14:*87, 1963.
372. Coventry, M. B., Ghormley, R. K., and Kernohan, J. W.: The intervertebral disc: Its microscopic anatomy and pathology. Part. I. Anatomy, development and physiology. J. Bone Joint Surg., *27:*105, 1945.
373. Coventry, M. B., Ghormley, R. K., and Kernohan, J. W.: The intervertebral disc: its microscopic anatomy and pathology. Part II. Changes in intervertebral disc concomitant with age. J. Bone Joint Surg., *27:*233, 1945.
374. Coventry, M. B., Ghormley, R. K., and Kernohan, J. W.: The intervertebral disc: Its microscopic anatomy and pathology. Part III. Pathologic changes in intervertebral discs. J. Bone Joint Surg., *27:*460, 1945.
375. Crosett, A. D., Jr.: Calcification of the intervertebral discs in a child. Report of a case following poliomyelitis. J. Pediat., *47:*481, 1955.
376. Eyring, E. J., Peterson, C. A., and Bjornson, D. R.: Intervertebral disc calcification in childhood. J. Bone Joint Surg., *46–A:*1432, 1964.
377. Francon, F., and Legrand, P.: Deux cas de calcification cervicale du "nucleus pulposus." Presse Méd., *62:*1841, 1954.
378. Keyzer J. L.: Calcinosis intervertebral. Maandscr. Kindergeneesk., *8:*467, 1939.
379. Kohlmann, G.: Röntgendiagnostik der Wirbelsäule. Verh. Deutsch. Röntgenges., *23:*48, 1931.
380. Lasserre, C., and Phelippot, G.: Discite calcificante intervertébrale. Rev. Orthop., *33:*494, 1947.
381. Legré, J., Padovani, J., and Merjanian, R.: Calcification de disque intervertebral cervicale chez le jeune enfant. J. Radiol. Electr., *41:*194, 1960.
382. Lyon, E.: Kalkablagerungen in der Zwischenwirbelscheibe im Kindesalter. Z. Kinderheilk, *53:*570, 1932.
383. Mann, M. B.: Calcification of intervertebral discs in children. Report of a case. N. Carolina Med. J., *18:*195, 1957.
384. Melnick, J. C., and Silverman, F. N.: Intervertebral disc calcification in childhood. Radiology, *80:*399, 1963.
385. Morris, J., and Niebauer, J.: Calcification of the cervical intervertebral disc. Amer. J. Dis. Child., *106:*295, 1963.
386. Newton, T. H.: Cervical intervertebral-disc calcification in children. J. Bone Joint Surg., *40–A:*107, 1958.
387. Ongaro, M., and Ronconi, G. F.: Rilievi clinico-radiologica sulla calcificazione dei dischi intervertebrale nell'infanzia. Minerva Pediat., *14:*846, 1962.
388. Peacher, W. G., and Storrs, R. P.: Cervical disc calcification in childhood. Radiology, *67:*396, 1956.
389. Peck, F. C., Jr.: A calcified thoracic intervertebral disc with herniation and spinal cord compression in a child; case report. J. Neurosurg., *14:*105, 1957.
390. Pierce, F. T., Jr., and Hanafee, W.: Calcified cervical discs in a child. Calif. Med., *92:*282, 1960.
391. Rechtman, A. M., Hermel, M. B., Albert, S. M., and Boreadis, A. G.: Calcification of the intervertebral Disc: Disappearing, dormant and silent. Clin. Orthop., *7:*218, 1956.
392. Schorr, S., and Adler, E.: Calcified intervertebral disc in children and adults. Acta Radiol., *41:*498, 1954.
393. Sigman, C. C., Jr., and Silepstein, C. M.: Calcification of intervertebral discs in children. The report of a case and review of the literature. J. Med. Ass. Georgia, *51:*214, 1962.
394. Silverman, F. N.: Calcification of the intervertebral discs in childhood. Radiology, *62:*801, 1954.
395. Von Held, H. J.: Zur Frage der Zwischenwirbelscheibenverkalkung. Ein röntgenologisch-klinscher Beitrag. Deutsch Z. Chir., *242:*675, 1934.
396. Walker, C. S.: Calcification of intervertebral discs in children. J. Bone Joint Surg., *36–B:*601, 1954.
397. Wallman, I. S.: Radiological calcification of intervertebral discs in children. Arch. Dis. Child., *32:*149, 1957.
398. Weens, H. S.: Calcification of the intervertebral discs in childhood. J. Pediat., *26:*178, 1945.

DISCITIS

399. Böhmig, R.: Die Blutgefässversorgung der Wirbelbandscheiben, das Verhalten des intervertebralen Chordasegments und die Bedeutung beider für die Bandscheibendegeneration. Zugleich ein Beitrag zur enchondralen Ossification der Wirbelkorper. Arch. Klin. Chir., *158:*374, 1930.
400. Bremner, A. E., and Neligan, G. A.: Benign form of acute osteitis of the spine in young children. Brit. Med. J., *1:*856, 1953.
401. Butler, E. C. B., Blusger, I. N., and Perry, K. M. A.: Staphylococcal osteomyelitis of the spine. Lancet, *1:*480, 1941.
402. Compere, E. L., and Garrison, M.: Correlation of pathological and roentgenographic findings in tuberculosis and pyogenic infections of the vertebrae. Ann. Surg., *104:*1038, 1936.
403. Coventry, M. B.; Ghormley, R. K., and Kernohan, J. W.: The intervertebral disc: Its microscopic anatomy and pathology. Part I. Anatomy, development and physiology. J. Bone Joint Surg., *27:*105, 1945.
404. Doyle, J. R.: Narrowing of the intervertebral disc space in children. Presumably an infectious lesion of the disc. J. Bone Joint Surg., *42–A:*1191, 1960.
405. DuPont, A., and Anderson, H.: Non-specific spondylitis in children. Acta Pediat, *15:*361, 1956.
406. Flemming, C.: Chronic staphylococcal osteomyelitis of the spine. Proc. Roy. Soc. Med., *28:*897, 1935.
407. Ghormley, R. K.; Bickel, W. H., and Dickson, D. D.: A study of acute infectious lesions of the intervertebral disks. Southern Med. J., *33:*347, 1940.
408. Guri, J. P.: Pyogenic osteomyelitis of the spine. J. Bone Joint Surg., *28:*29, 1946.
409. Harbin, M., and Epton, J. W.: Osteomyelitis of the spine. Amer. J. Surg., *22:*244, 1933.
410. Jamison, R. C., Heimlich, E. M., Miethke, J. C., and O'Loughlin, B. J.: Nonspecific spondylitis of infants and children. Radiology, *77:*355, 1961.
411. Keyes, D. C., and Compere, E. L.: The normal and pathological physiology of the nucleus pulposus of the intervertebral disc. J. Bone Joint Surg., *14:*897, 1932.
412. Knutsson, F.: Fusion of vertebrae following a non-infectious disturbance in the zone of growth. Acta Radiol., *32:*404, 1949.
413. Kulowski, J.: Pyogenic osteomyelitis of the spine. An analysis and discussion of 102 cases. J. Bone Joint Surg., *18:*343, 1936.
414. Leigh, T. F., Kelley, R. P., and Weens, H. S.: Spinal osteomyelitis associated with urinary tract infections. Radiology, *65:*334, 1955.
415. Martin, P.: Pyogenic osteomyelitis of the spine. Brit. Med. J., *2:*688, 1946.
416. Mathews, S. S., Wiltse, L. L., and Karbelnig, M. J.: A destructive lesion involving the intervertebral disc in children. Clin. Orthop., *9:*163, 1957.
417. Menelaus, M. B.: Discitis: An inflammation affecting intervertebral discs in children. J. Bone Joint Surg., *46–B:*16, 1964.
418. Phemister, D. B.: Changes in articular surfaces in tu-

berculosis and in pyogenic infections of joints. Amer.
J. Roentgen.,*12:*1, 1924.

419. Saenger, E. L.: Spondylarthritis in children. Amer. J.
Roentgen., *64:*20, 1050.

420. Scherbel, A. L., and Gardner, W. J.: Infections involving
the intervertebral discs. Diagnosis and management.
J.A.M.A., *174:*370, 1960.

421. Smith, A. De F.: A benign form of osteomyelitis of the
spine. J.A.M.A., *101:*335, 1933.

422. Smith, N. R.: The intervertebral discs. Brit. J. Surg., *18:*
358, 1931.

423. Sullivan, C. R.: Diagnosis and treatment of pyogenic
infections of the intervertebral disc. Surg. Clin. N.
Amer., *41:*1077, 1961.

424. Wilensky, A. O.: Osteomyelitis of the vertebrae. Ann.
Surg., *89:*561, 731, 1929.

HERNIATED INTERVERTEBRAL DISC

425. Bradford, D. S., and Garcia, A.: Herniations of the
lumbar intervertebral disc in children and adolescents.

A review of thirty surgically treated cases. J.A.M.A.,
*210:*2045, 1969.

426. Day, P. L.: The teenage disc syndrome. Southern Med.
J., *60:*247, 1967.

427. Epstein, J. A., and Lavine, L. S.: Herniated lumbar intervertebral discs in teen-age children. J. Neurosurg.,
*21:*1070, 1964.

428. Key, J. A.: Intervertebral-disc lesions in children and
adolescents. J. Bone Joint Surg., *32–A:*97, 1950.

429. Lyons, H., Jones, E., and Quinn, F. E.: Changes in pro-
tein-polysaccharide fractions of nucleus pulposus from
human intervertebral disc with age and herniation.
J. Lab. Clin. Med., *68:*930, 1966.

430. Rand, R. W., and Rand, C. W.: Intraspinal Tumors of
Childhood. Springfield, Ill., Charles C Thomas, 1960.

431. Rugtveit, A.: Juvenile lumbar disc herniations. Acta
Orthop. Scand., *37:*348, 1966.

432. Wahren, H.: Herniated nucleus pulposus in a child of
twelve years. Acta Orthop. Scand., *16:*40, 1946.

433. Webb, J. H., Svien, H. J., and Kennedy, R. L. J.: Protruded lumbar intervertebral discs in children.
J.A.M.A., *154:*1153, 1954.

7. The Foot and Leg

The Foot and Ankle

The human foot has the dual function of *supporting* the body in stance and *propelling* it forward in gait.

Subdivided into parts, it consists of: (1) the *hindfoot*—the talus, calcaneus, and navicular; (2) the *midfoot*—the cuneiforms and the cuboid; and (3) the *forefoot*—the metatarsals and phalanges. Some anatomists include the navicular in the midfoot.

The skeletal components of the foot are grouped together architecturally to form a longitudinal arch, the function of which is to provide a resilient spring during locomotion. This longitudinal arch is highest medially, its apex being at the midtarsal joint, and shallow laterally, where it is limited by the lateral border of the foot that lies flat on the floor. The longitudinal arch is maintained by the structure and relationship of the bony parts, especially that of the calcaneus and talus; by the ligaments, particularly the spring, the interosseus, and the long and short plantar ligaments; and by the muscle tone of the four long plantar muscles, namely the posterior tibial, flexor digitorum longus, flexor hallucis longus, and peroneus longus.

It is not in the province of this book to describe in detail the embryologic development, normal anatomy, and mechanics of the human foot; for these the reader is referred to the cited literature.[1-16]

The components of the hindfoot and midfoot articulate in a complex system of multiplaned synovial joints that act as a functional unit. The anterior and middle subtalar articulations, the talonavicular joint, and the plantar calcaneonavicular (spring) ligament together form a ball-and-socket joint. The *socket* consists of the articular surface of the navicular anteriorly; the tibionavicular ligament, the capsule of the talonavicular joint, and the posterior tibial tendon dorsomedially; and the calcaneonavicular part of the Y or bifurcated ligament laterally. The head of the talus forms the *ball* of the ball-and-socket joint. The calcaneocuboid joint is slightly curved in two planes, permitting principally gliding motion and slight rotation.

The movements of the foot and ankle should be considered as a unit. During plantar flexion and dorsiflexion of the foot, motions take place at both the tibiotalar and the talocalcaneonavicular joints. Upon plantar flexion, the hindfoot rotates medially and the forefoot adducts, whereas on dorsiflexion, the midfoot and hindfoot rotate laterally and the forefoot abducts; most of the motion of eversion takes place at the calcaneocuboid joint in a gliding, rotary manner. As the calcaneus everts, it also moves posteriorly and its anterior portion is displaced laterally. As a result, the head of the talus loses its normal support, plantarflexes, and projects further anteriorly. The forefoot abducts as a consequence of the backward displacement of the calcaneus and forward displacement of the talus. The tibiotalar joint does not participate in the complex motions of eversion and inversion of the foot.

The skeletal elements of the foot are first recognized at the fifth postovulatory week as condensed mesenchymes, with chondrification taking place during the sixth and seventh weeks. Thus, in considering the pathogenesis of congenital deformities of the feet, it is important to keep in mind that the structure and skeletal components of the foot are determined prior to the seventh postovulatory week of intrauterine life.[13]

Ossification of the foot takes place in a more or less definite sequence. The distal phalanges are first to ossify, their distal ends showing signs of ossification as early as the seventh postovulatory week.

In the tarsus, at birth, the primary centers of ossification of the calcaneus, talus, and cuboid are usually present. The calcaneus is first to ossify (third fetal month), followed by the talus and then the cuboid. The three cuneiforms and the navicular ossify postnatally. The average age of appearance of the primary and secondary ossification centers in the ankle and foot is shown in Figure 1–30 (p. 43) and the average age of fusion of the ossification centers in Figure 1–31 (p. 44).

Growth of the Normal Foot

The pattern of longitudinal growth of the foot is an important consideration in the planning of surgical procedures. Blais, Green, and Anderson have provided normal standards for the length of the growing foot (Fig. 7–1 and Table 7–1).[2] The feet of both boys and girls grow at a sharply decreasing rate from infancy through the age of five years. Then from 5 to 12 years of age in girls and from 5 to 14 years of age in boys, the average increase in the length of the foot is 0.9 cm. per year. This rate of growth decreases markedly after 12 years of age in females and after 14 years of age in males, and the foot attains its mature length at the average age of 14 years in girls and 16 years in boys. Blais, Green, and Anderson also observed that at all times during the growth period, the size of the foot is relatively closer to its adult size than is the total height or the length of the femur and tibia of the same individual. For example, at the age of one year in girls and at one and one half years in boys, the foot has achieved half of its mature length. The femur and tibia, on the other hand, reach half their mature length at three years of age in girls and four years in boys. Thus, the factors that would disturb growth would affect the ultimate length of the foot proportionately less than they would the femur or the tibia. If, for example, the linear growth of the foot is completely arrested at the skeletal age of 10 years in girls or at 12 years in boys, the result would be an average reduction in adult length of the foot of only 10 per cent (about 2.5 cm.); if at the skeletal age of 12 years in girls and 14 years in boys, of only 3 per cent (or about 1 cm.).[2]

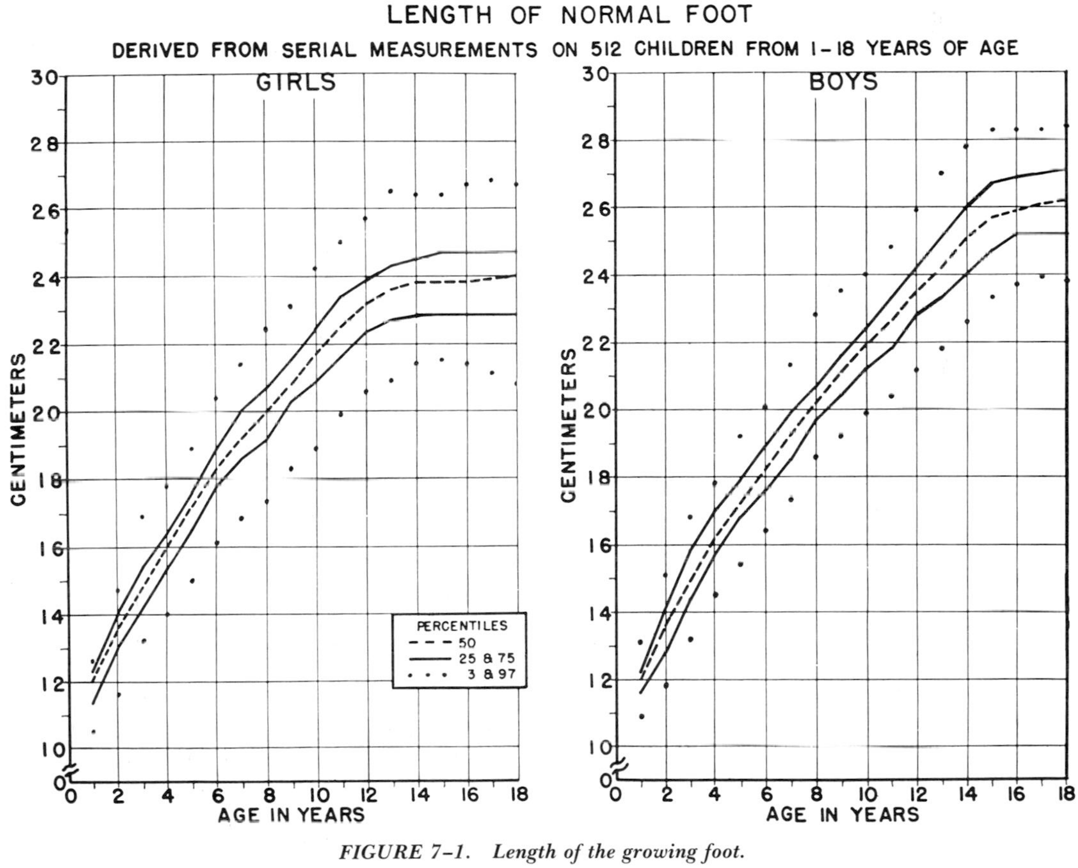

FIGURE 7–1. *Length of the growing foot.*

Length of normal foot derived from serial measurements on 512 children from 1 to 18 years of age. (From Blais, M. M., Green, W. T., and Anderson, M.: Lengths of the growing foot. J. Bone Joint Surg., *38–A*:998, 1956.)

Table 7–1. *Length of the Normal Foot**

	Girls Percentile				Age		Boys Percentile			
3	*25*	*50*	*75*	*97*	*Age*	*3*	*25*	*50*	*75*	*97*
10.5	11.4	12.0	12.3	12.6	1	10.9	11.6	12.0	12.2	13.1
11.6	13.0	13.6	14.0	14.7	2	11.8	12.8	13.6	14.1	15.1
13.2	14.3	14.8	15.4	16.9	3	13.2	14.4	14.9	15.8	16.8
14.0	15.4	16.0	16.4	17.8	4	14.5	15.7	16.2	17.0	17.8
15.0	16.5	17.2	17.6	18.9	5	15.4	16.8	17.2	17.9	19.2
16.1	17.8	18.3	18.9	20.4	6	16.4	17.6	18.2	18.9	20.1
16.8	18.6	19.2	20.0	21.4	7	17.3	18.5	19.2	19.9	21.3
17.3	19.2	20.0	20.7	22.4	8	18.6	19.7	20.2	20.7	22.8
18.3	20.3	20.8	21.5	23.1	9	19.2	20.4	21.1	21.6	23.5
18.9	20.9	21.7	22.4	24.2	10	19.9	21.2	21.9	22.4	24.0
19.9	21.6	22.5	23.4	25.0	11	20.4	21.8	22.6	23.3	24.8
20.6	22.3	23.2	23.9	25.7	12	21.2	22.8	23.5	24.2	25.9
20.9	22.7	23.6	24.3	26.5	13	21.8	23.3	24.2	25.1	27.0
21.4	22.8	23.8	24.5	26.4	14	22.6	24.0	25.1	26.0	27.8
21.5	22.8	23.8	24.7	26.4	15	23.3	24.7	25.7	26.7	28.3
21.4	22.8	23.8	24.7	26.7	16	23.7	25.2	25.9	26.9	28.3
21.1	22.8	23.9	24.7	26.8	17	23.9	25.2	26.1	27.0	28.3
20.8	22.8	24.0	24.7	26.7	18	23.8	25.2	26.2	27.1	28.4

*Caliper measurements in centimeters in weight-bearing position derived from semilongitudinal series of 227 girls and 285 boys.

From Blais, M. M., Green, W. T., and Anderson, M.: Lengths of the growing foot. J. Bone Joint Surg., *38-A*:999, 1956. Reproduced with permission of authors and publisher.

Normal Variations of the Bones of the Foot and Ankle

The growing tarsal and metatarsal bones are characterized by numerous variations that may simulate pathologic conditions. The orthopedic surgeon should be familiar with these normal anatomic variants in order not to misinterpret them as fractures, osteochondritis, or diseases of bone.

ACCESSORY BONES OF THE FOOT

Numerous accessory bones in the foot have been described. These are shown in the diagrams in Figure 7–2. In the feet of about 22 per cent of children under 16 years of age, one or more accessory bones may be found on roentgenograms.[29] The accessory navicular and os trigonum are described here in detail because of their clinical importance.

Accessory Tarsal Navicular

The accessory tarsal navicular (also referred to in the literature as *os tibiale externum* or *prehallux*) is present as a separate bone in about 10 per cent of human beings. It has been demonstrated in the fetus to be a separate center of ossification for the tuberosity of the navicular. In adolescence it frequently coalesces with the contiguous navicular; however, in about 2 per cent of the population, it persists as a separate ossicle. It is often bilateral, and may be bifid.

The accessory tarsal navicular is located at the medial end of the navicular. The posterior tibial tendon is attached to it, passing across the medial aspect of the navicular instead of underneath it. Thus, the dynamic support of the longitudinal arch of the foot normally afforded by the posterior tibial muscle is weakened. The result is planovalgus deformity of the foot. Following prolonged walking, the patient will complain of pain in the midfoot. Shoe pressure on the accessory bone may also cause the formation of an inflamed adventitious bursa with local swelling and tenderness (Fig. 7–3 A). There may be associated nonspecific tenosynovitis of the posterior tibial tendon.

In the roentgenograms, the accessory bone will be visible medially and proximal to the navicular bone (Fig. 7–3 B). Its smooth and rounded outline differentiates it from the irregular margin that characterizes a fracture. In later adolescence, the accessory navicular may fuse with the body of the tarsal bone and present as an abnormally prominent and curved medial end of the navicular (Fig. 7–4). This is referred to as a *cornuted navicular* and produces the same symptoms as the accessory navicular.

Initially, treatment should be conservative. A ⅜-inch felt longitudinal arch support is placed in the shoe. When pain is acute, hydrocortisone may be injected into the adventitious bursa and the inflamed posterior tibial tendon sheath, and the foot immobilized in a below-knee walking plaster cast for a period of three weeks.

If symptoms persist and do not respond to these measures, surgical excision of the accessory navicular with rerouting of the posterior tibial tendon to a point well on the plantar aspect of the navicular (Kidner procedure) is performed.[41, 42]

In the Kidner operation the incision is approximately 5 cm. long and begins 1 cm. inferior and 2 cm. distal to the distal tip of the medial malleolus and extends forward to the base of the first metatarsal bone. The subcutaneous tissue and deep fascia are divided and the wound margins are retracted to expose the posterior tibial tendon and the medial tip of the navicular bone. The posterior tibial tendon inserts into the tuberosity of the navicular bone, into the plantar surfaces of the three cuneiform bones and of the bases of the second, third, and fourth metatarsal bones, and into the cuboid bone. It is detached only from its insertion to the accessory navicular, leaving its other attachments intact.

The accessory navicular bone is excised and the medial surface of the navicular is resected until it is flush with the talus and cuneiform. Bleeding cancellous bone is coagulated with electrocautery. The pos-

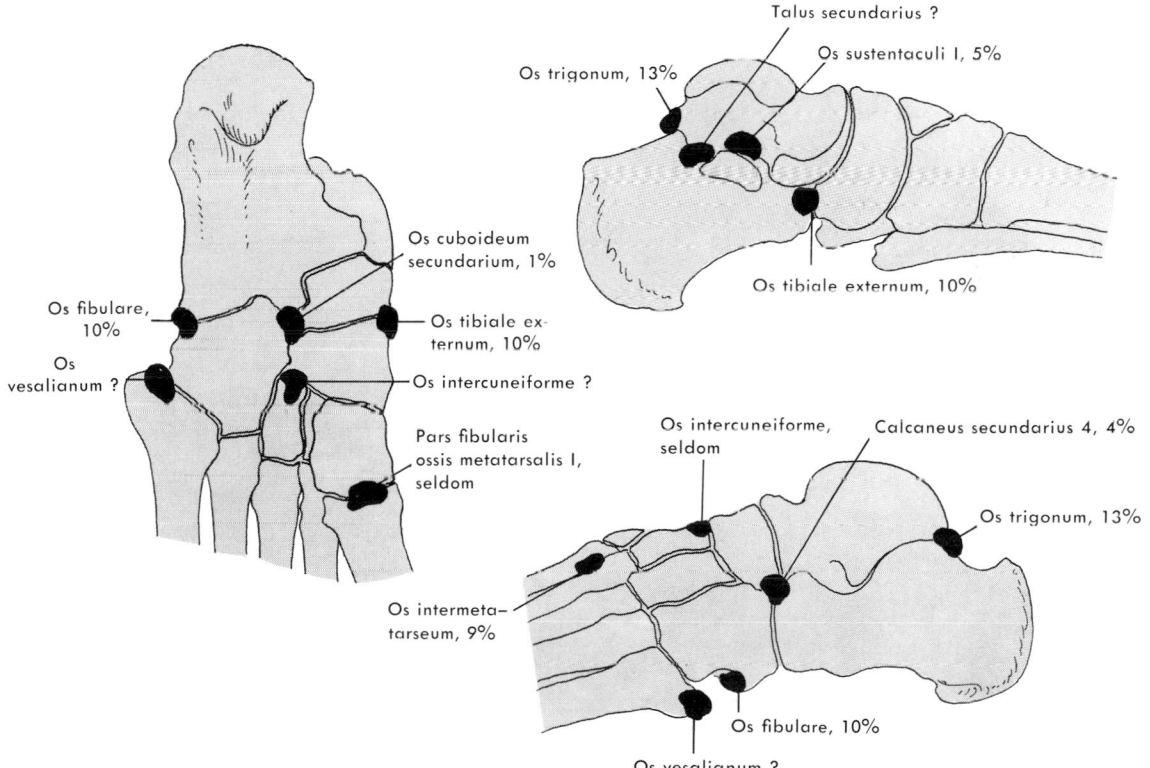

FIGURE 7–2. *Accessory bones in the foot.*

(Adapted from von Lanz, T., and Wachsmuth, W.: Praktische Anatomie, Band I, Teil 4, Bein und Statik. Berlin, Julius Springer, 1938, p. 359.)

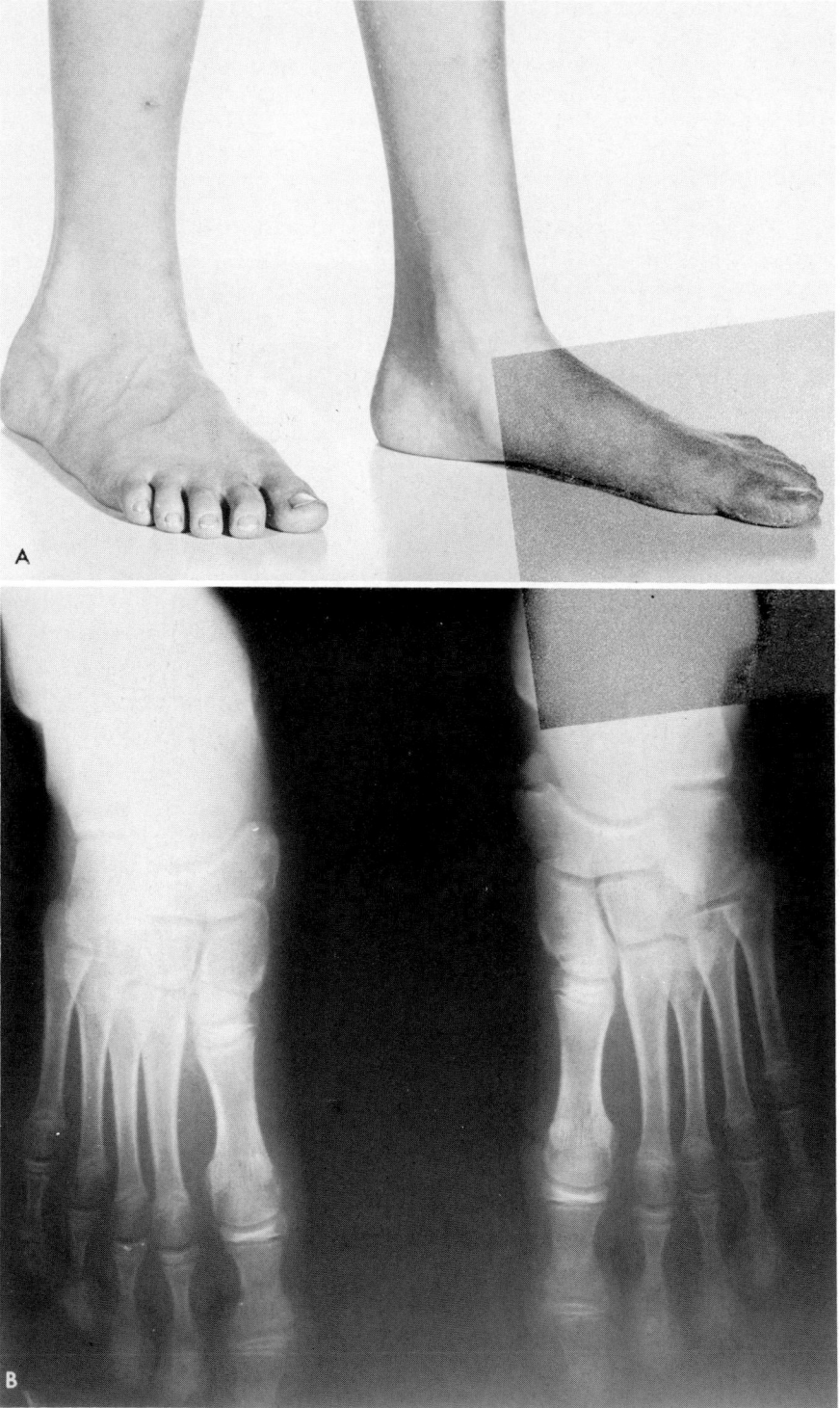

FIGURE 7–3. *Accessory navicular of left foot.*

A. Clinical appearance—showing the local swelling. **B.** Roentgenographic appearance. Note the smooth and rounded outline of the accessory ossicle.

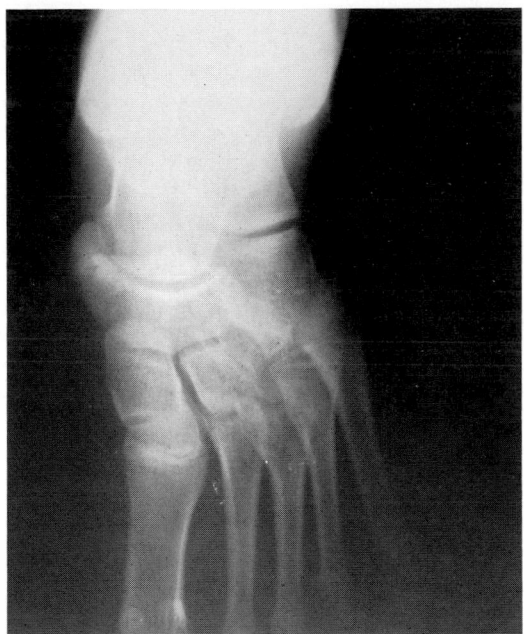

FIGURE 7-4. *Accessory navicular fused with the body of the tarsal bone (cornuted navicular).*

terior tibial tendon is transferred laterally and plantarward on the under surface of the navicular, where it is anchored under tension with two or three interrupted sutures to the periosteum and plantar ligaments. Usually it is not necessary to make drill holes through the navicular. The wound is closed and a below-knee walking cast is applied.

The cast is removed in three to four weeks, following which a longitudinal arch support is used. The result of the Kidner procedure is good. Pain will subside; one should not, however, expect correction of pes planovalgus deformity in the adolescent.

Os Trigonum

On the posterior aspect of the talus there is a groove for the flexor hallucis longus tendon. The bony tubercle lateral to this tendon groove is usually larger than the medial one, and if elongated, it is known as "Stieda's process." Between 8 and 11 years of age, separate centers of ossification appear for the medial and lateral tubercles, and they quickly (usually within a year) fuse with the main body of the talus. The posterior fibers of the lateral ligament of the ankle joint are attached to the lateral tubercle. When the ankle is in full plantar flexion the posterior tubercles of the talus come in full contact with the posterior edge of the distal end of the tibia, serving as a bony block. Repeated minor injury in an active person may cause failure of union of the posterolateral tubercle, which then persists as a separate center of ossification known as *os trigonum* (Fig. 7-5). A fused

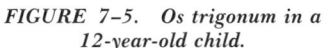

FIGURE 7-5. *Os trigonum in a 12-year-old child.*

Note also the accessory navicular visible in the lateral projection. The sclerosis of the apophysis of the os calcis is normal.

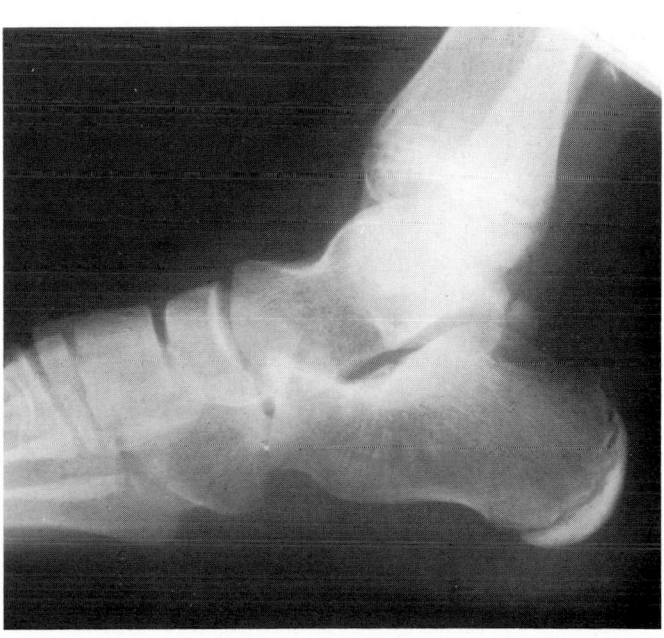

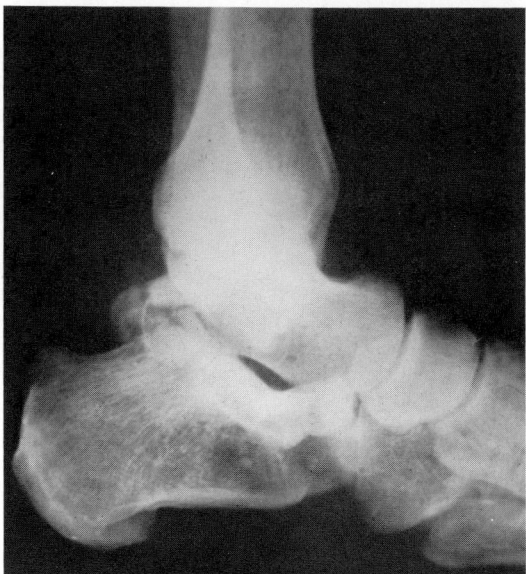

FIGURE 7-6.   Fracture of fused os trigonum.

but large ossicle may be detached by sudden violence, particularly when union of the ossicle to the talus is by synchondrosis (Fig. 7-6). The absence of irregularity between the os trigonum and the main body of the talus distinguishes synchondrosis from a fracture. In doubtful cases, an air arthrogram will settle the diagnosis (Fig. 7-7).[22]

Miscellaneous Accessory Bones

Only a brief listing of the accessory bones and normal anatomic variations of the foot and ankle is given here; for a detailed description the reader should consult the comprehensive reviews of Caffey, O'Rahilly, Trolle, and other cited references.[18, 24, 29, 32]

Medial Malleolus. This may have a separate ossification center (Fig. 7-8 A). In the literature, the reports of its incidence vary. Selby found it in 47 per cent of girls and 17 per cent of boys, whereas Powell reports 20 per cent.[25, 28] The average age of appearance of a separate center of ossification for the medial malleolus is 7.6 years for girls and 8.7 years for boys; by the twelfth year, the extra center of ossification fuses with the main center.

Distal End of Fibula. The lateral malleolus has a separate center of ossification in 1 per cent of cases. A small accessory ossicle is occasionally present in a notch in the distal fibular metaphysis and should not be mistaken for osteochondritis dissecans; also on oblique views of the lateral malleolus, an area of rarefaction in the medial surface of the distal fibular epiphysis should not be misdiagnosed as a destructive bone lesion.

Talus. In addition to os trigonum, an accessory bone may develop on the dorsal aspect of the head of the talus (os sustentaculare). A separate center of ossification for the head of the talus is a very rare anomaly. *Af(icoid talus* is a developmental anomaly in which the head and neck of the talus are tilted dorsally (Fig. 7-9).

Os Calcis. A triangular or circular area of radiolucency may appear in the interior half of the body of the calcaneus, suggesting a pseudocyst (Fig. 7-8 B). It is a normal variation and not a deficiency of spongy bone, occurring in about 10 per cent of children older than seven years.

The enlarged trochlea of the calcaneus may be mistaken for an exostosis.

The apophysis of the os calcis begins to ossify at four to six years of age in the female and at four to nine years in the male. Often a secondary center of ossification in the calcaneal apophysis develops in girls between 10½ and 12 years and in boys between 11½ and 13½ years; it quickly fuses with the body of the calcaneus. A secondary center of ossification may also be present in the tip of the trochlear process on the lateral wall of the calcaneus. Occasionally the body of the calcaneus may ossify from two centers of ossification instead of one, the cartilaginous juncture between the two ossific nuclei suggesting a fracture. Sclerosis and fragmentation of the apophysis of the calcaneus are common (see Fig. 7-5).

Cuboid, Navicular, Cuneiforms. Multiple fine ossification centers may be present in the cuboid. In addition to an accessory navicular there may be a small ossicle on the dorsum of the navicular—os supranaviculare. The edges of the cuneiforms may be irregular.

Metatarsals. An accessory ossicle at the base of the fifth metatarsal is quite common (Fig. 7-10); occasionally it may have a fish-scale appearance, simulating a

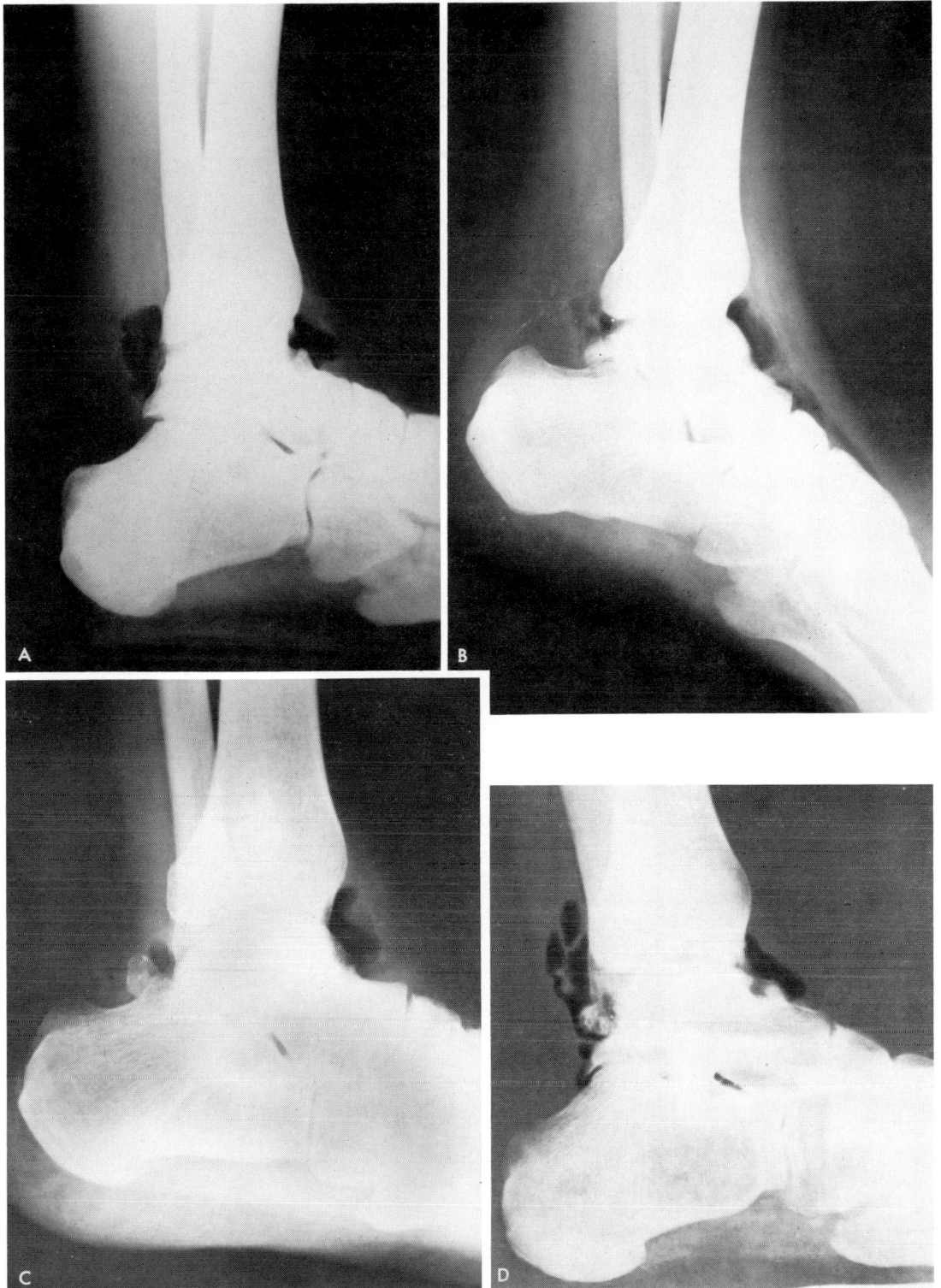

FIGURE 7–7. *Arthrogram of the ankle.*

A. A normal ankle. **B.** An ankle with os trigonum. Note the radiolucent shadow cast by the air is located superior to the os trigonum. **C.** In a fracture of a fused os trigonum, the air has sandwiched itself between the detached accessory bone and the main body of the talus. **D.** In an osteocartilaginous loose body of the ankle the air shadow surrounds the loose bone. (Courtesy of Dr. H. Kelikian.)

1271

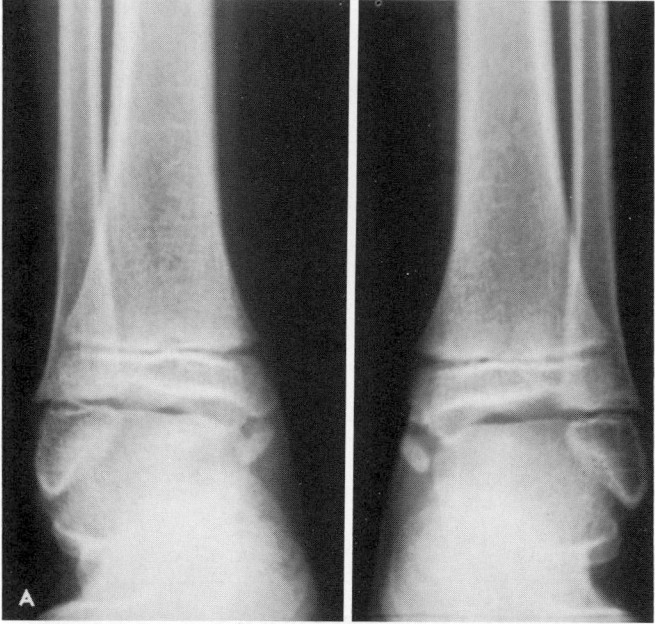

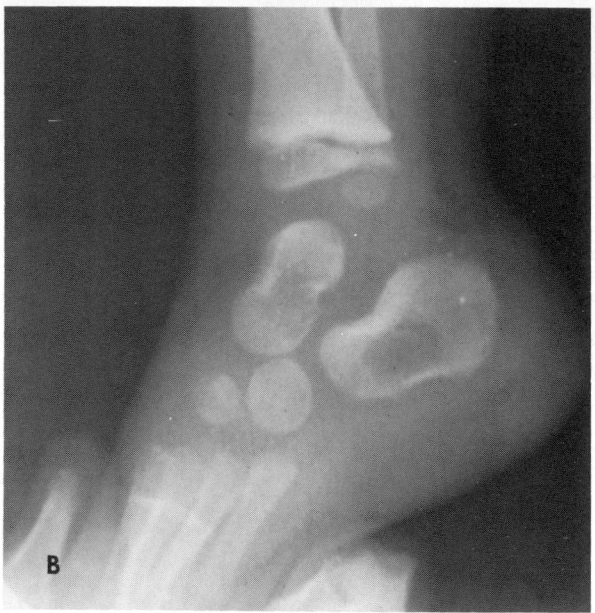

*FIGURE 7–8.   Normal anatomic
variations of the foot and ankle.*

A. Accessory ossification center of medial
malleolus. **B.** Area of rarefaction in body
of os calcis simulating cyst.

fracture. The distal end of the first metatarsal may have an incomplete synchondrosis.

Phalanges.   The skeletal variations of the
digits of the foot are numerous. The reader
is referred to the statistical study of Venning.[33]

In the hallux the number of phalanges is
almost always two, though occasionally a
three-phalangeal big toe may be encoun-

tered. The lesser toes usually have three
phalanges. Not infrequently the fifth toe
may have two phalanges, and occasionally
the second, third and fourth toes may have
a two-phalangeal form. With the exception
of the big toe, toes with two phalanges are
nearly always lateral to the toes having
three phalanges. The two-phalangeal lesser
toes are more preponderant in the female.

The middle phalanx may lack an epiphysis

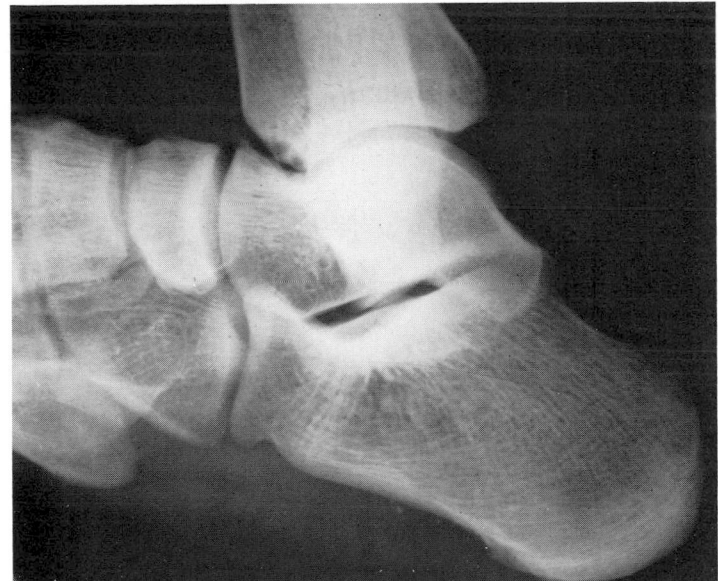

FIGURE 7-9. *Africoid talus.*

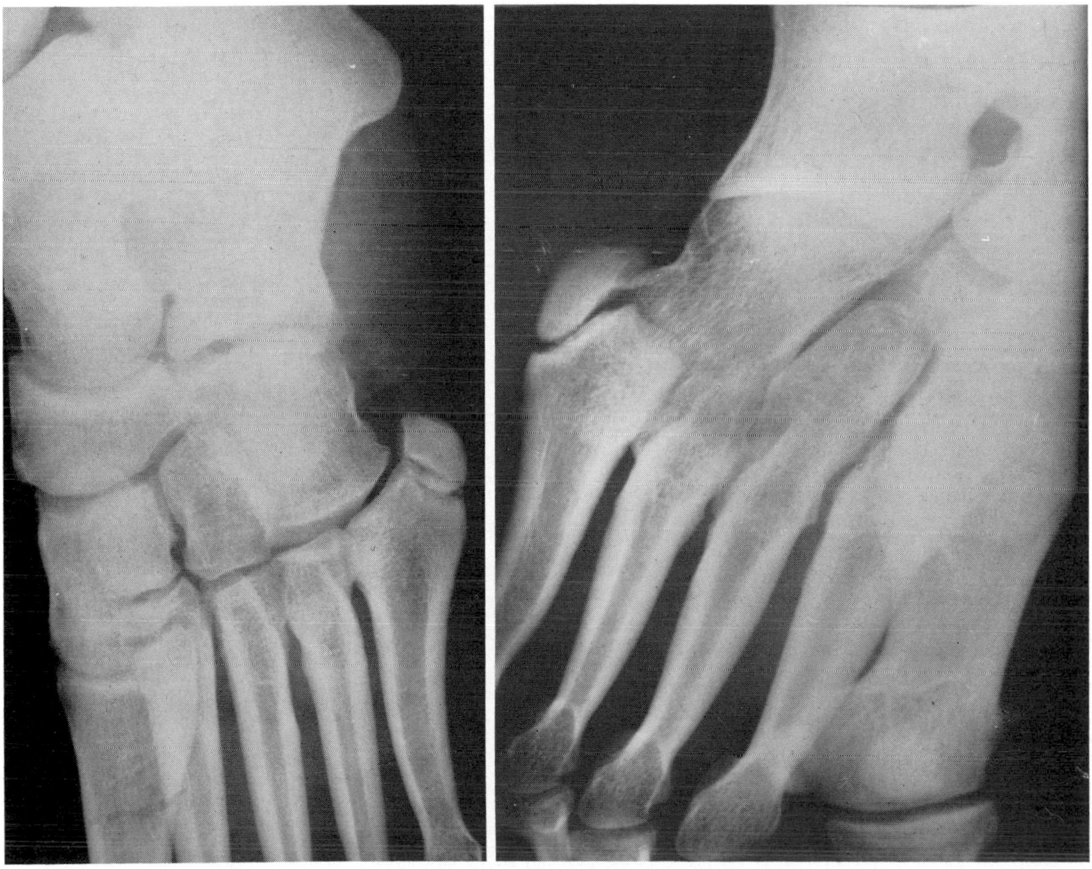

FIGURE 7-10. *Accessory ossicle at the base of fifth metatarsal (os vesalianum).*

or may be entirely absent. The ossification centers of the epiphyses of the phalanges, particularly the proximal phalanx, may be cone-shaped, invaginating into the diaph- ysis. Fissuring of the epiphyses of the proximal phalanx of the hallux is another variation. The sesamoid may be bipartite and have to be distinguished from fracture.

Congenital Deformities of the Foot

CONGENITAL CLUBFOOT

Clubfoot may be congenital or acquired. The word *talipes* is derived from the Latin *talus* (ankle bone) and *pes* (foot), and is the generic term used for foot deformities of congenital origin. Originally it was applied only to those deformities of the foot that caused the patient to walk on the ankles. Terms designating acquired deformities of the foot are preceded by the word *pes*.

The four primary deformities of the foot and ankle are described as: *varus*—the heel is inverted, and the forefoot is adducted and inverted; *valgus*—the heel is everted and the forefoot is abducted and everted; *equinus*—the foot is plantar-flexed, and the toes are at a lower level than the heel; and *calcaneus*—the foot is dorsiflexed, and the heel is at a lower level than the toes (Fig. 7–11).

Combinations of these deformities are equinovarus, equinovalgus, calcaneovalgus, and calcaneovarus.

TALIPES EQUINOVARUS

Talipes equinovarus is one of the commoner congenital deformities of the foot and has been known since ancient times. It occurs in approximately one in 1,000 live births.[137, 181, 195]

Etiology

The exact cause of talipes equinovarus has not been determined. It has, in the past,

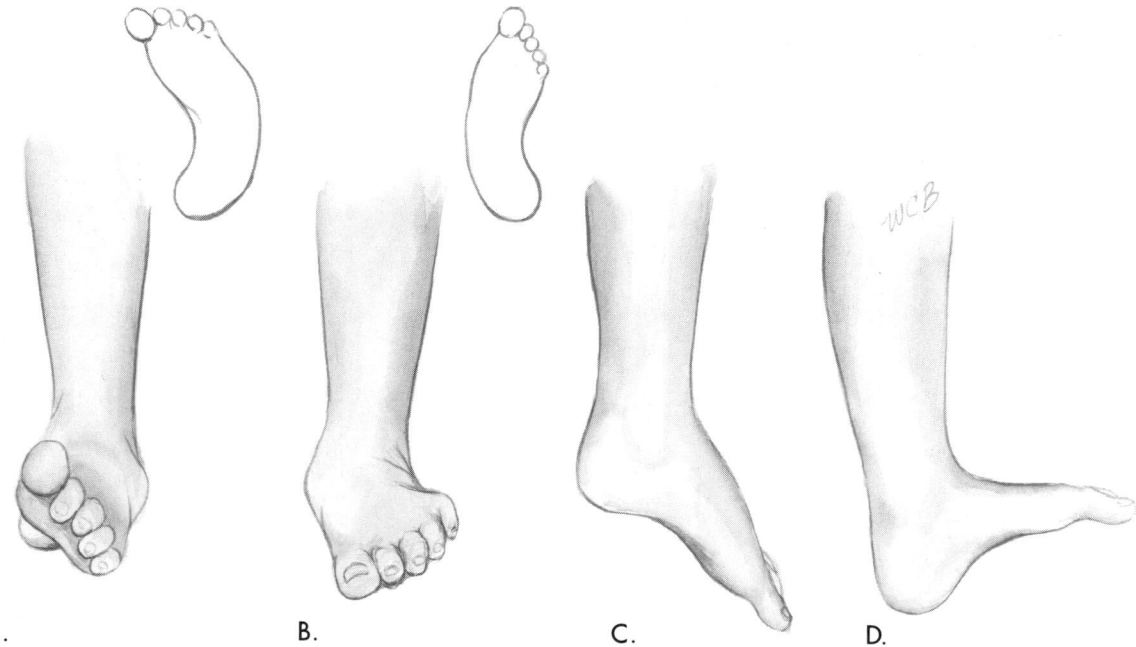

FIGURE 7–11. *Primary deformities of the foot and ankle.*

A. Varus. **B.** Valgus. **C.** Equinus. **D.** Calcaneus.

been the subject of much speculation and theorizing characterized by a striking paucity of facts.

Over 100 years ago, Hüter regarded talipes equinovarus to be the result of an arrest of development of the foot in one of the physiologic phases of its embryonic life.[125] That there are physiologic positions in the embryologic development of the foot that are similar to talipes equinovarus has been demonstrated by Henke and Reyher, Schomburg, Bardeen, and Böhm.[57, 69, 118, 175] The four stages in the evolution of the human foot in the first half of prenatal life were delineated by Böhm.[69]

First Stage (Second Month). The form of the foot is characterized by marked equinus inclination (about 90 degrees of plantar flexion) and by severe adduction of the hindpart and forepart of the foot, with the navicular lying in close proximity to the medial malleolus. The plane of the lower leg and the transverse axis of the knee and the plane of the foot (i.e., the one passing transversely through the long axis of the foot plate) are superimposed.

Second Stage (Beginning of Third Month). There is a new development—the foot rotates into a position of marked supination, but remains in 90 degrees of plantar flexion. The first metatarsal is markedly adducted; the lateral four metatarsals are adducted to a lesser extent (Fig. 7–12 A and B).

Third Stage (Middle of Third Month). The equinus inclination decreases to a mild degree, but the marked supination and metatarsus varus persist. In this stage, the long axis of the foot is perpendicular to the plane of the lower leg (Fig. 7 12 C)

Fourth Stage (Beginning at Fourth Month). The foot is in midsupination with slight metatarsus varus (Fig. 7–12 D). In this stage, the foot plate begins to rotate toward pronation on its long axis, the planes of the foot and lower leg gradually assuming the relative positions seen in the human adult.

It is obvious from the preceding observations that the three primary deformities of talipes equinovarus, namely plantar flexion, adduction, and supination, exist normally in the early stages of physiologic embryonic development of the human foot. This relationship is given in Table 7–2. Studies of the pathologic anatomy of severe talipes equinovarus have shown that it

resembles an embryonic foot at the beginning of the second month.[69]

Irani and Sherman and Settle believed talipes equinovarus to be the result of a primary germ plasm defect, developing in the foot in the first trimester of pregnancy.[128, 177]

Wynne-Davies, after studying the family history of 144 patients with talipes equinovarus, proposed that the cause of talipes equinovarus is partly genetic and partly environmental, owing to a factor acting on the fetus in utero. The chance of any individual having talipes equinovarus is one per thousand. If one child in a family has the deformity, the chances of a second child having it are one in 35. There is a definitely greater incidence among the male relatives of a female patient; it is very unlikely, however, that female relatives of a male patient will be affected. It is preponderant in boys, the male to female ratio being approximately two to one. Birth order, age of parents, and consanguinity were of no significance. No recognizable pattern of inheritance to indicate a dominant, recessive, or sex-linked gene was demonstrated.[195]

Idelberger examined 174 pairs of twins. In one in three of identical twin pairs, both had talipes equinovarus (33 per cent), as opposed to only one in 35 of nonidentical twin pairs (2.9 per cent).[126] Since the deformity is not invariably present in both identical twins, the cause of talipes equinus cannot be solely genetic; an environmental factor must act in utero, affecting one twin but not the other.[195]

Palmer, in a genetic study based on 108 unrelated families, each having at least one child under treatment for talipes equinovarus, found two recognizable groups of patients, one with and one without a positive family history. In the presence of a positive family history there is approximately a 10 per cent chance of the deformity appearing in additional children born to the same parents. It appears to be inherited as an autosomal dominant trait with about 40 per cent penetrance. In the group with a negative family history the risk of the deformity occurring in a subsequent sibling of the proband is no greater than in the general population, and the condition appears to be partially or totally nonheredi-

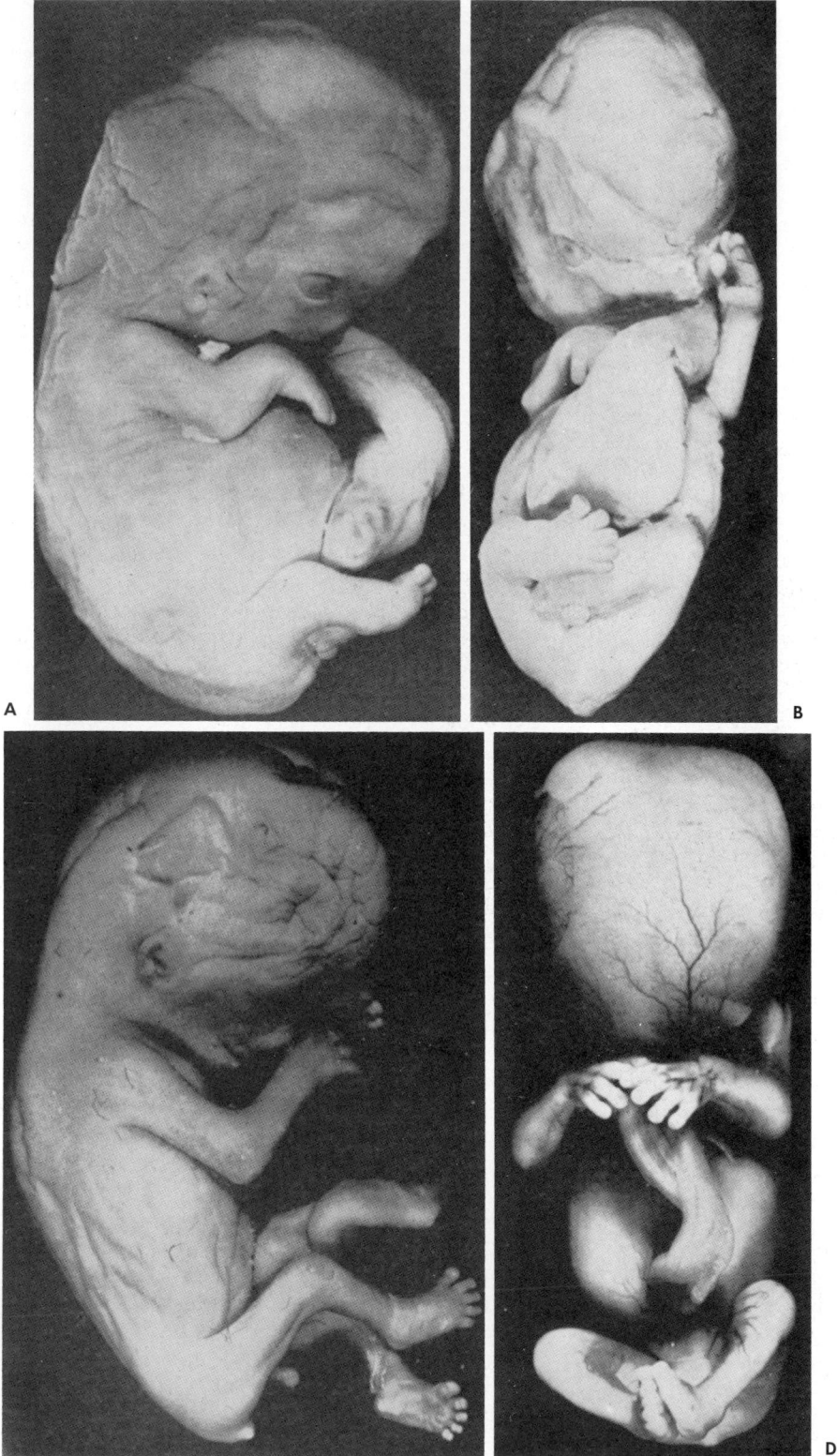

FIGURE 7–12. *Appearance of lower limbs of human embryo in first half of prenatal life. See opposite page for legend.*

Table 7–2

	Primary Deformities in Talipes Equinovarus					
	Plantar Flexion		Adduction		Supination	
Stages of Physiologic Embryonic Development	Marked	Slight	Tarsus	Metatarsus	Marked	Slight
First stage (second month)	+	−	+	+	−	−
Second stage (beginning of third month)	+	−	−	+	+	−
Third stage (middle of third month)	−	+	−	+	+	−
Fourth stage (beginning of fourth month)	−	−	−	+	−	+

From Böhm, M.: The embryologic origin of clubfoot. J. Bone Joint Surg., *11*:246, 1929. Reproduced with permission of the publisher.

tary. Talipes equinovarus in these children is perhaps due to new mutations like those that, in past generations, produced the current hereditary cases.[165]

Pathologic Anatomy

The characteristic deformity consists of the following components: (1) inversion and adduction of the forepart of the foot; (2) inversion of the heel; and (3) equinus fixation of the foot in plantar flexion at the ankle and subtalar joints (Fig. 7–13). Often there is associated cavus deformity, with the forefoot plantar-flexed on the hindfoot at the midtarsal joint.

The pathologic changes observed may be either primary (congenital) or secondary (adaptive). Irani and Sherman studied the pathologic anatomy of 11 fetal limbs with talipes equinovarus deformity; and Settle dissected 16 specimens from the late fetal period.[128, 177] The study of morbid anatomy in the fetus distinguished the primary from the adaptive changes. The findings of the

preceding 27 dissected fetal specimens and of the previously reported dissections in the literature are essentially the same.*

SKELETAL CHANGES

The primary deformity in talipes equinovarus is medial and plantar deviation of the anterior part of the talus. In the normal foot the angle formed by the long axis of the head and neck of the talus with the long axis of its body is between 150 and 155 degrees, whereas in talipes equinovarus, it is constantly decreased, measuring 115 to 135 degrees (Fig. 7–13 D). Normally, the articular surface of the talus in the talonavicular joint faces forward in the frontal plane of the body; in talipes equinovarus, it faces medially and plantarward. The talus is in equinus posture, with the anterior part of its superior articular surface displaced out of the ankle mortise.

The articular facets on the inferior surface of the talus are markedly distorted. Set-

*See References 53, 54, 64, 65, 68, 78, 79, 98, 101, 162, 168.

FIGURE 7–12. *Appearance of lower limbs of human embryo in first half of prenatal life.*

A and *B.* Lateral and anteroposterior view of 23 mm. long (vertex to buttocks) human embryo at nine weeks. Note the 90-degree pes equinus, marked supination of the feet, and adduction of the metatarsals. *C.* Lateral view of 35 mm. embryo (middle of third month). Note the slight pes equinus, marked supination of the entire foot, and moderate metatarsus varus. *D.* An anteroposterior view of 57 mm. long human embryo (end of third month). Note the midsupination of the feet and the slight metatarsus varus. (From Böhm, M.: The embryologic origin of clubfoot. J. Bone Joint Surg., *11*:246, 1929.)

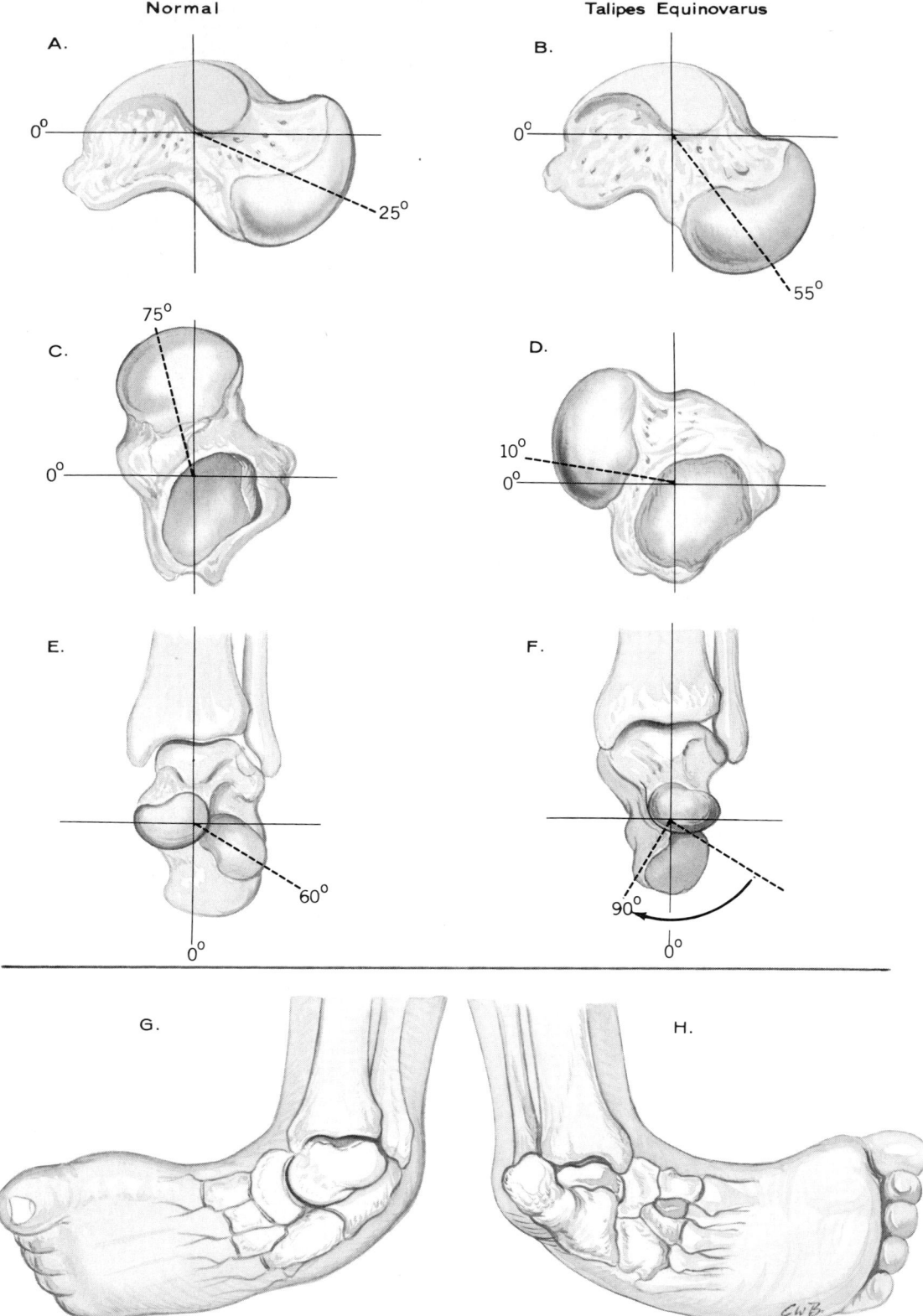

FIGURE 7–13. *Pathologic anatomy of talipes equinovarus — skeletal changes. See opposite page for legend.*

tle found a single misshapen articular surface, which was located on an axis slanted medially.[177] Irani and Sherman noted the posterior subtalar joint to be relatively normal, but the anterior portion to be deranged.[128] The medially deviated head of the talus articulates with the medial surface of the anterior part of the calcaneus. The sinus tarsi is widened.

The contour of the calcaneus in general is normal, with the articular facets normally oriented on its body. Since these facets articulate with those of the talus, the calcaneus is, of necessity, displaced in varus and equinus inclination and internal rotation. In severe deformities the calcaneus may be somewhat bowed, with its concave aspect facing medially. The varus position of the heel disappears upon release of its capsular and ligamentous attachments, indicating that it is a secondary positional deformity.

The talonavicular and calcaneocuboid articular surfaces face medially and plantarward. With the calcaneus rolled in under the talus, the talonavicular and calcaneocuboid joints lie beneath one another instead of in their normal side-by-side position (Fig. 7–13 E and F). As a result of this skeletal relationship, the forepart of the foot rests on its lateral side.

The navicular is smaller than normal and its proximal articular surface is inclined toward the medial and plantar surface of the foot to articulate with the medially deviated head of the talus (Fig. 7–13 H). This contributes to the shortening and increased concavity of the inner border of the foot. The cuboid, cuneiforms, and metatarsals are essentially normal.

In severe deformity, the navicular becomes markedly displaced medially and may rest against the anterior portion of the medial malleolus, the posterolateral portion of the calcaneus may be in close apposition to the posterior aspect of the lateral malleolus, and the sustentaculum tali may be in contact with the tip of the medial malleolus. Accessory articulations in these three locations may develop.

If the deformity is severe, the body of the talus is tilted medially, so that its medial surface is pressed against the medial malleolus, and the upper border of its lateral surface is pressed against the fibular malleolus. Irani and Sherman could not demonstrate rotational deformity in the coronal section.[128]

The tibia is essentially normal. Settle found a minimal degree of increased internal tibial torsion in 4 of the 16 clubfoot specimens; however, this variation is considered normal and is not pathologic.[177] There is some disagreement in the literature concerning rotational deformity of the tibia and talus in the ankle mortise in talipes equinovarus. Kite states that excessive internal tibial torsion is a common associated finding.[137] This is not correct, and the old concept of exaggerated internal tibial torsion as the fourth element of the complex deformity of talipes equinovarus should be disregarded. Posterior displacement of the fibular malleolus despite alleged internal tibial torsion was noted by Ober.[163] Curtis and Butterfield believed the talus to be internally rotated in the ankle mortise.[88] External rotation of the hindfoot on the tibia was found by Wynne-Davies.[196]

Swann, Lloyd-Roberts and Catterall pro-

FIGURE 7–13. *Pathologic anatomy of talipes equinovarus – skeletal changes.*

At upper left are normal specimens; on the right, are specimens of tali and hindfoot in talipes equinovarus. **A** and **B** are medial views. In talipes equinovarus (**B**) the neck of the talus and its articular surface are markedly deviated plantarward. **C** and **D** show the tali from below. In the normal foot (**C**) the neck of the talus is deviated medially 15 degrees, whereas in the clubfoot the angle of its medial deviation is 80 degrees (i.e., the angle formed by the long axis of the head and neck of the talus with the long axis of its body measures 100 degrees). **E** and **F** show the anterior articular surfaces of the calcaneus and talus. In talipes equinovarus (**F**) note the medial rotation of the calcaneus under the talus. In the normal foot (**E**) the articular surface of the calcaneus for the cuboid is well to the lateral side of the long axis of the leg, whereas in talipes equinovarus (**F**) this articular surface is displaced medially.

G and **H.** These are anterior and posterior views of a specimen of a foot and ankle with talipes equinovarus, showing the general skeletal relationships. (Adapted from Settle, G. W.: The anatomy of congenital talipes equinovarus: Sixteen dissected specimens. J. Bone Joint Surg., *45–A*:1341, 1963.)

posed that in uncorrected clubfeet, the distal part of the talus and forefoot are laterally rotated in the ankle mortise on the tibia, which has no rotational deformity. In talipes equinovarus the soft tissues (musculotendinous units, capsule, and ligaments) are shortened both medially and posteriorly. If both yield to primary stretching forces of passive manipulation and corrective cast, the deformity will be corrected; but if either or both remain unyielding, a spurious correction will be obtained. A transverse breach in the midtarsal joint will result in the familiar "rocker-bottom" deformity. A longitudinal breach may also take place when the midtarsal deformity does not yield in the horizontal axis. The abduction-eversion correcting force (applied on the anterior lever of the forefoot) is transmitted to the hindfoot, which, being tethered medially by the posterior tibial muscle, rotates into lateral position at the ankle joint, thus displacing the fibular malleolus backward. The resulting deformity is referred to by Swann et al. as the "bean-shaped foot." They further support their observation by citing four clinical signs: (1) Without lateral rotation of the hindfoot, the foot might lie almost at a right angle to the leg when the talonavicular joint is dislocated. This does not occur. (2) In uncorrected clubfoot, the head of the talus is palpable laterally below and in front of the outer side of the ankle. Only lateral rotation could thus modify its normal alignment, for if it rotated inward, it would lie on the medial side of its normal position. (3) The lateral malleolus is palpable posterior to and the medial malleolus anterior to their normal position when the proximal tibial tubercle is pointing directly forward. (4) Medial rotational osteotomy of the tibia not only accentuates the varus deformity of the forefoot but improves the alignment of the hindfoot clinically and radiographically as well.[183] It should be emphasized that the lateral rotation of the hindfoot in the ankle mortise on the tibia is an *acquired* deformity, not a primary one, and that it results from inadequate treatment of clubfoot.

SOFT-TISSUE CHANGES

In talipes equinovarus there are no primary abnormalities of the muscles, tendons, nerves, or vessels. The soft-tissue alterations are adaptive in nature, conforming to the skeletal deformity. The nerves and muscles are normal grossly and histologically. There are no primary abnormal insertions.

The soft tissues on the medial and posterior aspect of the foot and ankle are shortened. All the components of soft tissue participate in the shortening—the skin, adipose tissue, muscles, tendons, capsule, ligaments, and nerves and vessels. Initially, the decrease in length is not due to fibrotic contracture; they simply have grown to that length, conforming to the contours of the bones. Later on, however, repeated forceful manipulations and bruising of the foot may lead to fibrosis of the soft parts.

The soft-tissue contractures are categorized as posterior, medial, subtalar, or plantar.[190]

Posterior Contractures. The posterior part of the capsule of the ankle and subtalar joints, the calcaneofibular ligament, the posterior talofibular ligament, and the triceps surae muscle are shortened. The medial fibers of the tendo Achillis insert more medially and anteriorly on the calcaneus, thereby pulling the heel into varus position.

Medial Contracture. The deltoid, tibionavicular, and calcaneonavicular ligaments are shortened; and the posterior tibial, flexor digitorum longus, and flexor hallucis longus musculotendinous units are contracted. The contracted posterior tibial tendon, the deltoid and spring ligaments, and the talonavicular capsule are usually fused into a dense mass of scar tissue, pulling the navicular toward the medial malleolus and sustentaculum tali.

Subtalar Contractures. These involve the talocalcaneal interosseous ligament and the bifurcated (or Y) ligament that extends from the calcaneus to the lateral border of the navicular and to the medial border of the cuboid.

Plantar Contractures. When there is associated equinus deformity of the forefoot, the plantar fascia, abductor hallucis, short toe flexors, and abductor digiti quinti muscles are shortened.

Clinical Picture

The degree and severity of talipes equinovarus vary from a mild deformity to one in which the toes touch the medial side of the lower leg. Talipes equinovarus may be of the rigid or the flexible type; it is important to distinguish between the two. In the *rigid type* the deformity is very severe. The heel is small and is markedly equinus and in inversion, while the forefoot is markedly varus. The skin is stretched and thin on the dorsolateral aspect of the ankle and hindfoot; and it is creased on the inner side of the ankle and instep of the foot. The deformity is fixed and can be corrected only minimally by passive manipulation. It is usually accompanied by moderate atrophy of the leg. Hersh refers to this form as the *intrinsic type* of talipes equinovarus.[119]

In the *flexible type*, the deformity is less severe and can be readily corrected to neutral position by passive manipulation. There are skin creases on the dorsolateral aspect of the ankle and foot. The heel is of normal size and the leg is of normal circumference or minimally atrophied. Hersh uses the term *extrinsic type* to describe this form.[119] It is probably a static deformity associated with intrauterine malposture.

The clinical findings depict the anatomic deformities. In the typical case, the affected foot and leg have a clublike appearance (Fig. 7–14). The hindfoot points downward, and draws up the heel, which is rolled in under the talus in an inverted position. The heel appears small, and there are deep creases at the ankle joint posteriorly. The forefoot is adducted and inverted. The body of the talus is partially displaced forward out of the ankle mortise between the malleoli. With inversion of the entire foot underneath the talus and adduction of the forefoot, the head of the talus is the most prominent subcutaneous bone on the lateral side of the dorsum of the foot. The skin in this convex area of the foot is stretched and thinned, and its creases have disappeared. The lateral malleolus is more prominent than the medial malleolus. The medial displacement of the navicular bone can be palpated on the inner side of the head of the talus. The skin creases are deeply furrowed on the concave medial side of the foot.

On passive dorsiflexion and eversion of the foot, the taut triceps surae and posterior tibial muscles can be palpated. One can also feel the thickened and shortened ligaments and joint capsule on the medial side of the foot and the posterior aspect of the ankle and subtalar joints. If the forefoot is in equinus position, the plantar fascia and the intrinsic muscles on the plantar aspect of the foot will be contracted. Circumference of the calves and leg lengths should be measured. As stated previously, atrophy of the leg is usually severe with the more rigid type of clubfoot.

The hips must be carefully examined for subluxation or dislocation. All other joints and limbs are checked to rule out the presence of arthrogryposis multiplex congenita. The spine should be carefully examined for abnormalities, and the neuromuscular system assessed to rule out paralytic disease.

If talipes equinovarus remains untreated, the deformity will progressively increase and the contractures will become more rigid. The child will bear weight on the lateral border of the foot and on the fibular malleolus (Fig. 7–15). Ambulation will be difficult and the gait awkward. Soon painful callosities and bursae will develop over the lateral side of the foot.

It is important to differentiate the congenital from the acquired type of clubfoot. In the newborn this is usually easy, but in older children it may be more difficult. Paralytic clubfoot is seen in myelomeningocele, intraspinal tumors, poliomyelitis, peroneal type of progressive muscular atrophy, and cerebral palsy. Growth disturbances of the distal tibial epiphyses secondary to fracture or infection are other causes of acquired equinovarus deformity.

Roentgenographic Findings

The primary value of roentgenograms is not in the diagnosis of clubfoot but in the determination of the degree of varus and equinus deformity, the demonstration of the deranged mechanics of the hindfoot, and as a device for accurate assessment of the amount of correction obtained.

In the infant, the primary centers of ossification of the talus, calcaneus, and cuboid are well developed and are visible on the roentgenogram; frequently that of the third cuneiform may also be present. The ossification center of the navicular, however, does not appear until three years of age. The metatarsals and phalanges are also os-

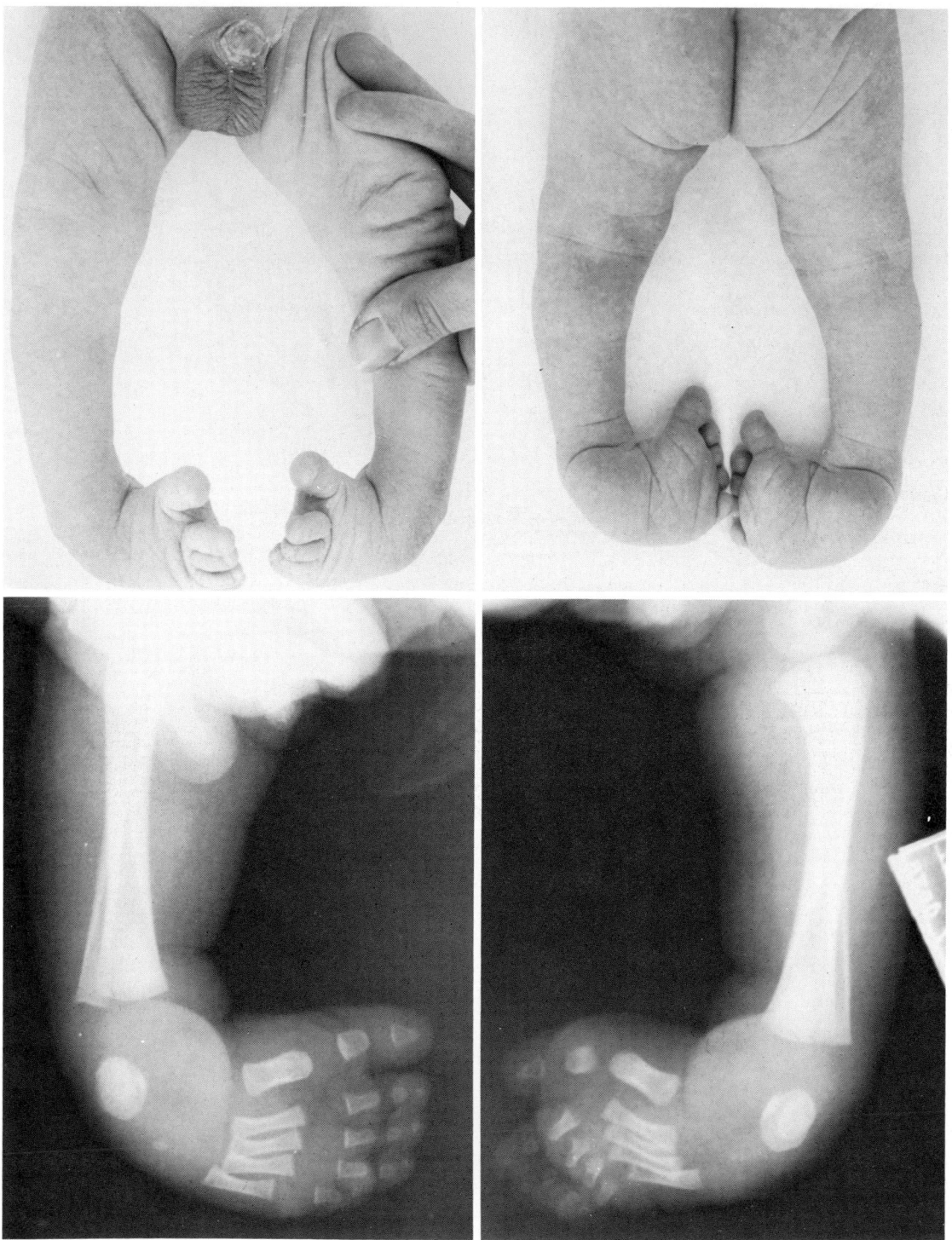

FIGURE 7–14. Bilateral talipes equinovarus of the rigid or intrinsic type in a newborn infant.

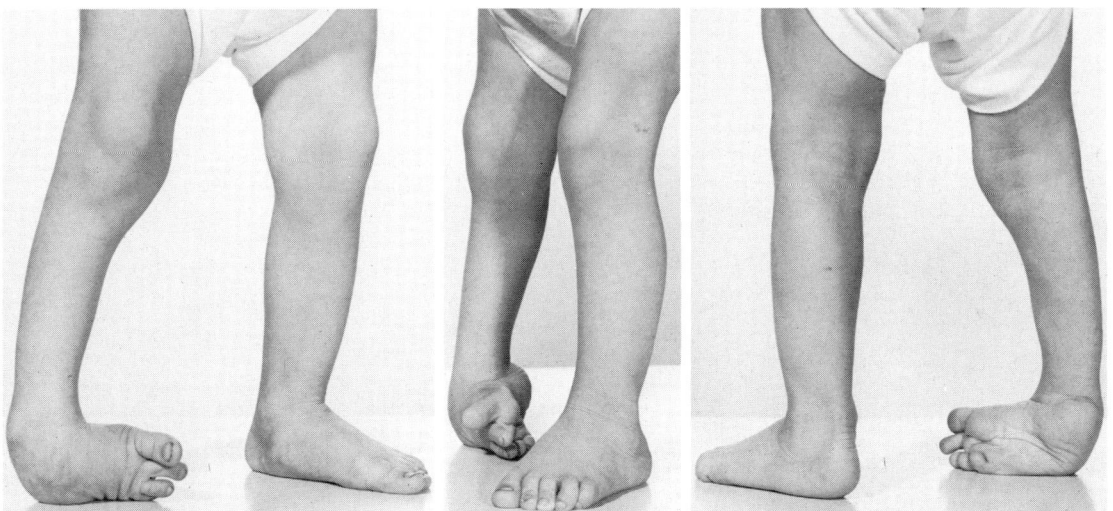

FIGURE 7–15.   *Untreated severe talipes equinovarus on the right in a three-year-old boy.*

The body weight is borne on the lateral border of the foot.

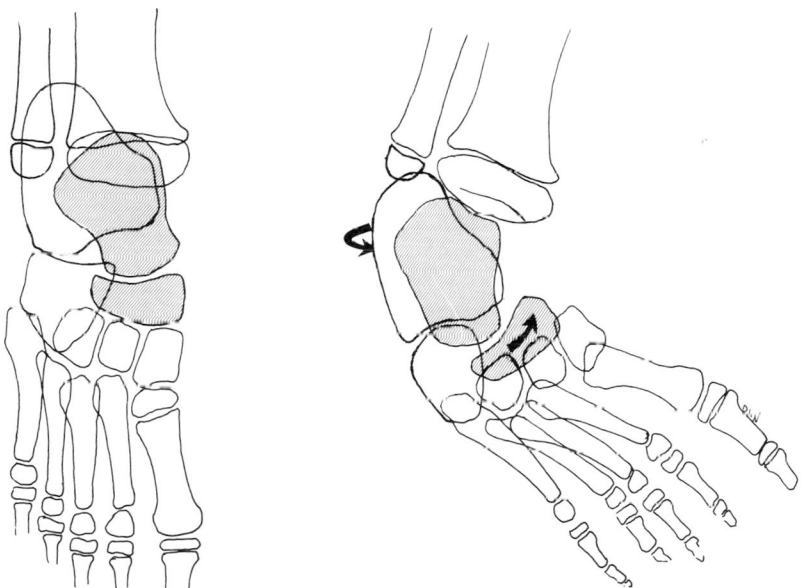

FIGURE 7–16.   *Diagram of anteroposterior roentgenograms of a normal foot and talipes equinovarus.*

A. In the normal foot, the radiopaque shadows of the anterior end of the calcaneus and the head of the talus are separated, the talus pointing to the first metatarsal and the calcaneus toward the fourth and fifth metatarsals. **B.** In talipes equinovarus the shadows of the anterior end of the calcaneus and the head of the talus are superimposed and point laterally to the fifth metatarsal. Also, note the medial displacement of the navicular bone on the head of the talus. In the infant, the navicular bone is not ossified.

sified. It must be remembered that the entire bone is not observed, only the small center of ossification surrounded by a large mass of cartilage having the same density as the soft tissues. The feet should be placed in identical positions during different examinations. In the literature a number of methods of roentgenologic assessment of primary and residual deformity of clubfoot are described.

The *anteroposterior roentgenogram* is made with the foot in 30 degrees of plantar flexion with the tube directed cranially 30 degrees from the perpendicular. The foot is placed flat on the cassette. Lines are drawn through the center of the longitudinal axis of the talus parallel to its medial border, and through that of the calcaneus parallel to its lateral border. In the normal foot, the direction of the long axis of the talus points toward the first metatarsal and that of the

calcaneus toward the fifth metatarsal, forming a "V" (Fig. 7–16 A). This talocalcaneal angle normally measures 20 to 40 degrees. In talipes equinovarus with inversion of the heel, the talocalcaneal angle diminishes and may approach zero. In severe inversion of the hindfoot, the longitudinal axes of the talus and calcaneus become superimposed and point laterally to the fourth and fifth toes (Fig. 7–16 B). Attention to the malalignment of the long axis of the talus and calcaneus in clubfoot was drawn by Kite and by Wisbrun and was also later stressed by Kandel.[132, 134, 194] As the inversion of the hindfoot begins to be corrected, the head of the talus no longer lies on top of the calcaneus, but projects medially, producing the normal talocalcaneal angle. Hindfoot correction should be verified roentgenographically before termination of stretching cast treatment.

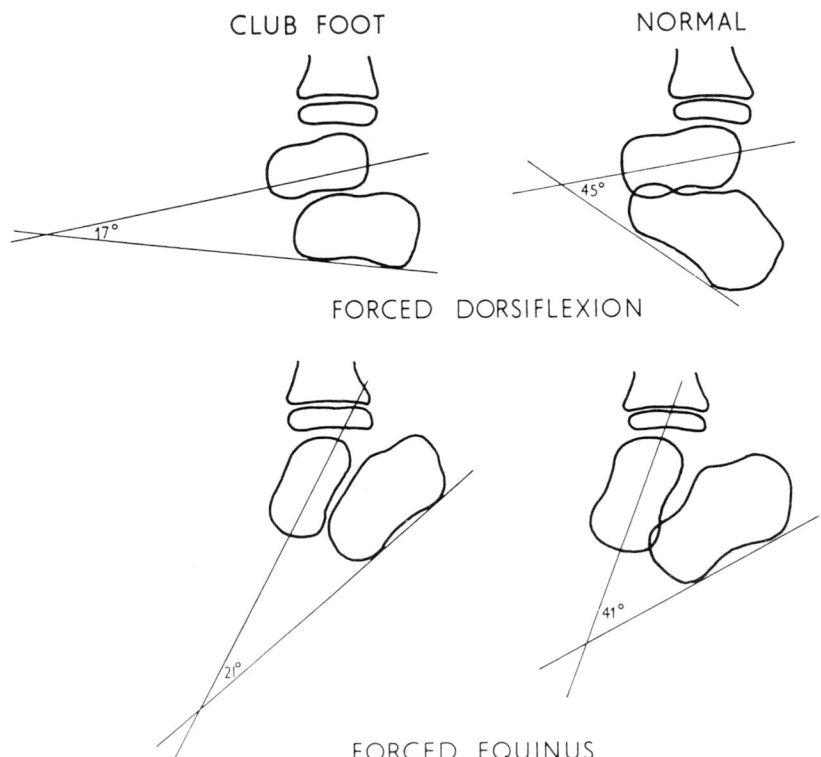

FIGURE 7–17. *The talocalcaneal angle in the lateral roentgenogram in the normal foot and in talipes equinovarus.*

The axis of the talus is the line joining the midpoints of the head and body of the talus. The axis of the calcaneus is the line joining the calcaneal tubercles and the anterior plantar convexity of the calcaneus. The normal talocalcaneal angle is between 35 and 50 degrees, and it increases in forced dorsiflexion, whereas in talipes equinovarus, it is less than 35 degrees, and is often decreased further by forced dorsiflexion. (From Heywood, A. W. B.: The mechanics of the hindfoot in clubfoot as demonstrated radiographically. J. Bone Joint Surg., *46–B*:105, 1964.)

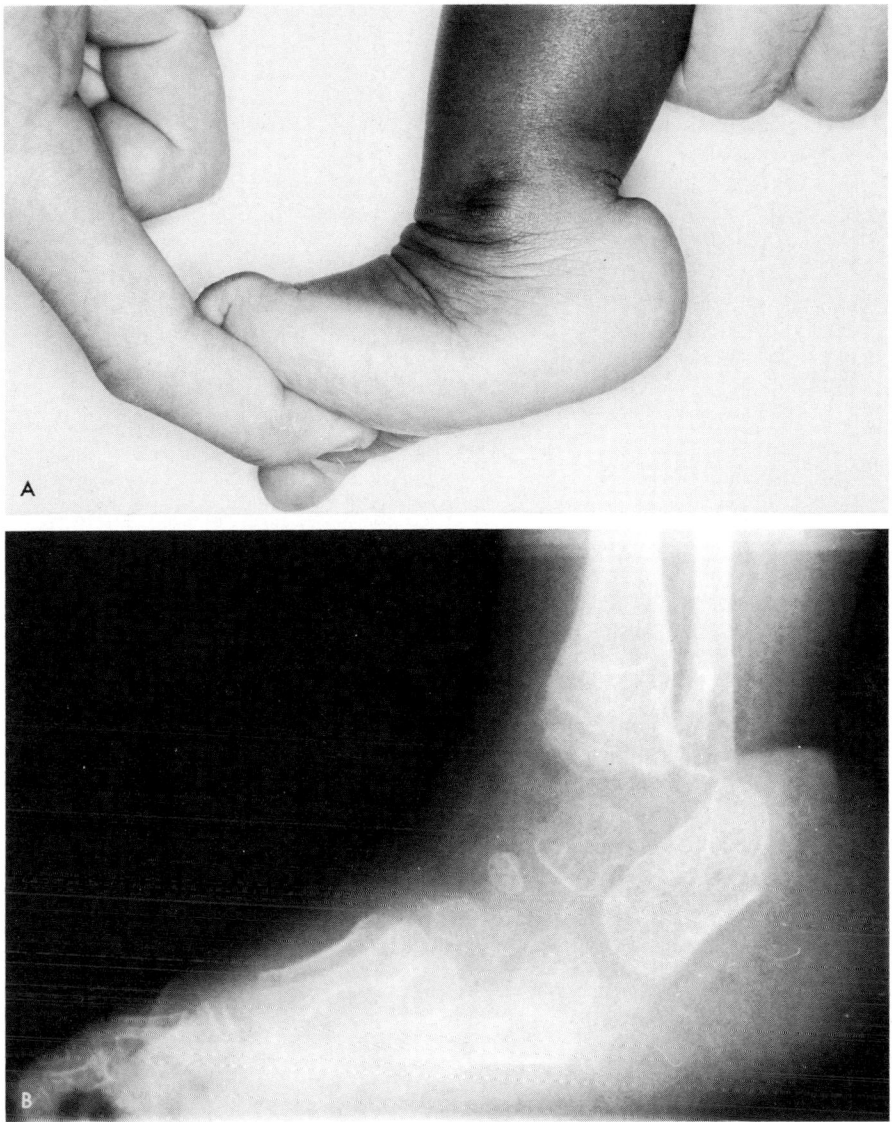

FIGURE 7-18. *Rocker-bottom deformity in talipes equinovarus.*

Deformity is the result of a transverse breach in the midtarsal area. **A.** Clinical appearance. **B.** Lateral roentgenograms of the foot and ankle.

A *lateral roentgenogram* is made with the infant lying on the affected side with his knee flexed and the lateral malleolus and the fifth metatarsal on the cassette. The x-ray tube is centered on the hindfoot. With a translucent splint on the sole of the foot, roentgenograms are made with the foot in 30 to 45 degrees of plantar flexion and then in maximal dorsiflexion. In the older patient, standing weight-bearing roentgenograms are also made. It is important to align the ankle mortise correctly by 30 to 60 degrees of internal rotation of the leg, depending upon the severity of the varus deformity of the foot.

In the standing roentgenogram (or on tracings of it) lines are drawn through the longitudinal axes of the talus, the calcaneus, and the sole of the foot. The axis of the talus is the line joining the midpoints of the head and the body; the axis of the calcaneus joins the calcaneal tubercles and the anterior

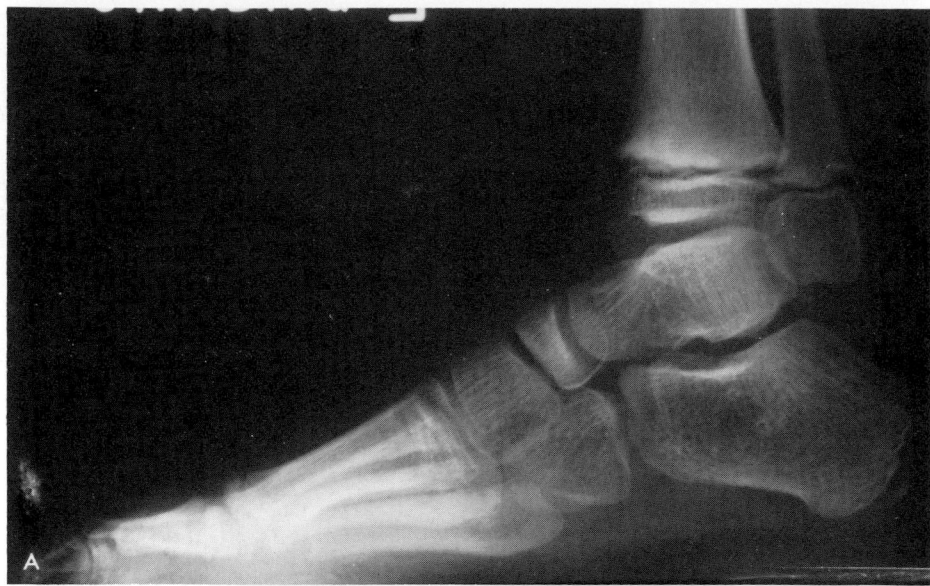

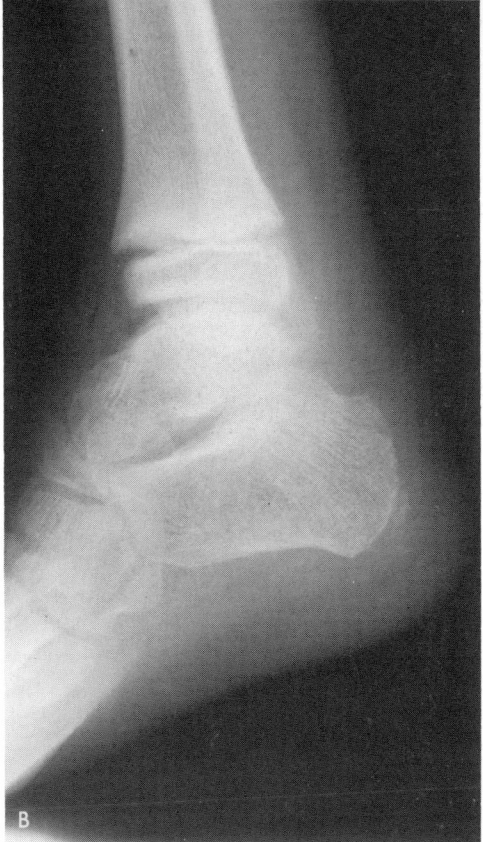

FIGURE 7–19.   Talipes equinovarus—lateral rotation of the distal part of the talus and the forefoot in the ankle mortise on the tibia.

This acquired deformity results from a longitudinal breach when the midtarsal deformity does not yield in the horizontal axis. **A.** Lateral roentgenogram showing posterior displacement of the lateral malleolus. Note the spurious flat-topped appearance of the talus. **B.** Lateral roentgenogram made with the leg internally rotated. Note the summit of the talus is dome-shaped. The forefoot varus deformity is increased as shown by the overlap of the cuboid and navicular on the calcaneus and talus.

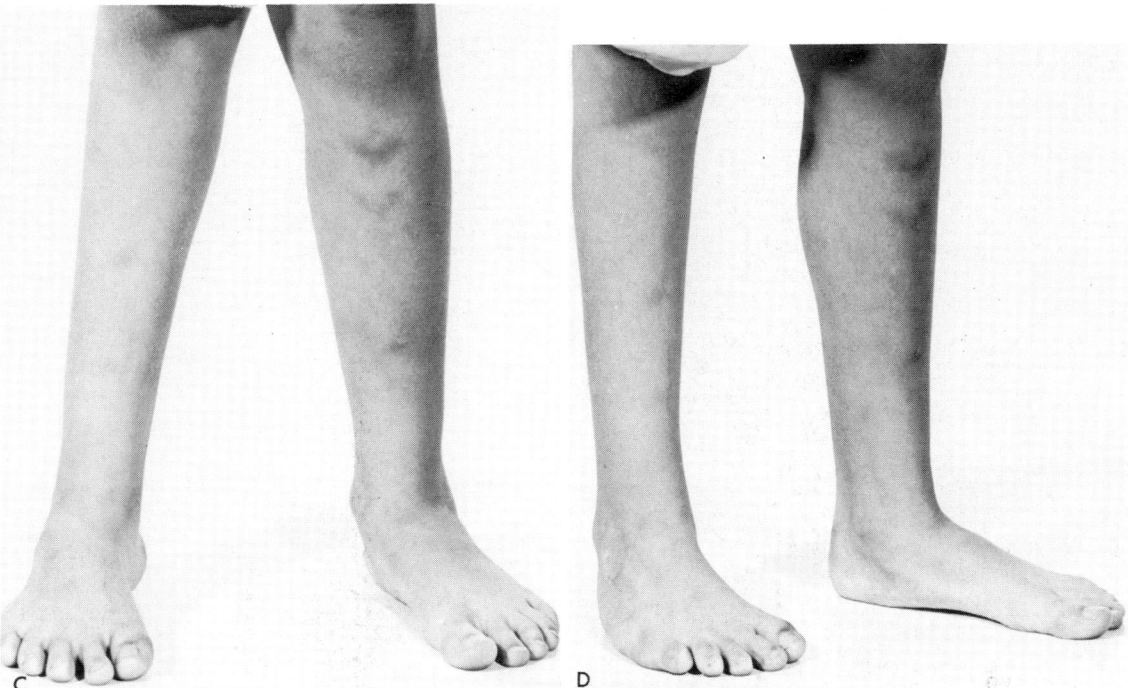

FIGURE 7–19 Continued. *Talipes equinovarus — lateral rotation of the distal part of the talus and the forefoot in the ankle mortise on the tibia.*

C and **D.** Standing photographs of same patient demonstrating exaggeration of forefoot varus deformity when the leg is internally rotated.

plantar convexity of the calcaneus. The axis of the sole is the line joining the calcaneal tubercle and the head of the third metatarsal (Fig. 7–17).

The talocalcaneal angle in the lateral roentgenogram of the normal foot measures between 35 and 50 degrees, whereas in talipes equinovarus it is less than 35 degrees and may reach minus 10 degrees. On forced dorsiflexion the talocalcaneal angle is increased in the normal foot (the mobile heel is pulled forward and upward by the plantar fascia), whereas in talipes equinovarus it is often decreased still further (as the calcaneus is fixed in equinus position by the contracted posterior soft tissues) (Fig. 7–17). It is obvious, therefore, that the determination of the talocalcaneal angle in the lateral roentgenogram is an invaluable guide to the degree of correction achieved.

The sole line normally passes below the calcaneocuboid joint; if it passes through it, a rocker-bottom deformity is being produced. Rocker-bottom deformity is the result of a transverse breach in the midtarsal area (Fig. 7–18).

Wynne-Davies and, more recently, Swann, Lloyd-Roberts, and Catterall have emphasized the possibility of a longitudinal breach that may occur when the midtarsal deformity remains uncorrected in the horizontal plane. The corrective abduction forces are transmitted to the hindfoot, which is rotated spuriously into lateral rotation. Thus a longitudinal breach is produced by premature eversion of the hindfoot prior to correction of the midtarsal varus inclination.[183, 196] This is evidenced in the lateral roentgenogram by posterior displacement of the lateral malleolus (Fig. 7–19 A). To detect it, the x-ray tube should be centered on the hindfoot and ankle, with the foot as nearly as possible at a right angle in relation to the leg.

True *flat-topped talus* may occur if forced manipulation causes osteochondral compression fracture or ischemic necrosis. Often, however, the flat-topped appearance of the talus is spurious, the result of its lateral rotation and projection in a frontal profile in the lateral roentgenogram. The calcaneus will appear shortened and the forefoot will look relatively normal. If another roentgenogram is taken with the leg internally rotated, the summit of the talus will be dome-shaped, and the length and contour of the calcaneus will improve. The forefoot varus inclination will be increased, as shown by the overlap of the cuboid and navicular on the calcaneus and talus (Fig. 7–19 B, C, and D).

With lateral rotation of the talus, the medial side of its dome comes to lie outside the ankle mortise, in contact with the edge of the tibia. Dorsiflexion of the ankle is prevented by contact at this point, and not by widening of the anterior part of the talus.

Treatment

Treatment should be started as soon as possible, preferably immediately following birth. A frequently quoted adage is that the prognosis in a breech delivery is better than that in a vertex presentation because exercises and treatment can be begun earlier while awaiting the after-coming head.

It is best for the orthopedist to talk to the parents shortly after the baby is born and to explain to them the nature and course of the treatment and what they can expect.

Conservative measures should always be employed first, and treatment begins in the nursery. First, the foot is gently and firmly manipulated out of forefoot adduction, heel and forefoot inversion, and equinus position (Fig. 7–20). In stretching the tendo Achillis, the physician should pull the os calcis distally with one hand (bringing the heel down), while using the other hand to push the calcaneocuboid area into dorsiflexion. One must not stretch the midfoot by forced dorsiflexion of the forefoot, or a "rocker-bottom" foot will result (Fig. 7–20 A and B).

The varus deformity of the hindfoot is corrected by pushing the heel into eversion with one thumb as counterpressure is applied by forcing inward the dorsolateral aspect of the head of the talus. Varus deformity of the forefoot is corrected by pushing it firmly outward into abduction and twisting it out into eversion. Pressure is exerted on the first metatarsal head, not on the great toe. The hindfoot is stabilized with the opposite hand. The corrected position is maintained to the count of 10 and then released. Passive stretching exercises are repeated for 10 to 15 minutes, and the correction obtained is then maintained by adhesive strapping or a plaster of Paris cast.

Forcible manipulation with wrenches or by other methods should be condemned because it will cause fractures of the tarsal bones and injury to the distal tibial epiphysis (Fig. 7–21).

During the first few days of life, adhesive strapping is applied to hold the foot in the corrected position (Fig. 7–22 A). The skin is painted with a nonirritating adhesive liquid, such as tincture of benzoin, and 1/2-inch-wide adhesive tape is applied directly on the skin, beginning in the middle of the dorsum of the foot, passing from the lateral to the medial side under the sole, and then obliquely upward and backward on the outer side of the leg. Three or four partially overlapping strips of adhesive tape are applied. The strapping is completed by several pieces of adhesive tape halfway around the leg. The tape should never be applied circumferentially around the leg or foot, as it will act as a constrictor and obstruct circulation to the distal part; it should be applied only on the outer side of the leg and ankle so as not to obstruct further correction by manipulation. The nurse, and later the mother, is shown how to manipulate the foot at regular intervals at each feeding time, 20 repetitions of each exercise at each period. If the strapping loosens, it may be changed or reinforced by an additional layer of adhesive tape.

After a few days, the adhesive strapping is removed, the foot is remanipulated, and a plaster of Paris clubfoot cast is applied from the toes to the groin with the knees flexed so as to control the heel and the rotation of the leg (Fig. 7–22). The skin is usually painted with a nonirritating adhesive liquid, such as tincture of benzoin or Ace Adherent, to prevent slipping of the cast and loss of correction. The successive plaster casts are changed at four- to seven-day intervals in the very young infant, and later at two-week intervals. With each change of cast, the foot is gently manipulated to obtain further correction. This is promoted by the relaxation and atrophy produced by the immobilization.

During manipulation all elements of the deformity are corrected; this is in contrast to

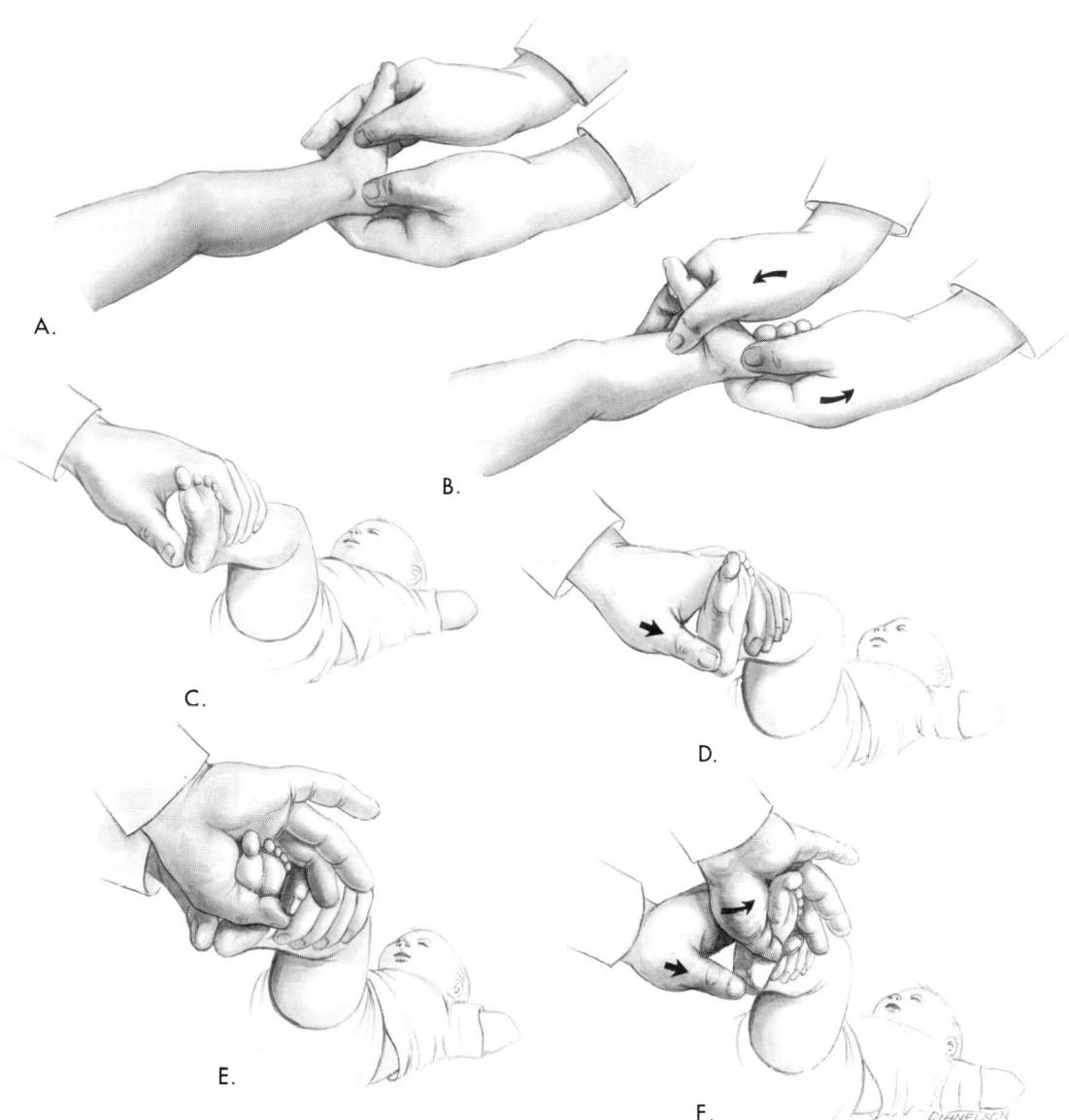

FIGURE 7–20.   *The technique of manipulation for correction of talipes equinovarus.*

A and **B.** *Manipulation of the foot to correct equinus deformity.* The os calcis, held between the index finger and thumb of one hand, is pulled distally, bringing the heel down; with the other hand, the calcaneocuboid area is pushed into dorsiflexion. The midfoot should not be stretched by forced dorsiflexion of the forefoot, or a "rocker-bottom" foot will be obtained.

C to **F.** *Manipulation of the forefoot and hindfoot to correct varus deformity.* The surgeon's left thumb pushes the heel into eversion as the pulp of the left index finger applies counterpressure by forcing the dorsolateral surface of the head of the talus inward; the remaining digits of the surgeon's left hand are used to stabilize the infant's leg. **E** and **F** show how the forefoot is pushed firmly outward into abduction and twisted out into eversion. Pressure is applied on the first metatarsal head and *not* on the big toe. (In the older infant, manipulations to correct varus forefoot and varus hindfoot are performed as separate steps.) The corrected position should be maintained to the count of 10 and then released. The passive stretching exercises are repeated for 10 to 15 minutes, and then the correction obtained is maintained by adhesive strapping or plaster of Paris cast. Before manipulation, the small heel of a newborn infant is painted with a nonirritating adhesive liquid to improve the surgeon's grip.

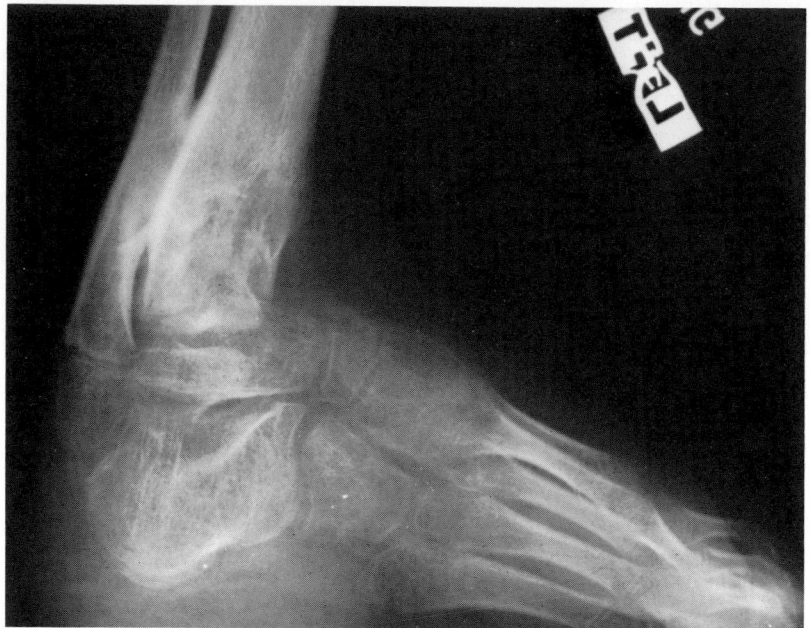

FIGURE 7–21. *Damage to the distal tibial epiphysis and growth arrest caused by forceful manipulation to correct talipes equinovarus.*

Multiple osteochondral compression fractures have resulted in flat-topped talus. Note the overgrown fibular malleolus.

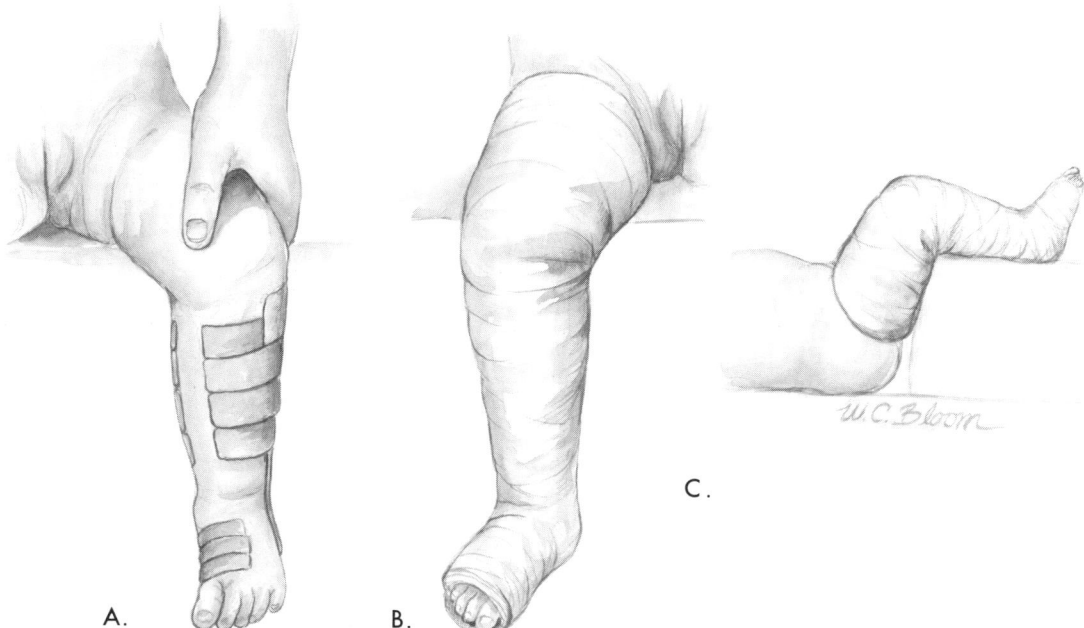

FIGURE 7–22. *Adhesive strapping and plaster of Paris cast in treatment of talipes equinovarus.*

the traditional teaching of Kite that the clubfoot should be corrected in sequence from front to back and that one should not proceed to the next stage until any distal deformity has been fully corrected. Kite first corrects the varus forefoot, then the hindfoot inversion, and last, the equinus ankle and subtalar joints.[134-138] We have been constantly alerted to the dangers of premature dorsiflexion as a cause of transverse breach at the midtarsal joint, resulting in "rocker-bottom" foot. Recently Wynne-Davies, and Swann, Lloyd-Roberts, and Catterall have warned us that a longitudinal breach of the foot may be produced by premature eversion of the hindfoot prior to correction of the varus forefoot.[183, 196]

Leaving the hindfoot in equinus position until the deformity is corrected, however, allows the posterior capsular and triceps surae contracture to become more rigid and is an important factor in the causation of "rocker-bottom" foot. Another anatomic factor to consider is that full plantar flexion of the foot is accompanied by varus deformity and full dorsiflexion by valgus deformity. While the hindfoot is left in equinus position, the subtalar joint and the forefoot are kept inverted unless the foot is forcibly breached at the midtarsal joint.

Dorsiflexion of the hindfoot takes place in two stages: (1) at the ankle joint, which requires relaxation of the triceps surae muscle; and (2) at the subtalar joint, around which the remainder of the foot rotates as the posterior tibial muscles relax. In clubfoot, both these muscles are shortened, causing the hindfoot to be fixed in equinovarus position. If both yield to initial stretching, normal dorsiflexion of the hindfoot will be obtained, but if either or both remain contracted, full dorsiflexion cannot be obtained.

In the literature it is often stated that it is difficult, if not impossible, to manipulate the small heel of an infant with clubfoot. A common error is to apply the dorsiflexion force on the long anterior lever of the forefoot. It is imperative to paint the small heel with an adhesive liquid and hold it with an opened 2 × 2 inch surgical gauze and *pull it down*. The posterior tibial muscle is then stretched by everting the hindfoot as the anterior end of the calcaneus is pushed into dorsiflexion.

Various methods of immobilization to maintain the correction achieved by manipulation are available. The author prefers the plaster of Paris cast, as it is simple to apply, maintains correction effectively, and causes less difficulty with skin and circulation. Serial adhesive strapping is recommended by Brockman, by Fripp and Shaw, and by Clark.[71, 82, 105] If one chooses such a method, he should study the details of technique as described by Fripp and Shaw.[105] Orthopedic white felt is used for padding bony prominences. The strapping on the forefoot should pass over the knee and then over the medial side of the leg, while the heel is held in eversion and dorsiflexion by strapping that begins on the medial side of the leg, passes under the heel, then up the lateral side of the leg over the knee. The author does not recommend the use of adhesive strapping in the rigid type of talipes equinovarus because he finds that it does not maintain correction as effectively as a plaster of Paris cast; also, skin irritation is a greater problem. In the flexible type of talipes equinovarus, however, it can be used as effectively as the cast, if the surgeon so prefers.

Once the deformity is fully corrected, one should hold it in the overcorrected position in a solid cast for three to six weeks. Roentgenograms are made at the time the cast is removed to ensure that correction is complete. Then bivalved casts are made with the foot in slightly overcorrected position for use at night, and a prewalker clubfoot shoe is worn during the day (Fig. 7–23). The mother is taught passive stretching exercises for manipulating the forefoot into abduction and eversion, the heel into eversion, and the foot into dorsiflexion (see Fig. 7–20). The parents should be cautioned not to stretch the midfoot by forced dorsiflexion of the forefoot. The exercises should be performed 15 times slowly in each direction, four times a day. Active exercises promoting eversion and dorsiflexion of the foot are added when the child is older.

The treatment of clubfoot must be continued until the child is able to walk normally and until the wear on several pairs of shoes demonstrates that there has been no recurrence of deformity. Straight last shoes or tarsal pronator shoes with a $1/8$- to $3/16$-inch outer side heel and sole wedges promote walking in overcorrection (Fig. 7–24).

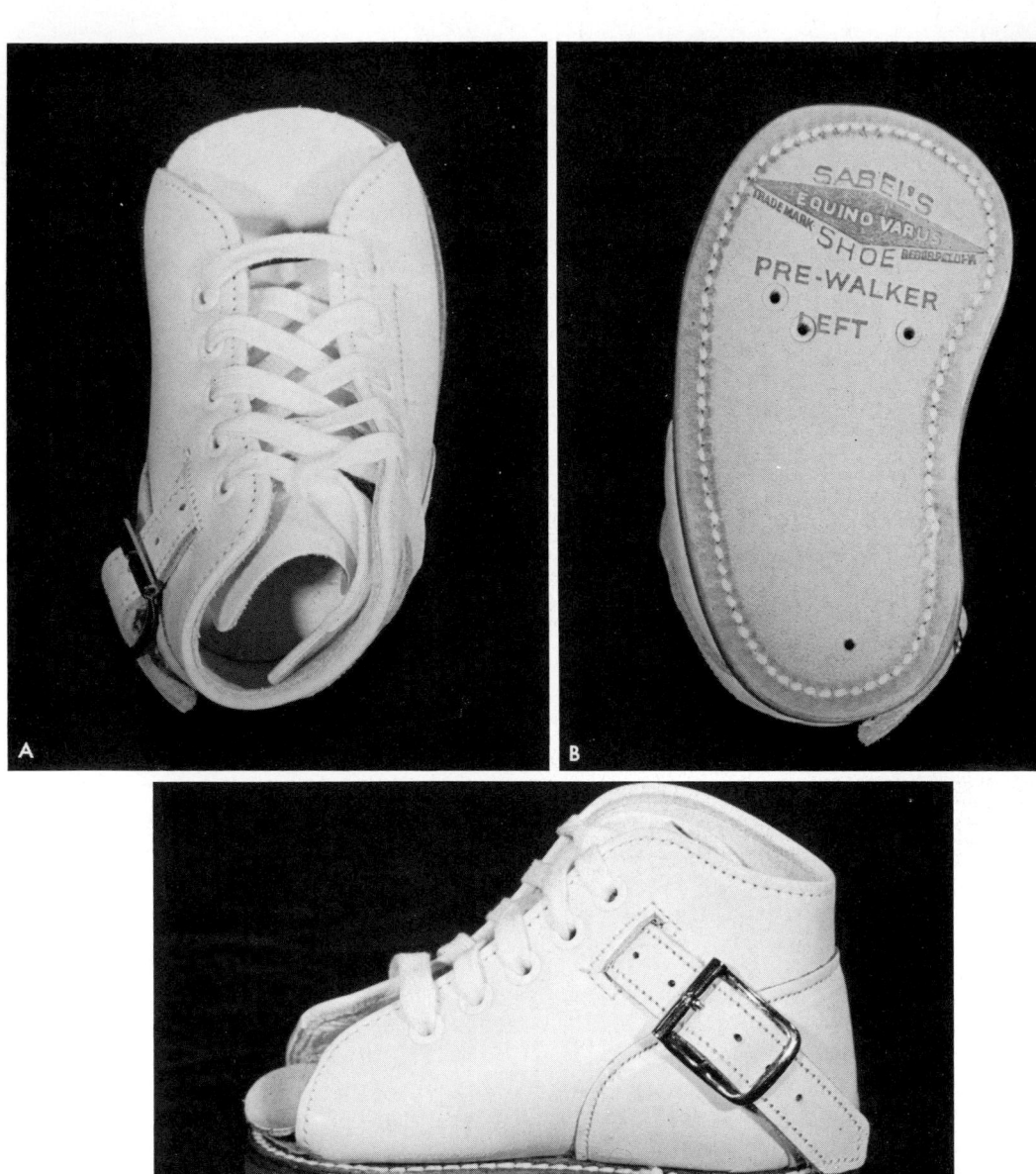

FIGURE 7–23.   Prewalker shoe with valgus strap.

A. Dorsal view. **B.** Plantar view. **C.** Lateral view.

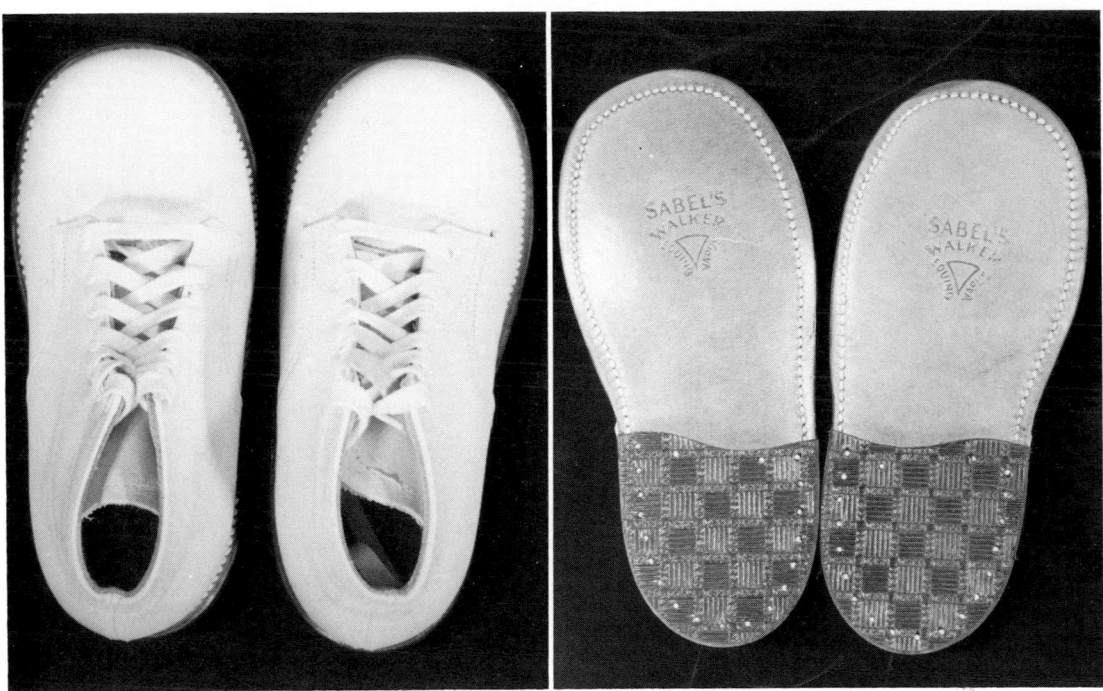

FIGURE 7–24.   Tarsal pronator shoes.

Surgical Measures

Operative treatment is indicated when conservative methods of management fail to correct the deformity, or when the deformities in the older child are so severe and rigid that it becomes obvious they will not respond to nonsurgical measures.

Approximately 50 per cent of children with clubfoot develop rigid fixed deformity that is resistant to correction by conservative means. Persistence or recurrence of deformity of 46 per cent was reported by Brockman in 1930, and of 56 per cent by Ponseti and Smoley in 1963; these statistics demonstrate the failure of improvement in the results of conservative management over this period of 30 years.[71, 170]

The *intrinsic type* of clubfoot is rigid and often requires surgery for full correction. Failure to recognize this fact and procrastination will do more harm than good. Recurrence or relapse of talipes equinovarus is often a reflection of either inadequate initial correction or failure to maintain correction, owing to poor postoperative care, casual supervision by the surgeon, or parental neglect. Acquired muscle imbalance is occasionally a factor in the older patient.

The literature on operative management of talipes equinovarus is extensive, and there is considerable difference of opinion as to the indications for surgery and the procedure to be used. In general, bony procedures are rarely, if ever, indicated in the infant and young child, as they would disturb the normal growth and development of the foot; if surgery is performed in this age category, it should consist only of soft tissue procedures.

In the older child, the tarsal and metatarsal bones become deformed and resist correction; in these patients, various bony procedures are performed. These may include: Dwyer osteotomy of the os calcis for correction of inversion of the heel, cuboid decancellation or wedge resection and arthrodesis of the calcaneocuboid joint for shortening the lateral column of the foot, or osteotomy at the base of the metatarsals to correct varus forefoot. In the fully grown foot, tarsal reconstruction and triple arthrodesis are performed to correct the deformity. Table 7–3 gives the various methods of treatment of talipes equinovarus in different age groups, and Table 7–4, a brief resumé of the operations.

The various categories of operative pro-

Table 7–3. *Methods of Treatment of Talipes Equinovarus in Different Age Groups*

Method of Treatment	1 day to 2 mo.	3 to 9 mo.	10 to 18 mo.	1½ to 3 yr.	4 to 8 yr.	9 to 11 yr.	Over 12
Conservative							
Manipulation—passive stretching	+	+	+	+	+	+	+
Adhesive strapping	+	−	−	−	−	−	−
Corrective cast	+	+	±	+	+	±	±
Dynamic splinting	−	+	−	−	−	−.	−
Bivalved cast or other night splint to maintain part in corrected position	−	+	+	+	+	−	−
Dynamic below-knee orthosis (dorsiflexion assist, valgus strap, tarsal pronator shoe)	−	−	−	+	+	+	
Special shoes							
Prewalker clubfoot	−	+	+	−	−	−	−
Tarsal pronator (reversed Thomas heel, ⅛″ outer sole and heel wedges)	−	−	−	+	+	+	−
Straight last shoe (⅛″ outer sole and heel wedges)	−	−	−	+	+	+	−
Operative—Soft-Tissue Procedures							
Posterior release							
Heel cord lengthening	−	+	+	+	+	+	+
Post. tibial lengthening	−	+	+	+	+	+	+
Capsulotomy (posterior ankle and subtalar)	−	+	+	+	+	+	+
Section calcaneofibular, posterior part of deltoid, and talofibular ligaments	−	+	+	+	+	+	+
Medial release hindfoot and midfoot	−	±	+	+	+	+	±
Mediodorsal release metatarsotarsal joints (Heyman-Herndon)	−	−	−	+	+	−	−
Plantar release	−	±	+	+	+	+	+
Posterior tibial transfer (anterior through interosseus route)	−	−	−	−	±	±	±
Anterior tibial transfer laterally	−	−	−	−	−	−	−
Operative—Bony Procedures							
Cuboid decancellation	−	−	−	+	+	−	−
Evans procedure (resection and fusion of calcaneocuboid joint)	−	−	−	−	+	+	+
Dwyer osteotomy of os calcis (open-up)	−	−	−	−	+	+	+
Dwyer osteotomy of os calcis (close-up)	−	−	−	−	±	+	+
Metatarsal osteotomy (at their bases) for correction of metatarsus varus	−	−	−	−	−	+	+
Triple arthrodesis, tarsal reconstruction by wedge resection and fusion of midtarsal and subtalar joints	−	−	−	−	−	+	+
Astragalectomy	−	−	−	−	±	+ (severe untreated)	+ (severe untreated)
Dorsal angulation osteotomy of distal tibia and fibula	−	−	−	−	+ (rigid equinus)	+ (rigid equinus)	+ (rigid equinus)
Derotation osteotomy of tibia	−	−	−	−	−	+	+

cedures for correction of talipes equino-varus are next discussed separately; some are combined in selected cases.

PROCEDURES ON SOFT TISSUES

Posterior Release. If, after a six- to ten-week period of adequate conservative treatment, the equinus position of the os calcis still persists (as demonstrated clinically and roentgenographically), a posterior release operation is performed. In the opinion of Swann, Lloyd-Roberts, and Catterall, another indication for posterior release may be posterior displacement of the lateral malleolus.[183]

First, a sliding lengthening of the Achilles tendon is performed; a Z-plastic lengthening of the tendo Achillis is indicated only if the tendon is scarred and sliding lengthening is not feasible. If full normal dorsiflexion of the hindfoot is not obtained (as demonstrated by roentgenograms made in the operating room), the posterior part of the capsule of the ankle and subtalar joints and the calcaneofibular ligament are sectioned by horizontal incisions. The posterior talofibular ligament is divided by a vertical incision. The details of operative technique are described and illustrated in Plate 50. The importance of placing a Kirschner wire transversely in the os calcis cannot be over-emphasized; at the end of the operation, the wire transfixing the calcaneus is incorporated in the cast to hold the correction.

Mild equinus deformity in early infancy may be corrected by subcutaneous tenotomy of the tendo calcaneus; often, however, these cases will respond to stretching by well-molded casts. The more severe equinus deformities require the extensive open posterior release.

The posterior tibial muscle is often taut, in which case it should be lengthened by the sliding technique simultaneously with the heel cord lengthening.

Medial and Subtalar Release for Hindfoot and Midfoot Varus Deformity. The commonest residual deformity of talipes equinovarus is persistence of the varus hindfoot. In the long-term follow-up study of 84 patients by Wynne-Davies, about half the cases had only false correction of the deformity, in that the foot was "broken" at the talonavicu-

lar level and the forefoot was plantigrade, but the heel was in inversion. None of her cases had "rocker-bottom" foot; i.e., the feet were "broken," not around a transverse axis, but around a longitudinal one.[196] To avoid this pitfall in correction and resultant fixed deformity, it behooves us to correct varus deformity of the hindfoot surgically at an early age.

If, after six months of diligent and thorough conservative management, varus deformity of the hindfoot cannot be fully corrected (as demonstrated in the roentgenogram), medial and subtalar release should be performed. Other indications for the procedure are demonstration of a persistent tendency to lose the correction once gained, or occasionally, a patient in whom the outlook for success is doubtful and in whom application of corrective casts would require an especially lengthy period of time (Fig. 7–25).

The various techniques of medial and subtalar soft-tissue release described in the literature are summarized in Table 7–3. The technique used by the author is described and illustrated in Plate 51.

Turco has reported a surgical technique in which all the elements of talipes equinovarus are corrected at the same operation. The method is derived from the procedures previously described by Codivilla, Brockman, McCauley, and Bost.[70–72, 83, 84, 148–153, 189, 190]

Turco observed that it is impossible to correct the hindfoot equinus deformity completely without correcting the varus and adduction components of the deformity. Posterior release alone decreases the equinus deformity of the talus, but it does not correct that of the calcaneus when it is locked in varus position under the talus. Both ends of the calcaneus and navicular must be released. For the posterior tuberosity of the calcaneus to move downward, its anterior end must be free to evert and move laterally with the navicular. He also noted that it is impossible to correct the varus and adduction components of the deformity without elimination of the equinus deformity.

Turco also emphasized the importance of transfixing the talonavicular joint with a fine Kirschner wire, ensuring maintenance of correction; a common pitfall is to use only a plaster cast to stabilize the reduction result-

(*Text continued on page 1314.*)

Table 7–4. *Operative Correction of Talipes Equino*

	Ober	Brockmann	McCauley	Bost, Schottstaedt, and Larsen
Posterior Release				
Achilles tendon	Subcutaneously Do it at end to assist in driving talus back into mortise	Lengthen by Z-plasty 2 weeks after medial release	Lengthen by Z-plasty 8 weeks after medial release	Lengthen (tri-cut method of Hoke)
Posterior capsule of ankle joint	——	Section 2 weeks after medial release	Section 8 weeks after medial release	Section
Posterior talofibular ligament	——	——	——	——
Posterior capsule of subtalar joint	——	Section 2 weeks after medial release	Section 8 weeks after medial release	Section
Calcaneofibular ligament	——	——	——	——
Posterior insertion of deltoid ligament on calcaneus	Section (whole attachment removed from medial surface of calcaneus subperiosteally)	Section	Section	Section
Flexor digitorum longus	——	——	Excise sheath Lengthen by Z-plasty (if necessary)	——
Flexor hallucis longus	——	——	Excise sheath Lengthen by Z-plasty (if necessary)	——
Kirschner wire in os calcis (to be incorporated in cast)	——	——	——	——
Medial Release				
Posterior tibial tendon	Lengthen	Z-plasty lengthening	Z-plasty lengthening	Detach from insertions (tuberosity of navicular, cuneiform, metatarsals)
Tibionavicular ligament (anterior part of deltoid ligament)	Section	Section	Section	Section
Talonavicular capsule	Section	Section	Section	Section
Calcaneonavicular (spring) ligament	Elevate subperiosteally from calcaneus	——	Section	Section
Deltoid ligament (superficial layer)	Elevate subperiosteally from calcaneus	Section	Section	Section
Deltoid ligament (deep layer)	Elevate subperiosteally from talus	Section	Preserve	Section (sometimes)
Capsule of naviculo-cuneiform joint	——	——	Section (if necessary)	Section
Subtalar Release				
Capsule of medial side of subtalar joint	Lengthen by subperiosteal elevation from calcaneus	Section	Section	Section
Talocalcaneal interosseus ligament	——	——	Section	Section
Bifurcated (Y) ligament (extends from calcaneus to lateral border of navicular and medial border of cuboid)	——	——	——	Section

varus by Soft-Tissue Release and Bony Procedures

Gelman	Turco	Evans	Dwyer
Lengthen 2 months after medial release	Z-technique Detach medial half of insertion on os calcis	Lengthen by Z-plasty	Lengthen by Z-plasty
Section 2 months after medial release	Section	Section	——
Section 2 months after medial release	Section	Section	——
Section 2 months after medial release	Section	Section	——
Section 2 months after medial release	Section	Section	——
Section	Section (retract neurovascular bundle posteriorly, for exposure)	Section	——
——	——	——	——
——	——	——	——
——	——	——	——
Z-lengthening	Divide above medial malleolus (use distal stump for traction and identification of navicular, then reinsert)	Lengthen by Z-plasty	——
Section	Section	Section	——
Section	Section	Section	——
Preserve—will prevent rocker bottom deformity	Detach from sustentaculum tali	Section	Subperiosteally elevated from calcaneus
Section	Section	Section	Subperiosteally elevated from calcaneus
Preserve	Preserve	——	——
——	Section (if necessary)	——	——
Section	Section	Section	Elevate subperiosteally and release
Section through medial approach above sustentaculum tali	Section through medial approach above sustentaculum tali	——	——
——	Section	——	——

(Table continued on following pages.)

	Ober	Brockmann	McCauley	Bost, Schottstaedt, and Larsen
Plantar Release				
Incision	Subcutaneously	Separate linear incision along interolateral border of os calcis	——	Medial
Plantar fascia	Section	Excise origin	——	Section
Abductor hallucis Intrinsic toe flexors Abductor digiti quinti	——	Detach all muscles	Superior origin of abductor hallucis detached and displaced downward	Section at origin
Long and short plantar ligaments	——	——	——	Section at the calcaneocuboid joint
Capsule of cal- caneocuboid joint	——	——	——	Section
Procedures on Tarsal Bones	No	No	No	No
Internal Fixation	No	No	No	No
Postoperative Care	Change cast at 2 weeks and manipulate foot into overcorrection	Posterior release and heel cord lengthening 2 weeks after medial release	Change cast in 2 weeks and manipulate foot into further correction	Foot held in relaxed position until wound healed
	Change cast monthly, each time manipulating foot into corrected position	Change casts to obtain full correction	Posterior release and heel cord lengthening at 8 weeks (if necessary)	Repeated changes of casts at 2 week inter- vals to obtain gradual correction
	Total of 4–5 mo. immobilization	Total of 3–5 mo. immobilization	Total of 2–4 mo. immobilization	Total of 5 mo. immobilization
	Some form of clubfoot brace worn night and day 8 months longer	Below-knee orthosis with medial bar and outside T-strap at night	Cross bar splint at- tached to shoes at night; ¹/₈″ outer sole and heel wedges on shoes during day	Brace at night to hold foot in corrected position
		Outside sole and heel wedges on shoe		Shoe wedges
		Active exercise to strengthen	Active exercises to strengthen peroneals and dorsiflexors	Periodic cast treatment if necessary
Remarks	Subperiosteal elevation of contracted capsule and ligaments (par- ticularly deltoid) pro- vides stability of ankle joint as they heal and reattach in lengthened position Overcorrect every ele- ment of deformity Cure not complete until patient actively can put his foot in a position of overcorrection		Release abductor hallucis to decrease its deforming force More extensive section- ing of capsules and ligaments (particu- early of interosseous talocalcaneal ligament, which binds talus and calcaneus in varus posi- tion) Following sectioning, marked release of deformity occurs	Thorough plantar dis- section and release Section of talocalcaneal interosseus and of bifurcated ligament stressed

Table 7–4   *Continued. Operative Correction of Talipes Equino*

varus by Soft-Tissue Release and Bony Procedures

Gelman	Turco	Evans	Dwyer
Medial	Separate (3 cm. long on plantar surface of hindfoot)	Medial	Medial
Section	Excise origin	Section	Section
Section at origin	Strip subperiosteally from os calcis	Section	Section
——	——	——	——
——	——	——	——
No	Excise elongated tuberosity of navicular after reduction (to prevent pressure necrosis of skin)	Shorten lateral column of foot by resection and fusion of calcaneocuboid joint	Osteotomy of calcaneus lever inferior segment inferiorly and laterally (held open by wedge of bone graft)
No	Kirschner wire to transfix talonavicular joint	Two staples across calcaneo-cuboid joint	——
In long leg cast for 2–3 mo.	Cast change under general anesthesia 3 mo. after operation	Immobilize in long leg cast for 5 mo. Walking in plaster cast permitted in 6 weeks	Immobilize in cast 8 weeks
Posterior release 2 mo. following medial release if necessary to correct equinus deformity	Remove sutures and Kirschner wire at 6 weeks Total of 4 mo. immobilization (last 2½ months can be walking cast in older child) Pronator walking shoes during day Denis Browne splint (25 cm. everting crossbar) at night for 2 yr.		
Preserve calcaneonavicular ligament to prevent rocker-bottom deformity Preserve deep layer of deltoid ligament (tibiotalar position)	Preserve deep layer of deltoid ligament (it inserts on the body of the talus) Tilting of the talus and pes valgus will develop if tibiotalar ligament is sectioned Calcaneus must be released at both ends to obtain complete correction Internal fixation of talonavicular joint Note: Ingram divides in-terosseus talocalcaneal ligament and capsule of calcaneocuboid joint through lateral incision He transfixed calcaneocuboid joint with Kirschner wire in addition to talonavicular joint	Shorten lateral column of foot	Corrects fixed bony varus deformity of hindfoot

Z-Lengthening of Tendo Achillis and Posterior Capsulotomy of Ankle and Subtalar Joints

Note: Sliding lengthening of the tendo Achillis should be performed whenever possible, as it preserves function of the triceps surae muscle; but if previous surgery has resulted in scarring of the Achilles tendon, a Z-plastic lengthening of the tendon is required.

THE PROCEDURE

A. A longitudinal incision is made medial to the tendo calcaneus, beginning at the heel and extending proximally for a distance of 7 to 10 cm. The subcutaneous tissue and tendon sheath are divided in line with the skin incision, and the wound flaps are retracted, exposing the Achilles tendon.

B. Z-plastic lengthening is performed in the anteroposterior plane. With a knife the Achilles tendon is divided longitudinally into lateral and medial halves for a distance of 5 to 7 cm. The distal end of the medial half is detached from the calcaneus to prevent recurrence of varus deformity of the heel; the lateral half is divided proximally. Often posterior tibial tendon lengthening is required. Its technique is illustrated in Figure 5–11.

C. If the posterior capsules of the ankle and subtalar joints are contracted, a varying degree of equinus deformity will persist following sectioning of the tendo Achillis. Posterior capsulotomy of the ankle and subtalar joints is indicated if the foot cannot be dorsiflexed to 5 degrees beyond neutral. If in doubt, one should take roentgenograms to determine the exact degree of correction of the equinus deformity. The flexor hallucis longus tendon is retracted medially and the peroneal tendons are retracted laterally to expose the posterior part of the ankle and subtalar joints. Neurovascular structures behind the medial malleolus should be protected from injury.

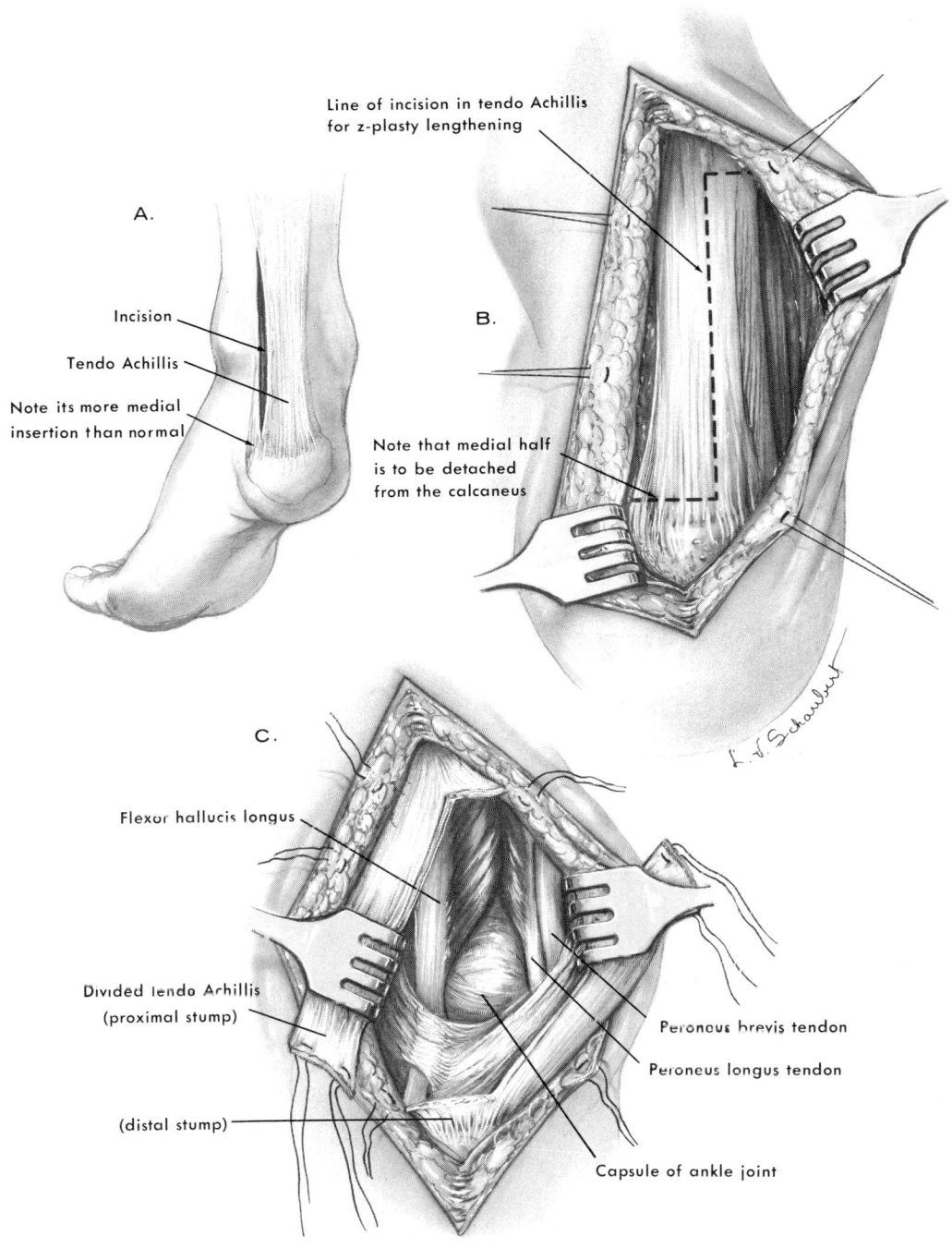

A.

Incision

Tendo Achillis

Note its more medial insertion than normal

Line of incision in tendo Achillis for z-plasty lengthening

B.

Note that medial half is to be detached from the calcaneus

C.

Flexor hallucis longus

Divided tendo Achillis (proximal stump)

(distal stump)

Peroneus brevis tendon

Peroneus longus tendon

Capsule of ankle joint

1301

Z-Lengthening of Tendo Achillis and Posterior Capsulotomy of Ankle Subtalar Joints (Continued)

D. Next, using Mayo or Madsenbaum scissors, completely divide the posterior capsules of the ankle and subtalar joints. A knife should not be used, as it may damage the articular cartilage. Caution should be exercised; the distal tibial epiphyseal plate must not be injured.

E. Laterally, the calcaneofibular and talofibular ligaments are sectioned, with care not to injure the peroneal tendons. Medially the posterior part of the deltoid ligament is divided immediately next to its attachment to the os calcis; in this way, the likelihood of injury to the posterior tibial vessels and tibial nerve is minimized. With a blunt periosteal elevator, any remaining capsular fibers across the ankle and subtalar joints are freed.

F. Next, lateral roentgenograms of the ankle and hindfoot are made with the foot held in maximal dorsiflexion to determine exactly the degree of correction achieved. Occasionally, fractional lengthening of the flexor hallucis longus and flexor digitorum longus may be required. The longitudinal halves of the tendo Achillis are sutured in the lengthened position. A Steinmann pin is inserted transversely across the os calcis. The tourniquet is released and hemostasis is secured.

The edges of the skin are observed; if they are blanched and under tension when the foot is maximally dorsiflexed, a primary full-thickness skin graft may be indicated to prevent sloughing of the wound, secondary infection, scarring, and recurrence of fixed equinus contracture.

A long leg cast is applied in which the Steinmann pin is incorporated. Failure to fix the os calcis to the cast with a pin is a common error; the heel will slip upward in the cast, correction will be lost, and a "rocker-bottom" deformity will result.

POSTOPERATIVE CARE

After four weeks, the Steinmann pin and sutures are removed, the foot is manipulated, and a new above-knee cast is applied. The cast is changed every three to four weeks while the foot and ankle are immobilized for a total of three months.

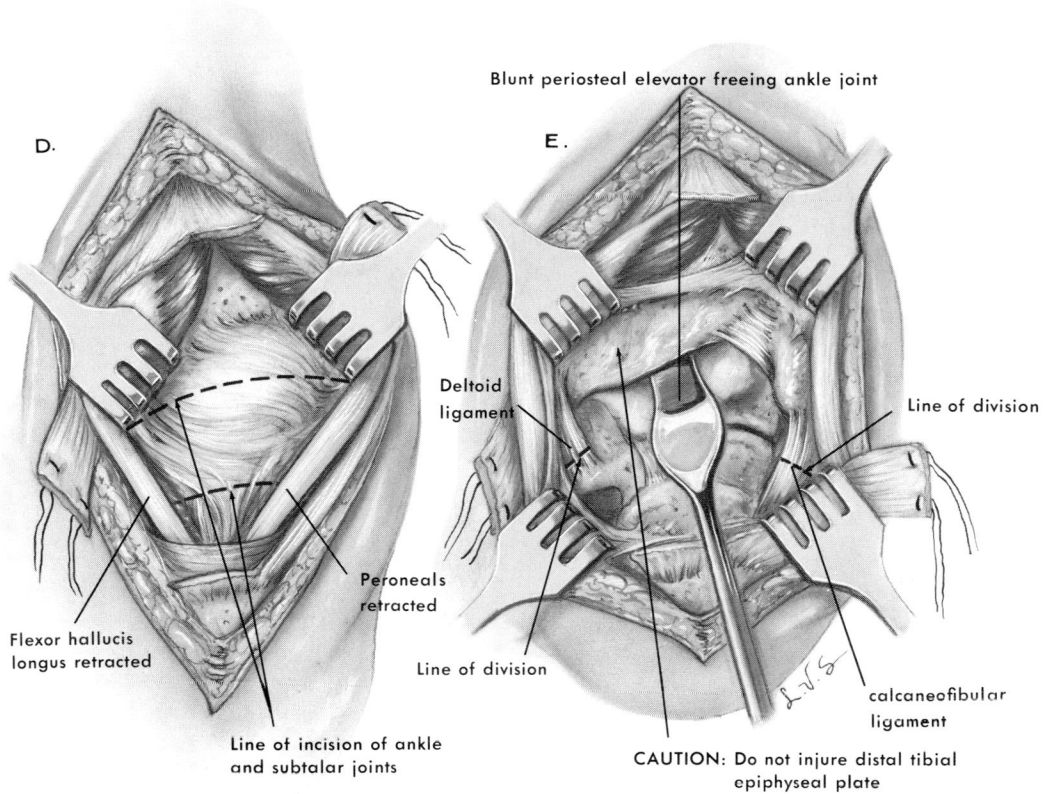

D.

E.

Blunt periosteal elevator freeing ankle joint

Deltoid ligament

Line of division

Flexor hallucis longus retracted

Peroneals retracted

Line of incision of ankle and subtalar joints

Line of division

calcaneofibular ligament

CAUTION: Do not injure distal tibial epiphyseal plate

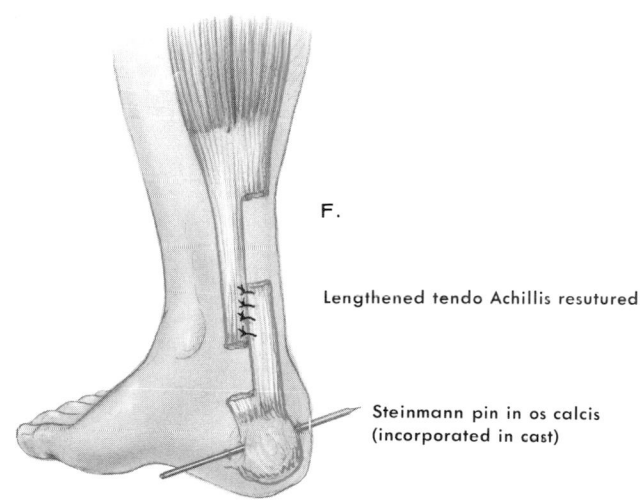

F.

Lengthened tendo Achillis resutured

Steinmann pin in os calcis (incorporated in cast)

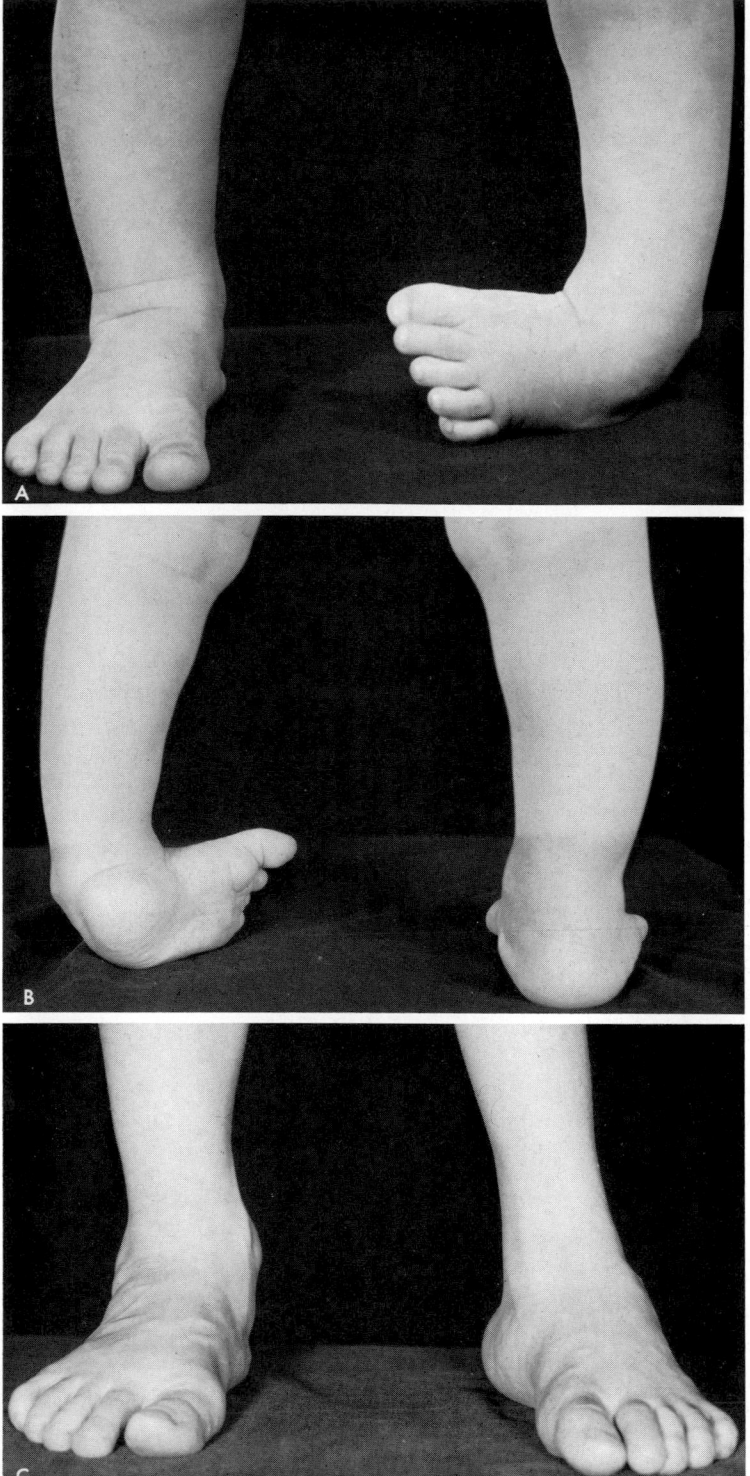

FIGURE 7–25. Talipes equinovarus on the left.

Deformity was untreated until patient was three and one half years of age. A series of stretching casts was applied continuously for one year and then intermittently. **A** and **B.** These are initial photographs showing the deformity. **C.** Photograph taken at seven years of age.

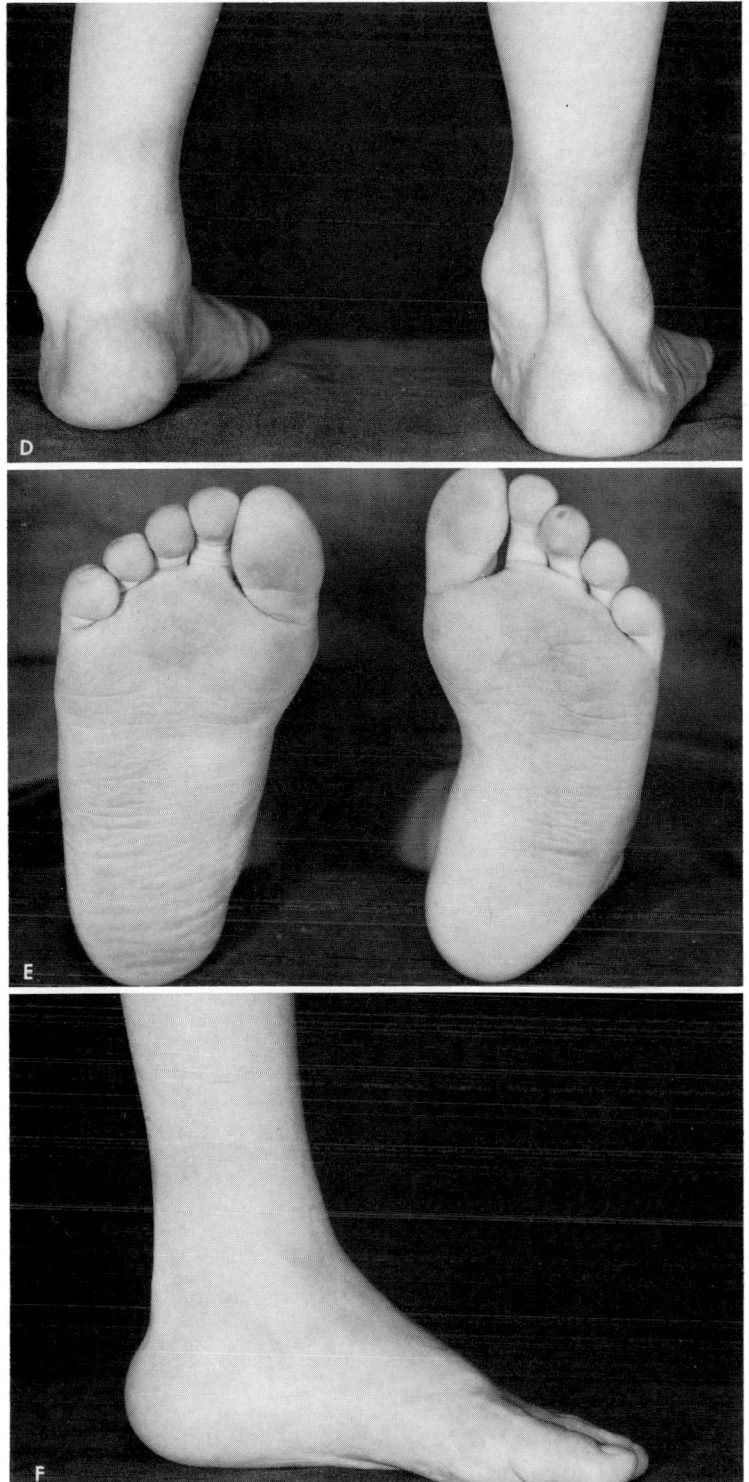

FIGURE 7–25 Continued. Talipes equinovarus on the left.

D to **F.** Photographs taken at seven years of age (F is medial view of left foot). Note the persistence of varus deformity. Following posteromedial and plantar soft-tissue release, a close-up Dwyer osteotomy of the os calcis was performed to correct hindfoot varus deformity, and metatarsal osteotomy at their bases to correct that of forefoot.

Medial and Plantar Release for Correction of Resistant Talipes Equinovarus

THE PROCEDURE

A. A medial incision is made convex dorsally, starting at the middle of the first metatarsal shaft and continuing proximally along the first cuneiform and the tuberosity of the navicular; at the sustentaculum tali it is swung plantarward to terminate at the medial aspect of the tuberosity. The subcutaneous tissue is divided and the veins are clamped and coagulated. The wound flaps are undermined and retracted with 0 silk traction sutures. Damage to soft tissues by excessive traction with rakes should be avoided.

B. On the medial aspect of the midfoot and hindfoot, the following structures are identified: (1) the *tuberosity of the navicular,* which is displaced medially in relation to the head of the talus; (2) the *posterior tibial tendon;* (3) the *flexor digitorum longus tendon;* (4) the *posterior tibial neurovascular bundle* (vein, artery, and nerve); (5) the *flexor hallucis longus tendon;* and (6) the *abductor hallucis muscle.*

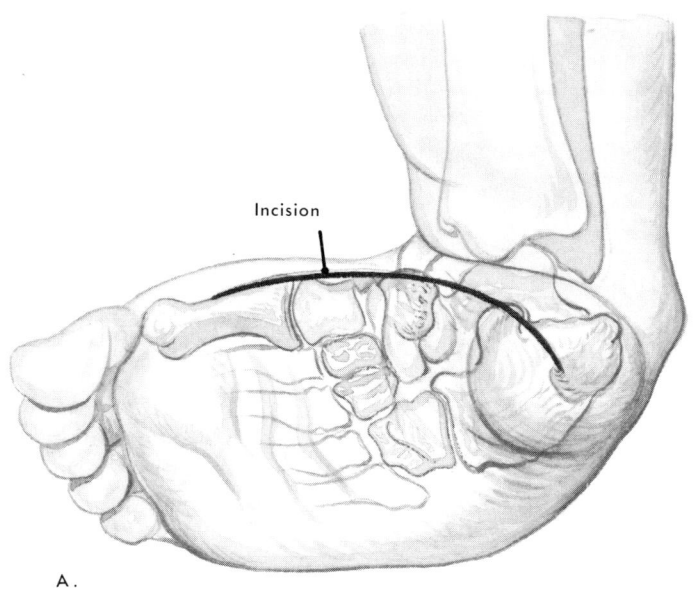

Incision

A.

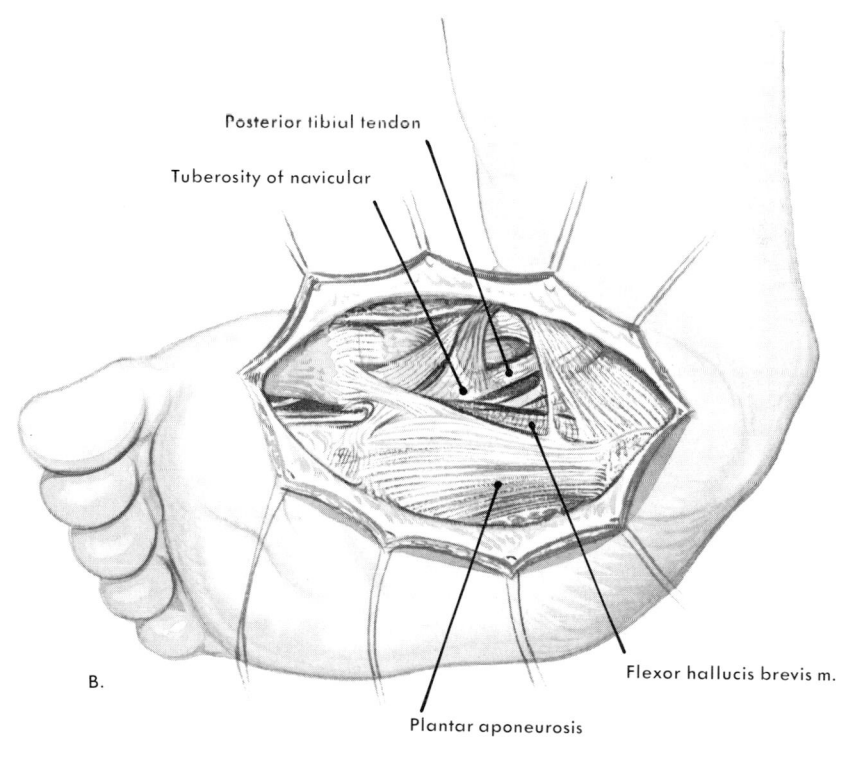

Posterior tibiul tendon

Tuberosity of navicular

Flexor hallucis brevis m.

Plantar aponeurosis

B.

Medial and Plantar Release for Correction of Resistant Talipes Equinovarus (*Continued*)

C and **D.** The tendon of the abductor hallucis is identified; by blunt and sharp dissection it is separated from the adjacent flexor hallucis brevis muscle, from its fascial attachments with the tuberosity of the navicular bone, and posteriorly from the laciniate ligament and medial aspect of the tuberosity of the navicular bone. The motor branches of the medial plantar nerve to the abductor hallucis should not be damaged.

The tendons of the flexor digitorum longus and flexor hallucis longus are identified: their sheaths and the master knot of Henry are divided. The tendons are dissected free and retracted plantarward. The origin of the flexor hallucis brevis muscle is sectioned and all the plantar intrinsic muscles are retracted plantarward with the neurovascular bundle. In order to mobilize the navicular, it is important to divide the master knot of Henry. The posterior tibial tendon is split longitudinally for Z-lengthening, and the proximal end of the tendon is marked with 00 silk suture. Traction is applied on the distal portion of the posterior tibial tendon for opening up of the talonavicular joint.

Plate 51. Medial and Plantar Release for Correction of Resistant Talipes Equinovarus

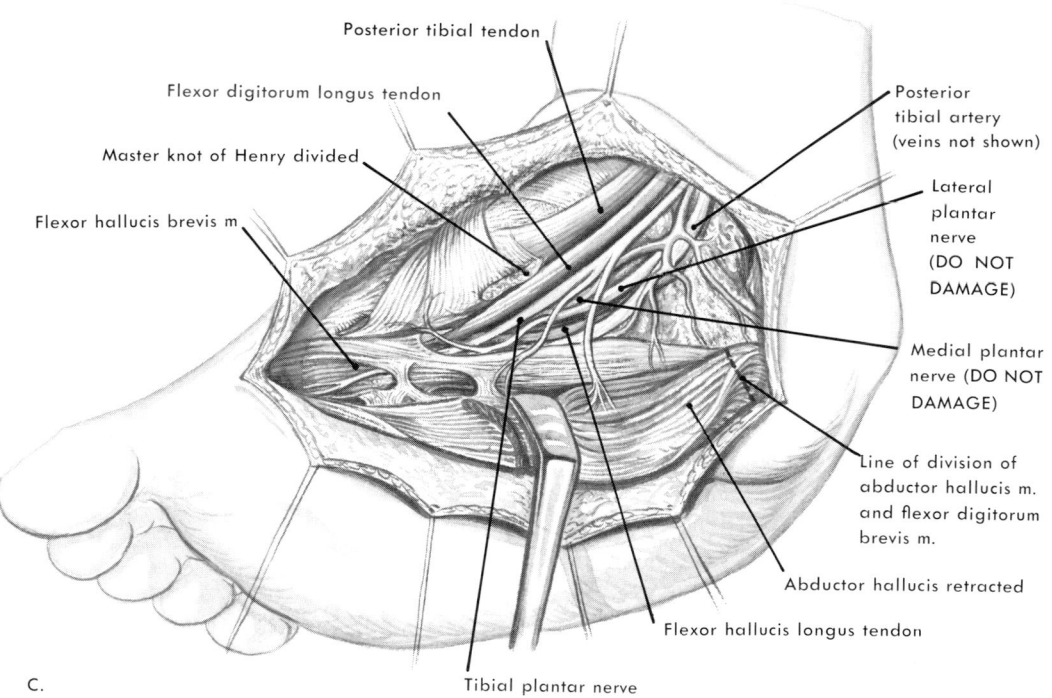

Posterior tibial tendon

Flexor digitorum longus tendon

Master knot of Henry divided

Flexor hallucis brevis m.

Posterior tibial artery (veins not shown)

Lateral plantar nerve (DO NOT DAMAGE)

Medial plantar nerve (DO NOT DAMAGE)

Line of division of abductor hallucis m. and flexor digitorum brevis m.

Abductor hallucis retracted

Flexor hallucis longus tendon

Tibial plantar nerve

C.

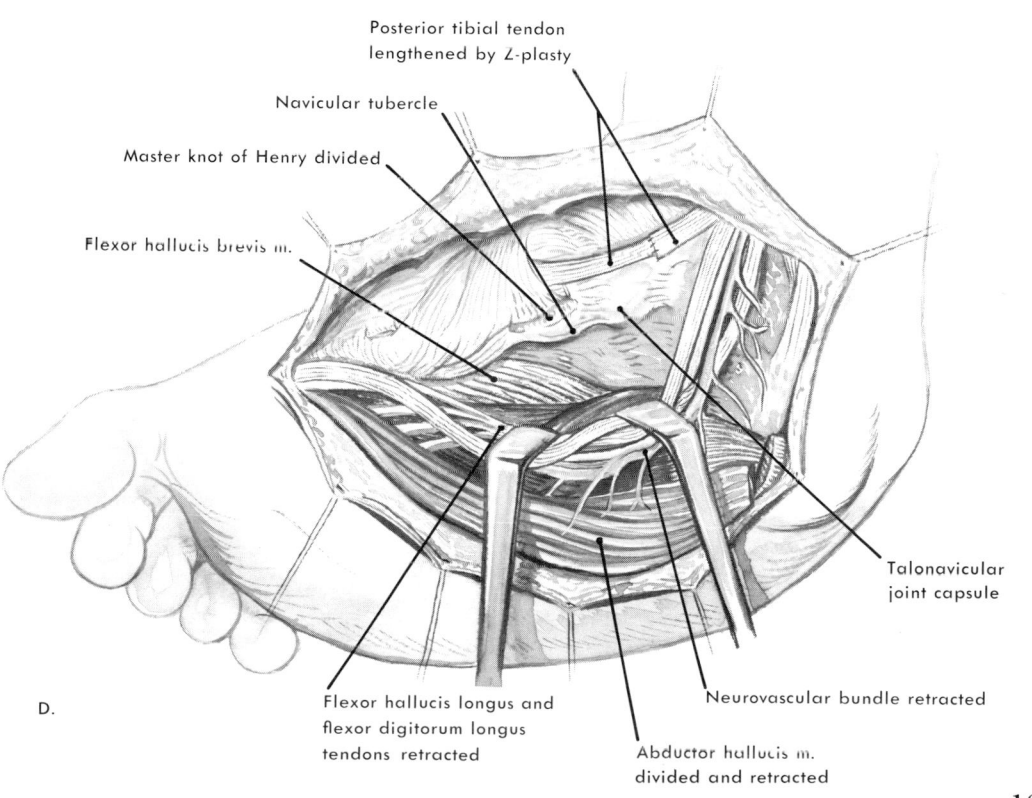

Posterior tibial tendon lengthened by Z-plasty

Navicular tubercle

Master knot of Henry divided

Flexor hallucis brevis m.

Talonavicular joint capsule

Flexor hallucis longus and flexor digitorum longus tendons retracted

Neurovascular bundle retracted

Abductor hallucis m. divided and retracted

D.

1309

Medial and Plantar Release for Correction of Resistant Talipes Equinovarus *(Continued)*

E and **F.** The adherent and contracted capsule of the talonavicular joint is incised on its dorsal, medial, and plantar aspects. The tibionavicular component of the deltoid ligament and the plantar calcaneonavicular ligament are sectioned. Following this, the medially displaced navicular is mobilized, the false articular facet on the proximal and medial aspect of the head of the talus is identified. The head of the talus is tilted slightly medially toward the medially displaced navicular. Next, the superficial layer of the deltoid ligament (i.e., the tibiocalcaneal component) is sectioned from the calcaneus. The deep portion of the deltoid that inserts into the body of the talus must be left intact because, if it is divided, a pes planovalgus deformity with tilting of the talus may develop. The capsule of the naviculocuneiform joint is divided on its medial and plantar aspects.

G. Next, the hindfoot is everted and the interosseous talocalcaneal ligament located above the sustentaculum tali is sectioned.

H. Next, the plantar fascia, flexor digitorum brevis, and abductor digiti quinti are sectioned at their origin from the tuberosity of the calcaneus.

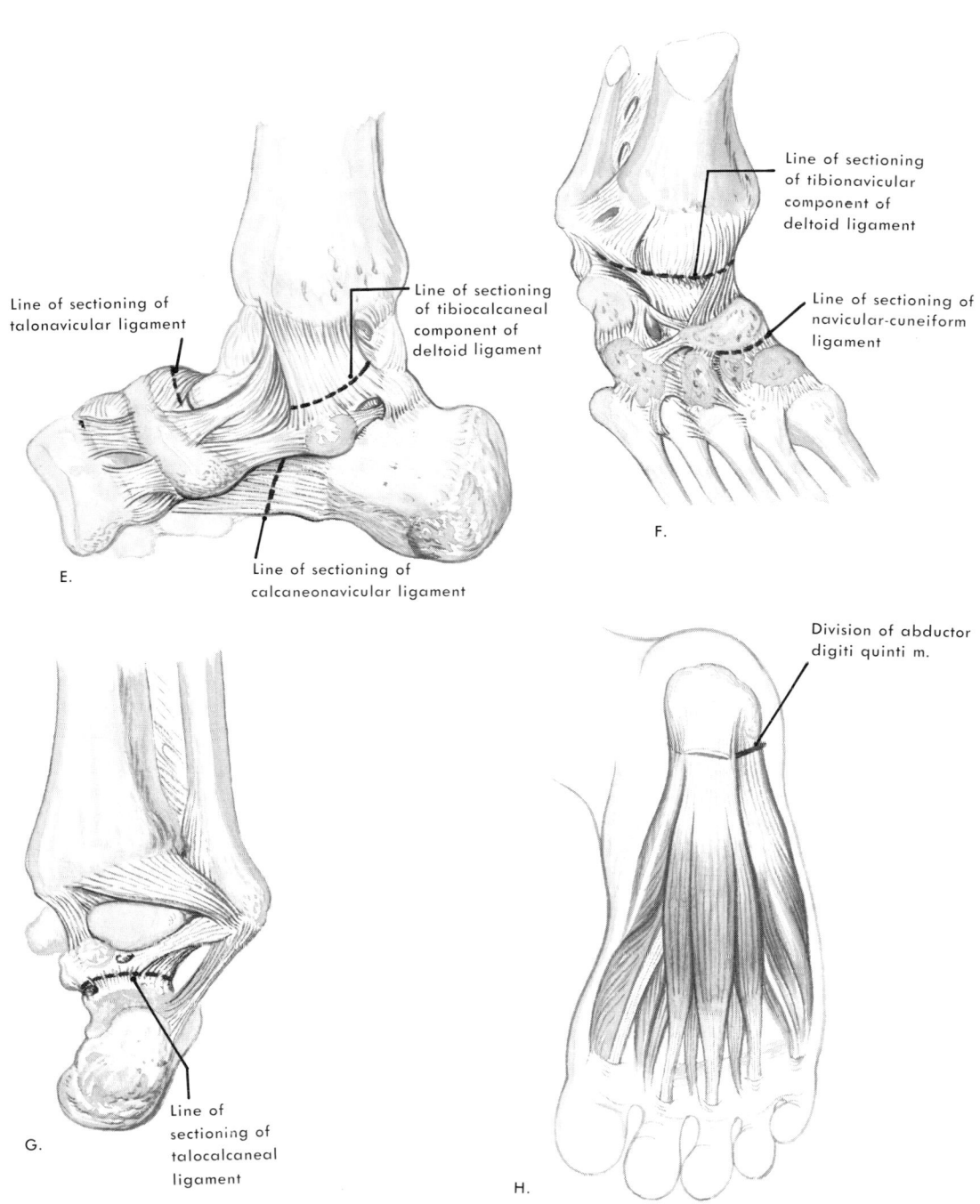

Line of sectioning of talonavicular ligament

Line of sectioning of tibiocalcaneal component of deltoid ligament

Line of sectioning of calcaneonavicular ligament

E.

Line of sectioning of tibionavicular component of deltoid ligament

Line of sectioning of navicular-cuneiform ligament

F.

Line of sectioning of talocalcaneal ligament

G.

Division of abductor digiti quinti m.

H.

Medial and Plantar Release for Correction
of Resistant Talipes Equinovarus *(Continued)*

I and **J.** The quadratus plantae and long plantar ligament are also divided. Injury to neurovascular structures is avoided by keeping close to the calcaneal tuberosity.

K. The calcaneonavicular and calcaneocuboid ligaments are sectioned on the plantar aspect of the foot.

L. The foot is manipulated, and reduction is maintained by a heavy Kirschner wire transfixing the talonavicular joint. If necessary, a Kirschner wire is also placed across the calcaneocuboid joint. Roentgenograms are made to determine the thoroughness of correction of equinovarus deformity. The tourniquet is released, and after complete hemostasis, the wound is closed with interrupted sutures in the usual manner. A well-molded above-knee cast is applied.

POSTOPERATIVE CARE

The cast is changed three weeks postoperatively. It is best not to remove the sutures at this time. Six weeks after the operation, the cast, sutures and Kirschner wires are removed. The foot is manipulated and a new above-knee plaster cast is applied. Immobilization is continued for a total of 16 weeks, changing the cast as necessary. Then correction is maintained in a bivalved cast that is worn during the night for a period of two years. Tarsal pronator shoes with a ⅛-inch outer sole and heel wedges are worn during the day for 6 to 12 months. Passive stretching exercises are performed daily to maintain normal range of motion of ankle and foot. In the older child, active exercises are carried out to strengthen the motor power of the peroneals.

Plate 51. Medial and Plantar Release for Correction of Resistant Talipes Equinovarus

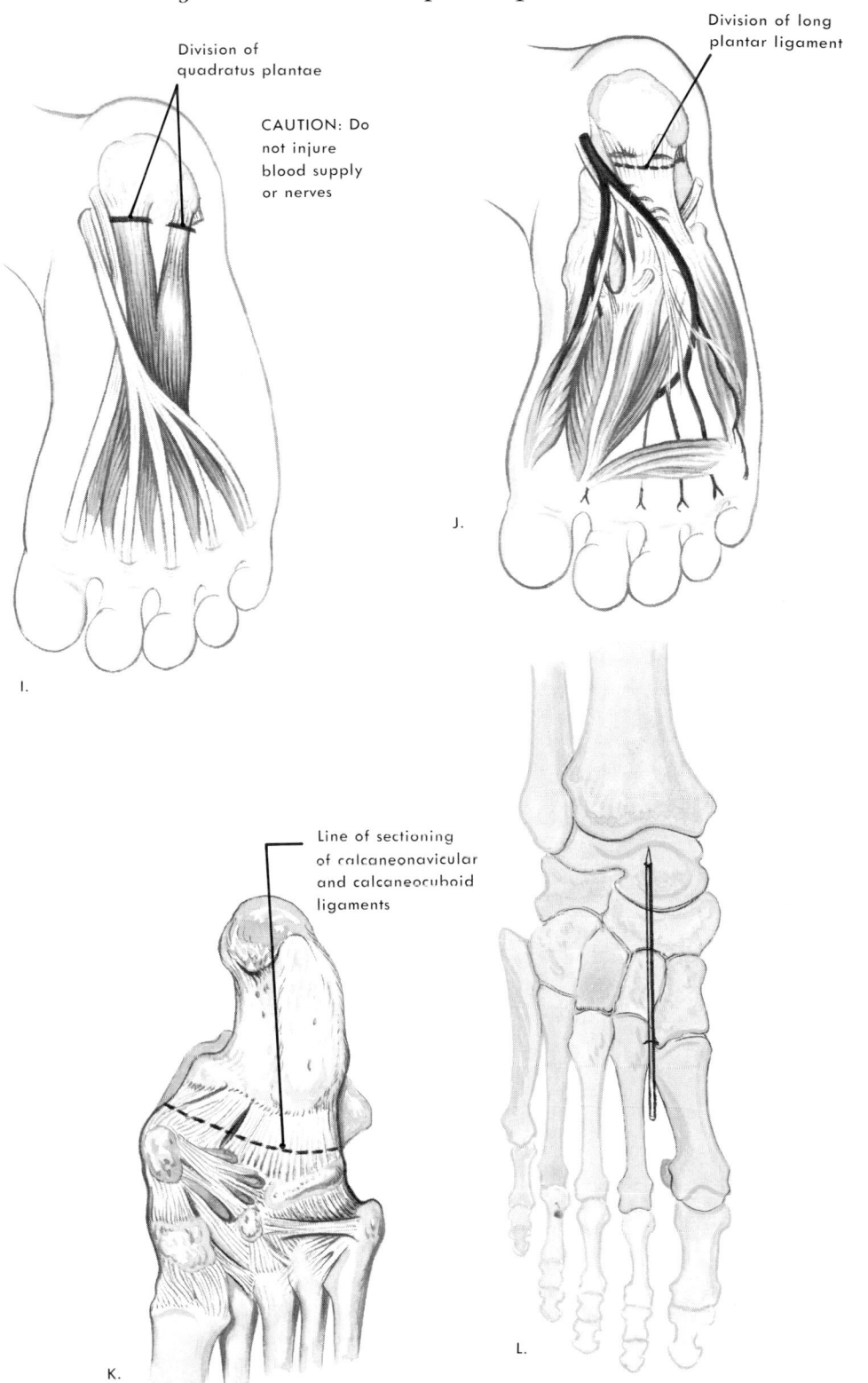

Division of quadratus plantae

CAUTION: Do not injure blood supply or nerves

Division of long plantar ligament

I.

J.

Line of sectioning of calcaneonavicular and calcaneocuboid ligaments

K.

L.

Pin engaging navicular and talus

ing in loss of initial correction. He used a straight medial incision extending from the base of the first metatarsal to the tendo Achillis posteriorly, curving slightly under the medial malleolus in its course. He advised that the incision not extend vertically along the tendo Achilles and also recommended that the sutures be left in place for at least six weeks following surgery, as the skin on the medial side of the foot is contracted and noted as being poorly nourished and subject to delayed healing. The use of a Kirschner wire for stabilization eliminates the need for cast pressure to maintain correction and decreases the likelihood of skin necrosis. Excision of contracted soft tissues under direct vision prevents damage to the articular surfaces and consequent stiffness of the foot. In a preliminary report with a follow-up of two years or more, Turco reports the results of operation on 31 feet as follows: *excellent* or *good*, 27 feet (about 90 per cent); *fair*, 3 feet; and *failure*, 1 foot, his conclusions being that complete correction is best attained with a one-stage posterior and medial soft-tissue release, and that lasting correction is achieved if it is complete at operation and temporarily stabilized by internal fixation.[190]

With the exception of a few modifications, the author concurs with Turco. First, in order to correct hindfoot equinus deformity completely, the incision described by Turco is not adequate. It is recommended that a longitudinal incision be made on the medial side of the tendo Achillis; this surgical exposure allows sectioning of the calcaneofibular and talofibular ligaments under direct vision and capsulotomy of the posterior parts of the ankle and subtalor joints. Second, the medial incision recommended by the author is different from that of Turco; as the heel is everted, with Turco's incision, the skin flaps are under tension and may gape; by making the incision perpendicular to the varus deformity on eversion of the heel, the wound flaps are approximated. Third, to maintain correction of the hindfoot equinus deformity and inversion, a threaded Steinmann pin is inserted from the lateral side and incorporated in the cast.

Plantar Soft-Tissue Release is performed when the forefoot is in equinovarus position (Fig. 7–26). The operative technique of plantar soft-tissue release is described and illustrated in the section on pes cavus (see Plate 57). When combining plantar soft-tissue release with medial and subtalar release, soft tissues should be handled gently, and extensive wound flaps should be avoided to prevent sloughing of the skin (Fig. 7–27). If necessary, a lateral incision on the plantar aspect of the foot is made.

The surgical correction of forefoot varus deformity is described in the discussion of congenital metatarsus varus. Between the ages of three and seven years, tarsometatarsal and intermetatarsal soft-tissue release is performed; in children eight years or older, the fixed bony deformity requires correction by osteotomy of the metatarsals at their bases (Fig. 7–28).

TENDON TRANSFERS

The equinovarus position of the foot provides a mechanical advantage to the invertors and plantar-flexors of the foot, and places the evertors and dorsiflexors in a position of relative weakness as they are stretched over the convexity of the dorsolateral aspect of the foot.

Muscle imbalance with motor weakness of the peroneals and toe extensor muscles may be a factor in recurrence of equinovarus deformity, and occasionally tendon transfers may be indicated to balance the dynamic forces acting on the foot and ankle.

Anterior Tibial Tendon Transfer. Lateral transfer of the anterior tibial tendon was recommended by Garceau.[106-109] Critchley and Taylor and Singer and Fripp have also reported their experience with tibialis anterior transfer in congenital clubfoot.[87, 179] In his last report Garceau stated that the operation is indicated if there have been multiple recurrences of all components of the deformity, if there is weakness or absence of the peroneus longus and brevis muscles, and if "bowstringing" of the anterior tibial tendon and supination of the forepart of the foot are evident in the swing phase of gait. He stressed the importance of correcting fixed deformity prior to tendon transfer. Roentgenograms of the foot should be taken, as clinical evaluation of the foot is not necessarily an adequate assessment of the amount of correction. Garceau

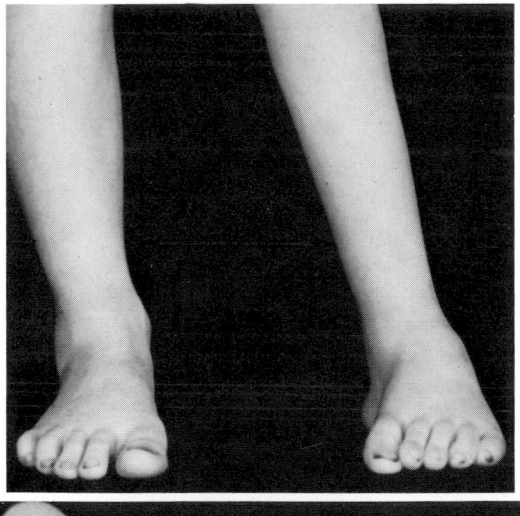

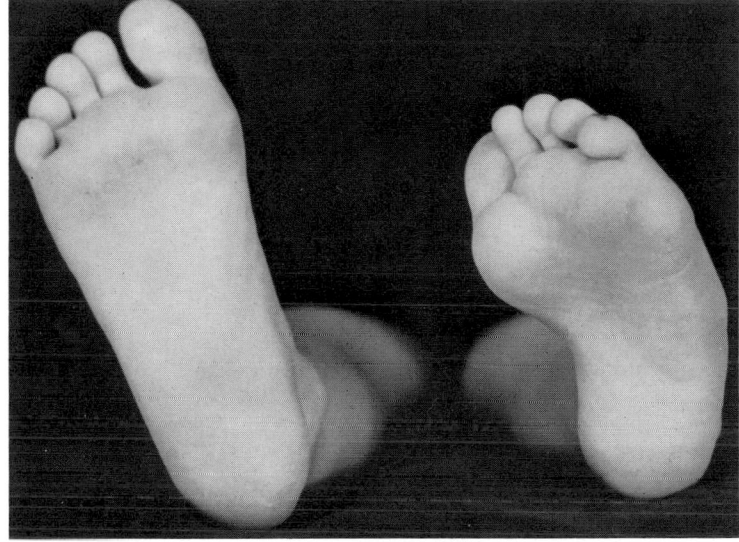

FIGURE 7–26.   Talipes equinovarus on the left.
Note the associated forefoot equinus deformity, which requires a plantar soft-tissue release for correction.

also suggested the possible use of electromyographic studies of the peroneus longus and brevis muscles in order to permit a more accurate assessment of the potential power of these muscles and minimize the risk of overcorrection.[109] Singer and Fripp found that lateral transfer of the anterior tibial tendon does not increase dorsiflexion power, and that relapse occurred 52 times in 76 feet on which the procedure had been performed.[179]

The author does not recommend lateral transfer of the anterior tibial tendon in talipes equinovarus for the following reasons: (1) with anterior tibial tendon transfer, a varying degree of loss of power of ankle dorsiflexion occurs and causes recurrence of equinus deformity of the ankle; (2) equinus posture of the first metatarsal and clawing of the great toe result because of the unopposed action of the peroneus longus muscle; and (3) when the varus deformity is corrected, peroneal muscle power returns and provides active eversion of the foot. Even when the anterior tibial tendon is transferred only to the third metatarsal, overcorrection and pes valgus deformity are frequent complications.

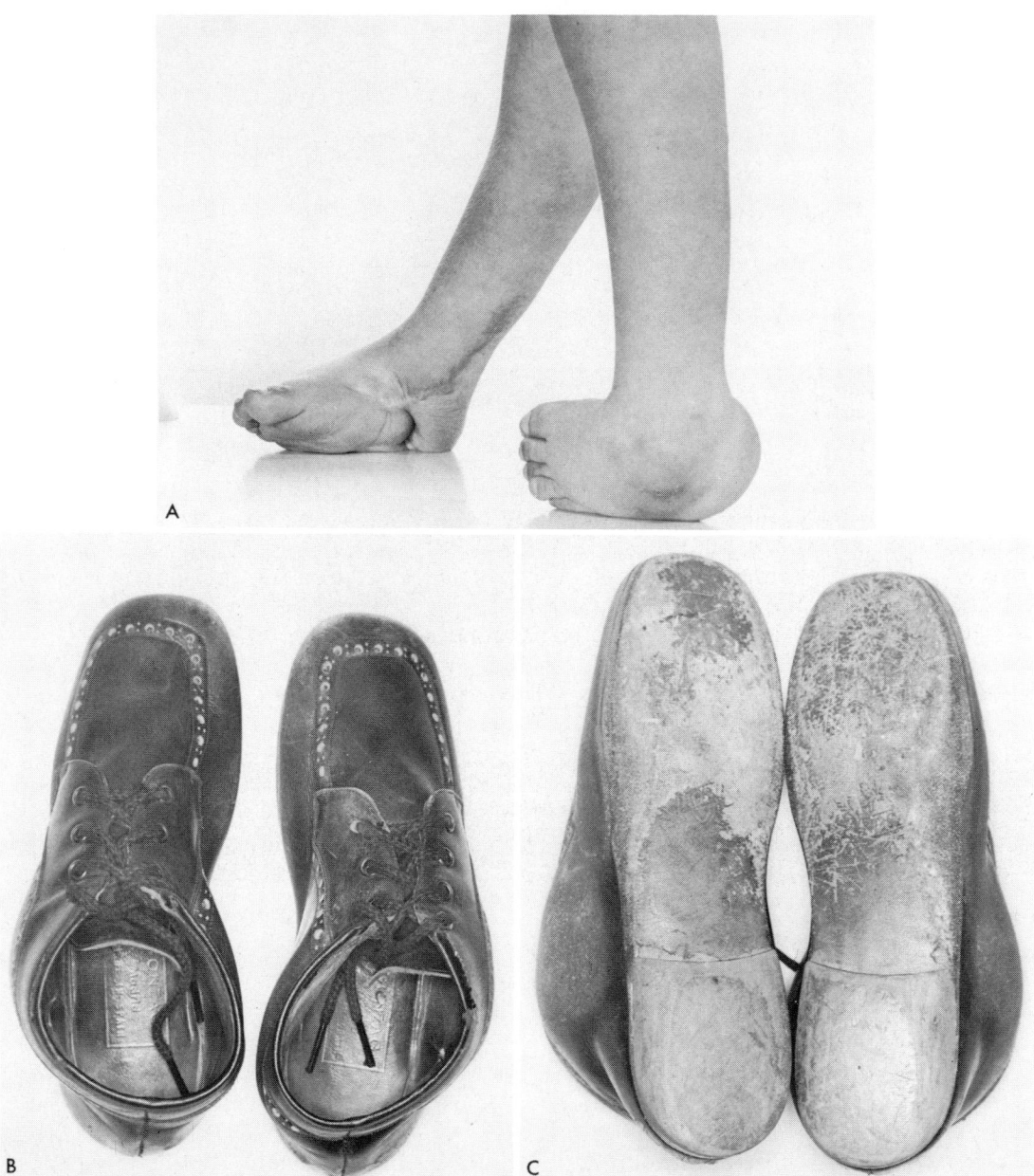

FIGURE 7–27. *Talipes equinovarus—bilateral.*

A. Sloughing of skin following extensive posteromedial and plantar soft-tissue release. **B** and **C.** Shoe wear of same patient.

Lateral transfer of the anterior tibial tendon is indicated only very occasionally under the following conditions: (1) when there is unquestionable motor weakness of the peroneals; (2) when there is definite evidence of motor weakness of the triceps surae muscle as a result of overzealous heel cord lengthening; (3) when the foot is completely flexible, with no fixed varus or equinus deformity (i.e., the passive range of ankle dorsiflexion is 10 to 20 degrees, forefoot abduction is 10 degrees, and eversion of the forefoot and hindfoot is 10 to 20 degrees). A tendon transfer will not correct a fixed deformity. (4) The anterior tibial tendon should be normal in motor strength, and (5) the child should be at least four years of age and in a family situation such that there will be adequate postoperative training and care.

To prevent overcorrection the tendon should not be transferred more laterally than the base of the third metatarsal.

Posterior Tibial Tendon Transfer. Fried dissected the insertions of the posterior tibial tendon in 54 clubfeet with recurrent deformity and in two clubfeet that had had no previous treatment. In all the cases the insertions were abnormal. Beginning at the level of the medial malleolus, the tendon changed to a thick, hard, fibrous mass that encompassed the entire medial side of the tarsus and inserted with thick strands of fibrous tissue to other parts of the foot; namely, to the cruciate ligament, plantar fascia, deep plantar ligaments, os calcis, scaphoid, anterior tibial tendon, navicular, and the bones of the midfoot. Fried believed the deformity of the posterior tibial muscle to be the principal cause of clubfoot. Following excision of the abnormal distal attachments, he recommended transferring this muscle to the dorsum of the foot via the interosseous route and suturing it to the third cuneiform bone. Lengthening of the Achilles tendon and capsulotomy of the posterior parts of the ankle and subtalar joints were performed at the same time to achieve correction of equinus deformity. Capsulotomy of the talonavicular, navicular first cuneiform, and first cuneiform–first metatarsal joints was also carried out. He reported the results to be good in 12 of the 13 patients who were followed for at least four years. In seven patients, the results

were excellent with full correction of deformity and satisfactory function. In five patients, there was persistence of minor residual deformity and walking on tiptoes was still not feasible. In one patient, the result was unsatisfactory because of overcorrection resulting from a too lateral transfer of the tendon to the cuboid rather than only as far as the third cuneiform.[102]

Gartland suggested that muscle imbalance was the primary cause of relapse in clubfoot, and he recommended anterior transfer of the posterior tibial tendon through the interosseus membrane. He believed that when indicated, the procedure should be performed by the age of two or three years in order to avoid adaptive bone changes. The results of the operation on 20 feet were excellent in 10, satisfactory in 6, and unsatisfactory in 4. The failures were due either to transfer of the tendon to the cuboid instead of the third cuneiform, as recommended, or else the result of adherence of the tendon in a small hole in the interosseus membrane. In the experience of Gartland, inadequate surgical performance rather than any basic fault of the procedure was the cause of his poor results.[110]

The author disagrees with Fried and Gartland. As stated previously, there are no primary abnormalities of the muscles and tendons in talipes equinovarus. Apart from directional changes, Wiley could find no regular pattern of abnormality of the tendons or their insertions.[193] If the posterior tibial muscle is contracted and is a deforming force, it should be fractionally lengthened at its muscle tendon juncture and should not be transferred anteriorly through the interosseus route. The contractural deformity on the medial aspect of the foot is released by sectioning of the shortened soft tissues. The author finds that in a two- or three-year-old child it is very difficult, if not impossible, to train an out-of-phase tendon transfer (e.g., an invertor and plantar-flexor to function as evertor and dorsiflexor). It is only in paralytic equinovarus deformity of the foot that anterior transfer of the posterior tibial muscle is indicated, and then only when the child is old enough to cooperate in the postoperative muscle re-education program.

The Switch Operation on the Tendo Achillis. Stewart proposed that inversion

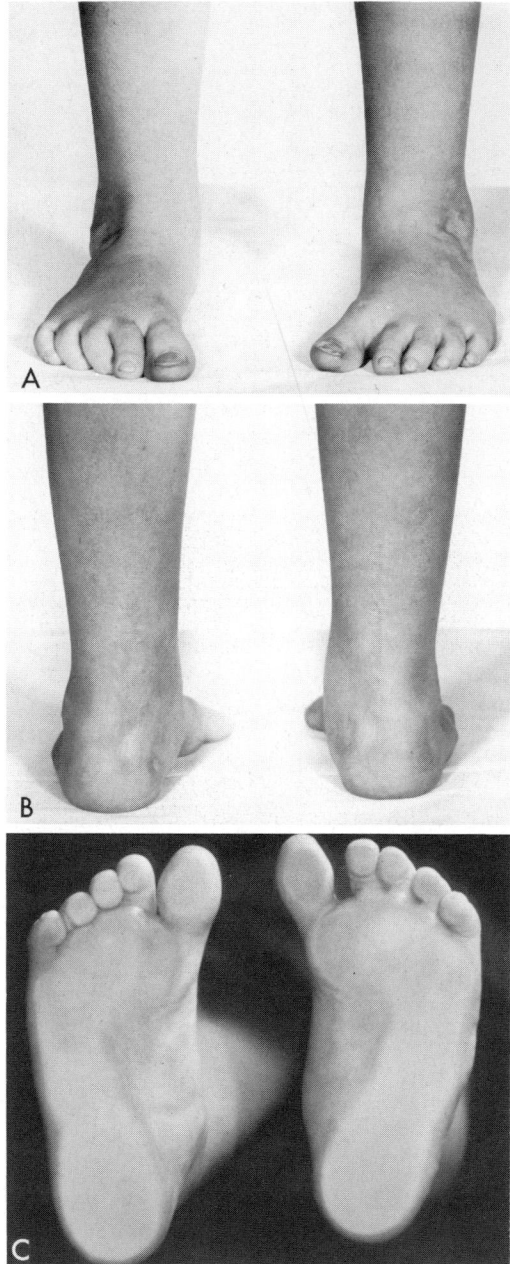

FIGURE 7–28. *Residual varus deformity of forefoot in bilateral clubfoot.*

A to **C.** Clinical appearance of deformity.

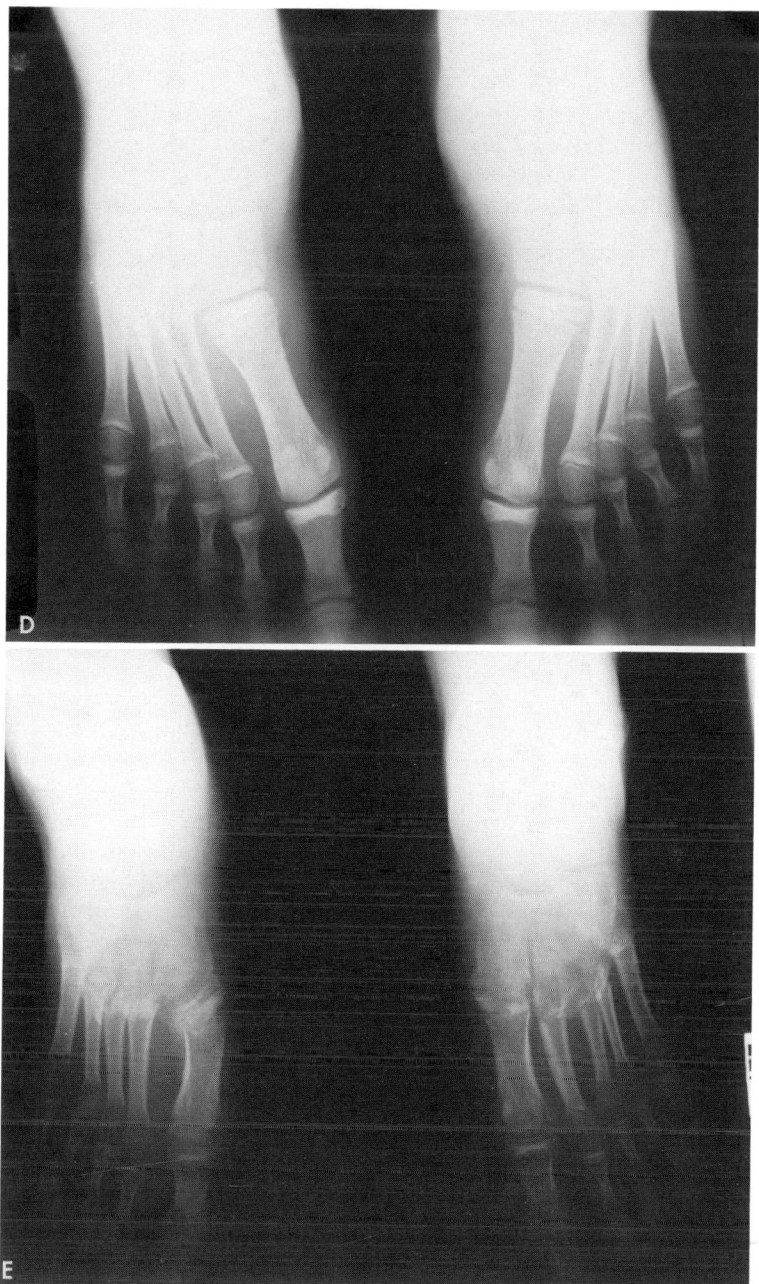

FIGURE 7–28 Continued. *Residual varus deformity of forefoot in bilateral clubfoot.*

D. Standing roentgenogram of both feet. **E.** Postoperative roentgenogram showing correction of deformity by osteotomy of metatarsals at their bases.

of the heel in talipes equinovarus is caused by malinsertion of the tendo Achillis, which is attached on the calcaneus more medially and farther forward than normal. This acts as a positive deforming force, inverting the heel and twisting the os calcis during its growth period. He recommended sectioning the medial and anterior attachments of the tendo Achillis to the calcaneus, leaving a small lateral attachment. Then the tendon is split longitudinally and its free tendinous part transferred to the lateral side of the attached remnant and sutured to the os calcis. Stewart states that he has performed this procedure more than 20 times and was surprised at the degree of eversion and dorsiflexion of the foot obtained. In only two instances was subsequent lengthening of the tendo Achillis necessary.[181]

Settle, in his dissections, found the fibers of the Achilles tendon to be inserted vertically into the calcaneus, which was rotated into a markedly varus position. When the heel was everted into neutral position, the medial fibers of the Achilles tendon were tighter than the lateral ones.[177] Irani and Sherman noted the tendo Achillis to be inserted slightly on the medial side of the calcaneus as a result of the shift of position of the posterior part of the bone. When the os calcis was placed in neutral position following sectioning of its ligamentous attachments, the apparent medial shift of the insertion of the tendo Achillis disappeared completely.[128]

The author finds that he achieves the same results as Stewart by sectioning the medial half or two thirds of the tendo Achillis insertion to the os calcis during sliding lengthening of the heel cord. Correction of equinus deformity is almost always required at the same time as that of the varus heel. Shortening of the posterior tibial muscle is a prime factor in persistence of varus hindfoot; it should be lengthened at the same time as the heel cord.

PROCEDURES ON BONE

Shortening of Lateral Column of Foot. Evans, in 1961, proposed that the essential deformity in talipes equinovarus was medial displacement and rotation of the navicular on the talus, with all other elements of the deformity being secondary and adaptive.

To support his view, he quoted Elmslie, who believed that the deformity was primarily one of the midtarsal joint with displacement of the navicular and cuboid inward. The os calcis consequently rotated, with downward and medial shifting of its anterior end.[95, 96]

Brockman, in 1930, had arrived at the same conclusion, i.e., that the major deformity is medial displacement of the navicular on the talus, with all changes being adaptive. As previously mentioned, Irani and Sherman and Settle have refuted this theory and have demonstrated that the primary deformity consists of medial and downward angulation of the anterior end of the talus.[128, 177]

Evans believed relapse of the talipes equinovarus is caused by failure to correct this medial dislocation of the navicular on the head of the talus.[96] Abrams found medial displacement of the navicular on the head of the talus in the 31 relapsed clubfeet explored surgically. The medial column of the foot—consisting of the talus, navicular, medial cuneiform, and first ray—is relatively shortened and is held in varus position by the contracted soft tissues. The lateral column of the foot—composed of the calcaneus, cuboid, and fifth ray—gradually develops adaptive changes consisting of overgrowth in length and distortion in the shape of the calcaneocuboid joint, primarily medial obliquity of its articular surfaces. These adaptive changes provide a resistant barrier to manipulative correction.

The obstruction by the lateral column of the foot has been noted previously. Ogston, in 1902, advocated enucleation of the cuboid bone, of the anterior part of the calcaneus, and of the head of the talus.[164] His operation, however, was not successful, because it weakened rather than restored the medial column of the foot. Johanning, in 1958, proposed enucleating the cuboid bone alone.[131] Other procedures designed to shorten the lateral column of the foot included wedge resection of the midtarsal joints, cuboid, and calcaneus.

Evans described a procedure in which, following medial and posterior release of the contracted soft tissues, a wedge resection of the calcaneocuboid joint was performed. He claimed this resection shortened the lateral column of the foot, and permitted the released navicular to be placed on the head of the talus so that the axes of the first metatarsal and the talus are aligned. The varus heel was also corrected. Evans emphasized the importance of carrying out the total procedure in one stage.[96]

In the Evans procedure, a posterior and medial release of contracted soft tissues is performed first. A posteromedial incision is made, beginning at the medial cuneiform and extending posteriorly along the course of the posterior tibial tendon, inferior to the medial malleolus, and then proximally up the leg along the anterior border of the tendo calcaneus for a distance of 7.5 cm. A Z-plasty of the tendo calcaneus and capsulotomy of the posterior parts of the ankle and subtalar joints are performed, correcting the equinus deformity. The foot should be passively dorsiflexed, at least to neutral position, before proceeding further. The neurovascular bundle is identified and protected from injury. A Z-plasty of the posterior tibial tendon is carried out next. Abrams prefers to perform this above the medial malleolus. The talonavicular joint is exposed. It is best to utilize the distal segment of the posterior tibial tendon to locate the tuberosity of the navicular. Inadvertent creation of a false joint in the neck of the talus should be avoided. With medial displacement of the navicular, the talonavicular joint is distorted to an oblique inclination, which is very deceptive. Next, the capsule of the talonavicular joint is divided on its superior, medial, and inferior aspects. If necessary, the tight plantar structures are also divided.

A long lateral incision 4 cm. in length is centered over the calcaneocuboid joint, running parallel with the tendon of the peroneus brevis. The subcutaneous tissue is divided and the skin flaps retracted. The peroneus brevis tendon is retracted plantarward and the calcaneocuboid joint is fully exposed. A wedge of the calcaneocuboid joint based laterally is resected. If there is associated equinus distortion of the forefoot, the wedge is thicker dorsally; if the foot is rocker-shaped, the wedge is thicker on its plantar surface. With a periosteal elevator, a connection is made between the resected area of the calcaneocuboid joint and the talonavicular joint, ensuring free motion of the Chopart's joint as a unit. Next the foot is manipulated, shifting the middle and fore-

part of the foot laterally and aligning the axes of the first metatarsal and talus. Two staples are inserted to hold the calcaneus and cuboid securely together. One staple is not adequate to prevent rotation. The elongated tendons are then sutured, the incisions are closed, and the limb is immobilized in an above-knee cast, holding the foot in the corrected position. After four to six weeks, a below-knee walking cast is applied. Both Evans and Abrams recommend that immobilization be continued for about five months.

Initially, Evans routinely transferred the anterior tibial tendon to the lateral side of the foot (in 26 of 30 feet); however, this proved unsatisfactory because of the resultant passive dropping of the forefoot. In later cases he abandoned the tendon transfer as a part of the procedure. Abrams did not transfer the anterior tibial tendon routinely; he found, with the exception of three cases, that there was return of sufficient peroneal power to provide active eversion of the foot.

Evans reported the results of his procedure on 30 feet followed for four to eight years postoperatively. He did not attempt a statistical analysis of the results because the initial factors were too variable and the series was too small. The correction of deformity at operation was permanent, and in the experience of Evans, the procedure eliminated the need for all after-care. He also observed that all elements of the deformity, including varus heel, were corrected by the operation.[96]

Abrams reported the results of Evans's operation in 31 feet, with an average follow up of 44.5 months. The results of his series were roughly comparable to those of Evans: in 74 per cent, good; in 23 per cent, fair; and in 3 per cent, poor. The result was poor when marked scarring and stiffness of the foot were present consequent to extensive or multiple previous surgical procedures. Another important factor determining the outcome of the procedure was the age of the patient. The best age is between four and eight years. The operation should not be performed under the age of four, as in the immature tarsal bones, wedge resection of the calcaneocuboid joint may remove too much cartilage, and fusion at the site of joint resection may be difficult to achieve. Abrams also states that the operation should not be done after the age of nine years. In his experience, the results of this operation are so much better than those following previous soft-tissue procedures after the age of two years that he advises using conservative methods of holding the foot between the ages of two and four years, and then performing the Evans procedure. He also warns that the operation does not correct adduction of the forepart of the foot at the tarsometatarsal joints, and that this should be treated separately.[52]

The principal contribution of Evans in this procedure is wedge resection of the calcaneocuboid joint, shortening of the lateral column of the foot, and fusion of the calcaneocuboid joint in order to provide more permanent correction. Evans noted no ill effects on the mechanics of the foot following calcaneocuboid fusion.

The author recommends shortening of the lateral column of the foot in resistant clubfeet. In a child under six years of age, a cuboid decancellation should be performed, with care being taken not to disturb the calcaneocuboid and cuboid–fifth metatarsal articulations. A tenodesis of the peroneus brevis tendon will securely hold the base of the fifth metatarsal near the anterolateral end of the calcaneus. (See Plate 52 for description and illustration of the technique of cuboid decancellation.)

When the child is six years old or older, the author recommends wedge resection and fusion of the calcaneocuboid joint. In preference to staples, he inserts two Kirschner wires to hold the calcaneus and cuboid firmly together. The wires are drilled from the posterior aspect of the calcaneus into the cuboid bone and the fifth metatarsal.

Osteotomy of Calcaneus. Dwyer, in 1963, described an open-up medial osteotomy of the calcaneus with a wedge of bone graft for correction of hindfoot varus deformity in relapsed clubfoot. The results of the operation on 56 feet in 48 patients were good in 27 and fair in 29 feet. The operation was repeated on six feet.[94] This operation corrects the bony deformity of varus heel, and increases the height and length of the calcaneus. It is indicated in a child between four and eight years of age with a rigid

varus deformity of the heel that does not exceed 15 degrees. The operative technique is described and illustrated in Plate 53. When the varus deformity of the heel exceeds 15 degrees and the child is over eight years of age, it is best to perform a close-up lateral osteotomy of the calcaneus (see Plate 60).

Triple Arthrodesis. Tarsal reconstruction by wedge resection and fusion of the midtarsal and subtalar joints is indicated in the adolescent with persistent rigid equinovarus deformity (Fig. 7–29). The operative technique of triple arthrodesis is described and illustrated in Plate 43. It is best to add bone rather than resect an excessive amount, since the height of the foot is an important consideration. Low-riding malleoli will be irritated by the shoes and cause moderate disability in walking.

Osteotomy of the Tibia. Recent evidence has well demonstrated that excessive internal tibial torsion does not commonly exist and is not a principal feature of talipes equinovarus.[128, 177] As stated previously, Swann, Lloyd-Roberts, and Catterall have shown that in uncorrected clubfoot the distal part of the talus and forefoot are laterally rotated in the ankle mortise on the tibia, which has no rotational deformity. The fibular malleolus is displaced posteriorly. In the child under four years of age, this can be corrected by soft-tissue release. After the age of four years, when structural changes have taken place and the deformity has become fixed, internal rotation osteotomy of the tibia may be indicated for proper alignment of the ankle mortise in relation to the leg. This will exaggerate the midfoot and forefoot varus deformity, which is corrected at a later stage by Evans's procedure.[183]

Anterior wedge close-up osteotomy of the tibia and fibula (supramalleolar—in the metaphyseal area) is performed occasionally to correct fixed severe equinus deformity.

TALIPES VARUS

In this congenital deformity the forefoot is adducted and inverted and the hindfoot is inverted, but the range of dorsiflexion of the ankle and foot is normal, a feature that differentiates it from talipes equinovarus

(Fig. 7–30). It is best to treat these feet by manipulative stretching and a series of corrective casts, as outlined for talipes equinovarus. This is followed by use of a bivalved cast at night, or outflare high-top clubfoot shoes with a valgus strap, which holds the foot in the corrected position. Passive stretching exercises are performed by the mother. With this regimen of therapy, the prognosis is good and full correction of deformity can be expected.

TALIPES CALCANEOVALGUS

This deformity is characterized by the dorsiflexion and eversion of the entire foot. The soft tissues on the dorsum and lateral aspect of the foot are contracted and limit plantar flexion and inversion (Fig. 7–31). The degree of severity of deformity varies.

The incidence of talipes calcaneovalgus was found by Wynne-Davies to be approximately one per thousand live births. The incidence may be higher, however, as some cases may go unnoticed or ignored.[199] It is more common in girls, with a male to female ratio of 0.61 to 1. There is a significantly greater incidence of talipes calcaneovalgus among first-born children and children of young mothers. It is probably caused by intrauterine malposture—the environmental factor of compression acting particularly in the primigravida with a small "tight" uterus and strong abdominal muscles.

It is important to distinguish talipes calcaneovalgus from congenital convex pes planovalgus. In the latter, the talonavicular joint is dislocated, the talus is locked in vertical position, the forefoot is in eversion and abduction, but the hindfoot is fixed in equinus position, giving a "rocker-bottom" shape to the sole of the foot. Roentgenograms of the foot should be taken in doubtful cases. Neuromuscular diseases, particularly spina bifida occulta with neurologic deficit, must also be excluded. It is important to demonstrate function in the triceps surae, posterior tibial, and long toe flexor muscles.

Mild deformities tend to resume normal alignment in about two to four months, and usually the only treatment required is daily passive stretching exercises of the shortened dorsolateral soft-tissue structures by the mother. The foot is plantar-flexed and inverted 15 to 20 times in three daily sessions. Severe and resistant deformities are treated by stretching of the soft-tissue contractures in corrective plaster casts or by the use of Denis Browne splints, both of which hold the foot in equinovarus posture. When the infant begins to stand and walk, the feet will often be pronated; this pronation is treated by a Thomas heel, 1/8-inch raise on the medial side of the heel, and longitudinal arch support in the shoe.

TALIPES EQUINOVALGUS

In this type of clubfoot, the forefoot and hindfoot are everted and abducted, and the entire foot is fixed in plantar flexion at the subtalar and ankle joints. This deformity is very rare and is usually encountered in arthrogryposis (see Fig. 2–79, p. 238).

CONGENITAL METATARSUS VARUS

In this congenital deformity of the forepart of the foot, all five metatarsals are adducted and inverted at the tarsometatarsal joints; usually the hindfoot is in slight or moderate valgus position, though it may be neutral. The term *skewfoot* was suggested by McCormick and Blount to describe the complex deformity of the varus forefoot and valgus hindfoot.[210] The commonly used term, "a third of a clubfoot," is a misnomer, as the navicular is laterally displaced on the head of the talus and *not* on the medial side, as seen in talipes equinovarus. The term *metatarsus adductus* is used by the author when the forepart of the foot is adducted but not inverted.

The incidence of congenital metatarsus varus is about one per thousand live births, according to Wynne-Davies. It occurs more frequently in the female, with a female to male ratio of 100:76.[214] Approximately 4.5 per cent of first degree relatives of a person with metatarsus varus are similarly affected. Thus, if one child is affected, the risk of a second occurrence in a family is about 1 in 20. There is no clear pattern of inheritance, the cause being partly genetic and partly environmental.[214] Metatarsus varus has been

(Text continued on page 1331.)

Cuboid Decancellation

THE PROCEDURE

A. A longitudinal incision about 4 cm. long is made, centering over the dorso-lateral aspect of the cuboid bone. Subcutaneous tissue and deep fascia are divided in line with the skin incision.

B. The peroneus brevis tendon is identified and retracted laterally and plantar-ward. The extensor digitorum brevis muscle is elevated off the cuboid bone and retracted dorsally and medially.

C. With an osteotome, a wedge of bone, based *laterally*, is excised. The capsules and articular cartilage of the calcaneocuboid and fifth metatarsal–cuboid joints should not be damaged.

D. With a sharp curet, almost all the cancellous bone from the cuboid bone is removed.

E. The foot is then manipulated for five to ten minutes, bringing the forepart into marked abduction. The segments of the cuboid bone are compressed and closely approximated, shortening the lateral column of the foot. The peroneus brevis tendon is anchored under tension to the capsule and periosteum on the distal end of the calcaneus; the tenodesing effect will hold the base of the fifth metatarsal in abduction and the cuboid segments firmly together. If adequate soft tissue is not available for anchoring the peroneal tendon, a drill hole can be made in the distal end of the cuboid for secure fixation of the tendon. The author does not recommend use of staples, and he does not perform fusion of the calcaneocuboid joint. The wound is closed and a below-knee cast is applied, holding the forepart of the foot in marked abduction.

POSTOPERATIVE CARE

After two to three weeks, the cast is changed and a new below-knee walking cast is applied following manipulation of the foot. The foot is immobilized for a total period of six weeks. When cuboid decancellation is combined with mobilization of the tarsometatarsal and intermetatarsal joints, the below-knee cast should be worn for a minimum of three months.

Plate 52. Cuboid Decancellation

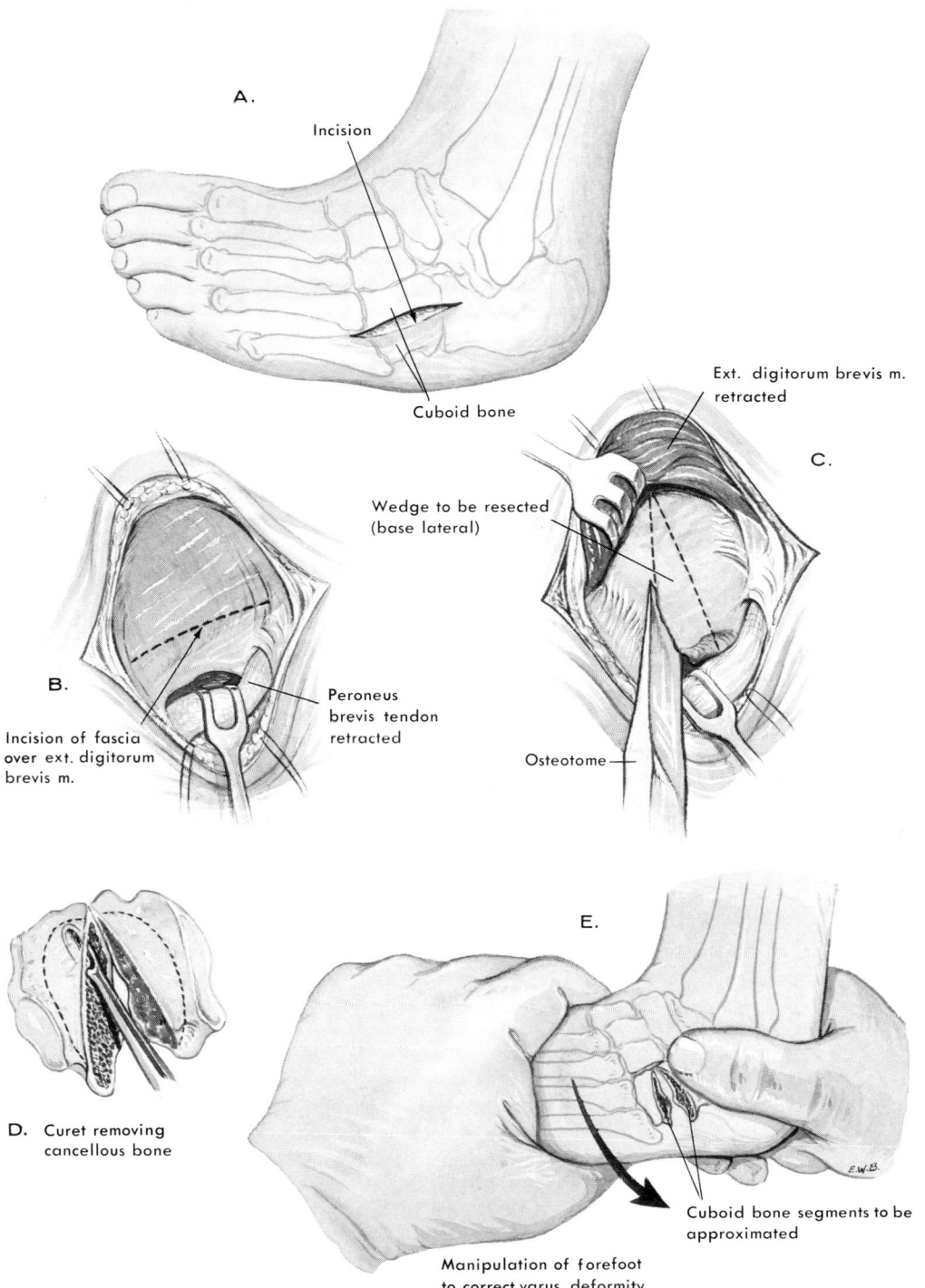

A.

Incision

Cuboid bone

B.

Incision of fascia
over ext. digitorum
brevis m.

Peroneus
brevis tendon
retracted

C.

Ext. digitorum brevis m.
retracted

Wedge to be resected
(base lateral)

Osteotome

D. Curet removing
cancellous bone

E.

Manipulation of forefoot
to correct varus deformity

Cuboid bone segments to be
approximated

E.W.B.

1325

Dwyer Open-Up Medial Osteotomy of Calcaneus with Bone Graft Wedge for Correction of Varus Hindfoot

Through a midline plantar incision, the plantar aponeurosis and short plantar muscles are sectioned near their origin from the tuberosity of the calcaneus, as shown in Plate 57.

THE PROCEDURE

A. The skin incision begins at a point in the midline in the posterior prominence of the heel, along the skin creases, and extends distally to the anterior border of the insertion of the tendo Achillis; then it swings obliquely, dorsally and distally, to a point 2 cm. distal to the lower tip of the medial malleolus. This incision differs from that described by Dwyer; as the varus heel is corrected, the skin margins are pulled together rather than apart, thus preventing delayed wound healing and slough. The subcutaneous tissue is divided in line with the skin incision. The elevated wound flaps are retracted and the plexus of veins is coagulated and divided to prevent bleeding later.

B. Next, the medial one third to one half of the insertion of the Achilles tendon to the calcaneus is sectioned. The lancinate ligament is divided near its insertion to the os calcis, at least 2.5 cm. inferior to the flexor hallucis longus tendon and neurovascular bundle. The medial surface of the calcaneus is subperiosteally exposed. The line of incision in the periosteum is 1.5 cm. inferior and in line with the flexor hallucis longus tendon. Injury to neurovascular structures should be avoided. Chandler elevator retractors are used to partially expose the superior and inferior aspects of the calcaneus.

C. With a wide osteotome, the calcaneus is sectioned just inferior to the flexor hallucis longus tendon. The lateral cortex of the calcaneus is left intact; however, its medial, inferior, and superior aspects should be completely divided.

D. Next, a Steinmann pin is inserted transversely into the os calcis. While the pin acts as a lever, with periosteal elevators and a laminectomy spreader, the site of osteotomy is opened. The width of the bone graft wedge is determined by inserting osteotomes of various sizes between the fragments. An appropriate bone graft wedge is taken from the ilium and, with its base medially, is placed in the gap in the calcaneus. The author finds that bone grafts from the upper end of the tibia are usually inadequate and not sturdy enough. The tension of the tissues will firmly hold the bone graft in position; the Steinmann pin is removed, as special fixation is not required. Roentgenograms are made in the operating room to ensure that the varus deformity of the hindfoot is corrected. The skin is closed with interrupted sutures, and a long leg cast is applied.

POSTOPERATIVE CARE

The cast and sutures are removed in two to three weeks, and a new long leg cast is applied. Approximately ten weeks is required for the bone graft to consolidate. Early weight-bearing will result in collapse of the graft and loss of correction. The importance of protecting the foot until the bone graft is fully incorporated cannot be overemphasized.

Plate 53. Dwyer Open-Up Medial Osteotomy of Calcaneus with Bone Graft Wedge for Correction of Varus Hindfoot

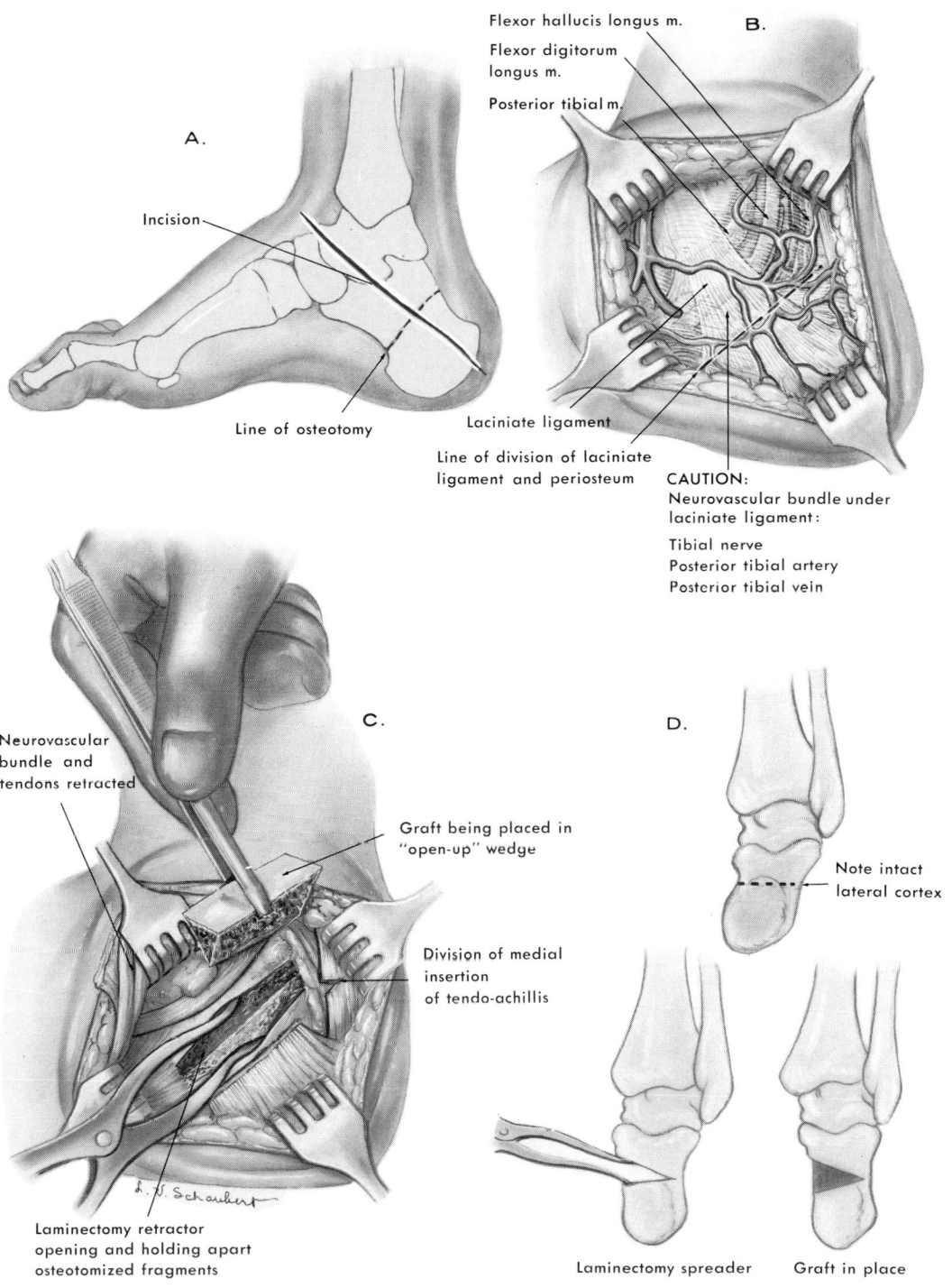

A.

Incision

Line of osteotomy

Flexor hallucis longus m.

Flexor digitorum longus m.

Posterior tibial m.

B.

Laciniate ligament

Line of division of laciniate ligament and periosteum

CAUTION:
Neurovascular bundle under laciniate ligament:

Tibial nerve
Posterior tibial artery
Posterior tibial vein

Neurovascular bundle and tendons retracted

C.

Graft being placed in "open-up" wedge

Division of medial insertion of tendo-achillis

Laminectomy retractor opening and holding apart osteotomized fragments

D.

Note intact lateral cortex

Laminectomy spreader

Graft in place

1327

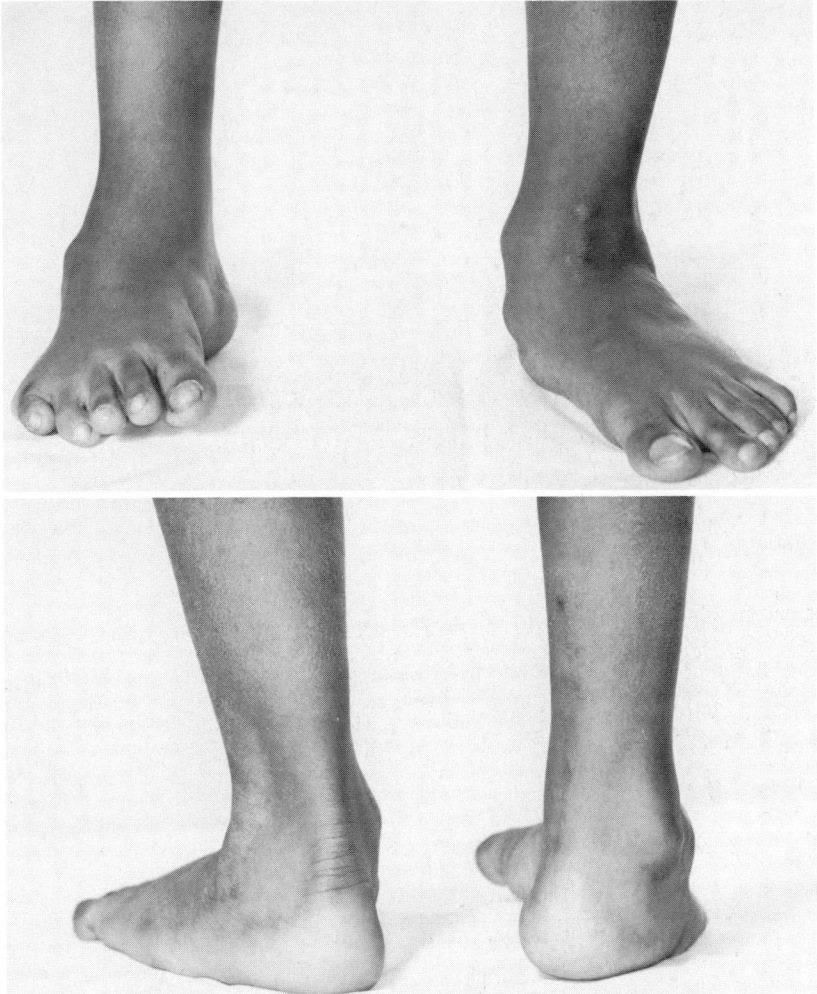

FIGURE 7–29.   *Talipes equinovarus on the right in a 12-year-old boy.*

The deformity is best corrected by tarsal reconstruction with wedge resection and fusion of the midtarsal and subtalar joints (triple arthrodesis).

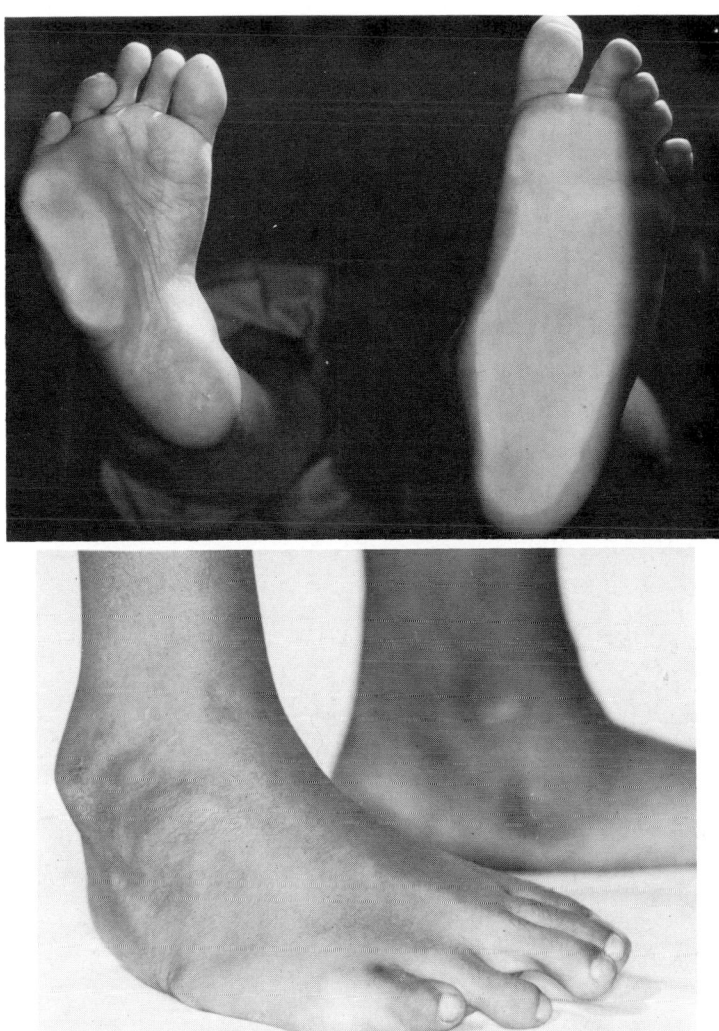

FIGURE 7–29 Continued.   Talipes equinovarus on the right in a 12-year-old boy.

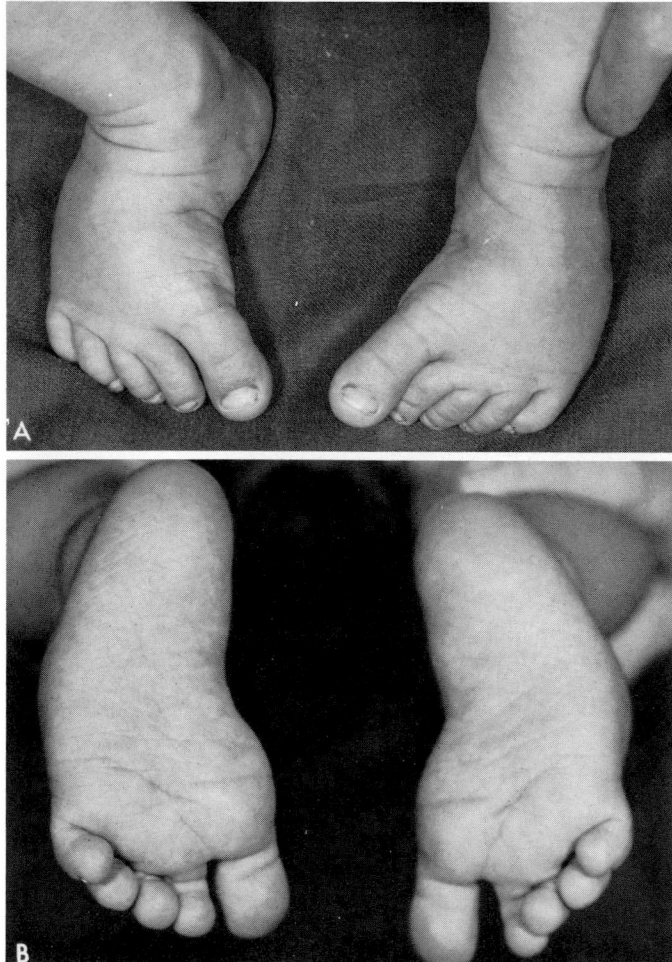

FIGURE 7–30. *Bilateral talipes varus.*

A. Dorsal view. **B.** Plantar view. The forefoot is inverted and adducted, the hindfoot is inverted, but the range of dorsiflexion of the foot and ankle is normal.

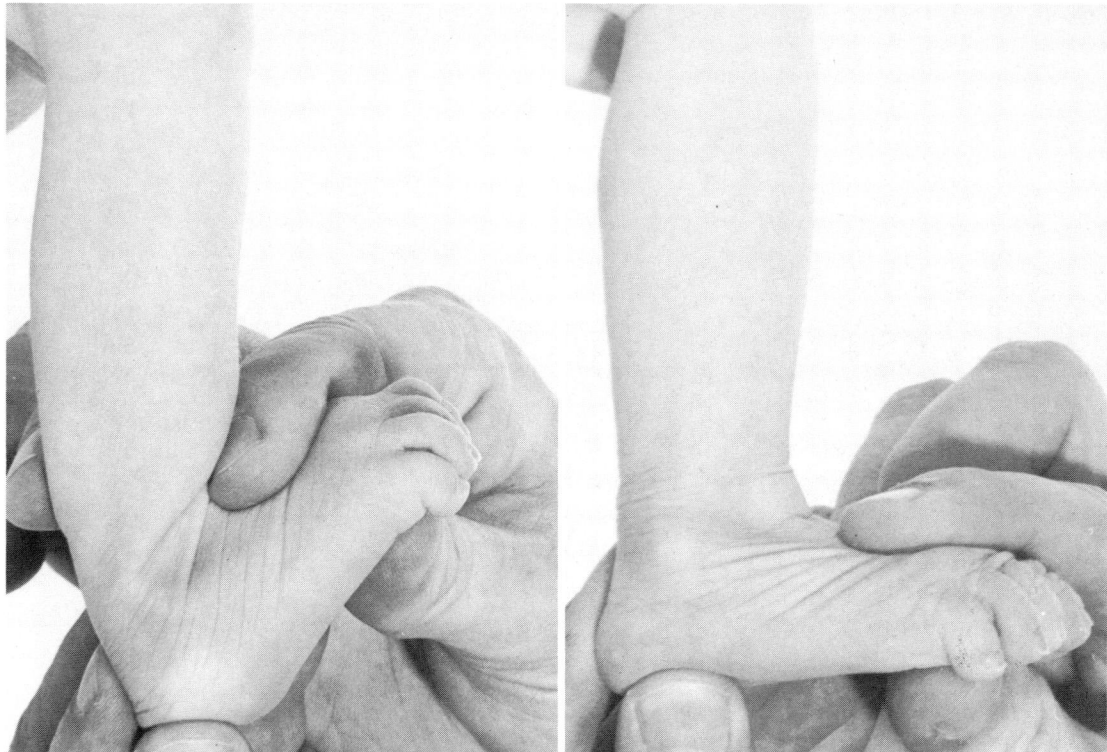

FIGURE 7-31. *Talipes calcaneovalgus on the right in an infant.*

Note the entire foot is dorsiflexed and everted.

observed with increasing frequency during the past three decades, and in the author's experience has been about ten times more frequent than talipes equinovarus.

Clinical Features

The deformity is present at birth, but may often go unnoticed for as long as several months to a year. Involvement may be unilateral or bilateral.

On inspection of the dorsal and plantar aspects of the foot, all the metatarsals are adducted and inverted, but the heel is in either valgus or neutral position. The great toe is usually widely separated from the second toe. The base of the fifth metatarsal is prominent. The medial border of the foot is concave and the lateral border convex. A high medial longitudinal arch is present; normally, an infant's foot appears flat because of the presence of a large fat pad under the medial longitudinal arch. Passively, the forepart of the foot cannot be ab-

ducted into neutral position. The invertor and adductor muscles pull the forefoot further into varus position, but on stimulation and contraction of the peroneal muscles, the foot fails to abduct or evert actively. Exaggerated internal tibial torsion is often present in metatarsus varus.[205-207, 209-212]

When the older child starts to walk, he toes in, his weight being borne on the lateral side of the sole. The fitting of shoes is difficult and shoe wear is noticeably abnormal, with early breakdown of the inner side of the upper of the shoe and the lateral side of the sole. Functional metatarsus varus is caused by hyperactivity of the abductor hallucis and short toe flexors; the foot is completely flexible and can be fully abducted. All infants have an active plantar grasp reflex and will actively hold their forefoot in adduction and the toes in flexion. The absence of *fixed* varus deformity of the forepart of the foot (i.e., actively and passively it can be brought to neutral position) should distinguish these normal conditions from congenital metatarsus varus.

Roentgenographic Findings

Routine roentgenograms are not required to establish the diagnosis. The roentgenograms will depict the adducted and inverted position of *all* the metatarsals at the tarso-metatarsal joints. The talocalcaneal angle in the anteroposterior view is normal or increased; in talipes equinovarus, the talocalcaneal angle is decreased. There is no deformity in the midfoot. When the child is over the age of three years, and the tarsal navicular is ossified, the navicular may be either in normal relationship to the head of the talus or lateral to it, whereas in talipes equinovarus, the navicular is displaced medially on the head. In the lateral roentgenogram, the talus and calcaneus are not plantar-flexed.

Treatment

When a pediatrician makes the diagnosis of congenital metatarsus, the infant should be referred to an orthopedic surgeon for immediate treatment. It is very unfortunate that often mild deformities are kept under observation by the pediatrician to see whether they will correct themselves spontaneously. During this period of procrastination the deformity increases and becomes more rigid and progressively more resistant to correction. The importance of treatment of true congenital metatarsus varus within the first week of life cannot be overemphasized.

Certain pitfalls of management should be avoided.[209, 212] (1) Stretching exercises are often poorly and improperly executed by the parents; the entire foot is abducted and pronated. The valgus inclination of the hindfoot is exaggerated, the navicular is displaced dorsolaterally on the head of the talus, which is plantar-flexed, and the metatarsals are fixed in varus position. The resultant "Z" deformity of the foot (fixed varus forefoot and valgus hindfoot) is then much more severe than the original metatarsus varus. (2) Reversing shoes—putting the left shoe on the right foot—will not correct the deformity. (3) "Swung-out" or tarsal pronator shoes or prewalker clubfoot shoes should not be used, as they accentuate the hindfoot valgus deformity by forcing the heel into eversion. (4) An abduction bar on the shoes (the usual Denis Browne splint or any of its modifications such as the Fillauer bar) should not be used as a corrective device, as the valgus force of the splint is exerted on the hindpart as well as the forepart of the foot.

The only effective way to correct fixed metatarsus varus deformity is by using serial stretching casts.

The technique of gentle manipulative exercises to stretch the soft-tissue contracture and application of corrective plaster cast is well described by Kite, by McCormick and Blount, and by Ponseti and Becker.[207, 210, 212] It is imperative that the details of technique be followed meticulously.

The tendency is to abduct and evert the whole foot during manipulation and application of the cast. This will increase the valgus deformity of the heel and provide only minimal corrective force at the tarsometatarsal joints (Fig. 7–32 A and B). The correct manipulation is as follows: (1) The hindfoot is placed in slight plantar flexion and the anterior process of the calcaneus is pushed medially beneath the head of the talus. (2) The metatarsals are forced into abduction while counterpressure is applied over the cuboid, immediately proximal to the base of the fifth metatarsal. The forepart of the foot is everted (Fig. 7–32 C and D). It is important not to produce an iatrogenic valgus deformity of the hindfoot. The corrected position is maintained to the count of 10 and then released. The exercises are performed for five to ten minutes. The manipulations should be gentle. Then an above-knee corrective cast is applied in two sections. First the plaster is wrapped over the foot and ankle, and is rolled against the deformity. Again, the hindfoot is maintained in inversion and slight plantar flexion, correcting the valgus deformity of the heel. With pressure over the cuboid bone, the metatarsals are pushed into maximal abduction, but not eversion. Pressure is exerted on the head and neck of the first metatarsal, not on the great toe. After the plaster sets, the cast is extended proximally to include the knee and thigh. Ponseti and Becker externally rotate the leg when applying the proximal part of the cast to correct the associated medial torsion of the tibia. There is no evidence that immobilizing the

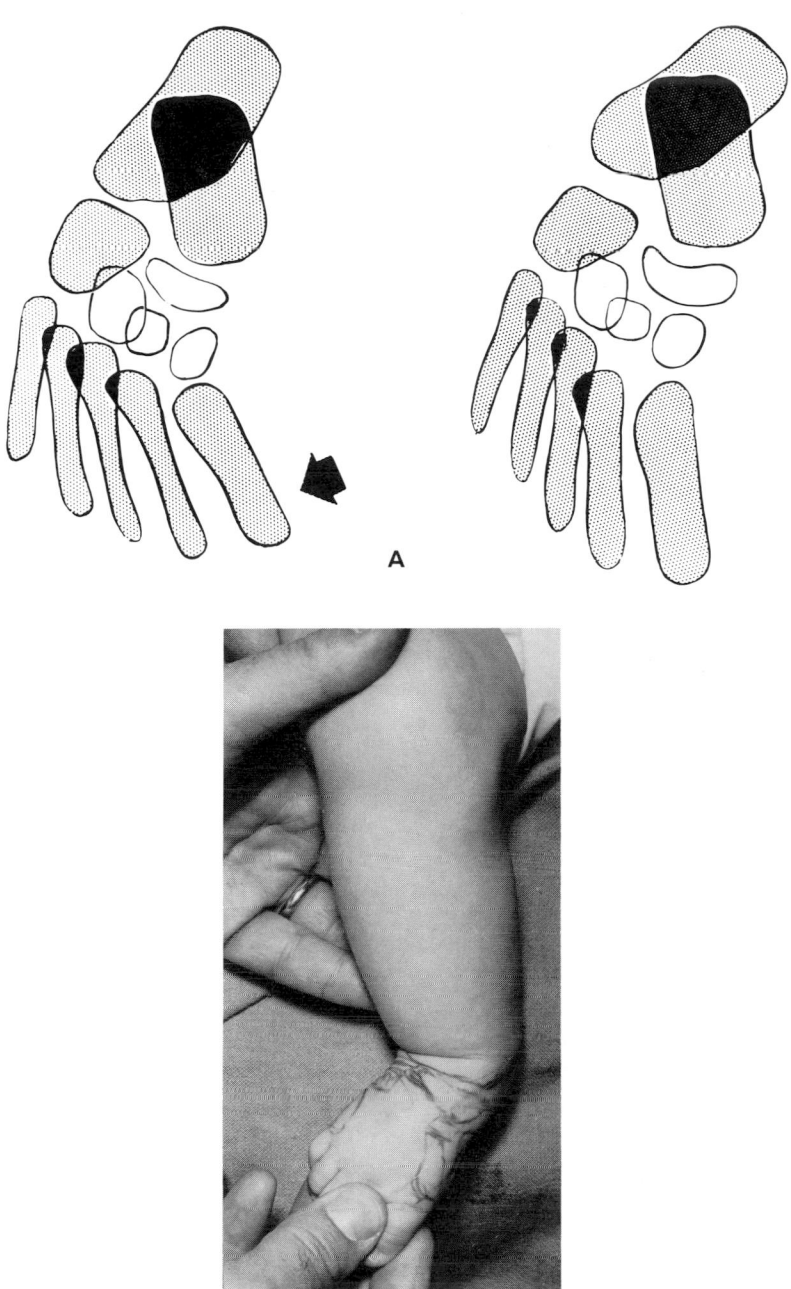

B

FIGURE 7-32. Correction of metatarsus varus by passive stretching.

A and **B.** *The incorrect method of manipulation.* The entire foot is abducted and everted by forcefully abducting and everting the forefoot without counterpressure on the hindfoot. The foot is simply being twisted at the ankle, with little corrective force being exerted at the metatarsotarsal joints. The diagram illustrates how the valgus deformity of the heel is increased and shows that the improved appearance of the varus deformity of the forepart of the foot is spurious and not real correction. (From Ponseti, I. V., and Becker, J. R.: Congenital metatarsus adductus: The results of treatment. J. Bone Joint Surg., *48–A*:706–707, 1966.

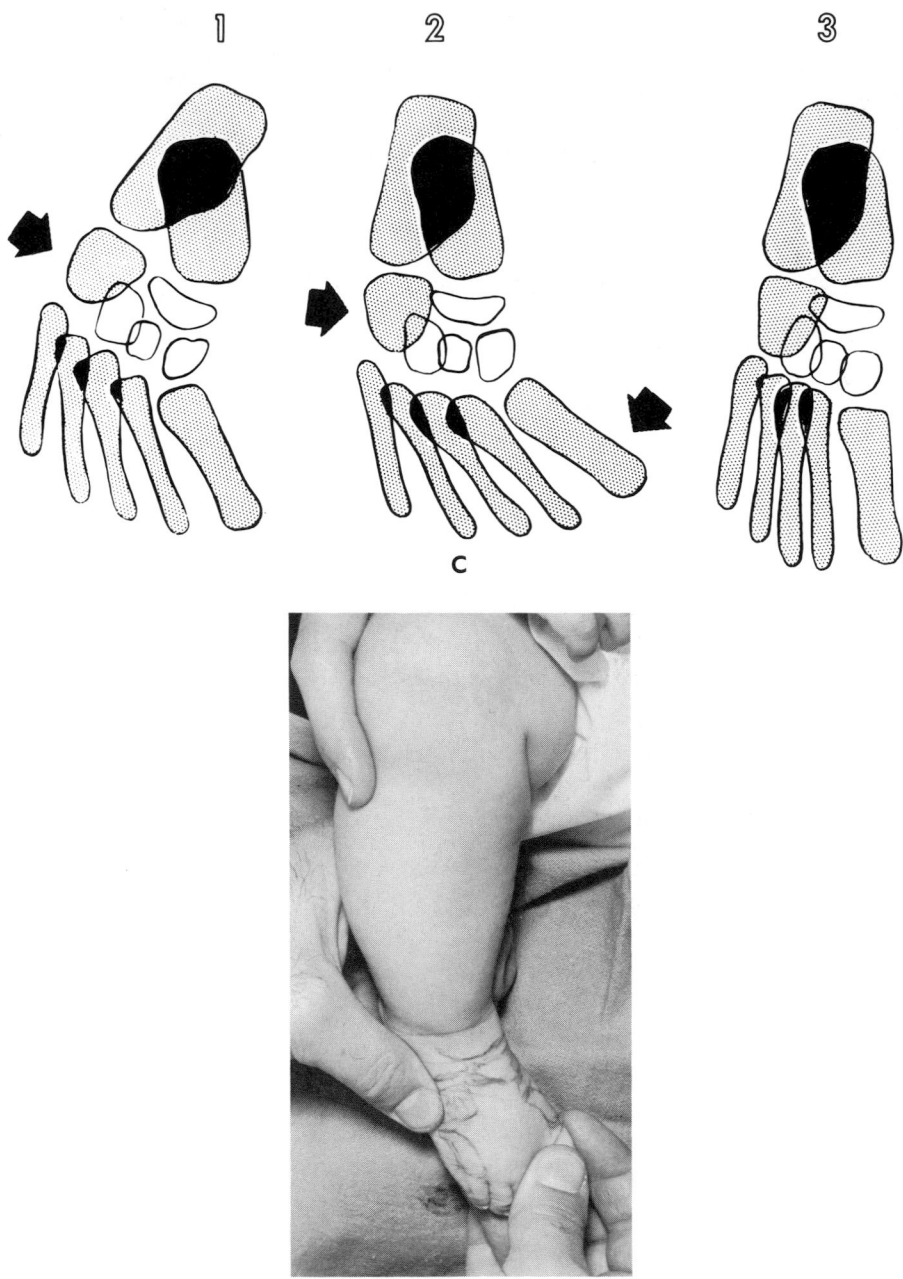

D

FIGURE 7–32 Continued.   Correction of metatarsus varus by passive stretching.

C and **D.** *The correct method of manipulation.* The hindfoot is slightly plantar-flexed, and the anterior process of the talus is displaced medially underneath the head of the talus; the metatarsals are pushed into abduction while counterpressure is applied over the cuboid. The diagram illustrates the proper method. (From Ponseti, I. V., and Becker, J. R.: Congenital metatarsus adductus: The results of treatment. J. Bone Joint Surg., *48–A*:706–707, 1966.)

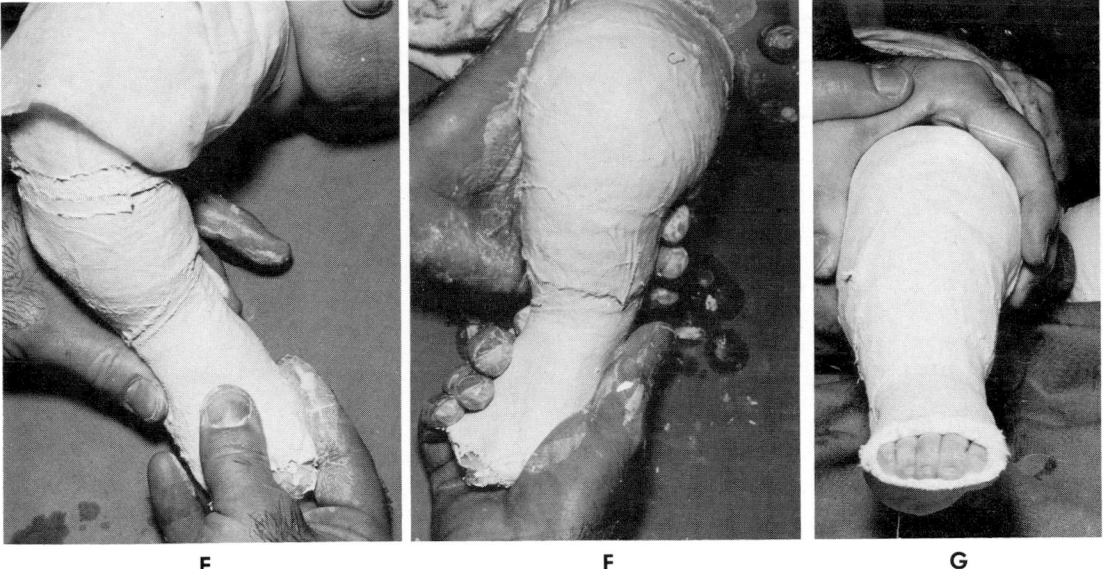

E   F   G

FIGURE 7–32 Continued.   Correction of metatarsus varus by passive stretching.

E. The foot points somewhat medialward while the first section of the plaster cast is applied. **F.** The foot and leg are in slight external rotation while the second section of the plaster cast is applied. **G.** Completed plaster cast. The heel and anterior part of the foot are immobilized in a position as near normal as possible. (From Ponseti, I. V., and Becker, J. R.: Congenital metatarsus adductus: The results of treatment. J. Bone Joint Surg., *48-A*:706–707, 1966.)

leg of an infant in external rotation for six to ten weeks will correct exaggerated medial tibial torsion; all it will accomplish is stretching of the soft tissues. If there is associated contracture of the invertors of the foot, the author externally rotates the leg. In children under the age of one year, below-knee casts are ineffective for controlling the heel in good correction. An above-knee cast that holds the knee in 60 to 90 degrees of flexion will provide much better control of the heel and will prevent the cast from slipping. Casts are changed at 10- to 14-day intervals, the total duration of cast treatment varying from four to ten weeks, depending upon the rigidity of the deformity and its resistance to correction.

According to Kite, the following three criteria must be met before cast treatment is discontinued: (1) Complete correction of the convexity of the lateral border of the foot must be achieved (in fact, it is preferable to obtain slight overcorrection so that the convexity is reversed to slight concavity). (2) The prominence at the base of the fifth metatarsal must be no longer palpable. (3) Muscular balance must be restored so that active abduction of the forefoot is just as strong as active adduction.[207] In children over one year of age, overcorrection is almost impossible, and in the small infant, it should be avoided, as it will produce a valgus foot. Following cast removal, corrective shoes usually are not required. When the deformity was severe initially or definitive cast treatment was delayed, it is best that the forepart of the foot be held in slight overcorrection in bivalved casts during sleep or in Orthoplast boots. Again attention should be paid to see that the heel is in slight inversion but without valgus distortion. Lusskin and Lusskin have devised a simple metatarsus varus aluminum splint that is taped to the foot to hold the correction.[208] A Denis Browne splint with reversed shoes should *not* be used for this purpose.

Surgical Treatment

When a patient with metatarsus varus is seen late, i.e., over one or two years of age, the deformity may be so fixed that it does not respond to conservative measures. Forceful manipulation in an attempt to correct the deformity of the forepart of the foot may force the heel into valgus posi-

(Text continued on page 1342.)

Mobilization of Tarsometatarsal and Intermetatarsal Joints by Capsulotomy and Ligamentous Release for Resistant Varus Deformity of the Forefoot
(Heyman, Herndon, and Strong)

THE PROCEDURE

A. A curved transverse skin incision is made, extending from the base of the first metatarsal to the lateral border of the cuboid bone. It runs obliquely across the dorsum of the forepart of the foot just distal to the tarsometatarsal joints.

An alternate method of exposure of the tarsometatarsal joints is to make three longitudinal incisions on the dorsum of the foot—the first overlies the first ray, the second is between the second and third rays, and the third overlies the fourth ray. In the young child, two instead of three linear skin incisions may be made—one between the first and second rays and the other overlying the fourth ray.

B. The subcutaneous tissue and deep fascia are divided. The skin flaps are mobilized and retracted with 00 silk sutures. By meticulous linear dissection the tendons of the extensor digitorum longus, extensor hallucis longus, anterior tibial, and peroneus brevis are exposed and freed. The dorsalis pedis vessels are identified. Meticulous care is taken not to injure the neurovascular structures.

C. The anterior tibial tendon is retracted medially and the extensor hallucis longus tendon with the dorsalis pedis vessels is retracted laterally. The intermetatarsal space between the first and second metatarsals is identified with a small hemostat and the intermetatarsal ligament is divided, beginning distally and progressing proximally. By this method the first metatarsocuneiform joint is located. The epiphyseal plate of the first metatarsal is proximally located; it should not be damaged. The medial and dorsal capsules are divided. The plantar capsule is not sectioned at this time. The anterior tibial tendon should be carefully protected in order to prevent its inadvertent sectioning. The articular cartilage should not be injured.

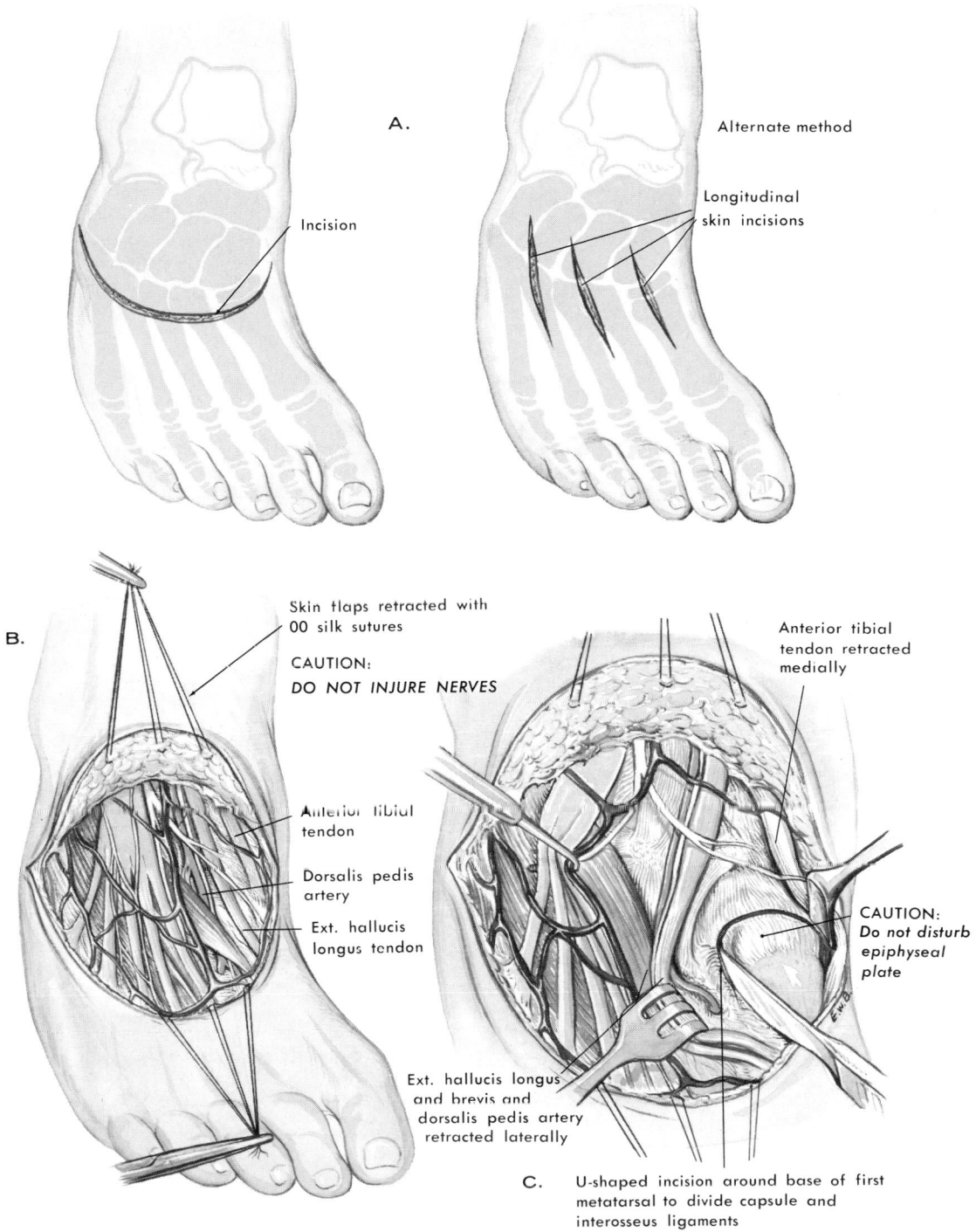

A.

Alternate method

Longitudinal
skin incisions

Incision

B.

Skin flaps retracted with
00 silk sutures

CAUTION:
DO NOT INJURE NERVES

Anterior tibial
tendon retracted
medially

Anterior tibial
tendon

Dorsalis pedis
artery

Ext. hallucis
longus tendon

CAUTION:
*Do not disturb
epiphyseal
plate*

Ext. hallucis longus
and brevis and
dorsalis pedis artery
retracted laterally

C. U-shaped incision around base of first
metatarsal to divide capsule and
interosseus ligaments

Mobilization of Tarsometatarsal and Intermetatarsal Joints by Capsulotomy and Ligamentous Release for Resistant Varus Deformity of the Forefoot (Heyman, Herndon, and Strong) *(Continued)*

D. Next, the second metatarsocuneiform joint is exposed; it is located slightly proximal to the first metatarsocuneiform joint. The intermetatarsal ligaments and dorsal capsule are divided. Then longitudinal dissection is carried out in a plane overlying the third ray, taking care to protect the neurovascular structures and the extensor tendons. Again, with a small hemostat, the intermetatarsal space between the second and third metatarsal is identified, and the intermetatarsal ligaments are sectioned. Dorsal capsulotomy of the second and third metatarsocuneiform joints is completed. The fourth metatarsotarsal joint is essentially at the same level as the second and third; the articulation is readily identified after division of the intermetatarsal ligaments. Dorsal capsulotomy is similarly carried out.

At the fifth metatarsocuboid joint the attachment of the peroneus brevis is protected and the lateral capsule is not disturbed; the latter will serve as a hinge that prevents lateral displacement of the fifth metatarsal as the foot is manipulated.

E. Attention is then directed to the plantar capsule and the plantar ligaments. The metatarsotarsal joints are opened by plantar flexion of the forefoot and distal traction on the individual metatarsals. The medial two thirds of the plantar capsule and ligaments at each joint are divided, leaving the lateral one third intact. This will provide sufficient stability to prevent displacement of the metatarsals while the forefoot is manipulated out of adduction. The intermetatarsal ligaments must be divided completely to permit gliding of the metatarsals as the deformity is corrected.

F and **G.** The forefoot is manipulated into abduction and eversion. After correction is achieved there will be considerable incongruity of the articular surfaces. If there is marked instability of the tarsometatarsal joints Kirschner wires may be inserted to fix the first metatarsal to the first cuneiform and the fifth to the cuboid. The author, however, has not found routine use of Kirschner wires to be necessary.

The tourniquet is released and complete hemostasis is secured. The wound is closed with *interrupted* sutures, and a well-molded long leg cast is applied, holding the foot in the corrected position.

POSTOPERATIVE CARE

For the first few days after surgery, the leg should be elevated to prevent excessive swelling. In 10 to 14 days when the reactive swelling has subsided, the cast is changed and a snug, well-molded cast is applied. It is best to carry this out under general anesthesia and manipulate the foot into the corrected position prior to application of the cast. The skin sutures should not be removed at this time, as the wound edges will separate.

Three weeks later (about four to five weeks after surgery) the cast and sutures are removed, and a carefully molded below-knee walking cast is applied. Immobilization in the cast is continued for a minimum of three to four months; this is important to allow adequate time for remodeling of articular surfaces. The casts are changed every three to four weeks (depending on how robust the child is, as walking is encouraged). Each time the foot is manipulated in the corrected position.

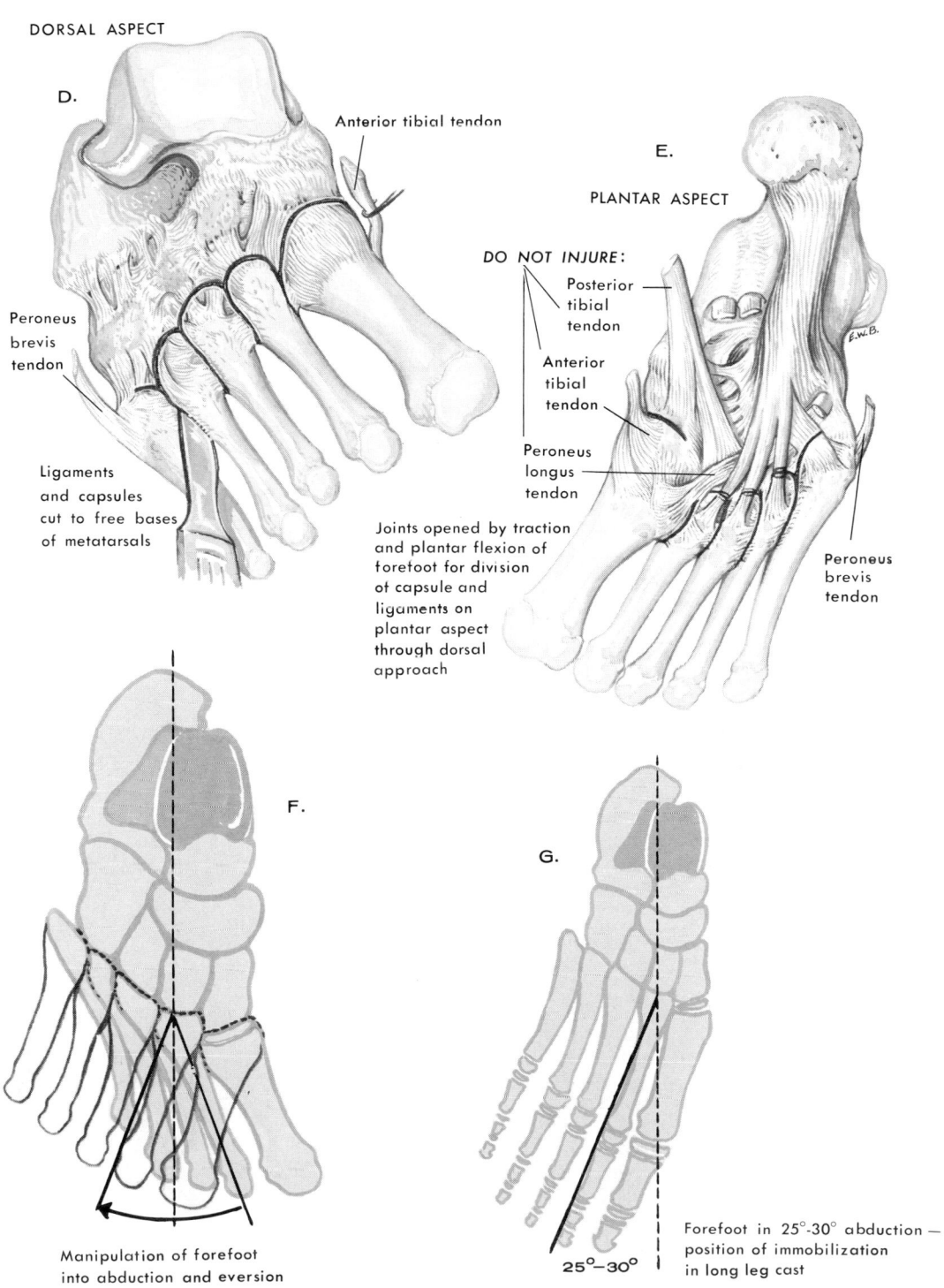

DORSAL ASPECT

D.

Anterior tibial tendon

Peroneus
brevis
tendon

Ligaments
and capsules
cut to free bases
of metatarsals

E.

PLANTAR ASPECT

DO NOT INJURE:

Posterior
tibial
tendon

Anterior
tibial
tendon

Peroneus
longus
tendon

Peroneus
brevis
tendon

E.W.B.

Joints opened by traction
and plantar flexion of
forefoot for division
of capsule and
ligaments on
plantar aspect
through dorsal
approach

F.

G.

Manipulation of forefoot
into abduction and eversion

25°-30°

Forefoot in 25°-30° abduction —
position of immobilization
in long leg cast

Osteotomy of Bases of Metatarsals for Correction of Varus Deformity of Forepart of Foot

THE PROCEDURE

A. The bases of all five metatarsals are exposed by three longitudinal skin incisions, all approximately 5 cm. long—the first on the medial side of the first metatarsal; the second, in the interval between the second and third rays; and the third, between the fourth and fifth rays. The subcutaneous tissue and fascia are divided in line with the skin incisions. The dorsal cutaneous nerves and the dorsalis pedis and metatarsal vessels should be protected from injury. The epiphyseal plate of the first metatarsal, in contrast to the lateral four metatarsals, is proximal in location and should not be damaged. By appropriate retraction of the extensor tendons and the anterior tibial tendon, the bases of all metatarsals are exposed.

B. The lines of osteotomy are marked with a small starter and drill holes. The osteotomies are dome-shaped, with their apices directed posteriorly. In the first four metatarsals the medial limb is longer than the lateral limb, whereas in the fifth metatarsal the lateral (fibular) limb is longer than the medial one in order to prevent lateral displacement of the distal fragment when the forefoot is manipulated into abduction. Often a laterally based wedge is excised from the lateral half of the base of the first metatarsal. The osteotomy is completed with a sharp dental osteotome.

C. A heavy Kirschner wire is inserted across the distal one fourth of the metatarsal shafts. The wound is closed and the foot is manipulated, swinging the forepart into abduction. An alternate method is internal fixation of the osteotomized fragments with two Kirschner wires—one inserted across the first metatarsal to the medial cuneiform and the other across the fifth metatarsal to the cuboid. A well-molded short leg cast is applied, holding the forepart of the foot in 5 to 10 degrees of abduction. The heel should be in neutral position.

Roentgenograms are made in the operating room with the patient under anesthesia to ensure that the desired degree of correction is achieved and that the osteotomized bone fragments are in satisfactory apposition.

POSTOPERATIVE CARE

At three weeks, the cast, Kirschner wires, and sutures are removed. A below-knee walking cast is applied, while the foot is held in the corrected position. Immobilization in the cast is continued for an additional three weeks.

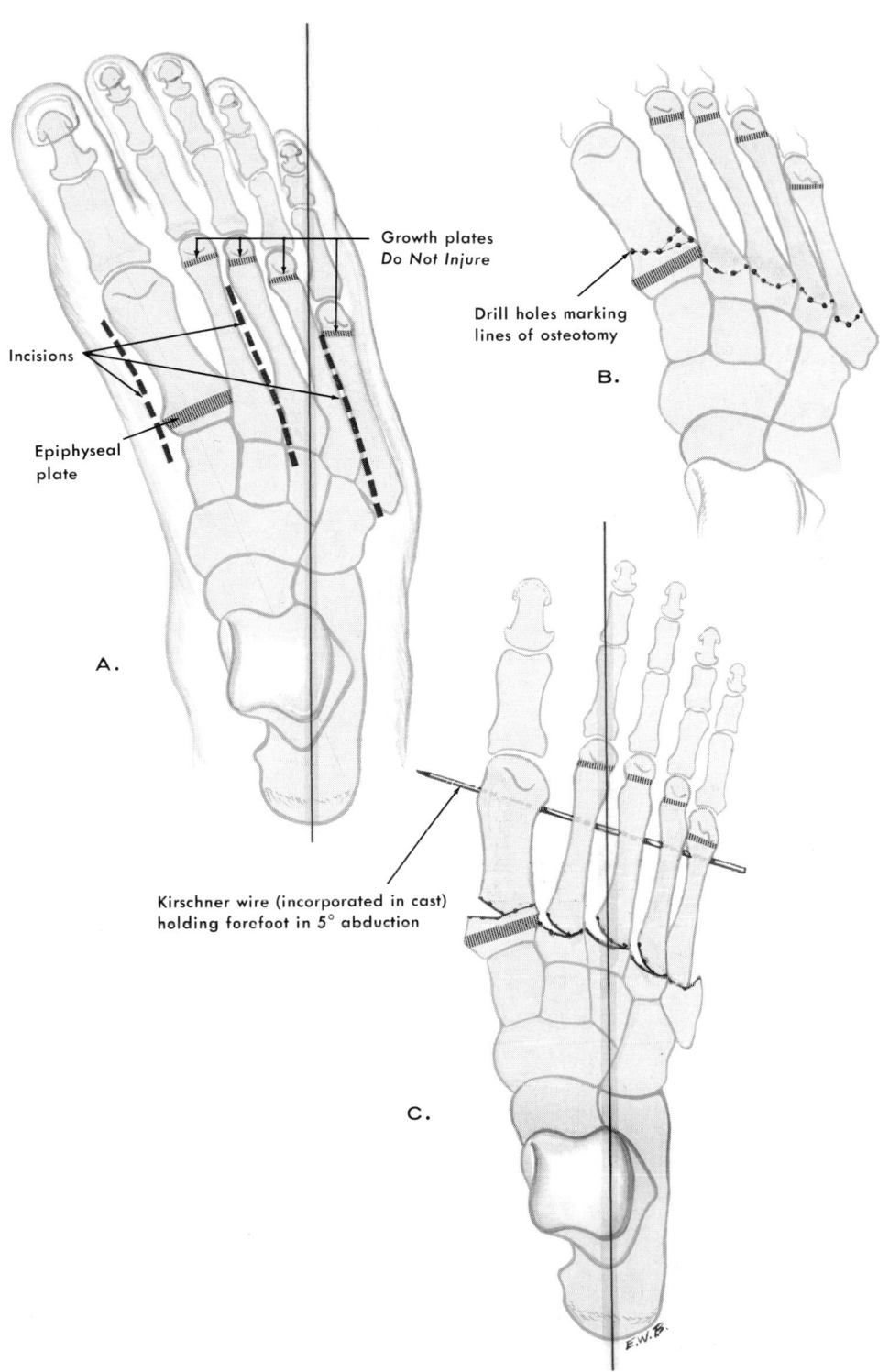

Growth plates
Do Not Injure

Drill holes marking
lines of osteotomy

B.

Incisions

Epiphyseal
plate

A.

Kirschner wire (incorporated in cast)
holding forefoot in 5° abduction

C.

E.W.B.

1341

tion, producing a skewfoot. In such an instance, surgical measures are indicated.

In children under two years of age, the deformity can be satisfactorily corrected by capsulotomy of the first metatarsocuneiform joint and soft-tissue release of the abductor hallucis and the short toe flexors, followed by a stretching plaster of Paris cast for six to eight weeks.

Tarsometatarsal and intermetatarsal soft-tissue release is performed in children between the ages of three and seven years. This is described and illustrated in Plate 54.

Osteotomies at the base of the metatarsals are performed in children over eight years of age. Operative technique is described and illustrated in Plate 55.

Unfortunately, walking on feet with rigid metatarsus varus forces the hindfoot into valgus position, producing a skewfoot. In such an instance, when only the varus deformity of the forepart of the foot is corrected, a severe pes valgus more disabling than the original skewfoot may be produced. If surgical correction is warranted, a two-stage procedure should be performed: first, a Grice extra-articular arthrodesis to correct the hindfoot valgus deformity; then correction of the forefoot varus deformity by soft-tissue release or metatarsal osteotomies, depending upon the age of the patient.

METATARSUS PRIMUS VARUS AND HALLUX VALGUS
Metatarsus Primus Varus

This is a congenital deformity in which the first metatarsal is deviated medially to an abnormal degree. The lateral four metatarsals have normal alignment (Fig. 7–33). In the standing anteroposterior roentgenogram of the foot, the angle between the first and second metatarsals measures about 7 degrees in the normal foot; an angle greater than 10 degrees is considered pathologic.

The condition is hereditary, with a marked preponderance in girls. Because of the trivial nature of this anomaly, it is often not recognized in infancy and early childhood. This is unfortunate because, in adolescence, the great toe will be gradually

pushed into abduction, and the secondary deformities of hallux valgus and bunion will develop (Fig. 7–34). When detected in infancy, metatarsus primus varus is treated by passive stretching and a corrective cast.

Hallux Valgus and Bunion

These two terms, commonly used synonymously, refer to separate elements of the same syndrome; namely, the lateral deviation of the great toe at the metatarsophalangeal joint and the prominence on the medial aspect of the forefoot produced by the bony deformity together with its acquired bursa. Since the deformity usually

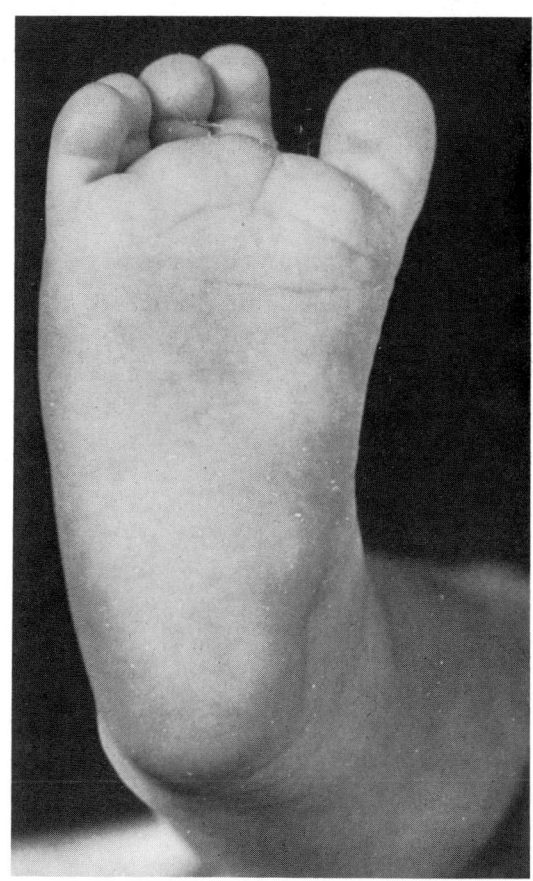

FIGURE 7–33. *Metatarsus primus varus.*

Note that only the first metatarsal is deviated medially to an abnormal degree. The lateral four metatarsals have normal alignment.

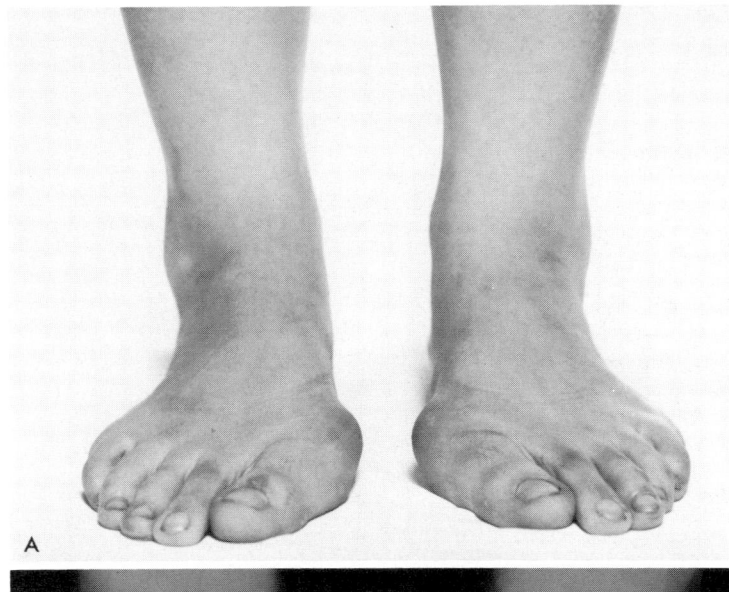

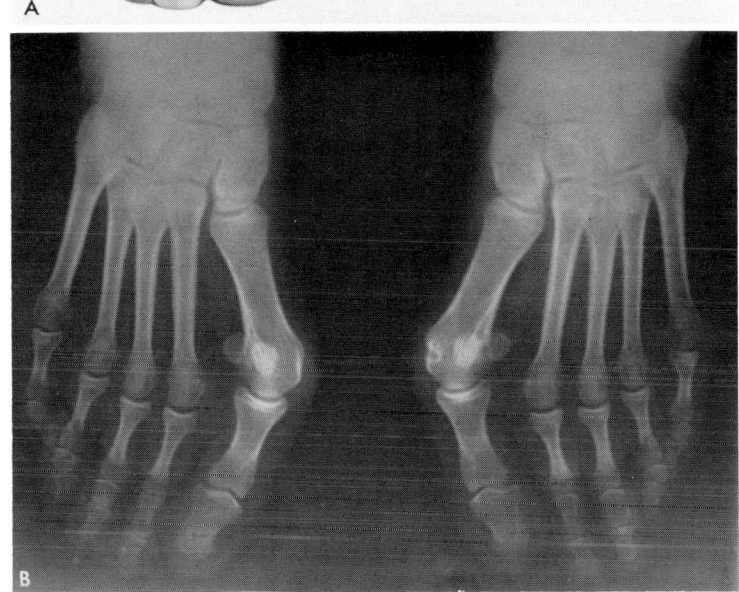

FIGURE 7–34. Severe bilateral metatarsus primus varus, hallux valgus, and bunion in an adolescent girl.

A. Clinical appearance. **B.** Standing anteroposterior roentgenograms.

causes disability in patients at or past middle age, the pathology is not discussed here and the presentation of treatment of hallux valgus will be very brief. The literature on the subject is voluminous; the reader is referred to the excellent monograph by Kelikian.[225]

The symptoms comprise those due to the bunion and those due to the secondary deformities and metatarsalgia. The initial presenting complaint is tenderness over the bunion from pressure and friction against the shoe. The adventitious bursa becomes inflamed and may also be secondarily infected and suppurate. Metatarsalgia and secondary deformities such as hammertoe and callosities are other causes of discomfort.

Treatment

Conservative measures will provide symptomatic relief, but they will not correct the primary deformity. Shoes of adequate width in the forefoot are provided, the bunion is protected with pads of felt, and a rubber wedge between the great and second toes or special bunion splints to hold the hallux straight are given to be worn at night. Metatarsal arch support in the form of appropriate insole pads is provided to treat metatarsalgia.

Operative treatment is indicated when conservative measures fail to give symptomatic relief and when the deformity is very severe. Surgical methods that have been described are many and include the following general technical features: (1) osteotomy of the first metatarsal at its base or neck to correct the metatarsus primus varus deformity; (2) soft-tissue procedures to correct the hallux valgus deformity at the metatarsophalangeal joint; (3) section and transfer of the adductor hallucis to the first metatarsal head; (4) partial excision of the medial prominence of the first metatarsal head; and (5) resection of the proximal two thirds of the proximal phalanx of the great toe.

In adolescents, degenerative changes in the first metatarsophalangeal joint are usually absent and arthroplasty by the Keller procedure is not indicated. If there is associated hallux rigidus with restriction of dorsiflexion of the great toe, osteotomy of the first metatarsal near its neck, displacing the metatarsal head plantarward as well as laterally, is advisable. One or two Kirschner wires are inserted to maintain alignment of the osteotomy. Otherwise, the author prefers the following technique for correcting metatarsus primus varus and hallux valgus (Fig. 7–35).

A dorsomedial incision is made, extending from the middle of the proximal phalanx of the great toe to the base of the first metatarsal. The subcutaneous tissue is divided in line with the skin incision; the digital nerves are identified, care being taken not to injure them inadvertently. Three sets of silk sutures are placed on the skin edges for retraction; the loops are passed distal to the toes and the ends of the sutures are tied on the lateral side of the forefoot. A U-shaped incision is made on the medial aspect of the capsule of the first metatarsophalangeal joint; the width of the U should be at least 2 cm. The capsule is divided as close to its metatarsal attachment as possible and is reflected distally, leaving its base attached to

the proximal phalanx. With an osteotome, the prominent nonarticular portion of the metatarsal head is resected in one piece, and kept sterile in a moist sterile sponge. The big toe is laterally displaced, and with Mayo or tenotomy scissors, the lateral part of the capsule of the metatarsophalangeal joint and the adductor hallucis tendon are sectioned. (The author has not found it necessary to transfer the adductor hallucis to the head of the first metatarsal, the only exception to this being in hallux valgus deformity in a spastic foot—in which instance a separate short dorsolateral incision is made and the adductor hallucis longus tendon is divided under direct vision and transferred to the first metatarsal head.) Then a whip 00 silk suture is inserted on the proximal end of the capsule, which is attached firmly to the distal shaft of the first metatarsal through two drill holes. If the abductor hallucis tendon is displaced plantarward, it is detached at its insertion and transferred to a more dorsal site on the medial aspect of the base of the proximal phalanx. Next, *without stripping the periosteum* the site of osteotomy is marked with a sharp starter and drill holes at the base of the first metatarsal. The lateral cortex is left intact. The bone is divided transversely with a thin osteotome, and the bone previously removed from the metatarsal head is shaped into a wedge and driven in between the osteotomized bone fragments—with care that the lateral cortex is not broken. Precautions should be taken to avoid elevating or depressing the first metatarsal unless this is indicated. This open-up osteotomy will only correct moderate medial divergence of the first metatarsal. If the metatarsus primus varus is severe, a modified dome-shaped osteotomy with a medial buttress in the proximal segment will more effectively correct the deformity. In such an instance, the alignment of the osteotomized fragments is maintained by fixation with an intramedullary heavy Kirschner wire. The wound is closed in the usual manner and a below-knee walking cast with a toe cap is applied. Ordinarily the osteotomy will heal in six weeks, at which time the cast is removed and weight-bearing is permitted without restriction. Passive exercises of the first metatarsophalangeal joint are performed several times a day until full range of motion is obtained.

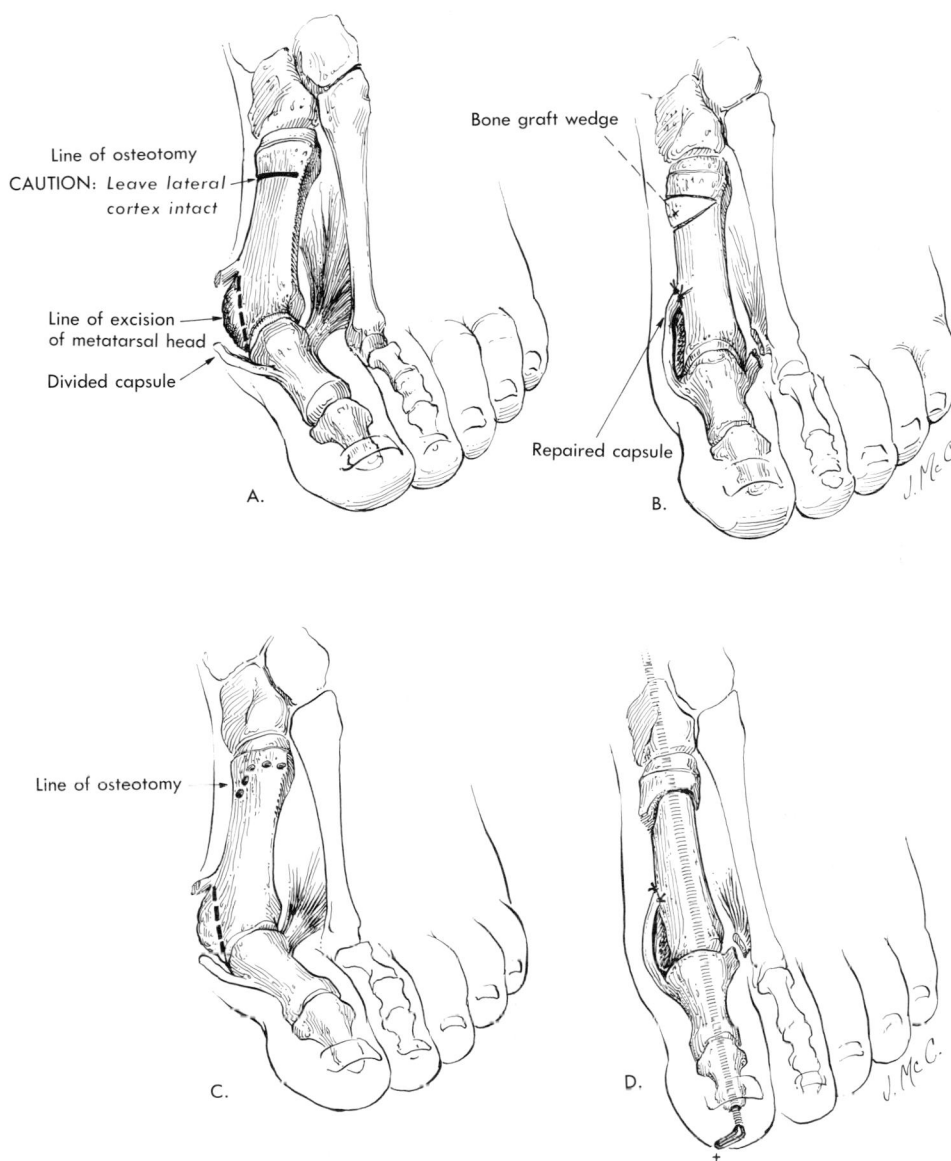

Line of osteotomy
CAUTION: *Leave lateral cortex intact*

Line of excision of metatarsal head

Divided capsule

A.

Bone graft wedge

Repaired capsule

B.

Line of osteotomy

C.

D.

Kirschner wire

FIGURE 7–35. *Correction of hallux valgus and metatarsus primus varus.*

Diagrams showing the deformity (**A**) and the postoperative correction (**B**). The hallux valgus is corrected by medial capsular tightening and sectioning of the adductor hallucis longus tendon and lateral capsule. The medial prominence of the first metatarsal head is excised and is used for bone graft. Metatarsus primus varus deformity is corrected by an open-up transverse osteotomy at the base of the metatarsal. The lateral cortex is left intact. **C** and **D.** Correction of metatarsus primus varus and hallux valgus by modified dome osteotomy of the first metatarsal at its base (note the medial buttress) and internal fixation with Kirschner wire.

TARSAL COALITION

In this congenital abnormality, varying degrees of union occur between two or more tarsal bones, producing a rigid plano-valgus foot.

The condition has long been recognized by anatomists. Cruveilhier, in 1829, reported the first recorded example of cal-caneonavicular coalition; Zuckerkandl is credited as being the first to give an ana-tomic description of talocalcaneal coalition; and Anderson that of talonavicular synos-tosis.[234, 250, 322]

The clinical significance of these intertar-sal bridges was not appreciated until 1880, when Holl proposed a possible relationship between flatfoot and intertarsal bar.[272] Sir Robert Jones gave the first clinical descrip-tion of peroneal spastic flatfoot in 1897; but it remained to Slomann and later Badgley to show that at least some cases of rigid pes planovalgus with peroneal spasm are caused by calcaneonavicular bar.[237, 277, 310] In 1948, Harris and Beath reported the correlation between medial talocalcaneal bridge and peroneal spastic flatfoot.[267]

Classification and Incidence

The coalition may be completely osseous (synostosis), or the connecting bone may be divided by a fissure of varying depth consist-ing of cartilage (synchondrosis) or fibrous tissue (syndesmosis). Involvement may be unilateral or bilateral.

The intertarsal fusions may be any of the following types:

Talocalcaneal
  Medial
  Posterior
  Anterior
Calcaneonavicular
Talonavicular
Calcaneocuboid
Cubonavicular
Multiple—various combinations of the preceding such as talocalcaneal and cal-caneonavicular
Massive tarsal—all major tarsal bones fused into a single block of bone

Medial talocalcaneal bridge may be present in a variety of forms:[265] complete, in which a bony bridge connects the talus and calcaneus (Fig. 7–36 A and Fig. 7–37); in-complete, in which a mass of bone projecting from the talus is united to a mass of bone projecting from the sustentaculum tali by a thin plate of fibrous tissue or cartilage (Fig. 7–36 B); or rudimentary, in which only one element of the bridge may be found, i.e., the bony mass either projects upward from the posterior margin of the sustentaculum tali or downward from the medial surface of the body of the talus posterior to the susten-taculum tali—in both instances, inversion of the os calcis being blocked (Fig. 7–36 C and D).

The complete and incomplete forms are readily recognizable, whereas the roentgen-ographic changes in the rudimentary form are equivocal.[265]

Harris reported the following distribution of the various types of intertarsal bridges found in 102 patients: medial talocalcaneal bridge in 62, calcaneonavicular bar in 29, posterior talocalcaneal bridge in 4, multiple intertarsal fusions in 4, talonavicular fusion in 1, calcaneocuboid fusion in 1, cubona-vicular fusion in 1.[265]

Of the intertarsal coalitions, medial talo-calcaneal bridge and calcaneonavicular bar are the more significant clinically, as they are responsible for the majority of cases of peroneal spastic flatfoot and cause the greater disability.

The incidence of tarsal coalition in the general population is unknown. In an ex-amination of 3,619 Canadian army recruits, Harris and Beath found 74 cases of peron-eal spastic flatfoot (about 2 per cent) and only one case of calcaneonavicular bar.[266]

Talonavicular coalition is very rare.[234, 243, 246, 275, 285, 302, 304] The total num-ber of reported cases in the world liter-ature is less than 40; however, Schreiber has suggested that it may be more common than the literature indicates.[305] Involvement may be unilateral or bilateral, with a definite he-reditary factor present in the latter.

Calcaneocuboid synostosis was first described by Wagoner in 1928, and isolated case re-ports have since appeared in the litera-ture.[238, 245, 283, 289, 316, 317] The condition is of academic interest only, as it is asymptomatic and does not require any orthopedic care.

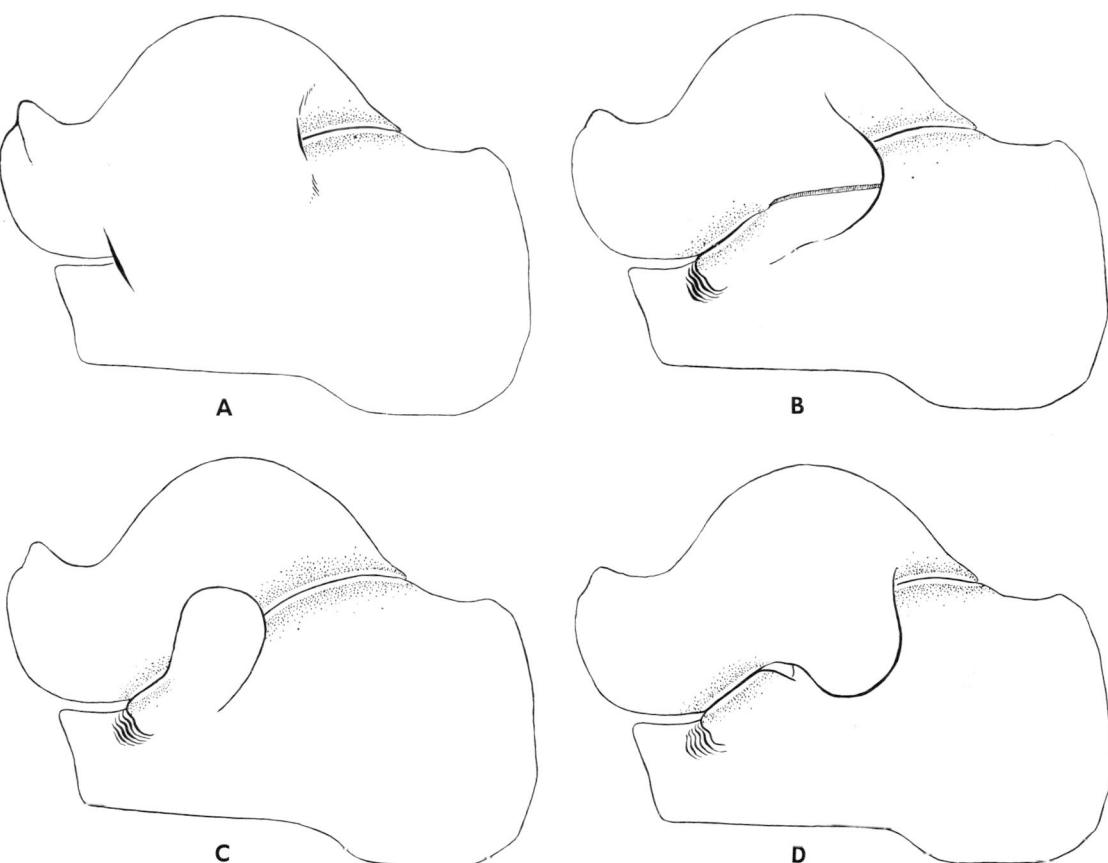

FIGURE 7–36. *Diagrams of variations in medial talocalcaneal coalition (bridge).*

A. Complete medial talocalcaneal coalition. **B.** Incomplete medial talocalcaneal coalition – syndesmosis and synchondrosis. **C.** Rudimentary medial talocalcaneal coalition – sustentacular element. (The bony mass projects upward from the posterior margin of the sustentaculum tali and impinges on the medial side of the body of the talus.) **D.** Rudimentary medial talocalcaneal coalition – talar element. (Bony mass projects downward from the medial surface of the body of the talus posterior to the sustentaculum tali. It impinges on the calcaneus on inversion, though not attached to it.) (From Harris, R. I.: Retrospect – Peroneal spastic flat foot (rigid valgus foot). J. Bone Joint Surg., 47–A:1661, 1965.)

Cubonavicular synostosis and *naviculocuneiform synostosis* are very rare.[251, 288, 318] Waugh reported a case of peroneal spastic flatfoot caused by cubonavicular coalition.[318]

Multiple and massive tarsal coalitions can occur; some cases have related carpal synostosis, symphalangism, and other deformities of the upper limbs (Fig. 7–38).* Nievergelt, in 1944, described a syndrome consisting of bilateral elbow dysplasia with subluxation of the radial heads, tarsal synostosis associated with clubfeet, and occasional fibular overgrowth and carpal coalition with associated brachydactylia and clinocamptodactylia. These deformities occurred in three successive generations of a family and involved both sexes.[293] Austin, in 1951, reported a 20-year-old man with symphalangism of the hands and feet and talonavicular and calcaneocuboid fusions; the same deformities were noted in his older brother, mother, maternal uncle, and maternal grandfather.[236] Pearlman, Edkin, and Warren reported another case of Nievergelt's syndrome occurring in a mother and daughter.[299]

---

*See References 239, 241, 253, 279, 284, 287, 291, 301, 309, 321.

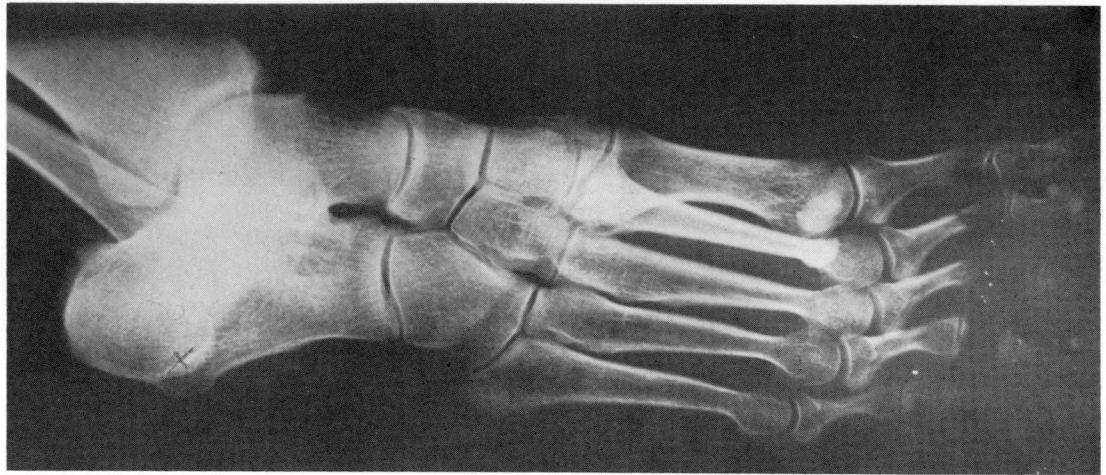

FIGURE 7–37. Complete medial talocalcaneal coalition.

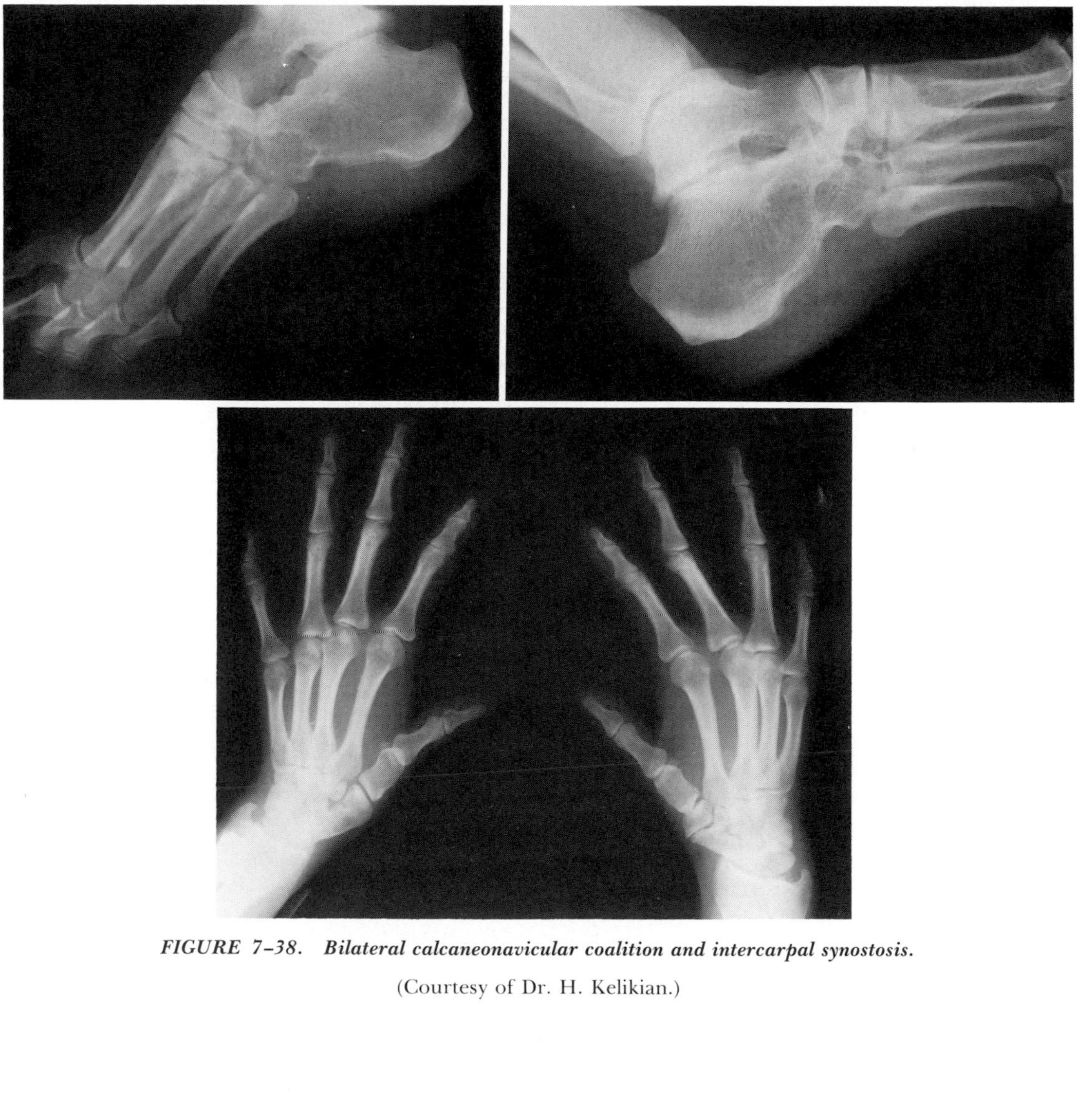

FIGURE 7–38. Bilateral calcaneonavicular coalition and intercarpal synostosis.

(Courtesy of Dr. H. Kelikian.)

Etiology

The exact cause of tarsal coalition is unknown. It seems to arise from failure of differentiation and segmentation of the primitive mesenchyme with resultant lack of joint formation.[265, 274] This theory is supported by the finding of intertarsal bridges in fetal feet (Fig. 7–39).[262, 312]

In the past, anatomists such as Pfitzner proposed that tarsal coalition was caused by incorporation of the accessory intertarsal ossicles into the adjacent major tarsal bones.[300] Thus calcaneonavicular coalition was believed to result from the union of the *os calcaneus secundarius* with the adjacent calcaneus and navicular bones; incorporation of the *os sustentaculare* with its neighboring os calcis and talus was proposed as the cause of medial talocalcaneal coalition. Similarly, one might implicate the os trigonum in posterior talocalcaneal fusion, the os tibiale externum in talonavicular synostosis, the os

peroneum in calcaneocuboid fusion, and multiple accessory ossicles in massive tarsal coalition. This attractive and popular hypothesis is not acceptable, however, as it fails to explain the presence of tarsal coalition in the fetus.

Hereditary transmission has been reported in the literature. For example, Wray and Herndon reported the occurrence of calcaneonavicular coalition in three generations of one family.[320] They proposed that at least some, perhaps all, cases of calcaneonavicular bar are caused by a specific gene mutation that is autosomally dominant, probably with reduced penetrance. Harris noted a pair of calcaneonavicular bars in identical twins and also in a father and son.[265] Talocalcaneal coalition in two sisters is reported by Webster and Roberts.[319] A definite hereditary factor in bilateral talonavicular synostosis is reported by Rothberg, Feldman, and Schuster; and familial incidence of synostosis involving several tarsal bones is described by Bersani and Samil-

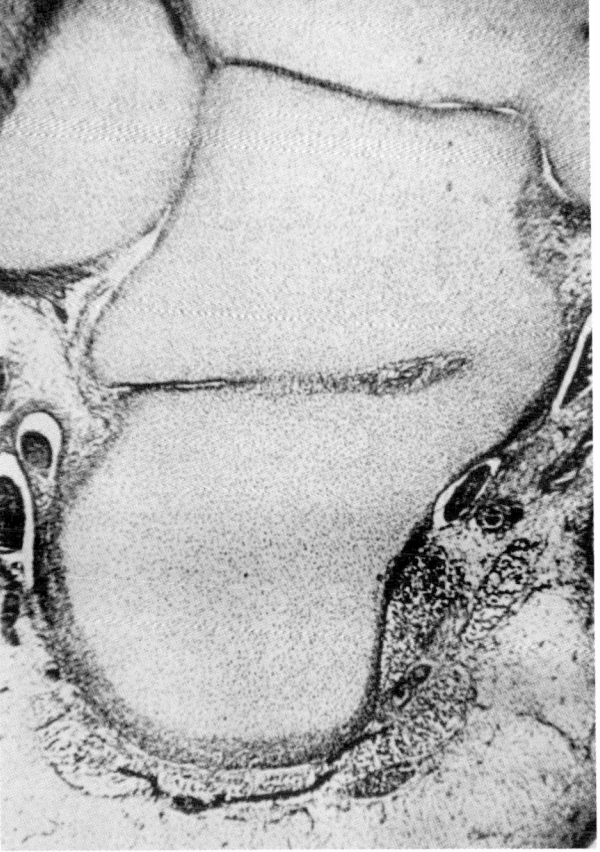

FIGURE 7–39. *Complete medial talocalcaneal bridge in the foot of a 72.3 mm. fetus (coronal section).*

(Courtesy of Barbara Anne Harris Monie; from Harris, R. I.: Retrospect—Peroneal spastic flat foot. J. Bone Joint Surg., *47–A*:1658, 1965.)

son.[241, 302] The literature on the hereditary aspects of tarsal coalition is scanty, however, and more data are needed to delineate a definite hereditary pattern. There may be several distinct genes causing the various intertarsal bridges. Roentgenographic examination of the feet and hands of apparently normal relatives of patients with tarsal coalition will augment our knowledge in this area.

Clinical Features

In infancy and early childhood the condition is usually asymptomatic and is seldom recognized. When the child begins to walk, varying degrees of restriction of motion between the involved tarsal bones may be apparent; during this period, however, the entity is not suspected, as pain is not a clinical feature, the bar is fibrous or cartilaginous, and the roentgenograms are normal.

Symptoms and signs usually tend to appear during the second decade of life, when stress and strain on the tarsus are increased with greater body weight and strenuous physical activity such as sports. At this time, also, ossification of the cartilaginous bar takes place.

The kinetic mechanism of the foot is disturbed by abnormal coalition and configuration of the tarsal bones. In addition to inversion-eversion motion of the subtalar joint, the calcaneus glides forward and backward on the talus. In the fibrous or cartilaginous stage of coalition, this gliding motion is not completely inhibited. With ossification of the medial talocalcaneal bridge, there is progressive restriction of motion on the medial aspect of the joint but not on the lateral aspect, which causes the calcaneus to be forced into valgus position. The longitudinal arch becomes obliterated and the navicular bone becomes displaced dorsolaterally over the head of the talus.

The degree of pes valgus varies greatly; it may be very marked or so minimal that it may be overlooked. In general, medial talocalcaneal bridges cause more deformity than do calcaneonavicular coalitions.

Restriction of motion at the subtalar and midtarsal joints is the characteristic physical finding. When the medial talocalcaneal coalition is complete, the hindfoot will be rigidly fixed in some degree of valgus deformity; midtarsal motion may also be restricted. In calcaneonavicular coalitions, motion at the subtalar and midtarsal joints is moderately limited, but usually not completely obliterated.

Pain in the subtalar or midtarsal area of the involved foot is quite common. It often develops in adolescence, though some patients have no symptoms until adult life. It is usually noted after some unusual activity or minor trauma, and is aggravated by walking over rough terrain, prolonged standing, jumping, or by participating in athletics. Rest relieves the pain.

Most patients develop spasm of the peroneal muscles at some time during the course of the disease. In severe cases, the extensor digitorum longus may also be in spasm. Muscle spasm may occur intermittently or it may be present continuously in varying severity; overactivity increases it, and rest relieves it. The exact pathogenesis of peroneal spasm is unknown. It seems to arise from irritation of the peroneal tendons that are in close proximity to the subtalar and midtarsal joints. Peroneal spasm increases valgus deformity of the foot.

Occasionally in tarsal coalition, the anterior tibial and posterior tibial muscles are in spasm and cause a varus deformity of the foot.[290, 308]

In talonavicular coalition, the presenting complaint is usually a hard prominence on the medial side of the foot, rather than pain. Some cases are discovered accidentally. The longitudinal arch is well maintained. Absence of the talonavicular joint, however, increases the strain of body weight between the fused bones and the cuneiforms. This excess stress may predispose the patient to arthritic changes in adult life.[243] Sanghi and Roby have reported a case of bilateral peroneal spastic flatfoot associated with talonavicular coalition.[304]

Roentgenographic Findings

Calcaneonavicular coalitions are best demonstrated in a 45-degree oblique view of the foot made with the patient standing on the film with the x-ray beam projected through the middle of the foot from the lateral to the medial side.[310, 311] Overlap of the tarsal bones may be mistaken for synostosis; in such instances, oblique projections at various angles are necessary for a definitive diagnosis (Fig. 7–40). The importance of these oblique views cannot be overemphasized, as often in the regular anteroposterior and lateral views of the foot, a calcaneonavicular bar may be entirely overlooked.

The bony bridge in calcaneonavicular synostosis is at least 1 cm. wide and will be clearly visible in the oblique roentgenogram; when the union is cartilaginous or fibrous, however, diagnosis is not that simple. Such a possibility should be suspected when the anterior medial end of the calcaneus and the navicular are in close proximity and their contiguous cortical surfaces are irregular and hazy. Hypoplasia and underdevelopment of the head of the talus is another associated finding. Fracture of the

anterior process of the calcaneus and the presence of an os calcaneus secundarius should be considered in the differential diagnosis. In chip fracture the bone fragment has a well-delineated trabecular structure and its surfaces are smooth and clearly demarcated.

Special projections are necessary to demonstrate talocalcaneal coalitions. Korvin, in 1934, was the first to describe use of the axial view of the calcaneus to reveal talocalcaneal coalition.[282] Harris and Beath, in 1948, emphasized the relation of peroneal spastic flatfoot with talocalcaneal bridge and recommended a 45-degree-angle axial view of the calcaneus for its demonstration (Fig. 7–41).[267] The subtalar joint is complex, consisting of anterior, middle, and posterior joints that are formed by three separate sets of facets on the superior surface of the calcaneus and the inferior surface of the talus.

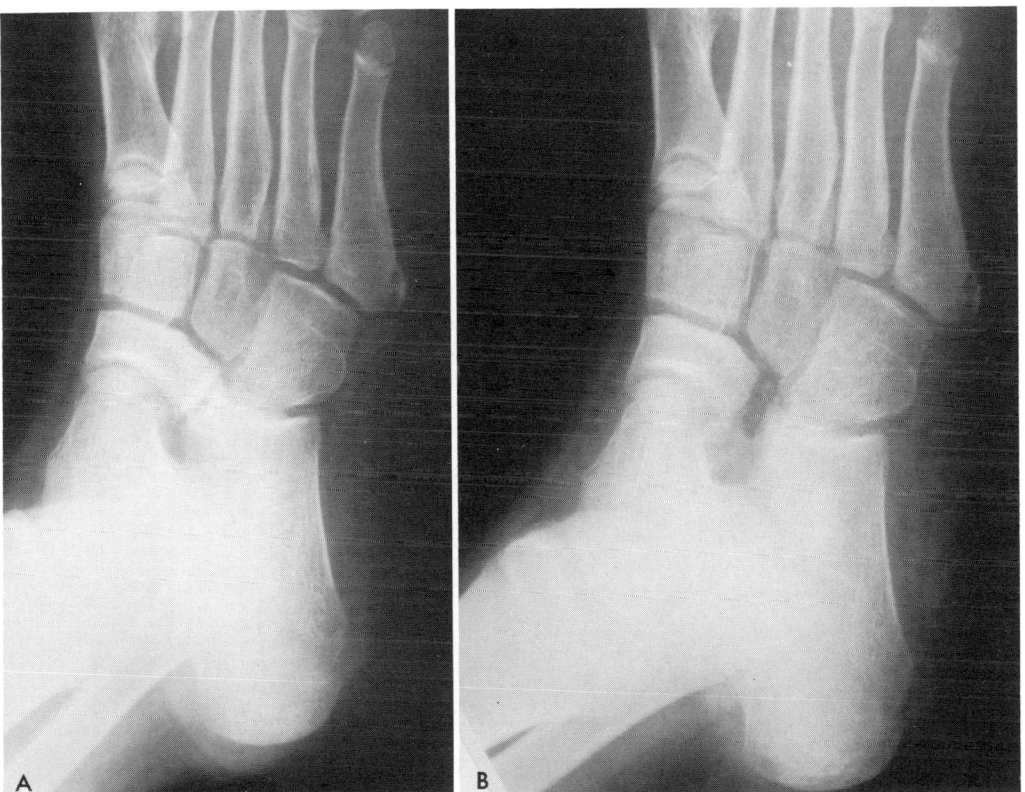

FIGURE 7–40. *Calcaneonavicular coalition treated by resection of bar and extensor brevis arthroplasty.*

A. Preoperative roentgenogram—45-degree oblique projection. Note the bony bridge divided by a fissure consisting of cartilage (synchondrosis). **B.** Postoperative roentgenogram after the bar was excised. Following surgery peroneal spasm disappeared and gradually almost full range of subtalar joint motion was achieved.

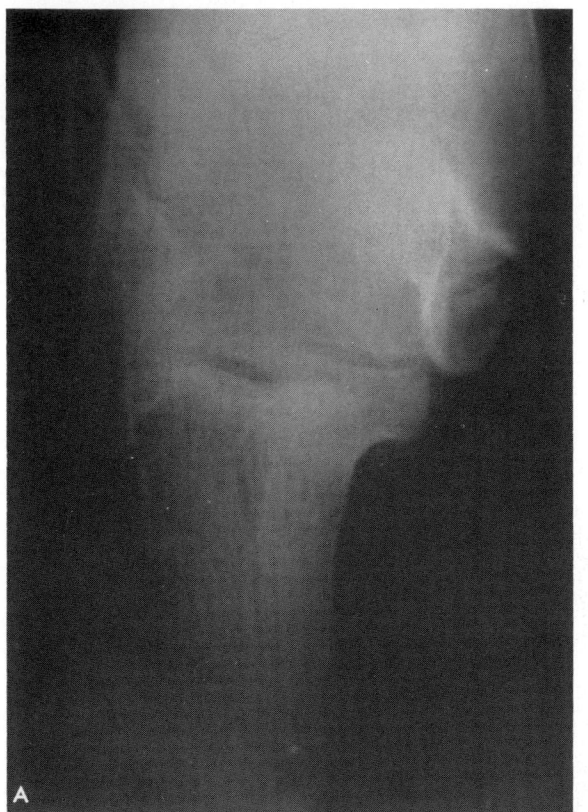

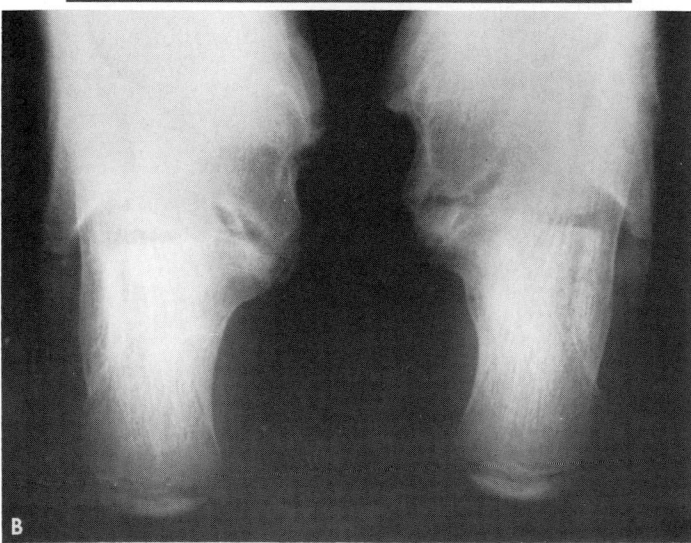

FIGURE 7–41.   Forty-five-degree axial view of the calcaneus for the demonstration of talocalcaneal bridge.

A. Axial view of the talocalcaneal joint in a *normal* foot. (Posterior facet is on the left and the middle facet is on the right of the photograph. Since the two facets are in different compartments, the articular cartilage spaces are not continuous on the roentgenogram.) **B.** Bilateral talocalcaneal coalition in the middle facet is shown in this axial view. (Courtesy of Dr. H. Cowell.)

The middle and anterior facets are located in the anterior compartment, whereas the posterior facet is in the posterior compartment (Fig. 7–42). All three parts of the subtalar joint should be studied to rule out the presence of talocalcaneal coalition. The middle and posterior facet joints usually lie within the same plane of the sustentaculum. In the standing lateral roentgenogram, the angle of the sustentaculum is determined and the axial view of the calcaneus is made at that angle (usually 30, 35, 40, or 45 degrees) (Figs. 7–43 and 7–44). The anterior facet joint is a variable structure; it may be separate and distinct, or may extend from the middle facet; on occasion, it may be absent. The oblique lateral (dorsoplantar) view will often demonstrate the anterior joint. The inner border of the foot is placed on the film, and the sole is tilted 45 degrees to the film. The tube is centered 2.5 cm. distal and 2.5 cm. anterior to the lateral malleolus.[273] Occult coalitions of the anterior and middle joints are best demonstrated by tomography (Figs. 7–45 to 7–47). For a description of tomographic technique for demonstrating the talocalcaneal joint, the reader is referred to Conway and Cowell.[248]

Distortion of movement between the talus above and the calcaneus, cuboid, and navicular below results in secondary degenerative changes visible in the roentgenogram. These vary in intensity, depending upon the type of coalition, whether the intertarsal bridge is complete or incomplete, and the age of the patient. They are best seen in standing lateral roentgenograms of the foot (i.e., the patient is standing, the film is vertical on the medial side of the foot, and the x-ray beam is projected from the lateral side with the rays parallel to the ground).

The most striking secondary change is beaking on the anteroposterior and lateral corner of the head of the talus (Fig. 7–47 B). There are no hypertrophic changes on the navicular. The articular cartilage space is not narrowed and there is no associated subchondral sclerosis or any cystic bony changes. Thus beaking of the talus should be regarded as a response to abnormal mechanics of the subtalar joint, not as a true degenerative arthritic process, though the latter may develop later in untreated cases of long standing.

Other secondary changes in talocalcaneal coalition are a narrowing posterior talocalcaneal facet joint space and broadening of the lateral process of the talus. Ball-and-socket ankle joint may be present.

Talonavicular coalition is readily diagnosed by the evident absence of the talonavicular joint, as seen on the anteroposterior roentgenogram.

Treatment

The method of treatment depends upon the type of coalition, the age of the patient, the severity of deformity, and the degree of disability caused by pain and muscle spasm.

Many patients with tarsal coalition may have little discomfort and will not require treatment. During the growing years, ⅛- to

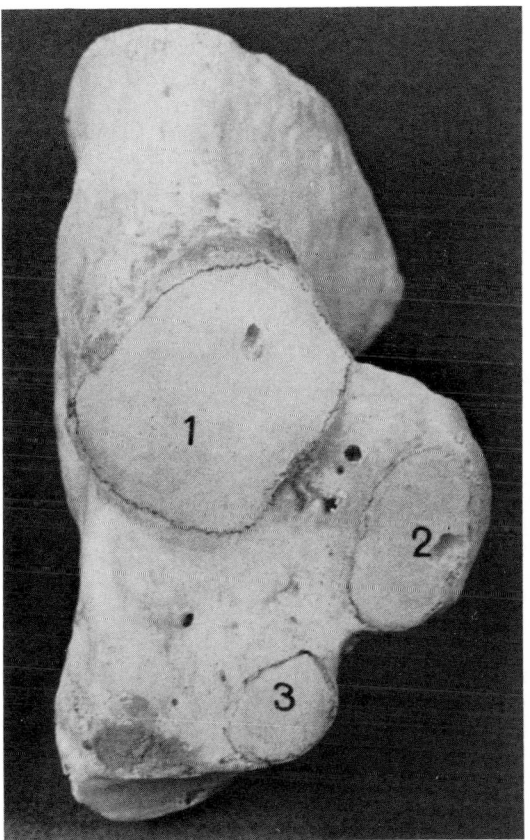

FIGURE 7–42. *The dorsal surface of the calcaneus.*

Note the three facets of the talocalcaneal joint. The posterior facet (1) is on the posterior compartment. The middle facet (2) and the anterior facet (3) are in the anterior compartment. (Courtesy of Dr. H. Cowell.)

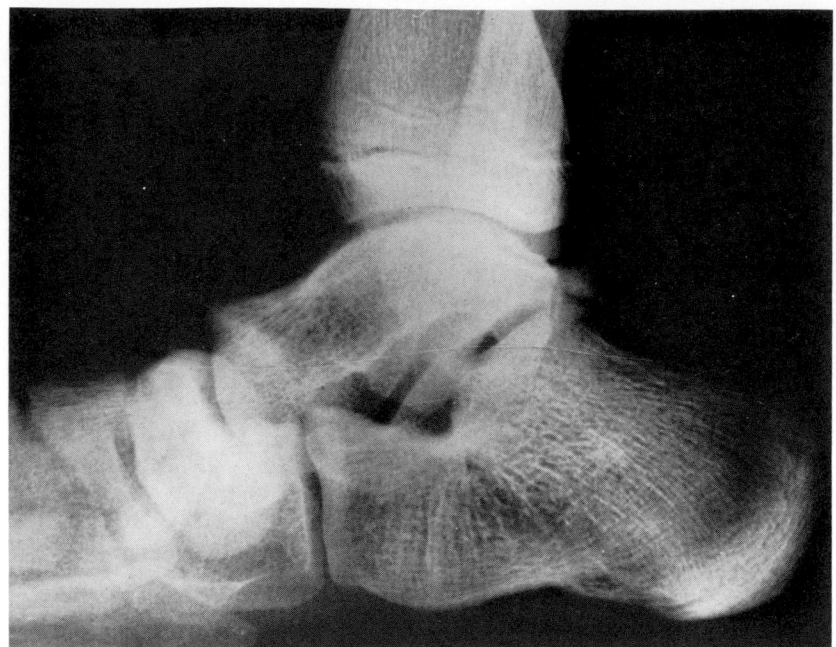

FIGURE 7–43. *The proper angle for the axial view of the talocalcaneal joint is determined in the standing lateral roentgenogram.*

Note in this extreme example the variation in the plane of the posterior and middle facets: an angle of 40 degrees is necessary to visualize the posterior facet and an angle of 55 degrees is required for the middle facet. (Ordinarily the middle and posterior facet joints lie within the same plane of the sustentaculum.) (Courtesy of Dr. H. Cowell.)

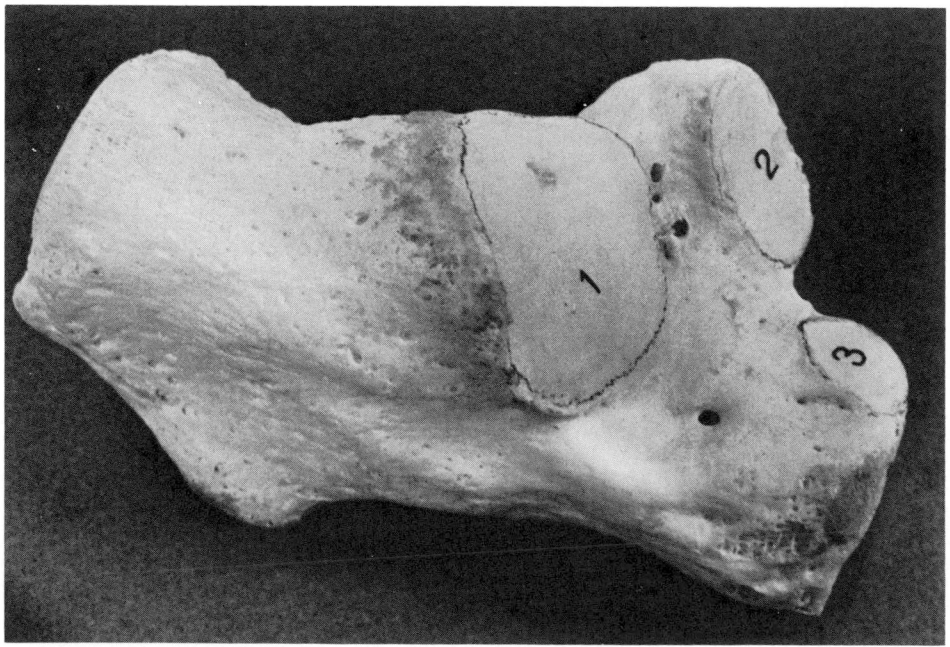

FIGURE 7–44. *Facets of the subtalar joint.*

In this anatomic specimen the posterior and middle facets (1 and 2) are in the same plane and can be easily visualized in the proper axial projection, whereas the anterior facet (3) is in a different plane and usually is obscured by the head of the talus in the axial view. (Courtesy of Dr. H. Cowell.)

1354

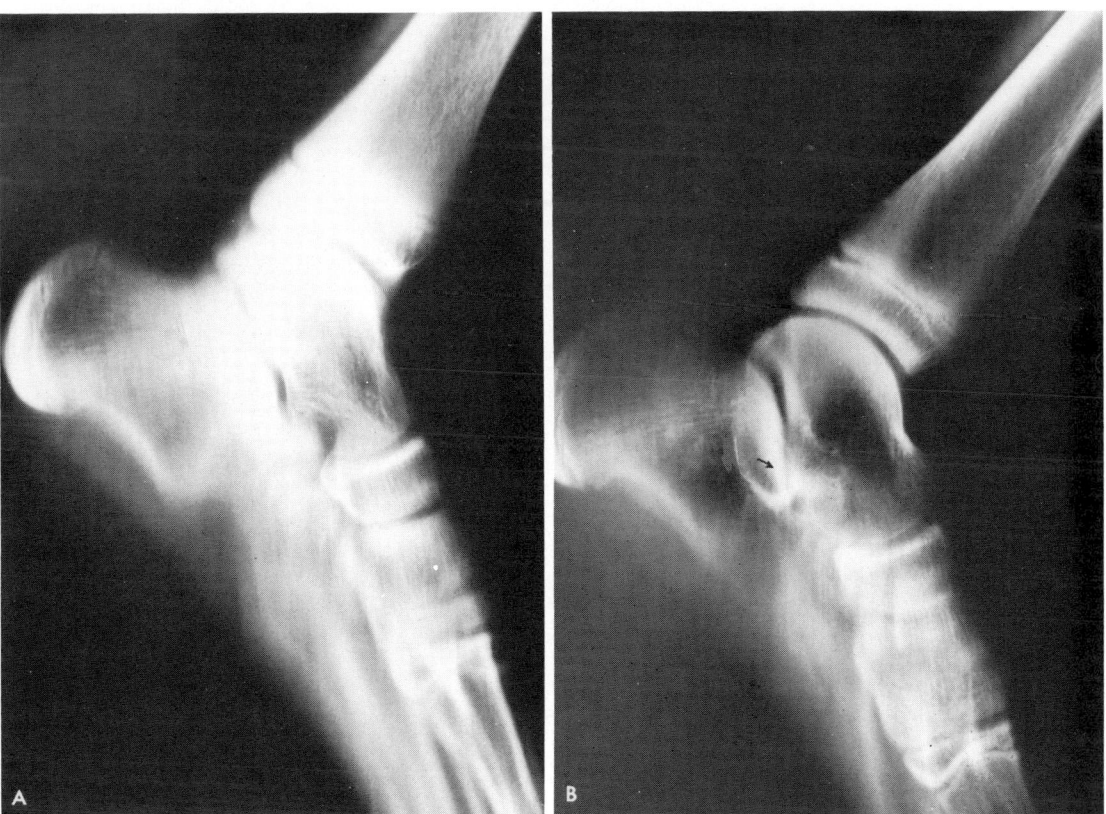

FIGURE 7–45. Tomograms of middle facet of talocalcaneal joint.

A. Normal foot. **B.** Foot with a middle facet coalition. (Courtesy of Dr. H. Cowell.)

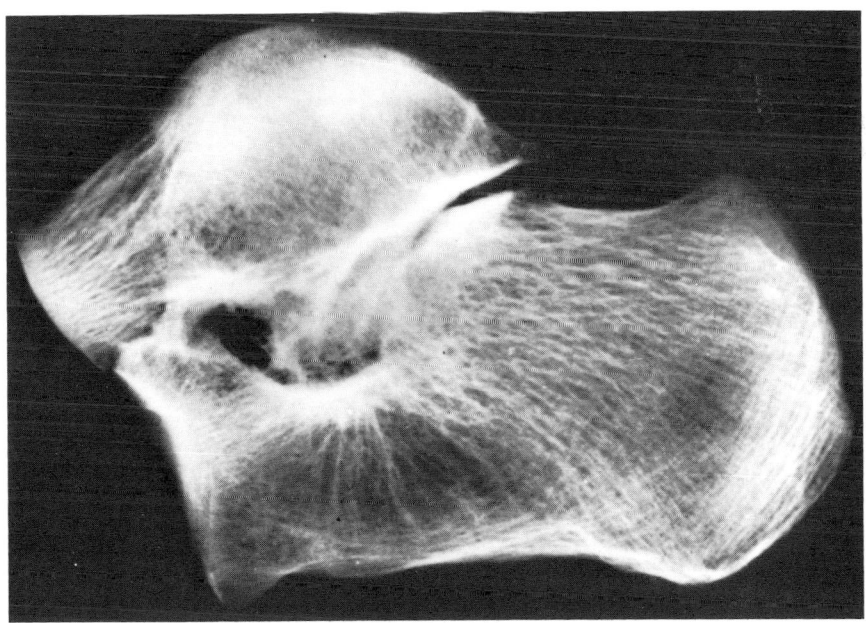

FIGURE 7–46. Roentgenogram of anatomic specimen showing coalition in the region of anterior facet of talocalcaneal joint.

(Courtesy of Dr. H. Cowell.)

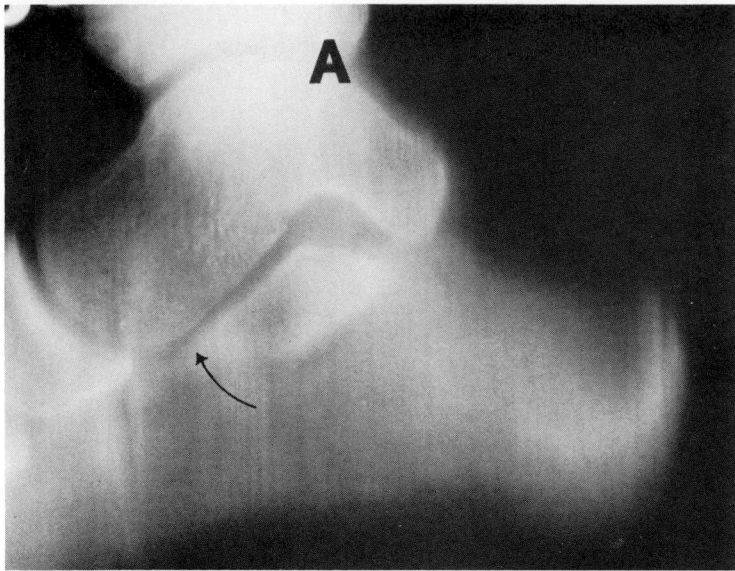

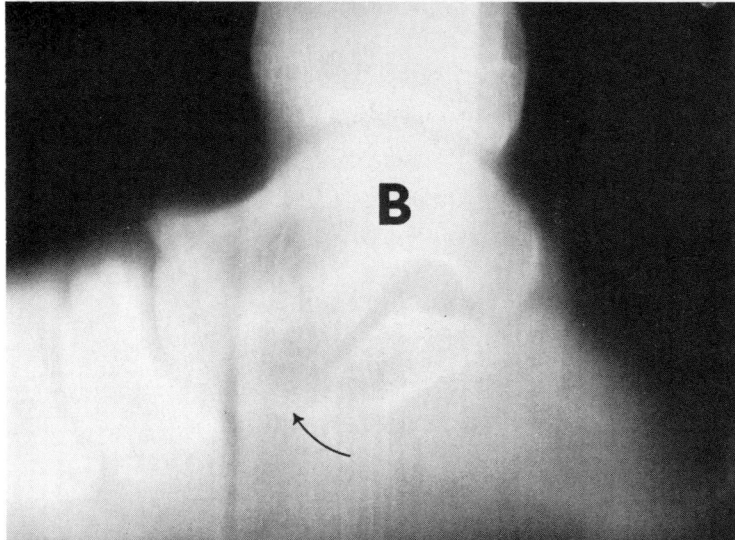

FIGURE 7–47. Tomograms of anterior facet of talocalcaneal joint.

A. Normal foot. **B.** Foot with talocalcaneal coalition. Note the talar beak and the irregularity and haziness of anterior facet indicating coalition. (Courtesy of Dr. H. Cowell.)

³/₁₆-inch inner heel wedges on the shoes and longitudinal arch support to the feet may be given; however, if the valgus deformity is of significant degree, a well-fitted Whitman plate with a lateral flange will prove more effective in diminishing stress on the rigid hindfoot.

If peroneal muscle spasm and pain do develop, more aggressive measures are indicated; initially these should be conservative. Acute symptoms following trauma or unusual stress may be relieved by immobilizing the foot and ankle in a below-knee walking cast for a period of three to four weeks.

It is doubtful whether manipulation of the foot under anesthesia is of any value. The hindfoot should not be forced into inversion while the cast is being applied, as it will be uncomfortable and cause more spasm. Occasionally the author injects hydrocortisone into the sinus tarsi when the peroneal spasm is severe and the foot is painful. Following removal of the cast the foot is supported in a below-knee orthosis (free ankle joint and valgus T-strap) for an additional three months.

Braddock studied the natural history of peroneal spastic flatfoot in 28 patients (15 with bilateral involvement, making a total of 43 feet). These patients (24 males and 4 females) first became symptomatic in adolescence. In 22 of the feet, tarsal coalition was disclosed in the roentgenograms. They were treated with manipulation under anesthesia, a below-knee walking plaster cast, or an orthosis with valgus T-strap. The average period of follow-up was 21 years, the longest being 34 years and the shortest 13 years. About half these patients continued to have minor symptoms for many years, but only 10 per cent were disabled with persistent pain and required operative treatment. An interesting finding in this report was that severe symptoms were more persistent in those patients without apparent tarsal anomalies than in those with obvious bars.[244] Probably more thorough roentgenographic examination including tomography (partic-

ularly of the anterior and middle facets of the talocalcaneal joint) would have disclosed partial or occult coalitions.

When pain and muscle spasm recur and become chronic or when the deformity is severe, surgical treatment is indicated. The operative procedure employed depends upon the type of coalition and the presence or absence of secondary changes in the talonavicular joint.

In *medial talocalcaneal coalition* a medial curvilinear incision is made, beginning at the base of the first cuneiform bone and terminating 2 cm. inferior and posterior to the tip of the medial malleolus. This medial approach, recommended by Harris, provides adequate exposure of the talonavicular and the medial aspect of the subtalar joints (Fig. 7–48). It also permits the surgeon to assess the pathologic anatomy of

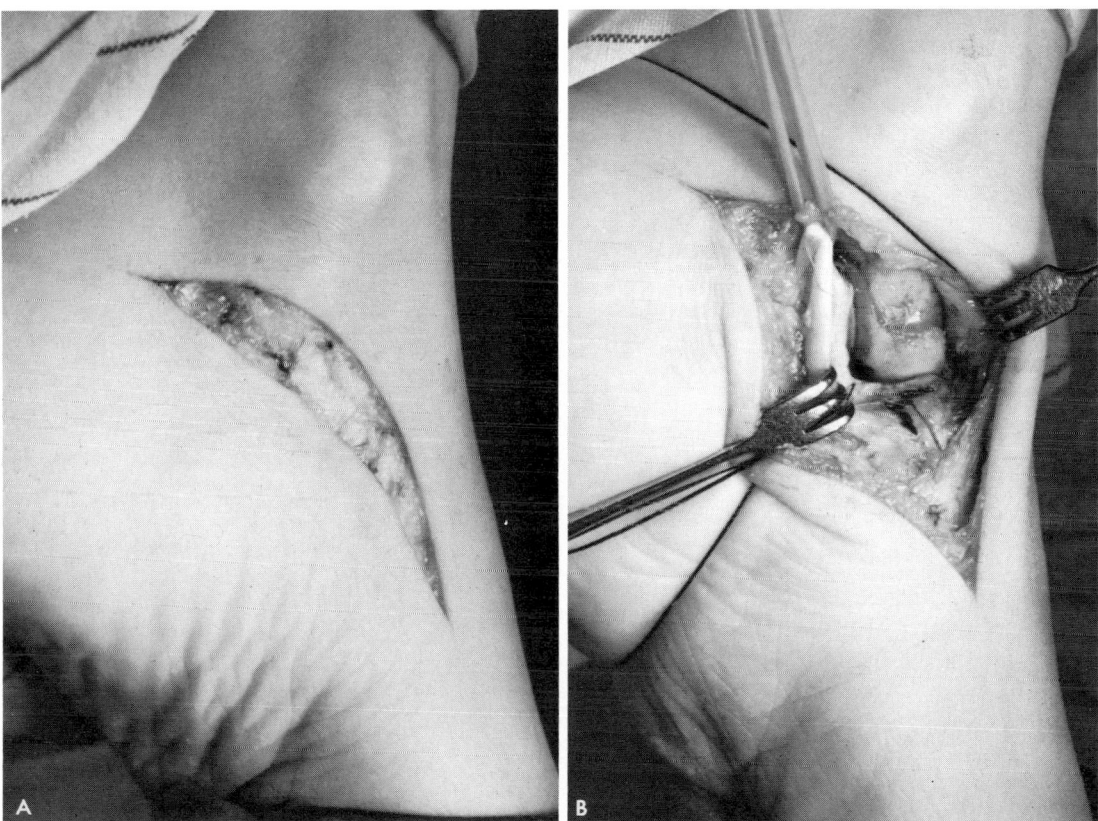

FIGURE 7–48. *Medial approach to subtalar joint.*

A. Skin incision begins at the base of the first cuneiform bone and ends 2 cm. inferior and posterior to the tip of the medial malleolus (the bony prominence in the photograph). **B.** Posterior tibial tendon is elevated and retracted inferiorly and posteriorly, exposing the subtalar joint.

the talocalcaneal coalition, the degree and rigidity of pes valgus, and the changes in the talonavicular joint.

If there is complete union of the medial talocalcaneal articulation and the fixed valgus deformity of the hindfoot is functionally acceptable (i.e., not exceeding 15 degrees), only the talonavicular joint is arthrodesed. It is not necessary to break apart the synostosis of the subtalar joints, nor is stabilization of the calcaneocuboid joint required. Occasionally the large bony mass of the medial talocalcaneal coalition is partially resected, which diminishes its prominence and prevents irritation from the shoe.

If the talocalcaneal coalition is incomplete, the subtalar joint should be stabilized. Harris recommends fusion of only the talocalcaneal and talonavicular joints; the author, however, prefers to include the calcaneocuboid joint in the fusion (i.e., triple arthrodesis). If the pes valgus exceeds 15 degrees, the intertarsal bony bridge is osteotomized and appropriate wedges are resected while triple arthrodesis is performed to provide a normal configuration of the foot. The peroneal muscles usually do not require lengthening, except in an occasional severe long-standing case with marked myostatic contracture. In such an instance, sliding lengthening of the peroneals is performed; i.e., through a separate incision on the lateral aspect of the middle third of the leg, the tendinous fibers are divided at two levels 3 to 4 cm. apart, and the sectioned fibers are slid over the underlying muscles by applying traction distally on the peroneal tendons.

The surgical treatment of the rare anterior and posterior talocalcaneal coalitions follows the same principles as those outlined for the medial one.

Calcaneonavicular bar will require surgical treatment similar to the medial talocalcaneal bridge when persistent pain, muscle spasm, and deformity do not respond to conservative measures. In calcaneonavicular coalition persistent disability is usually somewhat less as compared to talocalcaneal synostosis. There is a choice between two operative procedures, i.e., resection of the calcaneonavicular bar with extensor brevis arthroplasty and triple arthrodesis.

According to Cowell, bar resection and extensor brevis arthroplasty are indicated in a patient under 14 years of age who has pain in the foot, limited subtalar motion, and a cartilaginous bar. It should not be performed in the presence of degenerative changes in the talonavicular joint with accompanying talar beak or when there is an additional coalition between the talus and the calcaneus. Cowell reported the results of the procedure on 26 bars in 15 patients. Twenty-three of the twenty-six feet demonstrated no symptoms following surgery, and the patients were able to resume full activity, including participation in sports. According to Cowell, when proper indications are observed, satisfactory results may be expected in 90 per cent of the patients.[249] The author concurs with Cowell and also excises the calcaneonavicular bar when it is ossified in a patient over 14 years of age, provided there are no talonavicular degenerative changes.

The technique of resection of the calcaneonavicular bar with extensor brevis arthroplasty is as follows:

A lateral Ollier incision is made. The origin of the extensor digitorum brevis is elevated in one block and reflected distally. Following this, the entire bar is resected as a rectangle, not a wedge. Removing a rectangle will provide sufficient free space to prevent re-formation of bone. The articulation between the talus and navicular should not be disturbed. The raw cancellous bleeding bases of the excised bar are coagulated. The entire origin of the extensor digitorum brevis muscle is placed down into the defect with a chromic suture. Two Keith needles are used on each side of the suture; the needles are pulled out on the medial side of the foot, where the suture is tied over a well-padded button or over a rectangular piece of sterile felt. The wound is closed and the foot and ankle are immobilized in a below-knee cast. The chromic sutures will break in approximately three weeks, at which time the suture is completely removed. In about ten days, the cast is bivalved and passive and active exercises are performed to develop inversion and eversion of the hindfoot. Full weight-bearing is not permitted until full active subtalar motion is obtained by the patient. This will usually require eight to ten weeks.

A triple arthrodesis is performed when there are degenerative changes in the talonavicular joint or when excision of the bar fails to relieve the symptoms.

Talonavicular coalition usually does not require treatment, as the condition is asymptomatic. In adult life, naviculocuneiform fusion may be indicated if hypertrophic changes and pain develop. Subtalar and calcaneocuboid fusion is performed in the occasional case associated with painful and persistent peroneal spastic flatfoot.

Treatment of the other rare tarsal coalitions should be individualized.

CONGENITAL CONVEX PES VALGUS

Congenital convex pes valgus is a primary dislocation of the talonavicular joint, in which the navicular articulates with the dorsal aspect of the talus, locking it in a plantar-flexed vertical position. The condition is a teratologic anomaly of unknown etiology, probably developing in utero at some time during the first trimester of pregnancy. The subluxations of the adjacent joints—the subtalar, midtarsal, and ankle—are secondary and adaptive in nature, as are contractures of soft tissues.

The condition was first described by Henken in 1914.[339] The characteristic features of the deformity were reviewed by Lamy and Weissman, who also presented a comprehensive study of the literature up to 1939.[346]

The entity is known by various synonyms. Originally, congenital flatfoot due to vertical talus (pied plat congénital par subluxation sous-astragalienne congénitale et orientation verticale de l'astragale) was the name used by Rocher and Pouyanne.[356] The condition is now commonly referred to as *congenital vertical talus* or simply *vertical talus*—a usage to be discouraged, as it focuses attention upon only one facet of this severe deformity.[355] Congenital "rocker-bottom" flatfoot, "rocker-foot" due to congenital subluxation of the talus, and "rocker-foot" or congenital flatfoot due to talonavicular dislocation are other names given the condition. The term *congenital convex pes valgus* was initially proposed by Lamy and Weissman, and later adopted by Heyman and Herndon in preference to others.[340, 341, 346] Perhaps a more descriptive term that better portrays its pathogenesis and therapeutic implications would be *teratologic dislocation of the talonavicular joint.*

The condition may occur as an isolated primary deformity or it may occur in association with abnormalities of the central nervous and musculoskeletal systems. Sharrard and Grosfield found the incidence of congenital convex pes valgus to be 10 per cent in a large series of patients with myelomeningocele who had foot deformities.[357] Drennan and Sharrard proposed that a neuromuscular imbalance, i.e., a weak posterior tibial muscle and strong evertors of the foot, is responsible for the development of congenital convex pes valgus in myelomeningocele. They also noted the high incidence of abnormalities of the central nervous system in the reported cases of congenital vertical talus, and emphasized the importance of ruling out such associated anomalies prior to accepting the condition as being an isolated primary deformity.[331] Arthrogryposis multiplex congenita, pollex varus, dislocation of the hip, and neurofibromatosis are some of the associated abnormalities of the neuromusculoskeletal system.[336, 348] It may also be one of the numerous anomalies associated with autosomal trisomy, occurring both with trisomy 13–15 and with trisomy 18.[362, 363]

The cause of the primary isolated form is unknown. Heredity may be a factor. Familial incidence in parent and child has been observed by Ascher and Engelmann, and by Lamy and Weissman.[324, 346] Armknecht found congenital convex pes valgus in identical twins.[323]

The incidence of teratologic dislocation of the talonavicular joint is unknown. The deformity is very rare, as judged by the small number of case reports from major children's hospitals. It is more common in males. Involvement may be bilateral or unilateral; in the latter, the opposite foot may have a calcaneovalgus, equinovarus, or metatarsus varus deformity.

Pathologic Anatomy

The gross anatomic and histologic features of congenital convex pes valgus have been described by Patterson, Fitz, and Smith in a six-week-old female who succumbed to congenital heart disease, and by Drennan and Sharrard, who reported the findings in an 11-hour-old girl with myelomeningocele who died of cardiac arrest following spinal osteotomy.[331, 355] In the case of Patterson et al., the spinal cord was not examined. Observations at surgery have also contributed to our knowledge of its pathologic anatomy. The anatomic abnormalities may be subdivided into those of the bones and joints, of the ligaments, and of the muscles and tendons.

BONE AND JOINT CHANGES

The navicular will be found articulating with the dorsal aspect of the neck of the talus, locking it in a vertical position (Fig. 7–49). The proximal articular surface of the navicular is tilted plantarward. The head of the talus develops an abnormal shape, and is flattened superiorly, somewhat pointed, and oval rather than spherical. The neck of the talus is hypoplastic, and may have an abnormal facet on its dorsal surface that articulates with the navicular. The calcaneus is displaced posterolaterally in relation to the talus and is tilted into equinus posture. The anterior part of the calcaneus is deviated laterally and the talocalcaneal angle (formed by the longitudinal axes of the talus and the calcaneus) is abnormally increased. The sustentaculum tali is blunted, offering no support to the head of the talus. The calcaneus may be convex on its plantar aspect. There are abnormalities in the facets of the subtalar joint; the anterior articular facet is absent, the middle one is hypoplastic, and the posterior one is misshapen and has an increased lateral tilt. These changes are most

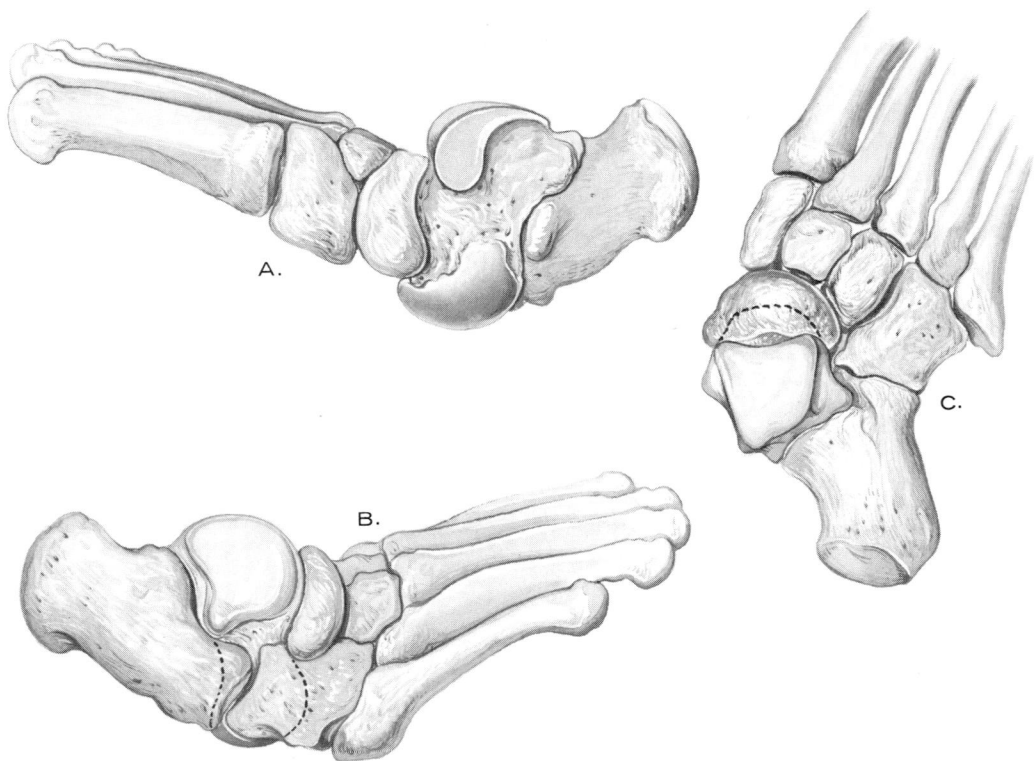

FIGURE 7–49. *Bone and joint changes in congenital convex pes valgus.*

A. Medial aspect of right foot showing dorsiflexion of forefoot at midtarsal joint; vertical talus producing a rocker-bottom convexity; subluxation of the navicular upon the neck of the talus, locking talus vertically; calcaneus 20 to 25 degrees equinus. **B.** Lateral aspect of right foot. Dotted lines indicate displaced head of talus. **C.** Dorsal aspect showing abducted forefoot beginning at midtarsus. Dotted lines indicate head of talus subluxated below navicular bone. (From Tachdjian, M. O.: Congenital convex pes valgus. Orthop. Clin. N. Amer., *3*:133, 1972.)

probably produced by the lack of contact between the normally congruent surfaces of the talus and calcaneus. There may be a varying degree of dorsolateral subluxation of the calcaneocuboid joint. The normal anatomic relationship of the navicular and cuboid with the cuneiform and the metatarsals is not disturbed.

LIGAMENTOUS CHANGES

As shown in Figure 7–50 A and B, the tibionavicular ligament (which is a part of the anterior portion of the deltoid ligament) and the dorsal talonavicular ligament are markedly contracted and present a major obstacle to successful reduction. The calcaneocuboid ligament is shortened, causing the forefoot to be held in abduction. Contracture of the interosseous talocalcaneal and calcaneofibular ligaments takes place, preventing reduction of the posterolaterally subluxated os calcis. In untreated cases, the posterior capsule of the ankle and subtalar joints is also shortened.

The plantar calcaneonavicular ligament or spring ligament is stretched and moderately attenuated.

MUSCLE AND TENDON ABNORMALITIES

The anterior tibial, extensor hallucis longus, extensor digitorum longus, peroneus brevis, and triceps surae muscles are contracted. The posterior tibial and peroneal tendons are usually anteriorly displaced, lying in grooves on the malleoli and acting as dorsiflexors rather than plantar flexors. In severe cases, they may "bowstring" across the ankle joint (Fig. 7–50 C). Patterson et al. found these muscles to be grossly and histologically normal, and proposed their contracture to be secondary to length deficit.[355] Drennan and Sharrard reported moderate atrophy of the posterior tibial and quadratus plantae muscles and hypertrophy of the extensor digitorum longus muscle; it should be remembered, however, that their anatomic specimen was that of a myelomeningocele child.[331] In an arthrogrypotic child with congenital convex pes valgus, the author has observed fibrosis of the anterior tibial, long toe extensor, and peroneal muscles.

Clinical Features

The rigid deformity of the foot is present at birth and is so distinct that the condition can be diagnosed at that time. The sole of the foot is convex and has a rocker-bottom appearance (Fig. 7–51). The head of the talus is markedly prominent on the medial and plantar aspects of the foot. The forefoot is abducted and dorsiflexed at the midtarsal joint. The long toe extensors, anterior tibial, and peroneal muscles are markedly shortened. The calcaneovalgus deformity of the forefoot is fixed; the taut muscles and the contracted tibionavicular and talonavicular ligaments resist plantar flexion and inversion of the forefoot. The hindfoot is equinovalgus; the triceps surae muscle is contracted and the calcaneus is everted and tilted downward in plantar flexion. The dislocated navicular may be palpable on the dorsum of the neck of the talus. Deep creases appear on the dorsolateral aspect of the foot near the ankle joint.

Walking is usually not delayed. The older child stands with the involved hindfoot markedly valgus and the posterior end of the heel not touching the floor. The forefoot is abducted and most of the body weight is borne on the head of the talus. The deformed foot is so rigid that its appearance remains the same, whether or not weight is being borne on it. The gait is awkward, clumsy, and almost peglike. The shoes rapidly become distorted, with the medial part of the heel and the upper part over the longitudinal arch wearing down within a few weeks. Pain is not a symptom in childhood; it usually becomes a complaint in later adolescence.

Roentgenographic Findings

The roentgenographic findings are characteristic, even in the newborn. The talus is vertical, lying parallel with the longitudinal axis of the tibia, and the calcaneus is in equinus position, whereas the forepart of the foot is dorsiflexed and deviated laterally at the midtarsal level. The outline of the soft tissues of the sole of the foot is convex. The talocalcaneal angle is abnormally increased.

To make a definitive diagnosis of congenital convex pes valgus, it is imperative to

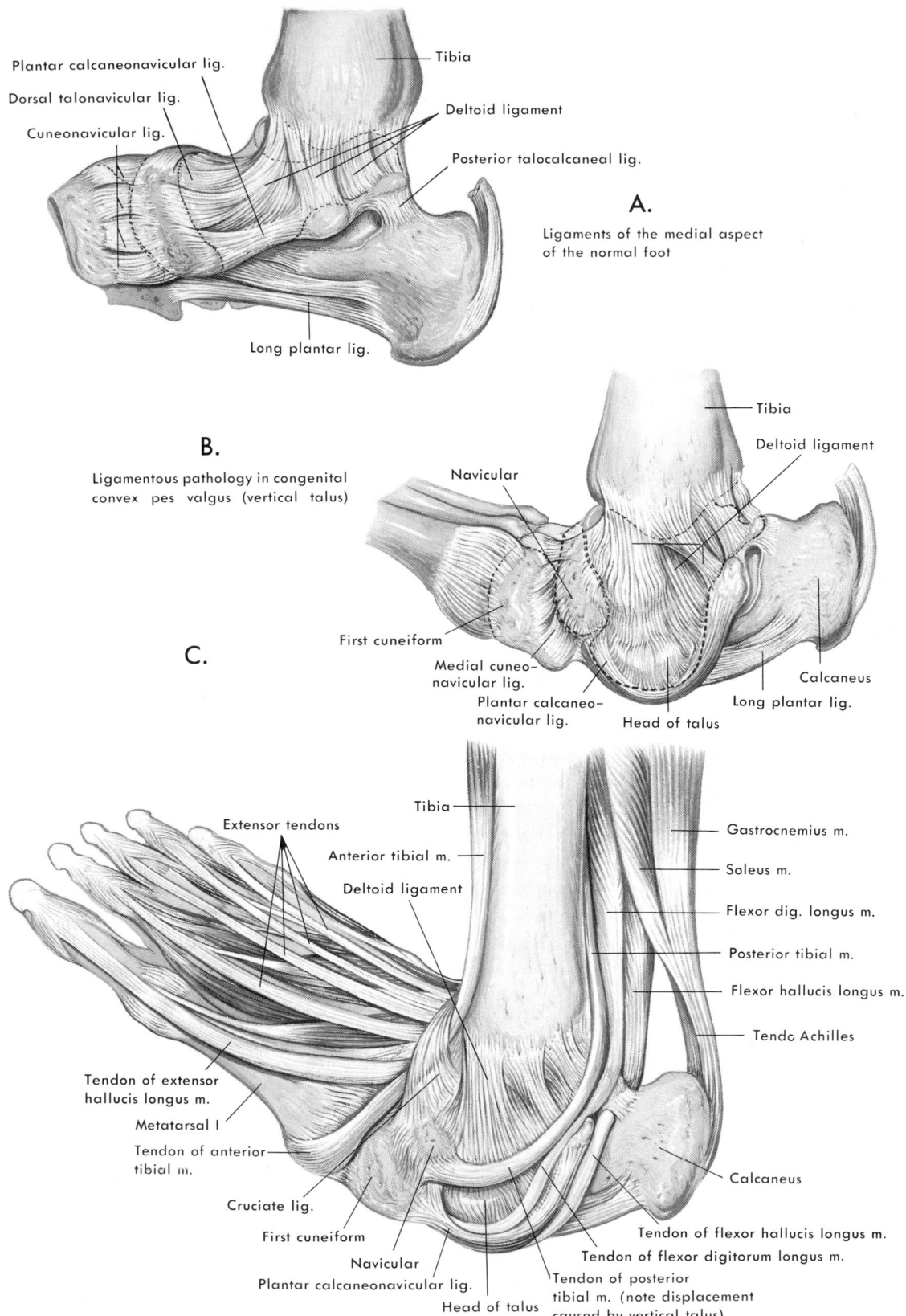

A.

Ligaments of the medial aspect of the normal foot

Plantar calcaneonavicular lig.
Dorsal talonavicular lig.
Cuneonavicular lig.
Tibia
Deltoid ligament
Posterior talocalcaneal lig.
Long plantar lig.

B.

Ligamentous pathology in congenital convex pes valgus (vertical talus)

Navicular
Tibia
Deltoid ligament
First cuneiform
Medial cuneo-navicular lig.
Plantar calcaneo-navicular lig.
Head of talus
Calcaneus
Long plantar lig.

C.

Extensor tendons
Tibia
Anterior tibial m.
Deltoid ligament
Gastrocnemius m.
Soleus m.
Flexor dig. longus m.
Posterior tibial m.
Flexor hallucis longus m.
Tendo Achilles
Tendon of extensor hallucis longus m.
Metatarsal I
Tendon of anterior tibial m.
Cruciate lig.
First cuneiform
Navicular
Plantar calcaneonavicular lig.
Head of talus
Tendon of posterior tibial m. (note displacement caused by vertical talus)
Tendon of flexor digitorum longus m.
Tendon of flexor hallucis longus m.
Calcaneus

FIGURE 7–50. Soft-tissue pathology in congenital convex pes valgus. See opposite page for legend.

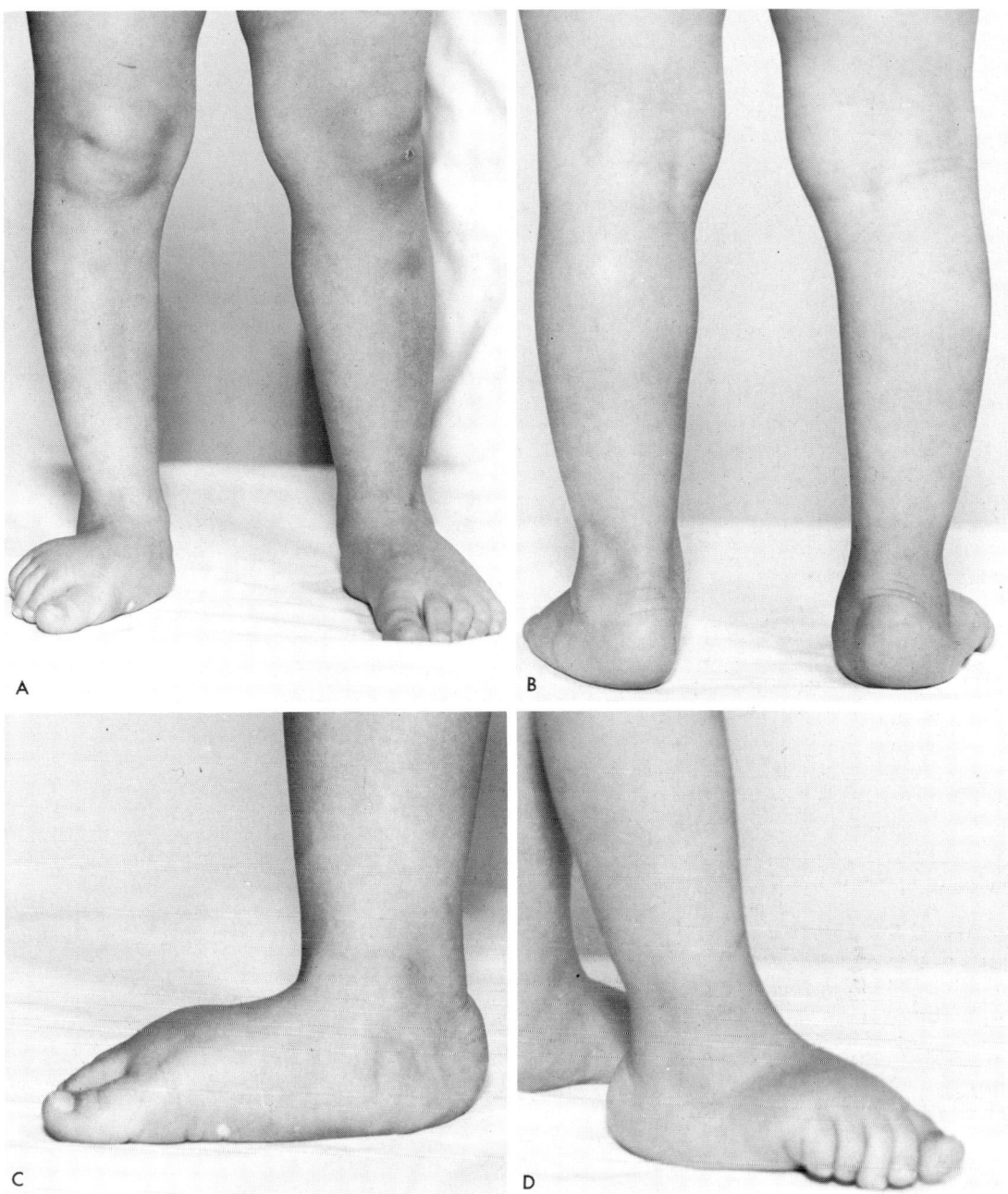

FIGURE 7–51. *Congenital convex pes valgus on the right in a two-year-old girl.*

A to **D.** Clinical appearance of the deformity.

FIGURE 7–50. *Soft-tissue pathology in congenital convex pes valgus.*

A. Ligaments of the medial aspect of the normal foot. **B.** Pathologic changes in ligaments in congenital convex pes valgus. **C.** Abnormalities of the muscles and tendons. (From Tachdjian, M. O.: Congenital convex pes valgus. Orthop. Clin. N. Amer., *3*:134, 1972.)

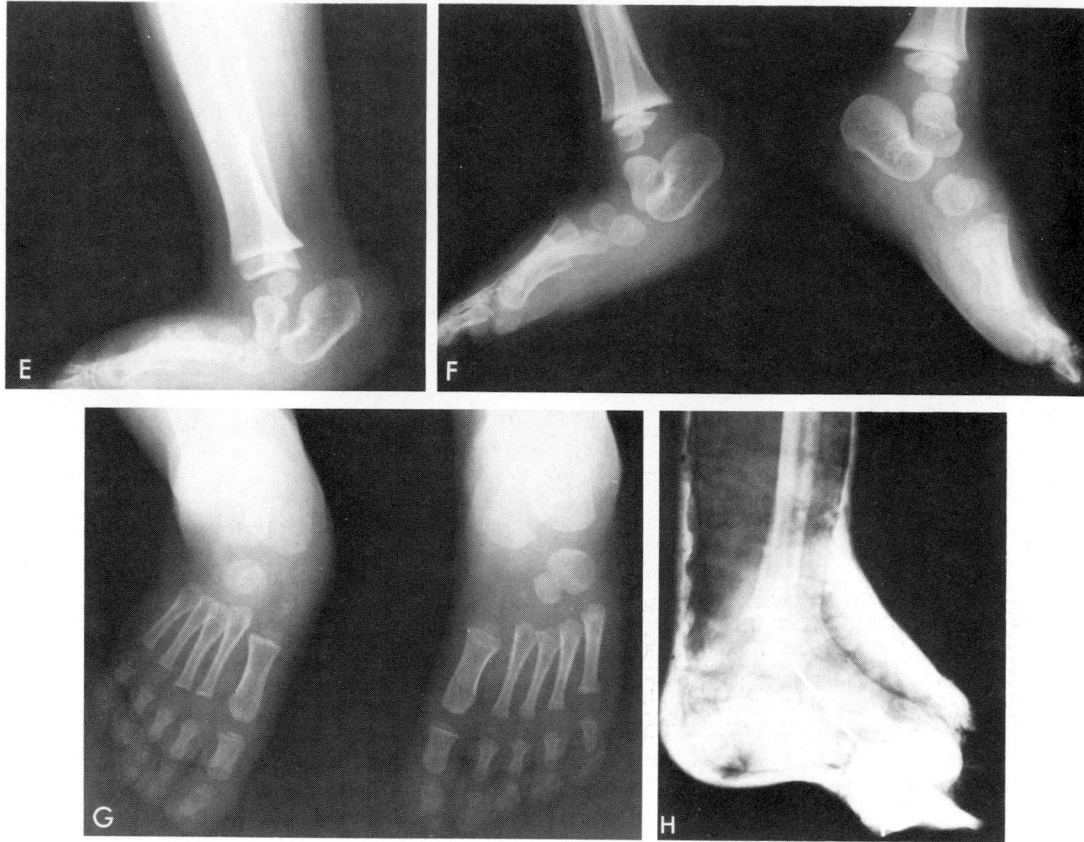

FIGURE 7–51 Continued.   *Congenital convex pes valgus on the right in a two-year-old girl.*

E to H. Roentgenographic appearance. **E** is standing. lateral view; **F** is lateral view with both feet in extreme plantar flexion; **G** is standing anteroposterior roentgenogram. In **E** note the vertical position of the talus, almost parallel with the longitudinal axis of the tibia. The calcaneus is in equinus position. The navicular is not visualized (since it is cartilaginous) but its location can be determined because it is normally situated between the ossified medial cuneiform and the head of the talus. In **F** it is shown that when the foot is maintained in marked plantar flexion the navicular is still dislocated dorsally on the neck of the talus. In **G** the lateral subluxation of the forefoot and the abnormal increase of the talocalcaneal angle is demonstrated. **H** is a lateral roentgenogram of the foot and ankle, made with the cast on. Open reduction and capsular repair as described in Plate 56 was performed two days before.

demonstrate that the navicular is dislocated dorsally on the neck of the talus when the foot is maintained in extreme plantar flexion. The ossific center of the navicular does not appear until three years of age; hence, it cannot be seen in the roentgenogram; but its location can be determined, as it is normally situated between the ossified medial cuneiform and the head of the talus (Fig. 7–51 E to G). At the age of three years, the navicular ossifies and its complete dislocation over the dorsal surface of the neck of the talus is clearly visible.

In paralytic pes valgus and severely pro-

nated feet, the talus may be tilted into vertical position (particularly if there is contracture of the triceps surae) and the navicular will sag on the head of the talus, suggesting subluxation of the talonavicular joint. On close scrutiny, however, it is evident that there is definite contact between the articular surfaces of the navicular and the head of the talus. In congenital convex pes valgus, the navicular bone may be irregularly ossified, suggesting Köhler's disease. With increasing age, the navicular becomes wedge-shaped toward its plantar surface. The calcaneus gradually develops a

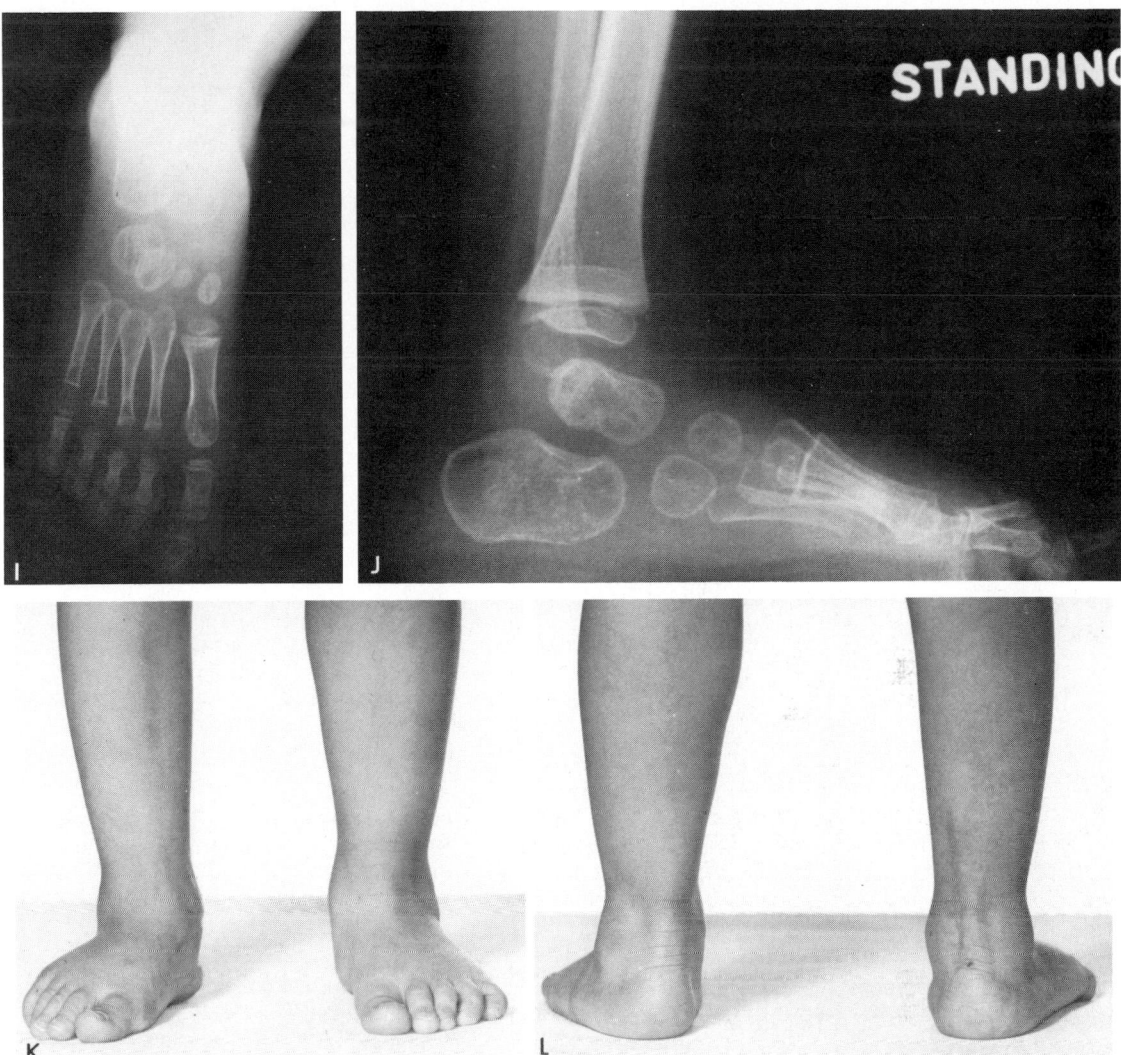

FIGURE 7–51 Continued. *Congenital convex pes valgus on the right in a two-year-old girl.*

I and **J.** Postoperative standing roentgenograms made 12 months later. **K** and **L.** Clinical appearance showing normal alignment of the foot.

convexity on its plantar aspect with upward tilting of its anterior end that gives it a beak-shaped appearance. With dorsal and lateral displacement of the forepart of the foot, dorsolateral subluxation of the calcaneocuboid joint is evident. The first metatarsal is dorsiflexed and the hallux is plantar-flexed at the metatarsophalangeal joint, compensating for the elevated first metatarsal bone.

The talus is underdeveloped, particularly at its waist, resembling an hourglass. In the lateral projection it will be seen that only the posterior portion of the superior surface of the talus is contained in the tibiofibular mortise.

Differential Diagnosis

In early infancy, congenital convex pes valgus is commonly mistaken for talipes calcaneovalgus. In both conditions, the forepart of the foot is dorsiflexed and everted, and there is limitation of plantar flexion and inversion. The heel in congenital convex pes valgus is in equinus position, the sole of the foot convex, and the deformity very rigid, whereas in talipes calcaneovalgus, the os calcis and talus are in dorsiflexion, and the deformity is quite flexible and responds rapidly to stretching exercises and treatment with corrective casts.

The presence of pes valgus with myostatic contracture of the triceps surae muscle may present a problem in differential diagnosis. In stance, the heel is equinovalgus and the talus is plantar-flexed with its head prominent on the medial and plantar aspects of the midfoot; however, the deformity is not rigid and when not bearing weight, the heel can be manipulated into neutral position and the head of the talus into dorsiflexion, giving a normal longitudinal arch to the foot. In congenital convex pes valgus, the deformity is fixed and does not improve on non-weight-bearing. Roentgenograms made with the foot in plantar flexion will establish the diagnosis.

Paralytic pes valgus due to cerebral palsy, myelomeningocele, or poliomyelitis should not be difficult to distinguish from congenital convex pes valgus. The clinical appearance of peroneal spastic flatfoot due to tarsal coalition may resemble congenital vertical talus; however, the roentgenographic findings are distinctive. An accessory navicular produces a prominence on the medial aspect of the foot, which is in a valgus position. Again, roentgenograms should settle the diagnosis.

Treatment

The objectives of therapy are to place the navicular and calcaneus in a normal anatomic relationship to the talus and to maintain the reduction by capsular and soft-tissue repair.

The method of treatment depends upon the age of the patient and the degree and severity of the deformity. A number of methods and techniques of treatment that have been proposed by various authors in the literature are summarized in Table 7–5. The principles of management of congenital dislocation of the hip might well be applied to teratologic dislocation of the talonavicular joint. These include:

Table 7–5. *Methods of Treatment of Congenital Convex Pes Valgus*

Procedures on Talus

Excision of head and neck of talus (Lange, 1912; Nové-Joseiand, 1923)

Curettage of talus with excision of its cuneiform portion (Camera, 1926)

Complete astragalectomy (Lamy and Weissman, 1939)

Open-up wedge osteotomy of neck of talus with insertion of bone graft on its plantar aspect (Hughes, 1957)

Procedures on Navicular

Excision of navicular (Stone, 1963)

Excision of dorsal wedge from navicular and placement of the wedge under elevated head of talus combined with open reduction, reefing of spring ligament, and shortening of posterior tibial tendon (Eyre-Brook, 1967)

Procedures on Talonavicular Joint

Open reduction with or without lengthening of Achilles tendon and release of shortened musculotendinous units, ligaments, and capsules on dorsolateral aspect of foot

Reduction maintained with plaster cast (Rocher and Pouyanne, 1934)

Reduction maintained with Kirschner wire across talonavicular joint (Hark, 1950; Heyman, 1959; Herndon and Heyman, 1963)

Reduction maintained with transfer of peroneus brevis tendon to neck of talus (Osmond-Clarke, 1956)

Reduction maintained with scarification of talonavicular joint with or without Kirschner wire through navicular into head of talus (Hughes, 1957)

Reduction maintained with reefing of capsule and rerouting of anterior tibial tendon under neck of talus and fixing to navicular (Grice, 1959)

Reduction maintained with subtalar arthrodesis (Grice, 1959; Coleman et al., 1966)

Reduction maintained with plication of calcaneonavicular ligament and reattaching of posterior tibial tendon with shortening (Eyre-Brook, 1967; Harrold, 1967; Støren, 1967)

Release of capsule of calcaneocuboid joint on its dorsolateral aspect (Coleman et al., 1966)

Closed reduction in young infant (under 3 mo. of age) following elongation of shortened soft tissues by serial stretching casts (Harrold, 1967; Støren, 1967)

Reconstructive or Stabilization Procedures on Tarsus

Triple arthrodesis (Hark, 1950; Lloyd-Roberts, 1958; and others)

Wedge tarsectomy (Lloyd-Roberts, 1958)

EARLY DIAGNOSIS AND IMMEDIATE TREATMENT

The condition may be diagnosed at birth by the characteristic rocker-bottom convex shape of the foot, the rigidity of the deformity, and its distinctive roentgenographic features. Treatment should begin at birth. Any delay in diagnosis will lead to a crippling deformity of the foot. The older the patient at the time treatment is initiated, the more rigid will be the ligamentous, capsular, and soft-tissue contractures and the greater the structural osseous changes. The pediatrician should examine the feet of every newborn infant in his practice for early recognition of this teratologic anomaly.

CORRECTION OF SOFT-TISSUE CONTRACTURE

In the infant, a preliminary period of manipulation and corrective casts are indicated to stretch the contracture of the skin and of soft tissues, which constitutes an extra-articular obstacle to closed reduction. First, the forefoot is gently but firmly manipulated, stretching it downward into plantar flexion, inversion, and adduction. The heel cord is then stretched by pulling the os calcis distally and inward with one hand while pushing the anterior end of the calcaneus (not the cuboid) into dorsiflexion with the other. This corrected position is maintained to the count of 10 and then released. The manipulations are performed for 15 minutes. The skin is painted with a nonirritating adhesive liquid such as tincture of benzoin to prevent slipping of the cast, and the limb is immobilized in a long leg cast with the foot and ankle in the corrected position—the forepart of the foot in equinus position and inversion and the heel well molded in the degree of dorsiflexion obtained by passive manipulation. During application of the cast on the foot, thumb pressure is applied on the anterior end of the os calcis. The successive plaster casts are changed at seven-day intervals; each time the foot is gently manipulated for 15 minutes to further stretch the soft-tissue contracture.

CLOSED REDUCTION

Following diagnosis of the condition at birth and stretching of the soft-tissue contractures by serial plaster of Paris casts over a period of six to eight weeks, closed reduction of the talonavicular dislocation should be attempted. This is performed by manipulating the forepart of the foot into equinovarus position with the hindfoot in plantar flexion and inversion. Restoration of the normal articular relationship of the navicular with the head of the talus should be verified by roentgenographic examination. As previously stated, the navicular is not ossified in infancy, and the anatomic relationship of the talonavicular articulation is difficult to establish. The exact location of the cartilaginous navicular between the ossified medial cuneiform and the head of the talus is determined. Arthrography of the talonavicular articulation may be attempted in borderline or doubtful cases.

Occasionally, closed reduction of teratologic dislocation of the talonavicular joint is successful.[337, 360, 361] In such an instance, the author recommends maintenance of reduction by "blind" pinning of the talonavicular joint. Image intensifier roentgenographic control will make the procedure a simple one. A heavy Kirschner wire is inserted in the web interspace between the great and second toes, and is then drilled proximally across the talonavicular joint, holding the forefoot in marked plantar flexion and inversion. Initially, the hindfoot and ankle joint are immobilized in plantar flexion. After two to three weeks, the cast is changed and the foot is brought into increasing dorsiflexion. Immobilization in the cast should be continued for at least three months.

OPEN REDUCTION

If closed reduction proves unsuccessful, open reduction should be performed at three months of age. First, a sliding lengthening of the tendo Achillis is performed. The distal transverse incision in the tendon is made laterally, as the heel is valgus. The calcaneofibular ligament should be sectioned to permit inversion of the os calcis. If necessary, posterior capsulotomy of the ankle and subtalar joints is performed. Next, roentgenograms of the ankle and foot are taken to ensure that the equinus deformity of the hindfoot is fully corrected, the importance of which cannot be overemphasized. The operative technique recommended by the author is described and illustrated in Plate 56.

TREATMENT IN AGE RANGE OF FOUR TO SIX YEARS

Corrective casts are applied as a preliminary measure to stretch the shortened extensor tendons and skin on the dorsum of the foot. Soft-tissue contracture, however, is

(*Text continued on page 1372.*)

Open Reduction of Congenital Convex Pes Valgus

THE PROCEDURE

A. The skin incision begins at a point 2 cm. posterior and 1 cm. distal to the tip of the medial malleolus and extends distally to the base of the first metatarsal. The subcutaneous tissue is divided. The skin margins are mobilized and retracted to expose the dorsal, medial, and plantar aspects of the tarsus.

B and **C.** The posterior tibial tendon is identified, dissected, and divided at its insertion to the tuberosity of the navicular. The end of the tendon is marked with 0 silk suture for later reattachment. The articular surface of the head of the talus points steeply downward and medially to the sole of the foot and is covered by the capsule and ligament. The navicular will be found against the dorsal aspect of the neck of the talus, locking it in vertical position. The pathologic anatomy of the ligaments and capsule is noted and the incisions planned so that a secure capsuloplasty can be performed and the talus maintained in its normal anatomic position. Circulation to the talus is another important consideration; it should be disturbed as little as possible by exercising great care and gentleness during dissection.[335] Avascular necrosis of the talus is always a potential serious complication of open reduction. The plantar calcaneonavicular ligament is identified and divided proximally from its attachment to the sustentaculum tali and a 0 silk suture is inserted in its end for later reattachment. The talonavicular articulation is exposed by a T-incision. The transverse limb of the T is made distally over the tibionavicular ligament (the anterior portion of the deltoid ligament) and over the dorsal and medial portions of the talonavicular ligament. A cuff of capsule is left attached to the navicular for plication on completion of surgery. The longitudinal limb of the incision is made over the head and neck of the talus inferiorly.

The articular surface of the head of the talus is identified and a large Kirschner wire inserted in its center. With the help of a skid and the leverage of the Kirschner wire, the head and neck of the talus are lifted dorsally and the forefoot is manipulated in plantar flexion and inversion, bringing the articular surfaces of the navicular and head of the talus into normal anatomic position.

Plate 56. *Open Reduction of Congenital Convex Pes Valgus*

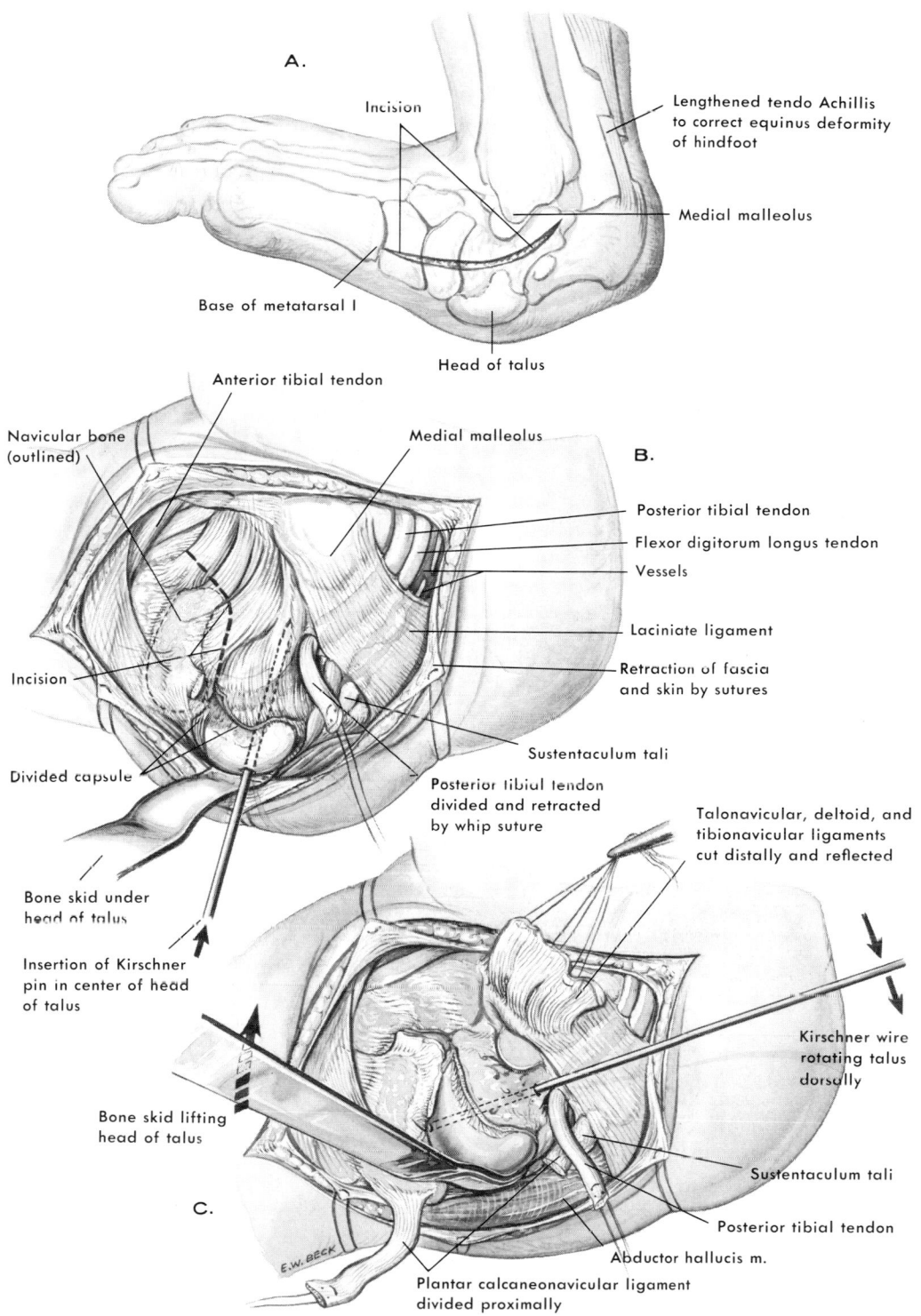

A.

Incision

Lengthened tendo Achillis
to correct equinus deformity
of hindfoot

Medial malleolus

Base of metatarsal I

Head of talus

Anterior tibial tendon

Navicular bone
(outlined)

Medial malleolus

B.

Posterior tibial tendon

Flexor digitorum longus tendon

Vessels

Laciniate ligament

Incision

Retraction of fascia
and skin by sutures

Divided capsule

Sustentaculum tali

Posterior tibial tendon
divided and retracted
by whip suture

Talonavicular, deltoid, and
tibionavicular ligaments
cut distally and reflected

Bone skid under
head of talus

Insertion of Kirschner
pin in center of head
of talus

Kirschner wire
rotating talus
dorsally

Bone skid lifting
head of talus

Sustentaculum tali

Posterior tibial tendon

Abductor hallucis m.

C.

Plantar calcaneonavicular ligament
divided proximally

E.W. BECK

A

(From Tachdjian, M. O.: Congenital convex pes valgus. Orthop. Clin. N. Amer., *3*:142, 1972.)

Open Reduction of Congenital Convex Pes Valgus (Continued)

D. The Kirschner wire is drilled retrograde into the navicular, cuneiform, and first metatarsal bones, maintaining the reduction. Roentgenograms of the foot are taken at this time to verify the reduction.

In the older child the calcaneocuboid and talocalcaneal interosseous ligaments may prevent reduction of the laterally subluxated Chopart's and subtalar joints. If necessary, they are divided through a separate anterolateral incision. The anterior tibial, extensor hallucis longus, extensor digitorum longus, and peroneal muscles may also be so shortened that they prevent reduction; if so, they are lengthened. The author prefers fractional lengthening of these muscles through a separate longitudinal incision over the anterior tibial compartment. Others prefer to lengthen them by a Z-plasty over the dorsum of the foot.[329, 330]

E and **F.** A careful capsuloplasty is very important for maintaining the reduction and the normal anatomic relationship of the talus and navicular. The redundant inferior part of the capsule should be tightened by plication and overlapping of its free edges. First, the plantar-proximal segment of the "T" of the capsule is pulled dorsally and distally and sutured to the dorsal corner of the inner surface of the distal capsule. Next, the dorsoproximal segment of the "T" is brought plantarward and distally over the plantar-proximal segment of the capsule and sutured to the plantar corner on the inner surface of the distal capsule. Then, by interrupted sutures, the capsule is tightened on its plantar and medial aspects by bringing the distal segment over the proximal segments.

The plantar calcaneonavicular ligament is sutured under tension to the sustentaculum tali. The posterior tibial tendon is tightened under the head of the talus by advancing it distally and suturing it to the inferior surface of the first cuneiform bone.

The anterior tibial may be transferred to provide additional dynamic force for maintaining the navicular in correct relationship to the talus.[333] The tendon is detached from its insertion to the medial cuneiform and first metatarsal bone, and dissected free proximally and medially for a distance of 5 cm. Then it is redirected to pass along the medial aspect of the neck of the talus and beneath the head of the talus, where it is fixed to the inferior aspects of the talus and navicular with silk sutures. Normally the lower end of the anterior tibial tendon may be split near its insertion. Often the author leaves intact the attachment to the first metatarsal, dividing only the insertion to the medial cuneiform. The tendon is split (if not normally bifurcated) and the portion to the medial cuneiform bone is transferred to the head of the talus and navicular. Frequently, following adequate capsuloplasty, the reduction of the talonavicular joint is so stable that anterior tibial transfer is not necessary to restore support to the head of the talus.

G. The wounds are then closed with interrupted sutures. The Kirschner wire across the talonavicular joint is cut subcutaneously. To maintain the normal anatomic relationship of the os calcis to the talus, a Kirschner wire is inserted transversely in the os calcis and incorporated into the cast. An alternate method is to pass the wire from the sole of the foot upward through the calcaneus into the talus. The author prefers the former, as it controls the heel in the cast and prevents recurrence of both equinus deformity and eversion of the hindfoot. A long leg cast is applied, with the knee in 45 degrees of flexion, the ankle in 10 to 15 degrees of dorsiflexion, the heel in 10 degrees of inversion, and the forefoot in plantar flexion and inversion. The longitudinal arch and the heel in the cast are well molded.

POSTOPERATIVE CARE

The Kirschner wires are removed in six weeks, but the foot and ankle are immobilized in a solid above-knee cast for a total period of 12 weeks. Then a below-knee walking cast is applied (with the walking heel placed posteriorly to prevent stretching of the triceps surae muscle) for another four weeks.

Plate 56. Open Reduction of Congenital Convex Pes Valgus

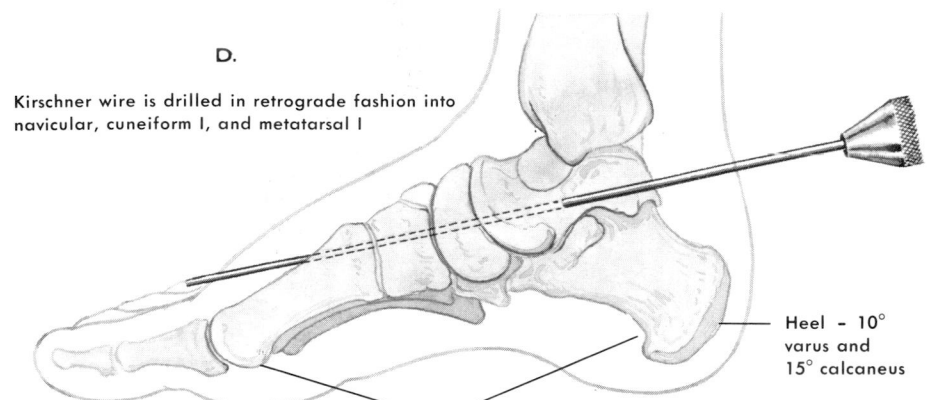

D.

Kirschner wire is drilled in retrograde fashion into navicular, cuneiform I, and metatarsal I

Heel – 10° varus and 15° calcaneus

Longitudinal arch is molded by plantar flexing heads of metatarsals and calcaneus as drilling of Kirschner wire proceeds

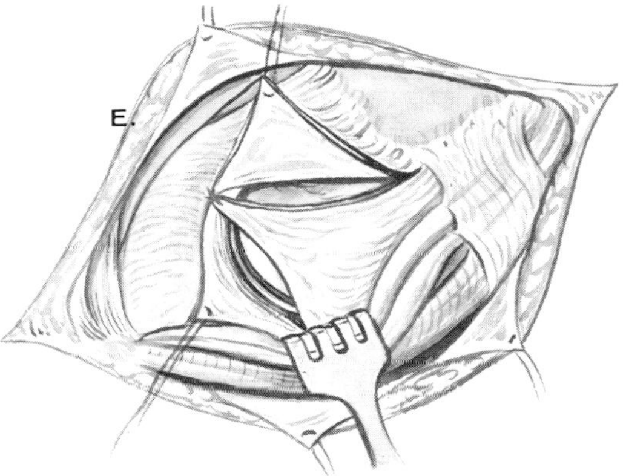

E.

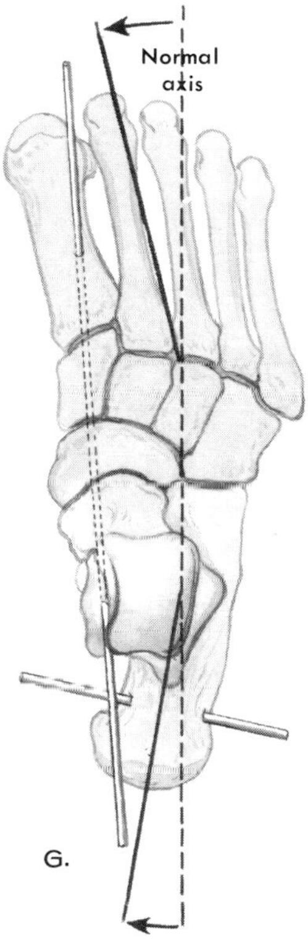

Normal axis

Tight closure of capsule

F.

G.

Calcaneus – 10° varus

Plantar calcaneonavicular ligament resutured under tension

Abductor hallucis m.

Posterior tibial tendon advanced distally and sutured to cuneiform I

Flexor digitorum longus tendon

E.W.B.

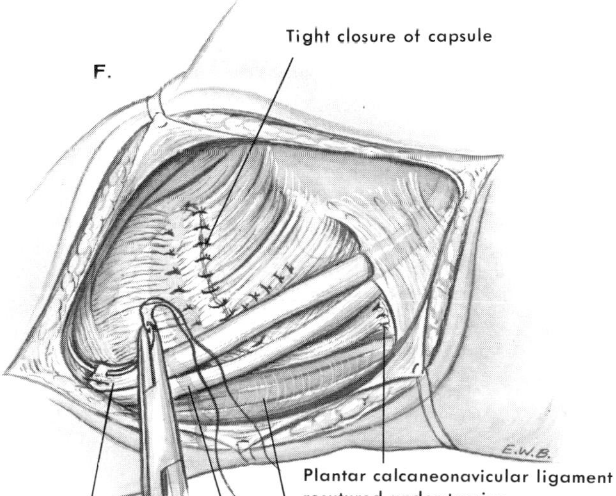

(From Tachdjian, M. O.: Congenital convex pes valgus. Orthop. Clin. N. Amer., 3:143, 1972.)

very fixed, and in order to achieve reduction, the talocalcaneal interosseous ligament must be sectioned. Often, it is also necessary to divide the dorsolateral part of the capsule of the calcaneocuboid joint and to lengthen the peroneus brevis, extensor digitorum longus, extensor hallucis longus, and anterior tibial muscles. Open reduction is carried out as just described. In addition, however, an extra-articular arthrodesis of the subtalar joint is performed, as recommended by Grice and by Coleman et al.[329, 330, 333] This will maintain the reduction and give stability to the subtalar joint. In the older child, surgery for correction of the deformity might be advisable and should be performed in two stages: (1) heel cord lengthening and posterior capsulotomy, and (2) open reduction and subtalar extra-articular arthrodesis three weeks later.

TREATMENT IN THE CHILD OVER SIX YEARS OF AGE

In this age group the deformity is very rigid and attempts at open reduction are usually unsuccessful. Avascular necrosis of the talus is a definite complication. It is best to wait until the patient is 10 or 12 years of age, at which time a reconstructive stabilization procedure on the foot is carried out. Following a preliminary period of corrective casts and soft-tissue lengthening, a triple arthrodesis is performed. Appropriate tarsal bone wedges are resected to correct the deformity. Often excision of the head and neck of the talus and part of the navicular is required. The height of the foot should be reduced as little as possible.

The recommended choice of operative procedure in relation to the age of the patient is summarized in Table 7–6.

CONGENITAL BALL-AND-SOCKET ANKLE JOINT

In this rare condition, the contour of the ankle joint is abnormal. The proximal articular surface of the normal talus is dome-shaped in the lateral, but not in the

Table 7–6.   *Choice of Operative Procedures in Relation to Age of Patient*

Procedure	Age of Patient at Initiation of Treatment				
	Birth to 2 mo.	*3 to 9 mo.*	*9 mo. to 3 yr.*	*4 to 6 yr.*	*Over 6 yr.*
Soft tissues					
Stretching cast	+	+	+	+	+*
Elongate contracted musculotendinous units (anterior tibial, toe extensors, peroneals)	−	±	+	+	+*
Heel cord lengthening	±	+	+	+	+*
Capsulotomy of posterior part of ankle and subtalar joints	−	±	+	+	+*
Section of calcaneofibular ligament	−	±	+	+	+*
Talonavicular joint					
Closed reduction	+	−	−	−	−
Open reduction	−	+	+	+	−
Medial incision	−	+	+	+	−
Maintain reduction by plication of capsule inferiorly and medially by tightening calcaneonavicular ligament and posterior tibial tendon	−	+	+	+	−
Internal fixation of talonavicular joint with Kirschner wire	±	+	+	+	+
May reroute anterior tibial tendon under head of talus	−	+	+	+	−
Both medial and lateral incisions (to release talocalcaneal ligament and calcaneocuboid capsule).	−	−	−	+	−
Reconstructive stabilization					
Triple arthrodesis with partial resection of navicular or head and neck of talus or wedge tarsectomy	−	−	−	−	+

Key: + Indicated
    − Not necessary
    ± May be required
    * Perform prior to triple arthrodesis when bony growth of foot is complete.

anteroposterior, view. In the ball-and-socket ankle joint the upper end of the talus is dome-shaped in both the anteroposterior and lateral projections, and articulates with the concave distal end of the tibia. The fibular malleolus may or may not participate in the ball-and-socket ankle. Lamb, in 1958, described five cases of this rare entity; in four of his patients, there was associated coalition of the tarsal bones; the fifth patient had congenital shortening of the lower limb without tarsal fusion.[367] Brahme reported another case with bilateral involvement and used the term "upper talar enarthrosis."[365] Congenital ball-and-socket joint may also be seen in association with congenital hypoplasia or absence of the fibula and failure of segmentation of the vertebrae.[370] Schreiber reported 27 congenital ball-and-socket ankle joints in 21 patients; the abnormality was found in 10 of 26 cases of congenital shortening of the leg (38 per cent), in 11 of 64 cases of tarsal coalitions (17 per cent), in 4 of 18 cases of congenital hypoplasia or absence of the fibula (22 per cent). In six of the 27 congenital ball-and-socket joints (22 per cent), no associated deformity of the lower limb could be found. The condition is twice as common in the male.[369] A familial case in father and daughter with bilateral involvement is reported by Jacobs.[366]

The condition is usually asymptomatic. The abnormal lateral mobility at the ankle may cause repeated sprains of the joint. Often the patients complain of weakness of the ankle. When there is associated loss of subtalar motion, degenerative arthritis of the ankle may develop in adult life because of excessive stress and repeated minor traumata to the joint.

The roentgenographic appearance is characteristic. The trochlear surface of the talus that is normally convex in the anteroposterior plane and gently concave from side to side loses its concavity in this deformity and becomes spheroid in shape. The lower end of the tibia becomes correspondingly molded into a cuplike cavity, forming a ball-and-socket joint. In infancy and early childhood, it is difficult to determine the exact shape of the ankle joint because of the great amount of cartilage in the unossified tibia, talus, and fibula. Treatment is not indicated, as the condition is asymptomatic. Ankle fusion is performed if degenerative arthritic changes in late adult life cause the deformity to become very disabling.

An acquired form of ball-and-socket ankle joint can be found; however, the rounding of the talus is not as smooth as in the congenital variety. It is reported to follow subtalar arthrodesis (Grice procedure) performed at an early age; it most probably represents an attempt to compensate for loss of subtalar motion. It is also found in congenital insensitivity to pain. Robins studied the ankle joints of 52 patients with poliomyelitis who had had arthrodesis of their feet: triple arthrodesis (42 cases), subtalar arthrodesis (4 cases), Lambrinudi arthrodesis (4 cases), and Campbell's bone block (2 cases). Eight feet (15 per cent) disclosed some compensatory increase in lateral movement of the talus within the tibiofibular mortise, and roentgenograms showed some rounding of the margins of the talus. Robins stated, however, that these structural changes in the proximal articular surface of the talus were noted in the operative films, when available; thus, they preceded the tarsal fusion and did not result from it.[368]

METATARSUS PRIMUS ATAVICUS (Congenital Short First Metatarsal)

The length of the first metatarsal in relation to that of the second metatarsal may show considerable variation in the normal foot. This was determined by Harris and Beath on standardized dorsoplantar roentgenograms of the foot that showed all the bones of the foot with equal clarity from the posterior end of the calcaneus to the tips of the distal phalanges. The distance from the posterior end of the calcaneus to the head of the first metatarsal and to the head of the second metatarsal was measured in 7,167 individual feet. In 2,878 feet (40 per cent), the first metatarsal was *shorter* than the second by 1 mm. or more; in 2,693 feet (38 per cent), the first metatarsal was *longer* than the second by 1 mm. or more; and in 1,596 feet (22 per cent), the first and second metatarsals were of equal length (within 1 mm.).[372]

Morton, in 1935, in his monograph *The Human Foot*, proposed that shortness of the first metatarsal can cause disability of the foot by disturbing transmission of weight and thrust forces through the forepart of the foot. According to his thesis, the head of the short first metatarsal does not reach the ground as readily as that of the longer second metatarsal. Hence, the greater part of the body weight that is borne through the forepart of the foot is shifted from the first metatarsal to the second, or to the second and third metatarsals. The forefoot pronates in an attempt to put the head of the first metatarsal into a weight-bearing position on the ground. This compensatory mechanism lowers the longitudinal arch, which is then subjected to undue strain. In response to this increased stress, callosities develop beneath the heads of the second and third metatarsals, and the shaft of the second metatarsal may thicken. Morton, however, emphasized that shortness of the first metatarsal is but *occasionally* the cause of foot disability, and then only in adult life.[373] Despite his observations, however, the presence of this anomaly was commonly believed to be the cause of symptomatic flatfoot.

The fallacy of this assumption was proved by Harris and Beath, who found in the Canadian Army Foot Survey that the short first metatarsal is seldom, if ever, the cause of foot disability.[371] They stressed that callus under the heads of the central metatarsals is not specifically related to the short first metatarsal, as it occurred almost as frequently in those feet in which the first metatarsal was longer than the second. That the first metatarsal is short does not necessarily indicate that it cannot reach the ground as readily or that less weight will be transmitted through this bone. The obliquity of the metatarsals in relation to the ground demonstrates that all can share equally in weight-bearing, provided the longer metatarsals are on a higher plane than the shorter. Depression of the central metatarsals and marked pressure under their prominent heads cause the callosity. Limitation of plantar flexion of the toes and fixation of the toes in dorsiflexed position will further exaggerate the depression of the metatarsal heads.

Primary marked shortening of the first metatarsal may be encountered as a rare isolated anomaly. It may also occur in association with metatarsus varus and talipes

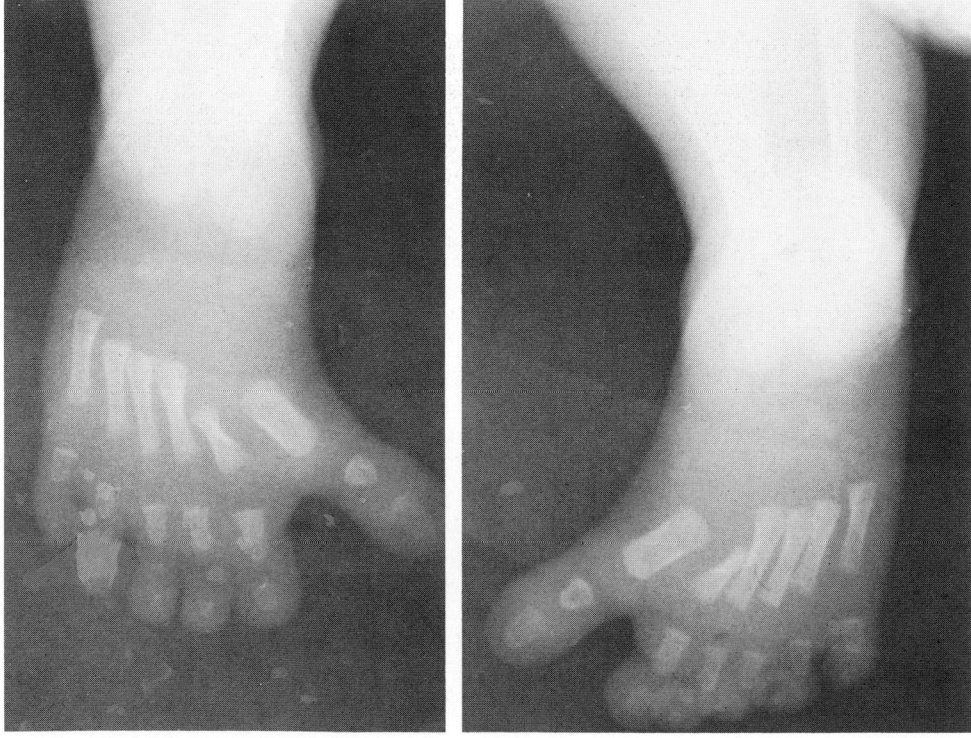

FIGURE 7–52. *Bilateral congenital hallux varus associated with supernumerary second toe and metatarsal.*

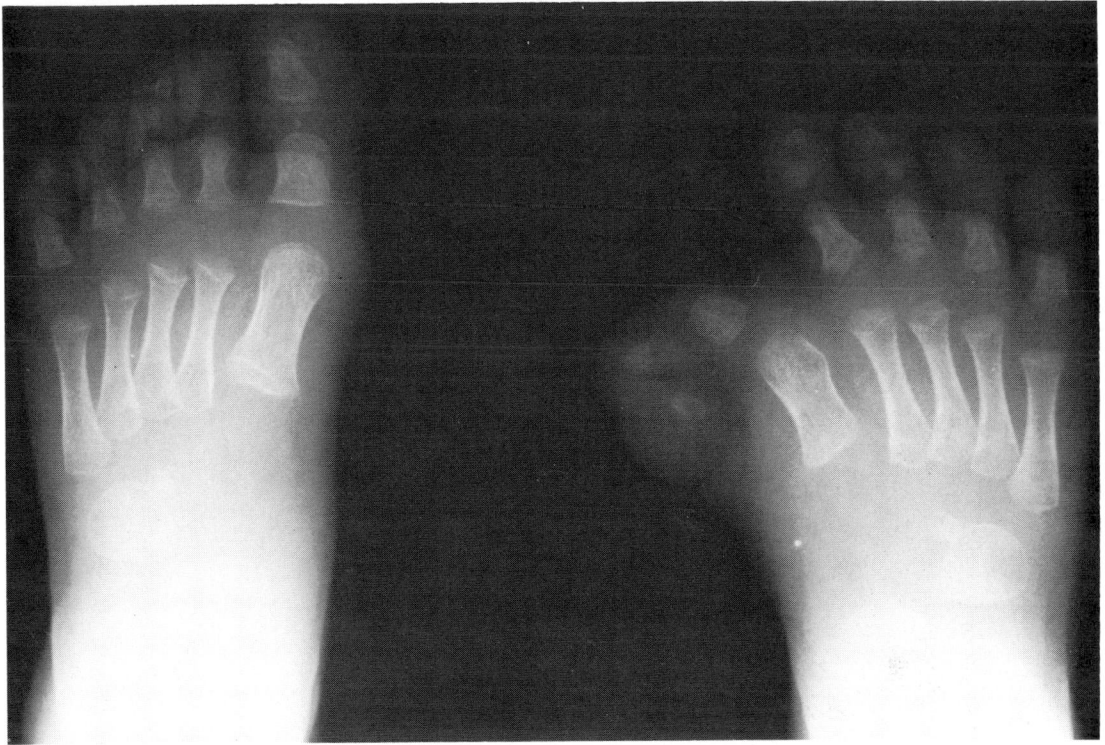

FIGURE 7-53.   Congenital hallux varus on the right associated with accessory hallux.

equinovarus. These may lead to abnormal stress and cause painful callosities under the remaining metatarsal heads. Treatment consists of fitting a metatarsal pad that is elongated medially under the first metatarsal to redistribute the body weight.

CONGENITAL HALLUX VARUS

In this deformity there is congenital medial angulation of the great toe at the metatarsophalangeal joint. There are several types of congenital hallux varus: (1) a primary type with no other associated congenital anomaly—in which a taut fibrous band extends from the medial side of the great toe to the base of the first metatarsal and progressively pulls the great toe toward the midline;[376] (2) those associated with congenital deformities of the forepart of the foot, namely, hallux varus with metatarsus varus, hallux varus associated with isolated congenital marked shortening of the first metatarsal, and hallux varus with accessory bones or toes (Figs. 7–52 and 7–53); and (3) hallux varus associated with extensive developmental affections of the skeleton, as in diastrophic dwarfism.

The method of treatment depends upon the type of hallux varus. The deformity is satisfactorily corrected by any one of the surgical methods of McElvenny, Farmer, or Kelikian.[371-376] The contracted fibrous band on the medial aspect of the great toe, the taut abductor hallucis, and shortened medial capsule of the metatarsophalangeal joint of the big toe are released. Any accessory phalanx or bone is excised and surgical syndactylism between the great and second toes is carried out to maintain correction. Capsuloplasty on the lateral side of the metatarsophalangeal joint and extensor hallucis tendon rerouting will assist in holding the hallux in proper anatomic alignment. A Kirschner wire is inserted into the great toe, across the metatarsophalangeal joint, and into the first metatarsal for three weeks to maintain correction.

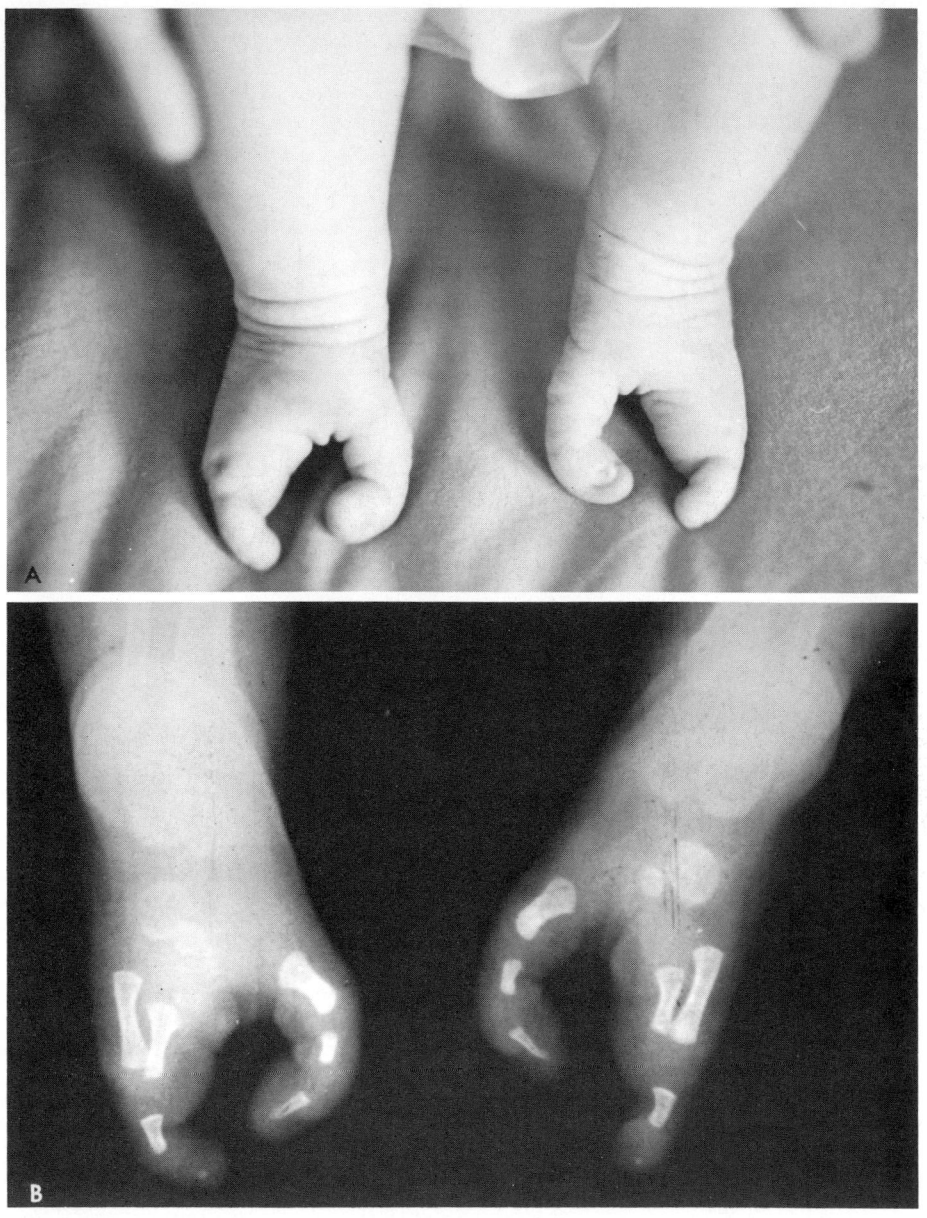

FIGURE 7–54. *Congenital split or cleft foot (lobster claw).*

A. Clinical appearance in six-month-old infant. **B.** Roentgenograms of both feet.

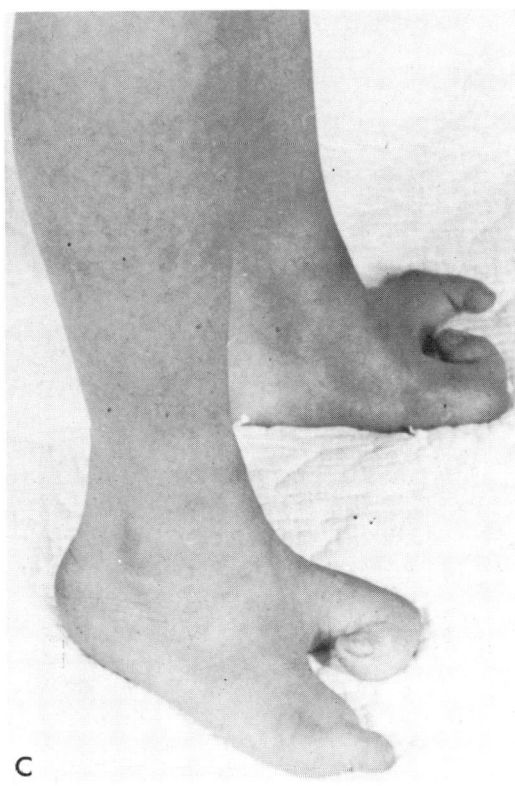

C

FIGURE 7–54 Continued. *Congenital split or cleft foot (lobster claw).*

C. Clinical appearance of a patient three years of age. To facilitate shoe wear, deformity is usually corrected before the child begins to walk.

CONGENITAL SPLIT OR CLEFT FOOT (Lobster Claw)

This rare congenital deformity is characterized by the absence of two or three central digital rays of the foot. The cone-shaped cleft in the forefoot tapers proximally. The first metatarsal may be of normal size, or it may be broad and connected with the intermediate cuneiform at its base, representing fusion of the first and second metatarsals. Valgus deformity of the great toe is common. The lateral digital ray may consist of only the fifth metatarsal or the fifth and fourth metatarsals. The phalanges of the lateral ray usually deviate toward the midline. The hindfoot is normal (Fig. 7–54).

Split foot (lobster claw) exists in two forms. In the less common atypical form, it occurs as a unilateral deformity with no evidence of familial inheritance. In the typical form the deformity is always bilateral and is inherited as an autosomal dominant trait with incomplete penetrance.[378, 381]

Although bilateral split foot may occur as an isolated deformity, it is usually associated with lobster clawing of the hand.[378, 385] Other associated abnormalities are cleft lip and palate, reduction in number and size of phalanges, syndactyly and polydactyly, triphalangeal thumb, and deafness.[380, 383, 384, 387]

Surgical correction of split foot is indicated to facilitate fitting of shoes and to improve the objectionable appearance. Surgery is performed between one and two years of age. The divergent metatarsals are approximated by osteotomy at their base, the deformed toes are normally aligned, and the split forefoot and toes are surgically syndactylized to maintain correction.

Pes Cavus

Pes cavus is a fixed equinus deformity of the forefoot on the hindfoot (Fig. 7–55). When associated with clawing of the toes, the term *clawfoot* is sometimes used to describe the condition.

Etiology and Pathogenesis

Cavus deformity of the foot is usually a manifestation of some underlying neuromuscular disease. The level of the lesion may be in (1) muscle (myopathic pes cavus); (2) peripheral nerves or lumbosacral spinal nerve roots; (3) anterior horn cells of the spinal cord; (4) spinocerebellar tracts; (5) pyramidal or extrapyramidal systems of the brain; or (6) cerebral cortex (hysterical). Examples of neuromuscular disease at these various levels are: (1) muscular dystrophy, particularly the distal type (at the muscular level); (2) Déjerine-Sottas interstitial hypertrophic neuritis, Charcot-Marie-Tooth disease, polyneuritis, and traumatic lesions of the sciatic nerve (peripheral nerve or spinal nerve root level); (3) poliomyelitis, myelomeningocele, diastematomyelia, and cord tumors (spinal cord level); (4) Friedreich's

ataxia and Roussy-Lévy syndrome (heredo-familial affections of spinocerebellar tracts); (5) cerebral palsy (spastic hemiplegia or athetosis) and dystonia musculorum deformans (pyramidal and extrapyramidal level); and (6) hysteria (cerebral level) in which, when the position of pes cavus is maintained constantly for prolonged periods, permanent contracture and fixed deformity may develop. Some cases of pes cavus are *congenital;* occasionally, a specific cause or neurologic deficit cannot be demonstrated, in which case the term *idiopathic pes cavus* is used.

In the pathogenesis of pes cavus, several factors should be considered:

Muscle Imbalance Between Weak Anterior Tibial and Strong Peroneus Longus Muscle. The medial cuneiform and the base of the first metatarsal are elevated by the action of the anterior tibial muscle and depressed by the peroneus longus muscle. Bentzon advanced the theory that when the anterior tibial muscle is weak, the first metatarsal is plantar-flexed by a strong peroneus longus muscle. The forefoot is pronated by the action of the peroneus longus muscle, which is further assisted by the valgus line of muscle pull of the long toe extensors. In attempting

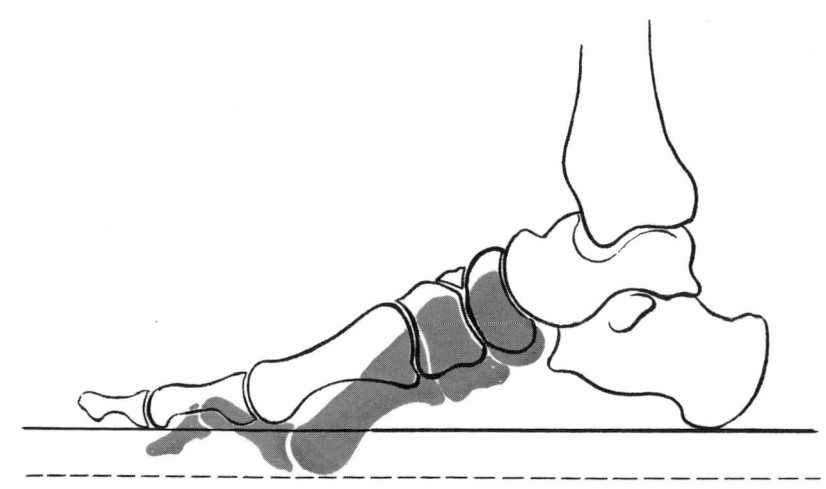

FIGURE 7–55. Pes cavus.

Note the fixed equinus deformity of the forefoot on the hindfoot.

to substitute for the dorsiflexing action of the weakened anterior tibial muscle, the long toe extensors pull the proximal phalanges of the toes into hyperextension; the tension on the long toe flexor muscle brings the distal two phalanges of the toes into plantar flexion.[391] This hypothesis of dynamic imbalance between a weak anterior muscle and a strong peroneus longus muscle sounds very plausible, but unfortunately, it fails to explain the actual clinical findings. In poliomyelitis, when the anterior tibial muscle is weak and the peroneal muscles are strong, a pes valgus deformity results. The os calcis is everted, the head of the talus is plantar-flexed, the medial longitudinal arch is flattened, and the toes are flat on the ground. In walking, however, the toe extensors do pull the toes into extension, but a fixed claw toe deformity does not develop. Another contradiction to the theory of Bentzon is the absence of definite anterior tibial muscle weakness in most cases of pes cavus.

Isolated Weakness of Peroneus Brevis Muscle. This is a very attractive theory. In an attempt to compensate for the paralysis of the peroneus brevis muscle, the peroneus longus hypertrophies and overpowers the action of the anterior tibial muscle. The first metatarsal and medial cuneiform are pulled into plantar flexion and the forefoot is pronated. The long toe extensors are hyperactive in compensation for dorsiflexion insufficiency caused by peroneus brevis muscle weakness; consequently, the proximal phalanges of the toes are pulled into hyperextension and their distal phalanx into flexion by the tension on the long toe flexors. The hindfoot inverts to compensate for eversion of the forefoot, enabling the first and fifth metatarsals to be placed evenly on the ground. The dynamic imbalance between a weak peroneus brevis and strong posterior tibial muscle may also be a factor in producing a varus heel. In support of this theory, one finds an occasional patient with poliomyelitis who has isolated paralysis of the peroneus brevis muscle and a deformity of the foot quite similar to pes cavus.

Paralysis of Intrinsic Muscles of Foot. Duchenne described a cavus clawfoot with atrophy of the muscles that insert into the sesamoids of the great toe and the interossei of the foot. The proximal phalanges are hyperextended so that they are subluxated on the metatarsal heads, and the middle and distal phalanges are flexed. The result is clawing of the toes and a considerable increase in the curvature of the plantar arch. Duchenne proposed the following theory of the pathogenesis of cavus clawfoot:

When the interossei are paralyzed or weakened, the force of the muscles which extend the proximal phalanges and the muscles which flex the middle and distal phalanges lose the moderating action of the interossei. The clawing of the toes sets in and gradually increases. The bases of the proximal phalanges progressively depress the heads of the metatarsals with increase of the degree of subluxation of the proximal phalanges; the curvature of the plantar arch increases considerably and the plantar aponeurosis contracts in time. Following this, all the joints, especially the mediotarsal joints and their ligaments, become deformed in a manner characteristic of all cavus feet.[398]

Duchenne believed the mechanism of the clawing of the foot to be similar to that of the clawhand seen following paralysis of the intrinsic muscles of the hand, i.e., "the heads of the medial four metacarpals are equally pushed by the proximal phalanges of the fingers, resulting in a form of cavus of the palm and of the hand."[398] It should be noted, however, that the interossei in the foot insert mainly into the bases of the proximal phalanges, an anatomic fact that contradicts the theory of Duchenne of the "moderating action of the interossei" on the middle and distal phalanges in preventing flexion at the interphalangeal joints.[411]

Also, paralysis of the intrinsic muscles of the foot produces pes planovalgus, *not* pes cavus. Coonrad, Irwin, Gucker, and Wray observed that persistent function of the short toe flexors and other intrinsic muscles of the foot in an otherwise flail foot resulted in the development of cavovarus deformity of the foot.[397] Garceau and Brahms demonstrated the importance of functioning intrinsic muscles in the production of pes cavus and cavovarus; they recommended resection of the motor branches of both the medial and lateral plantar nerves. In their experience the results of 47 operations in 40 patients were encouraging.[402] Electromyographic studies of the intrinsic muscles of the foot and the extrinsic muscles of the foot and leg in patients with pes cavus have been performed by Bertrand and Ingelrans. Both authors have demonstrated definite abnormality in the short toe flexors and other intrinsic muscles of the foot. Ingelrans also observed abnormal activity in the long toe extensors and peroneus longus muscles.[392, 408] The author has repeatedly observed such changes, but has found it difficult to interpret electromyographic findings in pes cavus in relation to dynamic muscle imbalance and abnormal forces causing cavus deformity.

Lambrinudi supported Duchenne's theory of interosseus insufficiency as the cause of clawfoot and devised an operation consisting of arthrodeses of both interphalangeal joints and sectioning of the long toe extensors. Stiffening the interphalangeal joints brings the entire action of the long toe flexor to bear on the metatarsophalangeal joint; thus, during locomotion, the toes are pressed on the ground and the metatarsal heads are supported.[413]

Triceps Surae Muscle. The triceps surae muscle has been blamed as a factor in the pathogenesis of pes cavus. When the gastrocnemius-soleus muscles are paralyzed, during the push-off phase of gait the normal long toe flexor muscles substitute for the lost action of the triceps surae, with resultant clawing of the toes. The forefoot becomes plantar-flexed secondary to the depressing action of the claw toes. In paralytic neuromuscular disease, calcaneocavus deformity may result from such a mechanism.

Hyperactivity of Intrinsic Muscles of Foot. This is considered by Coonrad et al. and by Garceau and Brahms to be a cause of pes cavovarus.[397, 402] However, this theory fails to explain the hyperextension deformity of the proximal phalanges of the toes.

Muscle Fibrosis and Contracture. Fibrosis and permanent contracture of the short toe flexors and other intrinsic muscles of the foot and plantar aponeurosis have been repeatedly demonstrated at surgery in pes cavus. Is it a primary or secondary deformity? As stated previously, the intrinsic muscles of the foot insert into the bases of the proximal phalanges, not into the metatarsal heads. The proximal phalanx of the toes in pes cavus is hyperextended and not flexed.

Genetic Factors. In idiopathic pes cavus there is a high rate of familial incidence; however, an exact method of hereditary transmission has not been delineated. The genetic aspects of degenerative diseases of the spinocerebellar tracts and spina bifida are discussed in Chapter 5.

In summary, the exact pathogenesis of pes cavus is not known. In some cases, equinus forefoot may be the primary deformity; in others, clawing of the toes, and occasionally inversion of the hindfoot. Every case of pes cavus should have the following studies to determine various possible etiologic factors: (1) a thorough family history (which should include foot examinations and neurologic assessments of the siblings and parents); (2) a muscle examination to rule out paralytic disease; (3) a thorough neurologic evaluation; (4) roentgenograms of the *entire* spine; (5) nerve conduction and electromyographic studies; and (6) lumbar puncture and myelography in selected cases when indicated.

Clinical and Roentgenographic Features

There are various types of pes cavus that should be distinguished: In *simple pes cavus*, the plantar flexion deformity of the forefoot is equal in its medial and lateral columns, with even distribution of weight on the first and fifth metatarsal heads. The heel is in neutral position or a few degrees valgus, which is normal. In *pes cavovarus* only the medial column of the forefoot is dropped in plantar flexion; consequently, the longitudinal axis of the first metatarsal is in markedly equinus, while that of the fifth metatarsal is in normal horizontal, position (Fig. 7–56 A). On examination of the non-weight-bearing foot (with the patient sitting and his leg hanging at the edge of the table), it will be found that the fifth metatarsal can easily be dorsiflexed into neutral position, whereas the first metatarsal is fixed in equinus position and cannot be passively manipulated into neutral extension. Closer scrutiny and analysis will disclose that the forefoot, particularly the first metatarsal, is in 20 to 30 degrees of pronation (Fig. 7–56). In the early stages the hindfoot is in neutral position, and in stance and locomotion there is excessive pressure on the pronated first metatarsal head. In order to relieve the excessive pressure on the first metatarsal head, the whole foot (forefoot and hindfoot) is inverted (Fig. 7–56 F and I). Initially, the varus deformity of the hindfoot is reducible, and can be expected to disappear when the fixed equinus and pronation deformities of the first metatarsal are corrected. With time, however, the varus deformity of the hindfoot becomes fixed and cannot be corrected by aligning the forefoot (Fig. 7–57). *Calcaneocavus* deformity of the foot usually occurs in flaccid paralysis, such as that in poliomyelitis or myelomeningocele. The triceps surae muscle is paralyzed. The hindfoot is in calcaneus position and the forefoot is fixed in equinus position. *Pes equinocavus* is usually secondary to talipes equinovarus.

On examination the soft tissues in the plantar aspect of the foot are taut, fixing the forefoot in plantar flexion. The contracted structures are the plantar aponeurosis, abductor hallucis, flexor hallucis brevis, flexor digitorum brevis, abductor digiti quinti, the interossei, the tendinous insertions of the posterior tibial tendon on the plantar aspect of the cuneiform and the base of the metatarsals, the Y-ligament (calcaneocuboid and calcaneonavicular), the capsule on the plantar aspect of the naviculocuneiform, and the cuneiform-metatarsal joints.

Bony deformities gradually follow the soft-tissue contracture. The articular and osseous changes are best depicted in a standing lateral roentgenogram of the foot. In the normal foot, the distal and proximal articular surfaces of the first cuneiform bone are almost parallel to each other. In pes cavus the forefoot equinus inclination is usually maximal at the first cuneiform bone, and the articular surfaces of the first cuneiform bone converge in the plantar aspect of the foot. Less often the tarsal navicular is at the apex of the cavus deformity; in such an instance, the navicular bone presents as a hard prominence on the dorsum of the foot. An adventitious bursa develops from shoe irritation. Occasionally the forefoot will drop into equinus posture at the tarsometatarsal joints more distally. Lateral roentgenograms of the foot—both weight-bearing and non-weight-bearing—and maximal forefoot dorsiflexion views to demonstrate the apex of the cavus deformity are taken.

Different methods may be used to measure the degree of pes cavus. Hibbs measures the angle formed between two lines drawn through the centers of the longitudinal axes of the calcaneus and the first metatarsal (Fig. 7–58 C).[406] Méary measures the angle formed between two lines drawn through the centers of the longitudinal axes of the talus and the first metatarsal (Fig. 7–58 B).[415]

THE TOES

In pes cavus the toes may be normal, but usually they become progressively retracted and clawed, with hyperextension of the metatarsophalangeal joints and flexion of the interphalangeal joints. The great toe and the fifth toe are ordinarily the most severely deformed (see Fig. 7–57 D). A painful adventitious bursa may develop over the dorsum of the interphalangeal joint as a result of irritation by the shoe; with dorsal subluxation of the metatarsophalangeal joints, the bases of the proximal phalanges press against the metatarsal heads and exaggerate the forefoot equinus deformity. In severe claw toe deformity, the toes do not touch the ground at all and lose their function of propulsion in gait; consequently, most of the body weight is transmitted to the metatarsal heads, and plantar keratosis develops.

THE HINDFOOT

Depending upon the type of pes cavus, the hindfoot may be in neutral position, inversion or equinus or calcaneus position. In pes cavovarus, the heel is inverted and the talocalcaneal angle is decreased in the roentgenogram. Routine standing roentgenograms of the ankle should be made to detect any medial tilting of the ankle mortise, which may be the cause of varus deformity of the hindfoot.

Contracture of the triceps surae muscle causes the hindfoot to be fixed in plantar flexion, and in stance the heel does not touch the floor (Fig. 7–57 C). Most of the body weight is transmitted to the metatarsal heads. If the equinus deformity is not corrected, painful callosities develop on the plantar aspect of the metatarsal heads. The keratotic skin eventually ulcerates and secondary infection sets in.

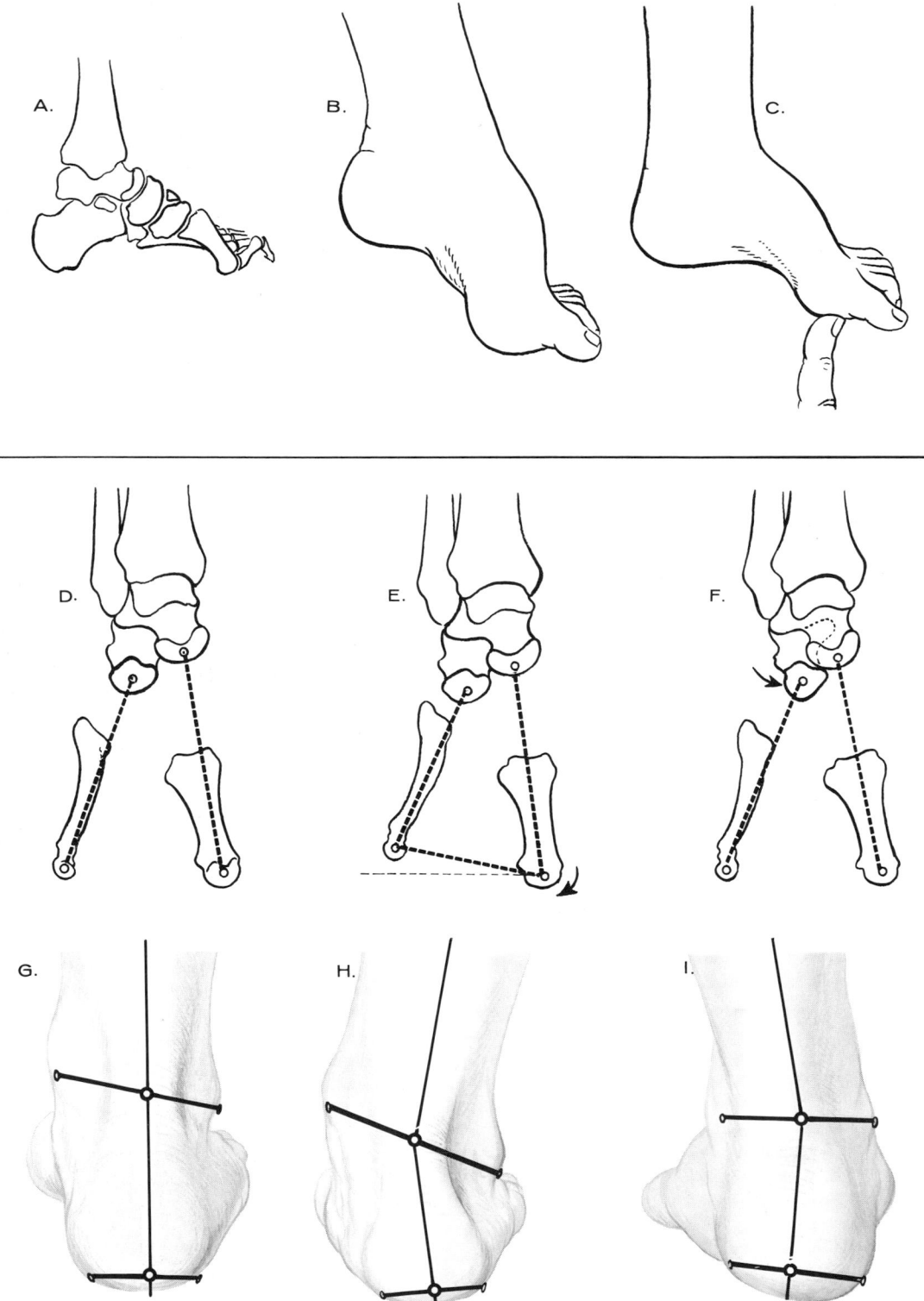

FIGURE 7–56. *Pes cavovarus. See opposite page for legend.*

Treatment

Conservative measures are indicated in early and mild cases; these consist of passive stretching of the contracted plantar fascia and the short plantar muscles, and elevation of the metatarsal heads by a supporting insole with a 3/8 inch pad placed just behind the metatarsal heads (Fig. 7–59). The toe portion of the shoes should be of adequate width in order not to press on the toes. A 1/8- to 3/16-inch wedge on the lateral side of the heel is given if the hindfoot tends to go into inversion.

Surgical measures are indicated when the deformity is severe and disabling. In general, operative treatment should be delayed until several periodic examinations have ruled out progressive neuromuscular deficit. The type of procedure depends upon the age of the patient and the rigidity and severity of the deformity.

SOFT-TISSUE PROCEDURES

These are indicated in children before fixed bony changes have taken place.

Release of Contractures on Plantar Aspect of Foot

SUBCUTANEOUS SECTION OF PLANTAR APONEUROSIS. This is carried out when contracture of the plantar fascia is moderate and that of the short plantar muscles is minimal. The technique is illustrated in Plate 57. It is imperative to apply a series of stretching casts to obtain full correction. Fibrositis of the plantar fascia is an occasional complication of this simple procedure; should it develop, local injection of hydrocortisone will relieve the condition.

SECTION OF PLANTAR APONEUROSIS AND SHORT PLANTAR MUSCLES NEAR THEIR ORIGIN FROM TUBEROSITY OF CALCANEUS. In 1920, Steindler described a stripping operation for pes cavus in which a longitudinal incision is made on the medial side of the calcaneus, and the long plantar ligament is transversely sectioned. The flexor digitorum brevis, abductor digiti quinti, and abductor hallucis brevis are also subperiosteally stripped and released from the calcaneus.[425] The Steindler procedure should not be performed because the operative scar in the instep contracts, hypertrophies because of irritation from the shoe, and acts as a deforming force. Other drawbacks of the Steindler plantar fascial stripping are the potential injury to neurovascular structures and the inadequate correction of forefoot equinus deformity.

The author prefers a midline incision on the sole of the foot. The resultant scar is minimal and not bothersome, and the exposure is adequate for the complete release of contracted plantar soft tissues as described in Plate 57. It is imperative postoperatively, to apply a series of stretching casts for a total period of at least 12 weeks.

If more extensive soft-tissue release is indicated, the procedure described by Bost, Schottstaedt and Larsen is carried out.[70] The contracted tendinous expansions of the posterior tibial tendon should be sectioned at their metatarsal and cuneiform attachments because they fix the first metatarsal in equinus posture. The Y-ligament (the calcaneocuboid and calcaneonavicular ligaments), and the plantar portion of the capsule of the cuboid–fifth metatarsal and cuneiform-metatarsals are sectioned. Again,

FIGURE 7–56. Pes cavovarus.

A to **C.** Diagrams of mediolateral view of the foot demonstrating that only the medial column of the forefoot is dropped in plantar flexion. Note the longitudinal axis of the first metatarsal is markedly equinus, whereas that of the fifth metatarsal is in normal alignment. On push-up test, the first metatarsal cannot be passively manipulated into neutral extension. **D** to **F.** Diagrams of the mechanism of inversion of the hindfoot in pes cavovarus. In the normal foot, the weight-bearing forces are equally distributed on the first and fifth metatarsal heads (D). In pes cavovarus the first metatarsal is fixed in equinus and the forefoot is in 20 to 30 degrees of pronation. In stance and locomotion, there is excessive pressure on the pronated first metatarsal head (E). Excessive pressure on the first metatarsal head is relieved by inverting the whole foot (both forefoot and hindfoot) (F). **G** to **I.** Posterior views of the ankle and foot, showing the normal, pronated, and inverted hindfoot. The hindfoot assumes a varus inclination as the forefoot is inverted.

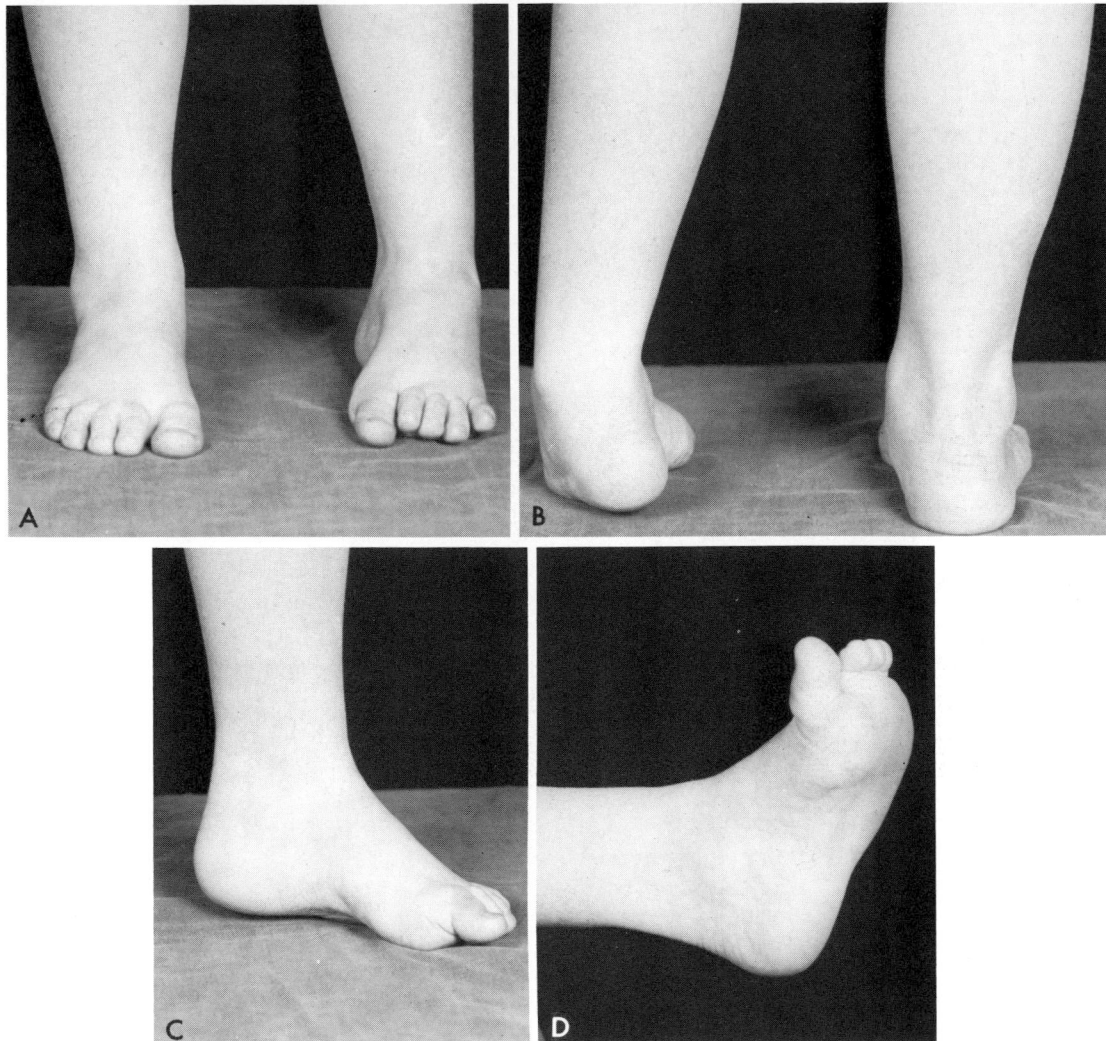

FIGURE 7–57.   *Cavovarus deformity of left foot.*

A and **B.** Anterior and posterior views showing varus deformity of both forefoot and hindfoot. **C.** Medial view of left foot showing the equinus forefoot. Note also that the heel is not touching the floor, indicating associated contracture of the triceps surae muscle. **D.** Range of active dorsiflexion of ankle and foot. Note the clawing of the great toe.

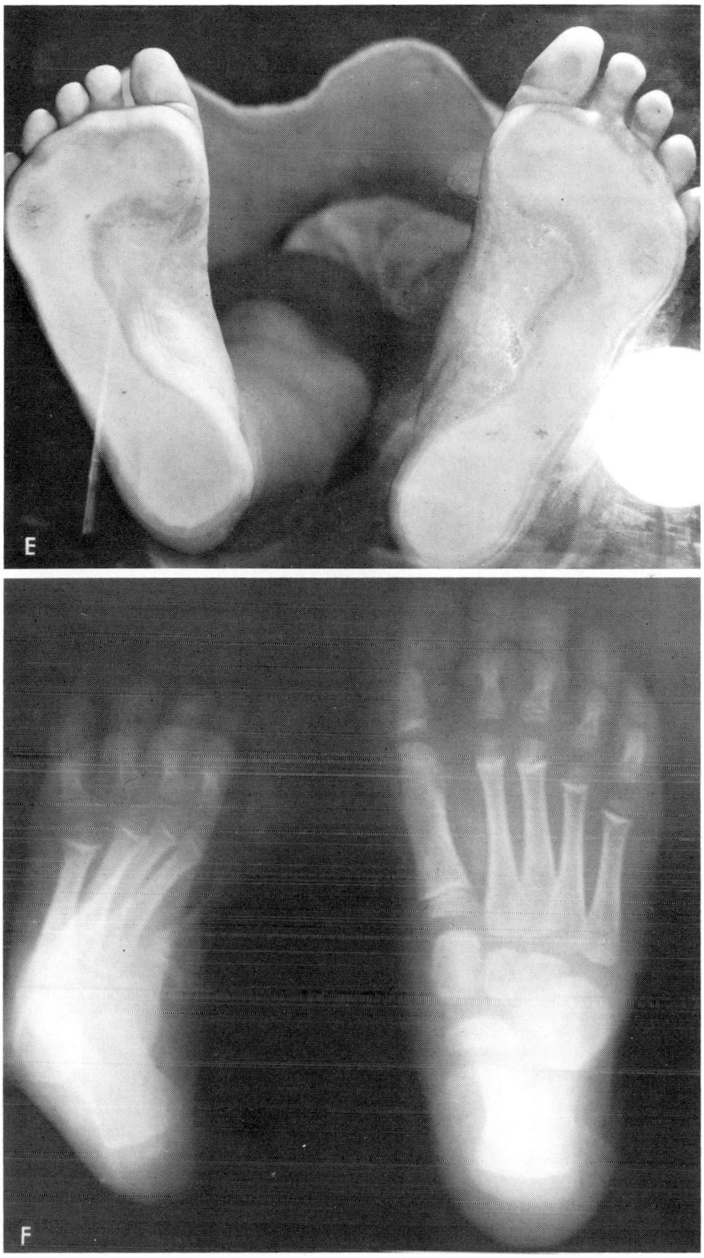

FIGURE 7–57 Continued.   *Cavovarus deformity of left foot.*

E. Plantar standing view. **F.** Weight-bearing anteroposterior roentgenogram of both feet, depicting the varus deformity of forefoot and hindfoot on the left.

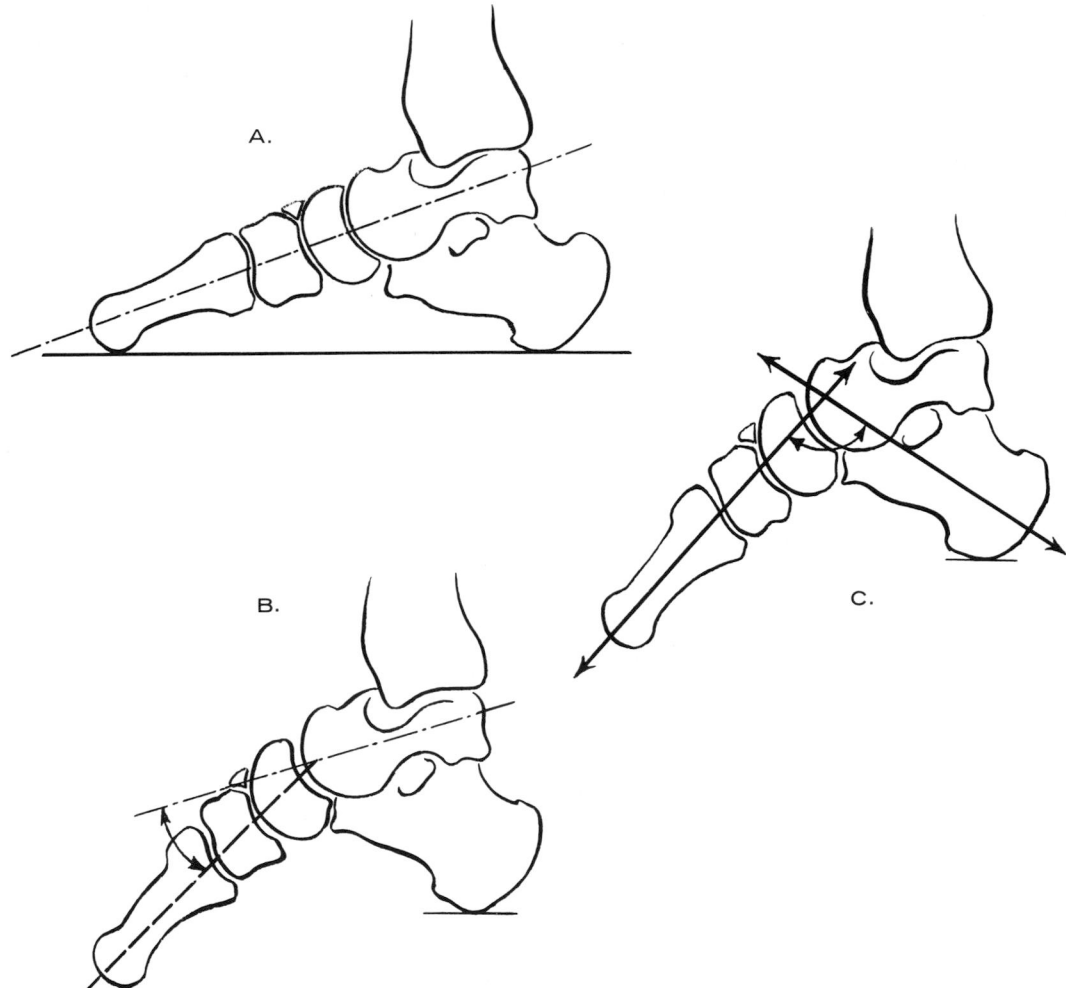

FIGURE 7–58. *Methods of measuring the degree of pes cavus in the standing lateral roentgenogram of the foot.*

A. In the normal foot, the longitudinal axis of the talus is parallel with that of the first metatarsal. **B.** *Méary* measures the angle formed between lines drawn through the center of the longitudinal axis of the talus and of the first metatarsal. **C.** *Hibbs* measures the angle formed between two lines drawn through the center of the longitudinal axis of the calcaneus and of the first metatarsal.

a series of stretching below-knee walking casts is applied postoperatively to be worn for at least three months.

Transfer of Long Toe Extensors to Heads of Metatarsals.[401, 410, 423] This procedure is particularly indicated in paralytic pes cavus. When there is associated clawing of the toes, it is combined with fusion of the interphalangeal joints. The tendon transfer will increase the power of dorsiflexion of the foot and elevate the metatarsal heads, providing a dynamic force against forefoot equinus deformity. By routing the tendons from the medial to the lateral side, the transfer will also be given some inversion power, which acts against the pronation deformity of the forefoot in pes cavovarus.

For the tendon transfers to function effectively, the foot should be flexible. First, a release of contracted soft tissues on the plantar aspect of the foot is carried out. In cases of moderate deformity the two procedures can be combined at the same operation; however, in severe deformity, the use of stretching casts for a period of three months is essential to correct the fixed equinus forefoot. Tendon transfers are performed *only* when fixed cavus deformity is fully corrected—the importance of this prerequisite cannot be overemphasized.

In 1919, Hibbs described an operation for correction of clawing of the lesser toes. The tendons of the extensor digitorum longus were divided as far distally as possible and anchored en masse into the third cuneiform bone.[406] The Hibbs operation should *not* be performed for pes cavus, as it fails to provide a dynamic force to elevate the metatarsal heads.

The operative technique of transfer of the long toe extensors to the metatarsal heads is described and illustrated in Plate 58.

Miscellaneous Soft-Tissue Procedures. Selective neurectomy of the motor branches of plantar muscles in pes cavus is not recommended by the author, as, in his experience, the results have been poor. The procedure was described by Garceau and Brahms for the treatment of paralytic cavovarus deformity of the feet following poliomyelitis;

they reported encouraging results.[402] Coonrad et al. recommend neurectomy of the motor branches of the lateral plantar nerve and partial excision of the short toe flexors and plantar fascia in paralytic pes cavovarus.[397] Such a procedure is indicated only when the short toe flexors and other intrinsic muscles of the foot are functioning in an otherwise flail foot.

Transfer of the anterior tibial tendon to the dorsum of the head of the first metatarsal is recommended by Fowler et al.[400] They combine the procedure with a vertical osteotomy of the medial cuneiform; the osteotomy site is opened on its plantar aspect and held by a triangular wedge of autogenous bone based plantarward. Plantar fasciotomy is usually necessary. The procedure elongates and elevates the medial ray of the foot. The transferred anterior tibial tendon acts as a dorsiflexor of the first metatarsal. In Fowler's experience, in the flexible cavovarus foot with satisfactory extrinsic muscle balance,

(*Text continued on page 1396.*)

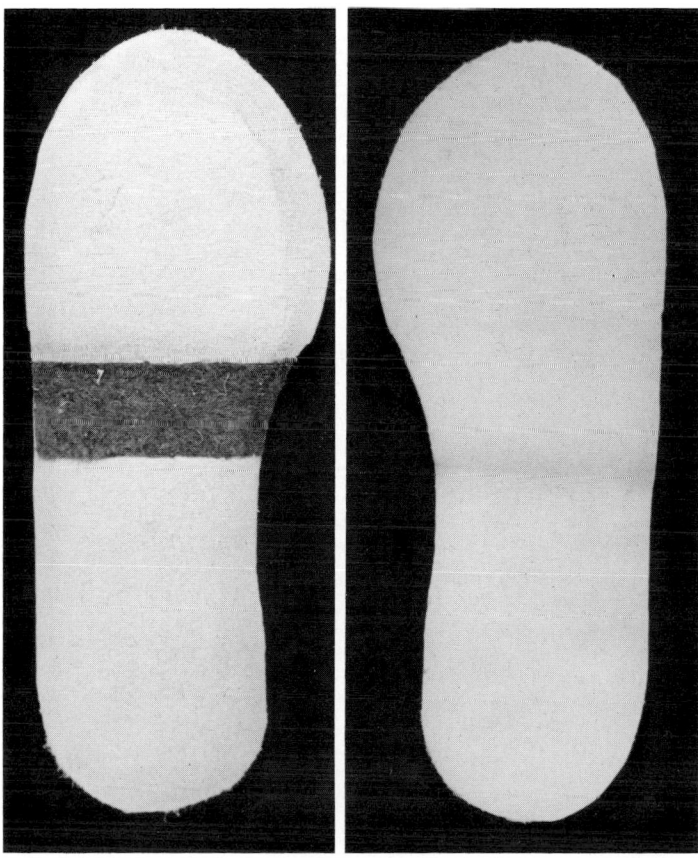

FIGURE 7–59. Insole with a ³/₈-inch pad placed just behind metatarsal heads.

Plantar Fasciotomy and Release of Contracted Soft Tissues on Plantar Aspect of Cavus Foot

SUBCUTANEOUS SECTION OF PLANTAR APONEUROSIS

A. The procedure is performed when contracture of the plantar fascia is moderate, but that of the short plantar muscles is minimal.

A sharp Ryerson knife is inserted deep to the plantar fascia with the blade flat to the skin. Then the sharp edge of the blade is rotated 90 degrees, bringing its sharp edge toward the plantar fascia. By pushing it against the knife with the index finger of the opposite hand, the plantar fascia is completely divided. It is sectioned at two levels about 2.5 cm. apart, and stretched by holding the heel steady and bringing the forefoot into dorsiflexion. A below-knee walking cast is applied. The cast is changed every two to three weeks, each time manipulating the forefoot into further dorsiflexion. The metatarsal heads and the heel should be adequately padded and the cast well molded to prevent pressure sores.

The total period for which stretching casts should be used should be 8 to 12 weeks, depending upon the severity and fixity of deformity. At night, following removal of the solid cast, the forefoot is held out of equinus and in neutral position in a bivalved cast. The night casts are worn for several years, depending upon the cause of pes cavus and the severity of deformity. Metatarsal pads are worn in the shoes during the day. Passive stretching exercises of the plantar fascia are performed several times a day.

SECTION OF PLANTAR APONEUROSIS AND SHORT PLANTAR MUSCLES THROUGH MIDLINE INCISION

B. The Steindler stripping operation for pes cavus should not be performed because of its possible inherent complications of contracture of the scar in the instep, injury to neurovascular structures, and inadequate correction of equinus forefoot. The author recommends the following technique:

A midline incision is made on the sole of the foot, extending from 1 cm. distal to the tuberosity of the calcaneus to the base of the metatarsals. The subcutaneous tissue is divided and the wound flaps are undermined and elevated. The central, medial, and lateral portions of the plantar aponeurosis are widely excised. The abductor hallucis is sectioned at its origin from the medial process of the tuberosity of the calcaneus and the laciniate ligament. The flexor digitorum brevis, abductor digiti quinti, and quadratus plantae muscles, and the long plantar ligaments are detached from their origin on the tuberosity of the calcaneus. By keeping the dissection immediately adjacent to bone, injury to neurovascular structures is avoided. The pneumatic tourniquet is released and after complete hemostasis the skin is approximated by interrupted sutures. A below-knee walking cast is applied. Postoperative care is similar to that for subcutaneous section of plantar aponeurosis, but the period of immobilization in a cast is longer, about 12 to 16 weeks.

Plate 57. Plantar Fasciotomy and Release of Contracted Soft Tissues on Plantar Aspect of Cavus Foot

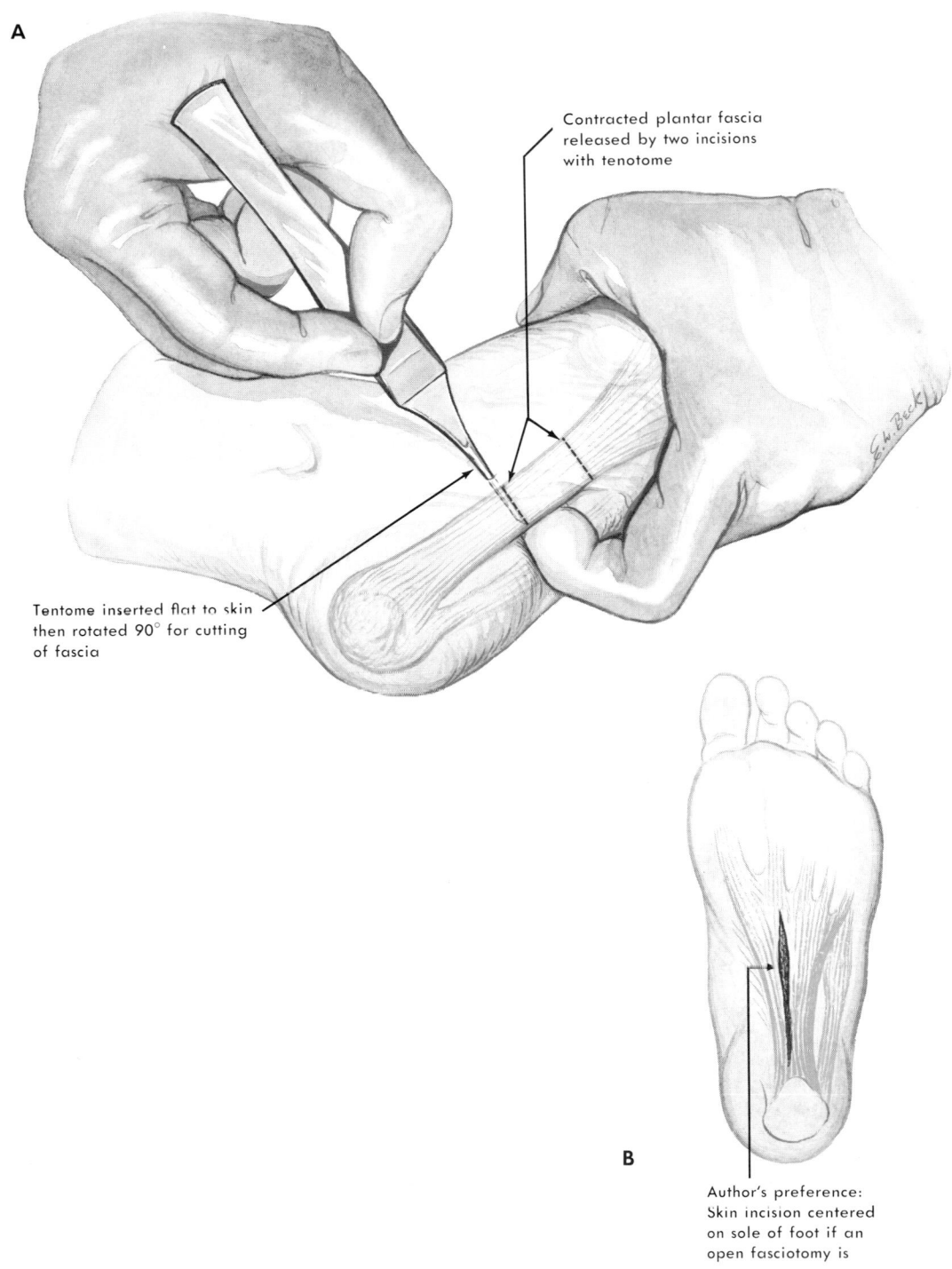

A

Contracted plantar fascia released by two incisions with tenotome

Tentome inserted flat to skin then rotated 90° for cutting of fascia

B

Author's preference: Skin incision centered on sole of foot if an open fasciotomy is necessary

Transfer of Long Toe Extensors to Heads of Metatarsals

A. A longitudinal incision is made on the dorsomedial aspect of the first metatarsal, extending from the base of the proximal phalanx to the proximal one fourth of the metatarsal shaft. The incision should be placed medial to the extensor hallucis longus tendon, toward the second metatarsal. The subcutaneous tissue is divided and the wound flaps are retracted with 0 silk sutures. The digital nerves and vessels should not be injured.

B. The extensor hallucis longus and brevis tendons are identified and sectioned at the base of the proximal phalanx. An alternate technique is to leave the insertion of the extensor hallucis brevis tendon intact; the stump of the extensor hallucis longus tendon is sutured to the intact brevis tendon. (This latter method is faster and is utilized by the author when the long toe extensors of all five toes are to be transferred to the heads of the metatarsals.)

C. Silk whip sutures (00) are inserted to the ends of the long and short toe extensors. The long toe extensor is dissected free, and with a sharp scalpel its sheath is thoroughly excised as far proximally as possible.

D. The epiphyseal plate of the first metatarsal is proximal, whereas that of the lateral four metatarsals is distal in location. The extensor hallucis longus tendon is transferred to the head of the first metatarsal. The long toe extensors of the lesser toes are transferred to the distal one third of the metatarsal shafts, with care taken not to disturb the growth plate. When the patient is over the age of 10 to 12 years, the tendons are transferred to the heads of the metatarsals, as by then, growth of the foot is almost complete.

With small Chandler elevator retractors, the soft tissues are retracted. The periosteum is not stripped. Through a stab wound in the periosteum, a hole is drilled in the center of the first metatarsal head and is enlarged to receive the tendon. The extensor hallucis longus tendon is passed through the hole in the first metatarsal in a medial to lateral direction and sutured to itself, with the forefoot in maximal dorsiflexion.

E. The extensor hallucis brevis tendon is then sutured to the stump of the long toe extensor, holding the toe in neutral extension or in 10 degrees of dorsiflexion.

A similar technique is employed to transfer the long extensor tendons of the lesser toes. Longitudinal incisions are made between the second and third metatarsals, and between the fourth and fifth metatarsals. The extensor brevis tendon of the little toe is either absent or not of adequate size to transfer to the stump of the longus.

The tourniquet is released and complete hemostasis is obtained. The wounds are closed with interrupted sutures. A below-knee walking cast is applied, to be worn for four to six weeks. A sturdy well-padded toe plate is made in the cast. The plantar aspect of the metatarsals should be well padded.

Special muscle training for the transferred tendons is not required, as the transfer is in phase.

Plate 58. Transfer of Long Toe Extensors to Heads of Metatarsals

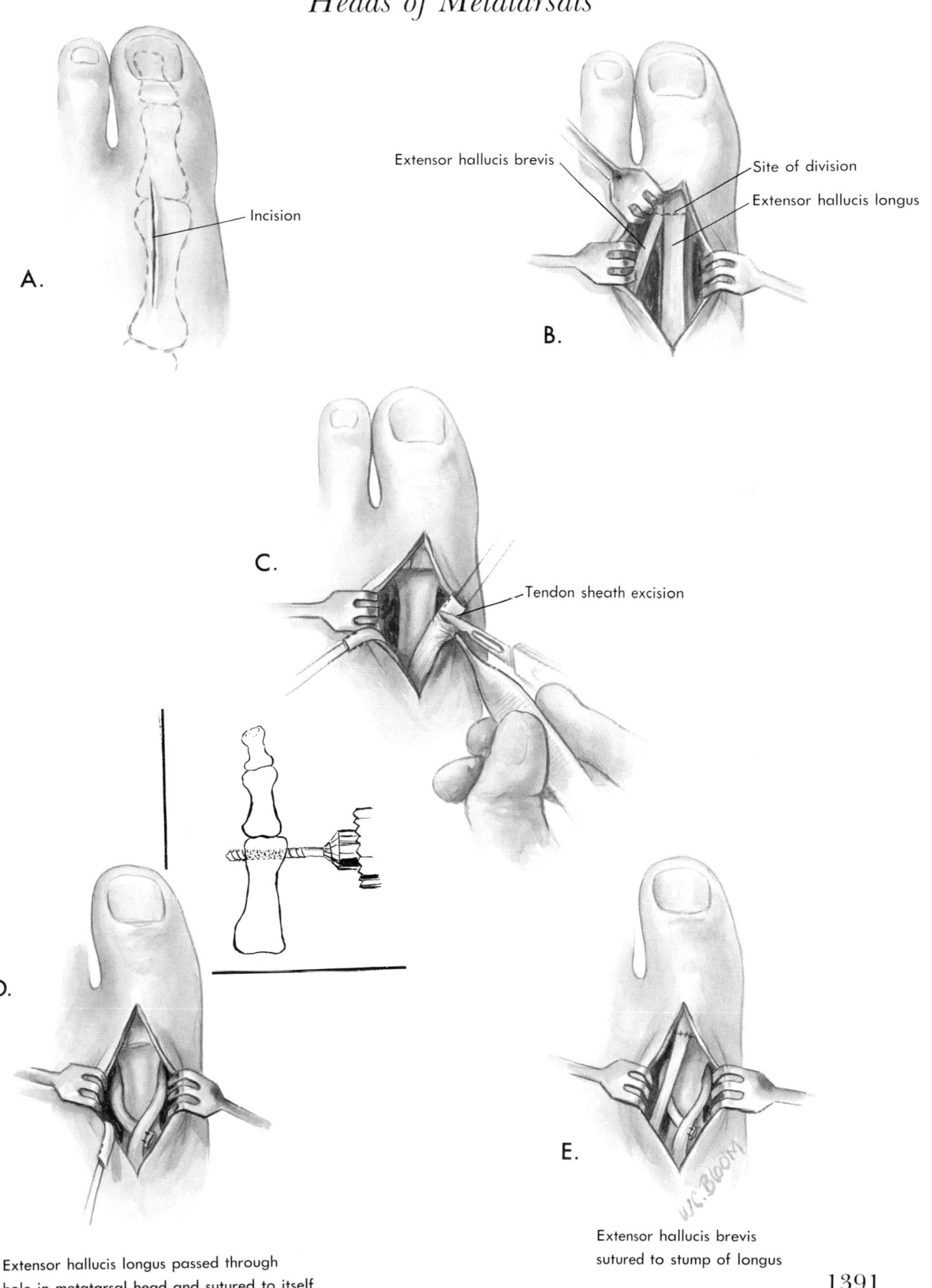

A.

Incision

B.

Extensor hallucis brevis

Site of division

Extensor hallucis longus

C.

Tendon sheath excision

D.

E.

Extensor hallucis longus passed through
hole in metatarsal head and sutured to itself

Extensor hallucis brevis
sutured to stump of longus

1391

Dorsal Wedge Resection for Pes Cavus

The dorsal aspect of the tarsal bones may be exposed by several means. Cole and Japas make a single dorsal longitudinal incision approximately 6 to 8 cm. long in the midline of the foot, centering over the midtarsal arch (naviculocuneiform junction). Subcutaneous tissue is divided, and the long toe extensors are identified and separated. The plane between the long extensor tendons of the second and third toes is developed, and the extensor digitorum brevis muscle is identified, elevated, and retracted laterally with the peroneus brevis tendon. The anterior tibial tendon and the long extensor tendons of the second and big toes are retracted medially. The periosteum is incised, longitudinally elevated, and retracted medially and laterally.[396, 409]

Méary makes two longitudinal incisions, each about 5 to 6 cm. in length on the dorsum of the foot. The medial incision is parallel to the longitudinal axis of the second metatarsal and is centered over the intermediate cuneiform bone. The extensor hallucis longus tendon, dorsalis pedis vessels, and the anterior tibial tendon are identified, dissected free, and retracted medially. The lateral incision is about 3 cm. long, and is centered about the cuboid bone. The peroneus brevis is identified and retracted laterally.

The author uses the following method of exposure of the dorsal and medial aspects of the foot:

THE PROCEDURE

A and **B.** Two longitudinal skin incisions are made. The medial incision, about 5 cm. long, is over the medial aspect of the navicular and first cuneiform bones in the interval between the anterior tibial and posterior tibial tendons. The subcutaneous tissue is divided. The anterior tibial tendon is retracted dorsally; the posterior tibial tendon is partially detached from the tuberosity of the navicular and is retracted plantarward to expose the medial and dorsal aspects of the navicular and first cuneiform bones. The lateral incision, about 4 cm. long, is centered over the cuboid bone. The extensor brevis muscle is identified, elevated, and retracted distally and laterally with the peroneus brevis tendon. The long toe extensors are retracted medially.

C. Next, through the medial wound, the capsule and periosteum of the navicular and first cuneiform bones are incised and elevated. The soft tissues are retracted dorsally and plantarward with Chandler elevator retractors. The capsule of the talonavicular joint should not be disturbed. If in doubt, one should take roentgenograms to identify the tarsal bones with certainty.

D and **E.** With osteotomes, a wedge of bone is excised, including the naviculo-cuneiform articulation. The base of the wedge is dorsal, its width depending upon the severity of the forefoot equinus deformity to be corrected. Through the lateral incision, the wedge osteotomy of the cuboid is completed.

F. The forefoot is then manipulated into dorsiflexion. If the plantar fascia is contracted, a plantar fasciotomy is performed. In severe cases the short plantar muscles are also sectioned. The first cuneiform bone should be dorsally displaced over the navicular bone. Two Steinmann pins are inserted to transfix the tarsal osteotomy. The medial pin is inserted into the shaft of the first metatarsal, directed posteriorly through the first cuneiform, across the osteotomy site into the navicular and the head of the talus. The lateral pin is started posteriorly along the longitudinal axis of the calcaneus, across the calcaneocuboid joint, into the cuboid and the base of the fifth metatarsal. (Méary uses staples to maintain position of the osteotomy.) Roentgenograms are taken to verify the position of the pins and the maintenance of correction of forefoot equinus deformity. The tourniquet is released and complete hemostasis is obtained. The incisions are closed. The pins are cut subcutaneously and a below-knee cast is applied.

POSTOPERATIVE CARE

The foot and leg are immobilized for eight weeks, at which time the cast, pins, and sutures are removed. A new below-knee walking cast is given—to be worn for another four weeks.

Plate 59. Dorsal Wedge Resection for Pes Cavus

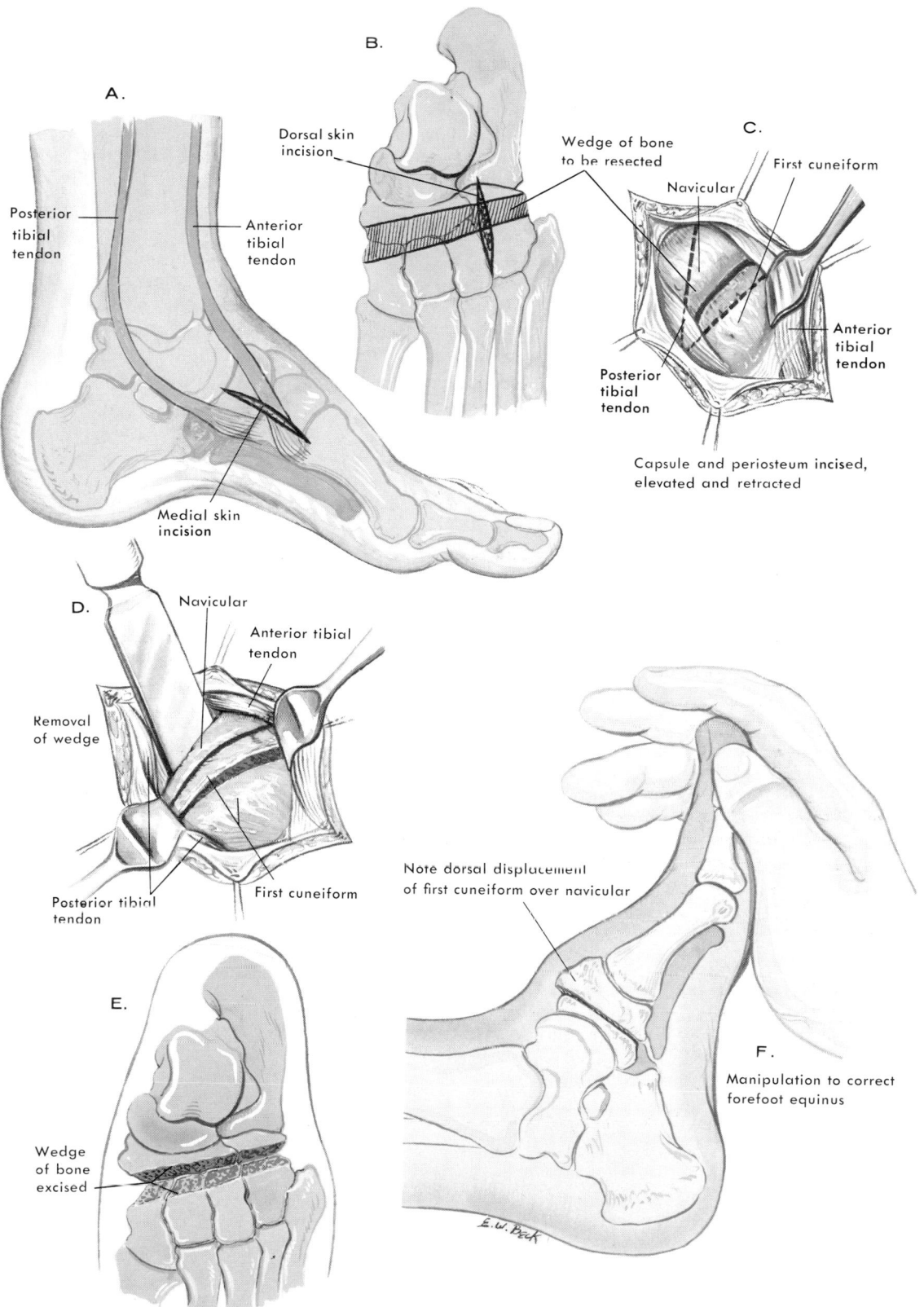

A.

Posterior tibial tendon

Anterior tibial tendon

Medial skin incision

B.

Dorsal skin incision

Wedge of bone to be resected

C.

First cuneiform

Navicular

Anterior tibial tendon

Posterior tibial tendon

Capsule and periosteum incised, elevated and retracted

D.

Navicular

Anterior tibial tendon

Removal of wedge

Posterior tibial tendon

First cuneiform

E.

Wedge of bone excised

Note dorsal displacement of first cuneiform over navicular

F.

Manipulation to correct forefoot equinus

E. W. Beck

1393

Dwyer Lateral Wedge Resection of Calcaneus for Pes Cavus

Forefoot equinus deformity is corrected first, either by plantar soft-tissue release or by dorsal wedge tarsal resection, depending upon the age of the patient and the severity of the deformity. Close-up wedge resection of the os calcis is designed to correct the varus deformity of the hindfoot in which the heel is of adequate height and size.

THE PROCEDURE

A. A 5 cm. long oblique incision is made on the lateral aspect of the calcaneus parallel to, but 1.5 cm. posterior and inferior to, the peroneus longus tendon. The subcutaneous tissue is divided and the wound flaps are retracted.

B and **C.** The peroneal tendons are identified and retracted dorsally and distally. The calcaneofibular ligament is sectioned and the periosteum is incised. The lateral surface of the calcaneus is subperiosteally exposed; with Chandler elevator retractors, the superior and inferior aspects of the calcaneus are partially exposed. With a pair of osteotomes of adequate width, a wedge of the os calcis with its base directed laterally is excised. The site of osteotomy is immediately inferior and posterior to the peroneus longus tendon. The medial cortex should be left intact. The width of the base of the wedge depends upon the severity of the varus deformity of the heel.

D. Next, a Steinmann pin is inserted transversely across the posterior segment of the calcaneus. The forefoot is dorsiflexed, putting tension on the Achilles tendon, and, the Steinmann pin serving as a lever, the bone gap is closed. The heel should be 5 degrees valgus. The wound is closed and a below-knee cast is applied, the pin incorporated in the cast.

POSTOPERATIVE CARE

The cast, pin, and sutures are removed in six weeks, by which time the osteotomy should be healed. A $\frac{1}{8}$- to $\frac{3}{16}$-inch lateral wedge on the heel (reverse Thomas) is worn for an additional 6 to 12 months.

Plate 60. Dwyer Lateral Wedge Resection of Calcaneus for Pes Cavus

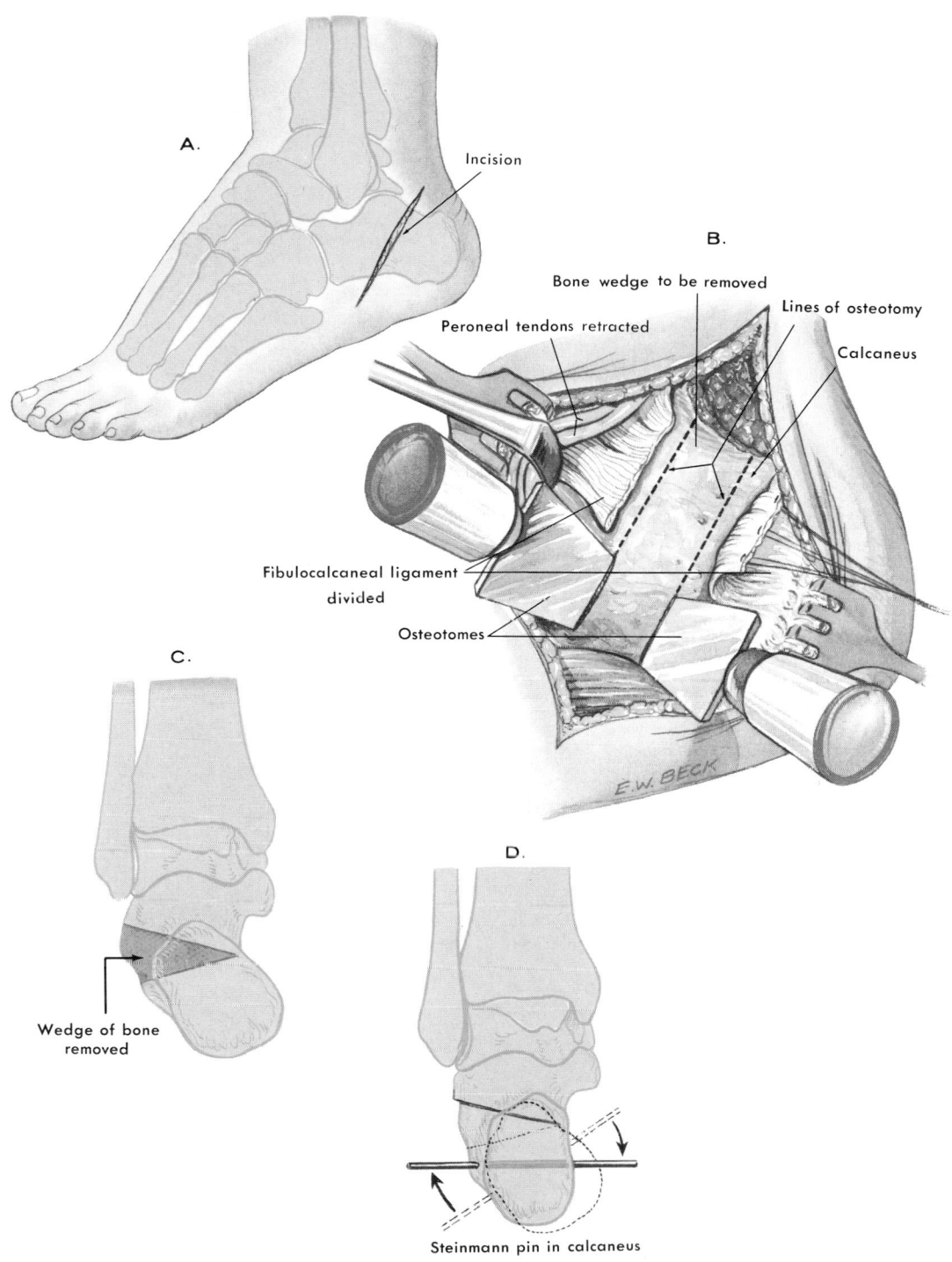

A.

Incision

B.

Bone wedge to be removed

Lines of osteotomy

Peroneal tendons retracted

Calcaneus

Fibulocalcaneal ligament divided

Osteotomes

C.

Wedge of bone removed

D.

Steinmann pin in calcaneus

E. W. BECK

the procedure will correct the deformity. Fowler's operation for pes cavovarus is based on sound principles, but the author has had no personal experience with it.

Lateral transfer of the anterior tibial tendon to decrease the inversion deformity in pes cavovarus should *not* be performed, because it will enhance the action of the peroneus longus as plantar-flexor of the first metatarsal.

PROCEDURES IN BONE

In the adolescent and adult patient with a skeletally mature foot, when structural changes have taken place in the tarsus and the forefoot is fixed in marked equinus position, bony procedures are indicated to correct the deformity. A number of operations have been described in the literature. As a rule, prior to performing bone operations, the contracted soft tissues on the plantar aspect of the foot should be released. These two procedures may then be combined, or may be performed in separate stages. Factors that determine the type of operation are the following:

1. *The location of the apex of cavus deformity,* whether at the midfoot, at the metatarsotarsal joints, or more posteriorly at the talonavicular and calcaneocuboid joints.

2. *The type of pes cavus.* Is it simple or is it a cavovarus foot? Is there pronation of the forefoot, particularly the first metatarsal?

3. *The nature of the hindfoot deformity.* Is the heel varus? How rigid is the inversion of the hindfoot? Or is there calcaneus or equinus deformity of the heel?

4. *The deformity of the toes.* Are they clawed? Is there painful plantar keratosis under the metatarsal heads?

5. *The degree and extent of associated muscle weakness.* Is it necessary to give stability to the foot when the deformity is corrected?

Procedures to Correct Forefoot Equinus Deformity

DORSAL TARSAL WEDGE OSTEOTOMY. Dorsal wedge resection at the level of the cuneiforms and cuboid bone was devised by Saunders and popularized by Cole.[396, 419] It is described and illustrated in Plate 59. The operation is based on sound principles. While preserving motion at the metatarsotarsal, midtarsal, and subtalar joints, it corrects the cavus deformity, provided the apex of the arch is at the midfoot. It should

always be combined with release of the contracted plantar soft tissues. Often equinus deformity of the first metatarsal will persist, necessitating a dorsiflexion osteotomy of the first metatarsal at its base or first metatarsocuneiform fusion for correction at a later stage. Wedge resection of the tarsus will shorten the foot — it should therefore never be performed in a skeletally immature foot. Circulatory insufficiency of the toes is a definite hazard, particularly when plantar soft-tissue release and dorsal wedge section are performed simultaneously. The procedure should not be combined with Dwyer osteotomy of the os calcis for correction of varus heel, since gangrene of the toes is a probable complication.

V-OSTEOTOMY OF THE TARSUS. This procedure for pes cavus is described by Japas.[409] The apex of the "V" is located proximally at the height of the curve; the lateral limb of the "V" extends to the cuboid, and the medial limb to the first cuneiform. The foot is not shortened by resection of a bone wedge. The forefoot is elevated by depressing the base of the distal fragment plantarward. The procedure lengthens the concave plantar surface of the foot. Japas recommends the operation in children six or more years of age. The author has had no personal experience with the procedure, and the reader is referred to the original article of Japas for technical details.[409]

Metatarsotarsal Wedge Resection and Fusion. This is indicated in the fully grown foot when the apex of the cavus deformity is located at the metatarsotarsal area. In the skeletally immature foot, osteotomies of the bases of the metatarsals are performed in order not to disturb growth. The surgical exposure of the bases of the metatarsals and the tarsometatarsal joints is described and illustrated in Plate 54. The shape of the osteotomy is cuneiform, with a buttress based plantarward. In order to avoid sloughing of the skin edges, the wound flaps should be retracted gently and the cast should be well padded on the dorsum of the foot. Hypercorrection will result in painful bony prominences at the bases of the metatarsals. Rotational malalignment or adduction or abduction of the distal fragments will produce deformities of the forefoot.

Fusion of the First Metatarsocuneiform Joint. McElvenny and Caldwell proposed that varus distortion of the hindfoot in pes cavovarus is caused by pronation of the first metatarsal. They recommended elevation and supination of the first metatarsal and fusion of the first metatarsocuneiform joint in this position. The naviculocuneiform joint is also fused if the forefoot drops into equinus position in this area. They stressed that only the first metatarsal should be supinated, not the entire forefoot. If the pes cavovarus deformity is fixed, they recommended plantar fasciotomy and a series of stretching casts to correct the hindfoot varus deformity and to provide flexibility to the forefoot.[414]

Dorsal Wedge Resection and Fusion of Talonavicular and Calcaneocuboid Joints. This is carried out when the apex of pes cavus is more posterior in the midtarsal area. It is usually combined with subtalar fusion to correct any hindfoot varus distortion if present. In paralytic pes cavovarus, triple arthrodesis will provide stability and at the same time correct the deformity.

Vertical Osteotomy of Medial Cuneiform. The vertical osteotomy with a wedge of bone graft based on the plantar aspect was recommended by Fowler et al. to elevate the first metatarsal into dorsiflexion as described earlier.[400]

Close-up Lateral Wedge Osteotomy of Calcaneus (Dwyer). This is combined with a release of contracted soft tissues on the plantar aspect of the foot for correction of varus hindfoot.[399] The vertical height of the hindfoot is an important consideration. The operation should only be performed in children over eight years of age; the operative technique is described and illustrated in Plate 60.

Sesamoidectomy. In the adult patient, irritation of the sesamoids under the first metatarsal head causes them to hypertrophy and become inflamed. Axial views demonstrate enlargement of the sesamoids and irregularity on their plantar surface. In such an instance, excision of one or both sesamoid bones affords complete symptomatic relief.

Subtotal Excision of the Talus. This may be indicated in a paralyzed cavovarus foot. Occasionally *amputation of the toes* is carried out if they are so deformed and inflamed that fitting shoes poses a formidable problem.

Pronated Feet

Pronated feet are feet that, on weight-bearing, assume a valgus deformity caused by ligamentous laxity, which is often a familial trait. When not bearing weight, the pronated feet have normal contour and longitudinal arches; however, under the incumbent body weight, the heel everts and the forefoot is twisted outward, with the center of gravity of the body over or medial to the first metatarsal bone (Fig. 7–60 A). Normally the weight falls on the second ray, which is the center of the foot. The associated generalized ligamentous laxity is also evident in hyperextensibility of the elbows, wrists, thumbs, and knees.

Pronated feet are very common in children. The condition is frequently referred to as "flatfoot," a loose term used to denote any deformity of the foot in which there is lowering of its longitudinal arch; however, there are many causes of pes planovalgus and one should be more exact in his terminology.

The pronated foot is mechanically weak, as the ligaments that support the tarsal bones are under excessive stress because of the medial displacement of body weight. It is not the flatness of the longitudinal arch, but rather the medial shift in weight-bearing that is the important factor in producing foot strain.

The child with pronated feet toes-in actively so that the center of gravity of the body is shifted laterally toward the center of the foot (Fig. 7–60 B). That such toeing-in is Nature's way of protecting a child's foot and is therefore good for him should be explained to the parents, who may find it difficult to comprehend, especially when they have sought medical advice because their child is toeing-in. The toeing-in is not a fixed forefoot adduction like metatarsus varus. In stance, however, the foot is valgus. Prolonged standing is likely to give rise to foot strain, with pain in the longitudinal arch, abnormal fatigue, and discomfort extending upward on the legs.

When there is associated myostatic con-

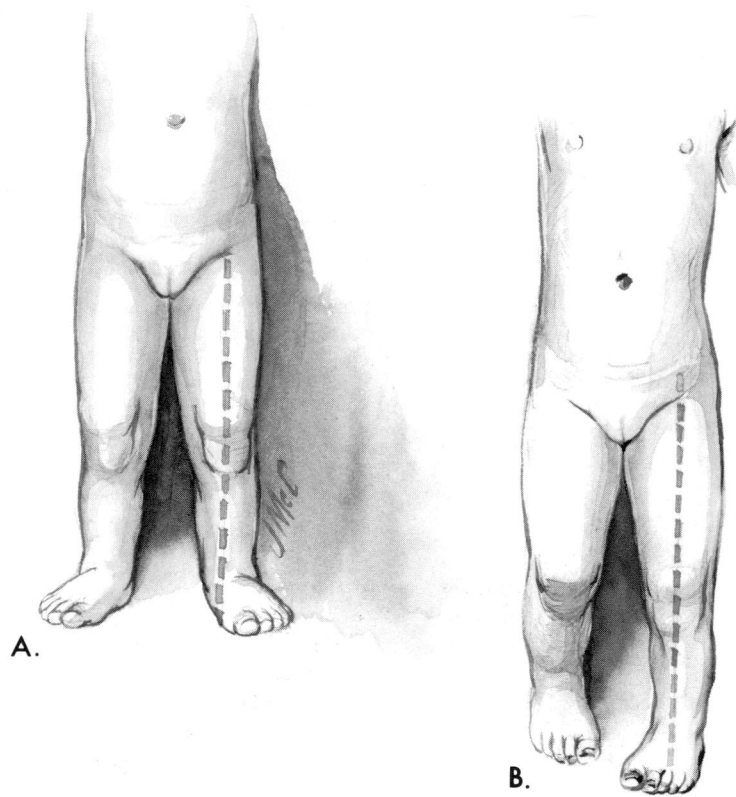

FIGURE 7–60.   *Pronated feet.*

A. In stance, the center of gravity of the body is over or medial to the first metatarsal bone. **B.** Protective toeing-in—so that the body weight is shifted laterally toward the center of the foot.

tracture of the triceps surae muscles (the hypermobile flatfoot with short tendo Achillis of Harris and Beath[437]), foot pronation will be more severe and the child will be unable to protect his feet naturally by toeing-in. This permanent shortening of the triceps surae muscle (the so-called "tightness of heel cords") is best demonstrated by testing the range of passive dorsiflexion of the ankle with the hindfoot in slight inversion or neutral position (never valgus) and the knee in neutral extension. The angle that the plantar aspect of the foot makes with the longitudinal axis of the leg is observed from the fibular side. During this test, the dorsiflexors of the ankle should not be made to contract actively, as their contraction will cause reciprocal relaxation of the gastrocnemius-soleus muscles.

Discomfort or pain of any consequence is unusual in the child with pronated feet, though faulty shoes or abusive use of the feet may give rise to symptoms. Prolonged bed rest due to ill health will increase the ligamentous laxity and consequently exaggerate pronation of the feet.

In adult life, structural changes gradually develop in the tarsal bones and the planovalgus deformity becomes rigid. Eventually foot strain and pain become disabling symptoms. Adult women tend to have more pain in the forepart of the foot (the so-called anterior or transverse arch) because of wearing shoes with high heels, which causes the weight to be transmitted to the metatarsal heads cramped in the narrow forepart of the shoe.

Treatment

Measures are directed toward making the child stand and walk more efficiently. The shoes should support the heel well and provide adequate room for the forefoot. The weight-bearing forces should be shifted laterally to prevent foot strain. A common practice is to use a wedged raise (1/8 to 3/16 inch) on the medial side of the heel, the aim of which is to tilt the hindfoot into inversion; however, this will not be accomplished if the uprights of the heel of the shoe do not grasp the heel snugly, as the hindfoot will simply twist into eversion. Additional support to the longitudinal arch may then be desirable, in the form of a 3/8-inch-thick flexible felt, leather, or rubber pad. In the older child with severe pes valgus, more rigid and effective support is indicated in the form of a modified Whitman plate with a lateral flange (Fig. 7–61), or the Helfet, Schwartz, Rose, or UCB shoe inserts.[438, 452]

The child with markedly pronated feet should not be permitted to walk barefoot on hard terrain; however, he can go without shoes on sand at the beach or on grass. Active exercises such as toe curling or picking up objects with the toes or tip-toe walking have no therapeutic value unless there is weakness of the muscles that control the foot. The shortened triceps surae muscle is stretched by passive exercises, manually or against the wall (Fig. 7–62).

Surgical Management

Operative correction of pes planovalgus is indicated when the deformity is so marked that it causes rapid abnormal wear of the shoes (Fig. 7–63), or the discomfort in the foot persists despite proper conservative measures and limits the patient from taking part in normal activities. However, surgery should not be considered before the age of ten years.

In the literature a number of operative procedures have been described for correction of pes planovalgus.* The author does not recommend ligamentous tightening and tendon advancement operations, as, in general, they do not stand the stresses of body weight, and the deformity recurs.

Hoke, in 1931, introduced naviculocuneiform fusion for correction of flexible pes planus.[442] Butte, in 1937, reported unsatisfactory results in 50 per cent of the cases of naviculocuneiform fusion for "flatfoot."[430] Crego and Ford, in 1952, condemned the

*See References 430, 431, 434–436, 442–447, 449, 450, 453, 456, 457.

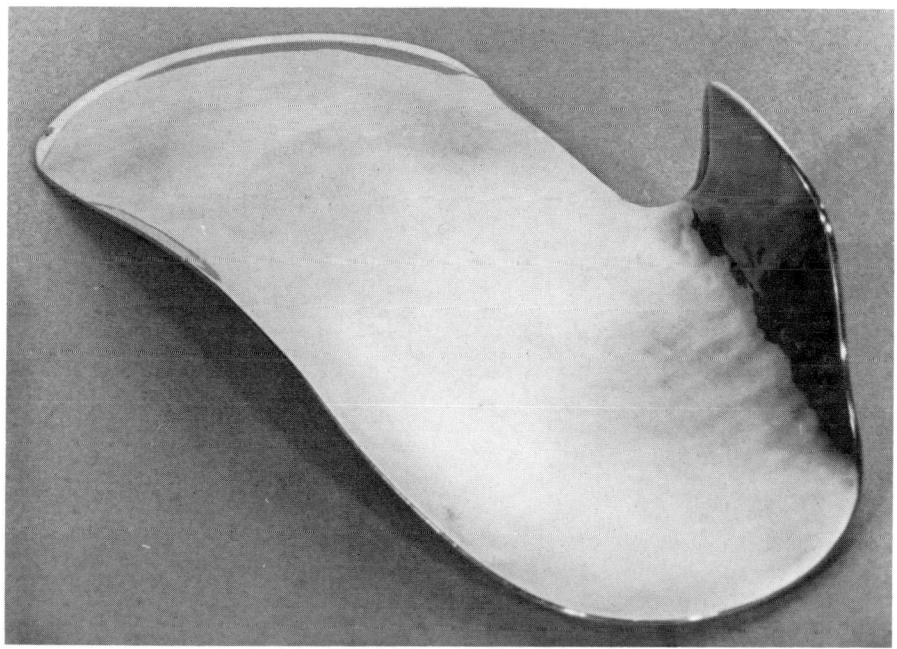

FIGURE 7–61. Modified Whitman foot plate with a lateral flange.

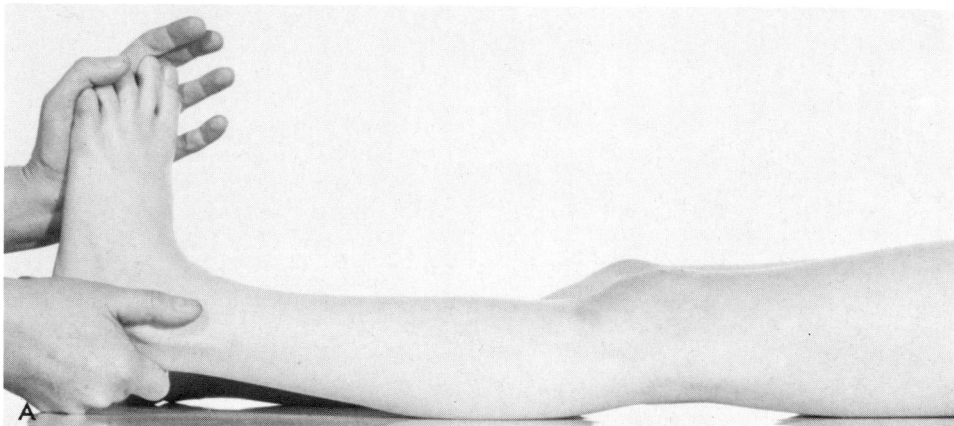

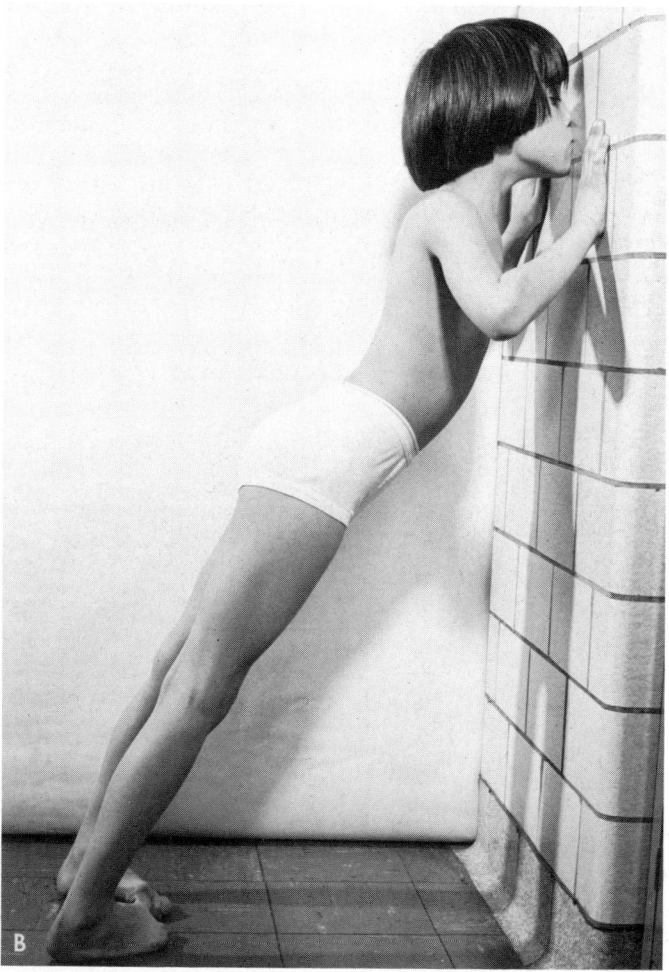

FIGURE 7–62.   *Passive stretching of contracted triceps surae muscle.*

A. Manual stretching by the parents. Note the knee should be in extended position and the hindfoot slightly in-verted. The child should not actively dorsiflex the ankle, as contraction of the anterior tibial muscle will relax the gastrocnemius-soleus muscles—its reciprocal antagonists. The maximally dorsiflexed position is maintained to the count of 10 and then relaxed. Exercises are performed 20 times each at three sessions a day. **B.** Passive stretching of triceps surae muscles against the wall is indicated in the older cooperative child. Note the feet are in inversion. The knees should not be hyperextended.

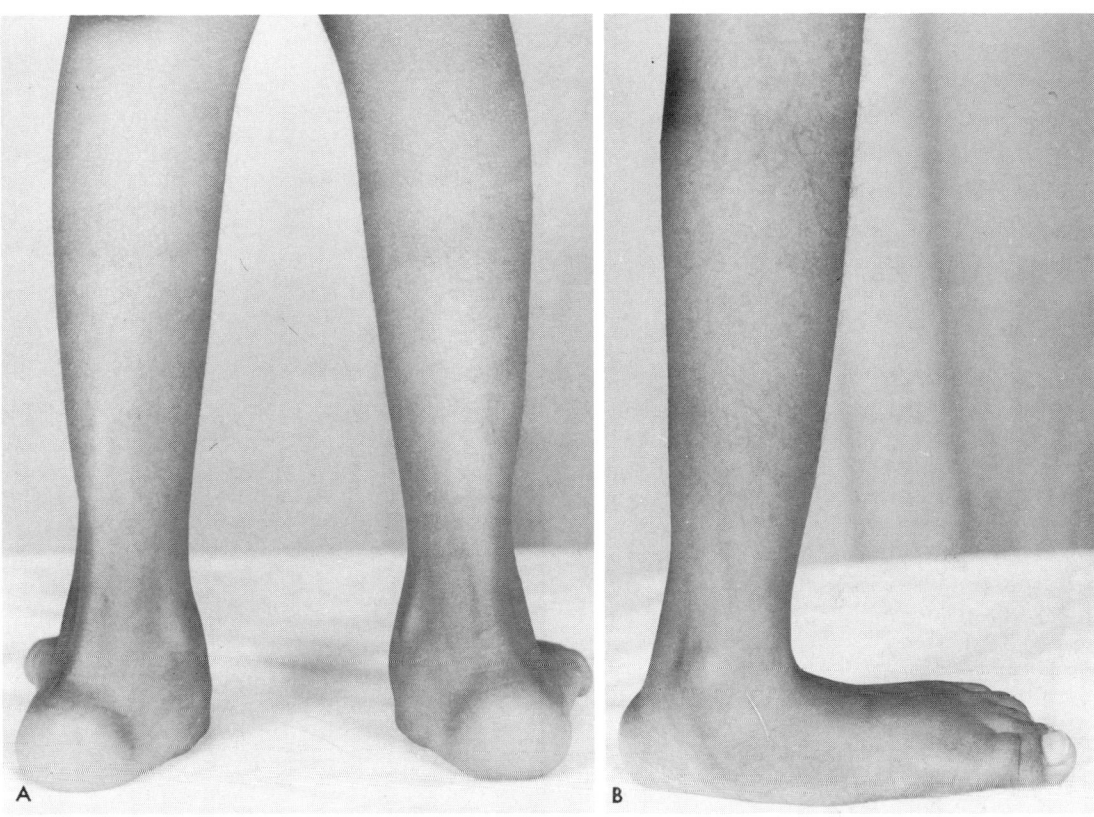

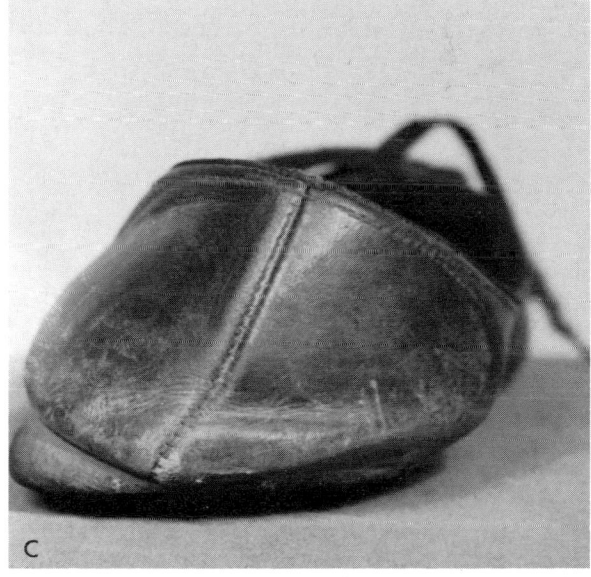

FIGURE 7-63. *Severe pronation of both feet in an eight-year-old girl.*

Surgical correction of deformity is indicated in such a case. **A.** Posterior view of both feet and legs. **B.** Medial view of left foot. **C.** Abnormal wear of the left shoe.

operation as being insufficient to support the flattened longitudinal arch.[434] Jack, in 1953, reported the results of naviculocuneiform fusion in 46 feet in 25 patients, aged 11 to 14 years, with flexible "flatfoot" with a break at the naviculocuneiform joint;15 months to five years after operation, the results were excellent in 54 per cent, good in 28 per cent, and unsatisfactory in 18 per cent. Jack stressed the importance of proper selection of patients.[443] Seymour, in 1967, reassessed 17 of the 25 patients on whom Jack had operated, 16 to 19 years after surgery. The results were excellent in 31 per cent, good in 19 per cent, and unsatisfactory in 50 per cent. Seymour pointed out that it is unlikely that only naviculocuneiform ligaments are affected and solely responsible for the flattening of the medial longitudinal arch, and that stabilization of only one segment of the complex cannot be expected to prevent collapse of the entire arch. He also cautioned that the procedure will cause degenerative arthritis in the adjacent joints, which are subjected to additional load and stress following naviculocuneiform arthrodesis.[454]

Miller described an operation in which the articulations between the navicular and medial cuneiform, and between the medial cuneiform and first metatarsal are fused in corrected position, and in which the calcaneonavicular ligament and posterior tibial tendon are transferred distally, thus tightening the "sling" that supports the medial longitudinal arch and holds up the head of the talus in normal relationship with the anterior end of the calcaneus.[449] In the standing lateral roentgenogram, if the location of the sag is at the naviculocuneiform and medial cuneiform–first metatarsal joint, and the hindfoot valgus inclination does not exceed 10 to 15 degrees, one can expect a satisfactory result from the Miller operation in the majority of cases, provided the patient is not overweight. In the experience of the author, however, the adolescent patient who has disabling pes valgus that requires surgical correction rarely meets the criteria for the Miller procedure. It is almost always the severe valgus deformity of the hindfoot that causes abnormal wear of the shoes and disability.

Lowman fuses the talonavicular joint and transfers the anterior tibial tendon dorsally to the navicular bone, providing a dynamic force to elevate the apex of the medial longitudinal arch.[447] Young transfers the anterior tibial tendon to the dorsal aspect of the navicular without fusion of the talonavicular joint.[456] The author has had no experience with the Lowman or Young operations.

As stated before, in the severely pronated foot, it is the valgus hindfoot that causes disability and requires surgical correction. The recommended procedure is Grice subtalar extra-articular arthrodesis; if there is significant valgus deformity in the midfoot, a triple arthrodesis is performed when the foot is skeletally mature.[435, 445, 453] The author has had no experience with the Chambers or reverse Dwyer operations.

Affections of the Toes

HALLUX RIGIDUS

Pain and stiffness in the metatarsophalangeal joint of the great toe are quite common in adults, but occur in children only very occasionally. The condition is referred to by a variety of terms—hallux rigidus (Cotterill), hallux flexus (Davies-Colley), hallux dolorosus (Walsham and Hughes), and metatarsus primus elevatus (Lambrinudi).[462, 463, 471, 477]

Etiology

In adolescent patients, hallux rigidus is often a familial affliction. Bonney and MacNab report that 50 per cent of patients with onset of symptoms prior to the age of 20 had a positive family history.[459] The condition is more preponderant in females. Hallux rigidus may be caused either by intrinsic disorders of the metatarsophalangeal joint or by extrinsic mechanical abnormalities acting on the joint.

ELEVATION OF FIRST METATARSAL

Lambrinudi observed that hallux rigidus is associated with dorsal hyperextension of the first metatarsal.[471] In about two thirds of the cases of Jack, and of Bonney and Mac-Nab, metatarsus primus elevatus was found in hallux rigidus.[459, 466] Kessel and Bonney reported two adult patients with acquired metatarsus primus elevatus (one resulting from an osteotomy of the first metatarsal done for hallux valgus and the other following triple arthrodesis) who developed typical hallux rigidus later. Thus evidence was presented that in some patients, hyperextension of the first metatarsal is the primary deformity and hallux rigidus secondary; however, it must be added that cases have been seen in which metatarsus primus elevatus developed following the operative production of a stiff and painful first metatarsophalangeal joint.[469] The question of which is the cause and which the effect in adolescent hallux rigidus has not, as yet, been answered.

RELATIVE LENGTH OF FIRST AND SECOND METATARSALS

Nilsonne observed that most of his adolescent patients with hallux rigidus had long narrow feet with a first metatarsal that was longer than the second.[474] This finding was also noted by Bonney and MacNab in 22 of the 53 feet examined, with the discrepancy in length of 0.5 cm. or more.[459] The common association of a long great toe with hallux rigidus was also noted by McMurray.[472]

STRESS ON FIRST METATARSOPHALANGEAL JOINT

A number of conditions predispose to excessive pressure on the base of the proximal phalanx of the great toe. In hallux rigidus, the feet are frequently pronated and the center of gravity of body weight is shifted toward the first metatarsal head.[467] Bingold and Collins proposed that the cause of hallux rigidus is an abnormal gait developed either to protect an injured or inflamed metatarsophalangeal joint from the pressure of weight-bearing, or to stabilize a hypermobile first metatarsal. As a result, excessive pressure is transmitted from the flexor hallucis brevis tendon and the two sesamoids to the base of the first phalanx and the great toe. They found evidence of this abnormal gait in the peculiarities of wear seen in old shoes and observed a high correlation between unilateral hallux rigidus and the patient's footedness.[458]

LOCAL INFLAMMATION OF THE JOINT

In some cases, a definite history of injury precipitates these symptoms and traumatic arthritis may be a factor. In other patients, hallux rigidus may be a local manifestation of generalized rheumatoid arthritis or pauciarticular arthritis.

OSTEOCHONDRITIS DISSECANS OF FIRST METATARSAL HEAD

This may be an occasional cause of hallux rigidus (Fig. 7–64). Increased density and fragmentation of the epiphysis of the proximal phalanx of the great toe was considered by Glissan to represent aseptic necrosis of bone, similar to Legg-Perthes disease of the femoral head.[464] Pathologic studies by Bingold and Collins have demonstrated that the increased density of the epiphysis of the proximal phalanx is caused by close packing of live trabeculae, and that fragmentation of the epiphysis represents irregular ossification, not aseptic necrosis. Similar changes are observed in normal feet of adolescents; they are of no etiologic significance in hallux rigidus.[458]

Clinical Features

The presenting complaint is pain in and around the metatarsophalangeal joint of the great toe. Usually the symptoms are of gradual onset, developing in adolescence. Occasionally pain occurs suddenly, precipitated by acute trauma. It is aggravated by walking or rising on the toes and is relieved by rest.

Abnormal patterns of wear in the shoes is suggestive of hallux rigidus. The shoes are often too narrow and short, and show excessive wear on the outer side of the heel, the posterior half of the sole, and under the terminal phalanx of the great toe. The uppers are bulged outward over the outer side of the heel and the posterior half of the sole.

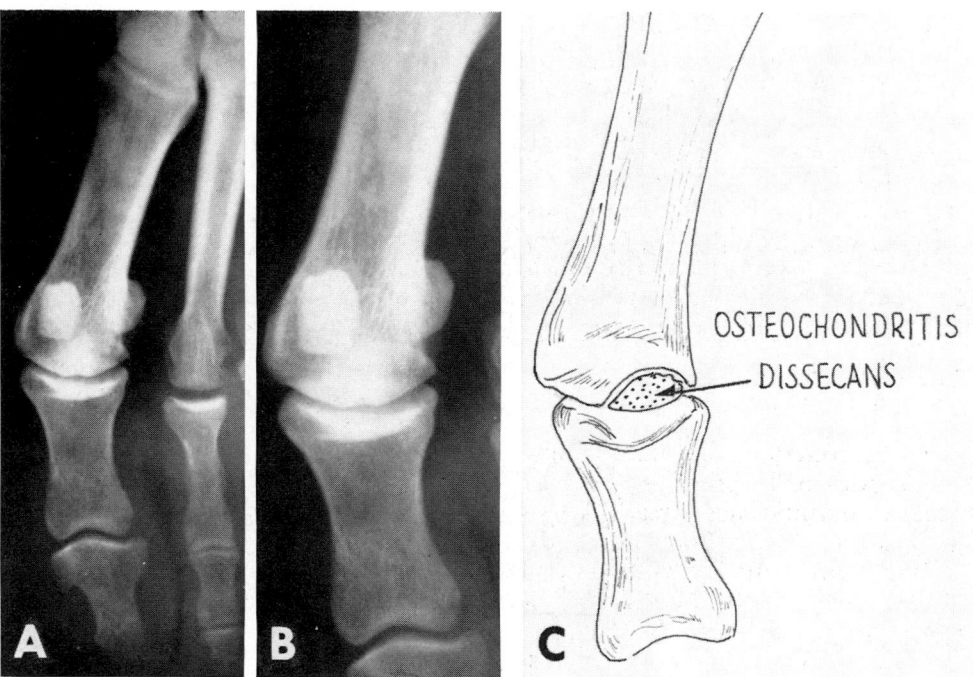

FIGURE 7–64. *Osteochondritis dissecans of the first metatarsal head.*

This condition is an occasional cause of hallux rigidus. (From Kelikian, H.: Hallux Valgus, Allied Deformities of the Forefoot and Metatarsalgia. Philadelphia, W. B. Saunders Co., 1965, p. 273.)

Their toe spring is shortened, and there are furrows over the medial side of the toe cap caused by the hypermobile interphalangeal joint of the great toe.[458]

The feet of these patients are long and narrow, and are usually pronated. The base of the first metatarsal is pushed plantarward and its head is tilted dorsally. The first metatarsophalangeal joint is enlarged and the great toe is held in a varying degree of flexion (hallux flexus). There is a callosity underneath the base of the proximal phalanx of the great toe, but the skin on the plantar aspect of the first metatarsal head is smooth (lacking its normal thickness). On palpation the metatarsophalangeal joint of the great toe is found to be tender and thickened. In severe cases one may palpate osteophytes at the articular margins. Active extension of the metatarsophalangeal joint is markedly restricted, but in the early stages of the disease, flexion is within normal range. Attempted passive dorsiflexion of the great toe is very painful and limited in range (Fig. 7–65). Passive motions of the joint may be accompanied by crepitus. A taut flexor hallucis brevis may be palpated on the plantar aspect. The interphalangeal joint of the great toe is hypermobile in adolescents; in adults, it may be restricted and somewhat painful.

There is a rare variety of hallux rigidus referred to as *hallux extensus* in which the first metatarsal is plantar-flexed and the great toe is fixed in hyperextension at the metatarsophalangeal joint (Fig. 7–66).

Roentgenographic Features

Early in the course of the disease, thickening of the soft tissues around the affected joint is observed. In the standing lateral roentgenogram of the foot, the first metatarsal is hyperextended, with its head tilting dorsally. Later on, the articular cartilage space becomes narrowed and eventually obliterated. Soon osteophytes form at the joint margins (Fig. 7–67).

Treatment

Initially conservative treatment should always be tried. The sole of the shoe between the shank and toe portions medially

under the first metatarsal head is stiffened. A slightly larger shoe with its leather softened dorsally over the first metatarsophalangeal joint will give symptomatic relief. Passive manipulative exercises are performed several times a day to increase the range of dorsiflexion of the great toe. In most cases, with conservative management, the symptoms will regress if the joint is protected for a few weeks or months. If the symptoms persist and disability remains moderately severe, operative correction of the deformity is required.

In these resistant cases, Kessel and Bonney (following an earlier suggestion of Bonney and MacNab) perform an extension osteotomy at the base of the proximal phalanx of the great toe, converting the normal range of plantar flexion at the metatarsophalangeal joint to a functional range of dorsiflexion and plantar flexion (Fig. 7–68).

The operative technique is as follows:

A curved dorsal incision about 4 cm. long is made, centering over the base of the proximal phalanx. The subcutaneous tissue is divided. The extensor hallucis longus tendon and digital nerves are retracted to one side to expose the proximal phalanx and metatarsophalangeal joint of the great toe. With small osteotomes, a wedge of bone with a dorsal base of predetermined width is resected from the phalanx as far proximally as possible. The cortex and periosteum on the plantar aspect are left intact. It is best to use drill holes to mark and control the extent of osteotomy. The phalanx is angulated dorsally to close the gap. One or two Kirschner wires are placed obliquely to keep the osteotomized fragments firmly together. The wound is closed and a below-knee walking cast with a sturdy toe plate is applied. The great toe should be held in extension by appropriate padding underneath. In four to six weeks the osteotomy will heal.

Kessel and Bonney report satisfactory results following surgery, with a mean improvement of dorsiflexion from 5 degrees before operation to 44 degrees afterward.[469]

Watermann, in 1927, recommended a cuneiform osteotomy of the head of the first metatarsal with the base of the wedge directed dorsally and including the hypertrophic spurs (Fig. 7–68 A) [478] Kelikian recommends the Watermann osteotomy in growing children in order to avoid injury to the growth plate of the proximal phalanx.[468]

(*Text continued on page 1410.*)

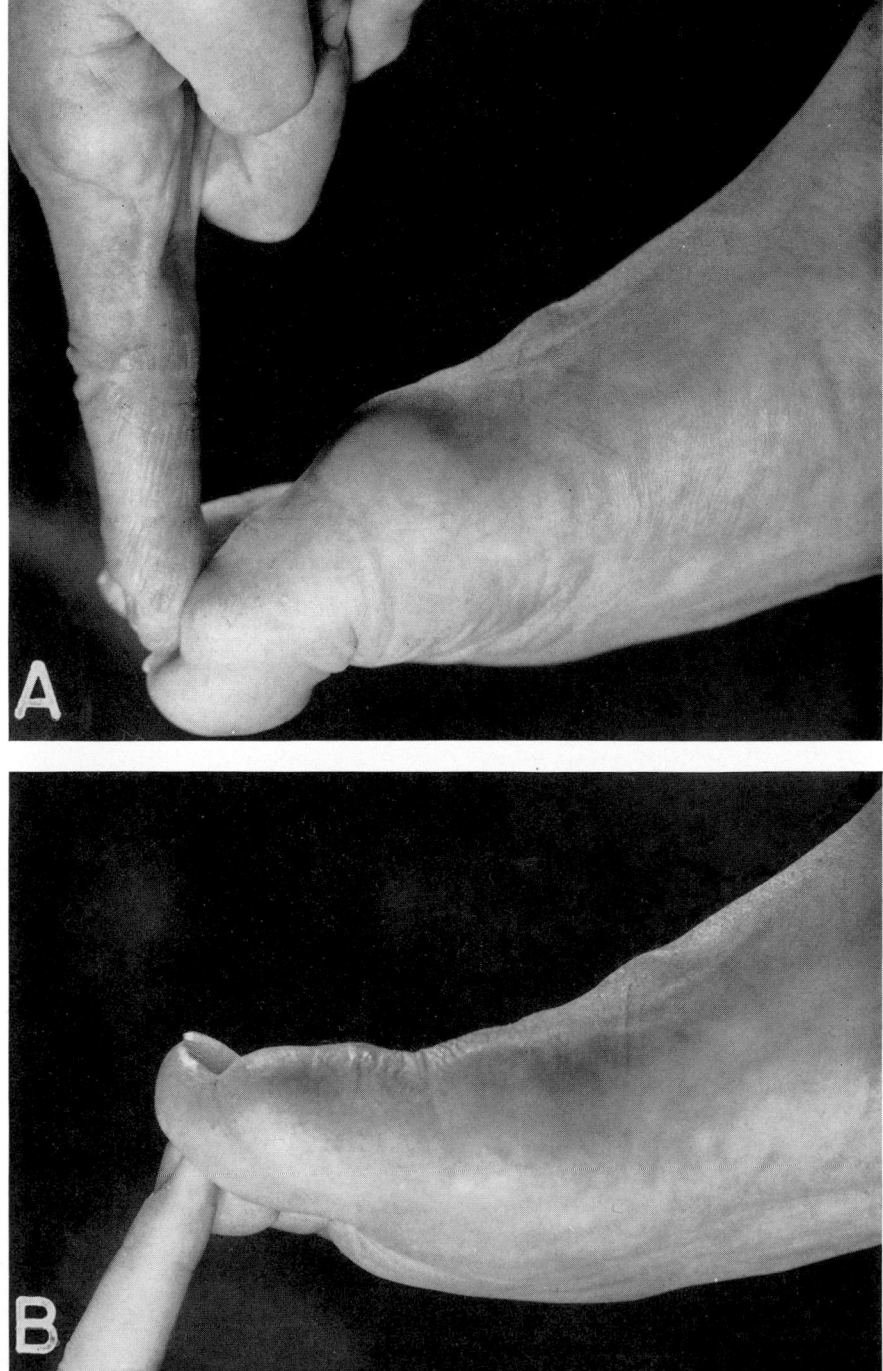

FIGURE 7–65.   Hallus rigidus.

The metatarsophalangeal joint is enlarged, and dorsiflexion of the great toe is markedly limited. (From Kelikian, H.: Hallux Valgus, Allied Deformities of the Forefoot and Metatarsalgia. Philadelphia, W. B. Saunders Co., 1965, p. 268.)

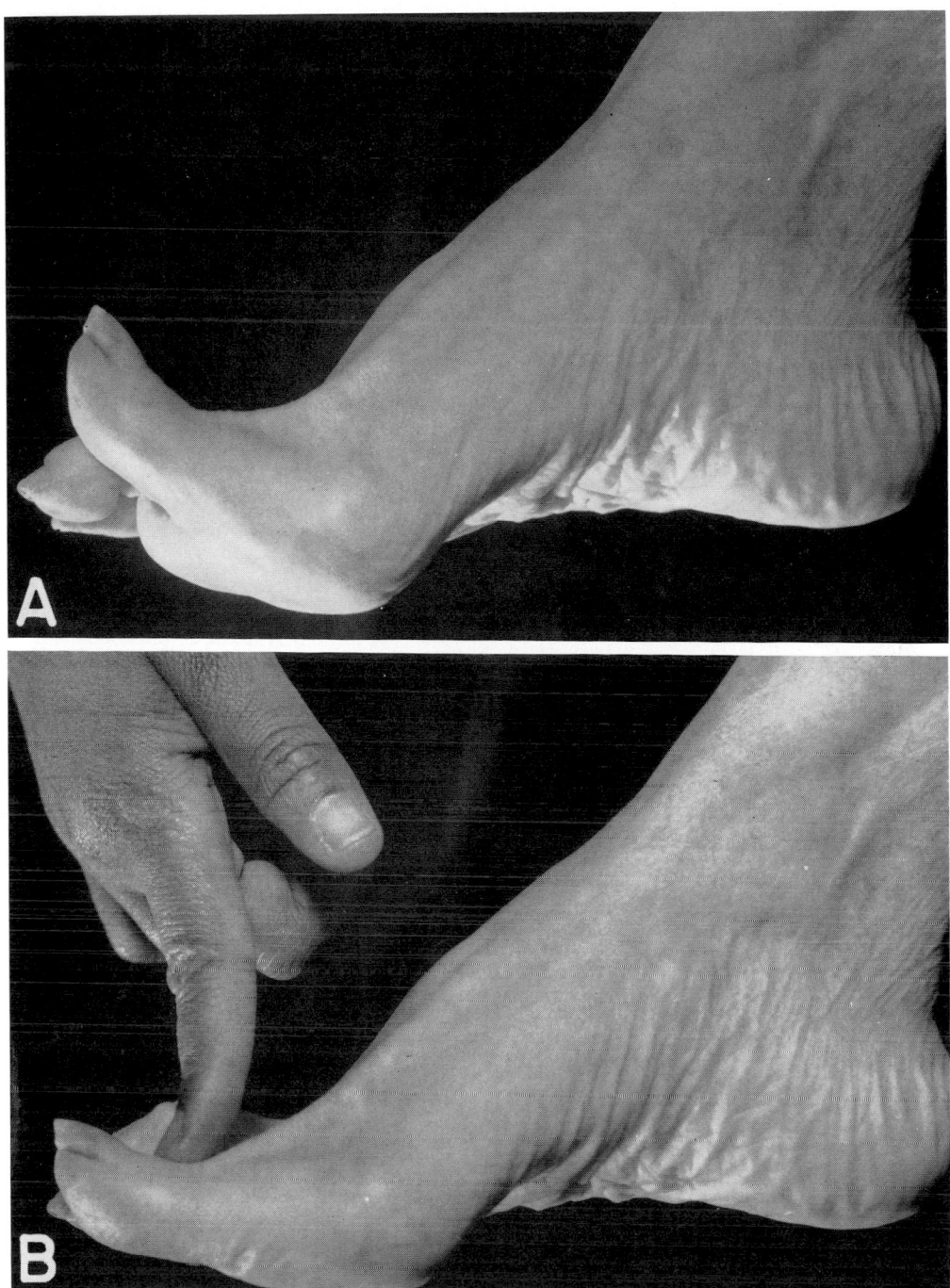

FIGURE 7–66. Hallux extensus.

A rare variety of hallux rigidus in which the first metatarsal is plantar-flexed and the great toe is held in hyperextension at the metatarsophalangeal joint. Note the hallux cannot be pushed plantarward. (From Kelikian, H.: Hallux Valgus, Allied Deformities of the Forefoot and Metatarsalgia. Philadelphia, W. B. Saunders Co., 1965, p. 269.)

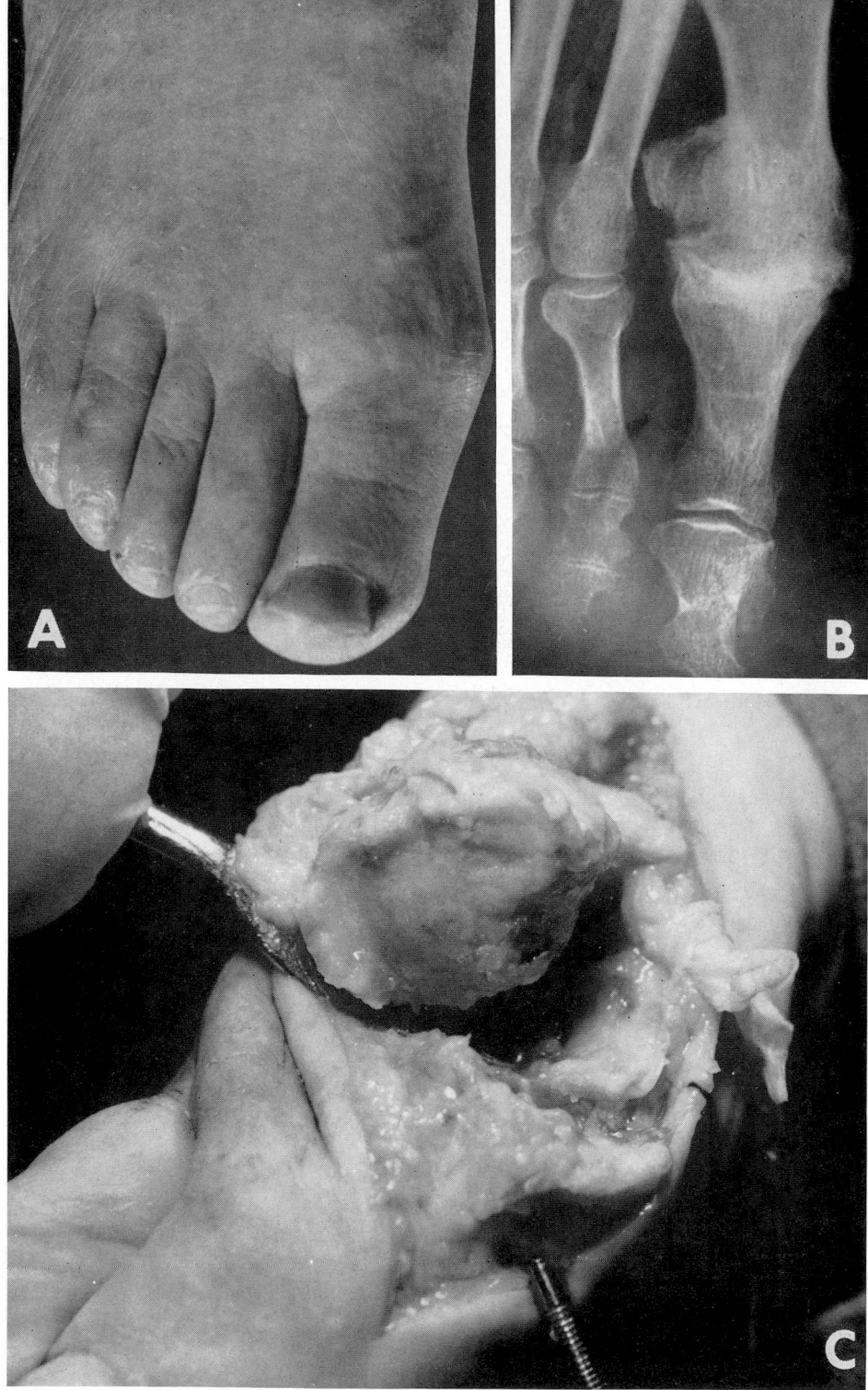

FIGURE 7–67. Hallux rigidus. *See opposite page for legend.*

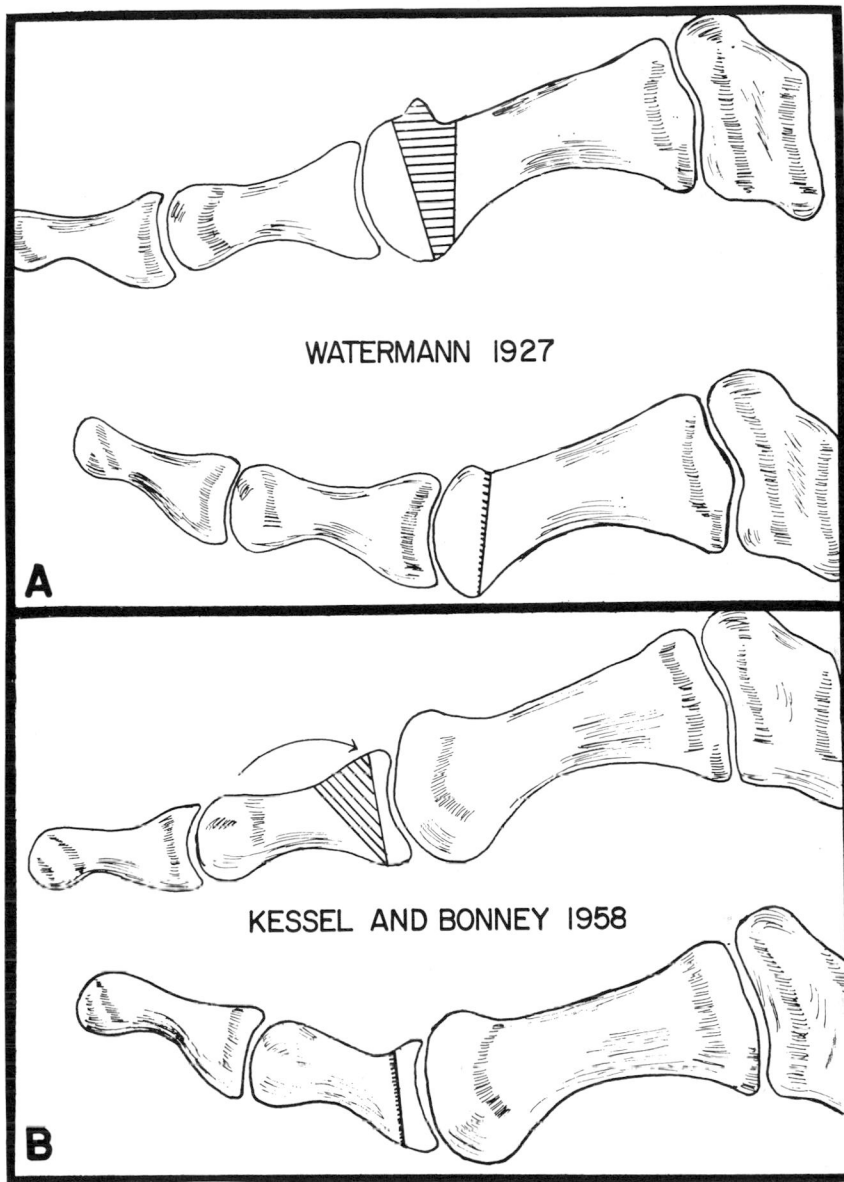

FIGURE 7–68. Operative treatment of hallux rigidus.

A. Watermann's cuneiform osteotomy of the first metatarsal head. Base of the wedge is directed dorsally and includes the hypertrophic spurs. **B.** Kessel and Bonney osteotomy. (From Kelikian, H.: Hallux Valgus, Allied Deformities of the Forefoot and Metatarsalgia. Philadelphia, W. B. Saunders Co., 1965, p. 280.)

FIGURE 7–67. Hallux rigidus.

A. Photograph of the forefoot, showing enlargement of the first metatarsophalangeal joint. **B.** Roentgenograms. Note the degenerative changes — the articular cartilage space is obliterated and osteophytes have formed at the joint margins. **C.** Findings at operation. The hyaline articular cartilage is eroded, the synovium is thickened, and there is marked proliferation of new bone. (From Kelikian, H.: Hallux Valgus, Allied Deformities of the Forefoot and Metatarsalgia. Philadelphia, W. B. Saunders Co., 1965, p. 271.)

A plantar capsulotomy of the first metatarsophalangeal joint is performed if it is contracted and limits extension. One may have to release the flexor hallucis brevis from the proximal phalanx.

Whether extension osteotomy of the base of the proximal phalanx or the first metatarsal head will prevent the development of hallux rigidus in adult life has not been determined, as long-term follow-ups are not available. If metatarsus primus elevatus is the primary cause of hallux rigidus, the symptoms being due to restriction of dorsiflexion of the first metatarsophalangeal joint, extension osteotomy of the base of the first phalanx is worth a trial.

Depression of the first metatarsal head by a wedge osteotomy (with its base on the plantar aspect) was recommended by Jack.[466] This may prevent the development of hallux rigidus; however, experience with this procedure is limited.

In the adult in whom hallux rigidus is symptomatic and disabling, resection of the proximal half of the first phalanx of the great toe is recommended. If the sesamoid bones are involved in the arthritic process, they are also excised.

When hallux valgus is accompanied by metatarsalgia, Kelikian recommends fusion of the metatarsophalangeal joint of the great toe; in such an instance, the distal third of the second metatarsal is resected and its digit is syndactylized with the first or third toe.[468]

HAMMER TOE

Hammer toe is a deformity characterized by flexion contracture of the proximal interphalangeal joint. The distal interphalangeal joint may be in flexion, in neutral extension, or in slight hyperextension. Eventually, with depression of the metatarsal head, the metatarsophalangeal joint becomes hyperextended. Painful calluses develop under the metatarsal heads. The capsules and ligaments on the plantar aspect of the flexed joints and on the dorsal aspect of the hyperextended joints become contracted. The interosseus tendons become shifted dorsally. Constant irritation caused by shoe pressure may cause calluses to develop over the dorsum of the flexed interphalangeal joint and on the end of the toe. An adventitious bursa may also appear between the indurated skin and subjacent bone.

Hammer toe is often bilateral and symmetrical. There is a very high familial incidence. The second toe is most frequently affected, and less often the third and fourth toes. The deformity is usually congenital; acquired cases are ordinarily caused by mechanical pressure of a small shoe on an abnormally long toe that is forced to flex at its interphalangeal joints. Hammer toe may occur in association with hallux valgus.

Treatment

In infants and children, the deformity should be treated conservatively. Passive stretching exercises are performed by the parents. The deformity is usually not fixed; if it is marked, the interphalangeal joint is manipulated into extension and strapped with adhesive tape in the corrected position. When the child begins to walk, it is important to provide him with shoes that have adequate room. Pain from inflamed calluses over the dorsum of the flexed interphalangeal joint is alleviated by protective pads.

In the adolescent, if the deformity is severe and disabling, surgical correction is indicated. Various operative procedures are available. A simple and very satisfactory method is resection of the proximal interphalangeal joint and arthrodesis of the joint in neutral position. This was first reported by Soule, in 1910, and later was popularized by Sir Robert Jones.[482, 490] The operative correction of hammer toe by resection and fusion of the proximal interphalangeal joint is described and illustrated in Plate 61. The procedure is combined with dorsal capsulotomy of the metatarsophalangeal joint if the latter has developed fixed hyperextension contracture. In the presence of marked depression of the metatarsal head, the long toe extensor is transferred to the metatarsal head.

When the hammer toe deformity is severe with *irreducible* dorsal subluxation of the metatarsophalangeal joints, partial proximal phalangectomy is preferred and the adjacent digits are syndactylized surgically (Fig. 7–69).

The Girdlestone operation was designed

to provide active plantar flexion of the proximal phalanx by transfer of the toe flexor to the extensor hood. The author is dissatisfied with the procedure and does not recommend it because of the frequent development of lateral deformities of the toes following the transfer; also, because it does not always correct the deformity.

CLAW TOES

Clawing of the toes is characterized by hyperextension of the metatarsophalangeal joint and flexion of both the proximal and distal interphalangeal joints (Fig. 7–70 and 7–71). The deformity may be secondary to pes cavus, or it may be paralytic in its pathogenesis. During the push-off phase of gait, when the long toe flexors contract to substitute for the paralyzed triceps surae muscle, the interphalangeal joints of the toes are flexed, and the metatarsophalangeal joints are hyperextended. A reverse mechanism by which clawing of the toes may also occur acts when the anterior tibialis muscle is weakened or zero in motor strength, and the extensor hallucis longus and extensor digitorum longus muscles are used to substitute for its action. In this latter type, clawing of the toes is produced during the swing phase of the gait. The great toe is usually more severely affected than the lesser toes. Painful callosities gradually develop over the dorsum of the interphalangeal joints, which become fixed in flexion. Pressure keratoses under the metatarsal heads aggravate the disability.

Treatment

Treatment is dependent upon the type of claw toes, the degree of flexibility of the interphalangeal and metatarsophalangeal joints, and the age of the patient. The Girdlestone-Taylor operation (in which the long toe flexor is transferred to the dorsal expansion of the long toe extensors) should *not* be performed for clawing of the toes, as it causes rotational malalignment of the toes.[495,499] The experience of Taylor, who obtained good results in 27 of the 38 patients, is not shared by others. Pyper, reviewing the results of the Girdlestone-Taylor operation in 45 feet with clawing of the toes, found that in approximately 20 per cent of cases, the extensor tendons regenerated and the deformity recurred. The interphalangeal joints were stiff in 60 per cent, and in no case was there significant improvement in metatarsal pain and callosities. Worthwhile improvement was achieved in about 50 per cent of the cases, with the best results in those with only the mildest symptoms. The advantages observed by Pyper were: improvement in the shape of the toes with consequent easier fitting of shoes; disappearance of corns over the interphalangeal joints; and general improvement in walking.[498]

For clawing of the great toe, Dickson and Dively advise transfer of the extensor hallucis longus tendon to the flexor hallucis longus tendon, and resection and arthrodesis of the interphalangeal joint in normal alignment.[494] The author has had no experience with this operation.

In paralytic claw toes, the dynamic imbalance causing the deformity should be corrected whenever feasible. In the presence of anterior tibial muscle weakness, the motor power of ankle dorsiflexion should be restored by appropriate tendon transfer. First, associated equinus deformity is corrected by stretching casts; then the peroneal muscles are transferred to the base of the second metatarsal, or in the presence of peroneal muscle weakness, the long toe extensors are transferred to the metatarsal heads. The fixed flexion deformity of the interphalangeal joints is corrected by wedge resections and arthrodesis. If the primary cause of claw toes is triceps surae muscle weakness and hyperactive long toe flexors, posterior transfer of the appropriate muscles to the os calcis is performed to restore active power of plantar flexion. If the claw toes represent triceps surae muscle weakness and hyperactive long toe flexors, posterior transfer of the appropriate muscles to the os calcis is performed to restore active power of plantar flexion. If the claw toes are secondary to pes cavus, equinus deformity of the forefoot is corrected. Fixed claw toes are treated by dorsal capsulotomy of the metatarsophalangeal joints and transfer of the long toe extensors to the metatarsal heads and fusion of the in-

(*Text continued on page 1415.*)

Correction of Hammer Toe by Resection and Arthrodesis of Proximal Interphalangeal Joint

THE PROCEDURE

A. A longitudinal incision 3 to 4 cm. in length is made over the dorsal aspect of the proximal interphalangeal joint parallel to and at the lateral border of the extensor digitorum longus tendon. The subcutaneous tissue is divided and the skin flaps are retracted.

B. The long extensor tendon is split and retracted to expose the capsule of the proximal interphalangeal joint. The digital vessels and nerves are protected from injury. A transverse incision is made in the capsule and the joint surfaces are widely exposed.

C and **D.** With a rongeur, wedges of bone based dorsally are resected from the head of the proximal phalanx and the base of the middle phalanx. Enough bone should be removed to allow correction of deformity.

E and **F.** The proximal and middle phalanges are held together by internal fixation with a Kirschner wire that is inserted retrograde. The Kirschner wire should not cross the metatarsophalangeal joint. The cancellous bony surfaces of the middle and proximal phalanges should be apposed, and the rotational alignment should be correct. The capsule is resutured tightly by reefing. The wound is closed in routine manner. With a pair of nose pliers, the end of the Kirschner wire is bent 90 degrees and cut, leaving 0.5 cm. protruding through the skin.

POSTOPERATIVE CARE

A below-knee walking cast is applied with a band of plaster of Paris protecting the toe. The wire and cast are removed in six weeks, when the roentgenograms show fusion of the interphalangeal joint.

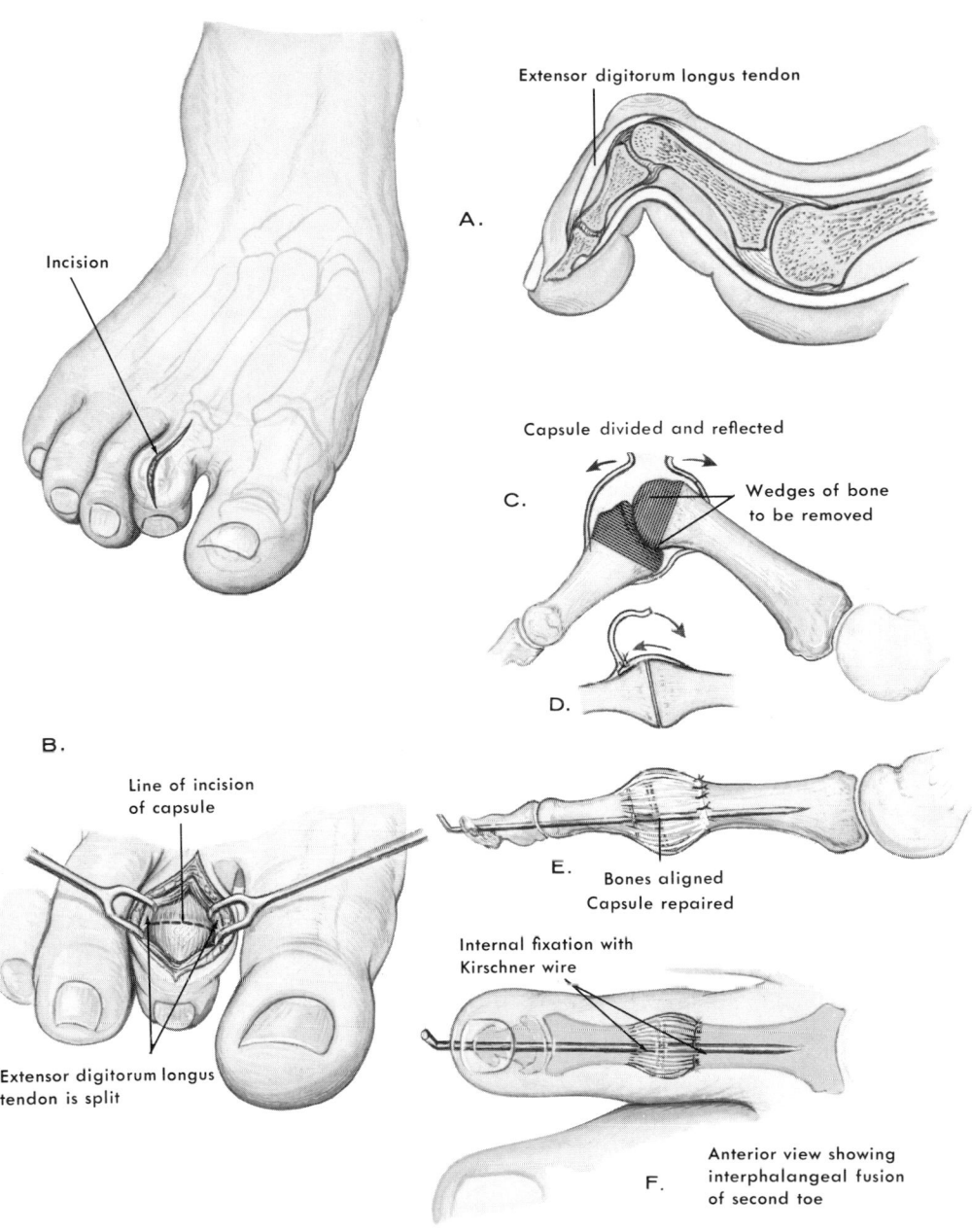

Incision

Extensor digitorum longus tendon

A.

Capsule divided and reflected

C.

Wedges of bone to be removed

D.

B.

Line of incision of capsule

Extensor digitorum longus tendon is split

E.

Bones aligned
Capsule repaired

Internal fixation with Kirschner wire

F.

Anterior view showing interphalangeal fusion of second toe

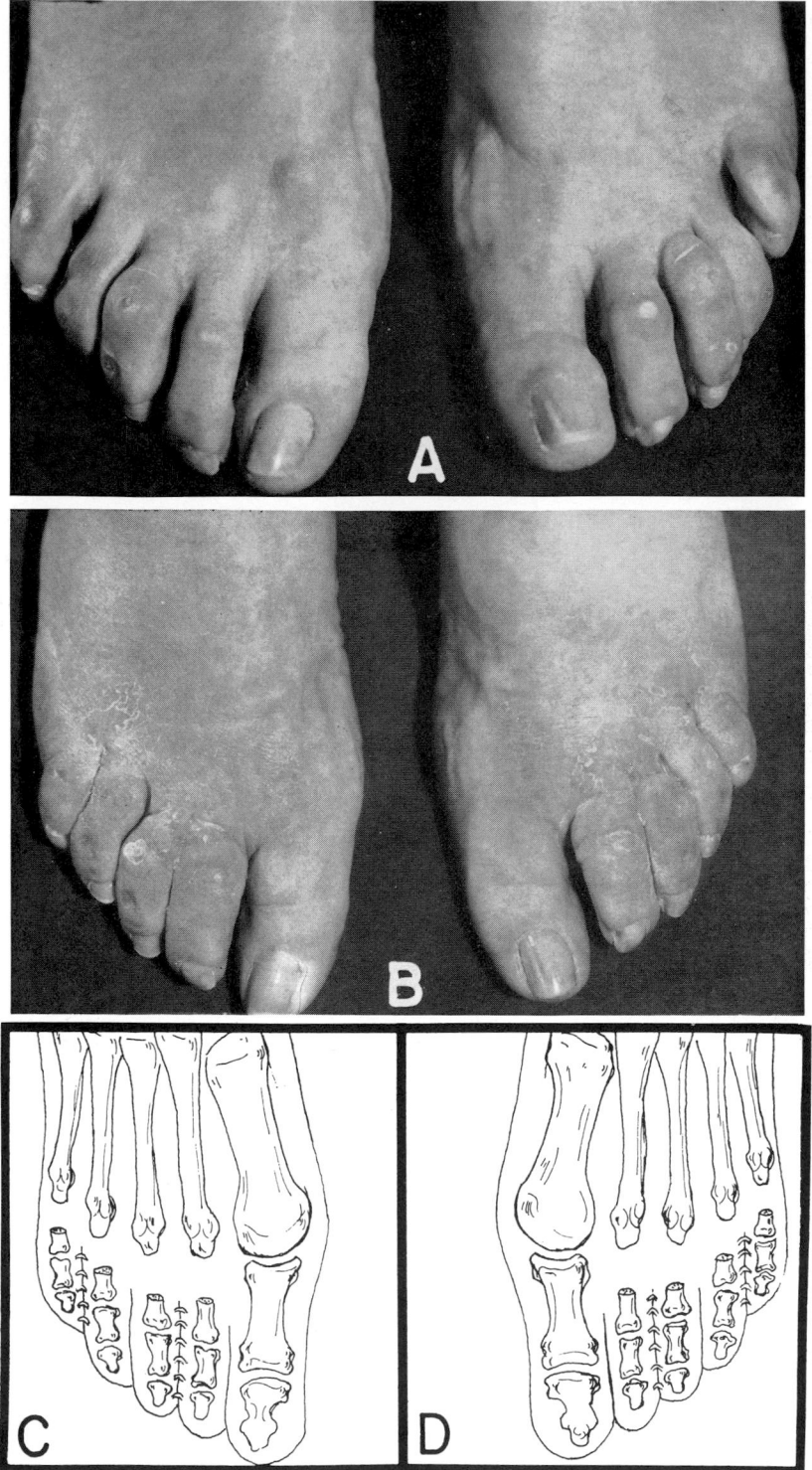

FIGURE 7–69. Multiple bilateral hammer toes.

The hammer toes were treated by partial proximal phalangectomy and surgical syndactylia of the adjacent digits. **A.** Preoperative photograph. **B.** Postoperative photograph. **C** and **D.** Diagrammatic illustration of the operative procedure. (From Kelikian, H.: Hallux Valgus, Allied Deformities of the Forefoot and Metatarsalgia. Philadelphia, W. B. Saunders Co., 1965, p. 304.)

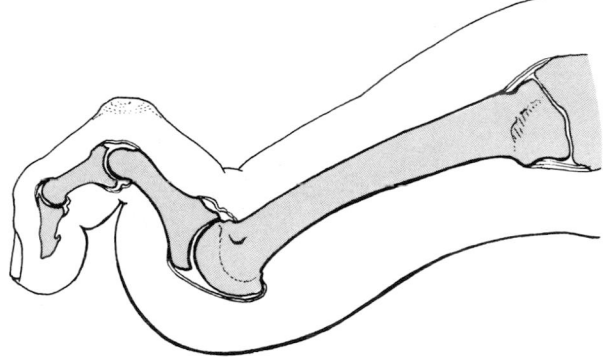

FIGURE 7-70. Claw toe.

The deformity is characterized by hyperextension of the metatarsophalangeal joint and flexion of both proximal and distal interphalangeal joints.

terphalangeal joints as described in Plate 61 for hammer toes.

MALLET TOE

This deformity is characterized by flexion deformity at the distal interphalangeal joint of any of the lesser toes. Usually a single toe or two neighboring ones are affected. The condition is less common than hammer toe, in which the flexion deformity is at the proximal interphalangeal joint. Mallet toes are asymptomatic in childhood, but in adolescence or early adult life, the development of a painful corn on the tip of the toe close to the nail may be very disabling.

Conservative measures such as adhesive strapping and passive stretching exercises do not correct the deformity. Shaving the corn and padding the toe will give symptomatic relief, but surgery is often preferred. Fusion of the distal interphalangeal joint in normal alignment and section of the long toe flexor corrects the deformity. A simpler method that provides immediate relief of symptoms is amputation of the distal phalanx, but this is esthetically undesirable.

CONGENITAL CURLY (OR VARUS) TOE

In this common congenital deformity one or more toes are bent plantarward, medially deviated, and laterally rotated at the distal interphalangeal joint (Fig. 7-72). The twisted terminal pulp then gradually begins to impinge upon and curl under the adjacent toe.

This affection is usually bilateral and symmetrical, and has a high familial incidence. It is most probably caused by hypoplasia of the intrinsic muscles of the affected toe. Trethowan regarded the anomaly as a congenital form of hammer toe.[504] Sweetnam coined the term *congenital curly toe*, and also observed that the deformity does not correct itself spontaneously and usually becomes exaggerated with growth.[502]

Treatment

If the deformity is mild and the curly toe does not impinge upon its adjacent toe, the

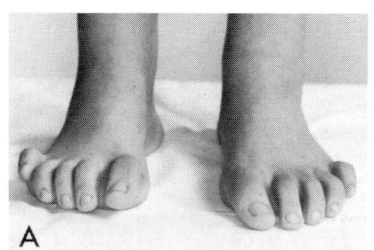
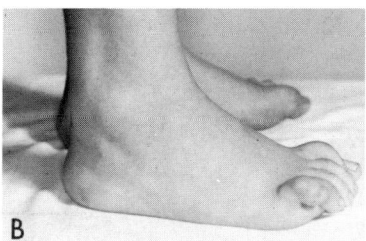
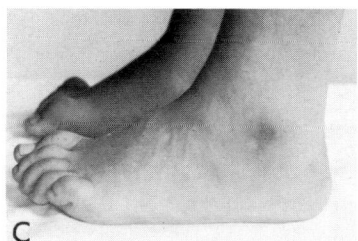

FIGURE 7-71. Bilateral clawing of the toes.

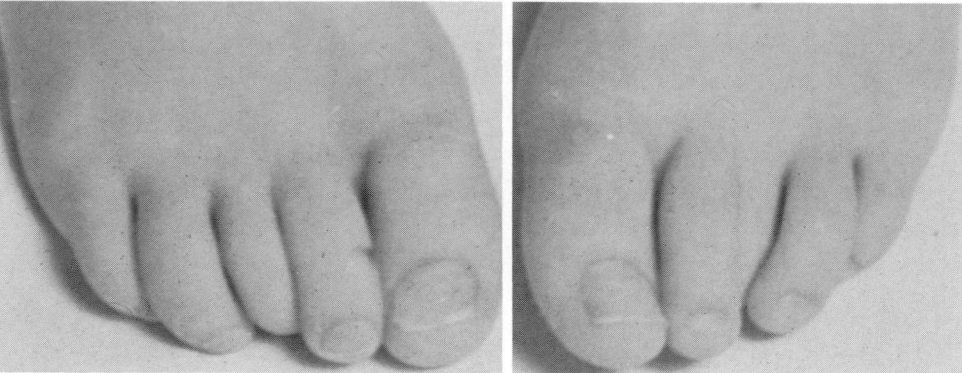

FIGURE 7-72.   Congenital curly toes.

condition can be ignored and no treatment is necessary. Over-and-under strapping is useless and has no permanent effect.

If the affected toe curls under the neighboring one, disabling symptoms are most likely to ensue later on in life, particularly in women, in whom discomfort results from the pressure of tight shoes. Pain under the adjacent medial metatarsal head develops as the underlying toe does not permit its neighboring medial toe to touch the floor; thus more body weight is transmitted to the metatarsal head. In children, Kelikian recommends surgical syndactyly of the curly toe with its normal neighbor on the medial side.[500] Another alternative is to transfer the flexor digitorum longus tendon of the affected toe to the dorsal and lateral aspect of the extensor hood.[501, 503] This is especially indicated in children in whom the deformity is not very severe or rigid. The operative technique is as follows:

A 3 cm. longitudinal incision is made on the dorsolateral aspect of the deformed toe. The subcutaneous tissue is divided and the digital nerve and long toe extensor tendon are pulled medially with a blunt retractor. The affected toe is acutely flexed, and on its plantar aspect the long toe flexor tendon is identified. A longitudinal incision is made in the flexor tendon sheath, and the long flexor tendon is pulled dorsally with a small hook and sectioned near its insertion. After manipulation of the distal interphalangeal joint into normal alignment, the long flexor tendon is sutured to the extensor expansion with the interphalangeal joints of the toe in

full extension and with the metatarsophalangeal joint in flexion. The tourniquet is released and the wound closed in the usual manner. Alignment of the affected toe is maintained by a smooth Kirschner wire drilled from the distal end of the toe into the base of the proximal phalanx. Adhesive strapping or a below-knee walking cast is applied. The cast and wire are removed three to four weeks after surgery.

In adults, Kelikian recommends partial proximal phalangectomy with surgical syndactyly of the toes.

CONGENITAL DIGITUS MINIMUS VARUS (Congenital Dorsal Overriding of Fifth Toe)

This is a common familial deformity in which the fifth metatarsophalangeal joint is subluxated dorsomedially. The fifth toe is hyperextended and adducted, lying across the base of the fourth toe (Fig. 7-73). The capsule of the metatarsophalangeal joint is contracted on its dorsomedial aspect. The extensor tendon is shortened, and the skin on the dorsum of the fifth and between the fourth and fifth toes is taut. In severe deformity, the fifth toe becomes rotated on its longitudinal axis with its nail pointing laterally. There is no flexion deformity of the interphalangeal joints. A hard callus often develops over the dorsum of the fifth toe because of irritation caused by the shoe.

The condition is usually bilateral. It causes disability in about half of the affected patients.

Treatment

In the infant and the young child conservative measures are indicated: passive stretching of the little toe into plantar flexion and abduction, and strapping of the little toe in normal alignment with adhesive tape. Usually these methods do not correct the deformity, and in the adolescent, if symptoms warrant it, operative correction is necessary.

Numerous surgical procedures have been proposed in the literature: (1) transfer of the extensor tendon of the fifth toe to the neck of the fifth metatarsal (Lantzounis);[512] (2) division of the extensor tendon of the fifth toe over the dorsum of the midfoot and transfer of its distal segment to the abductor digiti quinti by rerouting the tendon from the medial to the lateral side of the proximal phalanx (Lapidus);[513] (3) Z-plastic lengthening of the extensor tendon, dorsal and medial capsulotomy of the metatarsophalangeal joint, and plastic lengthening of the contracted skin fold (Goodwin and Swisher Y-plasty);[509] Wilson and DuVries V and Y-plasty);[507, 520] Thompson, Z-plasty;[509] (4) excision of the proximal phalanx of the fifth toe through a lateral incision (Gocht and DeBrunner);[508] (5) excision of the proximal phalanx and surgical syndactyly of the fourth and fifth toes;[510, 514, 516] (6) amputation of the fifth toe.

The author recommends tenotomy of the extensor tendon, dorsal and medial capsulotomy of the fifth metatarsophalangeal joint, excision of the proximal phalanx, and fusion of the skin (surgical syndactylism) of the fourth and fifth toes (Fig. 7–73). The operative technique is described and illustrated in Plate 62. In children the proximal phalanx is partially excised, leaving the

(*Text continued on page 1422.*)

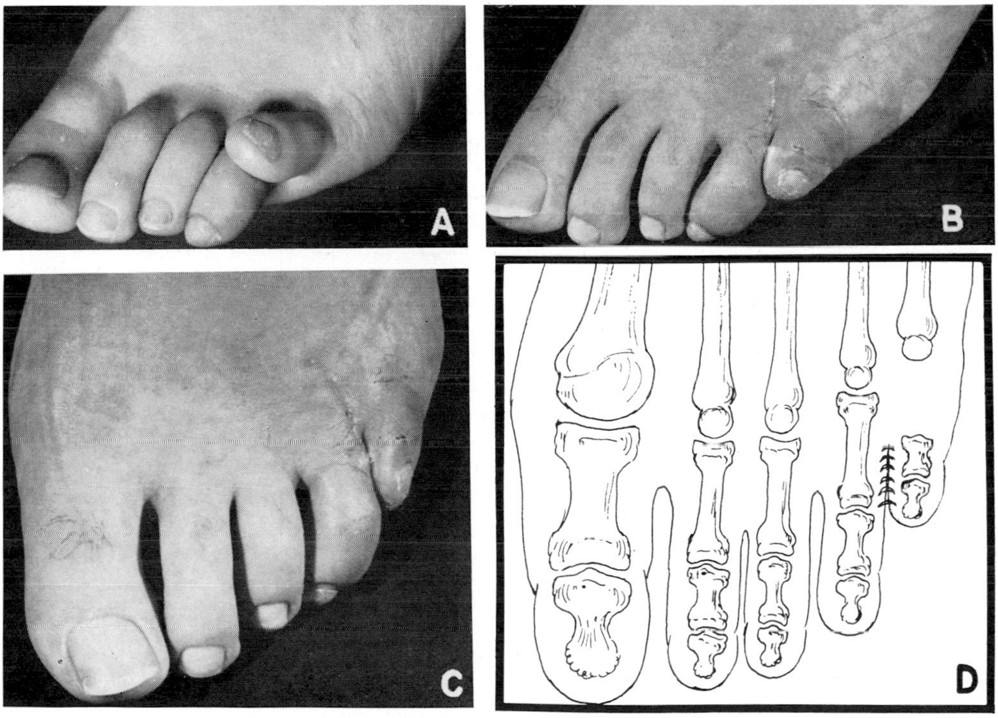

FIGURE 7–73. *Digitus minimus varus.*

Deformity was treated by excision of the proximal phalanx of the little toe, extensor tenotomy, dorsal capsulotomy of the fifth metatarsophalangeal joint, and surgical syndactyly of the fifth and fourth toes. **A.** Preoperative photograph. **B** and **C.** Postoperative photographs. **D.** Interpretative diagram. (From Kelikian, H.: Hallux Valgus, Allied Deformities of the Forefoot and Metatarsalgia. Philadelphia, W. B. Saunders Co., 1965, p. 328.)

Correction of Digitus Minimus Varus (McFarland, Kelikian)

THE PROCEDURE

A. First, a 00 silk whip suture is passed through each pulp of the fourth and fifth toes. The suture ends are clamped with hemostats and the toes are pulled apart, bringing the web space into full view.

B. Three sets of incisions are made: (1) a web-bisecting incision that starts on the dorsum of the forefoot in the groove between the metatarsal heads and extends distally to bisect the web, and then passes plantarward to terminate at about the same point posteriorly on the plantar aspect of the forefoot as it does on the dorsum; (2) two *paradigital incisions,* one for each toe, which begin at the point where the web-bisecting incision begins to dip plantarward and extend lengthwise along the adjacent side of each toe. The paradigital incision for the little toe ends on the side of the distal phalanx at a point plantar and just proximal to the base of the nail, whereas the incision for the fourth toe is the same length as that for the fifth. The paradigital incisions are placed slightly toward the plantar border of the toe to give a semblance of an interdigital groove after surgical syndactylism. (3) Two connecting oblique incisions extend from the terminal point of the paradigital incision on each side to the proximal end of the web-bisecting incision on the plantar aspect.

C. The triangular patches of skin between the paradigital and oblique connecting incisions are excised. In dissection of subcutaneous tissue in this area, care is taken not to injure the plexus of veins. The skin flaps are mobilized and retracted to their respective sides. The digital nerves and vessels should be identified and protected from injury.

D and **E.** The long extensor tendon of the fifth toe is divided at its insertion; a 00 silk whip suture is applied to its distal end. (This end is later transferred to the fifth metatarsal head according to the technique for the Jones procedure described in Plate 58.) Next, the long flexor of the fifth toe is dissected free of the proximal phalanx. Small retractors are placed on the dorsal and plantar aspects of the bone to protect the soft tissues. The capsules of the metatarsophalangeal and proximal interphalangeal joints of the little toe are divided, and the proximal phalanx is excised. The long fifth toe extensor is transferred to the fifth metatarsal head. The wound is packed with moist gauze, the pneumatic tourniquet is deflated, and bleeding vessels are clamped and coagulated.

F. The terminal points of the paradigital incisions are sutured together with 0000 nylon, bringing the toes together. The alignment of the toes is inspected. Care is taken to avoid eversion or inversion of the toes; if necessary, the terminal suture is removed and reapplied. The dorsal wound is closed with 0000 nylon and the plantar skin edges with 0000 plain catgut.

POSTOPERATIVE CARE

A below-knee walking cast is applied. Three to four weeks following surgery, the cast and sutures are removed. The patient is allowed to bear weight and resume normal activities.

Plate 62. *Correction of Digitus Minimus Varus (McFarland, Kelikian)*

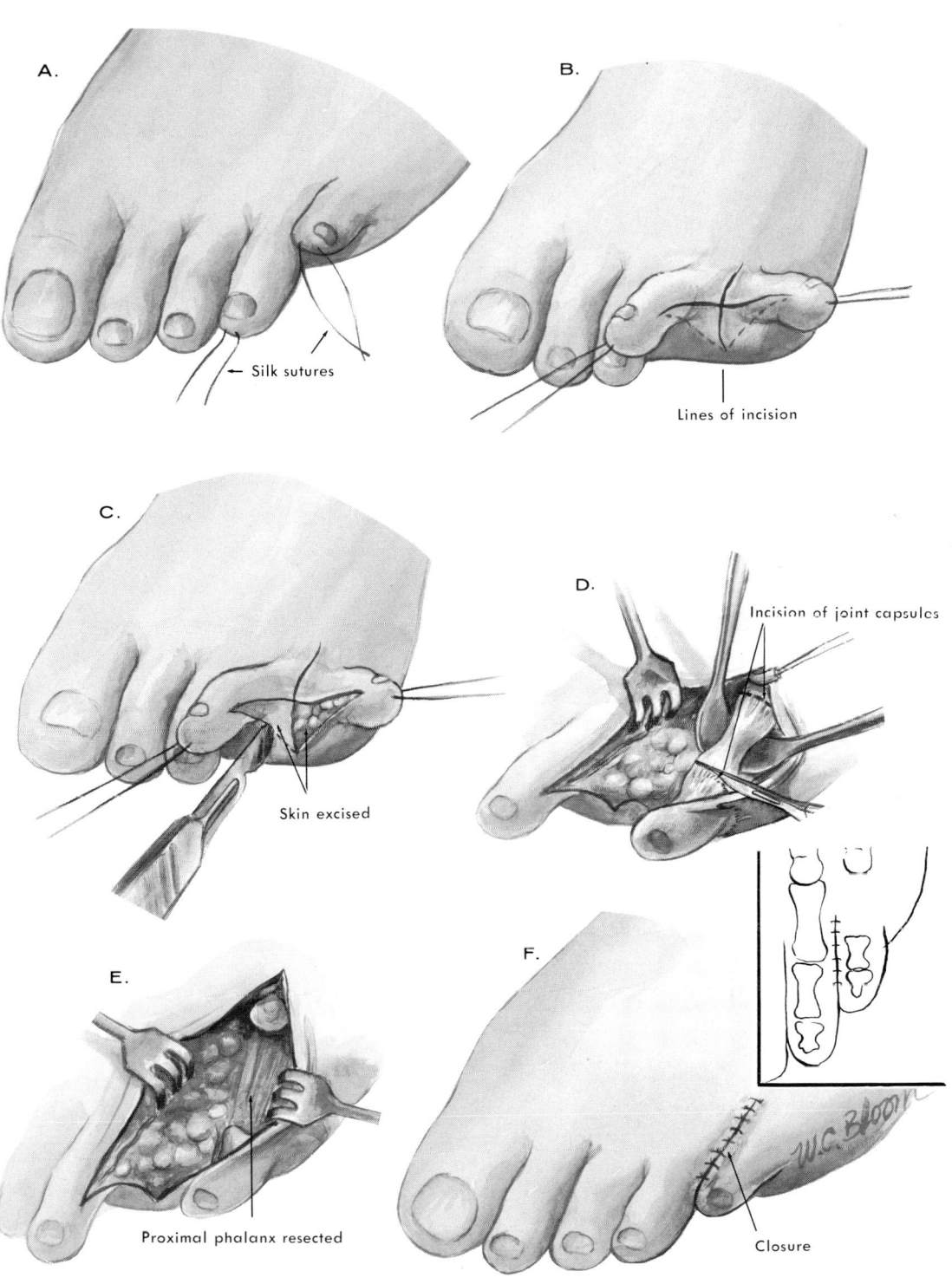

A.

← Silk sutures

B.

Lines of incision

C.

Skin excised

D.

Incision of joint capsules

E.

Proximal phalanx resected

F.

Closure

W.C.Bloom

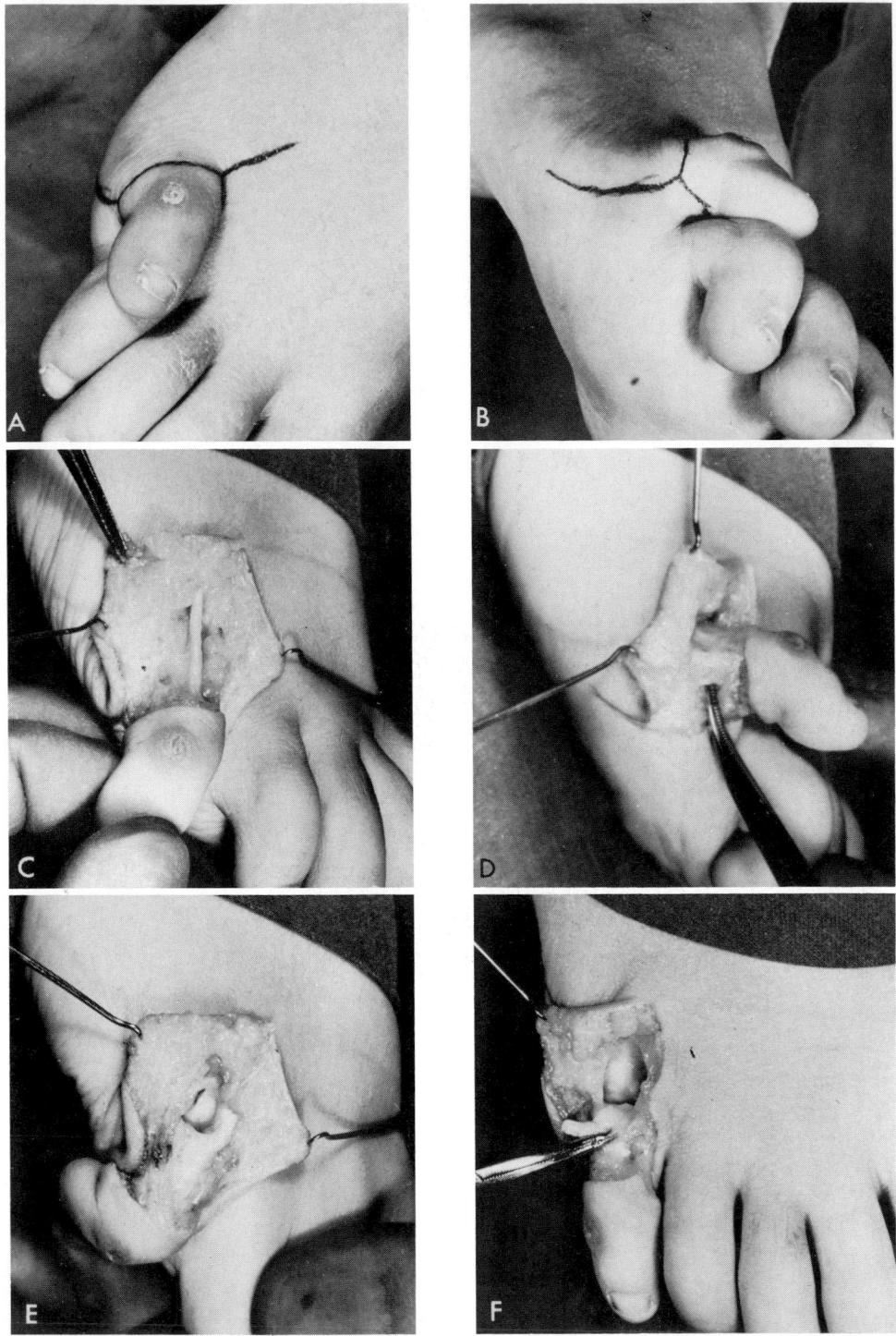

FIGURE 7-74. Butler's operation for an overriding fifth toe.

A and **B.** A dorsal racquet incision is made with a second handle added on the plantar aspect. The plantar handle is inclined laterally and is a little longer than the dorsal handle. **C** and **D.** The contracted extensor tendon to the fifth toe is exposed by elevating the skin flaps. The neurovascular bundles should be identified and carefully preserved. **E.** Sectioning of the extensor tendon and the dorsomedial part of the capsule of the metatarsophalangeal joint. **F.** In severe deformity, the articular surfaces of the metatarsophalangeal joints may be incongruous. This is due to plantar capsular adhesions. (From Cockin, J.: Butler's operation for an overriding fifth toe. J. Bone Joint Surg., *50-B*:78–80, 1968.)

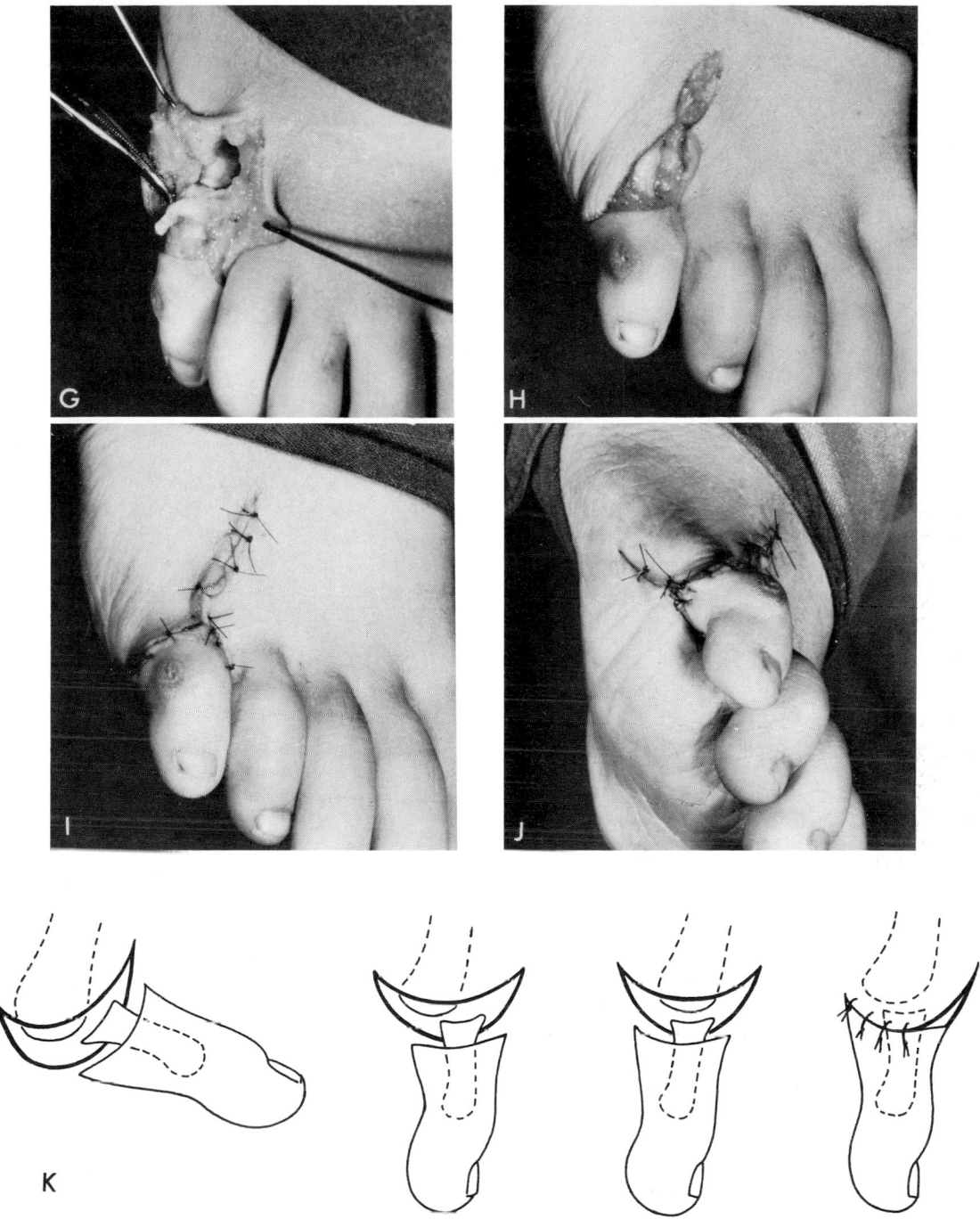

FIGURE 7–74 Continued. Butler's operation for an overriding fifth toe.

G. Adhesions on the plantar part of the capsule are freed by blunt dissection. Note the little toe now lies in the fully corrected position. **H.** Appearance of the toe before skin closure. It lies freely in normal alignment without tension. **I** and **J.** Closure of the wound. Skin sutures securely hold the toe in the correct position. **K.** Diagrammatic illustration of the mechanics of the operation. (From Cockin, J.: Butler's operation for an overriding fifth toe. J. Bone Joint Surg., *50–B*:78–80, 1968.)

growth plate at its base intact. The results of the McFarland operation are very satisfactory.

Plastic procedures involving V-Y elongation of the skin and soft tissues are not recommended by the author because they often result in an ugly scar that is cosmetically undesirable. Sometimes a keloid may form, which may be irritated by the shoe.

Cockin recommends the Butler operation, as it is safe and simple, and full correction of the deformity is obtained without tension.[506] He reported the results of 70 operations performed on 19 male and 36 female patients; the result was good in 91 per cent, fair in 6 per cent, and poor in 3 per cent. In the failures, the deformity recurred rapidly (within a year) and was then treated by amputation. Circulatory embarrassment to the little toe is prevented by avoiding traction on the neurovascular bundles. In the experience of Cockin, there has been no circulatory damage to the toe, and wound healing has not been a problem. The operative technique of the Butler operation is as follows:

A dorsal racquet incision is made on the skin; then a second handle is added to the racquet on the plantar aspect (the plantar handle inclined laterally and a little longer than the dorsal handle) (Fig. 7–74 A and B). The wound flaps are undermined and elevated, exposing the shortened extensor tendon of the fifth toe (Fig. 7–74 C). The neurovascular bundle is identified and carefully protected from injury (Fig. 7–74 D). The extensor tendon and the dorsomedial part of the capsule of the metatarsophalangeal joint are sectioned (Fig. 7–74 E). The toe can now be manipulated freely downward and laterally into correct alignment. Occasionally, in severe long-standing cases, adhesions on the plantar aspect of the capsule may prevent derotation of the little toe. In such instances, the adherent capsule is separated from the metatarsal head by blunt dissection (Fig. 7–74 F and G). Now the toe moves into the plantar handle of the incision and dangles in normal alignment without any tension (Fig. 7–74 H). The wound is closed, with the surrounding skin sutures holding the toe in the corrected position (Fig. 7–74 I and J). Figure 7–74 K is a diagrammatic illustration of the mechanics of the operation.

Skin dressing is applied. Splints to immobilize the toe in corrected position are not required. The sutures are removed in 10 to 14 days and normal activity is then allowed.

The author has utilized the Butler operation in children and has found it to be very satisfactory. In adolescents and adults, however, the potential embarrassment to circulation of the little toe is a definite drawback to the procedure.

POLYDACTYLISM

Supernumerary digits are common in the foot, and should be removed for cosmetic reasons as well as for the sake of comfort in wearing shoes (Fig. 7–75). In deciding which toe is to be excised, the general contour of the foot is the important consideration. Usually the most peripheral toe is amputated, despite the fact that it may be more normal than the one adjacent to it. Roentgenograms of the foot should also be considered in the decision. The extra toe is amputated through a racquet-shaped incision at its base and the tendons are divided near their insertion and sutured to the adjacent tendon. A transverse incision is made in the capsule of the metatarsophalangeal joint and the toe is disarticulated. Injury to the growth centers of the adjacent digits should be avoided. Any bony protrusion of the common metatarsal is excised; if there is a corresponding supernumerary metatarsal, it is excised through a proximal extension of the skin incision on the dorsolateral aspect of the foot. *The capsule and ligaments are reconstructed to prevent malalignment of the neighboring toes.*

MACRODACTYLISM

Gigantism of one or more toes is a rare deformity. The hypertrophy is frequently caused either by neurofibromatosis or by congenital hyperplasia of lymphatic and adipose tissue (Fig. 7–76). A grotesque ap-

(*Text continued on page 1426.*)

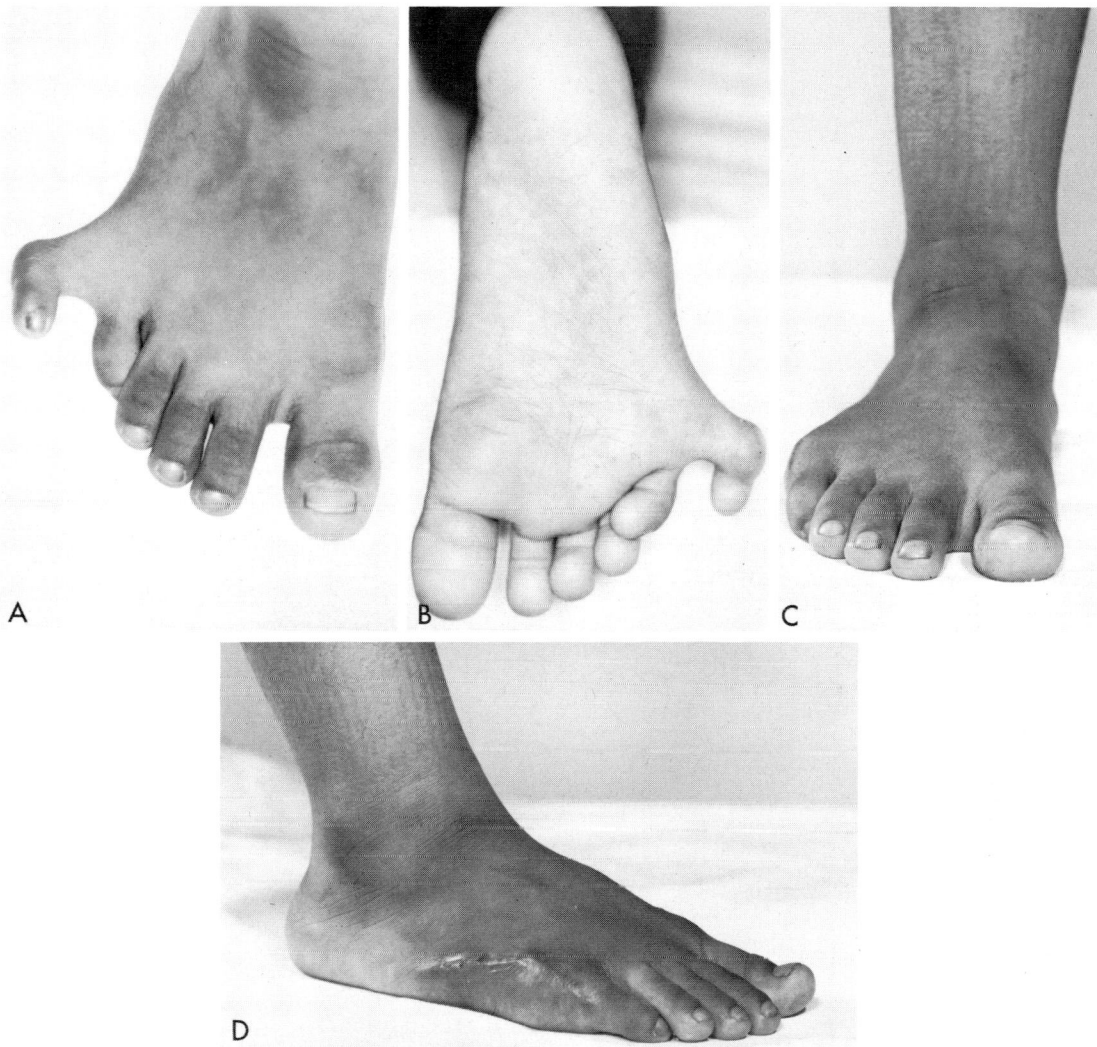

FIGURE 7–75. *Supernumerary sixth toe.*

A and **B.** Preoperative dorsal and plantar views. **C** and **D.** Postoperative views.

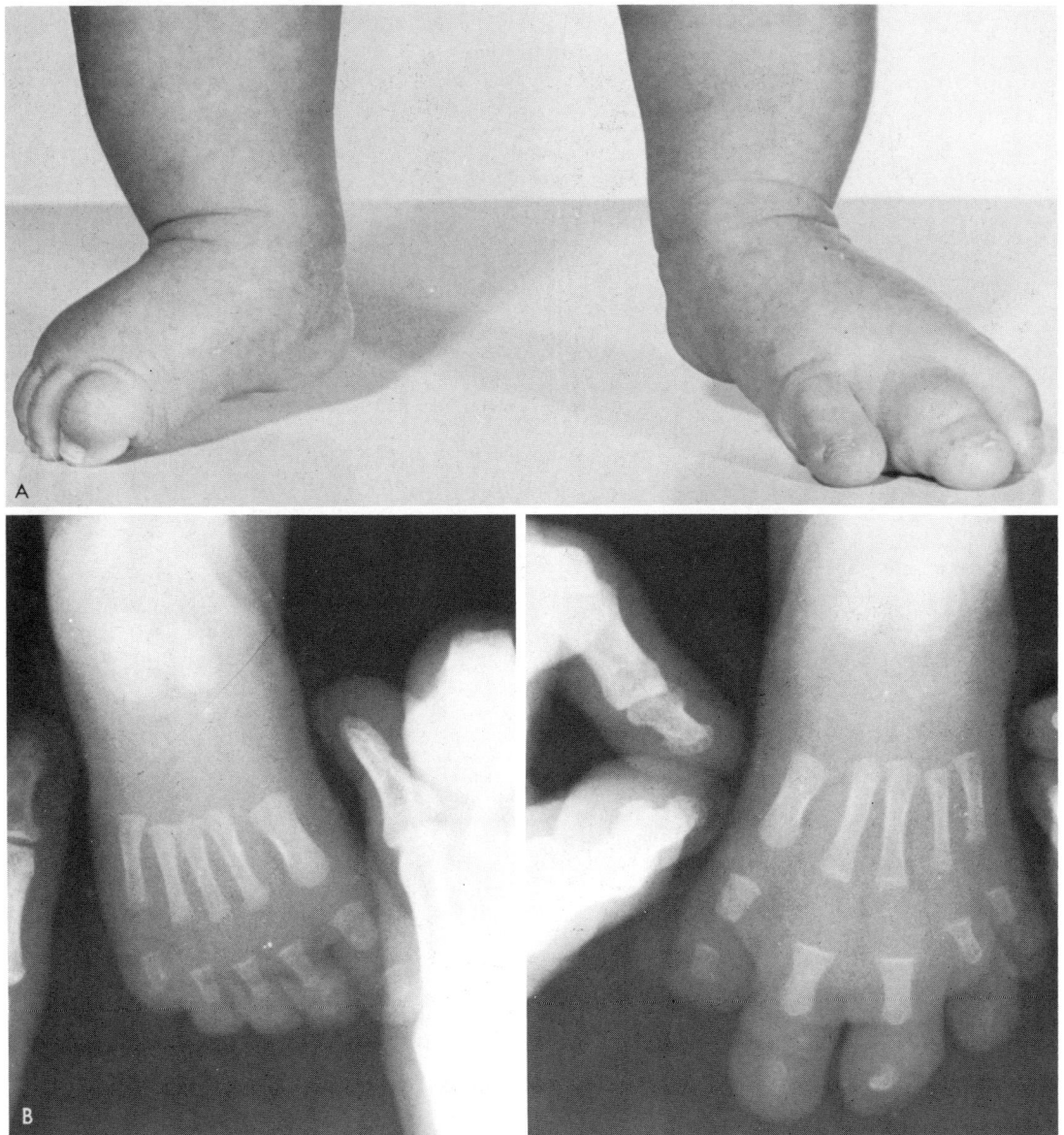

FIGURE 7-76.   Macrodactyly of the second and third digits of the left foot.

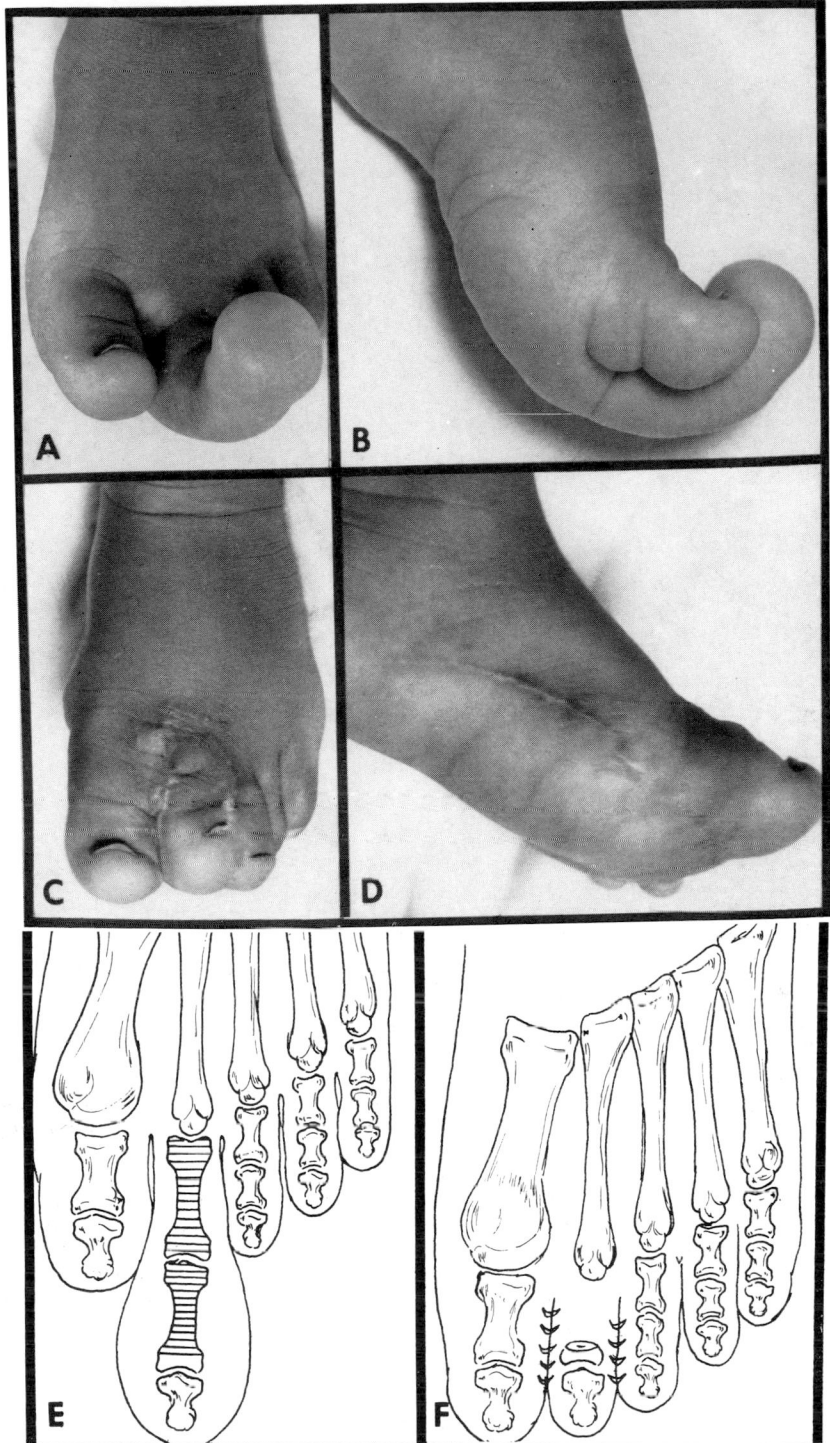

FIGURE 7–77. Severe macrodactyly of the second toe in a young girl.

A and **B.** Preoperative photographs. The deformity was treated in two stages: first the proximal phalanx of the second toe was excised, the toe was defatted from its medial side and syndactylized to the big toe; three months later, the middle phalanx of the second toe was excised, the toe was defatted from its lateral side and syndactylized with the third digit. The medial plantar nerve was normal on exploration. **C** and **D.** Postoperative photographs. **E** and **F.** Interpretative diagrams show the amount of bone resected. Amputation of the second toe should not be performed, as it will lead to hallux valgus. (From Kelikian, H.: Hallux Valgus, Allied Deformities of the Forefoot and Metatarsalgia. Philadelphia, W. B. Saunders Co., 1965, p. 332.)

pearance, difficulty in shoe-fitting, and interference with weight-bearing are indication for surgical treatment.

The operation is performed in two or three steps. First, the proximal phalanx is resected, and the toe is partially defatted on one side and is syndactylized with its neighboring toe on either side. Several months later, hypertrophied tissue is resected on the opposite side (Fig. 7–77). If the corresponding metatarsal is enlarged, its growth is arrested by epiphyseodesis at the appropriate age. Amputation of a gigantic second toe should not be performed, as it will lead to hallux valgus deformity. Severe macrodactyly of the third toe may be treated by amputation of the affected toe, partial resection of the corresponding metatarsal, and surgical syndactyly of the second toe to the fourth toe.

MISCELLANEOUS DEFORMITIES OF TOES

Microdactylism

Small toes may be an isolated deformity, with or without hypoplasia of the corresponding metatarsals, or may be associated with Streeter's dysplasia. Because they do not usually cause disability, treatment is not required.

Syndactylism

Congenital webbing of the toes neither causes disability nor does it interfere with function. Cosmetically it is usually not objectionable and no treatment is necessary (Fig. 7–78). If webbing is associated with poly-

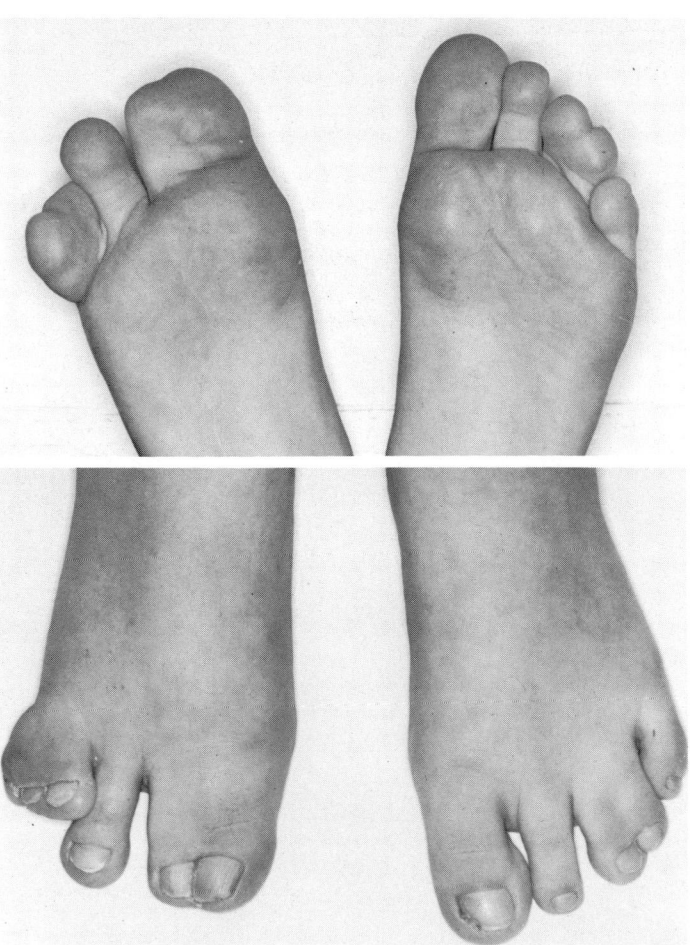

FIGURE 7–78. Congenital syndactylism of third and fourth toes on the left.

In the right foot, the great and second toes are congenitally webbed and there is a supernumerary sixth toe with complete syndactyly of the fourth, fifth, and sixth toes.

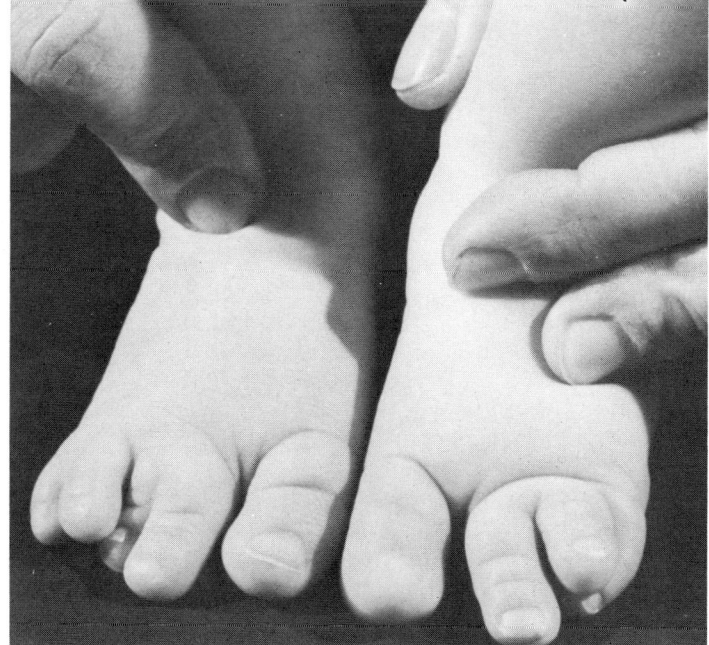

FIGURE 7–79. *Angular deformity of toes.*

Fourth toe on the right overrides the third toe. In the left foot, there are only three lesser toes and metatarsals.

dactylism, the most peripheral digit is excised to facilitate shoe wear.

Divergent or Convergent Toes

These may occur as an isolated angular deformity, without flexion contracture of the distal interphalangeal joint (Fig. 7–79). In minimal deformity, treatment is not necessary. In severe cases, when the angulated toe underrides or overrides the adjacent toe, surgical syndactylism of the affected toes is indicated; in adolescents, it is combined with proximal phalangectomy.

Valgus Deformity of Distal Phalanx of Hallux

This deformity may result from asymmetrical overgrowth of the medial portion of its epiphysis (Fig. 7–80). If symptoms warrant treatment, the bony protuberance is excised and growth of the medial half of the growth plate is arrested. In the skeletally mature foot, the interphalangeal joint of the great toe is fused in correct alignment following partial excision of the hypertrophied medial portion of the epiphysis.

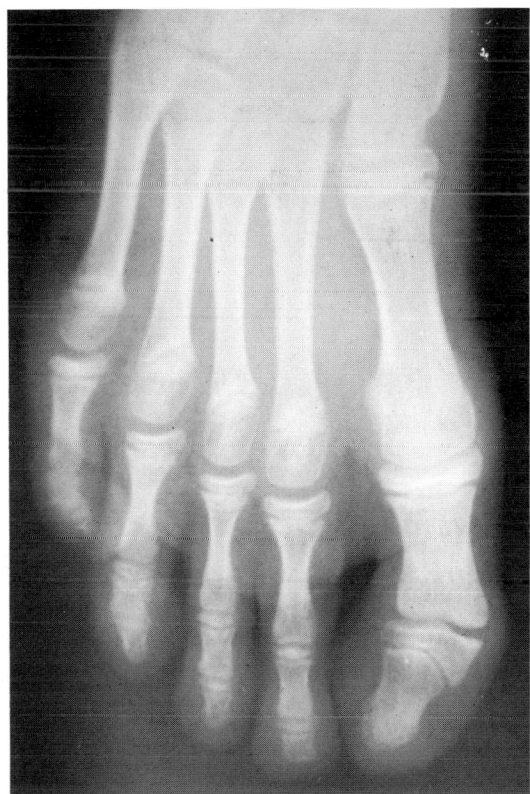

FIGURE 7–80. *Valgus deformity of the distal phalanx of the great toe caused by asymmetrical overgrowth of the medial half of its epiphysis.*

Tumors of the Foot

Tumors of the foot are uncommon in children. If they do occur, they may originate in the soft tissues or in bone, and may be either benign or malignant. Metastatic tumors distal to the knee are extremely rare.

The usual presenting complaints are a swelling or mass, difficulty in fitting shoes, local pain, or a limp. To detect minimal findings, it is essential to examine both feet, comparing the suspected pathologic limb with the contralateral normal limb. The exact site should be determined, whether it is in the soft tissues (subcutaneous tissue, fascia, muscle, tendon, or nerve), the joint, or the bone. Is the consistency of the swelling cystic, firm, or bony? Is it fixed to subjacent bone or is it freely movable? Are the boundaries of the mass well delineated or ill-defined and infiltrating adjacent tissues? Can it be transilluminated? What is the color of the overlying skin? Are the superficial veins dilated? Is there increased local heat? Does the mass pulsate? Upon tourniquet ischemia, does it decrease in size? The regional lymph nodes of the entire lower limb are also palpated for enlargement and tenderness. Roentgenograms of the foot are made to determine bony and soft-tissue al-terations. The more common tumors encountered in the foot are briefly described here.

SOFT-TISSUE TUMORS

Lipoma

Lipoma, one of the more common tumors in the foot, is seen in infants as well as in older children. It is usually located in the subcutaneous tissue of the instep of the foot, or deep to the plantar fascia (Fig. 7–81). Occasionally it may be found on the dorsum of the foot involving tendon sheaths or digital nerves. The mass is soft, generally lobulated, and surrounded by a definite capsule. The histologic picture varies, depending upon the amount of fibrous and myxomatous tissue associated with the fat.

On palpation, the mass has a soft flabby feeling, suggesting fluctuation. Its boundaries are usually not distinct. In the roentgenograms, the lipoma casts a soft-tissue shadow of "fatty density."

Treatment consists of surgical excision of the tumor. If the lesion is not completely

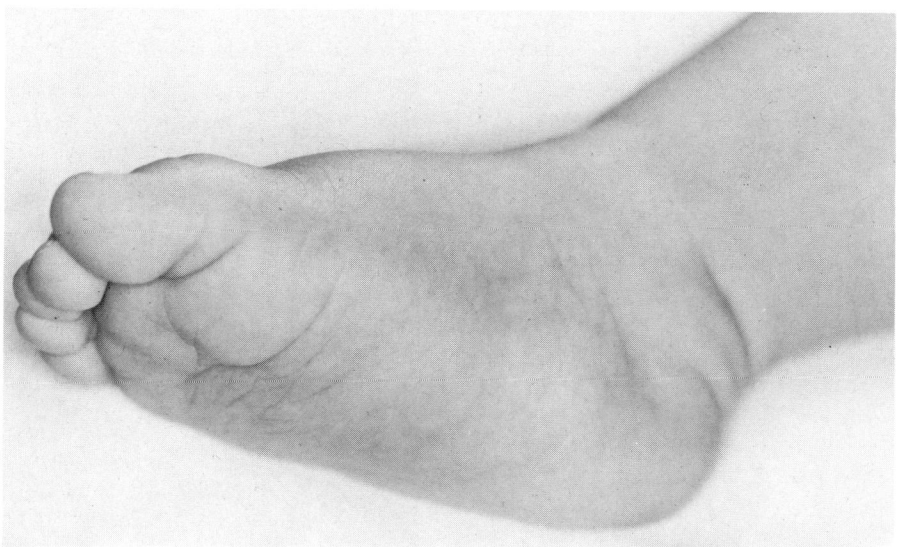

FIGURE 7–81. Lipoma of the right foot.

The mass was encapsulated and located deep to the plantar fascia.

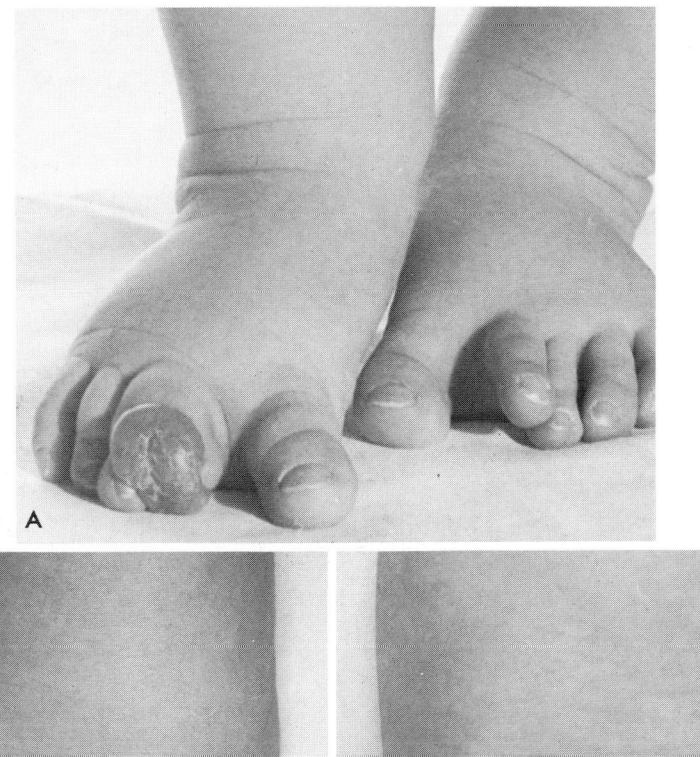

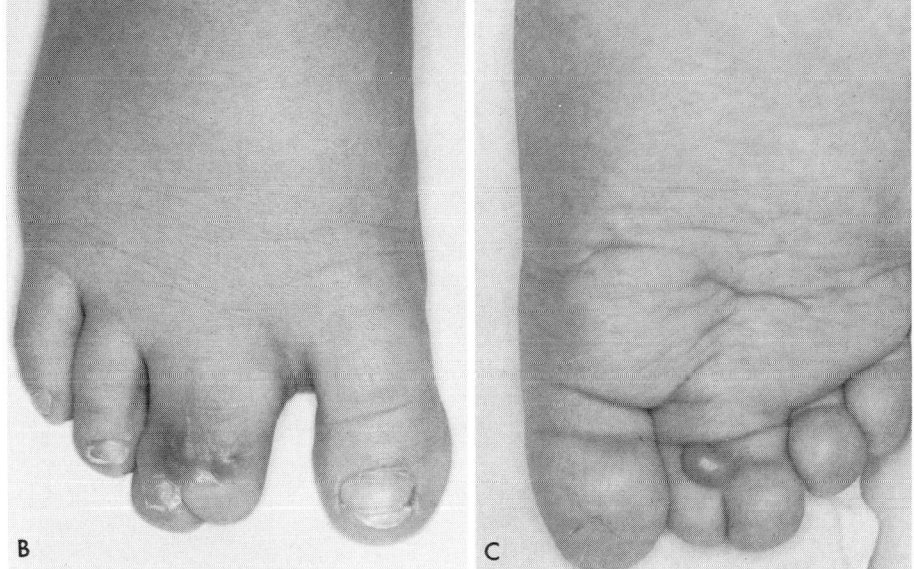

FIGURE 7–82. *Hemangioma involving skin and subcutaneous tissue of the second and third toes.*

A. Preoperative appearance. **B** and **C.** The lesion recurred one year following surgical removal. Again it was totally excised and the second and third toes were surgically syndactylized. Five-year follow-up showed no recurrence of the tumor.

removed, it may recur. It is best to perform the procedure with tourniquet ischemia with the child under general anesthesia.

Hemangioma

Angiomata may be of congenital origin, presenting at birth, or they may develop in childhood or adolescence. The cavernous type is more common. In the foot, hemangioma may involve the skin and subcutaneous tissue (Fig. 7–82), or it may involve the muscle and tendon (Figs. 7–83 and 7–84). The tarsal bones may be invaded. The instep and plantar aspect of the foot are favored locations. Occasionally the lesion affecting the foot may be part of multiple hemangiomatosis affecting the entire lower limb (Fig. 7–85).

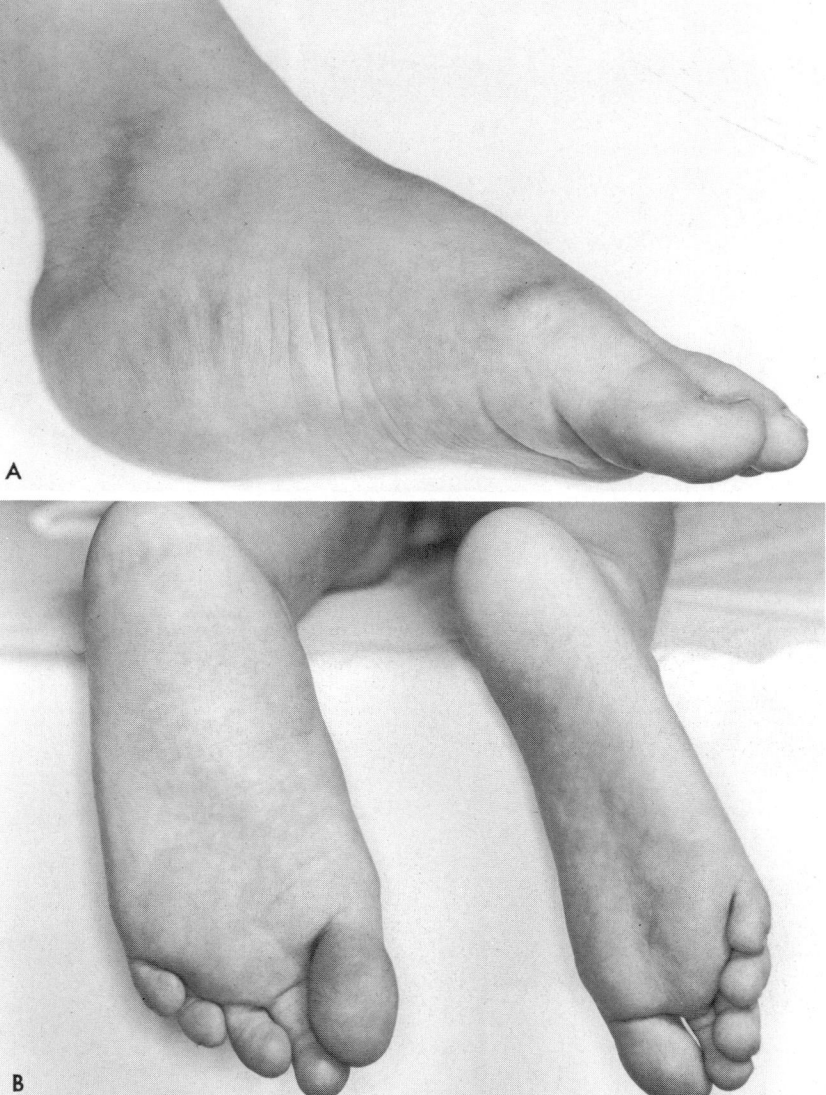

FIGURE 7–83. *Cavernous hemangioma involving the subcutaneous tissue of the instep and the short plantar muscles.*

A and **B.** Clinical appearance.

The presenting complaint is of a compressible mass, which may be irritated by the shoe. When one obstructs the venous return, the mass enlarges. Occasionally the lesion may be painful when it invades nervous tissue or when it is located in bone and expansion is taking place. When hemangioma involves the skin, its external appearance is characteristic and diagnosis is not difficult.

Treatment consists of meticulous and complete excision of the lesion. Large tumors may require surgical resection in two or three stages. Tourniquet ischemia controls hemorrhage, but it is disadvantageous because part of the lesion may be overlooked. Because the tissues often heal poorly, careful handling and hemostasis of the wound are required. Roentgen therapy should not be employed in the treatment of hemangioma in children, but cryotherapy may occasionally be indicated.

Aneurysm in the foot and ankle may result from blunt trauma, which weakens the vessel walls, or from penetrating wounds. During triple arthrodesis, aneurysm of the posterior tibial vessels may be caused by injury with an osteotome (Fig. 7–86).

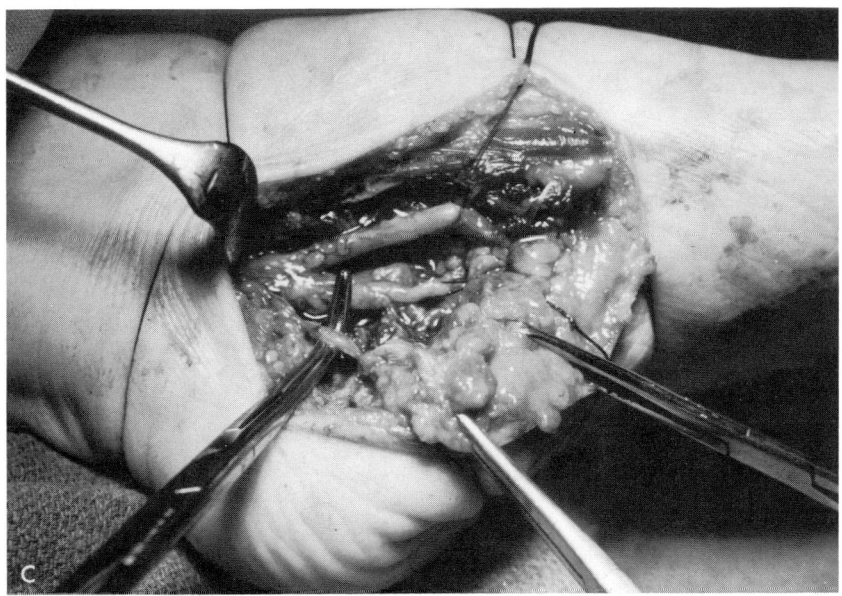

FIGURE 7–83 Continued.   Cavernous hemangioma involving the subcutaneous tissue of the instep and the short plantar muscles.

C. Gross appearance at surgery.

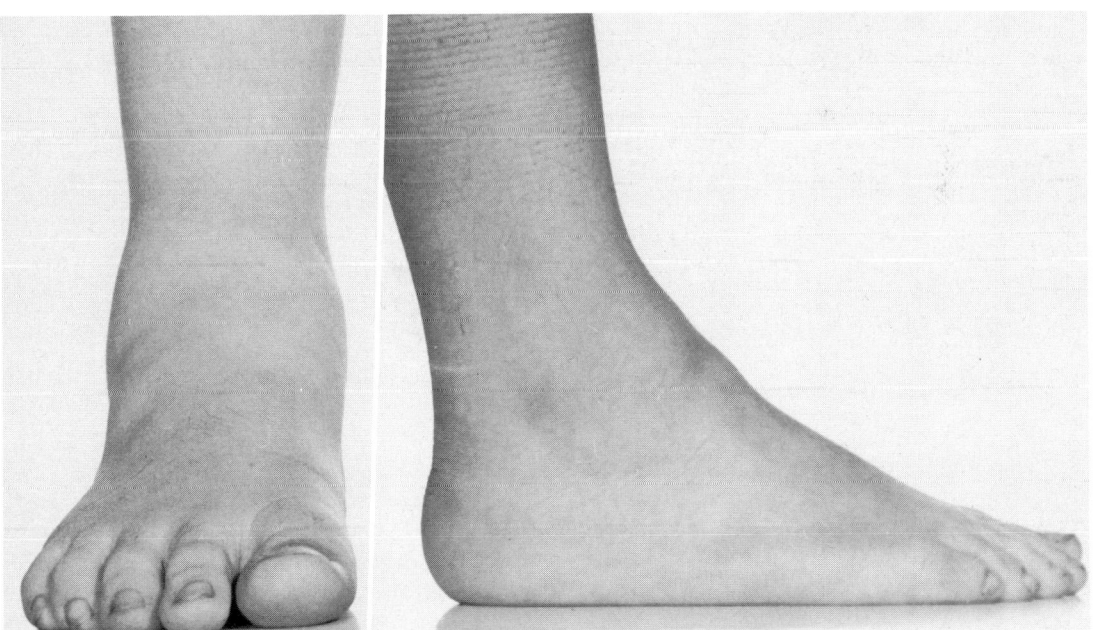

FIGURE 7–84.   Cavernous hemangioma of tendon sheaths.

It was misdiagnosed and the patient was treated for rheumatoid arthritis of the ankle and subtalar joints. Note the soft-tissue swelling.

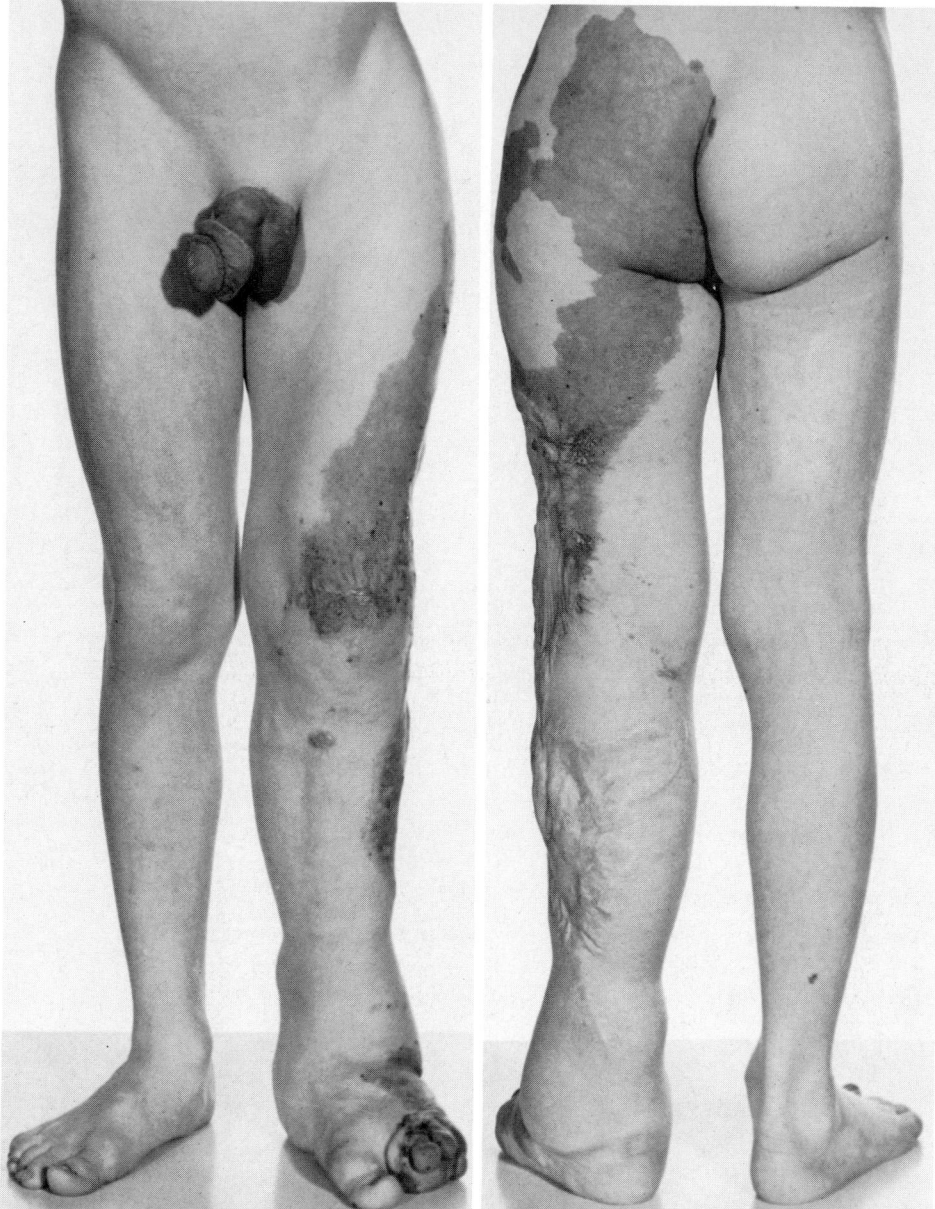

FIGURE 7–85. Massive hemangiomatosis involving the entire left lower limb.

Lymphangiectasis

In this condition the foot and often the entire lower limb are edematous and enlarged due to replacement of normal subcutaneous tissue by dilated lymphatics (Fig. 7–87). In later life, fibrous changes take place in the lesion. When the abnormality is familial, it is known as "Milroy's disease."

The condition should not be mistaken for a tumor; in doubtful cases, lymphangiography will establish the diagnosis.

Treatment consists of application of elastic bandages or stockings at night to shrink the dilated lymphatics. Excision of abnormal tissue is difficult, but possible. The resulting defects are covered by salvaged skin and skin grafts.

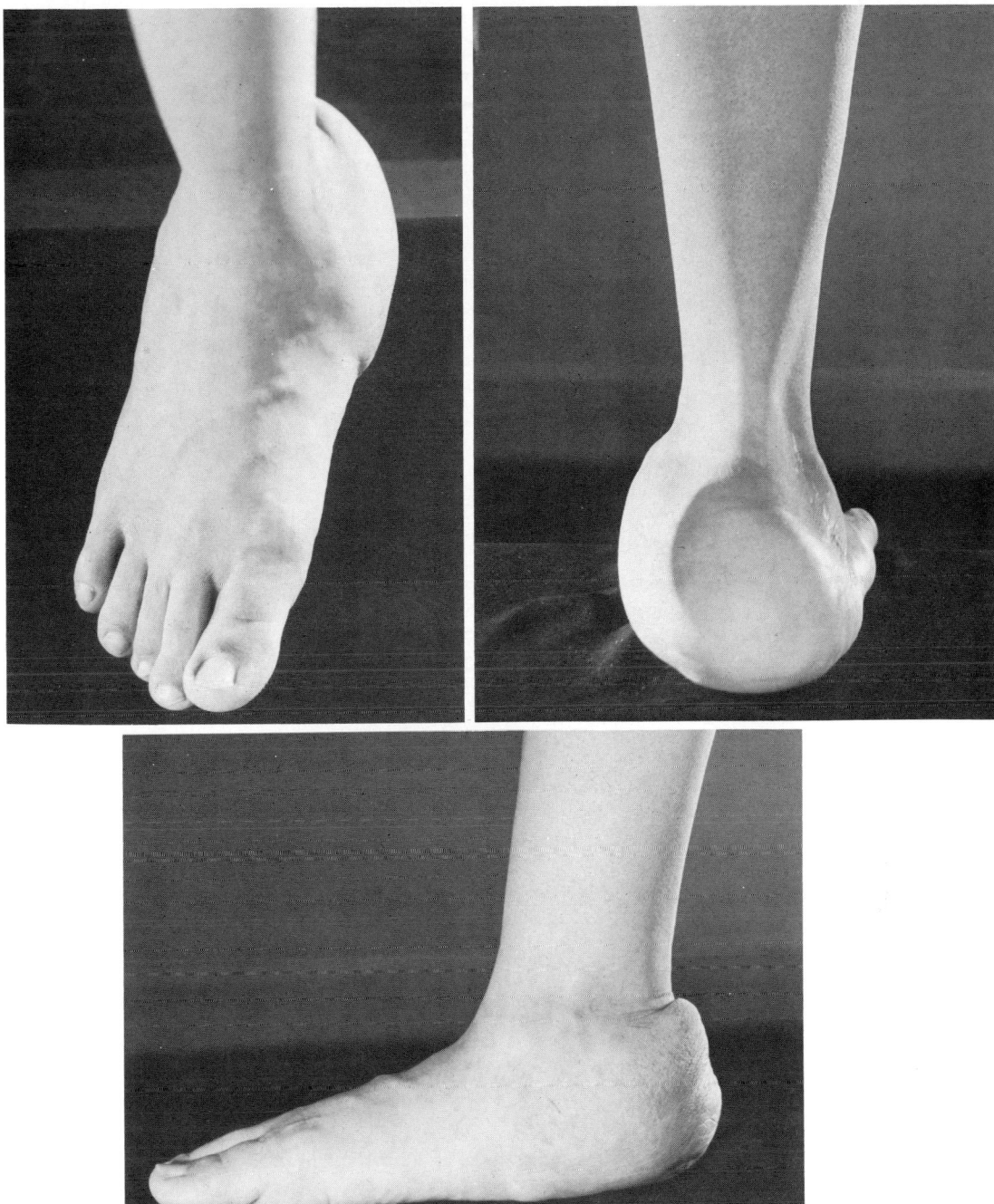

FIGURE 7–86. *Aneurysm of the posterior tibial vessels caused by injury during triple arthrodesis.*

Ganglion

The usual location of this common tumorous lesion is on the dorsum of the foot in the midtarsal area or in the region of the ankle adjacent to the lateral or medial malleolus (Fig. 7–88). The thin-walled cyst contains clear colorless gelatinous fluid, and seems to arise from tendon sheaths or from within the connective tissue of the subjacent

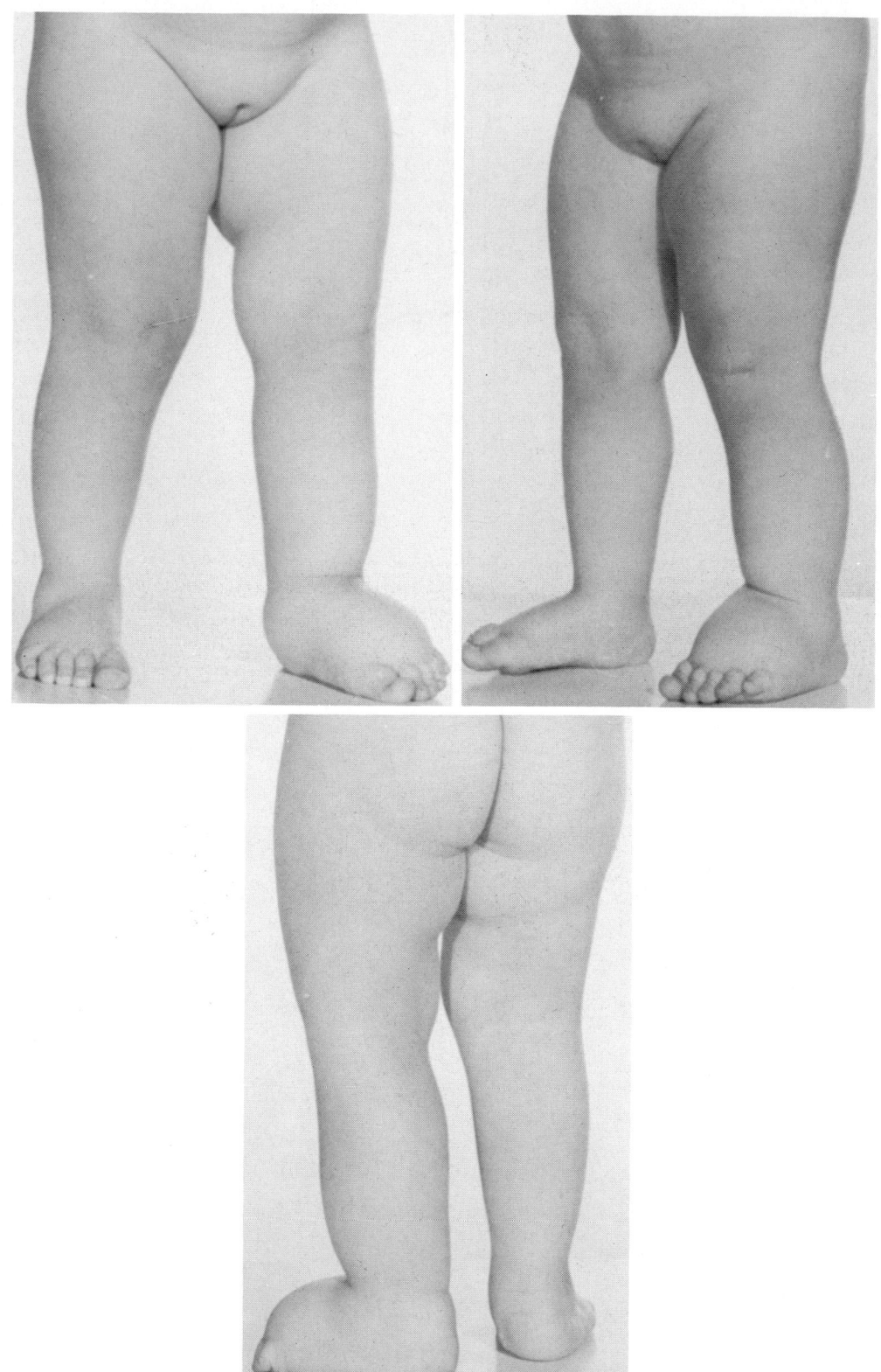

FIGURE 7–87. *Lymphangiectasis of the left foot and leg.*

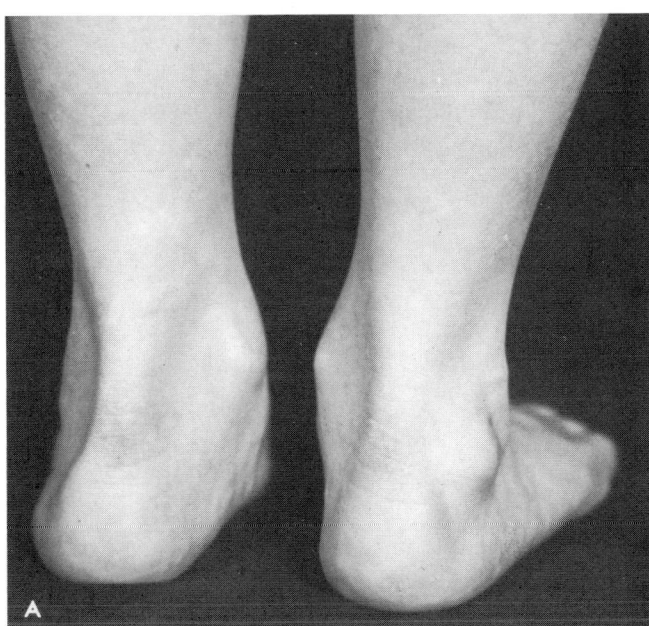

FIGURE 7–88. *Ganglion in the region of the right ankle behind the lateral malleolus.*

A. Photograph shows the mass behind the lateral malleolus. **B.** Gross appearance of the cyst at surgery.

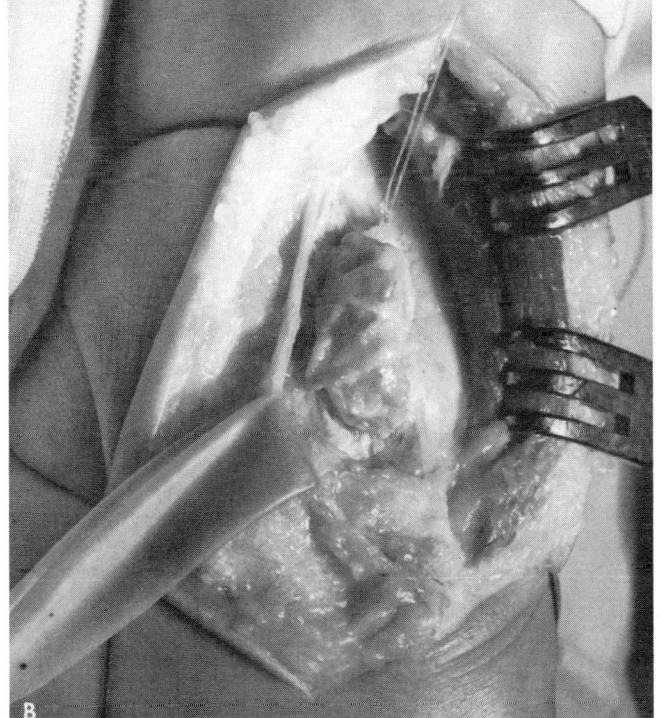

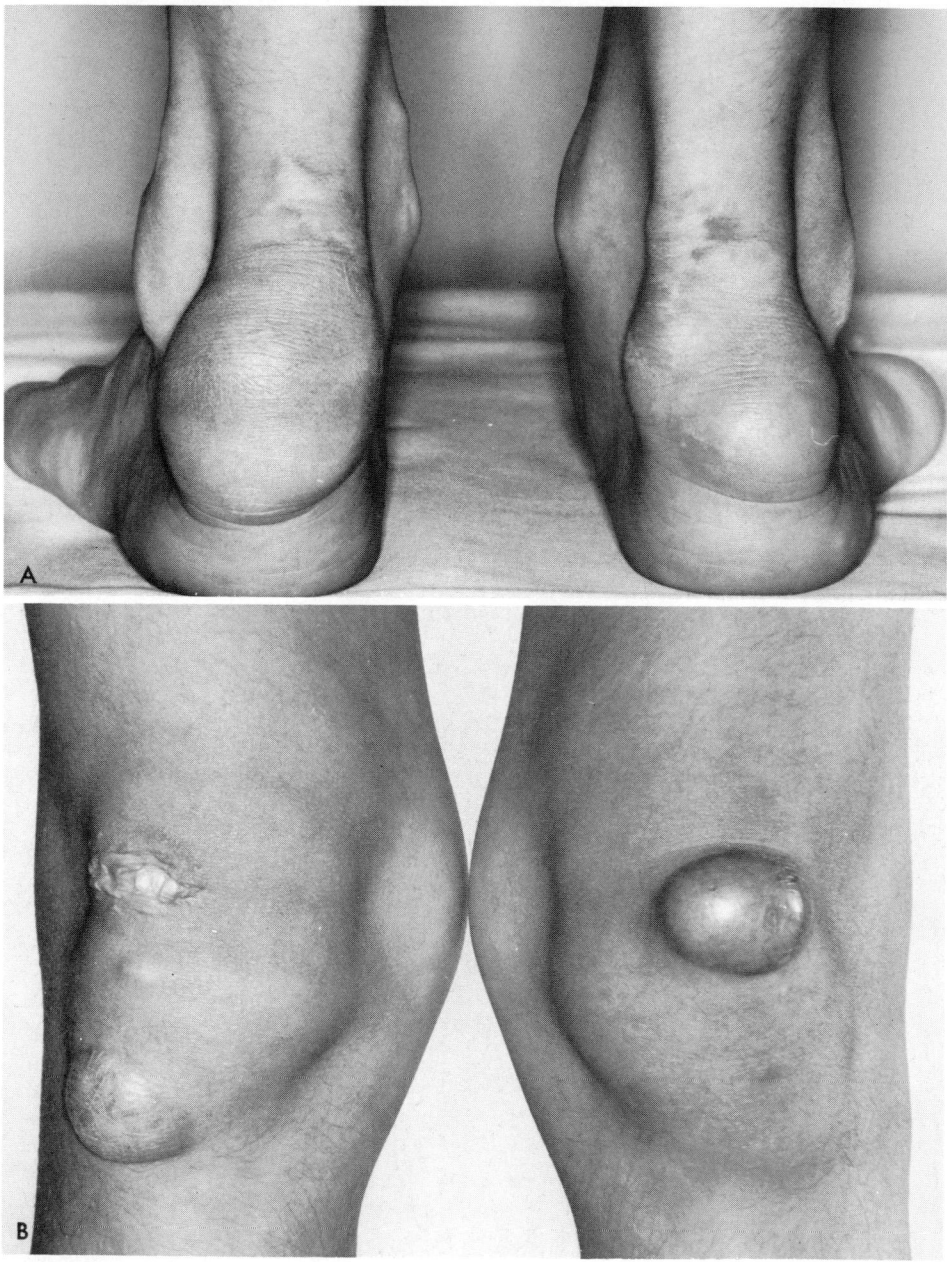

FIGURE 7–89. Multiple xanthomatosis involving both heels and the extensor surfaces of knees.

joint capsule. Surgical excision of the ganglia is usually indicated if they interfere with the normal fit of the shoe. Rupture of the cyst by external force or aspiration of its contents and injection of hydrocortisone are, as a rule, inadequate, and the ganglion eventually recurs. The best treatment is complete excision, which should be performed in the operating room under general anesthesia and tourniquet ischemia. The ligamentous tissue at the base of the stalk of the ganglion should be removed or scarified to prevent recurrence.

Fibroma and Fibromatosis

Solitary fibroma is rare, but may occur at any site in the foot and ankle; treatment is by surgical excision. Fibromata of plantar fascia does occur in adolescents, causing pain and disability; it is treated by excision of the plantar fascia. *Other soft-tissue tumors* that may affect the foot are multiple xanthomatosis (Fig. 7–89), tumoral calcinosis (Fig. 7–90), and pigmented villonodular synovitis (Fig. 7–91). Glomus tumor is rarely found in children.

TUMORS OF BONE

Tumors of bone occasionally occur in the foot, involving the tarsal and metatarsal bones. Osteoid osteoma, enchondroma, aneurysmal bone cyst, unicameral bone cyst, and multiple hereditary exostosis are some of the lesions encountered; they are discussed individually in Chapter 3.

A bony tumor characteristically found in the foot is *subungual exostosis.* It presents as a bony growth from the dorsal surface of the distal part of the terminal phalanx of a toe, usually the great toe. A history of previous injury may be obtained in some cases; however, its cause is unknown. The condition is usually encountered in adolescents or young adults and is preponderant in females. The tumor projects upward and forward between the tip of the nail and the terminal pulp. The nail is deformed, becomes elevated, and eventually undergoes degenerative changes. The tumor is very painful, especially when pressure is applied over the nail. Diagnosis is made by demonstration of the exostosis in the roentgenogram (Fig. 7–92). It is treated by excision through a transverse incision at the distal end of the nail.

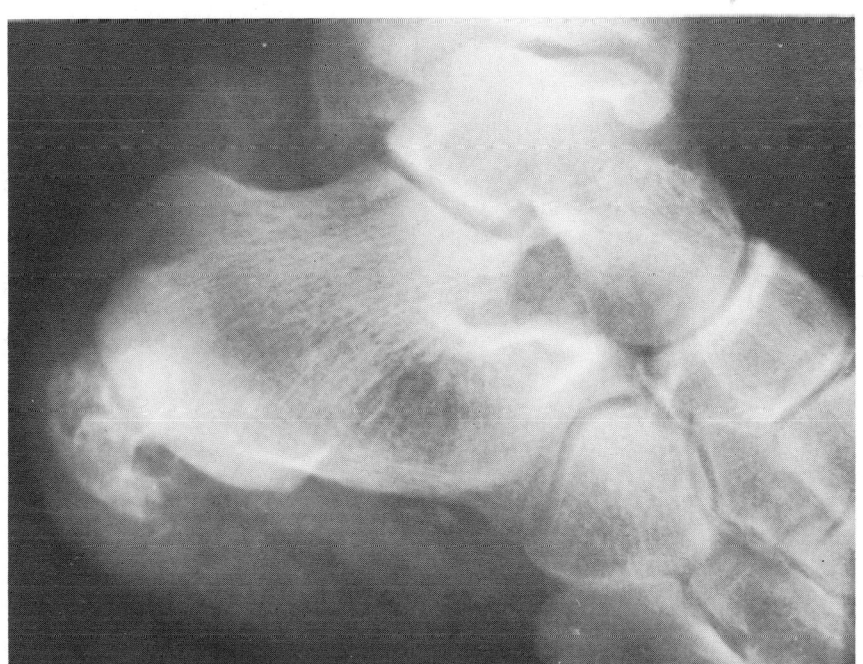

FIGURE 7–90.   Tumoral calcinosis presenting as firm calcified mass in the posterior aspect of the heel.

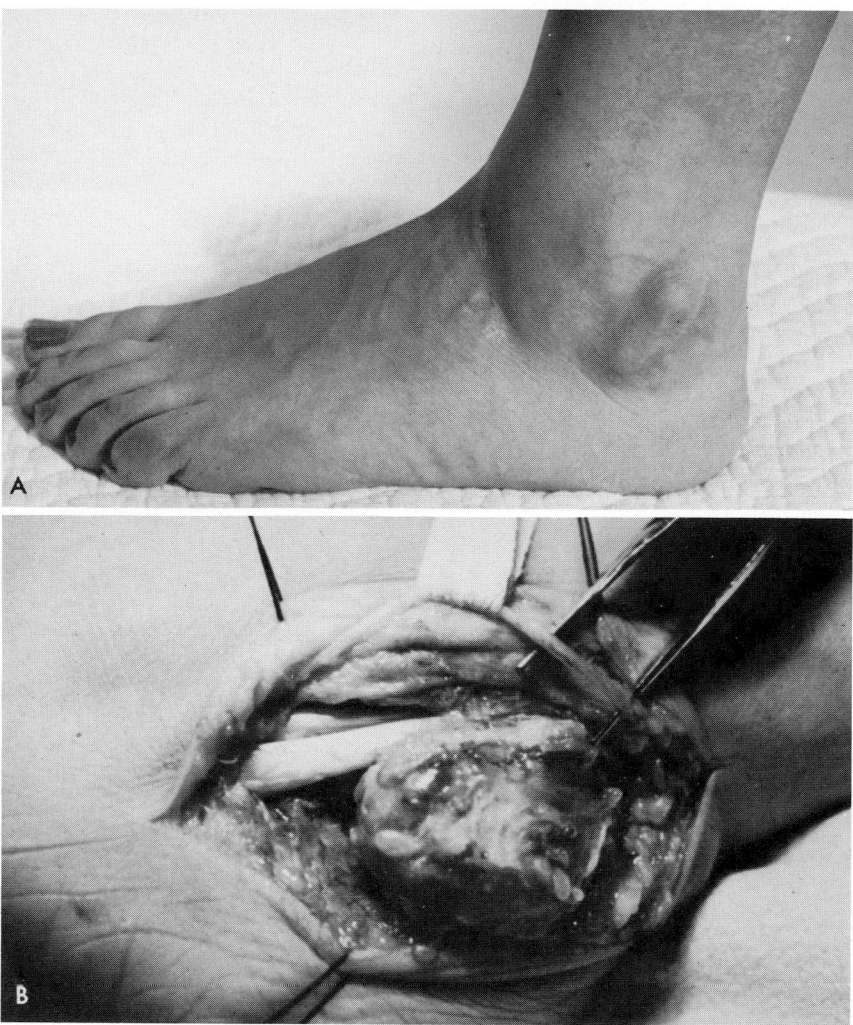

FIGURE 7–91.   *Pigmented villonodular synovitis of subtalar joint.*

A. Photograph showing soft-tissue mass below the lateral malleolus. **B.** Gross appearance at surgery.

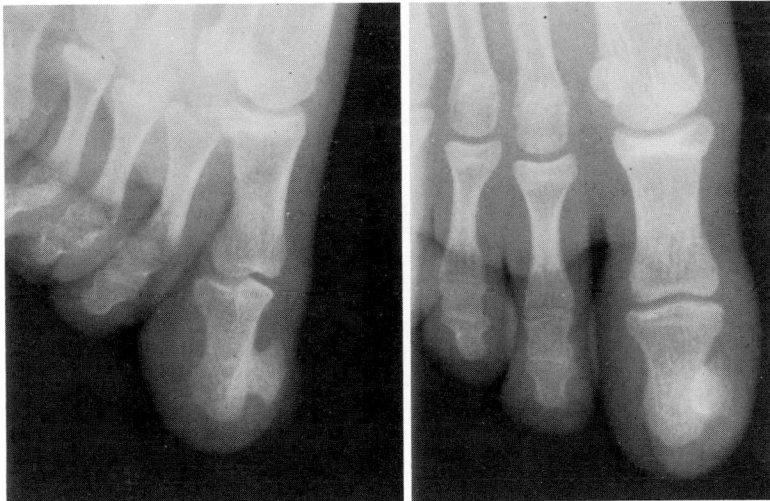

FIGURE 7–92. *Subungual exostosis of the distal phalanx of the great toe.*

Muscle Contracture and Tendinitis

CONGENITAL CONTRACTURE OF TRICEPS SURAE MUSCLE

Walking on tiptoes is normal when children first begin to walk. Within three to six months they "grow out" of the toe-toe or toe-heel gait pattern and learn to walk with a heel-toe gait. In some children, however, toe walking persists because of congenital short tendo calcaneus, an entity described by Hall, Salter, and Bhalla.[521] The affected children walk on their toes, though on volition, they are able to lower their heels to the ground. When they attempt heel-toe gait, their knees hyperextend and their gait is awkward; toe walking is naturally more comfortable. The range of dorsiflexion of the ankle is limited, with the degree of equinus deformity varying from case to case. On deep palpation, an abnormally low insertion of the hypertrophied soleus muscle may be palpated in the region of the tendo Achillis. Neurologic examination is completely normal.

In the differential diagnosis, one should consider an abnormally large soleus or accessory soleus muscle, hyperkinesia due to minimal brain damage syndrome, delayed maturation of corticospinal tracts, spastic paraplegia, diastematomyelia, and muscular dystrophy.

In delayed maturation of the corticospinal tracts in the early stages, there is no fixed equinus deformity. The deep tendon reflexes may be hyperactive and the Babinski sign may be equivocal. Other signs of spasticity cannot be elicited. The condition is usually familial, the toe walking normally disappearing between six and eight years of age.

Treatment

Conservative measures are indicated in the young child and consist of passive stretching exercises of the triceps surae muscle performed by the parents 15 to 20 times in several daily sessions. A splint or bivalved cast that holds the ankle in neutral position is worn at night.

If there is permanent contracture of the triceps surae muscle, a below-knee walking cast with an anterior walking heel is applied to stretch the triceps surae muscle. The cast is changed at two-week intervals, each time bringing the foot and ankle into further dorsiflexion. Usually two or three stretching casts are required to correct the equinus deformity. Following removal of the cast, gait training and passive stretching exercises of the triceps surae and active exercises to strengthen the anterior tibial function are important measures that will prevent recurrence of equinus deformity and toe walking. Occasionally a dorsiflexion assist below-knee orthosis is worn to establish the pattern of heel-toe gait.

When the child has reached the age of six to eight years and one or two trials of conservative management have failed, a sliding heel cord lengthening may be indicated (see Plate 28). An abnormally low insertion of the soleus muscle on the Achilles tendon or an accessory soleus is a common finding at surgery, in which instance, the accessory soleus or distal one fourth of the muscle belly of the soleus is excised. Postoperative care follows the same guidelines as outlined for cerebral palsy in Chapter 5. The presence of hyperkinesia and minimal brain damage should alert the orthopedist to undertake more aggressive measures during the postoperative period.

ACHILLES TENDINITIS

In children and adolescents, a painful heel is a common complaint that may arise from affections of any of the structures composing the heel. The most common cause, however, is nonspecific tendinitis of the heel cord. Symptoms usually develop following strenuous physical activity. The Achilles tendon is swollen and tender near its insertion. Roentgenograms demonstrate soft-tissue swelling. Fragmentation and irregular radiopacity of the calcaneal apophysis are normal findings, however, and the spurious diagnosis of calcaneal apophysitis or Sever's disease should not be made.

In mild cases, the counter of the heel of the shoe is softened and a $1/4$- to $3/8$-inch lift is added to the heel to decrease the tension of the triceps surae on the apophysis of the calcaneus. Sports, running, jumping, and prolonged walking are curtailed. These measures will usually relieve symptoms within three to four weeks. If tendinitis is severe, additional complete rest for the foot and leg is provided by immobilization for three weeks in a below-knee walking cast with the ankle joint at a 20-degree equinus angle; in the three-week period following cast removal, the patient is allowed to walk with a raised heel on the shoe.

Skin and Nail Lesions

The skin of the foot responds to stress of body weight and to external pressure applied by the shoes. The *epidermis*, the outermost layer of the skin, is an epithelial tissue derived from ectoderm; the *dermis*, the subjacent deeper layer, is of mesodermal origin and consists of dense connective tissue. In the sole of the foot, the epidermis is very thick. In the embryo, the nails first appear in the third lunar month as invasions of epidermis into the subjacent dermis over the distal ends of the toes. This epidermal plate forms the matrix of the nail from which the epidermal cells proliferate and gradually become transformed into hard keratinous nail tissue that is pushed distally over the nail bed. The matrix of the nail, extending from its root to the crescentic whitish lunula, is the only site where longitudinal growth of the nail takes place, normal growth being about 1 mm. per week. If the matrix of the nail is destroyed, longitudinal growth of the nail will be arrested, and instead of a hard smooth nail appendage, the nail bed will be covered with irregular, corrugated, horny tissue.

The skin and nails are affected by a great variety of lesions; only the commoner ones are briefly discussed here. For more extensive details, the reader is referred to general textbooks of dermatology and the cited references.

HARD CORN (CLAVUS DURUS)

A hard corn is a localized cornification of the skin resulting from shoe pressure on a bony prominence. It is most commonly seen over the dorsolateral aspect of the proximal interphalangeal joint of the fifth toe and over the tip of a flexed toe close to its nail. In the central area of the corn there is a deeply penetrating nucleus of hyperkeratosis, which is partly degenerated. Beneath this hyperkeratotic central nucleus, there may be a sac containing fluid; irritation and inflammation of this sac and consequent pressure on the nerve endings in the papillary layer of the dermis are the causes of pain.

The immediate cause of the corn must be removed to eliminate the possibility of recurrence; it may be a badly fitted shoe, deformed toes, or excessive use of the feet. The keratinized skin is softened with preparations containing salicylic acid; the horny layer and central nucleus will then eventually separate and fall away. Occasionally surgical excision of deep rooted corns is required; this should be done under strict aseptic conditions to prevent infection.

SOFT CORNS (CLAVUS MOLLIS)

Soft corns are rare in children. They usually occur between the toes, the most frequent sites being between the fourth and fifth toes, where they are caused by bony pressure from a small exostosis on the lateral aspect of the base of the proximal phalanx of the fourth toe. They are soft, of whitish appearance, and have a depressed central area.

The condition is painful and disabling. Treatment consists of excision of the interdigital clavus, resection of the exostosis or the proximal half of the proximal phalanx of the fourth toe, or surgical syndactylism of the fourth and fifth toes.

PLANTAR WART (VERRUCA PLANTARIS)

These are very common in children, and may be found on any part of the plantar aspect of the foot, on either weight-bearing or non-weight-bearing surfaces. Frequent sites are the heel, under the metatarsal heads, and the big toe. They may be single or may be surrounded by a whole crop of daughter warts, their size ranging from a few millimeters to two or three centimeters. A multitude of tiny warts may conglomerate into a large "mosaic wart." Plantar warts are infectious and may be transferred from one child to another by direct contact or by indirect means such as bath mats. Epidemics have been known to occur in schools.

Anatomically, a plantar wart is a papillomatous growth, but instead of projecting beyond the skin surface (like warts elsewhere), they are buried under the stratum corneum of the skin, with only the ends of the papillae showing through. They are extremely vascular and bleed profusely when trimmed. Plantar warts have a dark, punctate surface and are clearly demarcated from the surrounding skin. On direct pressure and lateral compression of the skin, the lesion is markedly tender.

Treatment

In children, a conservative approach is advised. Small lesions can be ignored, but if they are especially painful, the area is padded to relieve pressure of body weight on the wart. Larger or persistent lesions are destroyed by a caustic or keratolytic agent. Lapidus recommends applying 50 per cent salicylic acid ointment, covering the entire area of the wart with 40 per cent salicylic acid plaster (manufactured by Duke Laboratories, Inc.), and strapping it with adhesive tape. In three or four days, the dressing is removed and the foot is re-examined. The keratolytic medication may not be tolerated by some children and may produce irritation and aggravate the pain, in which case, the dressing is removed and the foot is soaked in pHisoHex solution and zinc oxide ointment is applied. Most patients do tolerate the salicylic acid ointment. At weekly intervals the macerated skin is debrided, bleeding vessels are cauterized with silver nitrate stick, and again salicylic acid and plaster are applied. Intractable plantar warts, particularly the mosaic warts, may require several weeks of treatment before being cured. Parents should be advised of the stubborn nature of the condition.[528]

Electrocoagulation of the plantar wart under local infiltration anesthesia may result in an intractable ulcer; it should be performed in only a few selected cases. Excision of the lesion may result in a disabling postoperative scar and is not recommended. Irradiation is contraindicated, as it may cause chronic indolent ulceration.

INGROWING TOENAIL

Ingrowing toenail most commonly involves the great toe. It is caused by external pressure from tight shoes or hose on an improperly trimmed nail that has been cut too short so that its corners dig into the pulp. The edges of the nail become thickened and press into the neighboring soft tissues, which respond by hypertrophy. Soon the overgrown soft tissues obliterate the medial or lateral nail grooves. This mechanical irritation is followed by infection of the skin fold. Pus then spreads around the edge of the nail and between the nail and the matrix, the great toe becoming red, swollen, locally tender, and painful.

Conservative treatment is indicated in mild and early cases. A pledget of cotton or gauze soaked in an antiseptic (such as aqueous Zephiran) is tucked beneath the corner of the nail so that it does not dig into the skin. This is done once or twice a day; then the nail is allowed to grow until its edges project beyond the skin folds. Local hot soaks may be used three or four times a day or continuously, depending upon the severity of infection. The toe nails should subsequently be cut with square corners and the child should be fitted with proper shoes and socks to prevent recurrence.

Surgery is indicated in long-standing cases or when conservative measures have failed, the simplest method being excision of a wedge of nail bed together with the margin of skin fold. In very severe or recurrent cases, permanent ablation of the nail by excision of the nail bed is indicated.

The Leg

TORSIONAL DEFORMITIES OF THE LOWER LIMBS

Torsion is defined as the twisting of a long bone on its longitudinal axis. In *tibial torsion* the distal segment of the tibia may be rotated toward the medial malleolus (internal or medial tibial torsion) or toward the lateral malleolus (external or lateral tibial torsion). As the tibia twists, the relative planes of the transverse axes of the knee and ankle joints are consequently altered. In *femoral torsion* the lower or condylar portion is the fixed end upon which the proximal part rotates on its longitudinal axis. In *anteversion* or *antetorsion* the femoral neck axis is twisted forward or anteriorly in relation to the frontal or coronal plane of the femoral condyles, whereas in *retroversion* or *retrotorsion* the plane of the femoral neck axis is rotated posteriorly or directed backward with reference to the coronal condylar plane.

In the past, the term "angle of declination" was used interchangeably with "femoral torsion." Such usage is misleading and should be discontinued, as the "angle of declination" is often confused with the "angle of inclination," which is that angle formed by the femoral neck axis with the femoral shaft axis (the so-called shaft-neck angle).

Pathophysiologic Considerations

The shape of a bone is determined by both intrinsic and extrinsic factors. In order to understand the pathogenesis and rationale of therapy of torsional deformities of the lower limb, certain basic facts and experimental work are reviewed here.

Deformation of growing bones by abnormal pressure has been known for centuries, as attested by the Chinese bound-foot deformities and the elongated skull of the Egyptians. This quality of bone was well portrayed by Nicholas André in his familiar picture of the crooked tree bound to the straight rod as a symbol of the plasticity of the skeleton of the growing child.

Abnormal pressure can alter the shape of the growing skeleton only when applied more or less continuously over a period of time. Osseus tissue, being a crystalline structure, is elastic rather than plastic in the true sense. The "plasticity" of the skeleton is biologic, apparent only after the passage of time and existing only during periods of growth.[587] According to Wolff, "Every change in the form and function of bones or their function alone is followed by certain definite changes in their external configuration in accordance with mathematical laws."[589]

The rate of epiphyseal growth is affected by pressures applied to its axes, i.e., increased pressure inhibits growth and decreased pressure accelerates it, a relationship that was originally noted by Delpech in 1829 and was later recognized by Hueter and Volkmann in 1862; it is often referred to as the Hueter-Volkmann law.[545, 554, 586]

There have been a number of experimental studies on the effects of pressure on epiphyseal growth:

Appleton, in 1934, demonstrated that minor degrees of pressure can slow growth without stopping it entirely. He applied abnormal pressures to the growing bones of young rabbits by creating postural abnormalities by surgical section of certain muscle groups; for example, by division of the external rotators of the hip, he could produce internal deformation of the femur. He also found that the opposite limb was held in lateral rotation and the femur became retroverted.[532] Haas caused total arrest of epiphyseal growth by means of compression with a wire loop.[559]

Arkin and Katz applied pressure over the growing epiphyses of young rabbits by means of plaster casts that immobilized the limbs in deformed positions. They demonstrated that when a growing epiphysis is subjected to a stress, the rate or the direction of growth of that epiphysis, or both, are modified by that stress. Epiphyseal growth is inhibited by pressure applied parallel to its direction of growth. Cartilaginous growth is completely arrested by considerable pressure, but pressure does not inhibit it by an all-or-none law. Rather, growth is retarded by slight or intermittent pressures—such as those from a plaster cast, postural stress, or gravitational and muscular forces. In vertical weight-bearing bones, the gravitational force of normal weight-bearing seems to slow cartilaginous growth, whereas lack of normal weight-bearing stresses results in overgrowth. Pressures applied perpendicularly to the direction of epiphyseal growth

deflect such growth, resulting in lateral or spiral (torsional) displacement of the newly laid-down bone. The diameter of a bone is a determining factor in the ease with which angular or torsional deformities are produced—the narrower the bone, the greater its "plasticity."[533]

The effect of splinting the hind limbs of immature animals in different positions, with particular reference to rotation, has been studied by a number of investigators. Bernbeck produced increased femoral anteversion by immobilizing the hindlegs of kittens in medial rotation.[536]

Wilkinson used six- to eight-week-old rabbits for his experiments, rabbits being chosen because of the similarity of the normal posture of their hindlimbs in flexion, abduction, and lateral rotation to the human prenatal and neonatal postures. He showed that: (1) prolonged medial rotation of the femur produces anteversion, whether the hip is in flexion or extension, abduction or adduction; (2) prolonged lateral rotation of the femur, with the hip flexed and abducted, increases retroversion; and (3) prolonged fixation of the femur in the Lorenz position corrects or prevents the development of retroversion. The deformity occurred mostly in the metaphyseal region and was twice as great in the distal metaphysis as in the proximal metaphysis, reflecting the relative growth in these areas.[588] Salter performed similar experiments and demonstrated that anteversion is produced by the strain of medial rotation on the femoral epiphysis, and retroversion is produced by the strain of lateral rotation.[578] The bone displacement in a rotational deformity is always in the direction opposite to that of the deforming force.

Salter, in a series of experiments in newborn pigs, also studied the effect on the acetabulum of maintained extension and flexion of the hip. A position of forced extension of the hip for a period of six to eight weeks resulted in dysplasia and maldirection of the acetabulum, whereas maintained flexion was associated with normal acetabular development. The restricting bandages were removed from one group of animals that were then allowed to run free; the acetabular dysplasia was reversed and the maldirection of the entire acetabulum reverted to normal.[577]

Brookes and Wardle studied the effect of muscle action on the shape of decalcified femora. They showed that an iliopsoas force acting at the lesser trochanter causes an immediate valgus deformity, posterior deflection of the neck, and lateral rotation of the shaft with an increase in its anterior convexity. Conversely, the effect of gluteal action at the greater trochanter produced coxa vara and anterior deflection of the neck with medial torsion and straightening of the shaft. The tendency to femoral deformity produced by the iliopsoas force was abolished by a gluteal force acting on the greater trochanter when these were in a ratio of 5:3. Adductor action causes medial deflection and torsion of the diaphysis with some varus deformity of the neck of the femur.[541]

Rotation of the Limb Bud

In humans, the evolution of upright posture requires the limb buds to rotate during embryonic development. The lower limbs originate in a laterally abducted and flexed position relative to the pelvis and acetabular anlage. Around the third month of intrauterine life, the femoral neck and shaft become adducted (almost 90 degrees) to a position parallel with the longitudinal axis of the trunk and rotate medially to allow the patella and leg to face forward.[535]

This rotation phenomenon of the lower limb necessitates certain adaptive changes in the direction in which the acetabulum faces. Dega studied 100 fetal skeletons and found the angle of forward inclination of the acetabulum to be 29.5 degrees and its angle of downward inclination in relation to the transverse plane to be 62.8 degrees.[544] With the change in the position of the hip from the intrauterine posture of flexion and abduction to that of erect posture of hip extension and neutral adduction, the forward inclination of the acetabulum decreases. Some degree of retention of fetal position of the lower limbs is common and normal in early infancy.

Etiologic Considerations

The exact cause of torsional deformities of the lower limb is not known. A number of possible factors should be considered.

PERSISTENT FETAL ALIGNMENT

Böhm observed that human beings have an inherent predisposition to certain infantile deformities of the ankles, knees, and hips, and he proposed these to be caused by an arrest of skeletal development. The proximal tibial epiphysis of the adult gorilla was noted by Böhm to have marked asymmetry — the lateral condyle is overdeveloped, whereas the medial condyle is underdeveloped. In the human fetus, the proximal tibial epiphysis has certain anthropoid characteristics — the lateral condyle is high and convex, the medial condyle is low and concave, and the tibial diaphysis is deviated medially, producing a genu varum.[540]

In the newborn child the fetal configuration of the tibia with a high lateral condyle, a low medial condyle, and varus inclination of the shaft is still present. This tibia vara deformity will gradually correct itself with growth. If the tibia retains its fetal shape, a genu varum deformity results. Böhm calls attention to the difference in the volume and height of the femoral condyles in the anthropoid knee; the medial femoral condyle is much larger and higher than the lateral condyle. In his studies of the human knee in different age groups, Böhm has observed underdevelopment of the lateral femoral condyle in the fetus, and believes that genu valgum results from persistence of underdevelopment of the lateral condyle.[540]

Somerville proposed that abnormal femoral anteversion represents a persistent fetal alignment of the hip due to failure of normal derotation of the femur in utero.[581] Embryologic evidence supports his theory.

HEREDITY

Abnormal femoral antetorsion and internal tibial torsion are familial afflictions. Blumel, Eggers and Evans reported eight cases of bilateral medial tibial torsion in four generations. In their pedigree they demonstrated a mendelian autosomal dominant type of inheritance.[539] That a genetic factor is partly responsible in the causation of abnormal femoral torsion is supported by the report of Crane — in 21 of his 72 patients (29 per cent), siblings or a parent were similarly affected. An exact clear pattern of inheritance could not be demonstrated, however.[543]

PERSISTENT MALPOSTURE IN POSTNATAL LIFE

That the sleeping, sitting, and play habits of the infant and child may disturb the normal developmental pattern of the lower limbs and even cause deformities has been much emphasized in the literature.[551, 555, 558–562] Fitzhugh reviewed the sleeping positions of children, and found that of 100 infants who slept in the knee-chest position, 84 per cent had a deviation of their lower limbs, either inward or outward, of more than 10 degrees.[551] The importance of intrauterine malposture as a factor in the causation of deformities of the newborn is well known. A logical corollary is that sleeping and sitting habits might well influence the persistence of these positional deformities, as well as increase their severity.

The following outline as given by Knight, shows the deformities of the lower limbs that are associated with certain habitual sleeping or sitting positions:

SLEEPING HABITS

I. Prone knee-chest position with:
  a. Extremities internally rotated, results in:
   (1) internal rotation deformity of the hips,
   (2) medial tibial torsion,
   (3) bow-leg,
   (4) ankle equinus,
   (5) adduction and varus of the fore part of the foot (may appear to be a metatarsus varus).
  b. Extremities externally rotated, results in:
   (1) external rotational deformity in the knees,
   (2) knock-knee,
   (3) ankle equinus,
   (4) valgus of the feet.
  c. Extremities neutral, results in:
   (1) ankle equinus (toe-walking of early childhood).

II. Frog-leg position, most frequently prone but occasionally supine, resulting in:
   (1) external rotation deformity of the hips,
   (2) external rotation deformity in the knee joints, in conjunction with shortening of the iliotibial band and of the biceps femoris,
   (3) knock-knee,
   (4) valgus and abduction of the feet.

III. Prone, with hips extended and:
  a. Internally rotated, may result in:
   (1) internal rotation contracture of the hips,
   (2) medial tibial torsion (to a lesser degree than that which results from the knee-chest position),
   (3) ankle equinus,
   (4) varus of the metatarsus, with or without adduction.
  b. Externally rotated, may result in:
   (1) external rotation contracture of the hips,
   (2) external rotation deformity in the knee joints,
   (3) ankle equinus,
   (4) valgus of the feet.

SITTING HABITS

I. Reversed tailor position with:
  a. Feet internally rotated beneath the buttocks (sitting on the feet), results in:
   (1) internal rotation contracture of the hips,
   (2) medial tibial torsion,
   (3) adduction of the fore part of the foot.
  b. Feet externally rotated, results in:
   (1) internal rotation contracture of the hips,
   (2) external rotation deformity in the knees,
   (3) knock-knee, with relaxation or stretching of medial collateral ligaments,
   (4) valgus deformity of the feet.
  c. One foot internally rotated and the other externally rotated.*

Crane cites two examples to support the postnatal malposition theory. Both these patients had cerebral atrophy, were unable to talk or walk, and were confined to mental institutions. The first patient was a seven-year-old boy who constantly sat in the reverse tailor's position with the feet externally rotated, a position that provided a broader base and greater stability. With the hips in extension, internal rotation of the hips was 75 degrees and external rotation only 5 to 10 degrees. The angle of anteversion was 50 degrees on the right and 57 degrees on the left (Fig. 7–93 A-C). The second patient, in the next bed, sat continually in the tailor's position. Upon straightening his lower limbs, he reverted to this position. With the hips extended, internal rotation of the hip was 10 degrees and external rotation

---

*From Knight, R. A.: Developmental deformities of the lower extremities. J. Bone Joint Surg., 36-A:521, 1954. Reprinted with permission.

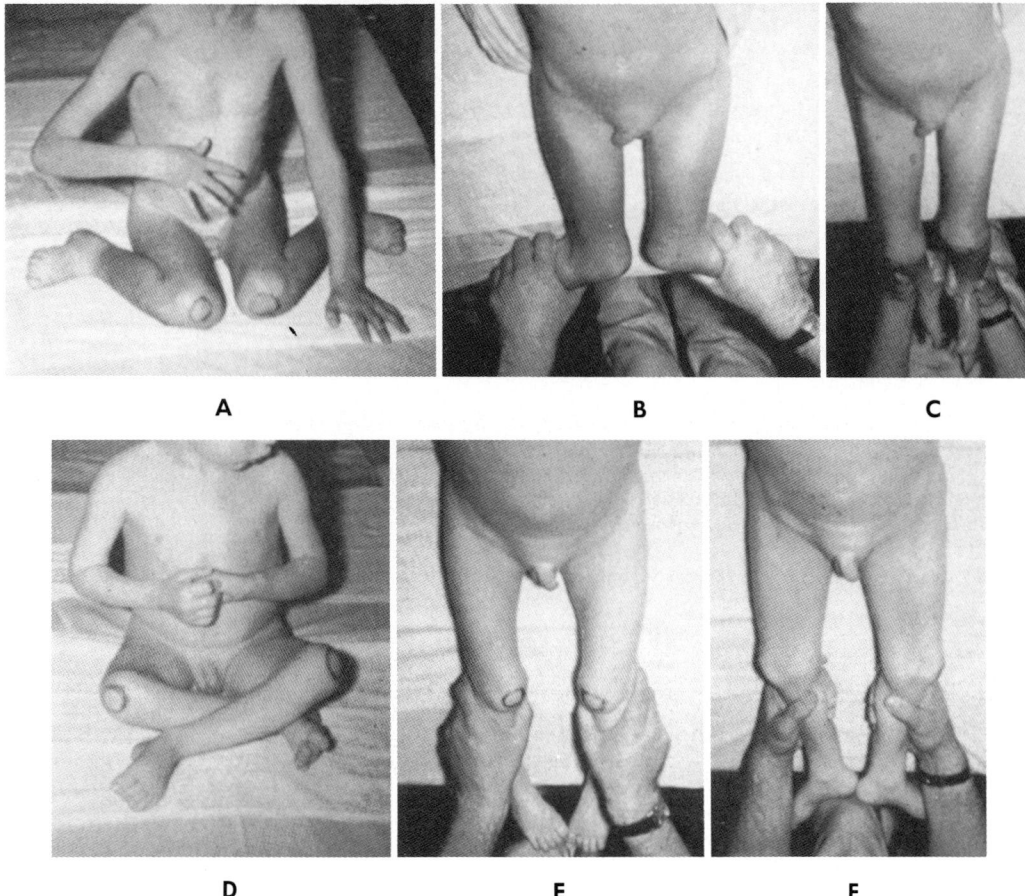

FIGURE 7–93. *Developmental deformities of the lower limbs due to persistent malposition.*

Both patients had cerebral atrophy, were confined to mental institutions, and could not talk or walk. **A** to **C.** A seven year old boy who sat constantly in the reverse tailor's position with the feet externally rotated (**A**). Maximum internal rotation of the hips (**B**) — 75 degrees; maximum external rotation of the hips (**C**) — 5 to 10 degrees; femoral antetorsion was exaggerated bilaterally — right. 50 degrees; left, 53 degrees. **D** to **F.** A five-year-old boy who persistently sat in the tailor's position. He always reverted to this posture after his legs were straightened (**D**). Maximum internal rotation of the hips (**E**) is 10 degrees and maximum external rotation is 80 degrees (**F**). Femoral anteversion was less than 10 degrees. (From Crane, L.: Femoral torsion and its relation to toeing-in and toeing-out. J. Bone Joint Surg., *41–A*:427, 1959.)

80 degrees. Femoral anteversion was less than 10 degrees (Fig. 7–93 D to F).[543]

There is no evidence that, in *normal* infants and children, static forces of malposition are of etiologic significance. Normal children constantly move around and do not remain in one position long enough for the force of gravity to be a factor in the causation of torsional or angular deformities of the lower limbs. Often they assume the tailor's or reverse tailor's position because it is more comfortable for them.

FEMORAL TORSION

Exaggerated anterior torsion of the femur is a common developmental deformity that affects rotational alignment of the lower limb and causes toeing-in. It occurs twice as frequently in girls as in boys.

Methods of Measurement

ROENTGENOGRAPHIC METHOD

A number of techniques are available for the measurement of upper femoral torsion.

The reader is referred to the original descriptions by Dunn, by Dunlap, Shands, Hollister, Gaul, and Streit, by Magilligan, and by Shands and Steele.[546, 547, 549, 567]

The essential features of roentgenographic technique are as follows: (1) The apparent angle of inclination or shaft-neck angle is measured in an anteroposterior or posteroanterior roentgenogram of the pelvis. The hips should be in full extension and neutral rotation, achieved by flexing the knees 90 degrees (over the end of the table when the patient is supine). (2) Torsion of the proximal femora is determined on a lateral roentgenogram of each hip. A frame is used to position the lower limbs — with the hips and knees each flexed 90 degrees and the thighs abducted 10 or 30 degrees. In the Dunlap and Shands technique, the transcondylar axis of the femur is determined by placing a radiopaque reference bar just lateral to the greater trochanter and attaching a second radiopaque bar at right angles to the first bar; the second bar represents the transcondylar axis of the femur (Fig. 7–94).[546] In the Ryder and Crane technique, the baseline of the lateral roentgenogram is used to represent the transcondylar plane, and a line parallel to this is drawn in the

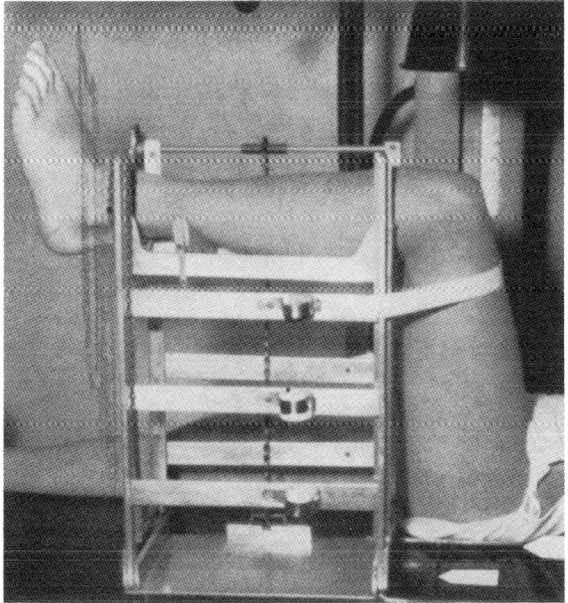
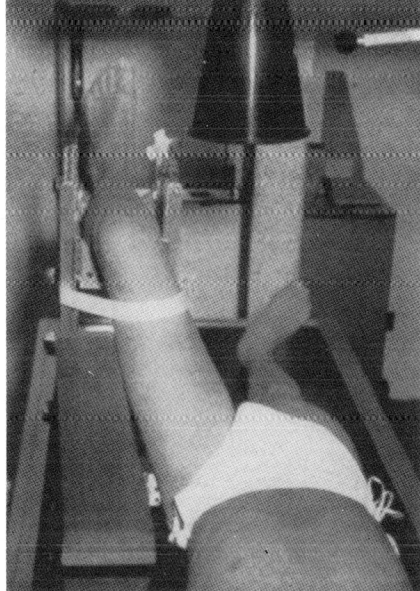

FIGURE 7–94. *The apparatus used by Dunlap et al. and Shands and Steele for making lateral roentgenograms of each hip.*

(From Shands, A. R., Jr., and Steele, M. K.: Torsion of the femur. J. Bone Joint Surg., *40-A*:804, 1958.)

region of the femoral shaft (Fig. 7–95).[576] The apparent angle of torsion is that angle formed by the intersection of the transcondylar plane with the neck axis. (3) The true angle of torsion is then determined from the angle of measured torsion and the angle of measured inclination by using a graph prepared from special mathematical formulas (Figs. 7–96 and 7–97).

The author employs a simple method to determine the degree of anteversion of the proximal femur. The patient is placed in prone position. Under image intensifier fluoroscopy, the length of the femoral neck (intertrochanteric line to capital physis) is determined with the hip in varying degrees of rotation. The hips should be in full extension; and flexion of the knees to right angles will assist in determining the degree of hip rotation. The degree of femoral anteversion is the degree of internal rotation of the hip beyond which the relative length of the femoral neck does not increase.

Shands and Steele determined the degree of femoral torsion in 238 normal children ranging in age from three months to 16 years.[579] The degree of femoral torsion in relation to age is shown in Figure 7–98. Between 3 and 12 months of age, the average degree of normal femoral torsion is 39 degrees; and at the end of the second year, 31 degrees. From that age on, the torsion decreases 1 to 2 degrees every two years until the tenth year, when the average is 24 degrees. From the fourteenth to the sixteenth year, it decreases from 21 to 16 degrees, the latter figure corresponding to the femoral torsion of +15.3 degrees found by Pearson and Bell in the English skeleton.[571] Shands and Steele consider a variation of 10 degrees above or below the average normal value to be within the limits of normal error.[579] The normal values of Ryder and Crane are almost identical to those of Shands and Steele (Fig. 7–99).[576]

CLINICAL METHOD

Femoral antetorsion can be assessed clinically by determining the relative positions of the midpoint of the lateral surface of the greater trochanter and the transverse axis of the femoral condyles.

The Ryder method of clinical estimation of femoral torsion is as follows: (1) The greater trochanter is palpated, (2) the lower limb is externally rotated until the greater trochanter reaches the most lateral position, and (3) the degree of rotation of the femoral transcondylar plane from 0 degrees (neutral position) is estimated—this is the angle of femoral torsion. In antetorsion the leg is externally rotated at the end of Step 2 and the greater trochanter lies posteriorly when the patella faces straight forward, whereas in femoral retroversion the leg is internally rotated at the end of Step 2.

Clinical Features

The condition is usually present at birth; however, this is usually overlooked until the child starts to walk, i.e., between one and two years of age. The chief presenting complaint is that the child is pigeon-toed. The gait is clumsy; the knees and patellae are turned inward. The appearance of the lower limbs is unsightly and disturbing, especially to a girl, while the primary concern of a boy is the loss of agility in athletic activities.

In stance also, the patellae face inward and the legs appear bowed when the feet are aligned so that they point straight forward with the knees in full extension (Fig. 7–100 A). When the thighs are rotated laterally at the hip joints so that the patellae are facing to the front, the feet and legs point outward and the bowleg appearance is corrected (Fig. 7–100 B). A compromise between the two positions is reached by slight flexion of the knees.

Limitation of lateral rotation of the hips in extended position is the principal physical finding. Internal rotation of the hip in extension is exaggerated and may be as much as 90 degrees, whereas lateral rotation is restricted, usually to neutral position (Fig. 7–101). When the hip is in 90 degrees of flexion, lateral rotation of the hip is increased to as much as 45 degrees. This is explained by the fact that in extension of the hip, the anterior capsule and Bigelow ligament become taut; in flexion they are relaxed, permitting lateral rotation of the hip. Thus, the importance of testing the degree of rotation of the hip in extension in femoral anteversion cannot be overemphasized. Crane has determined the normal

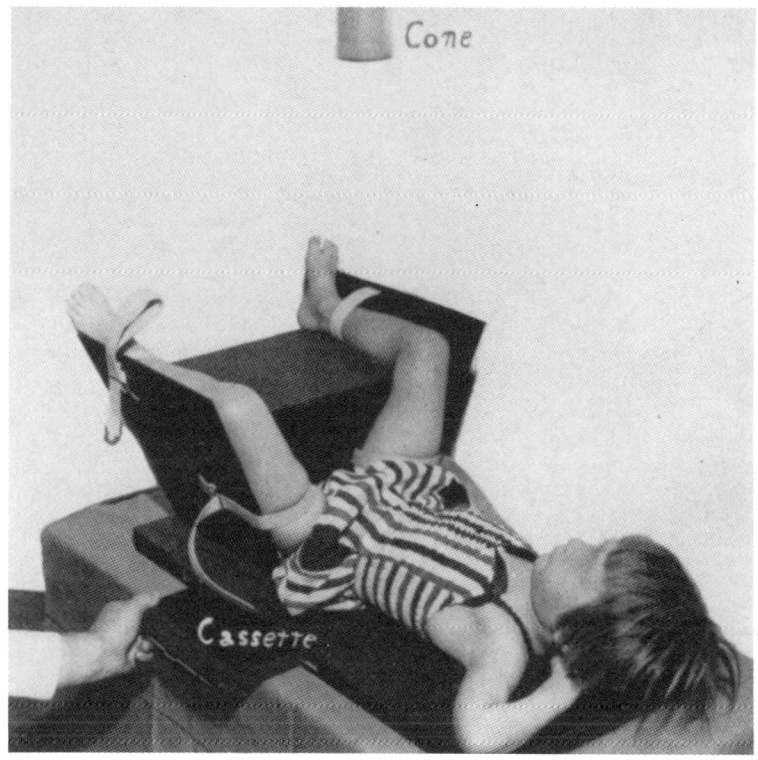

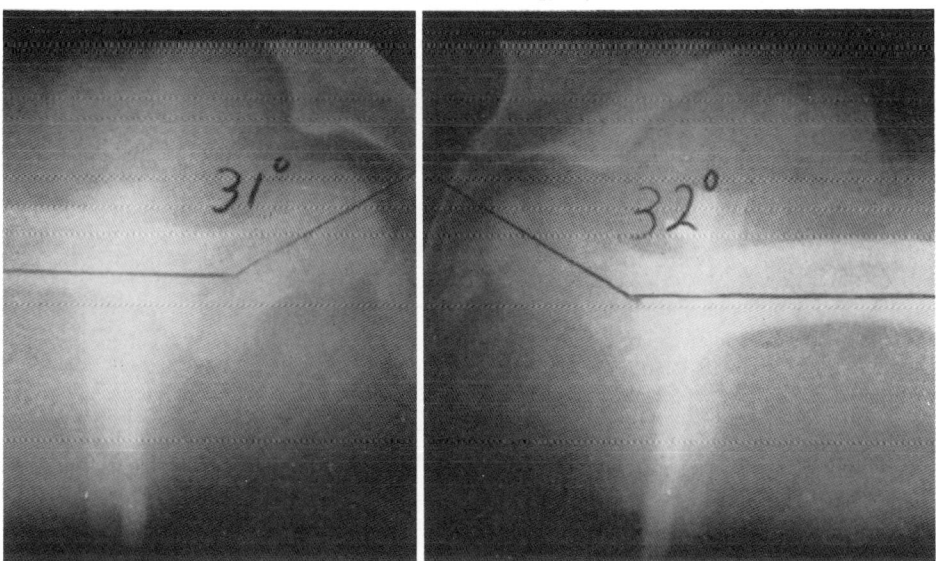

FIGURE 7–95. *Ryder and Crane method of measuring femoral torsion.*

A. Modified flexion-abduction frame. *B.* Roentgenograms of both hips made with the lower limbs positioned in the flexion-abduction frame. The baseline of the roentgenograms represents the transcondylar plane, and a line parallel to it is drawn in the region of the femoral shaft. The angle formed by the intersection of the neck axis and the transcondylar plane is the projected angle of anteversion. The true, or corrected, angle of torsion is determined from a special chart (see Fig. 7–97). (From Crane, L.: Femoral torsion. J. Bone Joint Surg., *41-A*:425, 1959.)

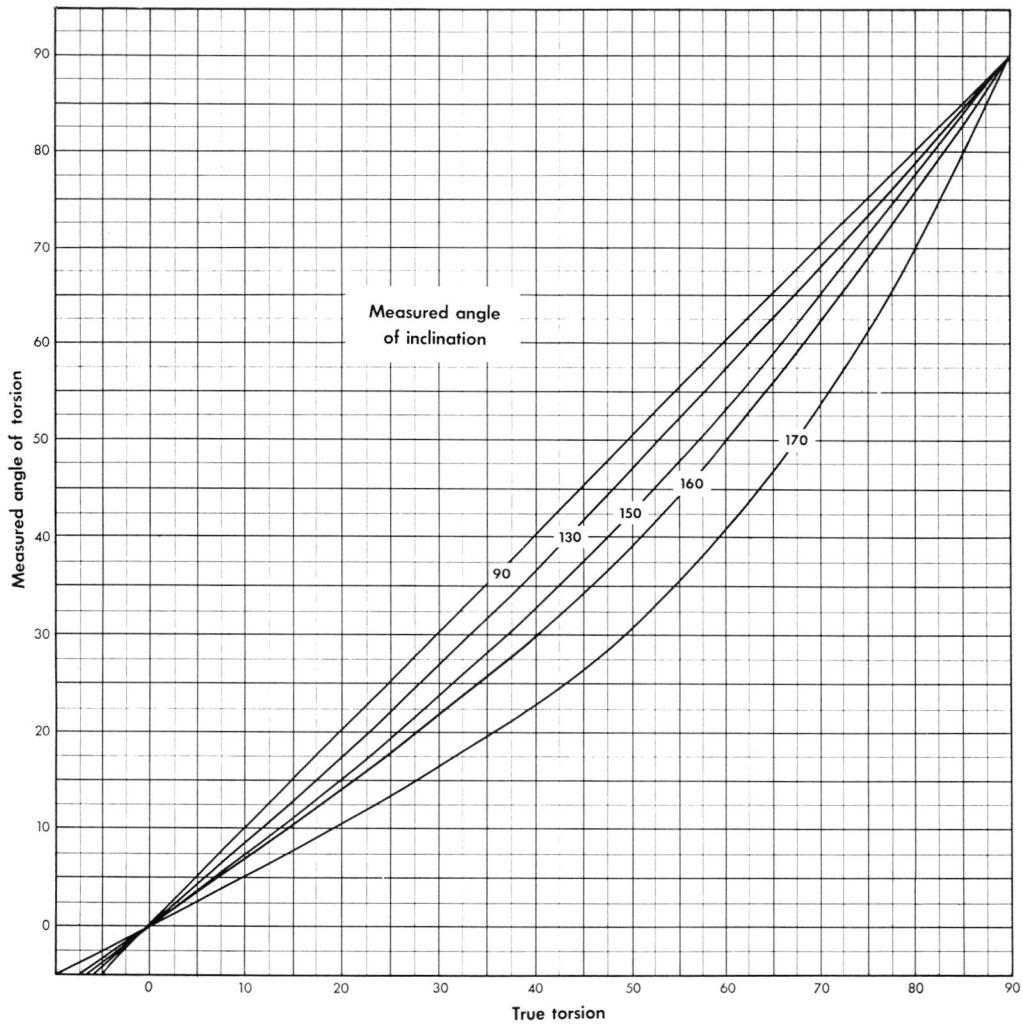

FIGURE 7–96. *Graph used by Dunlap et al. to determine true angle of femoral torsion.*

The measured angle of torsion and the measured angle of inclination are determined from the roentgenogram. The angle of hip abduction is 10 degrees. The graph is prepared from the Weber Formula No. 1. (From Dunlap, K., et al.: A new method for determination of torsion of the femur. J. Bone Joint Surg., *35-A*:299, 1953.)

range of rotation of the hip in extension in various age groups (Fig. 7–102).

The range of rotation of the hip in extension depends upon the inclination of the acetabulum, the angle of torsion of the proximal femur, and contracture of soft tissues—capsule, ligaments, and the muscles and fasciae about the hip, particularly the iliotibial band. It should be stressed that the degree of femoral torsion is only one factor in determining the range of medial and lateral rotation of the hip. To distinguish between soft-tissue and bony obstacles to joint motion, the hip is passively rotated laterally

20 to 30 times; by thus stretching soft-tissue contracture, the range of rotation will be increased. In childhood, internal and external rotation of the hips in extension range from about 35 to 45 degrees. In normal adults, external rotation of the hips exceeds internal rotation by approximately 10 degrees.

Certain adaptive changes take place in response to excessive abnormal femoral antetorsion. In an attempt to compensate for the lack of lateral rotation of the hips, the hindfoot develops a valgus deformity. Soon lateral torsion of the tibia also becomes evi-

projected inclination	projected anteversion 0	5	10	15	20	25	30	35	40	45	50	55	60	65	70	75	80	85	90
80	0	3	7	12	16	20	24	29	33	38	43	47	53	59	65	71	77	84	
90	0	4	9	13	17	22	27	31	36	41	46	51	56	62	67	73	79	84	
95	0	5	9	14	18	23	28	32	37	42	47	52	58	63	68	74	79	85	
100	0	5	10	14	19	24	29	34	39	44	49	54	59	64	69	74	80	85	90
105	0	5	10	15	20	25	30	35	40	45	50	55	60	65	70	75	80	85	90
110	0	5	10	16	21	26	31	36	41	46	51	56	61	66	71	76	80	85	90
115	0	5	11	16	22	27	32	38	43	48	53	57	62	67	72	76	81	85	90
120	0	6	11	17	23	28	34	39	44	49	54	59	63	68	72	77	81	86	90
125	0	6	12	18	24	30	35	41	46	51	56	60	65	69	73	78	82	86	90
130	0	6	13	19	25	31	37	42	47	52	57	62	66	70	74	78	82	86	90
135	0	7	14	20	27	33	38	44	48	54	58	63	67	71	75	79	83	86	90
140	0	7	14	21	28	34	40	46	50	56	60	64	68	72	76	80	83	87	90
145	0	8	16	23	30	36	42	48	53	58	62	66	70	74	77	80	84	87	90
150	0	9	17	25	32	39	45	50	55	60	64	68	72	75	78	81	84	87	90
155	0	10	19	27	35	42	48	54	58	63	67	70	73	77	79	82	85	87	90
160	0	11	22	31	39	46	52	58	62	65	70	73	76	78	81	83	86	88	90
165	0	13	26	36	45	52	57	62	66	70	73	76	78	80	82	84	86	88	90
170	0	18	33	45	53	60	65	69	72	75	77	79	81	83	84	86	87	89	90
175	0	29	48	59	67	71	75	77	79	81	82	84	85	86	87	88	88	89	90
180	0	90	90	90	90	90	90	90	90	90	90	90	90	90	90	90	90	90	90

(ANTEVERSION — right axis label)

FIGURE 7–97. *Chart used by Ryder and Crane to calculate the true angle of femoral torsion.*

(From Ryder, C. T., and Crane L.: Measuring femoral anteversion. J. Bone Joint Surg., 35-A:324, 1953.)

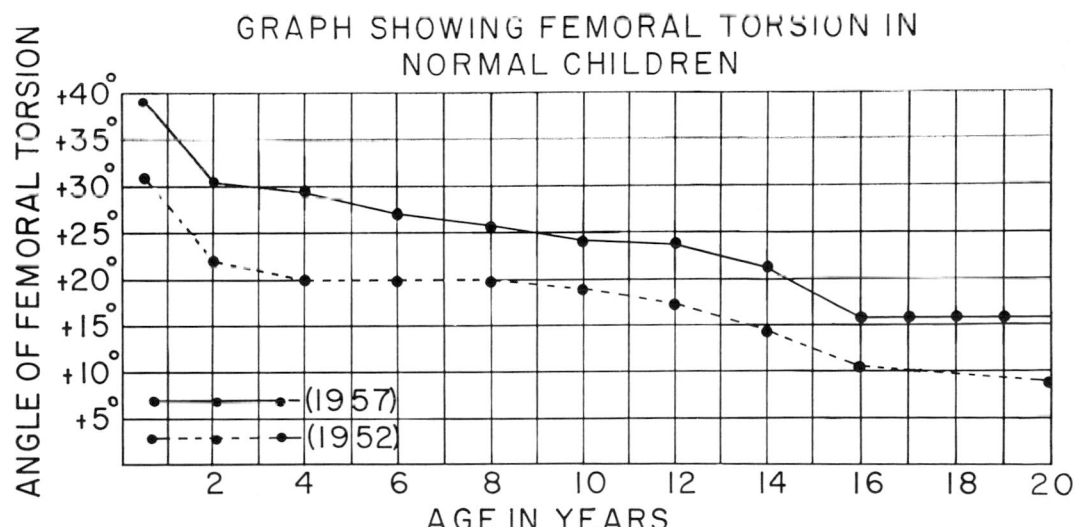

FIGURE 7–98. *The degree of femoral torsion in relation to age.*

The solid line on the graph (1957 study) represents the average values in 238 children with the roentgenograms made with the hips in 10 degrees of abduction. The broken line represents the average degree of femoral torsion determined in 215 normal children in 1952, when the roentgenograms were made with the hips in 35 degrees of abduction. The 1952 determinations are less accurate and their values are from 5 to 9 degrees lower than those in the 1957 study. (From Shands, A. R., Jr., and Steele, M. K.: Torsion of the femur. J. Bone Joint Surg., 40-A:806, 1958.)

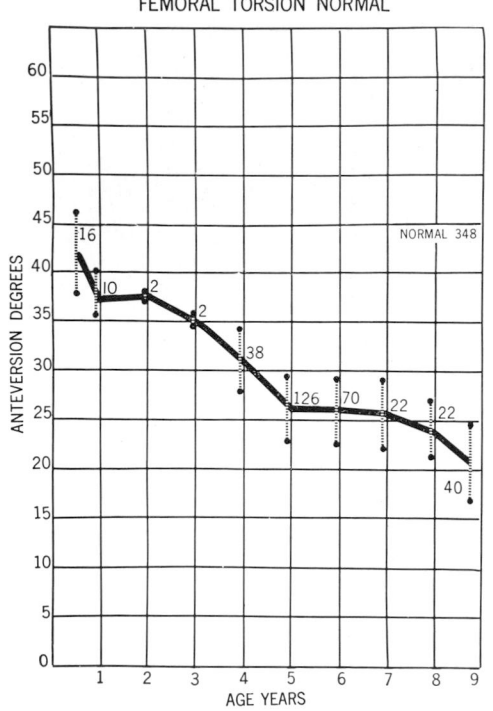

FEMORAL TORSION NORMAL

NORMAL 348

*FIGURE 7–99.   The degree of normal femoral torsion
in relation to age.*

The solid lines represent the mean; the vertical lines
represent standard deviation. (From Crane, L.: Femoral torsion and its relation to toeing-in and toe-
ing out. J. Bone Joint Surg., *41-A*:423, 1959.)

dent. As stated previously, in the fetus and
newborn, the acetabulum faces in a more
forward direction than in the adult. With
exaggerated femoral antetorsion, this fetal
direction of the acetabulum may persist,
and may itself be a cause of toeing-in. In the
series of McSweeny, femoral torsion was
found to be normal in one third of those
children whose in-toeing did not correct
itself, suggesting acetabular maldirection
at the cause of the toeing-in.[566]

The natural history of femoral anteversion is such that it will gradually undergo
spontaneous correction due to the forces exerted on the femoral neck by the taut capsule and Bigelow ligament. However, the
evidence is that an abnormal angle of
anteversion usually does not correct itself
after the age of seven years.[565]

The stresses of marked femoral anteversion may cause degenerative arthritic
changes of the hip in adult life.

Treatment

The type of treatment depends upon the
severity of deformity and the age of the patient.

In the young child passive stretching exercises are performed to elongate any associated soft-tissue contracture that is holding the hip in internal rotation. The child is
encouraged to sit in the tailor's position and
is not allowed to sit in reverse tailor's position. If in stance the hindfoot is valgus, a ⅛
to 3/16 inch inner heel wedge is put on the
shoe. Most important, the parents are reassured that excessive femoral antetorsion will
most probably correct itself spontaneously
by the age of seven or eight years. The child
is examined at six month intervals to assess
the improvement in the range of lateral rotation of the hip in extension. It is not necessary to make roentgenograms of the hip or
to perform antetorsion studies every six
months. If the initial studies showed the
degree of femoral antetorsion to exceed 45
degrees and if the hip could not be rotated
laterally beyond neutral position, periodic
roentgenograms once a year are sufficient.
If there is no spontaneous improvement,
splinting of the hips in forced external rotation should be considered. The author uses
bilateral above-knee bivalved hip spica
casts that hold the hips in 60 to 80 degrees
of external rotation, 90 degrees of flexion
and 45 to 60 degrees of abduction. These
bivalved casts are only used at night, and to
obtain any substantial improvement, they
should be used for at least one year.

Denis Browne splints should not be employed, as they will cause secondary deformities in the segments distal to the hip joint;
namely, pes valgus, lateral torsion of the
tibia, and genu valgum. The deforming influence and harmful effects of the Denis
Browne splint in the treatment of femoral
anteversion cannot be overemphasized.

In children over eight years of age, excessive femoral antetorsion probably will not
correct itself spontaneously and lateral rotation osteotomy of the femur is indicated if
the deformity is severe. The surgery should
not be postponed until late adolescence because of the possible development of increasing external tibial torsion and fixed pes
valgus deformity.

Somerville states that if lateral rotation of
the hip of more than 15 degrees is possible, the condition may be ignored.[580] It is

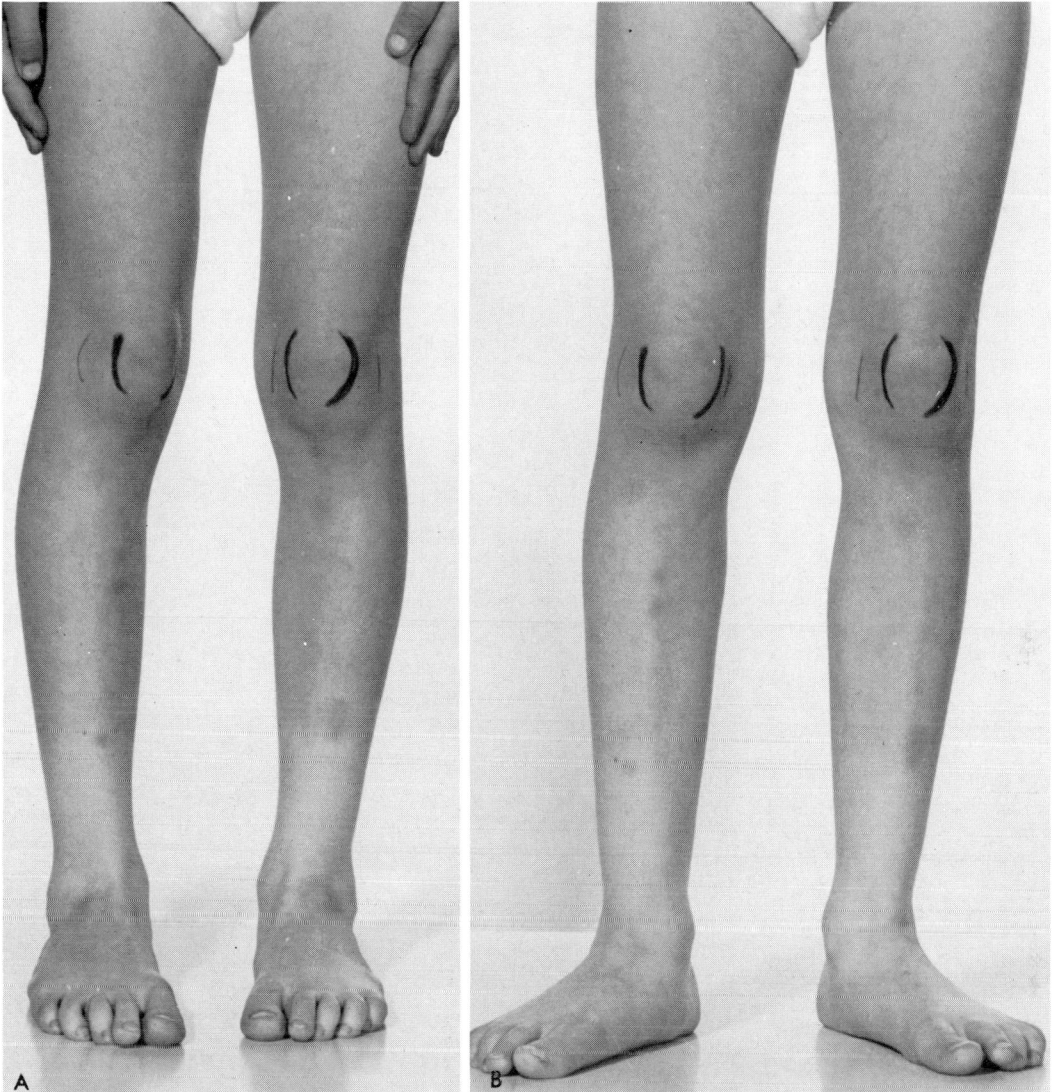

FIGURE 7-100. *Clinical appearance of excessive femoral torsion in a girl.*

A. With the knees in full extension and the feet aligned (pointing straight forward) the legs appear bowed and the patellae face inward. *B.* Upon lateral rotation of the hips so that the patellae are facing to the front, the feet and legs point outward and the bowleg appearance is corrected.

difficult to lay down definite guidelines for indications for surgery; each case should be individualized. The author recommends a derotation osteotomy of the femur if the child is eight years of age or older; if the hip cannot be rotated laterally beyond neutral position; if the degree of anteversion exceeds 40 degrees; and when the functional disability and unsightliness are so severe that parents demand that something be done.

It is preferable to perform the lateral derotation osteotomy at the subtrochanteric level. The technique of derotation osteotomy to correct excessive anteversion has been described in Plate 5 on pages 168–171. Some surgeons may prefer the level of osteotomy to be midshaft or supracondylar. The distal segment of the femur should be rotated laterally to such a degree that there is equal range of medial and lateral rotation of the hip.

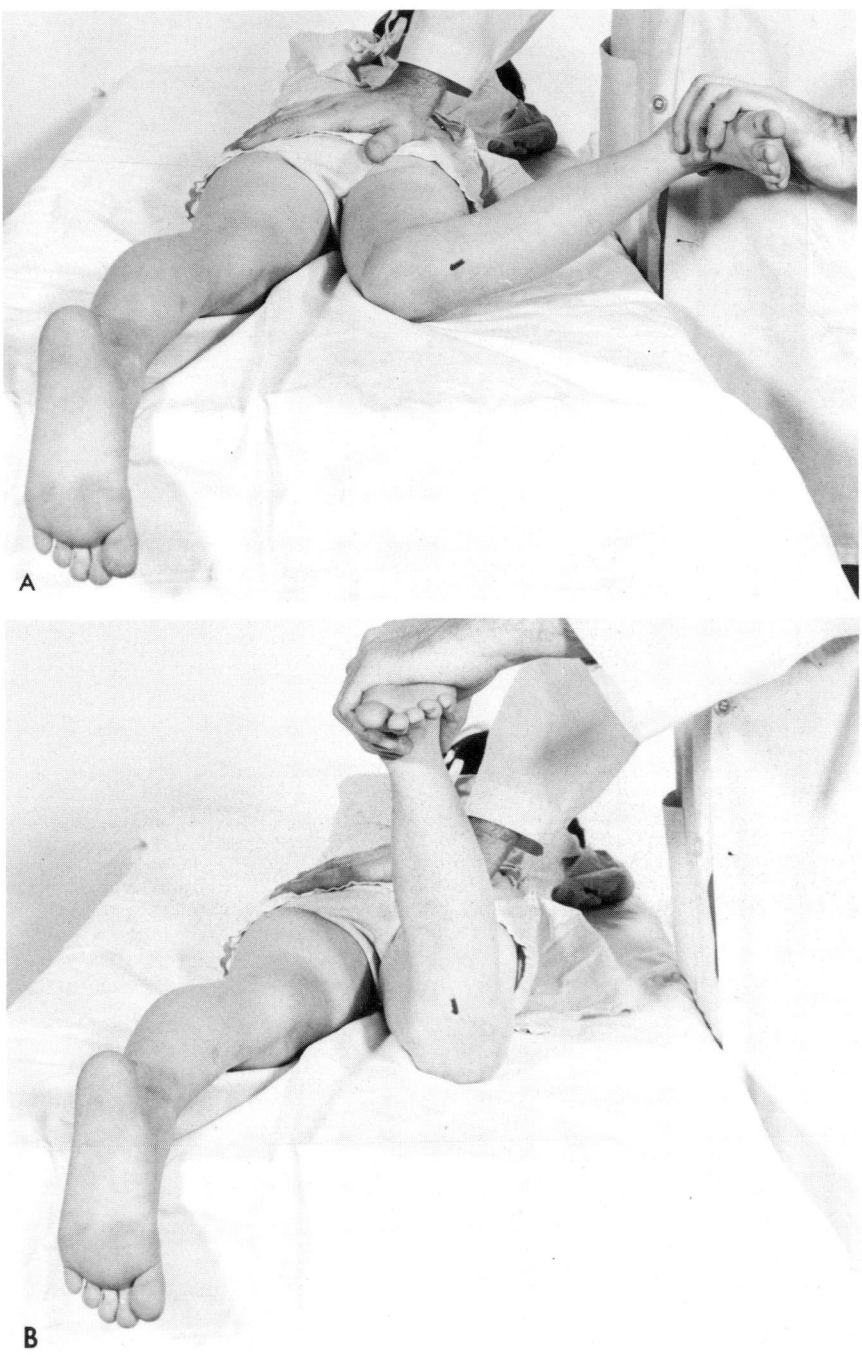

FIGURE 7–101.   *Range of rotation of the hip in excessive femoral antetorsion.*

A. External rotation of the hip in extension is limited to neutral. *B.* Internal rotation of the hip in extension is exaggerated.

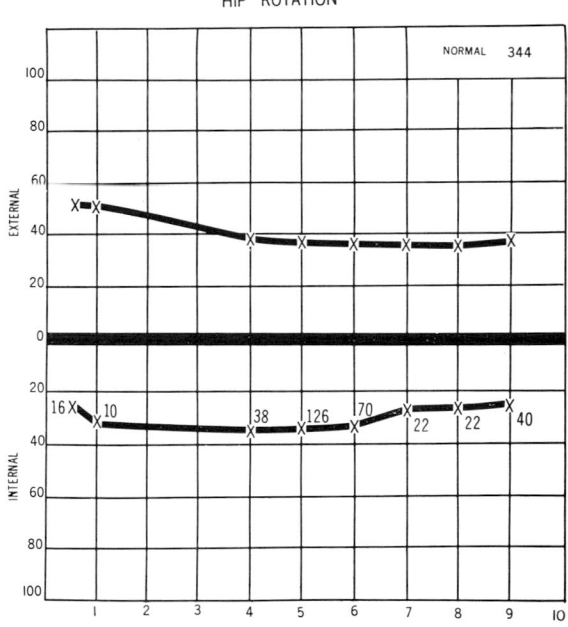

HIP ROTATION

NORMAL 344

FIGURE 7–102. *The range of internal and external rotation of the hips in extension in 344 normal hips.*

Figures on the chart designate the number of hips examined. (From Crane, L.: Femoral torsion and its relation to toeing-in and toeing-out. J. Bone Joint Surg., *41-A*:423, 1959.)

Medial rotation osteotomy of the tibia may be required if there is marked secondary external tibial torsion. It is best to delay this for one or two years following lateral rotation osteotomy of the femur to see how much correction can be obtained by the normal processes of growth and bone remodeling.

TIBIAL TORSION

The degree of tibial torsion depends upon the age of the child and is variable among different individuals. Le Damany measured the torsion of the tibia in anatomic specimens and found that in the fetus the medial malleolus was located behind the lateral malleolus and there was medial torsion of the tibia; at birth, the tips of the malleoli were level; and by the time walking was fully established, the medial malleolus was situated in front of the lateral malleolus and there was 20 degrees of lateral torsion of the tibia. In the normal adult tibia the average degree of torsion was +23.[564] Measurements of tibial torsion in various age groups by Dupuis and Wynne-Davies

have given approximately the same findings.[548, 590]

Khermosh, Lior, and Weisman measured tibial torsion in 230 normal newborn babies and young children up to five years of age. In the early postnatal period (birth to three months), most babies had mild external torsion with a mean value of 2.2 degrees; only 9 per cent had no torsion (0 degrees), and 12 per cent had internal torsion (0 to 8 degrees). A gradual increase in the torsional angle with age at an average rate of 1.3 degrees per year was noted. Tibial torsion was 3.5 degrees in the 4- to 9-month age group, 4.3 degrees in the 10- to 21-month age group. The angle increased at a greater rate in the 22- to 27-month age group in which the mean value was 6.1 degrees. There was no significant increase in the torsional angle in the 30- to 40-month age group; in the 41- to 60-month age group, it increased gradually to a mean value of 9.1 degrees. There was no statistically significant difference in the degree of torsion between the left and right tibiae in all age groups, or between the sexes.[556] Hutter and Scott measured tibial torsion in 40 adult skeletons and found an average measurement of 22.1 degrees of external tibial torsion.[555] Le Damany also measured torsion of the tibiae of human specimens dating from the prehistoric age when shoes did not exist; the average lateral tibial torsion was +25 degrees—apparently shoes played no role in the development of progressive external tibial torsion.[564]

The incidence of medial tibial torsion in 200 adults was determined by Hutter and Scott. They found internal tibial torsion in 5 per cent of the 100 women examined, and in 3 per cent of the men. The medial torsion was severe enough to cause difficulty in walking in 2 per cent of the female patients and in 1 per cent of the males.[555]

Measurement of Tibial Torsion

In anatomic specimens the degree of tibial torsion can be measured quite accurately by inserting a pin through the center of the condylar articulating surface of the proximal end of the tibia, and a second pin through the center of the distal end of the tibia, parallel to a line between the centers of

the medial and lateral malleoli. Rotation of the tibia on its longitudinal axis is assessed by means of a tropometer. One pin inserted in the distal end of the tibia holds it upright; another pin through the upper end of the tibia is fixed to the vertical standard, and the degree of tibial torsion is measured on a protractor placed underneath the distal pin (Fig. 7–103).[555] Inserting pins through the tibia of a living person to measure torsion is not justifiable.

ROENTGENOGRAPHIC METHODS

For the adolescent or adult patient several radiologic techniques are available to measure tibial torsion; roentgenographic methods cannot be applied to children, however, because of the lack of contrast shadows projected by their cartilaginous epiphyses.

Nachlas Method. With the proximal tibial tubercle maintained in neutral position, true anteroposterior and lateral roentgenograms of the tibia, including the knee and ankle joints, are made. The relative positions of the medial and lateral malleoli are

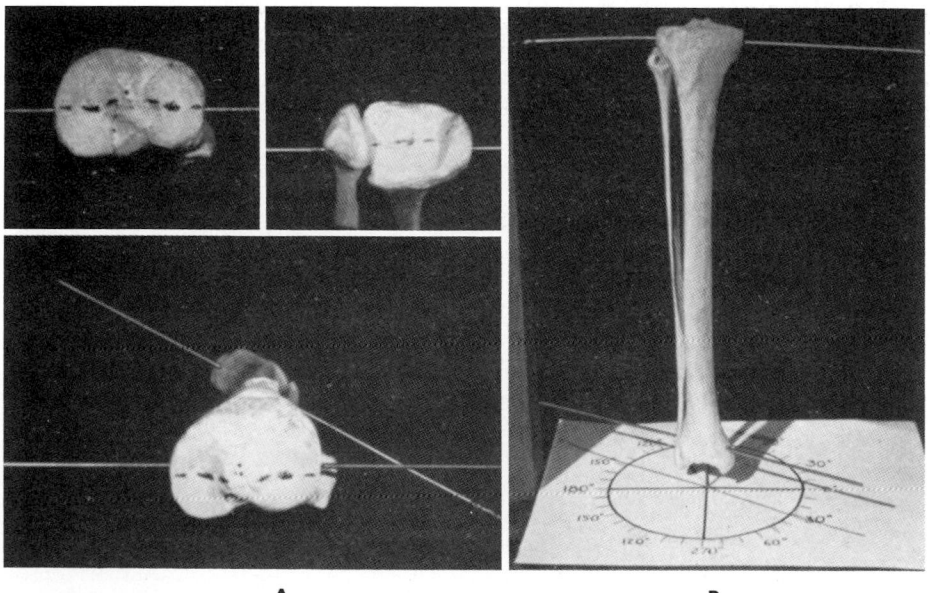

A   B

FIGURE 7–103. Method of determining the degree of tibial torsion in an anatomic specimen.

A. Pins are inserted through the articular axes of the upper and lower ends of the tibia. The angles formed by the two pins in the coronal plane is the degree of tibial torsion. *B.* A model demonstrating the method of obtaining tropometric measurements. (From Hutter, C. G., Jr., and Scott, W.: Tibial torsion. J. Bone Joint Surg., *31-A*:512, 1949.)

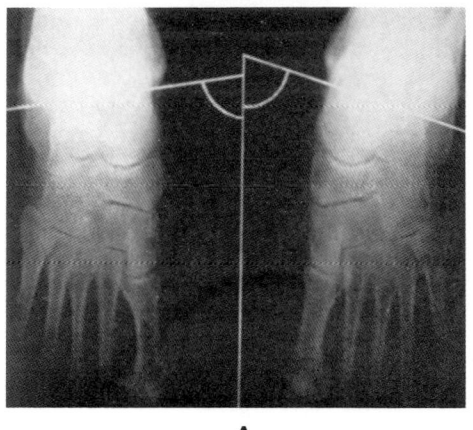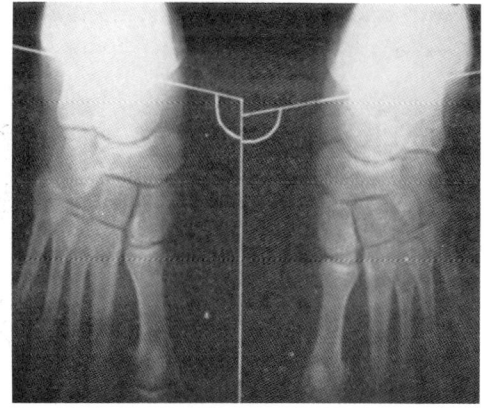

A   **B**

FIGURE 7–104.   Hutter and Scott roentgenographic method of measuring the degree of tibial torsion.

Roentgenograms made according to the technique described in the text. *A.* Internal tibial torsion; minus 10 degrees on the right and minus 18 degrees on the left. *B.* External tibial torsion: plus 13 degrees on the right and plus 12 degrees on the left. (From Hutter, C. G., Jr., and Scott, W.: Tibial torsion. J. Bone Joint Surg., *31-A*:515, 1949.)

compared. In internal tibial torsion, the medial malleolus lies posterior to the lateral malleolus, whereas in external tibial torsion it is located anterior to the fibular malleolus.[568] This technique only provides a rough estimate that is not inherently any more accurate than clinical methods of evaluation.

Hutter and Scott Method. The casette is placed beneath the soles of both feet. The patient sits with his knees flexed 90 degrees and the medial borders of his feet parallel to the medial borders of his thighs. The x-ray tube is placed above the knees and the exposure is made with the beam parallel to the longitudinal axis of the tibia. An image of the malleoli and the feet is projected on the film. Lines are drawn between the tips of the malleoli and along the medial border of the roentgenographic shadows of the bony structures of the foot, with the latter line approximately at a right angle to the articular axis of the knee. The intersection of these two lines forms an angle that, when subtracted from 90 degrees, will give the measurement of tibial torsion in degrees (Fig. 7–104).[555]

Rosen and Sandick Method. Two arbitrary pairs of points are marked on the leg: (1) The upper lateral point is marked at the prominent junction of the anterior and lateral aspects of the proximal end of the head of the fibula. (2) The upper medial point is marked at the most prominent medial part of the inner condyle. (3) The lower lateral point marks the prominence of the junction of the lateral and posterior margins of the fibular malleolus. (4) The lower medial point is made at the prominence of the junction of the anterior medial margins of the medial malleolus. Transverse lines are drawn between the upper two points (transcondylar axis) and between the lower two points (transmalleolar axis). The angle formed by these axes represents the degree of tibiofibular torsion.[575]

CLINICAL METHODS

Wynne-Davies designed an instrument for clinical measurement of tibial torsion.[590] Her apparatus was later slightly modified by Khermosh, Lior, and Weissman (Fig. 7–105).[556] The reader is referred to the original articles for description of the instruments. These clinical methods are not accurate, however, as the relative positions of the malleoli are used for measurement, not the tibia itself; thus, any motion between the tibia and fibula will give a false value.

A simple clinical method employed by the author is illustrated in Figure 7–106. The child is seated on the edge of a table with his knee flexed 90 degrees, or the infant is placed in prone position and his knee is flexed to a right angle. By proper posi-

A

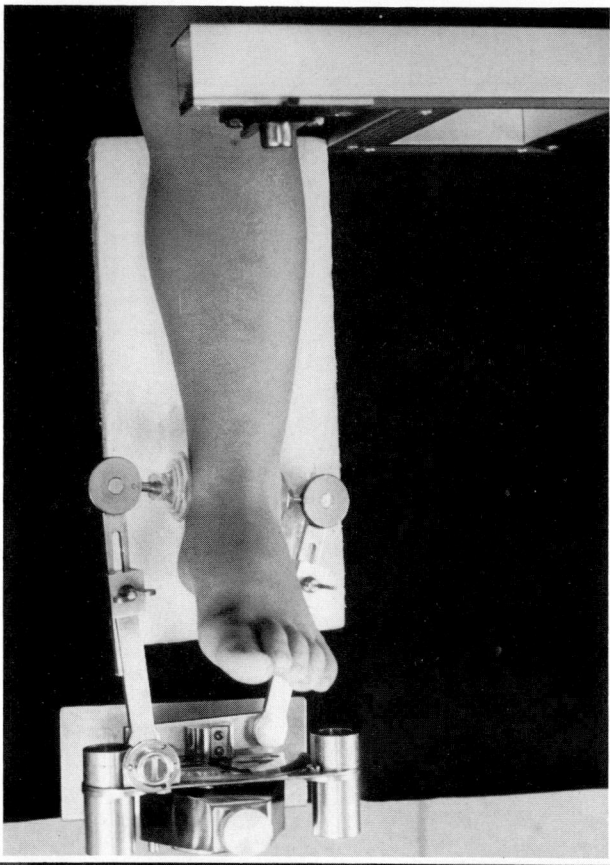

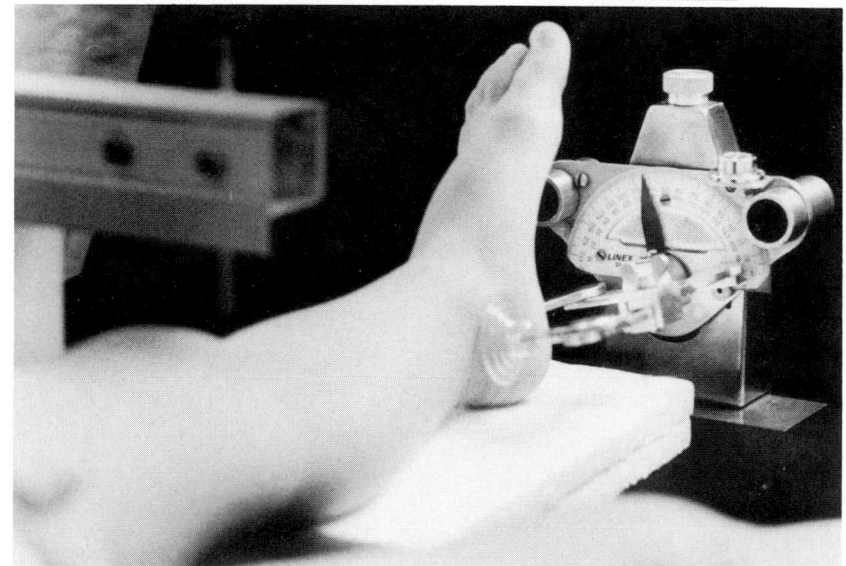

B

FIGURE 7-105. *Instrument used for measuring tibial torsion (designed by Khermosh et al.).*

A. The vertical pointer is directed toward the proximal tibial tubercle. The two distal discs are placed in contact with the center of the medial and lateral malleoli, while the leg is comfortably elevated and supported on a polyurethane foam plate. *B.* The pointer indicates the degree of torsion on the protractor, which is fixed at the end of the table. Internal torsion is recorded as minus (−), while external torsion is recorded as plus (+). (From Khermosh, O., Lior, G., and Weissman, S. L.: Tibial torsion in children. Clin. Orthop., 79:26, 1971.)

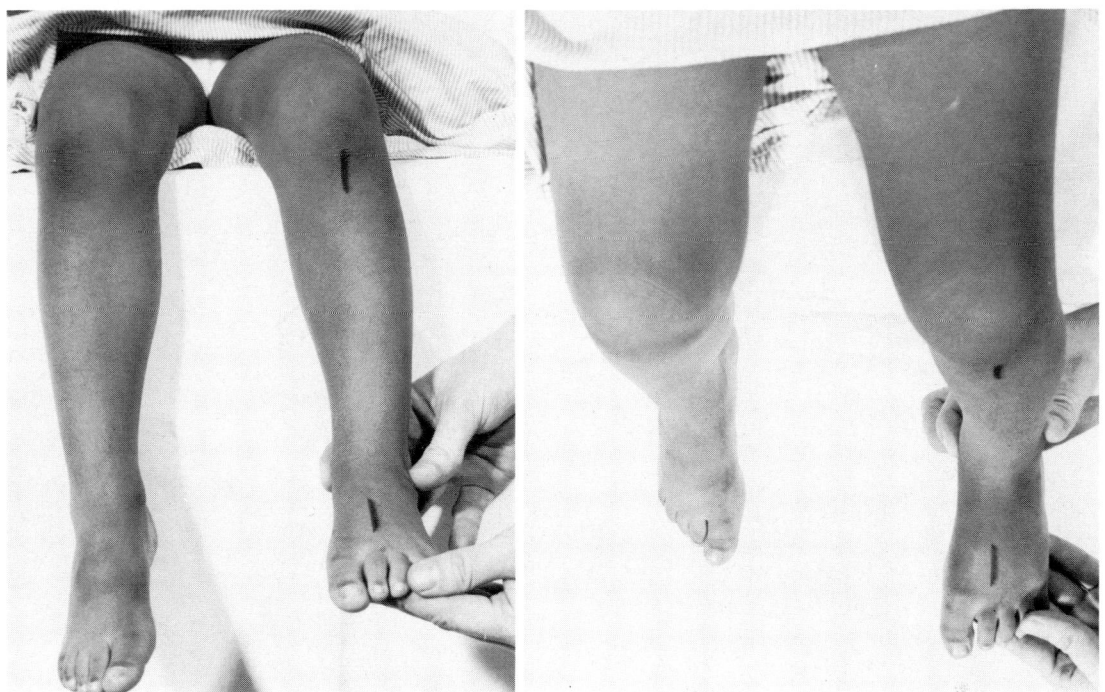

FIGURE 7–106.   Practical clinical method of measuring tibial torsion (see text for explanation).

tioning of the limb, the tibial transcondylar line (axis of the knee joint) is either made parallel to the edge of the table (when sitting) or to the top of the table (when lying prone). The transmalleolar line (axis of the ankle) is determined by placing the thumb on the distal tip of the medial malleolus and the index finger on the distal tip of the fibular malleolus. The degree of tibial torsion is determined by the angle formed between the transcondylar tibial axis and the axis of the ankle joint. The relationship between the proximal tibial tubercle and the midpoint between the medial and lateral malleoli is noted by observing the longitudinal axis of the tibia. The second metatarsal of a normal foot supported in neutral position may be another point of reference distally.

It is obvious that clinical methods of measurement of tibial torsion are only approximate and values should be measured only in 5-degree increments.

INTERNAL TIBIAL TORSION

In infants abnormal medial tibial torsion is usually associated with congenital metatarsus varus or developmental genu varum. As an isolated deformity, its incidence is not common. Exaggerated internal tibial torsion may occur in combination with or independent of abnormal femoral antetorsion.

The child is usually brought to the orthopedic surgeon between the ages of 6 and 19 months with the presenting complaint that he is pigeon-toed or bowlegged. Often the condition is overlooked until the child begins to walk; then the chief complaint is that he toes-in.

On examination, both in supine position and in stance the feet point inward. In the pure form there is no varus deformity of the metatarsals. The medial malleolus is located posterior to the lateral malleolus. Involvement is usually symmetrical. In stance, because the toes are pointed inward at an angle of from 35 to 15 degrees, the center of gravity of the body falls lateral to the second metatarsal, which is the center ray of the foot. The older child will compensate for this malalignment of the body's center of gravity by everting and abducting the forefoot.

Kite distinguishes between the congenital and acquired forms of medial torsion of the legs. In his rotation test, the ankles are grasped and the limbs rotated medially and laterally at the hip joints; in the congenital form of medial torsion, the patellae can be turned medially and laterally to the same degree as in the normal child, whereas in the acquired form of medial tibial torsion, the patellae can be turned medially 90 degrees or more, but they cannot be rotated laterally past neutral position.[558-561] It should be emphasized, however, that the determination made by Kite's rotation test is the range of rotation at the hip. As stated earlier, abnormal femoral anteversion or contracture of soft tissues in the medial and anterior aspects of the hip joint will restrict lateral rotation of the hip in extension. Kite also states that there is very little deformity of the femora in those with congenital medial torsion; also, the child with acquired medial torsion usually sits on his legs with his toes turned in; if his legs are unfolded, in a few seconds he will sit on his feet again because this is the position of comfort.[558]

It is very important to determine whether the older siblings and the parents have persistent abnormal internal tibial torsion, as the subdivision into hereditary and nonhereditary forms is of practical significance in the prognosis and treatment of internal tibial torsion. If the tibiae of the parents and the adolescent siblings have normal alignment, the probability of spontaneous correction by the age of seven to eight years of age is very great; however, if there is familial incidence of persistent abnormal internal tibial torsion, the prognosis for spontaneous correction should be guarded and aggressive therapeutic measures should be considered.

Differential Diagnosis

In-toeing may be due to a variety of abnormalities of congenital or acquired origin. It may stem from fixed bony deformity, soft-tissue contracture, muscle paralysis and imbalance, or a change in the planes of articulation. The level of pathologic involvement may be in the hip, femur, knee, leg or ankle, or the foot.

In Table 7–7 the various causes of toeing-in and toeing-out are listed. In the author's experience, the most common cause

Table 7–7. *Etiology of Toeing-In and Toeing-Out in Children*

Level of Affection	Toe-In	Toe-Out
Feet-ankles	Pronated feet (protective toeing-in) Metatarsus varus Talipes varus and equinovarus	Pes valgus due to contracture of triceps surae muscle Talipes calcaneovalgus Congenital convex pes planovalgus
Leg-knee	Tibia vara (Blount's disease) and developmental genu varum Abnormal internal tibial torsion Genu valgum—developmental (protective toeing-in to shift body center of gravity medially)	External tibial torsion Congenital absence or hypoplasia of the fibula
Femur-hip	Abnormal femoral antetorsion Spasticity of internal rotators of hip (cerebral palsy)	Abnormal femoral retroversion Flaccid paralysis of internal rotators of hip
Acetabulum	Maldirected—facing anteriorly	Maldirected—facing posteriorly

of toeing-in is protective in-toeing due to pronated feet and developmental genu valgum; next in order of decreasing frequency are abnormal femoral antetorsion, metatarsus varus, abnormal tibial torsion, forward inclination of the acetabulum, and paralytic acquired causes such as spasticity of the hip adductors or the posterior tibial muscle in cerebral palsy.

Abnormal lateral tibial torsion is usually an acquired deformity that is secondary to contracture of the iliotibial band, although it does occur occasionally as a congenital deformity. The deformity may be unilateral or bilateral. In the congenital forms, both tibiae are usually symmetrically affected.

In stance, with the patellae facing straight forward, the feet point outward (Fig. 7–107). The center of gravity is medial to the first metatarsal. The lateral malleolus lies posterior to the medial malleolus. Any associated knock-knee deformity is noted. Ober's test should always be performed for detection of iliotibial band contracture (see Fig. 1–9, p. 18). Lateral tibial torsion may be secondary to abnormal femoral antetorsion. The range of rotation of the hips is tested in full extended position; in abnormal femoral

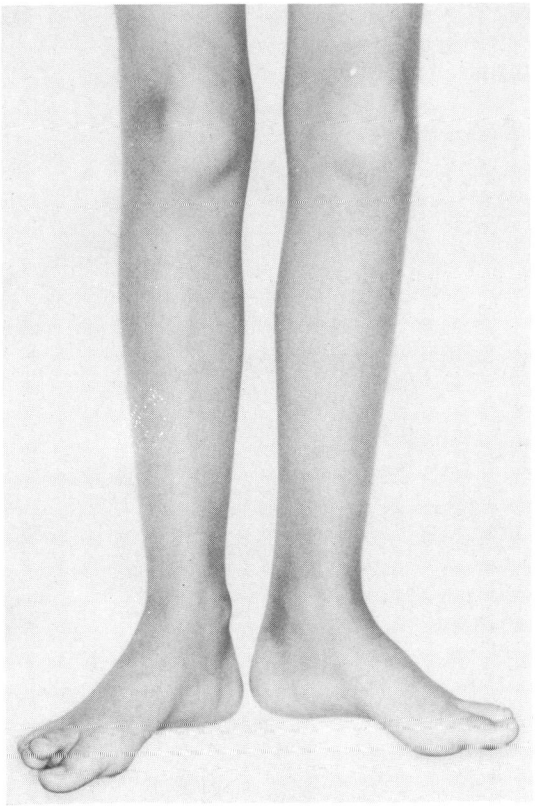

FIGURE 7-107. *Exaggerated tibial torsion.*

In stance, with the patellae facing straight forward, the feet point outward.

antetorsion, lateral rotation of the hip is restricted, whereas in iliotibial band contracture, it is the medial rotation of the hip that is limited.

In gait, the child toes out, the feet pointing in opposite directions. Triceps surae contracture, a common cause of toeing-out in children, is ruled out by testing the passive range of dorsiflexion of both ankles.

Treatment

The form of treatment is determined according to the patient's age, the severity of the deformity, and the presence or absence of familial incidence.

In infants, usually no treatment is required. With growth, the internal tibial torsion will correct itself spontaneously. Passive stretching exercises are indicated in some cases, primarily to appease the anxious parents or grandparents. The foot is manipulated into abduction and eversion 15 to 20 times in several daily sessions. These will help to correct any associated soft-tissue contracture, such as that of the posterior tibial muscle. More aggressive programs of therapy are ordinarily not indicated. As stated earlier, Denis Browne splints force the feet into abduction and cause genu valgum. Unfortunately they are indiscriminately used for treatment of toeing-in in children, most of whom do not have actual abnormal internal tibial torsion. The use of a Denis Browne splint is recommended only in cases in which internal tibial torsion exceeds 40 degrees in a child who has a positive family history of persistent abnormal internal tibial torsion and in whom spontaneous correction is *not* taking place. Often the author does not apply a Denis Browne splint until the child is 24 months of age. The length of the bar used to spread the legs should not exceed 10 cm., and tarsal supinator shoes should be used to prevent the development of pes valgus.

Some surgeons utilize corrective casts to force the legs and feet into external rotation. If the primary deformity is metatarsus varus, a corrective cast is indicated to correct the foot deformity. If there is associated soft-tissue contracture, particularly of the posterior tibial, gracilis, and medial hamstring muscles, a stretching cast may again be used. However, the torsional bony deformity in the tibia itself will not be corrected by maintaining the feet in forced eversion in an above-knee or below-knee cast for a period of four to eight weeks. At least 6 to 18 months are required for such passive force to change the shape of a bone. Immobilization of the limbs of a child for such a prolonged period is not justified. The only instance in which the author makes use of a corrective cast is for stretching soft-tissue contracture; later, bivalved casts or night splints are used during sleeping hours to correct the torsional deformity.

If abnormal tibial torsion persists past eight years of age, derotation osteotomy is indicated. The operative technique follows the same principles as those of correction of tibia vara illustrated in Figure 3–39 and described on page 352.

ANGULAR DEFORMITIES OF THE LONG BONES OF THE LOWER LIMBS

Mild to moderate medial bowing of the lower limbs—involving both the tibia and femur—is a common and normal finding in the newborn and the young infant. It proba-bly represents persistence of the in utero position of the lower limbs; however, severe genu varum may be atavistic in nature, re-sulting from intrauterine arrest of develop-ment. Bowlegs are usually associated with a varying degree of internal tibial torsion (Figure 7–108).

With the development of upright stance and locomotion, the medial deviation of the

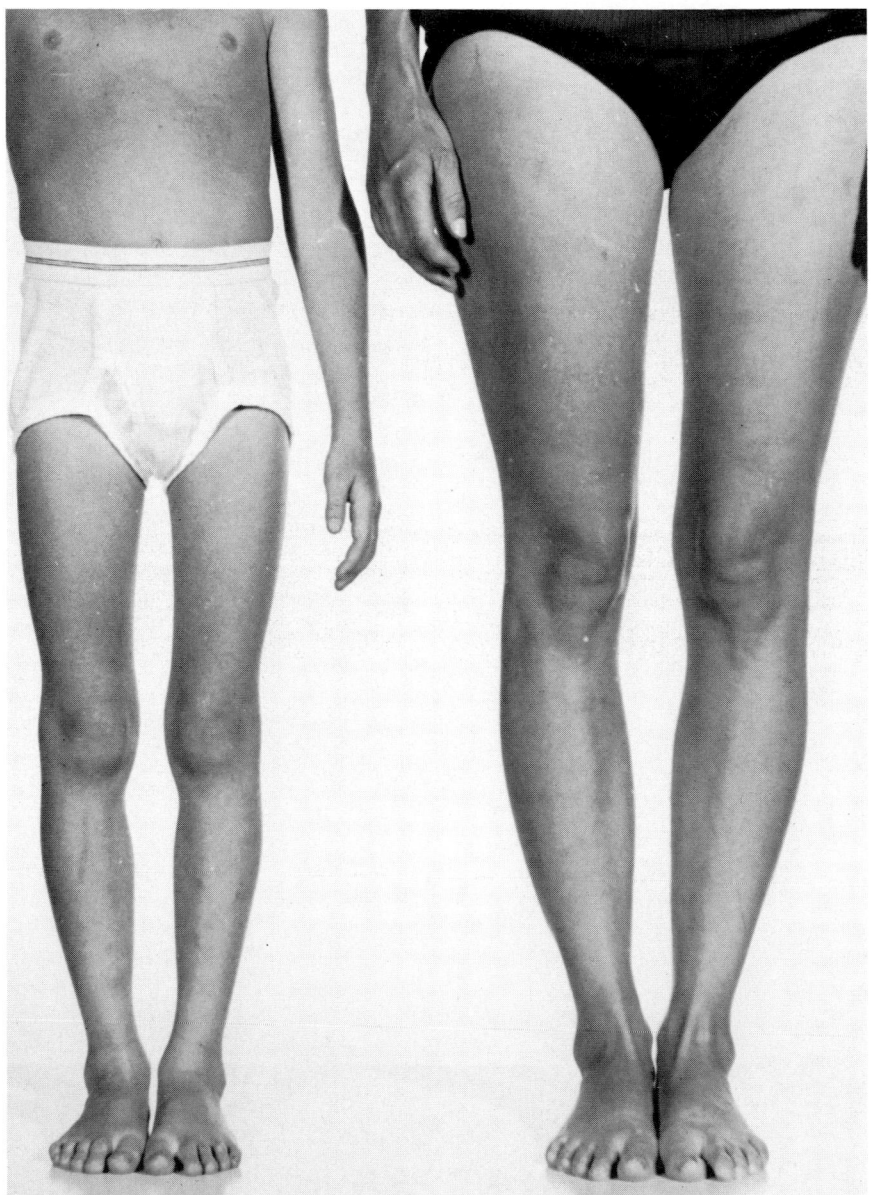

FIGURE 7–108. *Bilateral genu varum in mother and son.*

Note the associated internal tibial torsion. In the familial form prognosis should be guarded.

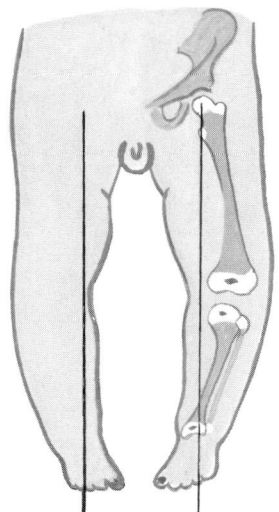 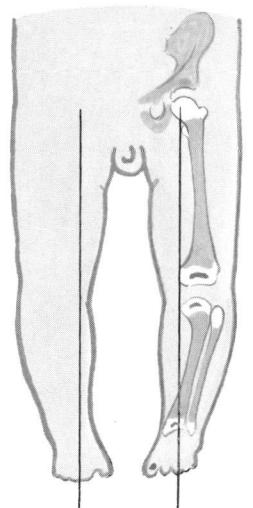 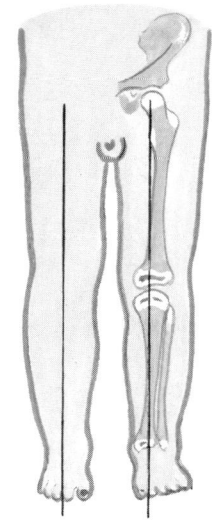

Newborn — Moderate genu varum   6 Months — Minimal genu varum   1 Year, 7 Months — Legs straight

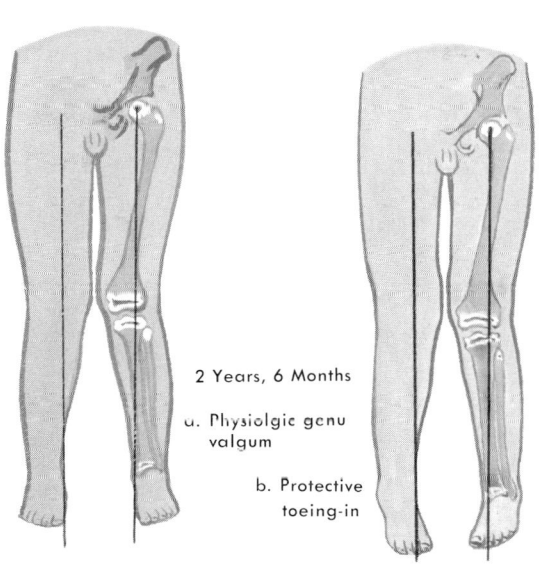

2 Years, 6 Months

a. Physiolgic genu valgum

b. Protective toeing-in

4 to 6 Years — Legs straight

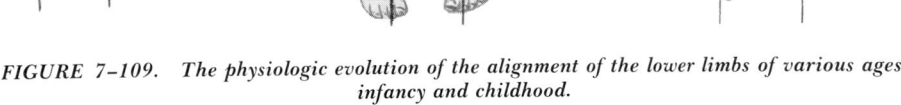

FIGURE 7–109. *The physiologic evolution of the alignment of the lower limbs of various ages in infancy and childhood.*

legs is spontaneously corrected, provided extraneous factors do not interfere. The "pendulum" swings toward genu valgum between two and three years of age; and finally the knock-knees are spontaneously corrected between the ages of four and ten years. Böhm, in 1933, was the first to describe this normal physiologic evolution of the shape of the lower limbs.[591] Figure 7–109 illustrates the physiologic evolution of the alignment of the lower limbs at various ages in infancy and childhood. Unfortunately, scientifically documented information on the natural history of bowlegs and knock-knees is not available.

Thirty infants with bowlegs were studied

by Sherman. The deformity corrected itself spontaneously. Only three infants had bowlegs at 16 to 18 months of age; one of these was corrected and the other two had slight knock-knees at five years of age.[609]

Morley studied the natural history of knock-knee by performing 1,000 examinations on unselected normal children (451 children aged 1 to 4 years, 318 children aged 5 to 11 years). The degree of knock-knee was measured by the distance between the medial malleoli (with the patellae facing straight forward, the medial surfaces of the knees just touching, and the ankles dorsiflexed to neutral position). Four grades of knock-knees were specified: *Grade I*—intermalleolar distance of less than 2.5 cm. (1 inch); *Grade II*—2.5 cm. (1 inch) but less than 5.0 cm. (2 inches); *Grade III*—5 cm. (2 inches) but less than 7.5 cm. (3 inches); and *Grade IV*—7.5 cm. (3 inches) and over.[604]

The incidence of genu valgum was found to increase until three to three and one half years of age, and then it declined. Between three and three and one half years of age, only 26 per cent of children had Grade I knock-knees; 52 per cent had Grade II, while 22 per cent had Grade III or IV (2 inches or more). Only 2 per cent of children aged seven years or older had an equivalent amount of genu valgum. There was no sex difference in the incidence of knock-knees in children under five years of age. The mean weight of children with knock-knees was greater than the mean weight of comparable children without knock-knees. Morley concluded that developmental genu valgum in children under seven years of age can probably be safely ignored unless it is very severe or unless an underlying cause such as renal rickets or epiphyseal damage from fracture is present.[604]

DEVELOPMENTAL GENU VARUM

As already stated, a minimal or moderate degree of bowlegs is normal in infancy. Internal rotation of the lower limbs exaggerates the appearance of bowlegs. It is important to align the legs so that the patellae face straight forward and to measure the degree of genu varum according to the distance between the medial femoral condyles with the medial malleoli touching. Usually orthopedic attention is not sought until the child begins to stand and walk. The parents are concerned because of the wide space between the knees, the rolling gait, and the toeing-in, which is due to associated internal tibial torsion and pronation of the feet. Ordinarily, roentgenograms are unnecessary. Radiologic findings, shown in Figure 7–110 are: (1) The transverse planes of the knee and ankle joints are tilted medially; (2) the tibia is angulated medially at the junction of its proximal and middle thirds, and the femur at its distal third; (3) the medial cortices of tibia and femur are thickened and sclerosed; (4) the epiphysis, physis, and metaphysis have a normal appearance and there is no evidence of intrinsic bone disease; (5) involvement is usually symmetrical.

In the differential diagnosis, rickets, tibia vara (Blount's disease), metaphyseal dysostosis, and various causes of asymmetrical growth disturbances of the physis (such as trauma) should be considered. Distinguishing features of these conditions are described in Chapter 3. One must differentiate between developmental genu varum and a severe form of tibia vara in which the angulation takes place at the junction of the middle and distal thirds; often in the latter there is a positive family history, with parents and siblings being similarly affected. In this form the prognosis for spontaneous correction should be guarded.

Treatment

No special treatment is necessary. Parents should be assured that the bowleg appearance is normal and that it will spontaneously correct itself with weight-bearing and growth. It should also be mentioned to the parents that the child will probably, at the age of three years, temporarily develop knock-knees that will be corrected spontaneously by the age of seven years. The use of Denis Browne splints for developmental genu varum is definitely contraindicated, as it will exaggerate the physiologic knock-knees and pronation of the feet that occur normally in these children.

If, in the older child with medial tilting of

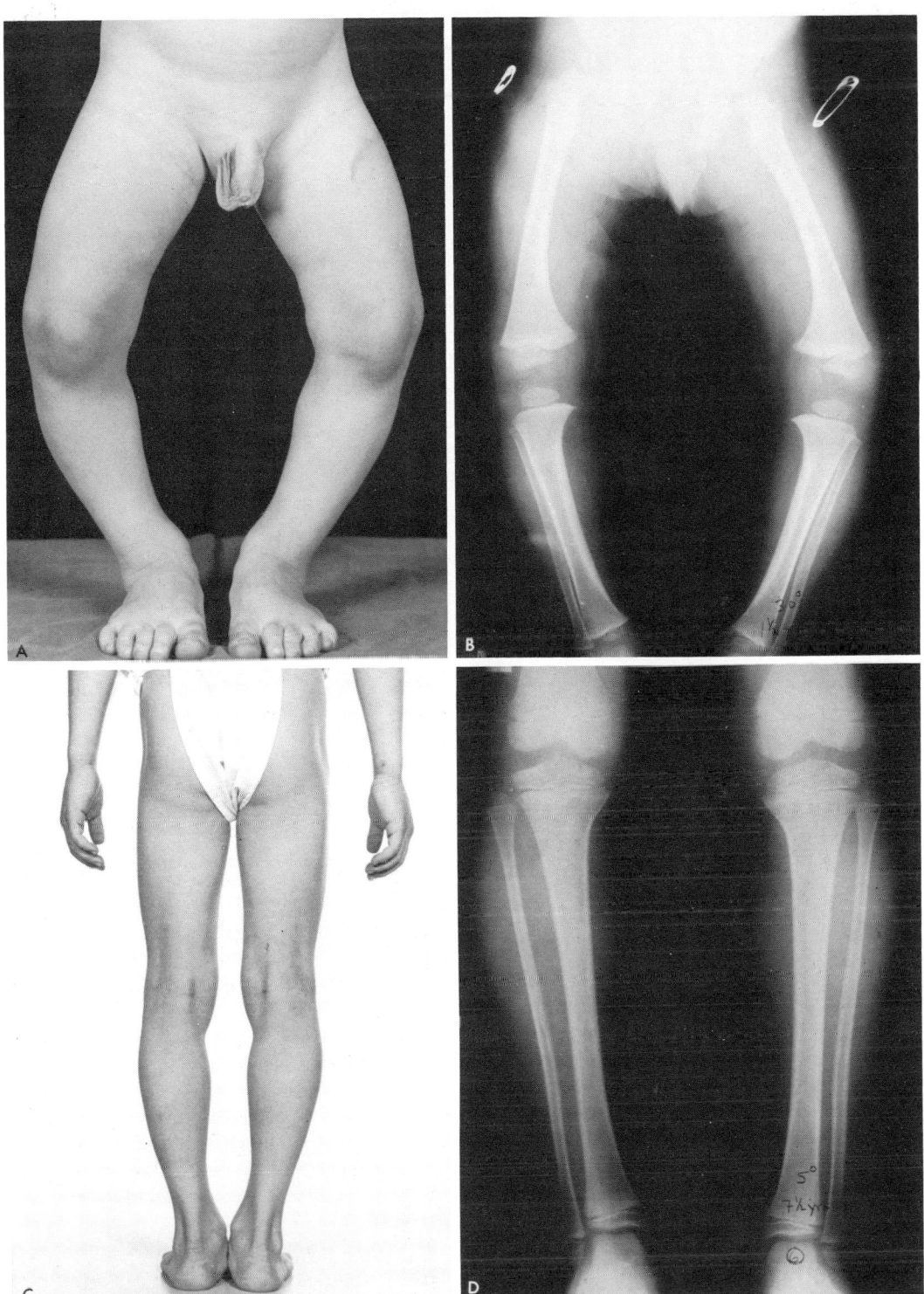

FIGURE 7–110. *Bilateral genu varum.*

A and **B.** At age one and one half years. **C** and **D.** At seven years, showing spontaneous correction without treatment.

the ankle mortise, compensatory pronation of the feet is marked and persistent, support of the feet by longitudinal arch pads is indicated. It should be made clear to the parents that this may temporarily exaggerate the child's toeing-in.

Osteotomy of the tibia or epiphyseal arrest of the lateral side of the distal femoral physis is not necessary in developmental genu varum. However, the familial severe form of tibia vara may fail to correct itself with growth, necessitating surgical intervention, which consists of osteotomy of the tibia and fibula at the apex of angulation—usually located at the junction of the middle and distal thirds of the tibia. As internal tibial torsion is commonly exaggerated in this form of tibia vara, the distal fragment is derotated as well as angulated laterally.

DEVELOPMENTAL GENU VALGUM

A minimal to moderate degree of knock-knees is a normal physiologic finding in children two to six years of age. When the genu valgum is *marked*, the child walks awkwardly, rubbing his knees and keeping his feet apart. He may swing one leg around the other to avoid banging his knees. He may be easily fatigued. The feet are pronated, and the uppers of the shoes bulge and collapse medially over the medial longitudinal arch. He will toe-in to shift the center of gravity of the body over the center of the foot, which is the second ray. If the triceps surae muscle and iliotibial band are contracted, he will toe-out. Pain in the calf and the anterior aspect of the thigh is common. In severe knock-knees, because of the malalignment of the quadriceps mechanism, the patellae may subluxate laterally. Because they are inactive, children with knock-knees are usually obese. Abnormal weight-bearing stretches the medial collateral ligaments of the knee, and in middle-aged or older adults, this excess wear and tear on the knees eventually leads to degenerative arthritis.

Intrinsic bone disease that is causing knock-knees should be ruled out if the condition is asymmetrical or unilateral; if it is excessive (the distance between the medial malleoli is greater than 9 or 10 cm.); if the child is of short stature for his age (suggesting the possibility of epiphyseal dysplasia or endocrine disease); or if there is a positive family history of marked genu valgum.

Treatment

In the two-to-six-year age group, the parents should be assured that in 95 per cent of cases the knock-knees will spontaneously correct themselves, making treatment unnecessary. This is particularly true if the child toes-in while walking. If the iliotibial band or triceps surae muscles are contracted and act as deforming forces, they should be stretched by passive manipulative exercises.

In the case of genu valgum and pronated feet, the center of gravity is medial to the first ray of the foot. To prevent foot strain, it is best to add a $1/8$ inch inner heel wedge to the shoes, which should be sturdy and well-constructed in order to resist distortion under the abnormal force of body weight. A longitudinal arch support will protect the feet from foot strain. These shoe alterations will also promote toeing-in. Developmental genu valgum in children is usually corrected spontaneously, provided the child toes-in. The use of an orthosis, night splints, or twisters is not indicated.

In adolescence, genu valgum requires more aggressive management. If the intermalleolar distance with the knees together exceeds 10 cm., operative correction of the deformity should be considered. Most often the valgus deformity is greater in the lower end of the femur than in the upper end of the tibia. Standing roentgenograms of the lower limbs should be made to verify this. Several methods of surgical treatment are available, namely, stapling or epiphyseodesis of the medial side of the distal femoral epiphysis, supracondylar osteotomy of the distal femur—either modified cuneiform or close-up wedge resection, and osteotomy of the proximal tibia and fibula.

Peroneal nerve palsy is a definite complication of osteotomy and occurs more frequently at the proximal tibial than at the distal femoral level. The advantage of osteotomy is that the deformity is fully corrected at the time of surgery. Stapling of the medial side of the distal femoral epiphysis is a

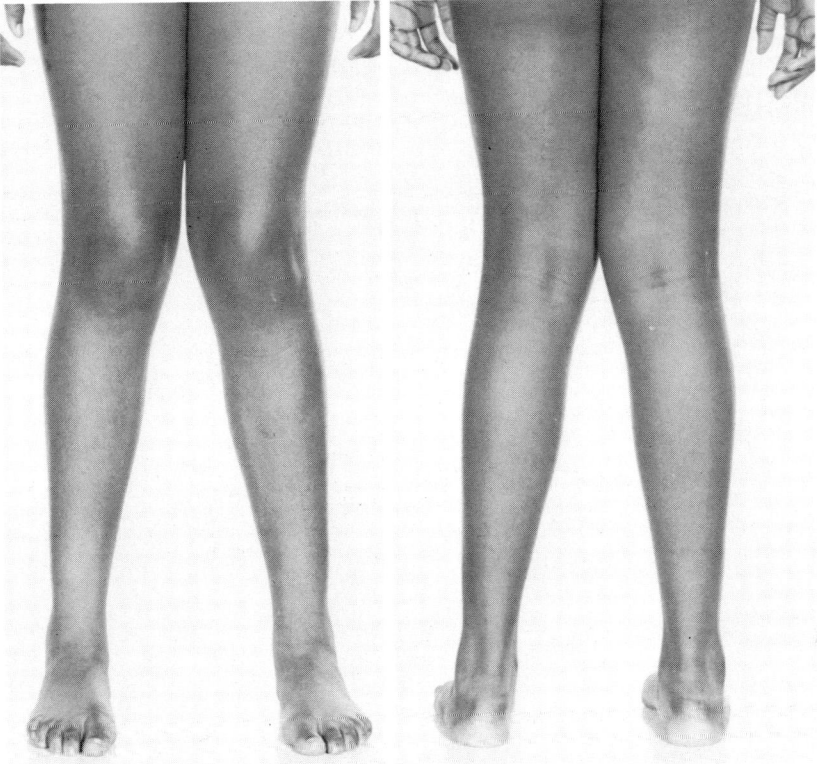

FIGURE 7–111. Bilateral genu valgum in an adolescent.

simple procedure, with no potential of injury to the peroneal nerve. The valgus deformity is corrected gradually over a period of one or two years. Unfortunately, the degree of correction that will be obtained at the end of the growth period cannot be predicted with surety; a second operation is often required to remove the staples. It is obvious that each case should be individually assessed. The author recommends the following plan of operative treatment:

Stapling or epiphyseodesis of the medial side of the distal femoral condyle is preferable when the physes are still open and there is sufficient longitudinal growth remaining to correct the deformity. Before considering stapling, it is important that the pattern of skeletal growth be observed and followed by anthropometric measurements. The skeletal age at which stapling should be performed depends upon the degree of genu valgum, the height of the patient, the length of the lower limbs, and the expected growth remaining in the distal femur. As a general rule, when the amount of knock-knee is 7.5

to 10 cm., medial stapling of the distal femur is performed between the skeletal ages of 10 and 11 years in girls, and in boys, 12 and 13 years. Precise methods of prediction for correction of genu valgum are not available at present.

Howorth gives the following rule of thumb to estimate correction: The ratio between the length of the leg from the distal femoral epiphyseal plate to the medial malleolus and the transverse diameter of the physis of the distal femur is determined; if the length of the leg is five times the width of the epiphysis, then the correction would be five times the amount of growth on the unstapled side of the epiphysis.[597] Thus if growth were completely arrested on the stapled side of the epiphysis, and the unstapled side of the condyle grew ¼ inch, the correction would be 1¼ inches for one leg, or 2½ inches for both legs. The operative technique of stapling of the medial side of the distal femoral condyle is as follows:

The medial approach to the distal femoral epiphysis is described and illustrated in Plate No. 63. The deep fascia and the patellar retinaculum are divided and each marked with 00 silk sutures for separate closure later. The epiphyseal plate is identified by probing with a straight skin needle; the plate is softer than adjacent cancellous bone. With the needle inserted in the growth plate, roentgenograms are made in the anteroposterior and lateral planes for definite localization of the site of the physis. Vitallium staples should be used because they cause less reaction, bend minimally, and almost never break. The growth plate of the distal end of the femur is convex distally and there is abrupt posterior tilting of the distal femoral condyle. With a staple holder, three staples are partially driven into bone, one in the center of the transverse diameter of the physis, one at the junction of the posterior one fourth and anterior three fourths, and another at the junction of the anterior one fourth and posterior three fourths.

The cross member of the staple must be parallel to the bone surface and perpendicular to the growth plate. The legs of the staple must be equidistant from the epiphyseal plate and point to the center of the bone. Both legs of the staple must be placed in bone; a common mistake is to leave the proximal leg of the posterior staple buried in the soft tissue. Meticulous attention should be paid to avoiding technical errors. The position of the staples is verified by anteroposterior and lateral roentgenograms of the distal femur; once this is established as being correct, the staples are securely driven into bone. The patellar retinaculum is closed with interrupted sutures; the deep fascia is closed separately with continuous sutures. The importance of separate closure of the patellar retinaculum and deep fascia cannot be overemphasized, as they should not be caught by the staples. Otherwise the patellar retinaculum will be bound down, with resultant restriction of knee motion, local swelling, and pain. The subcutaneous tissue and skin are closed in the usual manner and a long leg cylinder cast is applied. The cast is removed in two to three weeks and the patient is allowed to ambulate freely without restriction.

When, in addition to distal femoral stapling, retardation of growth of the medial aspect of the proximal tibia is indicated (because of skeletal maturity of the patient), the author prefers epiphyseodesis rather than stapling.

If the patient is seen at a skeletal age when one is sure that overcorrection cannot be obtained, the author prefers epiphyseodesis of the medial aspects of the distal femur and of the proximal tibia (see Plate 63 for operative technique).

SUPRACONDYLAR OSTEOTOMY OF THE DISTAL FEMUR

This is performed when the patient is seen late and it is too late to obtain correction by epiphyseal stapling or arrest (over 12 years in girls and 13 years in boys). A medial approach is used to expose the distal femur. The knee joint and suprapatellar pouch should not be opened. A close-up osteotomy at the distal metaphysis of the femur with resection of a wedge of bone based medially is preferred, the width of the wedge depending upon the degree of genu valgum to be corrected. Prior to completion of the osteotomy, two large threaded Steinmann pins are placed blindly from the lateral side, one in the distal fragment, and the other in the proximal segment. After completion of the osteotomy (and correction of the deformity), the two pins are connected with a Roger Anderson apparatus to maintain the alignment. A hip spica cast is used for immobilization. The osteotomy will usually heal in six weeks.

A modified cuneiform osteotomy with a lateral buttress is equally satisfactory. Symmetry of the lower limbs and equal leg lengths are important considerations in both techniques.

OSTEOTOMY OF PROXIMAL TIBIA AND FIBULA

This is indicated when the valgus deformity is below the knee joint. As already mentioned, peroneal palsy is a potential complication; this should be made very clear to the parents. Associated lateral torsional deformity is corrected at the same time. If the iliotibial band is taut, causing its attachments to subluxate the patella laterally, a Yount release is indicated.

Leg Length Inequality

Inequality of leg lengths is one of the commonest orthopedic problems. It is caused by a variety of conditions, as shown by the following list:

1. Congenital anomalies of skeletal system
   Congenital short femur
   Dysgenesis of proximal femur, congenital coxa vara
   Congenital dislocation of the hip
   Congenital absence or hypoplasia of the long bones in the lower limb
   Congenital hemihypertrophy, localized gigantism
2. Tumorous conditions of the skeleton
   Fibrous dysplasia
   Enchondromatosis
   Multiple hereditary exostosis
   Unicameral bone cyst
3. Infections of bones and joints (e.g., pyogenic osteomyelitis, tuberculosis, rheumatoid arthritis) may produce shortening by destroying the growth plate or may cause overgrowth by increasing the blood supply to the epiphyseal and metaphyseal regions
4. Legg-Perthes disease, slipped capital femoral epiphysis
5. Trauma
   Injury to the growth plate may cause its premature fusion and shortening
   Metaphyseal injuries may stimulate growth
   Fractures of the shaft of the femur or tibia (overlapping and malposition of fracture fragments cause shortening; stimulation of blood supply to epiphyseal areas causes overgrowth)
   Severe burns
6. Neuromuscular diseases (asymmetrical paralysis causes shortening)
   Cerebral palsy
   Poliomyelitis
   Myelomeningocele and other disorders affecting the spinal cord and spinal nerve roots
   Peripheral nerve injuries (e.g., sciatic or peroneal nerve palsy)
7. Soft-tissue abnormalities (usually malformations of vessels and nerves)
   Arteriovenous fistulae
   Hemangiomatosis of soft tissues
   Neurofibromatosis

Basic features of longitudinal growth of long bones and patterns of skeletal growth are reviewed next.

Longitudinal Growth of Long Bones

A long bone is divided into a middle portion (the shaft) and two end regions. The shaft is divided into the diaphysis and metaphysis; the end regions have an epiphysis and a physis (the cartilaginous growth plate).

Two types of epiphyses, *pressure* and *traction*, are found in the limbs. A *pressure epiphysis* is an articular epiphysis because it is located at the end of a long bone and enters into the formation of a joint. A greater portion of the longitudinal growth of a long bone takes place at the pressure epiphyses. *Traction epiphyses* are nonarticular; they serve as sites of origin or insertion for muscles, such as the lesser trochanter of the femur for the iliopsoas muscle; therefore, they are subject to traction rather than pressure, and their contribution to longitudinal growth of long bones is insignificant.

The major long bones—the femur, tibia, fibula, humerus, radius, and ulna—have an epiphysis and physis at both proximal and distal ends. In the short tubular bones (the phalanges, metatarsals, and metacarpals), there is only one epiphysis and one physis; these are located proximally in the phalanges, first metacarpal, and first metatarsal, whereas in the other metacarpal and metatarsal bones they are distal in location.

Long bones grow in length at the cartilaginous area of their extremities. This was shown by Stephen Hales in 1731. He marked the shafts of the limb bones of newly hatched chicks with two holes. Two months later when the chickens were sacrificed, the limb bones had increased considerably in length; however, the distance between the two "marker" holes had not increased.[728]

In 1736, Belchier discovered a new method of marking osseous tissue in pigs by feeding them madder root.[642, 643] Several years later, Duhamel, in his studies of bone growth, demonstrated that only the osseous tissue formed during the time when the animal was fed madder turned red, while that formed before and afterward was of normal color. In addition to confirming the findings of Hales that longitudinal growth of long bones takes place at the extremities, Duhamel proposed that interstitial growth also occurs to a varying extent in the diaphysis. He also demonstrated that transverse growth of the diaphysis occurs by appositional bone formation from the periosteum and not by interstitial growth in the bone tissue.[687-691] The experiments of Hales and Duhamel were repeated by John Hunter, who showed that appositional bone formation is accompanied by resorption of previously formed bony tissue.[744, 745] Flourens found that resorption of bony tissue is not confined to the endosteal aspect of the diaphysis, but also occurs in most parts of bony tissue.[697-700]

A discussion of normal bone growth and bone modeling is beyond the scope of this textbook. The reader is referred to Rubin, from whose textbook the following facts are quoted:

1. *Epiphysis.* Growth in the epiphysis at first extends in all directions, but for the most part of its development, the epiphysis grows as a hemisphere. The epiphysis, in contrast to the growth plate, adds little to the total length of the shaft.

2. *Physis or Growth Plate.* The zone of resting cartilage grows by appositional rather than interstitial growth, increasing the transverse diameter of the shaft only. The zone of proliferating cartilage grows by interstitial division and increases the vertical, but not the transverse diameter of the shaft. The zone of vacuolization and calcification does not contribute to any significant increase in the transverse or vertical dimensions of the shaft.

3. *Metaphysis.* This is the site between the cartilage growth plate and the diaphysis in which active bone absorption occurs and the normal tendency is toward a progressive reduction of shaft caliber. The metaphyseal segment is shaped like a funnel at the ends of the bone. The primary and secondary spongiosa are absorbed due to osteoclasis and vascular mesenchyme, and this serves to reduce the transverse diameter of the shaft.

4. *Diaphysis.* The shaft of the bone increases in diameter by thickening of the cortex and expansion of the marrow in an appositional manner. Remodeling of the shaft is eccentric in many instances. Increase in length of the periosteum is not synonymous with increase in length of the diaphysis. Remodeling of the cortical bone is a life-long process in which the ratio of bone deposition to bone resorption varies with age.*

Patterns of Skeletal Growth

A knowledge of the fundamental principles and factors that control future growth is a prerequisite in the management of leg length inequality. These are reviewed briefly here; the reader is advised to study carefully the writings of Green and Anderson, from whom the following information is taken.[626-629, 712-717]

RATE OF GROWTH

The rate of growth varies with each age level (Fig. 7–112). Growth during infancy is very rapid, but it progressively decreases during the years of the first decade until the period of the "adolescent growth spurt,"

*From Rubin, P.: Dynamic Classification of Bone Dysplasias. Chicago, Year Book Medical Publishers, Inc., 1964.

FIGURE 7–112.   Rate of growth at various ages.

A. Pattern of growth in a boy from the age of 1 to 18 years. Note, during the first decade, the decreasing rate of growth of stature and of length of femur, tibia, and trunk. In the second decade, there is a definite short period of accelerated growth—the "adolescent growth spurt." This general pattern of growth is similar in all children. (From Green, W. T., and Anderson, M.: A.A.O.S. Instructional Course Lectures, Vol. 17, p. 200. St. Louis, C. V. Mosby Co., 1960.)

B. Average yearly rates of growth derived from completely longitudinal series. (From Anderson, M., Green, W. T., and Messner, M. B.: Growth and prediction of growths in the lower limbs. J. Bone Joint Surg., *45-A*:5, 1963.)

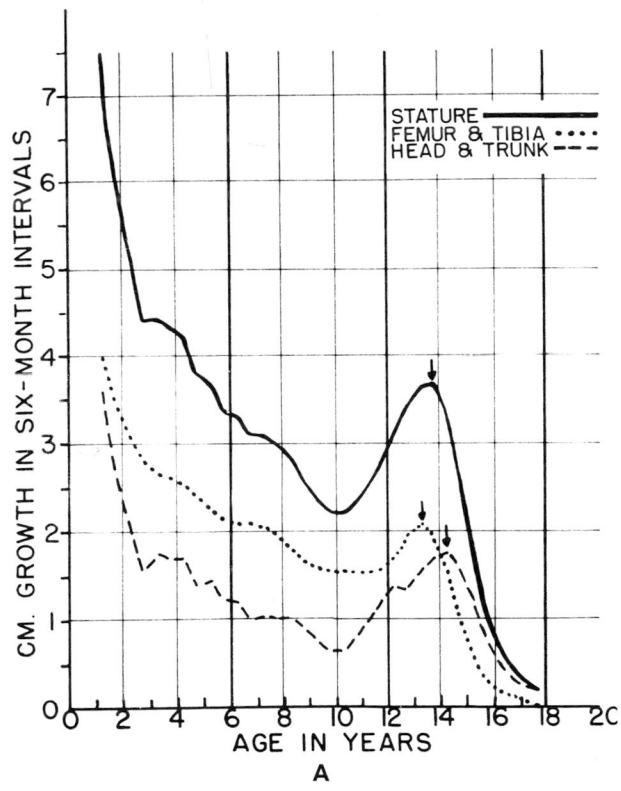

AVERAGE YEARLY RATES OF GROWTH
DERIVED FROM COMPLETELY LONGITUDINAL SERIES

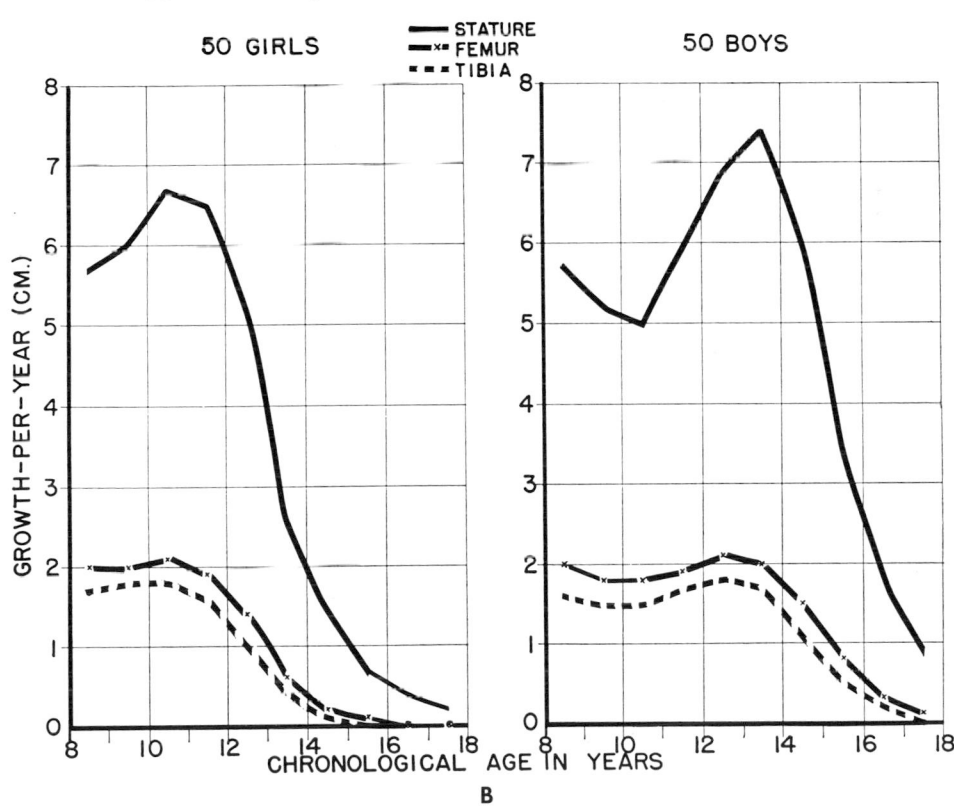

when it is again accelerated. The duration of this so-called adolescent growth spurt is one to two years, its age of occurrence depending primarily upon the sex of the child; in girls, it takes place between 10 and 12 years; in boys, it usually occurs between the ages of 12 and 14. During this rapid growth period in adolescence, the rates of growth of the long bones and of general total height often double; in the ensuing four years or so, the rate of growth tapers off to zero. During all the years preceding the adolescent growth spurt, the lower limbs grow at a more rapid rate than the trunk, whereas following this spurt, the trunk grows more rapidly than the lower limbs. After cessation of growth in the long bones, the vertebral column continues to grow for about two years.

In the first decade of life, the growth rate is similar in boys and girls; but during the adolescent growth spurt there are definite differences in the rates of growth between males and females. In general, girls are two years ahead of boys in the onset of their adolescent growth spurt and in the completion of growth. Significant growth in the lower limbs is usually terminated by the age of 14 years in girls and 16 years in boys.

Between the age of four years and maturity, in a normal lower limb, the femur usually increases its total length by 2 cm. per year, while the average rate of growth of the tibia is 1.6 cm. per year.

According to Digby, 65 per cent of the growth of the entire lower limb takes place around the knee (distal femoral epiphysis, 35 per cent; proximal tibial epiphysis, 30 per cent), and 35 per cent of the total growth occurs in the proximal femur (15 per cent) and the distal tibia (20 per cent). These figures are only approximate since Digby calculated the proportional growths from dry bones and did not consider sex, age, growth spurt, and relative height.[686]

Longitudinal bone growth has been studied by the temporarily arrested growth lines, which are sharply delineated transverse zones of increased radiopacity oriented parallel to the physis toward the end of the diaphysis. The mechanism of formation of growth arrest lines is as follows: In children, during periods of illness or starvation, there is a failure of cartilaginous growth and longitudinal columns of cartilage are not formed; osteoblasts, however,

continue to manufacture osseous tissue and the newly formed bone accumulates, depicted as radiopaque transverse striations in the roentgenogram.[731, 789] Green and Anderson, using growth arrest lines as points of reference, found that between 10 and 15 years of age on the average, 71 per cent of the total femoral increment occurred at its distal metaphysis, whereas 57 per cent of the total tibial growth arose at its proximal metaphysis.[627, 716] The mean percentage of growth of each epiphysis in the lower limb is given in Table 7–8.

RELATIVE SIZE

The relative height and length of the femur and the tibia in relation to skeletal age are important factors in the determination of a prediction of the amount of future growth (Tables 7–9, 7–10, and 7–11, Figs. 7–113 and 7–114). It is obvious that a child destined to be a tall adult has relatively greater yearly increments of growth; and consequently the ultimate leg length discrepancy will be greater in a tall child than in a short one.

The height of the parents or of the elder siblings is of some assistance in assessing the future adult size of a child, provided there is no variation in the family pattern.

RELATIVE MATURITY

This is determined by the skeletal age. Todd, and more recently, Greulich and Pyle, have thoroughly standardized the roentgenographic appearance of the bones in the hands and wrists for boys and girls from birth through 18 years.[718, 832] By

Table 7–8. *Mean Average of Percentage of Growth of Epiphyses of Major Long Bones in the Lower Limbs*

	Femur		Tibia	
	Proximal	Distal	Proximal	Distal
Green-Anderson (1947, 1963)	29	71	57	43
Gill-Abbott (1942)	30	70	60	40
Wilson-Thompson (1939)	30	70	60	40
Digby (1916)	31	69	57	43

Table 7–9. *Variation in Size and Relative Maturity at Consecutive Chronological Ages** *(Values for stature, length of femur and tibia, and skeletal age derived from completely longitudinal series of fifty girls and fifty boys)*

50 Girls

Age	Stature (cm)		Femur (cm)		Tibia (cm)		Skeletal Age (Years)	
	Mean	σ	Mean	σ	Mean	σ	Mean	σ
8	128.1	4.78	33.1	1.63	26.3	1.39	7.6	1.02
9	133.8	4.78	35.0	1.71	28.0	1.50	8.7	1.02
10	139.9	5.24	37.0	1.82	29.8	1.67	9.9	1.03
11	146.6	5.93	39.2	2.00	31.6	1.84	11.1	1.07
12	153.2	6.36	41.1	2.12	33.2	1.95	12.5	1.12
13	158.3	6.14	42.4	2.12	34.2	1.94	13.8	1.06
14	160.8	6.16	43.1	2.15	34.5	1.97	14.8	1.05
15	162.3	6.02	43.2	2.18	34.6	1.98	15.8	1.00
16	162.9	6.10	43.3	2.20	34.6	2.00	16.4	0.92
17	(163.8)	(6.37)	(43.3)	(2.21)	(34.7)	(2.00)	(17.1)	(0.85)
18	(164.9)	(6.10)	(43.3)	(2.21)	(34.7)	(2.00)	(17.8)	(0.46)

Figures in parentheses based on 21–42 girls only, since data were not available on all subjects at these ages.

50 Boys

Age	Stature (cm)		Femur (cm)		Tibia (cm)		Skeletal Age (Years)	
	Mean	σ	Mean	σ	Mean	σ	Mean	σ
8	127.6	5.94	(32.8)	(1.53)	(25.9)	(1.55)	(7.8)	(1.00)
9	133.3	6.15	(34.6)	(1.78)	(27.1)	(1.86)	(8.8)	(1.04)
10	138.5	6.58	36.4	1.87	28.6	1.89	9.9	0.96
11	143.5	6.94	38.2	2.07	30.1	2.07	11.0	0.88
12	149.4	7.72	40.2	2.23	31.8	2.27	12.1	0.76
13	156.3	9.13	42.3	2.52	33.6	2.49	13.1	0.80
14	163.7	9.54	44.3	2.58	35.3	2.54	14.1	0.93
15	169.8	8.68	45.8	2.38	36.4	2.34	15.1	1.14
16	173.2	7.74	46.6	2.27	36.9	2.21	16.3	1.20
17	175.0	7.41	46.9	2.30	37.1	2.21	17.3	1.10
18	175.9	7.37	47.0	2.35	37.1	2.22	(18.0)	(0.89)

Figures in parentheses based on 31–49 boys only, since data were not available on all subjects at these ages.

Bone lengths, measured from orthoroentgenograms, include both proximal and distal epiphyses. Skeletal ages read according to Greulich-Pyle Atlas (1950).

*From Anderson, M., Green, W. T., and Messner, M. B.: Growth and prediction of growth in the lower extremities. J. Bone Joint Surg., *45-A*:3, 1963.

comparing roentgenograms of the wrist and hand of a given child with standard films of the same area, the skeletal age is determined. Assessment of bone age from the knee may be of some help in borderline or difficult cases.[803]

Skeletal age is an excellent indicator of maturity, and in predictions of future growth, it is skeletal rather than chronological age that should be considered. Another clue to skeletal maturity is the development of secondary sexual characteristics, the appearance of pubic hair, voice change, breast development, and menarche. These outward physical indicators, however, do exhibit great individual variation in the order and significance of their appearance, and are only rough tools at best.

The rate of growth is another factor to consider in assessing maturation; the completion of the adolescent growth spurt indicates greater maturity.

(*Text continued on page 1482.*)

Table 7–10.   *Boys: Lengths of the Long Bones Including Epiphyses**
Orthoroentgenographic Measurements from Longitudinal Series of Sixty-seven Children
Femur

| No. | Age | Mean | σ_d | σ_m | Distribution | | | |
					$+2\sigma_d$	$+1\sigma_d$	$-1\sigma_d$	$-2\sigma_d$
21	1	14.48	0.628	0.077	15.74	15.11	13.85	13.22
57	2	18.15	0.874	0.107	19.90	19.02	17.28	16.40
65	3	21.09	1.031	0.126	23.15	22.12	20.06	19.03
66	4	23.65	1.197	0.146	26.04	24.85	22.45	21.26
66	5	25.92	1.342	0.164	28.60	27.26	24.58	23.24
67	6	28.09	1.506	0.184	31.10	29.60	26.58	25.08
67	7	30.25	1.682	0.205	33.61	31.93	28.57	26.89
67	8	32.28	1.807	0.221	35.89	34.09	30.47	28.67
67	9	34.36	1.933	0.236	38.23	36.29	32.43	30.49
67	10	36.29	2.057	0.251	40.40	38.35	34.23	32.18
67	11	38.16	2.237	0.276	42.63	40.40	35.92	33.69
67	12	40.12	2.447	0.299	45.01	42.57	37.67	35.23
67	13	42.17	2.765	0.338	47.70	44.95	39.40	36.64
67	14	44.18	2.809	0.343	49.80	46.99	41.37	38.56
67	15	45.69	2.512	0.307	50.71	48.20	43.19	40.67
67	16	46.66	2.244	0.274	51.15	48.90	44.42	42.17
67	17	47.07	2.051	0.251	51.17	49.12	45.02	42.97
67	18	47.23	1.958	0.239	51.15	49.19	45.27	43.31

Tibia

| No. | Age | Mean | σ_d | σ_m | Distribution | | | |
					$+2\sigma_d$	$+1\sigma_d$	$-1\sigma_d$	$-2\sigma_d$
61	1	11.60	0.620	0.074	12.84	12.22	10.98	10.36
67	2	14.54	0.809	0.099	16.16	15.35	13.73	12.92
67	3	16.79	0.935	0.114	18.66	17.72	15.86	14.92
67	4	18.67	1.091	0.133	20.85	19.76	17.58	16.49
67	5	20.46	1.247	0.152	22.95	21.71	19.21	17.97
67	6	22.12	1.418	0.173	24.96	23.54	20.87	19.46
67	7	23.76	1.632	0.199	27.02	25.39	22.13	20.50
67	8	25.38	1.778	0.217	28.94	27.16	23.60	21.82
67	9	26.99	1.961	0.240	30.91	28.95	25.02	23.06
67	10	28.53	2.113	0.258	32.76	30.64	26.42	24.30
67	11	30.10	2.301	0.281	34.70	32.40	27.80	25.50
67	12	31.75	2.536	0.310	36.82	34.29	29.21	26.68
67	13	33.49	2.833	0.346	39.16	36.32	30.66	27.82
67	14	35.18	2.865	0.350	40.91	38.04	32.32	29.45
67	15	36.38	2.616	0.320	41.61	39.00	33.76	31.15
67	16	37.04	2.412	0.295	41.86	39.45	34.63	32.22
67	17	37.22	2.316	0.283	41.85	39.54	34.90	32.59
67	18	37.29	2.254	0.275	41.80	39.54	35.04	32.78

*From Anderson, M., Messner, M. B., and Green, W. T.: Distribution of lengths of the normal femur and tibia in children from one to eighteen years of age. J. Bone Joint Surg., *46-A*:1198, 1964.

Table 7–11. *Girls: Lengths of the Long Bones Including Epiphyses**
Orthoroentgenographic Measurements from Longitudinal Series of Sixty-seven Children

Femur

No.	Age	Mean	σ_d	σ_m	Distribution			
					$+2\sigma_d$	$+1\sigma_d$	$-1\sigma_d$	$-2\sigma_d$
30	1	14.81	0.673	0.082	16.16	15.48	14.14	13.46
52	2	18.23	0.888	0.109	20.01	19.12	17.34	16.45
63	3	21.29	1.100	0.134	23.49	22.39	20.19	19.09
66	4	23.92	1.339	0.164	26.60	25.26	22.58	21.24
66	5	26.32	1.437	0.176	29.19	27.76	24.88	23.45
66	6	28.52	1.616	0.197	31.75	30.14	26.90	25.29
67	7	30.60	1.827	0.223	34.25	32.43	28.77	26.95
67	8	32.72	1.936	0.236	36.59	34.66	30.78	28.85
67	9	34.71	2.117	0.259	38.94	36.83	32.59	30.48
67	10	36.72	2.300	0.281	41.32	39.02	34.42	32.12
67	11	38.81	2.468	0.302	43.75	41.28	36.34	33.87
67	12	40.74	2.507	0.306	45.75	43.25	38.23	35.73
67	13	42.31	2.428	0.310	47.17	44.74	39.88	37.45
67	14	43.14	2.269	0.277	47.68	45.41	40.87	38.60
67	15	43.47	2.197	0.277	47.86	45.67	41.27	39.08
67	16	43.58	2.193	0.268	47.97	45.77	41.39	39.19
67	17	43.60	2.192	0.268	47.98	45.79	41.41	39.22
67	18	43.63	2.195	0.269	48.02	45.82	41.44	39.24

Tibia

No.	Age	Mean	σ_d	σ_m	Distribution			
					$+2\sigma_d$	$+1\sigma_d$	$-1\sigma_d$	$-2\sigma_d$
61	1	11.57	0.646	0.082	12.86	12.22	10.92	10.28
67	2	14.51	0.739	0.090	15.99	15.25	13.77	13.03
67	3	16.81	0.893	0.109	18.60	17.70	15.92	15.02
67	4	18.86	1.144	0.140	21.15	20.00	17.72	16.57
67	5	20.77	1.300	0.159	23.37	22.07	19.47	18.17
67	6	22.53	1.458	0.178	25.45	23.90	21.07	19.61
67	7	24.22	1.640	0.200	27.50	25.86	22.58	20.94
67	8	25.89	1.786	0.218	29.46	27.68	24.10	22.32
67	9	27.56	1.993	0.243	31.55	29.55	25.57	23.57
67	10	29.28	2.193	0.259	33.67	31.47	27.09	24.89
67	11	31.00	2.384	0.291	35.77	33.38	28.62	26.23
67	12	32.61	2.424	0.296	37.46	35.03	30.19	27.76
67	13	33.83	2.374	0.290	38.58	36.20	31.46	29.08
67	14	34.43	2.228	0.272	38.89	36.66	32.20	29.97
67	15	34.59	2.173	0.265	38.94	36.76	32.42	30.24
67	16	34.63	2.151	0.263	38.93	36.78	32.48	30.33
67	17	34.65	2.158	0.264	38.97	36.81	32.49	30.33
67	18	34.65	2.161	0.264	38.97	36.81	32.49	30.33

*From Anderson, M., Messner, M. B., and Green, W. T.: Distribution of lengths of the normal femur and tibia in children from one to eighteen years of age. J. Bone Joint Surg., *46–A*:1199, 1964.

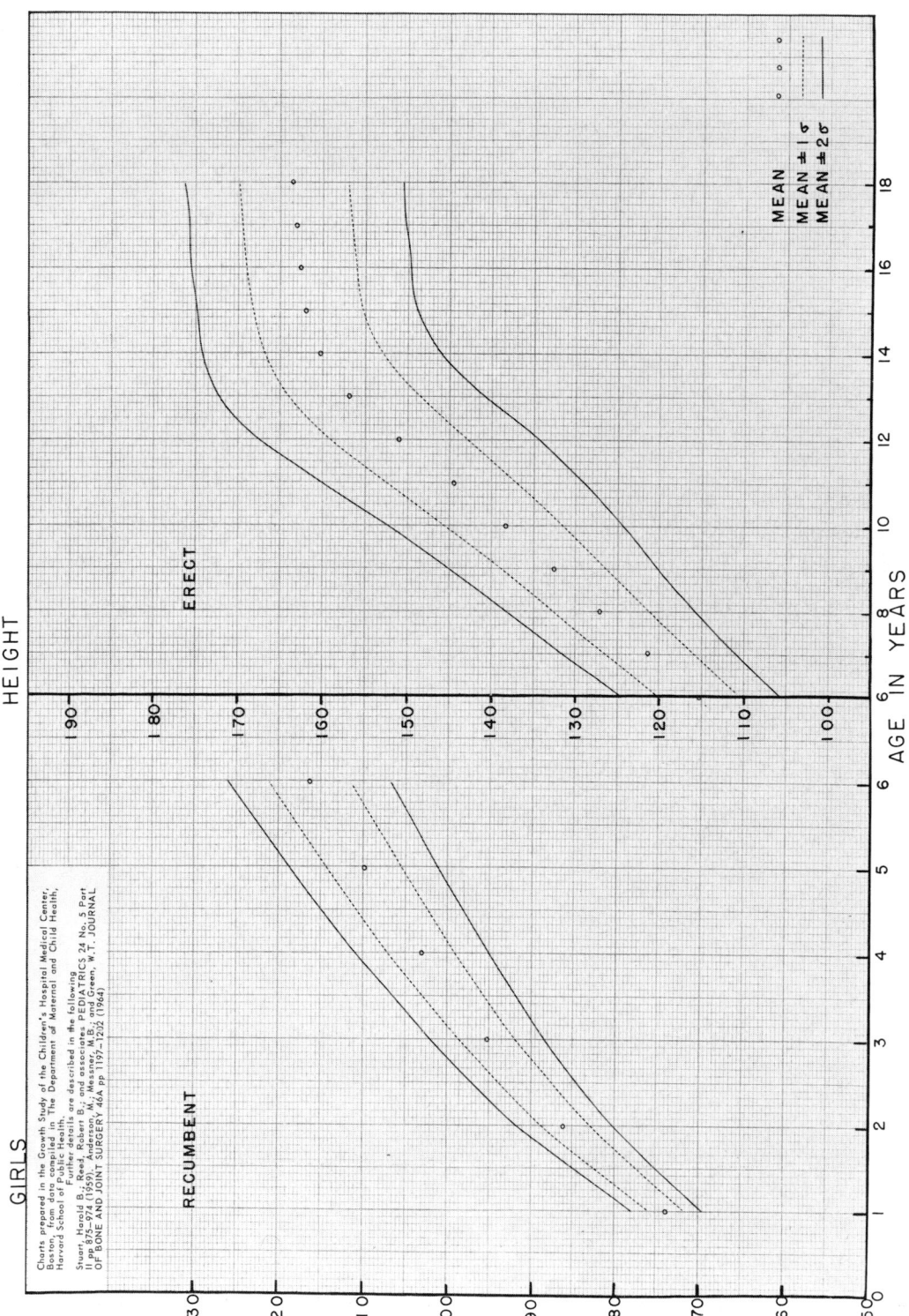

FIGURE 7–113. Total and sitting height between the ages of 1 and 18 years.

A. Total height in girls. (Chart prepared in the Growth Study of the Children's Hospital Medical Center, Boston, from data compiled in The Department of Maternal and Child Health, Harvard School of Public Health, Boston, Massachusetts. Courtesy of R. B. Reed, M. Anderson, et al.)

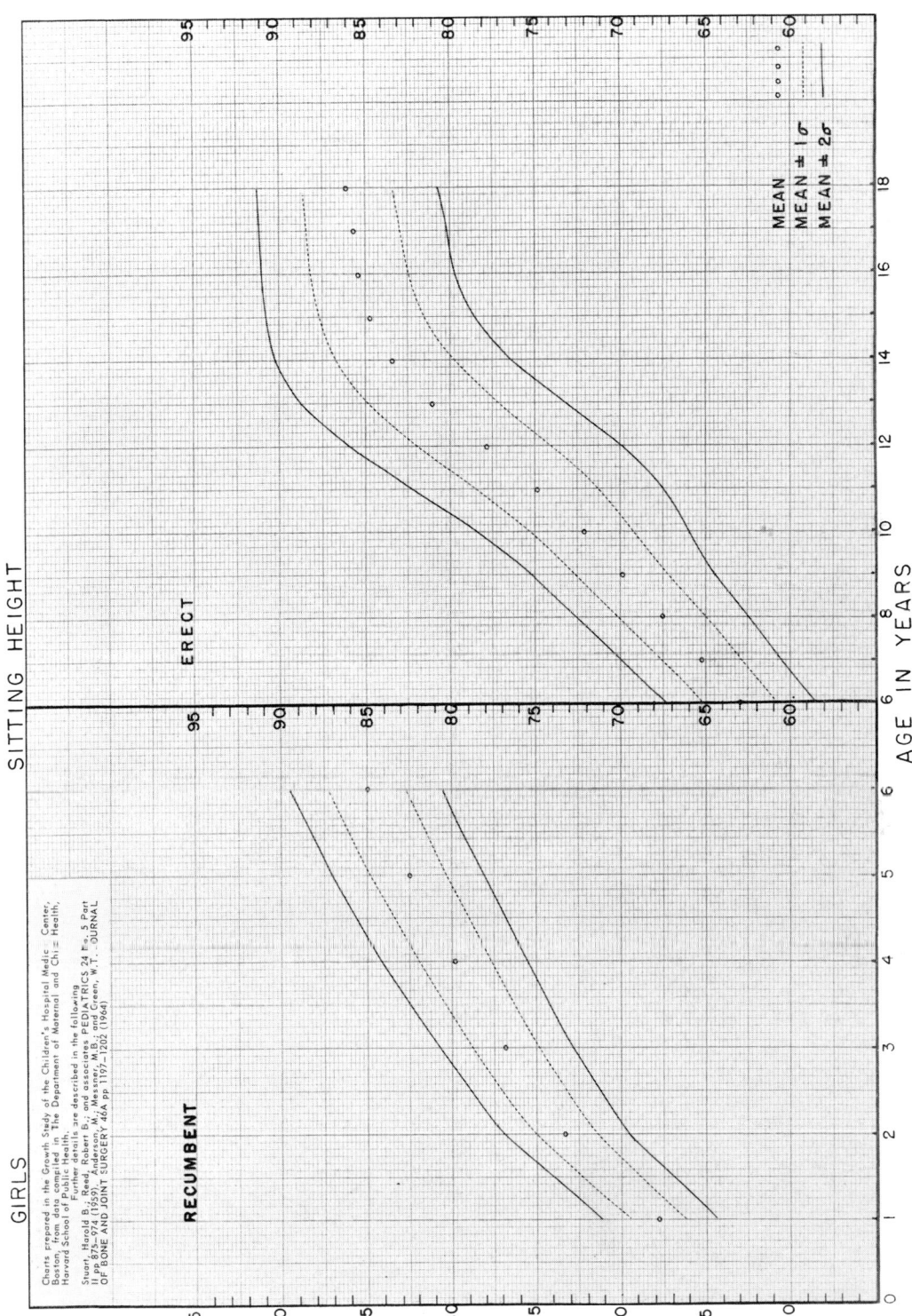

FIGURE 7–113 Continued.   Total and sitting height between the ages of 1 and 18 years.

B. Sitting height in girls. (Chart prepared in the Growth Study of the Children's Hospital Medical Center, Boston, from data compiled in The Department of Maternal and Child Health, Harvard School of Public Health, Boston, Massachusetts. Courtesy of R. B. Reed, M. Anderson, et al.)

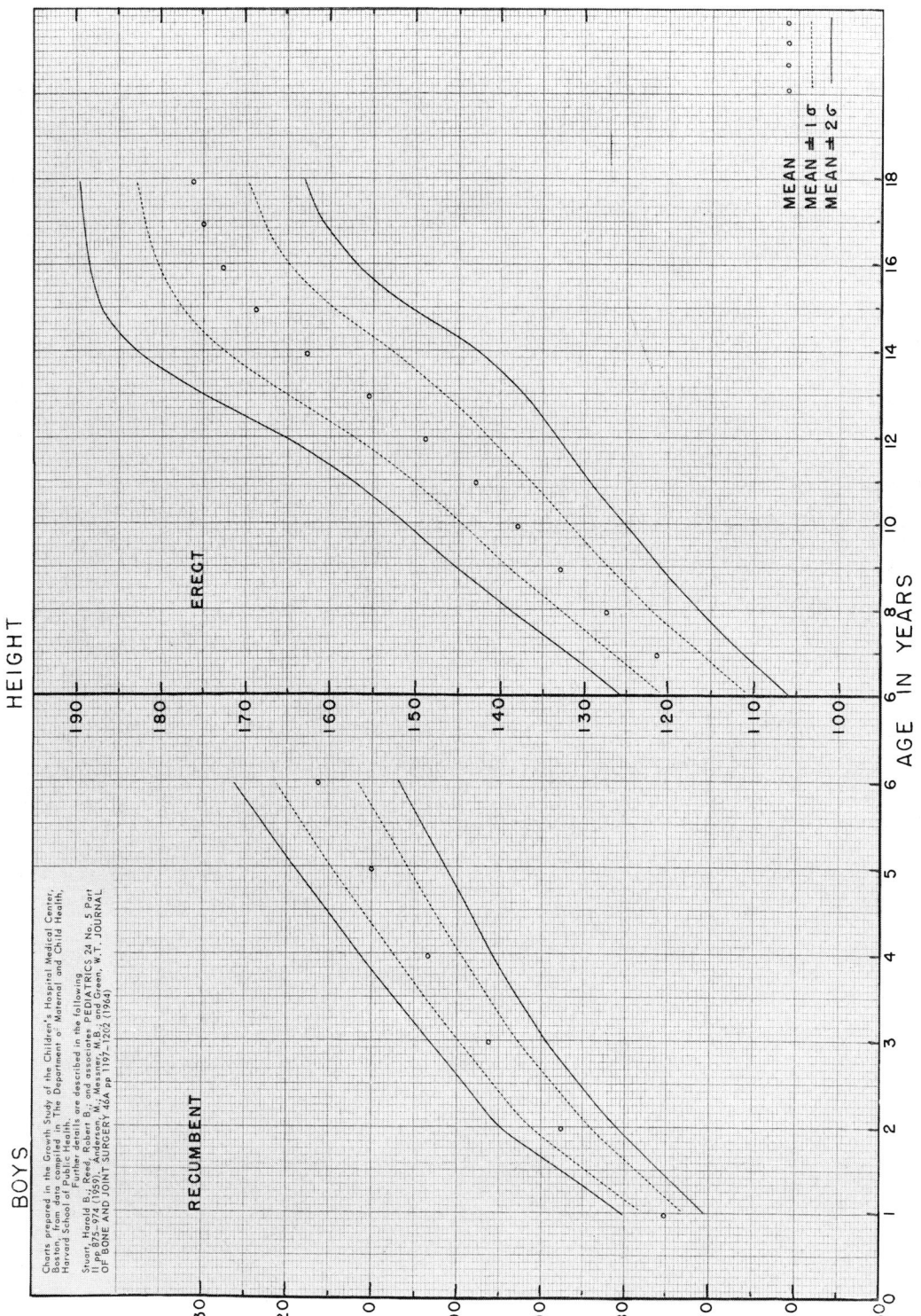

FIGURE 7–113 Continued. Total and sitting height between the ages of 1 and 18 years.

C. Total height in boys. (Chart prepared in the Growth Study of the Children's Hospital Medical Center, Boston, from data compiled in The Department of Maternal and Child Health, Harvard School of Public Health, Boston, Massachusetts. Courtesy of R. B. Reed, M. Anderson, et al.)

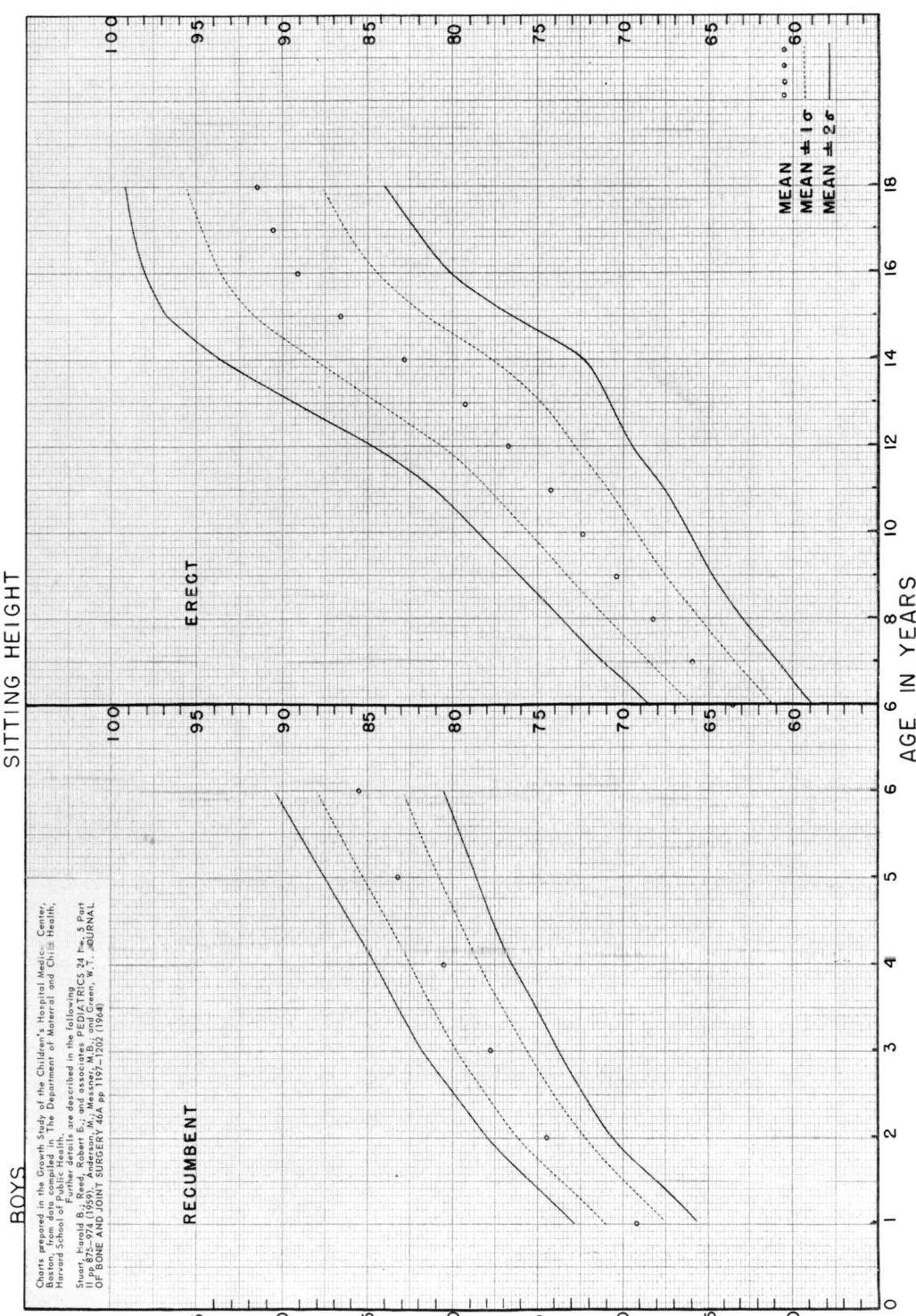

FIGURE 7–113 Continued. **Total and sitting height between the ages of 1 and 18 years.**

D. Sitting height in boys. (Chart prepared in the Growth Study of the Children's Hospital Medical Center, Boston, from data compiled in The Department of Maternal and Child Health. Harvard School of Public Health, Boston, Massachusetts. Courtesy of R. B. Reed, M. Anderson, et al.)

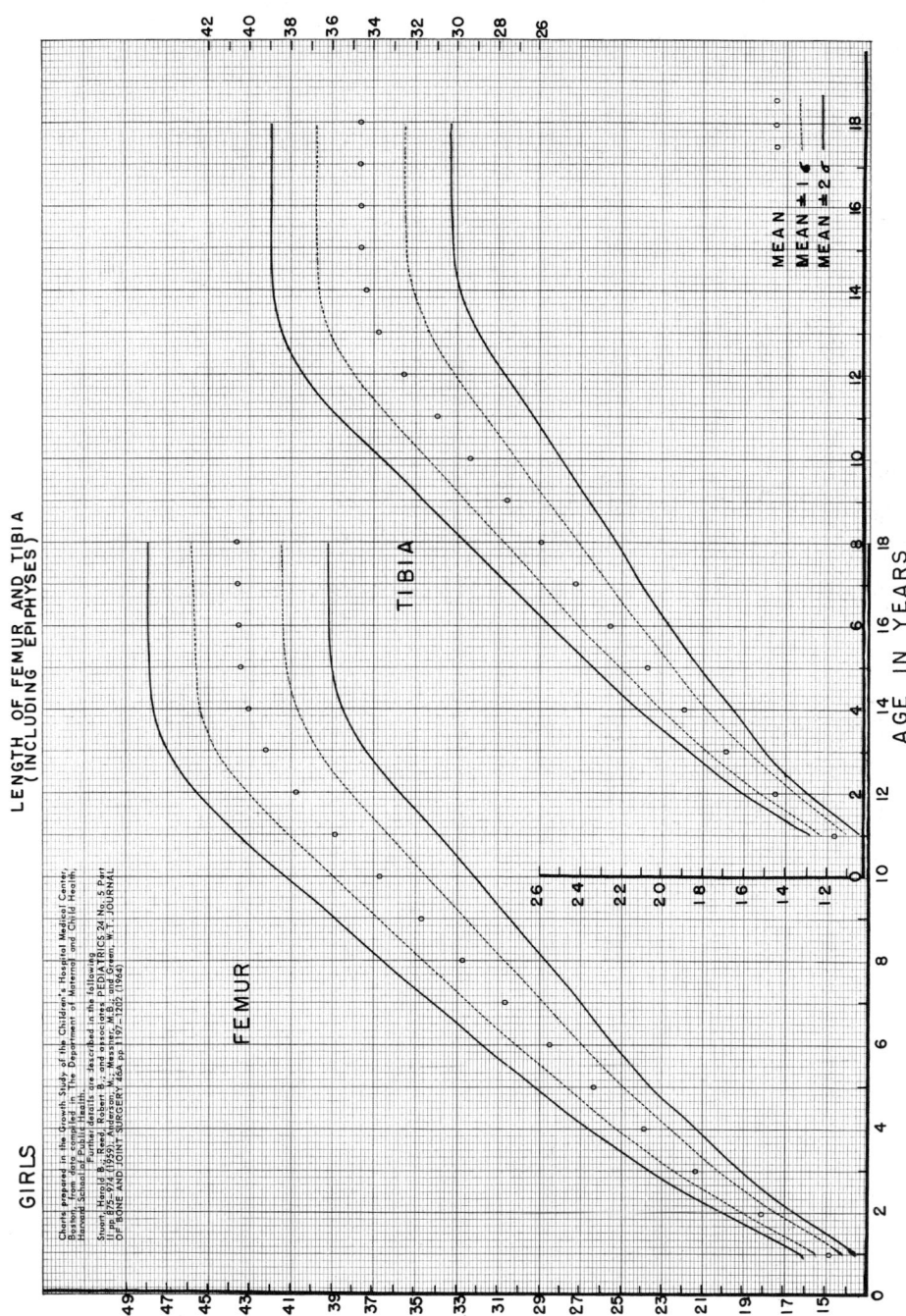

FIGURE 7-114. Values for lengths of the normal femur and tibia at consecutive chronological ages from 1 through 18 years.

A. In girls. (Courtesy of Drs. M. Anderson, M. B. Messner, and W. T. Green.)

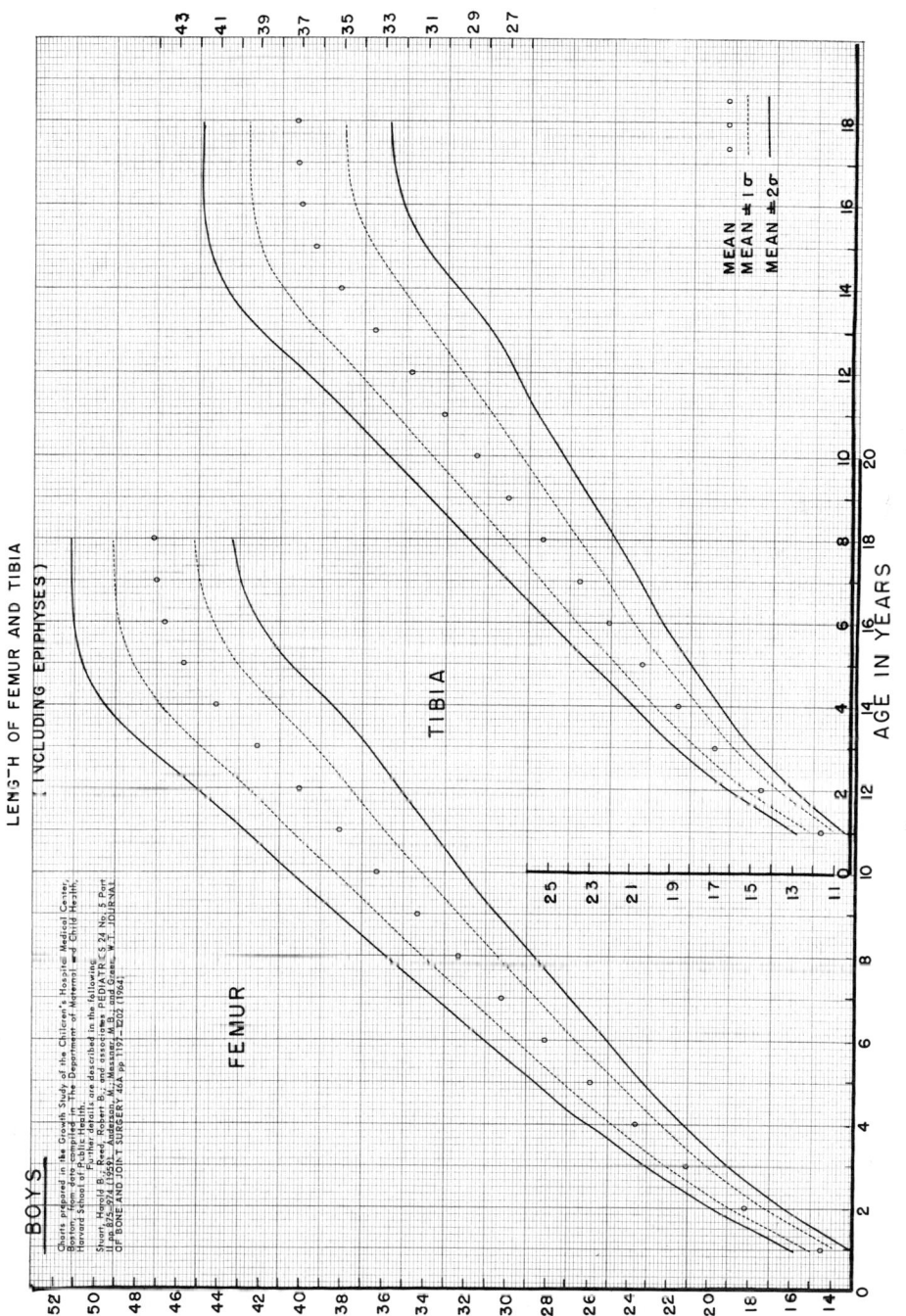

FIGURE 7–114 Continued. *Values for lengths of the normal femur and tibia at consecutive chronological ages from 1 through 18 years.* **B.** In boys. (Courtesy of Drs. M. Anderson, M. B. Messner, and W. T. Green.)

Growth Prediction Chart

Epiphyseodesis or stapling for retardation of growth should be carried out at a very carefully selected period in the child's growth if leg length discrepancy is to be corrected with any degree of accuracy. In order to do so, the amount of growth that may occur in a normal distal femur and proximal tibia following specific skeletal ages should be known. In 1947, Green and Anderson presented such a growth prediction chart, which was revised in 1963. The revision was derived from completely "longitudinal" data on 50 boys and 50 girls, each subject being represented at every consecutive skeletal age. The 1950 edition of the Greulich Pyle atlas was used for the assessment of the maturational levels.[627, 712]

In the new chart at each skeletal age, 8 $3/12$ to 15 $3/12$ years in girls and 10 $3/12$ to 17 $3/12$ years in boys, the mean values as well as the range of one and two standard deviations are given (Fig. 7–115). In Table 7–12 are shown the values for five percentile levels, the means, and the standard deviations. For example, the chart shows that the expected correction to be obtained from distal femoral epiphyseodesis in a boy at the skeletal age of 12 years on the mean average will amount to 5 cm. (fiftieth percentile); the broken lines on the chart indicate the range of *one standard deviation* (in 68 per cent of the boys at this age), which gives a correction between 4 and 6 cm.; the solid lines on the chart give the range of *two standard deviations* (in 95 per cent) and show an expected correction between 3 and 7 cm.

USE OF GROWTH PREDICTION CHART

It should be emphasized that this chart is to be considered as a guide rather than as an accurate prediction device.[627, 712] Various factors modify the actual correction of leg length discrepancy following epiphyseodesis. In addition to the effectiveness of the surgery itself, the sex, and the relative maturity of the individual, the following should be considered:

Growth of Long Bones of Contralateral Short Lower Limb. Correction of leg length discrepancy is provided by the growth of the short limb; if this is not normal, certain adjustments must be made. It is obvious that if leg length inequality is caused by premature fusion of the proximal tibial epiphysis following trauma, it will not be corrected by epiphyseodesis of the proximal tibia on the opposite normal side; all that will accomplish is to halt further shortening. Green and Anderson give the following method of computing the per cent of growth inhibition: The change in discrepancy in bone lengths in a given time interval is divided by the growth of the bone on the normal side during the same interval, and the resultant quotient is multiplied by 100, the formula being:

$$\text{Per cent of growth inhibition} = \frac{(\text{Growth normal}) - (\text{Growth involved})}{(\text{Growth normal})}$$

These computations should be based on a period of observation of at least three years' duration or on a measured growth of the unaffected side amounting to 5 cm. or more. The degree of inhibition is graded as follows: *mild,* 0 to 10 per cent; *moderate,* 11 to 20 per cent; *marked,* 21 to 30 per cent; and *severe,* over 31 per cent. Depending upon the rate of inhibition, individual adjustments should be made toward the lower value on the chart in the prediction of correction to be obtained from epiphyseal arrest. For example, in a girl with a skeletal age of 11 years with moderate (11 to 20 per cent) growth inhibition, 2.5 cm. rather than 3 cm. correction is predicted; if the degree of growth inhibition is marked (21 to 30 per cent), 2 cm. correction is predicted; and if it is severe, a maximum correction of only 1.5 cm. will be achieved at skeletal maturity.

Relative Size of the Individual. This also is an important consideration. It is obvious that a tall child will grow more over a number of years than a short child. The height and the femoral and tibial lengths as related with the standards are given in Tables 7–9 and 7–10 and Figures 7–113 and 7–114. In the growth prediction chart, adjustments are made for the upper value

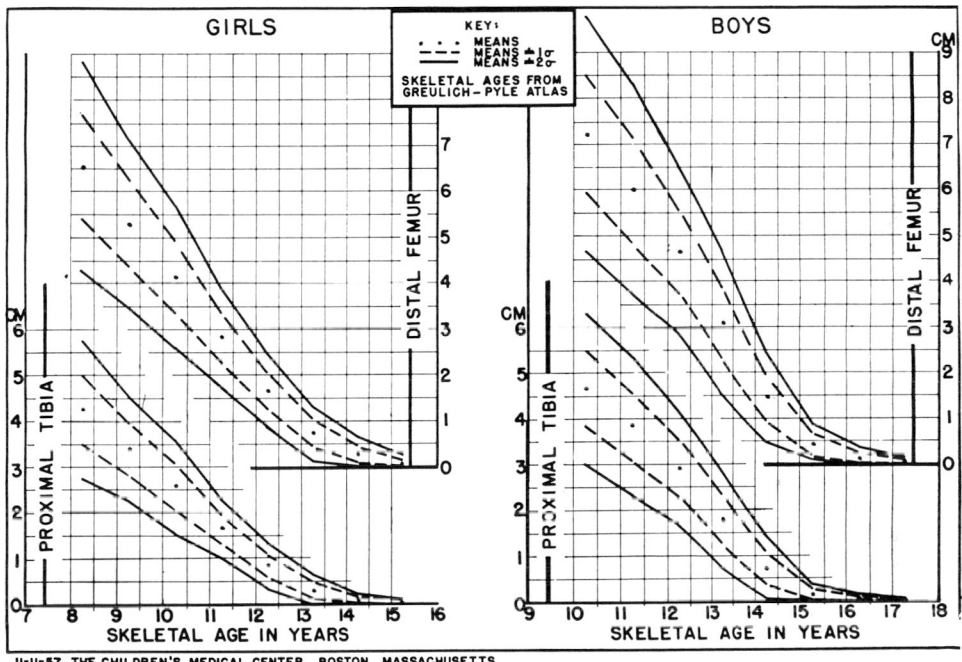

FIGURE 7-115. Growth prediction chart.

The chart is to be used as a guide in estimating the amounts of growth that may be inhibited in the distal end of the normal femur or the proximal end of the normal tibia by epiphyseal arrest at the skeletal ages indicated on the baseline. (From Anderson, M., Green, W. T., and Messner, M. B.: Growth and predictions of growth in the lower extremities. J. Bone Joint Surg., *45-A*:10, 1963.)

Table 7–12. *Growth in Distal End of Normal Femur and Proximal End of Normal Tibia Observed in Longitudinal Series Following Given Skeletal Ages†*
(Growth recorded in centimeters; skeletal ages assessed from Greulich-Pyle Atlas)

		50 Girls								**50 Boys**							
		8^3*	9^3	10^3	11^3	12^3	13^3	14^3	15^3	10^3	11^3	12^3	13^3	14^3	15^3	16^3	17^3
						Distal End of the Femur (Total Growth Femur $\times 71\%$)											
Mean		6.54	5.30	4.15	2.82	1.66	0.75	0.27	0.05	7.21	6.01	4.65	3.09	1.48	0.45	0.15	0.04
σ		1.14	0.92	0.78	0.53	0.40	0.30	0.18	0.08	1.28	1.14	0.91	0.78	0.50	0.23	0.12	0.06
Extreme		9.8	8.6	7.2	4.7	2.8	1.5	0.7	0.4	9.7	8.4	7.2	5.7	3.0	1.0	0.6	0.2
90th		8.4	6.7	5.0	3.4	2.1	1.1	0.6	0.1	8.9	7.8	5.7	4.2	2.2	0.8	0.3	0.1
Percentiles 75th		7.2	5.8	4.6	3.2	1.9	1.0	0.4	0.1	8.3	6.7	5.2	3.5	1.8	0.6	0.2	0.1
50th		6.5	5.2	4.1	2.8	1.7	0.7	0.3	0.0	7.2	6.1	4.8	2.9	1.4	0.4	0.1	0.0
25th		5.8	4.8	3.7	2.4	1.4	0.6	0.1	0.0	6.3	5.2	4.1	2.6	1.2	0.3	0.1	0.0
10th		5.0	4.3	3.3	2.2	1.1	0.4	0.0	0.0	5.3	4.4	3.4	2.3	1.0	0.2	0.0	0.0
Extreme		4.1	3.1	2.2	1.6	0.7	0.1	0.0	0.0	4.8	3.8	2.8	1.6	0.4	0.1	0.0	0.0
						Proximal End of the Tibia (Total Growth Tibia $\times 57\%$)											
Mean		4.25	3.39	2.58	1.65	0.86	0.32	0.09	0.02	4.65	3.83	2.92	1.80	0.74	0.16	0.04	0.01
σ		0.74	0.58	0.50	0.32	0.26	0.17	0.06	0.03	0.83	0.75	0.62	0.53	0.35	0.12	0.06	0.02
Extreme		6.0	5.1	4.3	2.8	1.5	0.8	0.3	0.1	6.7	5.6	4.7	3.4	2.2	0.7	0.3	0.1
90th		5.5	4.2	3.2	1.9	1.2	0.6	0.2	0.1	5.8	4.8	3.6	2.5	1.1	0.3	0.1	0.0
Percentiles 75th		4.6	3.7	2.7	1.8	1.0	0.4	0.1	0.1	5.3	4.3	3.3	2.0	0.8	0.2	0.0	0.0
50th		4.1	3.3	2.6	1.6	0.8	0.3	0.0	0.0	4.6	3.8	3.0	1.8	0.7	0.2	0.0	0.0
25th		3.8	3.0	2.3	1.5	0.7	0.2	0.0	0.0	4.0	3.2	2.6	1.4	0.5	0.0	0.0	0.0
10th		3.3	2.8	2.0	1.2	0.6	0.1	0.0	0.0	3.4	2.7	2.0	1.1	0.3	0.0	0.0	0.0
Extreme		2.5	1.9	1.1	0.9	0.3	0.0	0.0	0.0	3.0	2.3	1.6	1.0	0.1	0.0	0.0	0.0

*Figures indicate skeletal ages in years and months. Thus, 8^3 is eight years and three months.
†From Anderson, M., Green, W. T., and Messner, M. B.: Growth and prediction of growth in the lower extremities. J. Bone & Joint Surg., *45 A*:3, 1963.

in a tall child and for the lower value in a small child.

Clinical Factors. Several practical variables must be considered: Foremost is balance of the head, neck, and trunk over the pelvis. Any list of the spine toward the short side and the height of the lift needed under the short limb to correct it are noted. Is there any structural scoliosis? The important consideration is the provision of a compensated spine.

Is there any abnormality in the gait? How disabling is the short leg limp? How coordinated is the child? Does he walk and run well without a lift?

If the patient wears an above-knee orthosis on the short limb, it is preferable that the leg with the orthosis be 1 to 1.5 cm. shorter than the opposite limb, as the patient will clear the leg with the orthosis in the swing-through phase of gait with much more ease and less strain.

Is the leg length discrepancy increasing? An epiphyseodesis may be indicated to check further shortening only.

What is the predicted eventual total height of the child? This can be determined by the tables provided by Bayley and Pinneau for predicting adult height from skeletal age.[641] In a child destined to be of short stature, if the shortening of the affected limb exceeds 10 cm., it is undesirable to cause further reduction of limb length and height by epiphyseodesis. It is better to lengthen the short limb or to provide a prosthesis than to arrest growth on the long side. The total child should be assessed.

The importance of following the disparity in the rate of relative growth of the lower limbs prior to epiphyseodesis cannot be overemphasized. This is greatly facilitated by the establishment of leg length discrepancy (or growth study) clinics in children's hospitals. Any child with asymmetrical growth of lower limbs should be referred to such a clinic. Annual visits should coincide approximately with their chronological birth dates. An adequate record, preferably in the form of a work sheet, should be kept.

The following data are tabulated: (1) anthropometric measurements of height and leg lengths (both actual and apparent); (2) true lengths of the tibiae and femora as measured on the orthoroentgenograms; (3) the leg length discrepancy; total, femoral, and tibial, as measured clinically and on roentgenograms; (4) relative maturity as shown by the skeletal age (determined in roentgenograms of hands and wrists); roentgen appearance and maturity of each ossification center in the femur and tibia; (5) appearance of secondary sex characteristics; (6) lifts needed under the short leg to level the pelvis and to balance the trunk (centering of head, neck, and shoulders over pelvis); and (7) miscellaneous information such as wearing of an above-knee orthosis, or previous and future contemplated surgery on the lower limbs and for spinal deformity. Serial standing photographs of the child (anteroposterior and posteroanterior views) with and without a lift under the short leg are desirable.

Roentgenographic Methods of Measuring Length of Long Bones

Clinical measurements of leg lengths are by nature grossly inaccurate. More thorough determinations of the length of the femora and tibiae by the use of roentgenographic methods are essential in the treatment of significant leg length discrepancy. Various available methods are reviewed here. Each has its advantages and disadvantages.

Thoms, in 1929, described a method of roentgenometry of the pelvis in which a constant scale was obtained by superimposing a grid on the x-ray plate when the part is exposed to the rays.[601]

TELEOROENTGENOGRAPHY

In this technique, roentgenograms are made on one film with a single exposure for the entire lower limbs, or on two films with separate exposures for the femora and the tibiae (Fig. 7–116 A). The distance of the x-ray tube from the film is 6 feet. This method provides a fairly accurate measurement of the relative length of the two limbs at a single examination. Its disadvantages lie in the magnification produced by the divergent rays. Factors that give distortion are changes in position of centering of the tube, the length of the bone, and the distance of the bone from the film (as the posterior body structures get thicker, this decreases). Mathematical correction of magnification by triangulation is time-consuming and inaccurate. A radiopaque ruler placed on each side parallel to the bones may improve the accuracy of measurement of teleoroentgenograms. One of its advantages is that the entire length of the femora and tibiae of both lower limbs is visualized on a single film with minimal radiation to the patient, but the technique is not satisfactory for serial mensurations and bone detail is much less than that seen on spot orthoroentgenograms.

SLIT SCANOGRAPHY

This technique, developed by Millwee in 1937, reduced magnification to a minimum by rapid movement of the x-ray tube from one end of the table to the other.[778] Gill and Abbott, in 1942, described a technique in which teleoroentgenograms were made by the slit method with a tube-to-plate distance of 6 feet; the exact length of bones was determined by this technique, which also gave good bone detail.[707]

ORTHOROENTGENOGRAPHY

Green, Wyatt, and Anderson, in 1946, described the following method: On a single long film, three successive exposures are made, centered exactly over the hips, knees,

and ankles. The target-to-film distance is 6 feet, each exposure including about one third of the entire lower limb (Fig. 7–116 B). They had originally used a long casette tunnel that incorporated two sliding metal shields in order to restrict the area of film irradiated on the three successive exposures.[717] More recently they reported using a rectangular beam collimator that permitted the film to be made on the table top without the use of any casette tunnel or other special equipment (Fig. 7–117). With this latter method, measurements of bone length were strictly comparable to those made with the earlier used tunnel device; also, the patient received less radiation (total radiation, measured in air, varied from 35 mr for a young child to 84 mr for a young adult), and bone detail was greatly improved.[629]

The advantages of orthoroentgenography are that the true length of each bone can be measured, because magnification due to divergence of rays is eliminated by directing only perpendicular rays at the ends of the long bones. Details of the osseous structure, epiphyseal plates, and contour of the bones are visualized, enabling one to evaluate the factors of the deformity. Overlapping of the shadows at the junction of the shields obscures only the region of the midshafts, where it is of little consequence.

Certain precautions should be taken to ensure the accuracy of orthoroentgenography: (1) The tube should be centered over the articular ends of the long bones and the exact points of focus recorded on each film with a metal marker. (2) The position of the limbs should not change between exposures. Immobilization is secured by

---

FIGURE 7–116.   *Schematic representation of teleoroentgenogram and orthoroentgenogram.*

A. *Teleoroentgenogram* — roentgenograms are made on one film with a single exposure for both entire lower limbs (or on two films with separate exposures for the femora and the tibiae). In this one exposure technique the divergent rays produce magnification.

B. *Orthoroentgenogram* — on a single long film three successive exposures are made, centered exactly over the hips, knees, and ankles. Note the perpendicular rays intersect the ends of the bones, recording the true length.

C. Diagram of the cassette tunnel. The two sliding metal shields restrict the area of film irradiated on three successive exposures. (From Green, W. T., Wyatt, G. M., and Anderson, M.: Orthoroentgenography as a method of measuring the bones of the lower extremity. J. Bone Joint Surg., *28*:61, 1946.)

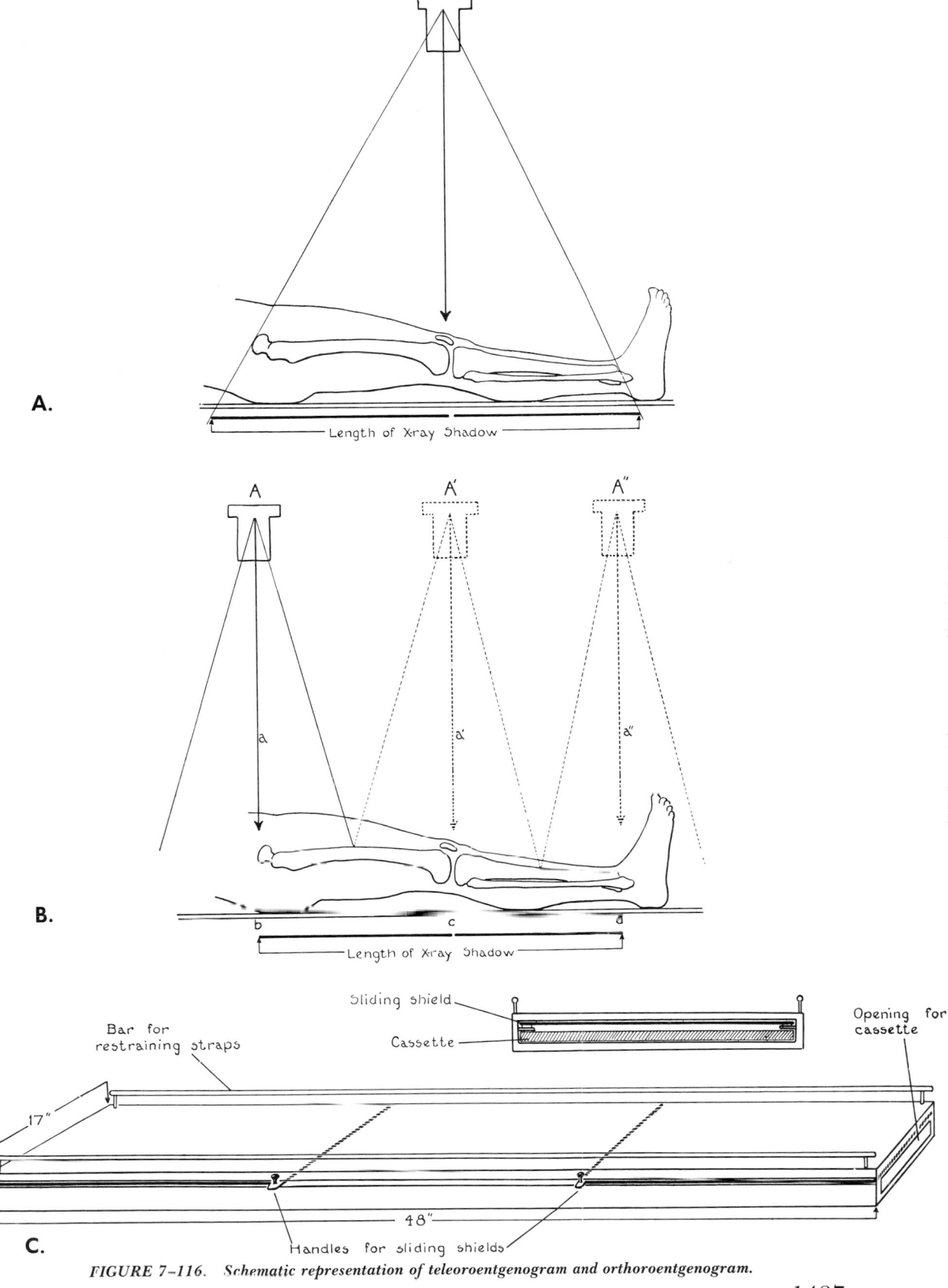

A.

Length of Xray Shadow

A   A'   A"

a   a'   a"

B.

b   c   d

Length of Xray Shadow

Sliding shield

Cassette

Opening for cassette

Bar for restraining straps

17"

48"

Handles for sliding shields

C.

FIGURE 7–116. *Schematic representation of teleoroentgenogram and orthoroentgenogram.*

See opposite page for legend.

1487

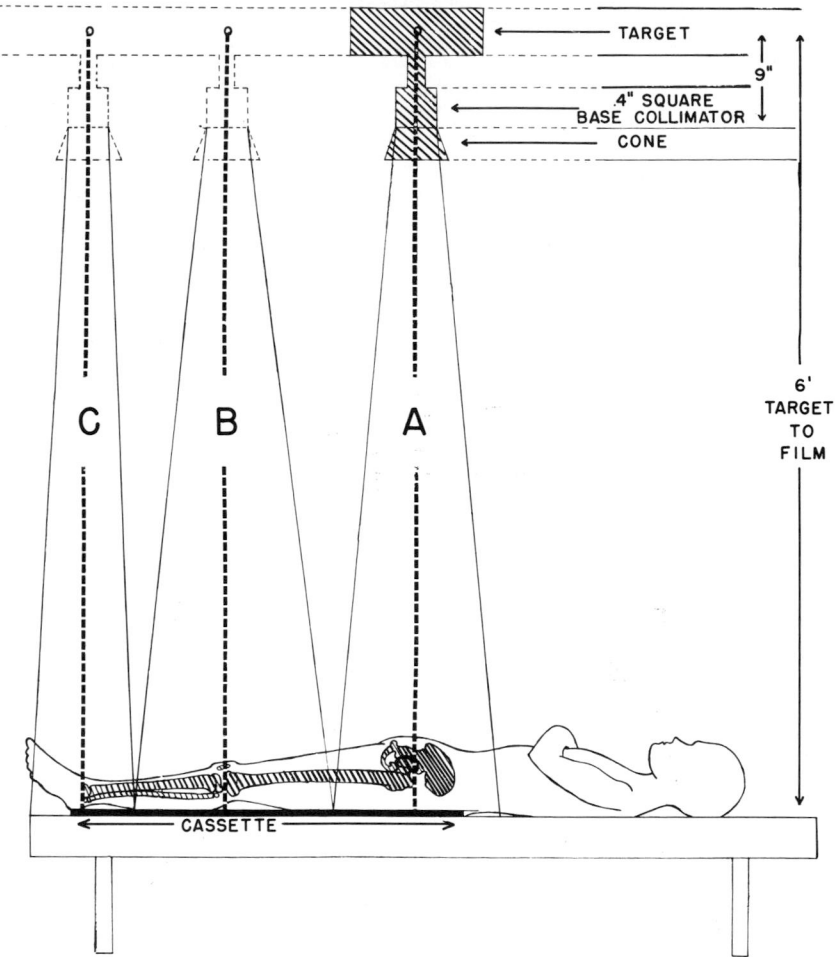

FIGURE 7–117. Diagram of the three consecutive exposures of lower limbs made on a single long film with the rectangular beam collimator.

The tube is focused precisely over the selected joint space so that the central ray passes directly through the end of the long bone. No metal is necessary to shield the parts of the film beyond the area of exposure. The size of each field can be varied according to the length of the child's limb and the desired portion of the shaft to be visualized. (From Anderson, M., Horton, B. G., and Green, W. T.: Orthoroentgenography for accurate long bone measurement. Personal communication, 1971.)

tightening the Velcro straps, one over the midthigh and the other over the midcalf. Sandbags are placed on each side of the feet. The technician should gently explain to the patient that he should not move and should be careful that movement does not occur. (3) The knees and hips should be in full extension. If there is fixed flexion contracture of the knee or hip, lateral roentgenograms of the femur and tibia are made; or two posteroanterior views are made, one of the femora by focusing over the hips and then the knees, and the other of the tibia, by

focusing over the knees and then the ankles. In either way, accurate length of the bones can be obtained. (4) In the presence of marked leg length inequality, proper centering of the x-ray rube may be difficult, with resultant divergence of rays and distortion. In such an instance, separate x-ray exposures of each limb are made.[717]

The author recommends orthoroentgenography as the method of choice for measuring leg lengths. The technique shows the entire length of both lower limbs from the iliac crests to the soles of the feet, with excellent detail of bone and soft tissue throughout; it gives an accurate measurement of true length of the bones; technically, the procedure is simple, both in making the exposure and in the measurement of the bones' shadows; radiation to the patient is minimal; and the cost is slight. Orthoroentgenography has been criticized because of the inherent difficulty of handling the long films and the matter of storage; if space is a problem, this objection can be eliminated by cutting the film into halves, taping the edges, and folding the films.

Treatment

Discrepancy in length of the lower limbs can be corrected by any one of the following methods: (1) permanent arrest of growth of the longer limb—by *epiphyseodesis*, (2) retardation of growth of the longer limb—by *epiphyseal stapling*, (3) *shortening* of the longer limb, or (4) *lengthening* of the shorter limb by osteotomy and distraction or by stimulation of epiphyseal growth.

When the leg length inequality is minimal, a simple lift in the shoe may suffice; when the discrepancy is very severe or the leg is deformed, prosthetic fitting with or without a Syme amputation may be the procedure of choice.

EPIPHYSEODESIS

In 1933, Phemister described his method of complete arrest of longitudinal growth at an epiphysis; premature fusion of one or more epiphyses of the longer limb allows the short limb to grow at a more rapid rate and corrects the length discrepancy by the normal growth process.[795] In the skeletally immature child, epiphyseodesis is a simple and safe method of equalizing leg lengths, provided the procedure is carefully timed and correctly executed. The principles involved in using the growth prediction chart have already been outlined. The operative technique of distal femoral epiphyseodesis is described and illustrated in Plate 63.

Epiphyseodesis of the proximal tibia and fibula is similar to that of the distal femur. Growth arrest of the proximal fibula is performed first, since this provides a more ade-

quate exposure and facilitates proper identification of the common peroneal nerve. After 20 to 30 minutes of tourniquet ischemia, stimulation of the common peroneal nerve will fail to produce contraction of the innervated muscles; and if the lateral side of the proximal tibial physis is arrested first, normal details of anatomy will be obscured by blood and distorted by the dissection.

The surgical approach is as follows:

Exposure of the Lateral Tibia and Fibula. A somewhat oblique longitudinal incision is made midway between the proximal tibial tubercle and the fibular head; it begins proximally 1 cm. inferior to the joint line and 1 cm. anterior to the fibular head and extends distally and forward for a distance of 5 cm. The subcutaneous tissue is divided, and the wound flaps are widely undermined and retracted. The head of the fibula is in line with the proximal epiphyseal plate of the tibia. The capsule of the knee joint, the insertion of the biceps tendon, and the fibular collateral ligament of the knee are identified. The origin of the toe extensors, extensor hallucis longus, and anterior tibial muscles with a cuff of periosteal flap are elevated from the arcuate line.

The common peroneal nerve lies close to the medial border of the biceps femoris muscle in the popliteal fossa; then it passes distally and laterally between the lateral head of the gastrocnemius and the biceps tendon. Behind the fibular head it is subcutaneous. In the gap between the origin of the peroneus longus muscle from the head and neck of the fibula, the common peroneal nerve winds anteriorly around the fibular neck and then passes deep to the peroneus longus muscle and branches into the superficial and deep peroneal nerves.

With a periosteal elevator, the origin of the peroneus longus muscle is detached from the head of the fibula; keeping the dissection anterior to the fibular head will prevent injury to the nerve. With a straight needle, the site of the growth plate of the proximal fibula is identified. Next, a longitudinal incision is made on the anterior aspect of the fibular head and is extended distally to include the epiphyseal plate. A rectangular piece of bone ($1/4''$ wide and $1/2''$ long) is removed from the proximal fibula, straddling the epiphyseal plate. Three fourths of the length of the bone graft

(*Text continued on page 1494.*)

Epiphysiodesis of Distal Femur
(Green Modification of Phemister Technique)

THE PROCEDURE

A. The knee is supported in 20 to 30 degrees of flexion and the joint line is identified. First, the medial aspect of the distal femur is exposed. Beginning 1 cm. superior to the joint line, a longitudinal incision about 5 to 7 cm. long is made midway between the anterior and posterior margins of the femoral condyles. The subcutaneous tissue and deep fascia are divided in line with the skin incision.

B. Following the anterior surface of the medial intermuscular septum, the vastus medialis muscle is lifted anteriorly with a blunt periosteal elevator. The suprapatellar pouch should not be entered. In the inferior margin of the wound, the capsule and reflected synovial membrane of the knee joint are gently elevated and retracted with blunt instruments distally—cautiously, in order not to open the joint. If inadvertently the synovial membrane is divided, which will be indicated by oozing of synovial fluid, it is closed by 0000 plain catgut continuous suture. The superior medial genicular vessels traverse the wound; it is best to coagulate them to prevent troublesome bleeding later.

C. A midline longitudinal incision is made in the periosteum, starting proximally and extending throughout the extent of the wound.

D. The epiphyseal cartilage plate is exposed by raising anterior and posterior flaps of periosteum by subperiosteal dissection; it appears as a white, glistening transverse line that is softer than adjacent cancellous bone. Some surgeons prefer to make a longitudinal I-shaped incision in the periosteum to expose the growth plate; the author, however, prefers a simple longitudinal incision as it permits a more taut periosteal closure. The periosteum is gently retracted by 00 silk sutures on its borders. Rough traction and shredding of the periosteum should be avoided. If necessary, Chandler elevators are placed subperiosteally on the anterior and posterior aspects of the distal femur for adequate exposure. Dull right-angled retractors are used for proximal and distal retraction.

E and **F.** With matched pairs of osteotomes, a rectangular piece of bone 1$\frac{1}{8}$ to 1$\frac{1}{2}$ inches long and $\frac{1}{2}$ to $\frac{5}{8}$ inch wide is excised. The epiphyseal plate should be at the junction of the distal one third and proximal two thirds of the length of bone graft resected, at a point equidistant between the anterior and posterior surfaces of the femur. The posterior cortex of the femur should not be broken. The depth of the bone graft is $\frac{1}{2}$ to $\frac{3}{4}$ inch (the blood at the tip of the osteotome will mark its depth of penetration into bone). Because of the flare of the femoral condyles, the anterior and posterior osteotomes should be tilted somewhat distally so that they are perpendicular to the medial surface of the femur. Following removal of the osteotomes, the completeness of osteotomy is checked with a thin ($\frac{3}{8}$- or $\frac{1}{4}$-inch) osteotome. Then with curved osteotomes the graft is removed. Breakage of the graft at the epiphyseal plate is prevented by straddling the plate with the osteotomes.

Plate 63.   Epiphysiodesis of Distal Femur
(Green Modification of Phemister Technique)

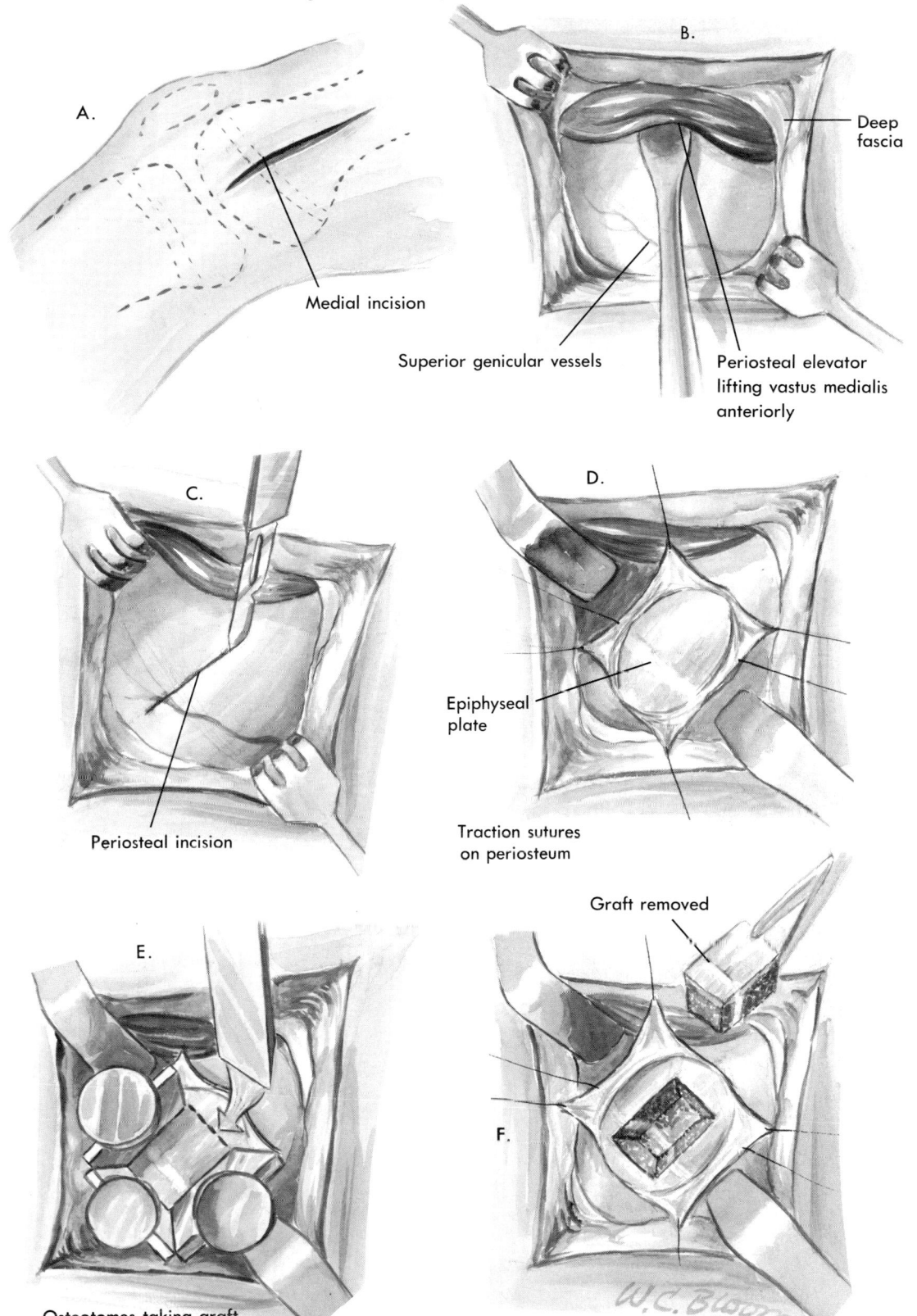

A.

Medial incision

B.

Deep fascia

Superior genicular vessels

Periosteal elevator lifting vastus medialis anteriorly

C.

Periosteal incision

D.

Epiphyseal plate

Traction sutures on periosteum

E.

Osteotomes taking graft

Graft removed

F.

W.C. Bloom

1491

Epiphysiodesis of Distal Femur
(Green Modification of Phemister Technique) *(Continued)*

G. The epiphyseal plate is drilled with diamond-shaped drills of increasing size in anterior, posterior, and distal directions. A hand drill provides better control and feel of depth. It should be remembered that the distal femoral epiphyseal plate is pointed inferiorly. The softness of the cartilaginous plate serves as a guide to its direction. Then, with a small curet, removal of the epiphyseal plate is completed, the debris of cartilage and bone being saved for later packing around the proximal end of the graft. Curettage should extend to the periphery of the growth plate, avoiding the popliteal vessels posteriorly.

H. Cancellous bone graft is taken from the proximal bed and packed into the defect created by removal of the epiphyseal plate.

I. The bone graft is then reinserted into its original bed, with its ends reversed by 180-degree rotation.

J. With an impacter and mallet, the bone graft is securely seated in the bony defect. It should be tapped in a distal direction, as the epiphyseal plate is inferior in location.

K. The periosteum is tightly closed with interrupted sutures. It is important not to include the patellar retinaculum with the periosteum, as this will bind it down, restricting knee motion.

L. The same procedure is repeated on the lateral side. Before closure of the wounds the position of the medial bone graft is checked to be sure it has not been dislodged by the tapping on the opposite side.

POSTOPERATIVE CARE

The limb is immobilized in a long-leg cylinder cast with the knee in neutral position or 5 degrees of flexion for a total of four weeks. The foot and ankle are left out of the cast and the patient is allowed to walk with crutches (three-point gait) as soon as he is comfortable. Because the long leg is in an extended position in the cast, appropriate lifts are placed on the shoe on the short side so that the patient can clear his leg with the cast.

Before the patient is discharged, it is best to make roentgenograms of the distal femur, taken through the cast, to record the integrity of bony continuity and the position of the reversed bone plugs. The cast usually becomes loose in 10 to 14 days. The cast and sutures are removed two weeks after surgery, and a new snug cast is applied. A common pitfall is the failure to extend the cast proximally enough on the thigh. Torsional stress on the distal femur should be prevented.

Following removal of the cast, the knee is mobilized by side-lying flexion-extension exercises to develop motor strength in the quadriceps femoris muscle. Crutch support is discontinued when there is 90 degrees of knee flexion and the quadriceps muscle is fair in motor power. Roentgenograms of the distal femur are made three months following surgery to be sure that fusion of the growth plate has taken place. Growth studies are performed at three-month intervals during the first year, and then at six-month intervals until completion of growth.

Plate 63. *Epiphysiodesis of Distal Femur (Green Modification of Phemister Technique)*

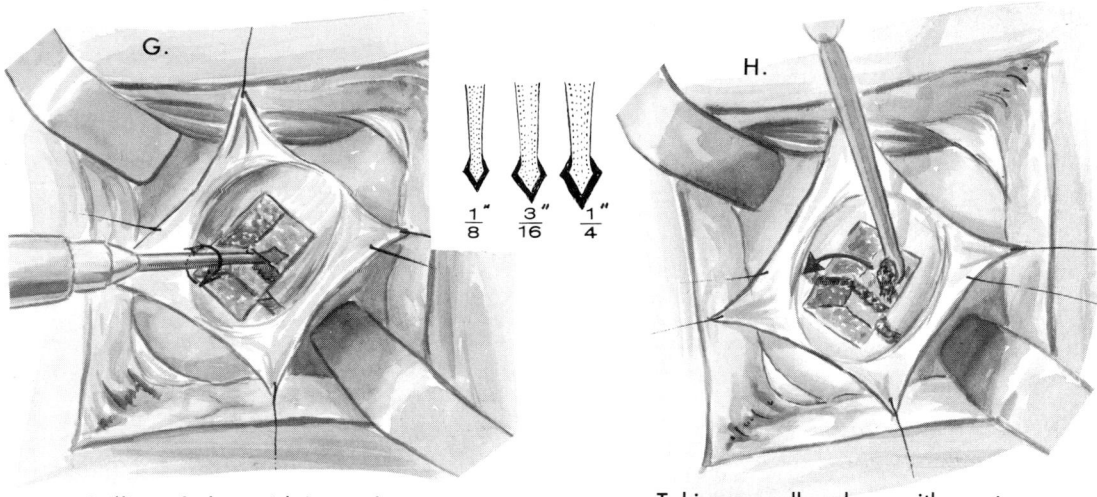

Drilling of plate with increasing
sizes of diamond-shaped hand drills

Taking cancellous bone with curet
to fill area of growth plate

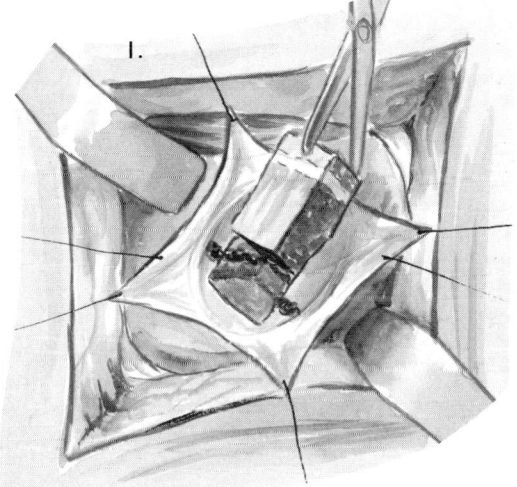

Placing of graft, which is rotated 180°

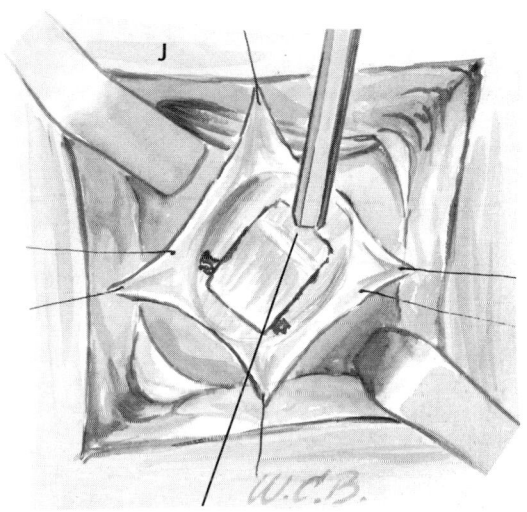

Impacting graft

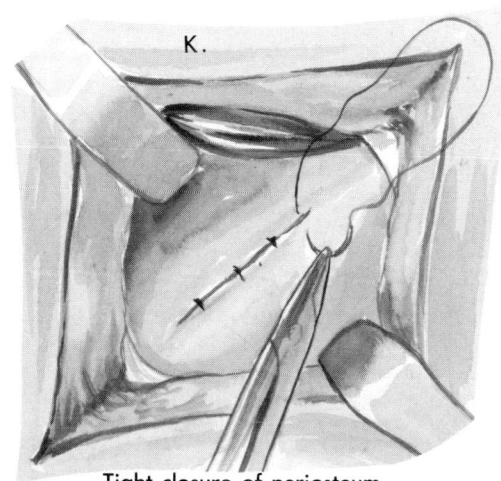

Tight closure of periosteum

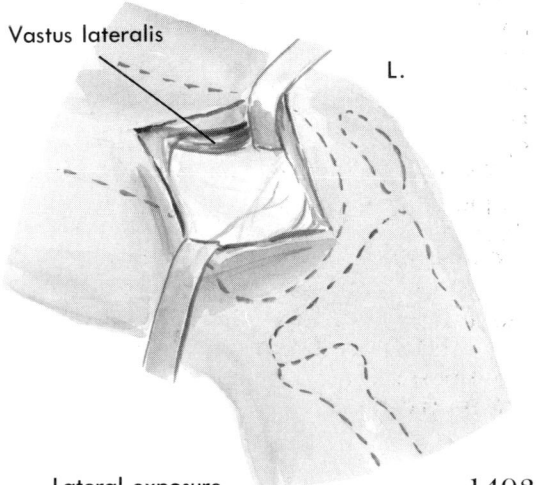

Vastus lateralis

Lateral exposure

includes the fibular head, and only fourth, the metaphysis. The growth plate is thoroughly curetted, the ends of the bone graft are reversed (180 degrees), and replaced securely in the graft bed. At times, the author curets the epiphyseal plate, but does not bother with the bone graft. A nerve stimulator should always be available in the operating room; if in doubt whether a strand of tissue is fibrous or neural, one should determine its nature positively by stimulation.

The lateral aspect of the proximal tibial physis is already exposed for the fibular epiphyseodesis. For the surgical approach to the medial side of the *proximal tibial physis,* a longitudinal incision about 5 cm. long is made, beginning 1 cm. distal to the joint line and continuing distally midway between the proximal tibial tubercle and the posteromedial margin of the tibia. The subcutaneous tissue and deep fascia are divided in line with the skin incision. The anterior margins of the sartorius tendon and tibial collateral ligament are partially elevated and retracted posteriorly.

The steps for growth arrest of the proximal tibial physis follow the same steps as described for distal femoral epiphyseodesis. The rectangular piece of bone graft removed from the tibia is smaller than that removed from the femur, usually $1/2$ inch wide and $3/4$ inch long. The tourniquet is always released and complete hemostasis is secured. Bleeding in the anterior tibial compartment will cause muscle ischemia and paralysis.

Following closure of the wound, the region of the fibular head is well-padded, and the limb is immobilized in an above-knee cast that includes the foot and ankle. The position of the knee is in 30 degrees of flexion and that of the foot-ankle in neutral position. The postoperative care is the same as that after distal femoral epiphyseodesis.

Figures 7–118 and 7–119 are two examples of adequate correction of leg length discrepancy by epiphyseodesis.

Complications. Significant complications occur in 5 to 10 per cent of cases of epiphyseodesis. They may result from miscalculation, technical errors during surgery, or from postoperative wound infection.

MISCALCULATION. Undercorrection will result if epiphyseodesis is performed too late. It occurred in 3 per cent (7 of 237 patients) in the series of Green and Anderson.[715] Overcorrection of discrepancy is caused either by overestimation of the growth potential of the longer limb or by underestimation of the growth potential of the shorter limb. It is imperative to follow the asymmetrical growth of the lower limbs prior to performing epiphyseodesis. In the series of Green and Anderson, overcorrecting occurred in 3 per cent; in five of these patients, distal femoral arrest on the originally short side was performed in order to prevent what appeared to be imminent overcorrection; in two patients of the entire group the original shorter limb became as much as $1/2$ inch longer than its opposite member.[715]

TECHNICAL ERRORS DURING SURGERY. Asymmetrical fusion will cause genu varum or valgum. It occurred in 2.6 per cent (6 of 237 patients of Green and Anderson).[715] Failure of fusion of the medial or lateral side can be detected by careful follow-up during the postoperative period and corrected by repeat epiphyseodesis. If the patient is seen too late with a disturbing angular deformity, an osteotomy is warranted for their correction.

Neuromuscular dysfunction is usually a complication of epiphyseodesis of the tibia and fibula. Paralysis may result either from laceration or compression of the common peroneal nerve or from ischemia of muscles in the anterior tibial compartment. Constant vigilance by the surgeon will decrease the incidence of this serious complication, which occurred in 0.8 per cent of the series of Green and Anderson.[715]

A stiff knee joint may result from the patellar retinaculum being sutured to the periosteum or from hemarthrosis. This usually takes place when epiphyseodesis of the distal femur and proximal tibia and fibula are performed simultaneously.

Partial extrusion of a loosely fitted graft may result in a bothersome bony prominence at the operative site.

POSTOPERATIVE WOUND INFECTION AND OSTEOMYELITIS. This complication occurred in 0.8 per cent of Green and Anderson's patients.[715] In one of their patients none of the limb-length discrepancy was corrected; actually, it increased

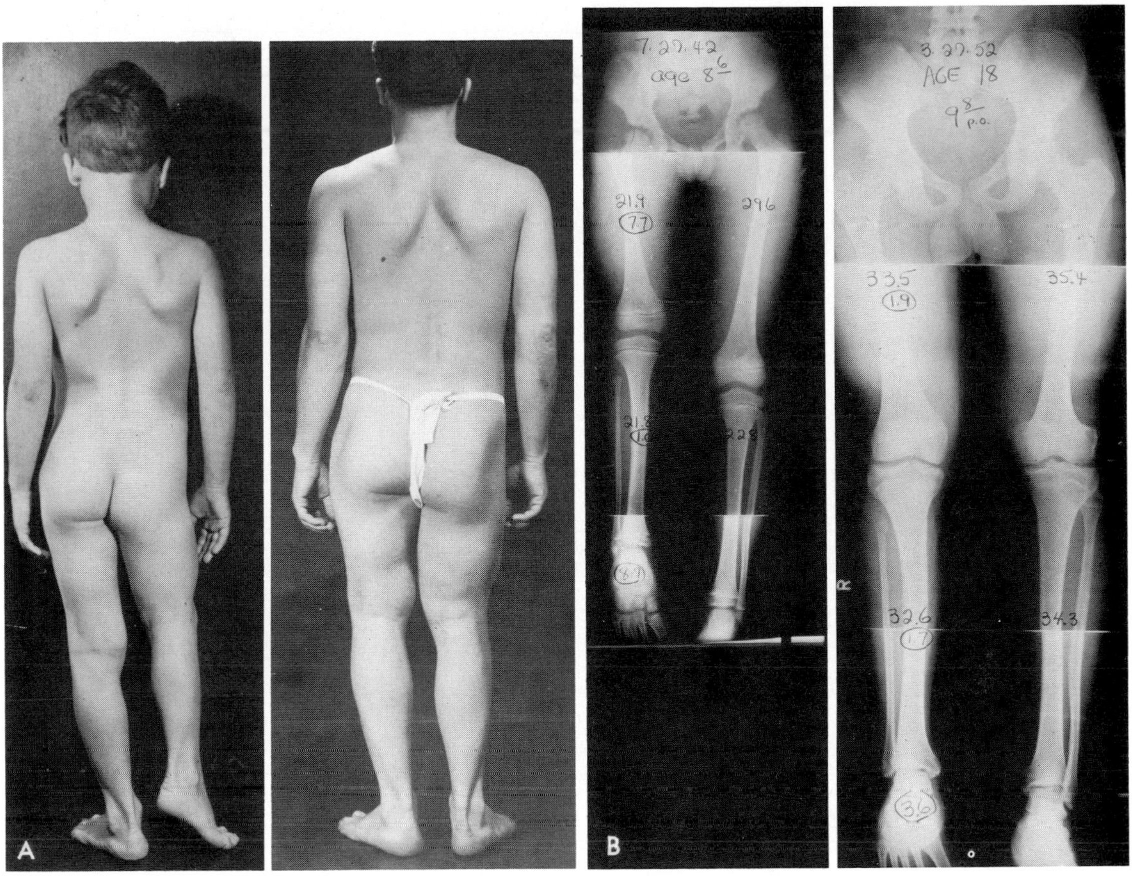

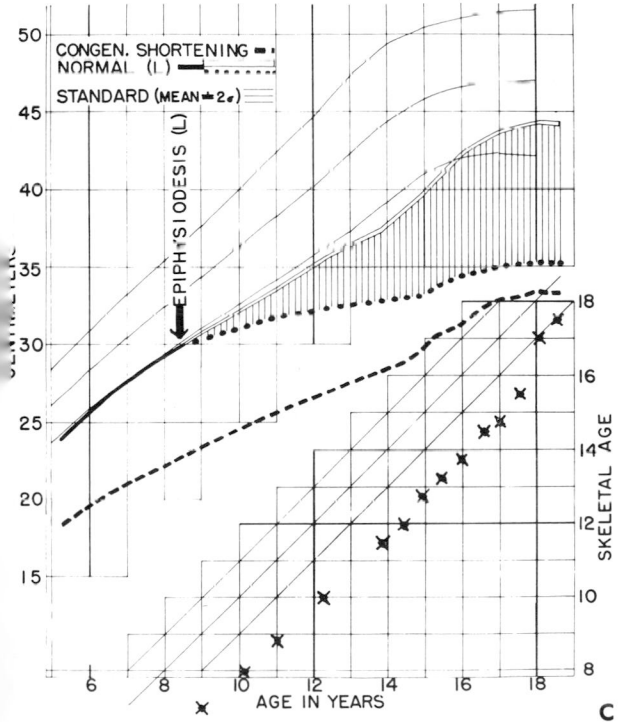

FIGURE 7–118. *A boy with a congenitally short right femur.*

Between the ages of five and eight years, the right femur as compared with the normal left femur had shown 26 per cent inhibition. The long bones in the normal side measured two standard deviations below average. At age eight years and five months, the total shortening of the long bones of the right limb measured 8.7 cm. (the femur 7.7 cm. short and the tibia 1 cm. short). The predicted total leg length discrepancy at skeletal maturity was 11 cm. His skeletal age was retarded two years. At age eight years and five months distal femoral epiphyseodesis of the normal left limb was performed.

A. Photographs taken at the age of eight years and at 26 years, showing the functional correction obtained. **B.** Orthoroentgenograms made at eight years and at skeletal maturity. **C.** Chart of progress in length of femora and skeletal age, demonstrating how distal femoral epiphyseodesis corrected the discrepancy in femoral lengths by 5.8 cm. At maturity, this boy still had 3.6 cm. shortening but he could get by with good gait without any lift in the shoe. (Figures from Green, W. T., and Anderson, M.: Skeletal age and the control of bone growth. A.A.O.S. Instructional Course Lecture, Vol. 17. St. Louis, C. V. Mosby Co., 1960, p. 209.)

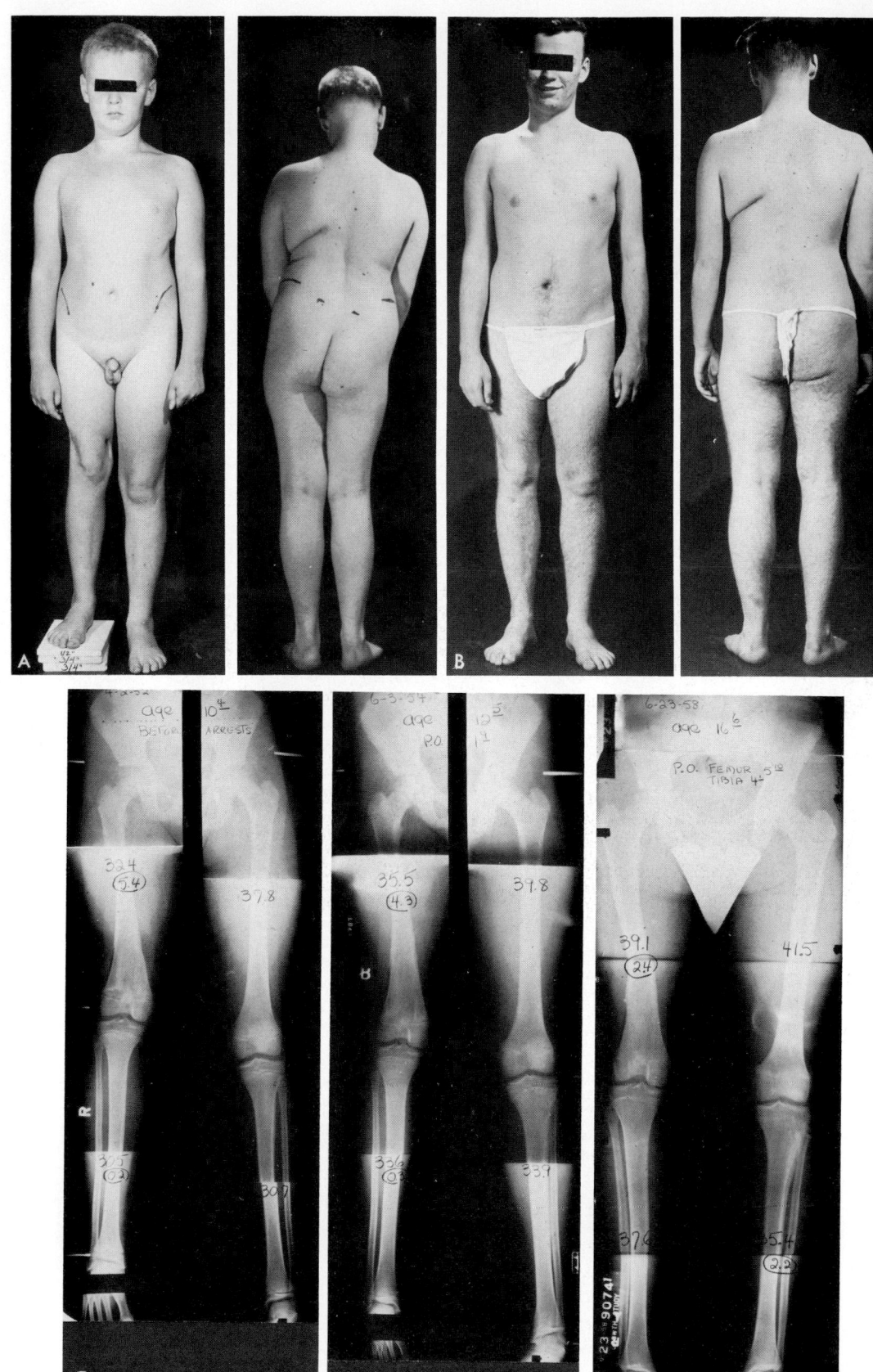

1496

FIGURE 7–119. *See opposite page for legend.*

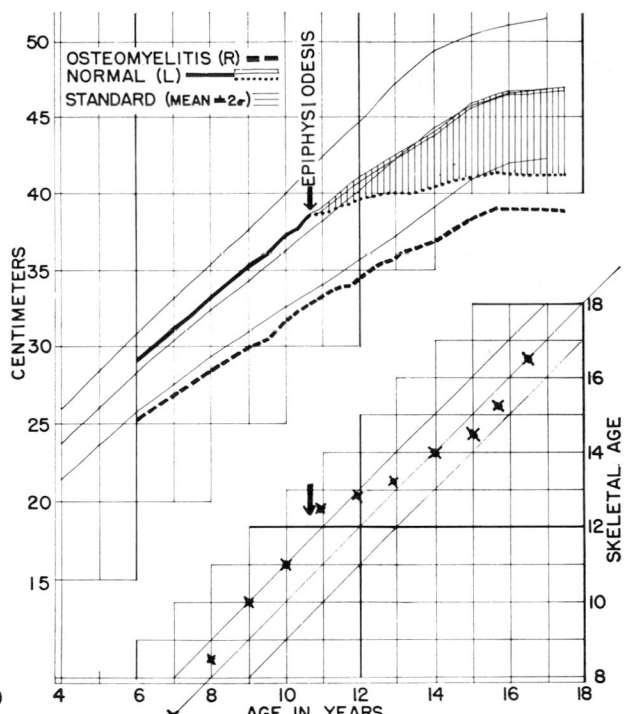

FIGURE 7–119 Continued.   *Short right femur due to marked growth inhibition following osteomyelitis of right lower femur in infancy.*

D. The composite chart showing the progress in length of femora and in skeletal age.

1 mm. When infection complicates epiphyseodesis, the wound is reopened, irrigated by closed suction, and appropriate antibiotics are given.

EPIPHYSEAL STAPLING

Retardation of longitudinal growth of limbs by the insertion of rigid staples across the epiphyseal plate was introduced by Blount.[656] Several years earlier, Haas had interrupted the growth of an epiphysis by a wire loop, and had demonstrated that growth resumed following removal of the wire. The principle of temporary arrest of linear growth was a good one, as the process was reversible; when the leg length discrepancy was corrected, the staples could be removed and growth would resume. The procedure was received with great enthusiasm. Unfortunately, many errors in surgical technique and judgment were committed. The original staples, made of 3/32 inch steel rod, were mechanically ineffective. The Vitallium staples, introduced several years later, proved to be far superior. The original technique suggested "blind nailing," but soon it was found that x-ray control was imperative to ensure correct positioning of the staples. Experience demonstrated that the periosteum and epiphyseal vessels should be left intact, if permanent interruption in growth were to be prevented. Sinking of the cross member of the staple into the bone will cause it to be buried, making its removal very difficult. During removal of the staple, the periosteum should not be incised and the epiphyseal plate should not be dis-

---

FIGURE 7–119.   *Short right femur due to marked growth inhibition following osteomyelitis of right lower femur in infancy.*

At 10½ years of age the total shortening on the right amounted to 5.8 cm. Left distal femoral epiphyseodesis was performed at 10 years and 8 months of age, followed by arrest of left proximal tibia and fibula 20 months later. The total correction of discrepancy from the two procedures was 5.9 cm. (3.4 cm. from the femur and 2.5 cm. from the tibia). **A.** Preoperative photograph. **B.** At 18 years of age when all growth is completed. Note the improved balance. **C.** Orthoroentgenograms before femoral arrest, before tibial arrest, and at skeletal maturity.

turbed. The incidence of complications of epiphyseal stapling is summarized in Table 7–13.

Green and Anderson observed that stapling does not inhibit growth as immediately as does epiphyseodesis. Complications of stapling of the proximal tibial epiphysis are much greater than after stapling of the distal femoral epiphysis. They also noted that one cannot have absolute faith in the resumption of growth following removal of the staples; in some cases, growth may resume normally, but in others premature fusion of the epiphysis may take place. For practical reasons, stapling must be considered as a method of complete arrest.[716] The author does not recommend epiphyseal stapling for equalization of leg lengths, as epiphyseodesis is more reliable, simpler, and has many fewer complications. In surgical management of leg length inequality, the only instance in which the author considers epiphyseal stapling is when there is marked irregularity of maturation, with two or more years of retardation of the skeletal age as compared to the chronological age. In order to minimize complications, meticulous attention should be paid to the technical details of the procedure (see p. 1468). During removal of the staples, the epiphyseal plate should not be injured by incising and elevating the periosteum.

SHORTENING OF THE LONG LIMB

Resection of a segment of the femur or of the tibia for equalization of limb lengths is performed after skeletal maturity is reached. It is not performed in a growing child, however; an epiphyseodesis at the appropriate age is a much simpler and safer method.

Leveling of the knees is an important cosmetic consideration. When leg length discrepancy is due to a short tibia, it is logical to shorten the tibia of the longer limb. Tibial shortening, however, is not recommended by the author for the following reasons: (1) If more than 3 cm. is resected from the tibia, the muscles of the leg controlling the foot and ankle become permanently relaxed and weakened. A 5 to 7 cm. long segment of the femur can be removed without residual weakness of the thigh muscles. Because of marked loss of tension of the leg muscles and the peculiar vascular anatomy of the tibia, delayed union or nonunion is common following tibial shortening. (2) In femoral shortening, only one bone is resected; whereas, in the lower leg, segments from both the tibia and fibula must be removed. (3) Ischemic necrosis of the muscles of the anterior compartment of the leg can occur following resection of the tibia.

When tibial shortening is performed it

Table 7–13. *Complications of Epiphyseal Stapling*

Author	Blount[655–657]	Brockway, Craig, Cockrell[665]	Green, Anderson[716]	May, Clements[775]	Pilcher[797]	Poirier[798]
No. of stapling operations	200	62	83	76	35	33
Complications			*Number of Patients*			
Asymmetric growth—genu valgum, varum, or recurvatum	7	13	2	11	30	15
Laxity of knee ligaments	—	?	—	—	6	20 (6 marked)
Stiff knee	—	—	—	—	—	—
Infection, metal reaction	—	—	1	3	12	—
Extrusion of staples	—	15	24	24	—	8
Buried staple	—	10	—	—	—	—
Broken staples	—	7	7	—	3	—
Failure to control growth	—	—	2	—	31	3
Slow arrest of growth	—	?	11	—	—	—
Loss of correction after removal of staples	—	?	—	4	—	—
Aneurysm	—	—	—	—	—	—
Peroneal nerve palsy	—	—	—	2	—	—

should not exceed 3 cm. A step-cut resection is performed in the proximal metaphyseal area through an anteromedial approach. The fibula is divided at the junction of the middle and distal thirds through a separate longitudinal incision, and its fragments are allowed to overlap. Two transfixing screws are used for internal fixation of the tibial fragments. The resected bone fragments are divided into matchstick bone grafts that will straddle the osteotomy site on the posterior and lateral surfaces of the tibia.

An above-knee plaster of Paris cast is applied with the knee in 30 degrees of flexion and the ankle in neutral position. In three weeks, the cast and sutures are removed, and an above-knee, snug, well-molded cast with a small walking heel is applied. The knee should be in 15 to 20 degrees of flexion and the ankle slightly equinus. Gradual weight-bearing is begun with the protection of a three-point crutch gait to stimulate osteogenesis. Periodic roentgenograms are taken to check alignment of the fragments and healing. Union is usually firm within 10 to 12 weeks. Following removal of the cast, the motor strength of the leg muscles is evaluated; temporary support by a below-knee dynamic orthosis may be indicated.

Femoral Shortening. Since Rizzoli's first report of femoral shortening by overriding (cited by Goff), many techniques of reduction in the length of the femur for equalization of leg lengths have been described in the literature (Fig. 7–120).[709] The principal methods are: (1) oblique osteotomy and resection of the medial two thirds of the upper end of the distal fragment, using its lateral cortex as an intramedullary bone peg (Calvé and Galland);[671] (2) simple overriding of the osteotomized fragments and internal fixation with three or four transversely inserted screws (White);[844] (3) step-cut osteotomy and resection of bone from both fragments and internal fixation with intramedullary rod and screws (Merle D'Aubigné and Dubousset);[776] (4) simple transverse osteotomy, resection of a segment of bone and intramedullary fixation with a rod;[230] (5) V osteotomy in which the "M" fragments are cut in half and the bone pieces are screwed to the shaft; (6) oblique, sliding osteotomy;[709] (7) shortening in the subtrochanteric region and internal fixation with a blade plate (Blount);[653, 655] and (8)

supracondylar shortening (R. D. Moore).[784]

In a growing child, the surgical procedure of femoral shortening may stimulate growth, increasing length by 1 to 1.5 cm. This is not absolute, however, and because of its uncertainty, it is best to postpone shortening of long bones until completion of growth. Although a 7.5 to 10 cm. segment of the femur can be resected without permanently weakening the thigh musculature, relaxation of the muscles during the period of bone healing may cause delayed union because of lack of compression of the osteotomized bone fragments. Thus, the importance of primary bone grafting and added support by a hip spica plaster of Paris cast is evident, whichever method of femoral shortening is used.

In the experience of the author, shortening of the femur, as advocated by White (simple lateral overlap, internal fixation with screws, and immobilization in a hip spica cast), by Blount (shortening in the subtrochanteric region, internal fixation with blade plate or other nail plate, and hip spica cast), and by Merle D'Aubigné and Dubousset (step-cut osteotomy and intramedullary fixation with a rod) are equally satisfactory. The reader is referred to the original articles for a description of operative technique.[653, 776, 846]

LENGTHENING OF THE SHORT LIMB

Theoretically, the ideal method of equalizing leg lengths is to lengthen the short limb. This can be achieved either by stimulation of epiphyseal growth or by osteotomy and mechanical stretching of the short femur or tibia.

In the literature many techniques of tibial or femoral lengthening by osteotomy and mechanical distraction of the short bone have been described.

Femoral Lengthening

It was first attempted by Codivilla in 1905. He performed an oblique osteotomy of the femoral shaft, and with the patient under anesthesia, applied skeletal traction through the calcaneus. A hip spica plaster cast was applied immediately to maintain the reduction. Codivilla reported the results in 26 cases, with a gain in length varying between 3 and 8 cm.[678]

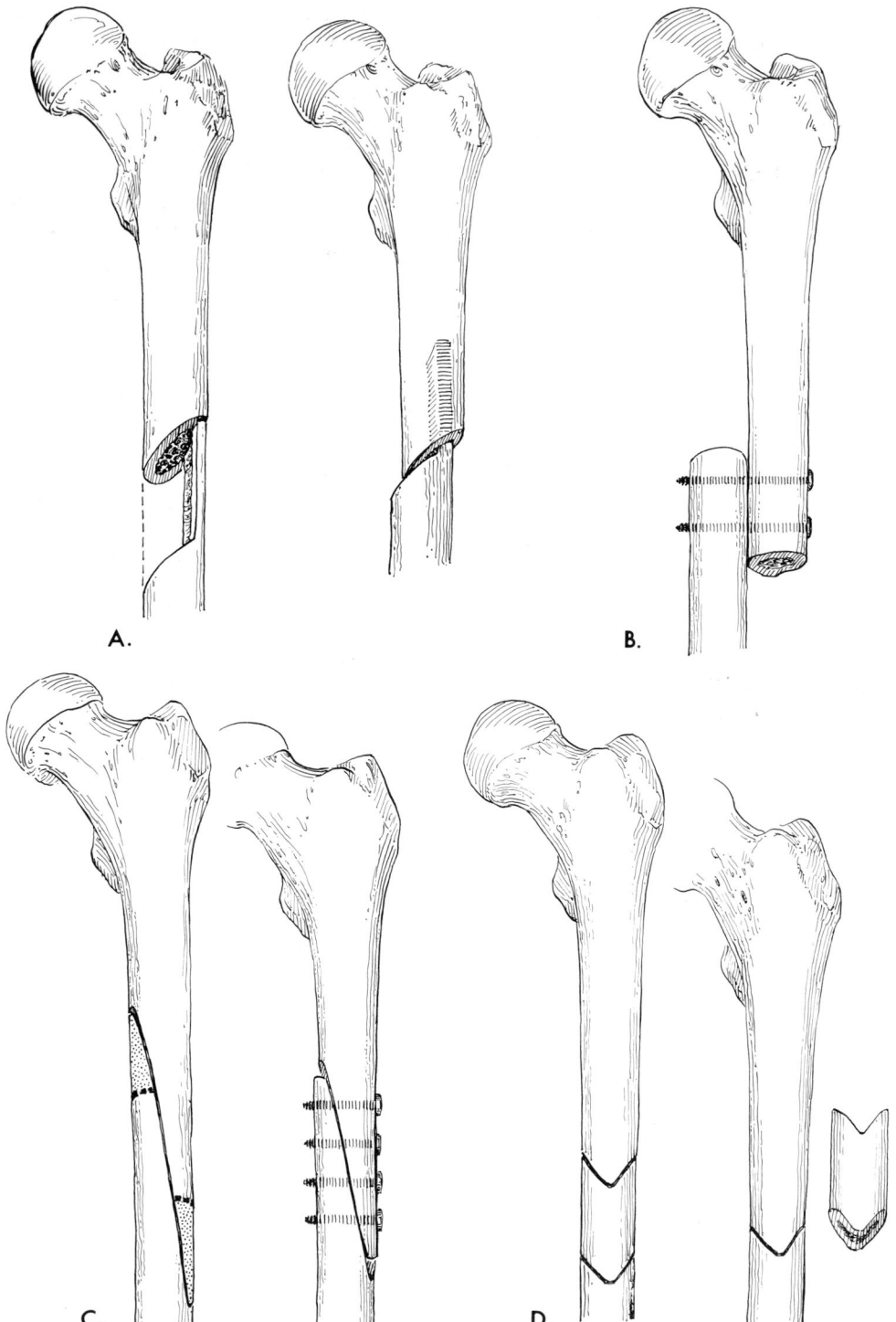

FIGURE 7–120. *Various methods of femoral shortening.*

    A. Oblique osteotomy and resection of medial two thirds of the upper end of the distal fragment, using its lateral cortex as an intramedullary bone peg (Calvé and Galland). **B.** Simple overriding of the osteotomized fragments and internal fixation with transversely inserted screws (White). **C.** Oblique sliding osteotomy. **D.** V-osteotomy in which the "M" fragments are cut in half and the bone pieces are screwed to the shaft.

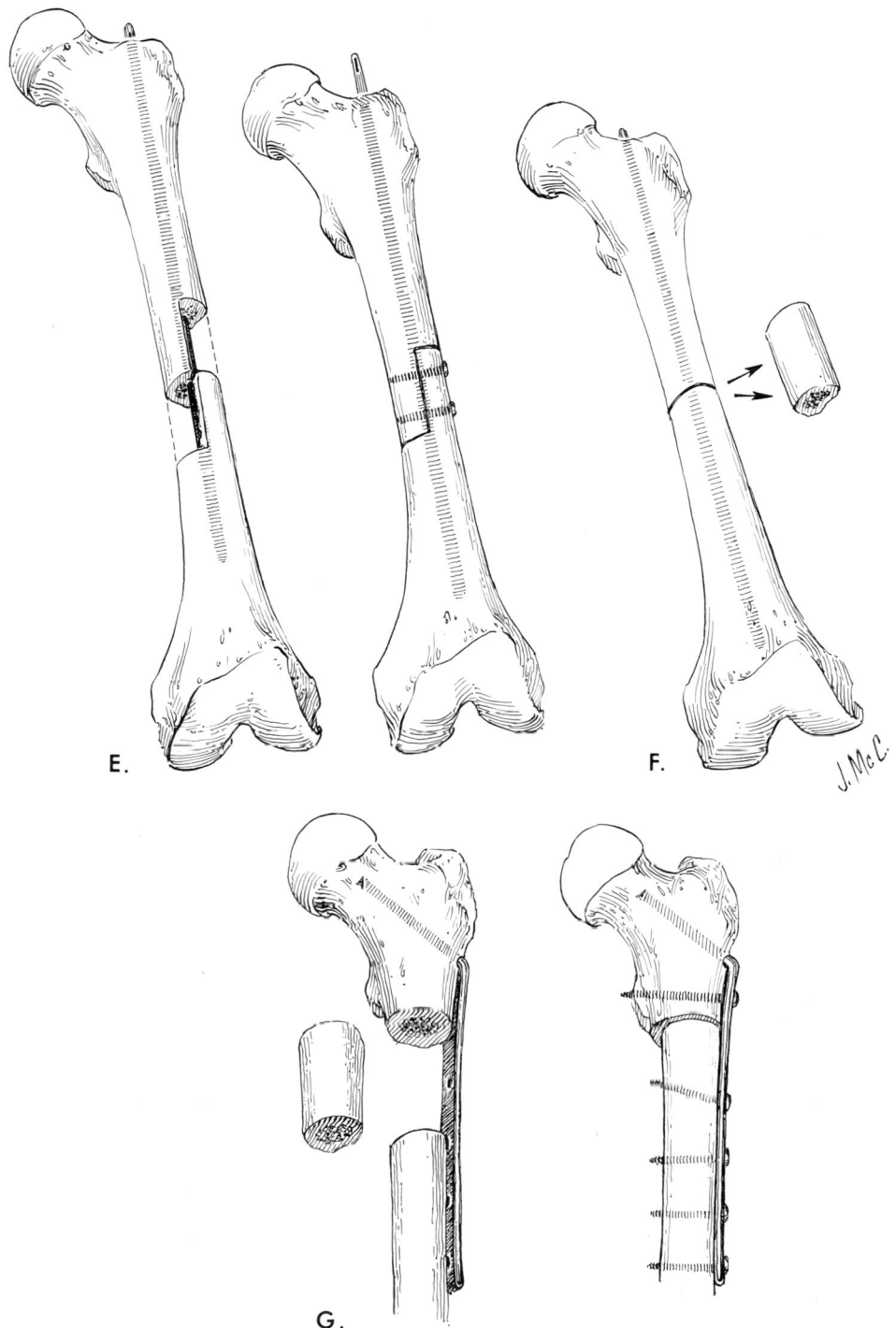

FIGURE 7–120 Continued. *Various methods of femoral shortening.*

E. Step-cut osteotomy with resection of bone from both fragments and internal fixation with intramedullary rod and screws (Merle D'Aubigné and Dubousset). **F.** Simple transverse osteotomy, resection of a segment of bone, and intramedullary fixation with a rod. **G.** Shortening in the subtrochanteric region and internal fixation with a blade plate (Blount).

Magnuson, in 1913, used a Hawley table to apply traction.[772] Putti, in 1921, applied traction and countertraction with one pin proximal to the site of osteotomy and one distal to it. In Putti's technique, the pin was inserted only through the lateral aspect of the thigh, but through both cortices of the femur. The two pins were connected with a telescoping tube and a spring extension mechanism.[801]

Abbott and Crego, in 1928, found control of the osteotomized fragments by Putti's technique unsatisfactory since the pins pulled out of the cortex. Better control of the fragments was secured by Abbott, who inserted four pins, two above and two below. The pins are inserted through the entire femur and thigh to prevent them from pulling out. The proximal pins are inserted in a vertical plane to avoid puncture of major vessels. Abbott also devised a single-unit extension mechanism by means of coil springs on parallel threaded bars.[613] Compere, in 1936, recommended simultaneous bone grafting to decrease the incidence of nonunion.[681]

McCarroll, in 1950, described a subtrochanteric Z-type of osteotomy and the use of a slotted blade plate for control of the fragments as length was increased. He also applied traction above and below the knee by means of one threaded pin through the distal femoral metaphysis and another through the upper portion of the tibia. This redistributed traction forces across the knee joint, protecting against compression of articular cartilaginous surfaces and over-stretching of the capsule, and provided ligamentous support of the knee, thus decreasing the possibility of a stiff or unstable joint.[768] Bost, in 1944, advised decreasing the resistance of these soft tissues by extensive release by lengthening of the hamstrings, hip adductors, and quadriceps femoris.[659]

Bost and Larsen, in 1956, used an intramedullary rod to control the alignment of the osteotomized fragments and in addition to the conventional step-cut or oblique osteotomies, they described a transverse osteotomy. The combination of intramedullary rod fixation and transverse osteotomy made the technique of femoral lengthening easy and afforded the best means for control of the fragments.[660] Wes-

tin, in 1967, constructed a periosteal sleeve to cover the gap in the bone.[842]

Merle d'Aubigné and Dubousset described a one-stage bilateral procedure for equalization of the femora, which they recommended as the best method to correct discrepancies of 10 cm. or more in older children and young adults with shortening primarily in the femur. The short femur is lengthened in two stages—first, an intramedullary rod is inserted in the short femur and, at a level 5 cm. distal to the lower margin of the greater trochanter, the femoral shaft is osteotomized. The fascia lata, the iliotibial band, the straight head of the rectus femoris, the intermuscular septa, and the muscles originating in the proximal segments are divided or lengthened to release the soft-tissue resistance to lengthening. Next, the osteotomized fragments are distracted with a spreader and a metal block is inserted to hold the fragments apart. The long femur is shortened over an intramedullary rod by a step-cut osteotomy and removal of two hemisegments of appropriate length; the bone fragments are impacted and transfixed with two screws, one anterior and the other posterior to the nail. Then the lengthening of the short femur is completed by spreading the osteotomized fragments further apart and by placing the hemisegments from the long femur in the defect (one anteromedially and the other posterolaterally).[776]

Merle d'Aubigné and Dubousset reported the results of their femoral equalization procedure in 13 patients with an average preoperative leg length inequality of 14.6 cm. Of the 13 patients, 5 had corrections of 9 cm.; 1 a correction of 8 cm.; 2, correction of 6 cm.; and 1, a correction of 5 cm. They caution that if this operation is performed, the technical details must be observed strictly. Oscillometry should be used to monitor circulation in the limb, and the knee should be maintained in flexion during and after the operation to avoid tension on the sciatic nerve. They also warn that very strict aseptic technique should be maintained during surgery, as the wounds are large and the operation is lengthy.[776]

Femoral lengthening is considered in the patient who is of unusually short stature and in whom leg lengths cannot be equalized by the simple procedure of epiphyseodesis, either because the leg length discrepancy is too great or the condition is encountered too late for correction by growth arrest. The shortening should be primarily in the femur, and the hip on the affected side should be normal or stable. These criteria are usually found in patients with congenitally short or dysgenetic femora or in those in whom the growth of the femur has been greatly disturbed at an early age, either by trauma or by disease.

Both the parents and patient should clearly understand that femoral lengthening is encumbered with serious possible complications and that a Syme amputation and prosthesis might conceivably be necessary. It should be explained, when recommending femoral lengthening, that the level of the knees is an important esthetic consideration. Details of postoperative care and the probable necessity of a second stage of bone grafting procedures should be meticulously outlined.

Operative Technique. The operative technique of femoral lengthening described here is that of Bost and Larsen as modified by Westin.[660, 842]

POSITION OF PATIENT. The patient is placed in lateral position, with the short limb to be lengthened in an upward position on a fracture table. A pelvic anchor sacral rest is used to lock the pelvis securely at three points, with the post against the ischium affording countertraction. The entire limb and gluteal region are prepared and draped sterile, so that the thigh can be moved about without contaminating the operative field. This lateral position is ideal for exposure of the femur, insertion of the intramedullary rod, and placement of Steinmann pins in a vertical-oblique direction in the proximal femur.

SKIN INCISION. A posterolateral longitudinal incision is made, beginning 2 cm. superior to the tip of the greater trochanter and extending distally parallel to the femoral shaft for a distance of 15 to 20 cm. In the superior aspect of the wound, the incision may be extended proximally to the iliac crest, if necessary.

EXPOSURE. The subcutaneous tissue, fascia lata, and gluteal fascia are divided in the same line as the skin incision. The upper half to two thirds of the femoral shaft is exposed extraperiosteally by anteriorly elevat-

ing and retracting the origins of the vastus lateralis, vastus medius, and intermedius muscles. The lateral and medial intermuscular septa are stripped longitudinally and extraperiosteally from the linea aspera, releasing the soft tissues from bone through the entire length of the operative wound. Perforating vessels are clamped and coagulated.

MAKING THE PERIOSTEAL SLEEVE. A lateral longitudinal incision about 12 cm. long is made in the periosteum, beginning 2 cm. proximal to the intended level of osteotomy. At the distal edge of the proposed periosteal sleeve, a circular incision is made in the periosteum. The periosteum is gently elevated from bone by stripping it upward and downward.

THE TRANSVERSE OSTEOTOMY. The level of osteotomy is usually at the junction of the proximal one fourth and distal three fourths of the femoral shaft, or about 3 cm. distal to the lesser trochanter. The femoral shaft is cut transversely, either with a motor saw or a Gigli saw.

THE INTRAMEDULLARY ROD. Proper selection of the intramedullary rod is important; it should have a diameter sufficiently small to allow distraction of the fragments, but yet heavy enough to prevent bowing and to control the alignment and the position of the osteotomized fragments. The intramedullary rod may be inserted from above through the greater trochanter, or retrograde into the proximal fragment and then driven in the opposite direction into the medullary canal of the distal fragment for a distance of 15 to 20 cm., depending on the length of the femur. The rod is securely anchored to the greater trochanter by means of a wire; this will prevent proximal migration of a loosened rod during lengthening.

The periosteal sleeve is closed longitudinally, leaving its distal margin free.

INSERTION OF TRACTION AND COUNTERTRACTION PINS. Threaded Steinmann pins $3/16$ or $1/4$ inch in diameter are used. In the introduction of the pins, it is important to avoid contact with the intramedullary rod or transfixing of the osteotomized fragments. The *countertraction pin* is placed in the proximal fragment at the level of the lesser trochanter; it is directed from the anterior aspect of the femur posterolaterally in the

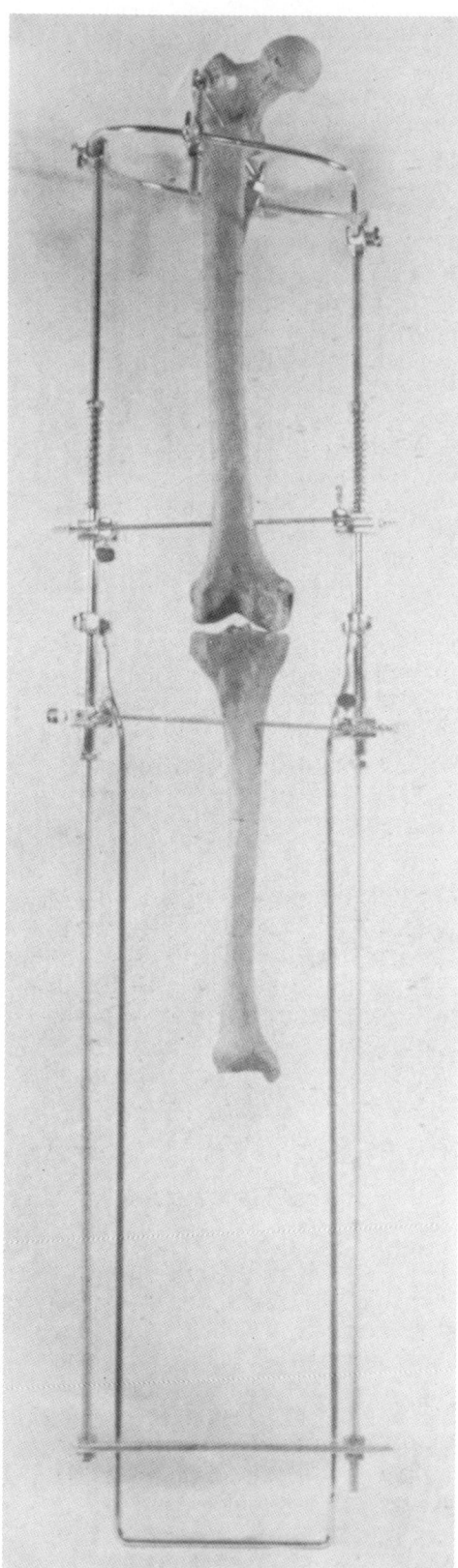

sagittal plane. Injury to the sciatic nerve and puncture of the hip joint capsule should be avoided. *Traction pins* are placed transversely through the distal femoral metaphysis and through the proximal metaphysis of the tibia at the level of the tibial tubercle. The distraction apparatus will apply traction upon both pins as a unit. It is important that the pins be parallel to each other and also that the proximal tibial pin does not puncture or press on the common peroneal nerve. Roentgenograms are then made to ensure proper placement of the pins and the position of the intramedullary rod.

COMPLETION OF SOFT-TISSUE RELEASE. The fascia lata is sectioned circumferentially at two levels above and below the level of osteotomy. The intermuscular septa are divided transversely. In some instances, fractional lengthening of the hamstrings and myotomy of the hip adductors are performed through separate incisions. Release or lengthening of the quadriceps femoris is usually unnecessary. The subcutaneous tissue and skin are closed in the usual manner.

The Steinmann pins are connected to the Bost femoral lengthening apparatus (Fig. 7–121), and a simple hip spica cast is applied on the affected side incorporating the pins. The perineum, ischium, sacrum, anterior superior iliac spines, and iliac crests are adequately padded to prevent pressure sores. The hip is in neutral position and the knee is in 40 degrees of flexion to relax the tension on the sciatic nerve. A circular segment from the cast is resected at the level of the osteotomy.

Lengthening of the femur begins on the operating table and is continued at a slow rate of one or two daily turns of the screw mechanism of the apparatus. Too rapid lengthening should be avoided. A maximum of 5 cm. should be attempted during a period of four weeks. To prevent complications, constant vigilance of the surgeon is required throughout the process of lengthening. Any occurrence of vascular or neuro-

FIGURE 7–121. Femoral lengthening apparatus (Bost).

(From Bost, F. C., and Larsen, L. J.: Experiences with lengthening of the femur over an intramedullary rod. J. Bone Joint Surg., *38–A*:572, 1956.)

logic complications obliges one to cease lengthening immediately.

When the desired amount of lengthening is obtained, traction is discontinued; however, the apparatus is left in place for three months or until bony union is sufficiently strong to permit substitution of a simple plaster hip spica support. Then the cast, Steinmann pins, and intramedullary rod are removed and a new single hip spica cast is applied. The cast immobilization is maintained until solid union of the femur has taken place, usually a total period of four to six months.

Complications. *Pin tract infection* is an almost universal complication; however, this will usually heal within several weeks following removal of the pins.

Delayed union is directly related to the lengthening obtained; the greater the lengthening, the longer the time required for the union. When over 5 cm. of lengthening is planned in an older child, primary autogenous iliac bone grafting should be considered. Westin recommends routine bone grafting at three months if the diameter of the bridging callus (as seen in the roentgenogram) is less than two thirds that of the femur.[842]

Unyielding soft tissues of the thigh constitute a frequent major problem in lengthening the femur. Sciatic nerve palsy is another serious complication. Bost and Larsen report one case of immediate and seven of late peroneal nerve palsy.[660] Vascular insufficiency and hypertension are other grave complications. Other problems are deformities of the knee joint (particularly posterior subluxation of the tibia on the femur), bending or breaking of the intramedullary rod, fracture of the lengthened femur, and consequent muscle weakness of the lengthened limb.

Tibial Lengthening

Abbott introduced the procedure for tibial lengthening in 1927, though various methods of femoral lengthening had been tried since the turn of the twentieth century.[612] The sound logic of lengthening the short limb rather than shortening the normal one initially stimulated great enthusiasm for the procedure. But in the ensuing two decades, the popularity of tibial lengthening waned and the operation fell into disrepute because of the numerous serious complications including shock, paralysis, sepsis, amputation, and even death. These complications were summarized by Compere in 1936.[681] Sofield, Blair, and Millar stressed another important drawback of the procedure—namely, the undesirable loss of muscle power in the lengthened limb.[223] Then, in 1952, Anderson modified Abbott's original technique. The essential features of his method are: (1) fibular osteotomy; (2) distal tibiofibular synostosis to prevent valgus deformity of the ankle; (3) subcutaneous division of the tibia into proximal and distal segments by percutaneous drilling and osteoclasis to minimize trauma to soft tissues; and (4) daily distraction of the tibial segments by means of transfixing pins held in a screw distraction apparatus.[630, 631] As a result of the encouraging results of Anderson's technique, interest in tibial lengthening was restimulated.

Anderson's method does have definite advantages: (1) soft-tissue damage is minimal; (2) stripping is avoided; (3) the periosteal tube is preserved; and (4) the hematoma remains localized.

The prerequisites initially set forth by Anderson for his procedure included: (1) The patient should be a child between 8 and 12 years of age with a predictable shortening of 4 cm. and (2) there should be sufficient muscle weakness in the leg that little can be lost by the procedure of leg lengthening. Coleman popularized Anderson's method of tibial lengthening in the United States, and the procedure was tried in various centers. It soon became obvious that Anderson's leg lengthening is certainly accompanied by marked increased morbidity as compared with simple epiphyscodesis. Thus Coleman and Noonan, reviewing their experience, added two further indications: (1) that the child should be close enough to skeletal maturity that satisfactory equalization cannot be achieved by epiphyseal arrest by completion of growth and (2) that it be understood that amputation may be required if acceptable equalization cannot be achieved by other means.[680] Gross, in a recent study of 26 patients on whom the Anderson tibial leg lengthening procedure was performed concluded that the principal usefulness of Anderson's method of limb lengthening is in selected cases of congenital short limb accompanied by muscle weakness and in which marked discrepancy in leg length is anticipated. In such an instance, a successful limb lengthening procedure performed when the child is seven or eight years old may prevent severe leg length discrepancy as the patient matures, and in early adolescence, less aggressive surgical procedures may give an acceptable functional result.[719]

The author, concurring with the conclusions of Gross, would like to stress further that tibial leg lengthening should be performed only in a few carefully selected patients and then only in special children's orthopedic centers. Both parents and patient should anticipate and accept the possibility of amputation and prosthesis, should the procedure fail. Anderson's first indication of predicted shortening of 4 cm. should be increased to 8 or 10 cm. It should also be realized that exaggeration of muscle weakness is more disabling in an already weakened limb than in a normal one.

Complications. It might be more appropriate to consider the complications of Anderson's leg lengthening prior to a detailed description of its technique. They may be subdivided into four groups: (1) overstretching; (2) interference with the blood supply; (3) insufficient fixation of fragments; and (4) problems of operative technique.[622, 623, 681, 753]

COMPLICATIONS DUE TO OVER-STRETCHING. *Articular and skeletal changes.* Equinovalgus deformity of the foot and ankle, and plantar flexion deformity of the toes commonly occur. These can be prevented by passive stretching exercises, by support of the foot in neutral position in a well-padded foot plate or plaster splint, and sliding lengthening of the Achilles tendon. Heel cord lengthening should *not* be performed indiscriminately, as overlengthening may result in triceps surae muscle weakness, calcaneus deformity, and greater functional disability. Eversion deformity of the ankle is obviated by distal tibiofibular synostosis (Anderson) or by transfixing the distal tibial and fibular segments with a transversely inserted screw.[630, 640, 680]

Proximal or distal fibular epiphyseolysis may occur as a result of premature union by scar or osteoid tissue of the osteotomized fibular fragments. It can be prevented by resection of a 3 cm. segment of the fibula at the level of osteotomy.

A flexible foot may become stiff during tibial leg lengthening. This is directly related to the speed at which the procedure is performed and the amount of lengthening. It may have its advantage in a flail foot, provided the foot does not become rigid in a deformed position. Compression of the talus may result in degenerative arthritis of the ankle.

Increasing genu valgum may occur during or following lengthening.

Muscular Changes. A decrease in motor strength of the muscles in the lengthened leg is a common complication and occurs to a varying degree in half to two thirds of the cases. In some limbs, ischemia of the affected muscles is a causative factor. Circulatory embarrassment results from hemorrhage and edema consequent to osteotomy of the tibia, from the trauma of mechanical stretching of the muscles, and from the application of the cast or splints for prevention of equinus deformity. After completion of lengthening, some degree of return of motor function can be expected; in a certain percentage of cases, however, motor loss is permanent. That correction of leg length inequality does not necessarily result in improved function has been well documented by Sofield et al.[823]

Neural Changes. Stretch paralysis of the common peroneal and plantar nerves is a definite potential complication that seems to be related to the amount and rapidity of lengthening. Sensory disturbance and motor weakness are often transient, though occasionally, permanent paralysis and numbness may occur.

COMPLICATIONS DUE TO INADEQUATE FIXATION OF FRAGMENTS. *Anterior angulation:* anterior bowing of the tibia took place frequently in earlier methods of tibial lengthening, with resultant sloughing of the overlying skin and protrusion of one or both tibial fragments through the skin, with secondary osteomyelitis necessitating amputation. Angular deformity is caused by improper placement of the pins and inadequate ossification and bone stability at the time the cast is applied or when the pins are removed. Another pitfall is windowing of the cast over the operative site for clear visualization of healing bone before sufficient stability of bone has developed.

Infected pin holes usually result from inadequate fixation and motion of the leg in the apparatus. It can be minimized by threading bilateral longitudinal strips of perforated plastic or solid padding with cork pieces over the pins. Septic pin tracts usually heal following removal of the pin.

COMPLICATIONS DUE TO INTERFERENCE WITH BLOOD SUPPLY. *Delayed union and nonunion* are common complications that can be anticipated when lack of adequate bone bridging is shown eight weeks after operation. Both Kawamura and Gross recommend early bone grafting (at eight weeks).[719, 753] Coleman and Noonan recommend bone grafting at four months, when there is definite roentgenographic evidence of delayed union: they obtained union in all four cases of nonunion after bone grafting.[680]

Failure of union of the tibiofibular synostosis can be prevented by internal fixation with a screw.

VASCULAR DISTURBANCES. Yosipovitch and Palti reported an increase of blood pressure of more than 20 mm. of mercury during Anderson's method of tibial lengthening in 20 of 24 patients. In experimental work done in dogs (in which the tibia was similarly distracted), an increase in blood pressure occurred, and the hypertension was shown to be caused by a reflex response to tension on the sciatic nerve in the upper part of the thigh. They suggested that elevation of blood pressure in human patients who had undergone femoral or tibial lengthening was due to the same cause.[854]

Soft tissues may be disturbed by a decrease of peripheral blood flow. Cyanosis and edema of the foot are not uncommon. Stretch necrosis of the skin and gangrene occasionally occur.

FRACTURE. Fracture at the osteotomy site results from early weight-bearing and torsional stress during the healing stage. The fractures usually heal, eventually, with immobilization in the cast.

OPERATIVE WOUND INFECTION. This occurs occasionally, with disastrous results. In the series of Gross, there was one case of superficial wound infection and one case of osteomyelitis.

Incidence of the complications encountered in Anderson's technique of tibial leg lengthening according to various authors is given in Table 7–14.

Operative Technique. Anderson's technique (as modified by Coleman and Noonan) is as follows:

The procedure can be performed in one (Coleman and Noonan) or two stages (Anderson). The author prefers the one-stage method because it spares the patient two months of the prolonged morbidity of the operation.

First, the ankle mortise is stabilized into a solid unit by creating a synostosis between the distal portions of the tibia and fibula. This allows both the tibia and fibula to be lengthened uniformly, prevents valgus deformity of the ankle, and protects the distal and proximal epiphyses of the fibula from shearing and slipping during the lengthening process.

A 5 cm. long linear incision is made over the lateral aspect of the distal third of the fibular shaft. The subcutaneous tissue is divided and the wound margins are mobilized and retracted to their respective sides. The deep fascia is divided in line with the skin incision, and the peroneal tendons are retracted posteriorly. Through an inverted "T" incision in the periosteum, the distal third of the fibular shaft is exposed subperiosteally. Next, using a Gigli saw, a 3 cm. long segment of the fibula is excised. The opposing surfaces of the lateral aspect of the tibia and upper half of the distal fragment of the fibula are partially decorticated and transfixed with a long screw inserted transversely from the lateral to the medial side. The screw should be placed proximally enough so as not to damage the distal tibial or fibular growth plate. The wound on the lateral aspect of the fibula is closed in routine manner.

Using the horizontal bars of the distraction apparatus as guides, four $5/32$-inch Steinmann pins are inserted transversely through the tibia. The upper two pins are placed parallel to the transcondylar axis of the knee joint; the lower two pins are parallel to the distal articular surface of the tibia. If there is equinus deformity, i.e., the foot cannot be passively dorsiflexed to neutral position, the tendo calcaneus is lengthened, preferably percutaneously.

Next, through a small puncture wound, at a site midway between the two sets of distraction pins, the tibia is weakened by multiple drill holes made through the anterior, posterior, medial, and lateral cortices. The

Table 7–14. *Complications Encountered in Anderson's Method of Tibial Leg Lengthening*

	Author		
		Coleman	
	Kawamura[753]	and Noonan[680]	Gross[719]
	(Total — 74 Patients)	*(Total — 32 Patients)*	*(Total — 26 Patients)*
Complication	*No. of Patients*	*No. of Patients*	*No. of Patients*
Due to overstretching			
Articular-skeletal			
Equinus	16	2	2
Pes valgus	3	2	1
Pes varus			2
Epiphyseolysis of fibula			
Proximal	2	—	—
Distal	1	—	—
Rigid or stiff joints of feet	Few cases	—	—
Osteoarthritis of talus	1	—	—
Genu valgum	1	8	—
Muscular — loss of muscle power	48		4 (1 due to Volkmann's ischemia)
Return to preoperative level	17	Some	
Some decrease remained	20		—
Permanent decrease	11		
Neural (peroneal and plantar nerve paralysis)			
Total	20	4	—
Permanent	4	—	—
Transient	16	4	—
Due to inadequate fixation of fragments			
Anterior angulation minimal	9	—?	4
moderate and severe with slough of skin	—	—?	—
Infected pin holes	7	1	2
Due to interference with blood supply			
To bone (delayed union, nonunion)	10	4	6
To soft tissues			
Cyanosis, edema	Some	Some	Some
Stretch necrosis of skin	—	—	—
Gangrene	—	—	—
Fracture at osteotomy site	2	2	1
Operative wound infection			
major (osteomyelitis)	—	—	1
minor (superficial)	—	—	1

drill holes are made transcutaneously with a $7/64$-inch drill point perpendicular to the longitudinal axis of the tibia.

The osteoclasis is completed over a sharp angled wedge. One or two sutures are placed over the stab wound. A Steinmann pin is placed through the os calcis if a heel cord lengthening was performed. Roentgenograms are made to check proper placement of the pins. Then a long leg cast is applied in two parts, with the knee in 15 degrees of flexion. The proximal segment of the cast incorporates the upper two pins, and the lower two pins and the pin in the os calcis are incorporated in the distal segment of the cast. The distraction apparatus is applied to the protruding parts of the Steinmann pins (Fig. 7–122).

Postoperative Care. Distraction is started immediately on the operating table. While the patient is under general anesthesia, 0.5 to 1 cm. of lengthening can be obtained. Following surgery, distraction is continued at a slow rate of $1/16$ inch per day. The surgeon who performed the operation should himself keep vigil throughout the process of lengthening. Careful attention is given to the onset of potential complications such as vascular or neurologic disturbances, the rate of lengthening, alignment of tibial fragments, pain, and pin tract sepsis.

When the total increment to be gained

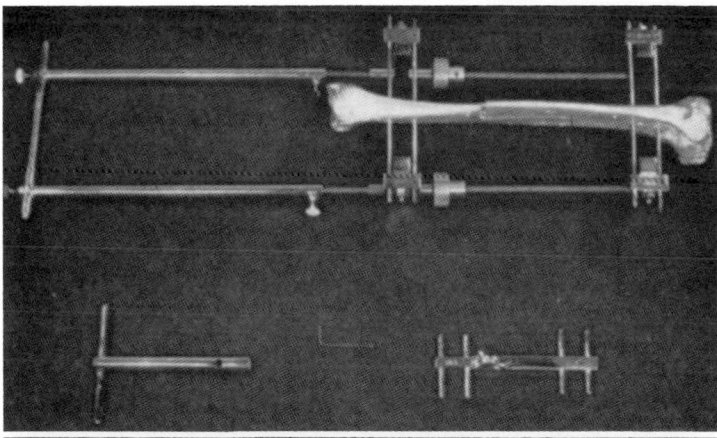

FIGURE 7–122. *The Anderson tibial lengthening apparatus.*

A. Semi-exploded view of the apparatus. The pin guide, Allen key, and box spanner form part of the kit. **B.** Lengthening of the tibia is demonstrated in this anatomic specimen. The amount of lengthening is reflected on the threaded side bar. **C.** The extension piece is attached to the lateral-distal block that bears the foot piece. **D.** Method of suspending frame. Active knee flexion and extension is encouraged. (From Anderson, W. V.: Lengthening of the lower limb: its place in the problem of limb length discrepancy. *In* Graham, W. D. (ed.): Modern Trends in Orthopedics, Vol. V. London, Butterworth & Co., 1967, pp. 10–11.)

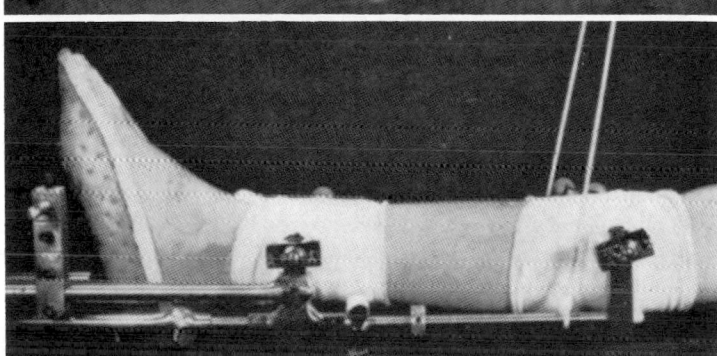

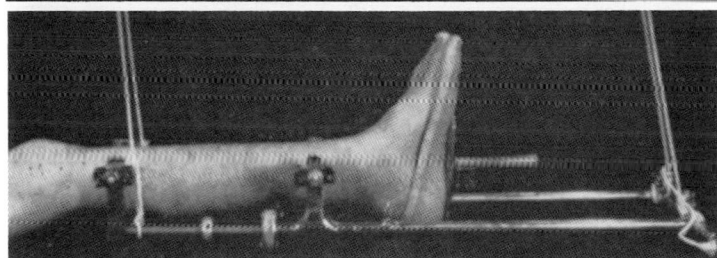

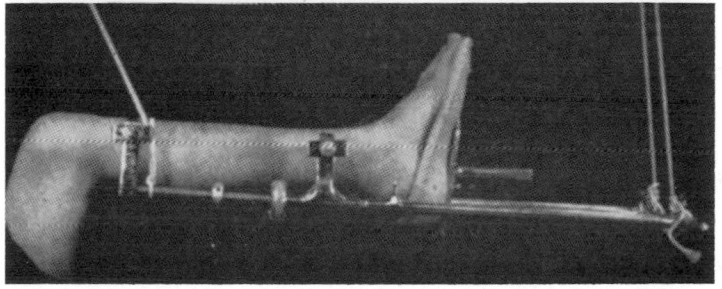

has been achieved and when there is sufficient callus and stability at the osteotomy site, a new long cast incorporating all the pins is applied. The distraction apparatus is removed. In an apprehensive child, it is safer to change the cast under general anesthesia.

Delayed union will be evident in the roentgenograms two to three months after completion of lengthening. At this time, if the roentgenograms disclose incomplete bone bridging, the lengthened area is bone grafted. When the bony union is adequate, the pins are removed and a snug above-knee walking cast is applied. Weight-bearing is not permitted until there is complete restoration of the medullary cavity at the site of osteotomy.

Amount of Lengthening. Anderson stated that 5 to 7.5 cm. of lengthening may be achieved without difficulty.[630] Coleman and Noonan recommended lengthening up to 5 cm. only.[680] Gross observed increased complications when lengthening exceeded 5 cm.[719]

Kawamura et al. performed histologic, histochemical, and microarterioradiographic studies in dogs, and observed that if tibial lengthening after tubelike elevation of the periosteum without tearing of the tube is limited to an amount equivalent to 10 per cent of the tibia's initial length, bony union progresses in a manner quite similar to that seen after a fracture. Electromyographic and enzyme studies in the elongated muscles indicated 10 per cent lengthening to be the safe limit, and that slow lengthening in several stages is far more advantageous than speedy lengthening. Clinical experiences of Kawamura et al. in 74 patients supported his conclusion that *lengthening of the tibia should be limited to 10 per cent of its initial length.*[753] Merle D'Aubigné and Dubousset recommend the following modification of Anderson tibial leg lengthening for adolescent or adult patients, as delayed union or nonunion is a likely complication in this age group. They give credit to Judet and associates for the development of the decortication technique.[776]

In the first stage, through a lateral incision, the distal fibula is fixed to the distal tibia with a screw inserted transversely immediately above the lateral malleolus (Fig. 7–123). Then the middle third of the tibia is

exposed through a separate anterior incision. A linear incision is made in the periosteum on the anteromedial surface of the tibia. With a sharp thin osteotome or periosteal elevator, the periosteum is elevated from the medial, lateral, and posterior aspects of the tibia in one piece. Next the periosteum is approximated with interrupted sutures. The wound is closed in routine fashion.

Three weeks later, the tibia is exposed through the old incision and the periosteal tube is opened and elevated as before. This is facilitated by the formation of soft new bone on the deep surface of the periosteum. The osteoperiosteal tube is sectioned circumferentially at its lower end. The fibula is divided transversely at the same level with a Gigli saw or an electric saw. A 2 to 3 cm. long segment of the interosseous membrane is resected at the same level,, exercising caution in order not to injure the deep interosseous nerve and anterior tibial vessels. Next, four Steinmann pins are inserted and the lengthening apparatus is applied, as described in the Anderson technique. A Gigli saw is inserted deep to the osteoperiosteal tube and the tibial shaft is sectioned at the proximal end of the osteoperiosteal tube. The periosteum and the wound are closed. While the patient is under general anesthesia, lengthening of 1 cm. may be obtained.

If there is equinus deformity, the Achilles tendon is lengthened at the same procedure. Other excessively tight soft tissues are also lengthened if necessary. Other details of postoperative care are similar to those outlined for Anderson's method of tibial leg lengthening.

Merle D'Aubigné and Dubousset report the results in three patients in whom the procedure was used. Union was clinically apparent at three months and solid union at four to five months. One month following surgery, the patients were discharged from the hospital, and at two months, the apparatus was removed and replaced by plaster of Paris cast. Weight-bearing was permitted in the cast at three or four months and full weight-bearing without the cast was permitted between four and five months. A lengthening of 5 to 6 cm. was achieved in all three patients with no complications.[776]

The series of Merle D'Aubigné and Dubousset is very small, but the procedure is

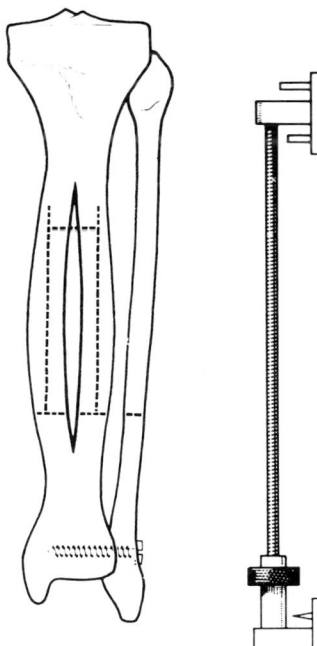

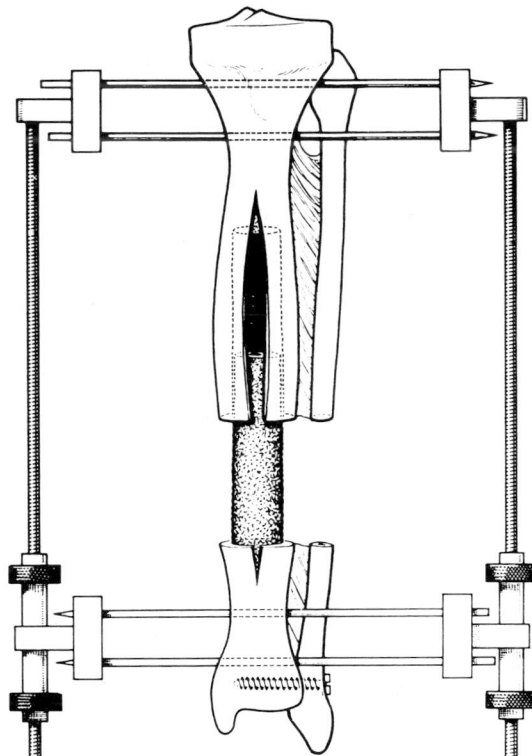

FIGURE 7-123. *Two-stage decortication method of tibial lengthening of Merle D'Aubigné and Dubousset (see text for explanation).*

(From Merle D'Aubigné, R., and Dubousset, J.: Surgical correction of large length discrepancies in the lower extremities of children and adults. J. Bone Joint Surg., 53-A:420, 1971.)

logical and physiologically sound. The author recommends that it be used in adolescents over 12 to 14 years of age.

Stimulation of Rate of Growth of Shorter Limb

The growth rate of a long bone may be increased when affected by a variety of pathologic conditions, such as fractures, chronic infections, and tumors. Ferguson proposed this to be caused by occlusion of the medullary arteries to the nutrient canal and diversion of the blood flow into the epiphyseal and metaphyseal vessels, with a consequent increase of circulation near the growth cartilage.[696]

Equalization of leg length discrepancy by stimulating the growth of the shorter limb has been the subject of intensive investigation. Theoretically, it is the ideal method, since discrepancy in limb length is commonly caused by shortening, and better symmetry of the body and contours of the limbs are provided by lengthening the short limb rather than by shortening the long limb. Unfortunately, a practical, reliable, and safe technique is not yet available. A survey of the literature on epiphyseal growth stimulation is given here to enhance our understanding of the problem of asymmetrical growth of the lower limbs.

Procedures on the Vascular System

CREATION OF ARTERIOVENOUS FISTULAE. That congenital and traumatic arteriovenous fistulae stimulate longitudinal growth of limbs has been observed clinically on numerous occasions.

Janes and Musgrove experimentally created arteriovenous fistulae in puppies, and observed that when the fistula was allowed to function from three to 15 months in 80 per cent of the tested puppies, there was an increased rate of longitudinal growth distal to the site of the fistula.[749] Kelly et al. reported more femoral than tibial overgrowth following formation of iliac arteriovenous fistulae in dogs, and more tibial than femoral overgrowth following creation of femoral fistulae.[755]

Weinmann, Kelly, and Owen studied blood flow in the femora, tibiae, and second metatarsals distal to a femoral arteriovenous fistula in immature dogs. The fistulae were allowed to function for from one hour to 25 weeks. They used short-term (10 minutes) clearance by the skeleton of ^{85}Sr and ^{47}Ca from the blood. The plasma flow per gram of bone decreased in these bones on the side of the fistula one hour following creation of the fistula; thereafter, the flow in the femur on the side of the fistula increased to a rate above normal, while in the tibae and second metatarsals, it increased but remained below normal limits when calculated on the basis of bone weight.[841]

Keck and Kelly determined the epiphyseal and diaphyseal intramedullary pressures and saphenous pressures in the hindlimbs of three groups of growing dogs: (1) normal, (2) with femoral arteriovenous fistulae, and (3) with selected venous ligation. Passive venous stasis did not stimulate bone growth, whereas arteriovenous fistulae induced bone growth and were associated with equalization of epiphyseal and diaphyseal intramedullary pressures.[754]

Clinical investigations by Janes and Jennings have demonstrated stimulation of bone growth in both length and thickness distal to the level of the fistula.[748] The procedure was abandoned, however, because of circulatory complications such as cardiac failure and hypertension and because of unpredictability of stimulation of the rate of growth.

LIGATION OF THE NUTRIENT ARTERY. That ligation of the nutrient artery does not stimulate growth was originally shown by Ollier and later confirmed by Wu and Miltner, and by Trueta.[786, 835, 836, 852] Brooks occluded the principal artery to the nutrient canal of the femur in one-day-old rabbits and observed the subsequent femoral growth. There was an initial shortening followed by equalization and final absolute shortening on the order of 3 per cent in occluded femora as compared with the experimental controls.[669] Troupp also demonstrated that growth retardation of both the femur and tibia resulted from proximal ligation of the femoral artery.[833]

IMPLANTATION OF ARTERIES. Experimentally, implantation of the femoral artery into the medullary cavity of the diaphysis or into the bony epiphysis increases blood flow to the physis, with consequent acceleration of growth.[662, 685]

Procedures on Bones

FRACTURE. That the length of a fractured limb in a growing child may exceed that of its opposite unfractured member has been observed in both clinical and experimental investigations. Bisgard and Compere and Adams concluded that hyperemia of the fractured bone leads to epiphyseal stimulation and overgrowth of that bone, its effect being limited to the fractured bone.[650, 682] Wray and Goodman studied postfracture vascular phenomena and long-bone overgrowth in the immature skeleton of the rat, and demonstrated that factors leading to growth changes are regional, rather than local in effect. Hyperemia following fracture is not confined to the fractured bone, but also involves the entire traumatized limb; also, the vascular changes vary according to the time after fracture, with the overgrowth response confined to a limited interval in the period after injury. Immediately following fracture of one tibia in the immature rat, femoral growth is temporarily retarded on both fractured and unfractured sides. This initial bilateral retardation of growth probably represents a reaction to the increased amount of cortisone liberated as a result of trauma. (The inhibitory effect of cortisone on epiphyseal growth is well documented.) Following this, there is a period in which both the fractured and unfractured limbs show overgrowth. Femoral overgrowth is significantly greater in the fractured limb than in the unfractured one. The occurrence of overgrowth on the unfractured side suggests the influence of a general factor such as the possible increased liberation of growth hormone in the period following the fracture.[851]

PERIOSTEAL STRIPPING. Ollier, in 1867, demonstrated that periosteal stripping of the tibia stimulated growth, the limb operated on being 2 to 5 mm. longer than the one not operated on three months following surgery.[786] This was later confirmed by numerous investigators.* The growth stimulating effect of periosteal stripping is greatest during the immediate postopera-

---

*See References 646, 666, 692, 757, 760, 761, 764.

tive period and decreases after a few weeks. Periosteal stripping of the proximal diaphysis of the tibia increases growth from the distal tibial epiphysis, but decreases growth from the proximal tibial epiphysis. Following periosteal stripping, Khoury Sola et al. observed an increase in longitudinal growth in 63 per cent of the stripped long bones as compared with corresponding unstripped bones. A second stripping operation further stimulated longitudinal growth; however, the amount of further growth stimulation from the second stripping was small and unpredictable. The high incidence of pathologic fractures after the second stripping procedure suggests that the two strippings have little, if any, clinical value.[757]

In an effort to make irritation of the periosteum more continuous and permanent, periosteal stripping has been combined with implantation of foreign material or organic tissue between the cortex and the periosteum; the result achieved has been a slight further increase in growth rate, though Khoury Sola has found the combined procedure to be inferior to stripping alone.[757]

Periosteal stripping has been tried clinically, and on the average, 1 cm. of additional growth has been obtained during the first year after operation.[646]

IMPLANTATION OF METALS IN MEDULLARY CAVITY. A variety of materials and metals have been introduced adjacent to the epiphyseal plate to stimulate linear growth. Von Langenbeck, in 1869, introduced ivory pegs into the left femora and tibiae of an eight-week-old dog. The animal was sacrificed 15 weeks later, and the femora and tibiae were removed and measured. There was 0.5 cm. overgrowth of the femur and 0.5 cm. overgrowth of the tibia in which the ivory pegs had been inserted.[762] Since then, numerous similar investigations have been carried out, using different substances.[677, 727, 739, 852] The reader is referred to the paper of Pease for a critical review of the literature.[792] The results in the literature have been varied, and sometimes growth was retarded, probably because the operation had injured the adjacent epiphyseal plate. Chapchal and Zeldenrust, in their experimental investigations, observed some lengthening of linear bone growth following insertion of various metals, metal alloys, and ivory adjacent to the epiphyseal plate—not only in the metaphyses, but also in the epiphyses. However, the amount of growth stimulation was minimal and uncertain. They also found various deformities of the bones to result from the procedure, concluding that this method of growth stimulation is not suitable for human practice.[677]

Pease, in 1952, gave a preliminary report of seven patients in whom stimulation of growth was attempted by inserting ivory screws adjacent to the epiphyseal plate. In five patients, the shortening was due to poliomyelitis; in one, due to congenital hypoplasia; and in another, a congenital dislocation of the hip with associated hypoplasia of the femur. The follow-up ranged from six months to 12 years. A variable degree of growth stimulation was obtained in all cases, and no severe consequent deformities were observed. Accelerated growth occurred during the first two postoperative years, becoming less as the epiphyseal plate grew away from the region of the foreign material. Pease emphasized that the report was merely preliminary, and that valid conclusions could not be drawn from so few cases.[793]

Trueta reasoned that to stimulate epiphyseal growth, the intramedullary circulation must be so altered that an increased blood flow is produced in and about the metaphyseal-epiphyseal junction. Thus he surgically blocked the medullary cavity with pieces of bone or inert metal. He claimed that the procedure resulted in definite stimulation of growth.[835, 836] Carpenter and Dalton blocked the intramedullary circulation of the distal femoral shaft immediately proximal to the flare of the femoral condyles by thorough curettage of the medullary canal, removal of the cancellous bone, and tight packing with small chips of ivory. They hoped provision of an irritative foreign body reaction would further increase the blood flow in the region of the epiphyseal plate. Some increase in growth was obtained in 26 of the 30 patients; however, in 70 per cent of the cases, the maximum gain was only $1/8$ to $1/4$ of an inch. They concluded the amount of increased growth was not sufficient to justify the procedure.[674]

For a critical review and study of the effect of the so-called growth stimulating operations on the rate of growth from different physes and their morphology, the reader is referred to Hansson.[729]

Procedures on Nervous System. Lumbar sympathectomy has been used in treatment of leg length inequality in poliomyelitis, with resultant insignificant or uncertain growth stimulation.[636, 648, 649, 732, 833]

Miscellaneous Methods. Roentgen ir- radiation, short-wave diathermy, ultrasonic therapy, direct heat, and injection of blood into the joint have been tried for local stimu- lation of growth. The results have been con- tradictory, with only slight, if any, stimula- tion of growth.[646, 765, 808, 849]

Congenital Hemihypertrophy

Congenital hemihypertrophy represents an asymmetrical overgrowth of one side of the body. The first clinical case of total hemihypertrophy was presented by Wagner in 1839;[880] however, asymmetry of the two sides of the body was well depicted by an- cient Egyptian and Greek sculptors. In the literature the condition is referred to by a variety of names, such as "congenital hemi- corporal disharmony," "megalosomia," "hemigigantism," "true hypertrophy," and "hemihypertrophy."

Classification

The extent and severity of hemihyper- trophy may vary greatly, and the condition may be congenital or acquired in type. Ward and Lerner gave the following classifica- tion:[883]

Congenital
  Total hypertrophy (all systems)
    segmental
    crossed
    hemihypertrophy
  Limited hypertrophy (not all systems involved)
    Muscular
    Vascular
    Skeletal
    Neurologic
Acquired
  Total
    Gigantism (hyperpituitarism)
  Limited
    Milroy's disease (familial lymph- edema)
    Elephantiasis
    Lipotomatosis
    Neurofibromatosis
    Vascular anomalies

The exact cause and mechanism of con- genital hypertrophy is still unknown. A number of possible etiologic factors have been suggested: endocrine abnormalities, vascular anomalies, lymphatic abnormali- ties, lesions of the brain (particularly of the hypothalamus), embryonic defects of the autonomic system, heredity, and em- bryogenic variants. Gesell believes hemihy- pertrophy to be the result of an imbalance of the normal process of twinning underly- ing all bilateral structures. It is essentially a developmental anomaly, antedating birth and arising in some way as a partial deflec- tion of the normal process of growth. For a more detailed discussion of his theory the reader is referred to his original paper.[863] Familial incidence has been reported by Scott, and Morris and MacGillivray.[869, 877]

Clinical Features

In hemihypertrophy one entire side of the body is enlarged, even to the point of af- fecting the size of the pupil in the eye on the involved side and the visceral organs of the thorax and abdomen. Growth of hair, erup- tion of teeth, and the texture of skin vary between the two sides. On the hyper- trophied side, the skin is thicker and there is increased hair. Pathologic examination will disclose true hypertrophy of all structures in the limbs, including blood vessels, muscles, and bones.

In crossed hypertrophy, an entire limb on one side and a limb on the opposite side, as well as several other organs, are involved.

In segmental hypertrophy, the skeleton and soft tissues in various parts of the body are involved. Usually there is a definite predilection for the limbs, however, with the lower limbs most frequently being involved. The left side appears to be more frequently affected than the right. In the foot, the first, second, and third toes are often involved.

Mental deficiency occurs in 15 to 20 per cent of cases. Other associated anomalies that have occurred in 50 per cent of cases are syndactylism, polydactylism, abnormal growth of nails, nevi, supernumerary nipples, congenital heart disease, and synostosis.

Leg length discrepancy is the primary concern of the orthopedic surgeon. Bryan, Lipscomb and Chatterton reviewed the literature and reported 11 cases of total congenital hemihypertrophy, 1 case of total crossed congenital hypertrophy, and 15 cases of total congenital segmental hypertrophy. Follow-up of these patients disclosed that the deformities did not disappear spontaneously. About 75 per cent of the cases required epiphyseodesis to correct leg length discrepancy.[855]

Hemihypertrophy is differentiated from hemiatrophy by estimating whether there is overgrowth or undergrowth of the involved limb, as compared with the normal one. For example, in hemiatrophy, there may be demonstrable muscle weakness and neurologic deficit that is not present in hemihypertrophy. Vascular and lymphatic abnormalities are ruled out by appropriate arteriograms or lymphangiograms.

Treatment

The disparity of growth is followed, and at the appropriate age, epiphyseodesis of the distal femur or proximal tibia is performed to equalize the leg lengths. Methods of treatment of increased girth of the limb, such as application of elastic bandages in the hypertrophied limb at night, are of doubtful value. Plastic surgical procedures may be indicated, particularly on the face.[866]

References

INTRODUCTION

1. Barnett, G. H., and Napier, J. R.: The axis of rotation of ankle joint in man. Its importance upon the form of the talus and the mobility of the fibula. J. Anat., *86*:1, 1952.
2. Blais, M. M., Green, W. T., and Anderson, M.: Lengths of the growing foot. J. Bone Joint Surg., *38-A*:998, 1956.
3. Elftman, H.: A cinematic study of the distribution of pressure in the human foot. Anat. Rec., *59*:481, 1934.
4. Elftman, H.: The transverse tarsal joint and its control. Clin. Orthop., *16*:41, 1960.
5. Elftman, H., and Manter, J. T.: The axes of the human foot. Science, *80*:484, 1934.
6. Elftman, H., and Manter, J. T.: The evolution of the human foot, with especial reference to the joints. J. Anat., *70*:56, 1935.
7. Feist, J. H., and Mankin, H. J.: The tarsus. Radiology, *79*:250, 1962.
8. Gardner, E., Gray, D. J., and O'Rahilly, R.: The prenatal development of the skeleton and joints of the human foot. J. Bone Joint Surg., *41-A*:847, 1959.
9. Hicks, H. J.: Mechanics of the foot. J. Anat., *87*:345, 1953.
10. Köhler, A.: (Revised by Zimmer, E. A., and edited by Case J. T.) Borderlands of the Normal and Early Pathologic in Skeletal Roentgenology. 10th Ed. New York, Grune & Stratton, 1956.
11. Lapidus, P. W.: Subtalar joint. Its anatomy and mechanics. Bull. Hosp. Joint Dis., *16*:179, 1955.
12. Manter, J. T.: Movements of the subtalar and transverse tarsal joints. Anat. Rec., *80*:397, 1941.
13. O'Rahilly, R., Gardner, E., and Gray, D. J.: The skeletal development of the foot. Clin. Orthop., *16*:7, 1960.
14. Steindler, A.: The pathomechanics of the static disabilities of the foot and ankle. A.A.O.S. Instructional Course Lectures, Vol. 9. Ann Arbor, J. W. Edwards, 1952, p. 327.
15. Straus, W. L., Jr.: Growth of the human foot and its evolutionary significance. Contrib. Embryol., *19*:93, 1927.
16. Wright, D. G., Desia, S. M., and Henderson, W. H.: Action of the subtalar and ankle-joint complex during the stance phase of walking. J. Bone Joint Surg., *46-A*:361, 1964.

NORMAL VARIATIONS OF THE BONES OF THE FOOT AND ANKLE

17. Bjornson, R. G. B.: Developmental anomaly of the lateral malleolus simulating fracture. J. Bone Joint Surg., *38-A*:128, 1956.
18. Caffey, J.: Pediatric X-ray Diagnosis. 5th Ed. Chicago, Year Book Medical Publishers, Inc., 1967, p. 744.
19. Gottlieb, C., and Berenbaum, S. L.: Pirie's bone, accessory ossicle on the dorsum of the astragalus—often bilateral. Radiology, *55*:423, 1950.
20. Harding, V. V.: Time schedule for the appearance and fusion of a secondary center of ossification of the calcaneus. Child Develop., *23*:181, 1952.
21. Hubay, C. A.: Sesamoid bones of the hands and feet. Amer. J. Roentgen., *61*:493, 1949.
22. McDougall, A.: The os trigonum. J. Bone Joint Surg., *37-B*:257, 1955.
23. Morrison, A. B.: The os paracuneiforme. Some observations of an example removed at operation. J. Bone Joint Surg., *35-B*:254, 1953.
24. O'Rahilly, R.: A survey of carpal and tarsal anomalies. J. Bone Joint Surg., *35-A*:626, 1953.
25. Powell, H. P. W.: Extra center of ossification for the medial malleolus in children. Incidence and significance. J. Bone Joint Surg., *43-B*:107, 1961.
26. Roche, A. F., and Sunderland, S.: Multiple ossification centers in the epiphyses of the long bones of the human hand and foot. J. Bone Joint Surg., *41-B*:375, 1959.
27. Ross, S. E., and Caffey, J.: Ossification of the calcaneal apophysis in healthy children: Some normal radiologic features. Stanford Med. Bull., *15*:224, 1957.
28. Selby, S.: Separate centers of ossification of the tip of the internal malleolus. Amer. J. Roentgen., *86*:496, 1961.
29. Shands, A. R., Jr.: The accessory bones of the foot. Southern Med. Surg., *93*:326, 1931.
30. Shands, A. R., Jr., and Wentz, I. J.: Congenital anomalies, accessory bones, and osteochondritis in the feet of 850 children. Surg. Clin. N. Amer., *33*:1643, 1953.
31. Sirry, A.: The pseudocystic triangle in the normal os calcis. Acta Radiol., *36*:516, 1951.
32. Trolle, D.: Accessory Bones of the Human Foot. Copenhagen, Munksgaard, 1948.
33. Venning, P.: Variation of the digital skeleton of the foot. Clin. Orthop., *16*:26, 1960.

ACCESSORY TARSAL NAVICULAR

34. Bautrier: Cited by Meyer, M., Cuny, J., and Trensz, F.: L'os tibial externe et ses divers aspects radiologiques. Strasbourg Méd., *85*:24, 1927.

35. Dwight, T.: Variations of the Bones of the Hands and Feet. Philadelphia, J. B. Lippincott, Co., 1907.

36. Faber, A.: Os tibiale externum bei erbgleichen Zwillingen. Erbartz, *4*:83, 1934.

37. Féré, C. H., and Deniker, M.: Note sur des exostosis symétriques des scaphoides tarsiens. Rev. Chir., *29*:544, 1904.

38. Francillon, M. R.: Untersuchungen zur anatomischen und klinischen Bedeutung des Os tibiale externum. Z. Orthop. Chir., *56*:61, 1932.

39. Geist, E. S.: The accessory scaphoid bone. J. Bone Joint Surg., 7:570, 1925.

40. Hohmann, G.: Fuss und Bein. 5th Aufl. München, J. F. Bergmann, 1951.

41. Kidner, F. C.: The prehallux (accessory scaphoid) in its relation to flatfoot. J. Bone Joint Surg., *11*:831, 1929.

42. Kidner, F. C.: The prehallux in relation to flatfoot. J.A.M.A., *101*:1539, 1933.

43. Kienböck, R., and Müller, W.: Os tibiale externum und Verletzung des Fusses. Z. Orthop. Chir., *66*:257, 1937.

44. Marti, T.: Kasuistischer Beitrag zum Studium des Os tibiale externum. Praxis, *51*:828, 1962.

45. Meyer, M., Cuny, J., and Trensz, F.: L'os tibial externe et ses divers aspects radiologiques. Strasbourg Méd., *85*:24, 1927.

46. Monahan, J. J.: The human pre-hallux. Amer. J. Med. Sci., *160*:708, 1920.

47. Niederecker, K.: Der Plattfuss. Stuttgart, Ferdinand Enke, 1959.

48. Pfitzner, W.: Beiträge zur Kenntnis des menschlichen Extremitätenskeletts. VII. Die Variationen im Aufbau des Fuffskeletts. Schwalbe's Morph. Arb., *6*:245, 1896.

49. Trolle, D.: Accessory Bones of the Human Foot. Copenhagen, Munksgaard, 1948.

50. Zadek, I.: The significance of the accessory tarsal scaphoid. J. Bone Joint Surg., *8*:618, 1926.

51. Zadek, I., and Gold, A. M.: The accessory tarsal scaphoid. J. Bone Joint Surg., *30–A*:957, 1948.

TALIPES EQUINOVARUS

52. Abrams, R. C.: Relapsed club foot. The early results of an evaluation of Dillwyn Evans' operation. J. Bone Joint Surg., *51-A*:270, 1969.

53. Adams, W.: A series of four specimens illustrating the morbid anatomy of congenital club-foot (talipes varus). Trans. Path. Soc. London, *6*:348, 1854–1855.

54. Adams, W.: Club Foot, its Causes, Pathology, and Treatment. London, J. and A. Churchill, 1866.

55. Alberman, E. D.: The causes of congenital club foot. Arch. Dis. Child., *40*:548, 1965.

56. Attenborough, C. G.: Severe congenital talipes equinovarus. J. Bone Joint Surg., *48-B*:31, 1966.

57. Bardeen, C. R., and Lewis, W. H.: Development of limbs, body-wall, and back in man. Amer. J. Anat., *1*:1, 1901.

58. Beatson, R. R., and Pearson, J. R.: A method of assessing correction in club feet. J. Bone Joint Surg., *48-B*:40, 1966.

59. Bechtol, C. O., and Mossman, H. W.: Club-foot. Embryological study of associated muscle abnormalities. J. Bone Joint Surg., *32-A*:827, 1950.

60. Bell, J. F., and Grice, D. S.: Treatment of congenital talipes equinovarus with the modified Dennis Browne splint. J. Bone Joint Surg., *26*:799, 1944.

61. Bentzon, P. G. K., and Thomasen, E.: On treatment of congenital clubfoot. Acta Orthop. Scand., *11*:129, 1940.

62. Berman, A., and Gartland, J. J.: Metatarsal osteotomy for the correction of adduction of the forepart of the foot in children. J. Bone Joint Surg., *53-A*:498, 1971.

63. Bertelsen, A.: Treatment of congenital club foot. J. Bone Joint Surg., *39-B*:599, 1957.

64. Bessel-Hagen, F. C.: Die Pathologie und Therapie des Klumfusses. Heidelberg, O. Peters, 1889.

65. Bissell, J. B.: The morbid anatomy of congenital talipes equinovarus. Arch Pediat., *5*:406, 1888.

66. Blockey, N. J., and Smith, M. G. H.: The treatment of congenital club foot. J. Bone Joint Surg., *48-B*:660, 1966.

67. Blumenfeld, I., Kaplan, N., and Hicks, E. O.: The conservative treatment of congenital talipes equinovarus. J. Bone Joint Surg., *28*:765, 1946.

68. Böhm, M.: Zur Pathologie und Röntgenologie des angeborenen Klumfusses. München. Med. Wschr., *55*:1492, 1928.

69. Böhm, M.: The embryologic origin of clubfoot. J. Bone Joint Surg., *11*:229, 1929.

70. Bost, F. C., Schottstaedt, E. R., and Larsen, L. J.: Plantar dissection. An operation to release the soft tissues in recurrent or recalcitrant talipes equinovarus. J. Bone Joint Surg., *42-A*:151, 1960.

71. Brockman, E. P.: Congenital Clubfoot (Talipes Equinovarus). Bristol, John Wright and Sons, Ltd., and New York, William Wood & Co., 1930.

72. Brockman, E. P.: Modern methods of treatment of clubfoot. Brit. Med. J., *2*:512, 1937.

73. Browne, D.: Talipes equinovarus. Lancet, *2*:969, 1934.

74. Browne, D.: Congenital deformities of mechanical origin. Proc. Roy. Soc. Med., *29*:1409, 1936.

75. Browne, D.: Congenital deformities of mechanical origin. Arch. Dis. Child., *30*:37, 1955.

76. Browne, D.: Splinting for controlled movement. Clin. Orthop., *8*:91, 1956.

77. Browne, D.: Talipes equinovarus. (Letter to the Editor.) Lancet, *1*:863, 1962.

78. Börnbeck, R.: Zur Pathologie des angeborenen Klumfusses. Orthop., *79*:521, 1950.

79. Burrell, H. L.: A contribution to the anatomy of congenital equino-varus. Ann. Surg., *17*:293, 1893.

80. Carpenter, E. B., and Huff, S. H.: Selective tendon transfers for recurrent club foot. Southern Med. J., *46*:220, 1953.

81. Cavanaugh, C. J.: Clubfoot and congenital hand anomalies. J. Hered., *44*:53, 1953.

82. Clark, J. M. P.: Treatment of clubfoot. Early detection and management of the unreduced clubfoot. Proc. Roy. Soc. Med., *61*:779, 1968.

83. Codivilla, A.: New procedure for surgical treatment of the congenital pes equinus varus. Arch. Soc. Ital. Chir., *18:* 1906.

84. Codivilla, A.: Sulla cura del piedo equino varo congenito. Nuovo metodo di cura cruenta. Arch. Ortop., *23*:245, 1906.

85. Compere, E. L.: Congenital talipes equinovarus. Surg. Clin. N. Amer., *15*:767, 1935.

86. Crabbe, W. A.: Aetiology of congenital talipes. Brit. Med. J., *2*:1060, 1960.

87. Critchley, J. E., and Taylor, R. G.: Transfer of the tibialis anterior tendon for relapsed clubfoot. J. Bone Joint Surg., *34-B*:49, 1952.

88. Curtis, B. H., and Butterfield, W. L.: Surgical treatment of congenital club-foot. *In* Delchey, J. (ed): Dixième Congrès International de Chirurgie Orthopédique et de Traumatologie. Paris, 4–9 Septembre, 1966. Bruxelles, Les Publications "Acta Medica Belgica," 1967, p. 1150.

89. Curtis, F. E., and Muro, F.: Decancellation of the os calcis, astragalus, and cuboid in correction of congenital talipes equinovarus. J. Bone Joint Surg., *16*:110, 1934.

90. Dangelmajer, R. C.: A review of 200 clubfeet. Bull. Hosp. Special Surg., *4*:73, 1961.

91. Denham, R. A.: Congenital talipes equinovarus. J. Bone Joint Surg., *49-B*:583, 1967.

92. Dittrich, R. J.: Pathogenesis of congenital club-foot. J. Bone Joint Surg., *12*:373, 1930.

93. Dunn, N.: The treatment of congenital talipes equinovarus. Brit. Med. J., *2*:1, 216, 1923.

94. Dwyer, F. C.: The treatment of relapsed clubfoot by the insertion of a wedge into the calcaneum. J. Bone Joint Surg., *45-B*:67, 1963.

95. Elmslie, R. C.: The principles of treatment of congenital talipes equino-varus. J. Orthop. Surg., *2*:669, 1920.

96. Evans, D.: Relapsed club foot. J. Bone Joint Surg., *43-B*:722, 1961.

97. Farill, J.: Tibioperoneal tenoplasty for congenital clubfoot with peroneal insufficiency. J. Bone Joint Surg., *38-A*:329, 1956.

98. Flinchum, D.: Pathologic anatomy in talipes equinovarus. J. Bone Joint Surg., *35-A*:111, 1953.

99. Forrester-Brown, M.: The treatment of congenital equinovarus (club-foot). J. Bone Joint Surg., *17*:661, 1935.

100. Forrester-Brown, M.: A clamp for stretching congenital club-feet. Lancet, *1*:897, 1936.

101. Fredenhagen, H.: Der Klumpfuss, Vorkommen, Anatomie, Behandlung und Spätresultate. Z. Orthop., *85*:305, 1954.

102. Fried, A.: Recurrent congenital club-foot. The role of the m. tibialis posterior in etiology and treatment. J. Bone Joint Surg., *41-A*:243, 1959.

103. Fripp, A. T.: The relapsed clubfoot. Proc. Roy. Soc. Med., *44*:873, 1951.

104. Fripp, A. T.: The problem of the relapsed clubfoot (editorial). J. Bone Joint Surg., *43-B*:626, 1961.

105. Fripp, A. T., and Shaw, N. E.: Club-foot. Edinburgh and London, E. & S. Livingstone, Ltd., 1967.

106. Garceau, G. J.: Anterior tibial transposition in recurrent congenital club-foot. J. Bone Joint Surg., *22*:932, 1940.

107. Garceau, G. J.: Recurrent clubfoot. Bull. Hosp. Joint Dis., *15*:143, 1954.

108. Garceau, G. J., and Manning, K. R.: Transposition of the anterior tibial tendon in the treatment of recurrent congenital club-foot. J. Bone Joint Surg., *29*:1044, 1947.

109. Garceau, G. J., and Palmer, R. M.: Transfer of the anterior tibial tendon for recurrent clubfoot. A long-term follow-up. J. Bone Joint Surg., *49-A*:207, 1967.

110. Gartland, J. J.: Posterior tibial transplant in the surgical treatment of recurrent club foot. A preliminary report. J. Bone Joint Surg., *46-A*:1217, 1964.

111. Gelman, W. B.: Soft-tissue releasing procedure for persisting heel varus in the uncorrected clubfoot. Clin. Orthop., *16*:177, 1960.

112. Gunn, D. R., and Molesworth, B. D.: The use of tibialis posterior as a dorsiflexor. J. Bone Joint Surg., *39-B*:674, 1957.

113. Hamsa, W. R., and Burney, D. W., Jr.: Open correction of recurrent talipes equinovarus. A study of end-results. Clin. Orthop., *26*:104, 1963.

114. Handelsman, J. E., Youngleson, J., and Malkin, C.: A modified approach to the Dwyer os calcis osteotomy in club foot. S. Afr. Med. J., *39*:989, 1965.

115. Harry, N. M.: Dennis Browne splints in the treatment of talipes equinovarus. Austr. New Zeal. J. Surg., *10*:117, 1940.

116. Hauser, E. D. W.: Cohesive bandage for clubfoot in newborn infants. J.A.M.A., *138*:19, 1948.

117. Hauser, E. D. W.: Origin and etiology of clubfoot. Quart. Bull. Northwest. Med. Sch., *28*:274, 1954.

118. Henke, W., and Reyher, C.: Studien über die Entwickelung der Extremitäten des Menschen insbesondere der Gelenkflächen. Sitzungsberichte d. k. Akademie d. Wissenschaften Wiener Math. Naturwissenschaftliche Klasse, Ed. 3. *50*:217, 1874.

119. Hersh, A.: The role of surgery in the treatment of club feet. J. Bone Joint Surg., *49-A*:1684, 1967.

120. Heyman, C. H.: Ober operation for congenital club-foot. End-results in fifteen cases. Surg. Gynec. Obstet., *49*:706, 1929.

121. Heyman, C. H., Herndon, C. H., and Strong, J. M.: Mobilization of the tarsometatarsal and intermetatarsal joints for the correction of resistant adduction of the forepart of the foot in congenital clubfoot or congenital metatarsus varus. J. Bone Joint Surg., *40-A*:299, 1958.

122. Heywood, A. W. B.: The mechanics of the hindfoot in clubfoot as demonstrated radiographically. J. Bone Joint Surg., *46-B*:102, 1964.

123. Hirsch, C.: Observations on early operative treatment of congenital club-foot. Bull. Hosp. Joint Dis., *21*:173, 1960.

124. Hoffa, A.: Lehrbuch der Orthopädischen Chirurgie. 5th Ed. Stuttgart, Ferdinand Enke, 1905, pp. 734–782.

125. Hüter, C.: Zu der Frage über das Wesen des angeborenen Klumpfüsses. Deutsch. Klinik, *15*:487, 1863.

126. Idelberger, K.: Die Ergebnisse der Zwillingsforschung beim angeborenen Klumpfuss. Verh. Deutsche. Orthop. Ges., *33*:272, 1939.

127. Inclán, A.: Las anomalias de las inserciones tendinosas en la pathogenia del pié bot varo equino congénito. Rev. Orthop. Traumatol., *5*:173, 1960.

128. Irani, R. N., and Sherman, M. S.: The pathologic anatomy of club foot. J. Bone Joint Surg., *45-A*:45, 1963.

129. Jansen, K.: Treatment of congenital club foot. J. Bone Joint Surg., *39-B*:599, 1957.

130. Jergesen, F. H.: The treatment of unilateral congenital talipes equinovarus with the Denis Browne splint. J. Bone Joint Surg., *25*:185, 1943.

131. Johanning, K.: Excochleatio ossis cuboidei in the treatment of pes equinovarus. Acta Orthop. Scand., *27*:310, 1958.

132. Kandel, B.: The suroplantar projection in the congenital clubfoot of the infant. Acta Orthop. Scand., *22*:161, 1952.

133. Kendrick, R. E., Sharma, N. K., Hassler, W. L., and Herndon, C. H.: Tarsometatarsal mobilization for resistant adduction of the forepart of the foot. A follow-up study. J. Bone Joint Surg., *52-A*:61, 1970.

134. Kite, J. H.: Non-operative treatment of congenital club-feet. Southern Med. J., *23*:337, 1930.

135. Kite, J. H.: The surgical treatment of congenital club-feet. Surg. Gynec. Obstet., *61*:190, 1935.

136. Kite, J. H.: Principles involved in the treatment of clubfoot. J. Bone Joint Surg., *21*:595, 1939.

137. Kite, J. H.: The Clubfoot. New York, Grune & Stratton Inc., 1964.

138. Kite, J. H.: Errors and complications in treating foot conditions in children. Clin. Orthop., *53*:31, 1967.

139. Kleiger, B.: Significance of tibiotalar navicular complex in congenital clubfoot. J. Hosp. Joint Dis., *23*:158, 1962.

140. Kocher: Zur Aetiologie und Therapie des pes varus congenitus. Deutsch. Z. Chir., *9*:329, 1879.

141. Kuhlman, R. F., and Bell, J. F.: A clinical evaluation of operative procedures for congenital talipes equinovarus. J. Bone Joint Surg., *39-A*:265, 1957.

142. Lange, M.: Orthopädische Chirurgische Operationslehre. Munchen, J. Bergman, 1951.

143. LeNoir, J. L.: Congenital Idiopathic Talipes. Springfield, Ill. Charles C Thomas, 1966.

144. Little, W. J.: A Treatise on the Nature of Club-Foot and Analogous Distortions. Including Their Treatment Both With or Without Surgical Operation. London, W. Jeffs, 1839.

145. Lucas, L. S.: Surgical procedures in treatment of chronic clubfoot. West. J. Surg., *56*:542, 1948.

146. Lusskin, H.: Nonrigid method of treatment for early clubfoot. J. Int. Coll. Surg., *14*:444, 1950.

147. MacEwen, G. D., Scott, D. J., Jr., and Shands, A. R., Jr.: Follow-up survey of clubfoot treated at Alfred I. Du Pont Institute. With special reference to the value of plaster therapy, instituted during earliest signs of recurrence, and the use of night splints to prevent or minimize the manifestations. J.A.M.A., *175*:497, 1961.

148. McCauley, J. C., Jr.: Operative treatment of clubfeet. N. Y. J. Med., *47*:255, 1947.

149. McCauley, J. C., Jr.: Surgical treatment of clubfoot. Surg. Clin. N. Amer., *31*:561, 1951.

150. McCauley, J. C., Jr.: A release operation for problem clubfoot. New York J. Med., *52*:2997, 1952.

151. McCauley, J. C., Jr.: Treatment of clubfoot. A.A.O.S. Instructional Course Lectures. Vol. 16. St. Louis, The C. V. Mosby Co., 1959, p.93.

152. McCauley, J. C., Jr.: Triple arthrodesis for congenital talipes equinovarus deformities. Clin. Orthop., *34*:25, 1964.

155. McCauley, J. C., Jr.: Clubfoot. History of the development and the concepts of pathogenesis and treatment. Clin. Orthop., *44*:51, 1966.

154. Mau, C.: Muskelbefunde und ihre Bedentung Beim angeborenen Klumfussleiden. Arch. Orthop. Unfallchir., *28*:292, 1930.

155. Menelaus, M. B.: Talectomy in equinovarus deformity in arthrogryposis and spina bifida. J. Bone Joint Surg., *53-B*:468, 1971.

156. Middleton, D. S.: Studies on prenatal lesions of striated muscle as a cause of congenital deformity. Edinburgh Med. J., N.S., *41*:401, 1934.

157. Morita, S.: A method for the treatment of resistant congenital clubfoot in infants by gradual correction with leverage-wire correction and wire-traction cast. J. Bone Joint Surg., *44-A*:149, 1962.

158. Morris, R. H.: Skeletal traction as a method of treatment for certain foot deformities. Arch. Surg., *46*:737, 1943.

159. Nagura, S.: Zur Ätiologie des angeborenen Klumpfusses. Z. Chir., *8*:187, 1956.

160. Nagura, S.: Zur Frage der Vererbung des angeborenen Klumpfusses. Arch. Orthop. Unfallchir., *52*:48, 1960.

161. Neel, J. V., Falls, H. T., and Test, A. R.: Pedigree of clubfoot. Amer. J. Dis. Child., *79*:442, 1950.

162. Nicholas, E. H.: Anatomy of congenital equinovarus. Boston Med. Surg. J., *36*:150, 1897.

163. Ober, F. R.: An operation for the relief of congenital equinovarus deformity. Preliminary report. J.A.M.A., *65*:621, 1915.

164. Ogston, A.: A new principle of curing club-foot in severe cases in children a few years old. Brit. Med. J., *1*:1524, 1902.

165. Palmer, R. M.: The genetics of talipes equinovarus. J. Bone Joint Surg., *46-A*:542, 1964.

166. Pansini, A.: Indications and results of Codivilla operation in treatment of congenital club feet. Minerva Ortop., *16*:158, 1965.

167. Parker, R. W.: Congenital Club-foot; Its Nature and Treatment. London, Lewis, 1887.

168. Parker, R. W., and Shattock, S. G.: The pathology and etiology of congenital club-foot. Trans. Path. Soc. London, *35*:423, 1884.

169. Penners, R.: Muskelanomalien bei angeborenen Klumpfüssen. Z. Orthop., *85*:103, 1954.

170. Ponseti, I. V., and Smoley, E. M.: Congenital club foot: The results of treatment. J. Bone Joint Surg., *45-A*:261, 1963.

171. Primrose, D. A.: Talipes equinovarus in mental defectives. J. Bone Joint Surg., *51-B*:60, 1969.

172. Salter, R. B.: Present trends in treatment of club feet. A.A.O.S. Sound-Slide Program, 1965, No. 7.

173. Scarpa, A.: A memoir on the congenital club foot in children. Translated from Italian by J. W. Wishart. Edinburgh, Constable & Co., 1818.

174. Scherb, R.: Zur Ätiologie Kongenitaler und Kongenital bedingter Fussdeformitäten mit besonderer Berücksichtingung des Pes equino-varus congenitus. Acta Chir. Scand., *67*:717, 1930.

175. Schomburg, H.: Untersuchung der Entwicklung der Muskeln und Knochen des Menschlichen Fusses an Serienschnitten und Rekonstruktionen und unter Zuhülfenahme Makrosko-pischer Präparation. Göttinger, Kaestner, 1900.

176. Sell, L. S.: Tibial torsion accompanying congenital clubfoot. J. Bone Joint Surg., *23*:561, 1941.

177. Settle, G. W.: The anatomy of congenital talipes equinovarus: Sixteen dissected specimens. J. Bone Joint Surg., *45-A*:1341, 1963.

178. Singer, M.: Tibialis posterior transfer in congenital club foot. J. Bone Joint Surg., *43-B*:717, 1961.

179. Singer, M., and Fripp, A. T.: Tibialis anterior transfer in congenital club foot. J. Bone Joint Surg., *40-B*:252, 1958.

180. Steindler, A.: Stripping of the os calcis. J. Orthop. Surg., *2*:8, 1920.

181. Stewart, S. F.: Club-foot: its incidence, cause and treatment. Anatomical-physiological study. J. Bone Joint Surg., *33-A*:577, 1951.

182. Steytler, J. C. S., and Van Der Walt, I. D.: Correction of resistant adduction of the forefoot in congenital clubfoot and congenital metatarsus varus by metatarsal osteotomy. Brit. J. Surg., *53*:558, 1966.

183. Swann, M., Lloyd-Roberts, G. C., and Catterall, A.: The anatomy of uncorrected clubfeet. J. Bone Joint Surg., *51-B*:263, 1969.

184. Templeton, A. W., McAlister, W. H., and Zim, I. D.: Standardization of terminology and evaluation of osseous relationships in congenitally abnormal feet. Amer. J. Roentgen., *93*:374, 1965.

185. Terry, R. J.: Sprengel's deformity and clubfoot; an anthropological interpretation. Amer. J. Phys. Anthrop., *17*:251, 1959.

186. Thomson, S. A.: Treatment of congenital talipes equinovarus with a modification of the Denis Browne method and splint. J. Bone Joint Surg., *24*:291, 1942.

187. Thomson, S. A.: The treatment of congenital club-foot. Nine years' experience with a modification of the Denis Browne method and splint. J. Bone Joint Surg., *31-A*:431, 1949.

188. Thomson, S. A.: Modified Denis Browne splint for unilateral club-foot to protect the normal foot. J. Bone Joint Surg., *37-A*:1286, 1955.

189. Turco, V. J.: Surgical correction of the resistant congenital club-foot—one-stage release with internal fixation. A.A.O.S. Film Library.

190. Turco, V. J.: Surgical correction of the resistant club foot. One-stage posteromedial release with internal fixation: A preliminary report. J. Bone Joint Surg., *53-A*:477, 1971.

191. Wagner, L. C., and Butterfield, W. L.: Surgical release of contracted tissues for resistant congenital clubfoot. Amer. J. Surg., *84*:82, 1952.

192. White, J. W., and Gulledge, W. H.: Skin-tight casts for treatment of club-foot. J. Bone Joint Surg., *33-A*:475, 1951.

193. Wiley, A. M.: Club foot. An anatomical and experimental study of muscle growth. J. Bone Joint Surg., *41-B*:821, 1959.

194. Wisbrun, W.: Neue Gesichtspunkte zum Redressement des angeborenen Klumpfusses und daraus sich ergebende Schlussfolgerungen bezüglich der Ätiologie. Arch. Orthop. Unfallchir., *31*:451, 1932.

195. Wynne-Davies, R.: Family studies and the cause of congenital clubfoot. J. Bone Joint Surg., *46-B*:445, 1964.

196. Wynne-Davies, R.: Talipes equinovarus. A review of eighty-four cases after completion of treatment. J. Bone Joint Surg., *46-B*:464, 1964.

197. Young, A. B.: Club foot treated by astragalectomy. 50-year follow-up of a case. Lancet, *1*:670, 1962.

198. Zadek, I., and Barnett, E. L.: The importance of the ligaments of the ankle in correction of congenital clubfoot. J.A.M.A., *69*:1057, 1917.

TALIPES CALCANEOVALGUS

199. Wynne-Davies, R.: Family studies and the cause of congenital clubfoot—talipes equinovarus, talipes calcaneovalgus and metatarsus varus. J. Bone Joint Surg., *46-B*:445, 1964.

CONGENITAL METATARSUS VARUS

200. Berman, A., and Gartland, J. J.: Metatarsal osteotomy for the correction of adduction of the forepart of the foot in children. J. Bone Joint Surg., *53-A*:498, 1971.

201. Herndon, C. H.: Discussion of paper by Berman, A., and Gartland, J. J. J. Bone Joint Surg., *53-A*:505, 1971.

202. Heyman, C. H., Herndon, C. H., and Strong, J. M.: Mobilization of the tarsotatarsal and intermetatarsal joints for the correction of resistant adduction of the forepart of the foot in congenital clubfoot or congenital metatarsus varus. J. Bone Joint Surg., *40-A*:299, 1958.

203. Jacobs, J. E.: Metatarsus varus and hip dysplasia. Clin. Orthop., *16*:19, 203, 1960.

204. Kendirck, R. E., Sharma, N. K., Hassler, W. L., and Herndon, C. H.: Tarsometatarsal mobilization for resistant

adduction of the forepart of the foot. J. Bone Joint Surg., *52-A:*61, 1970.

205. Kite, J. H.: Congenital metatarsus varus. Report of 300 Cases. J. Bone Joint Surg., *32-A:*500, 1950.

206. Kite, J. H.: Congenital metatarsus varus. A.A.O.S. Instructional Course Lectures. Ann Arbor, J. W. Edwards, 1950, p. 126.

207. Kite, J. H.: Congenital metatarsus varus. J. Bone Joint Surg., *49-A:*388, 1967.

208. Lusskin, R., and Lusskin, H.: A metatarsus varus splint for the prewalker. J. Bone Joint Surg., *41-A:*363, 1959.

209. McCauley, J., Jr., Lusskin, R., and Bromley, J.: Recurrence in congenital metatarsus varus. J. Bone Joint Surg., *46-A:*525, 1964.

210. McCormick, D. W., and Blount, W. P.: Metatarsus adductovarus. "Skewfoot" J.A.M.A., *141:*449, 1949.

211. Peabody, C. W., and Muro, F.: Congenital metatarsus varus. J. Bone Joint Surg., *15:*171, 1933.

212. Ponseti, I. V., and Becker, J. R.: Congenital metatarsus adductus: The results of treatment. J. Bone Joint Surg., *48-A:*702, 1966.

213. Thomson, S. A.: Hallux varus and metatarsus varus. Clin. Orthop., *16:*109, 1960.

214. Wynne-Davies, R.: Family studies and the cause of congenital club-foot—talipes equinovarus, talipes calcaneovalgus and metatarsus varus. J. Bone Joint Surg., *46-B:*445, 1964.

METATARSUS PRIMUS VARUS AND HALLUX VALGUS

215. Bonney, G., and MacNab, I.: Hallux valgus and hallux rigidus. A critical survey of operative results. J. Bone Joint Surg., *34-B:*366, 1952.

216. Carr, C. R., and Boyd, B. M.: Correctional osteotomy for metatarsus primus varus and hallux valgus. J. Bone Joint Surg., *50-A:*1353, 1968.

217. Cholmeley, J. A.: Hallux valgus in adolescents. Proc. Roy. Soc. Med. (Section of Orthopedics), *51:*903, 1958.

218. Ellis, V. H.: A method of correcting metatarsus primus varus. Preliminary report. J. Bone Joint Surg., *33-B:*415, 1951.

219. Haines, R. W., and McDougall, A.: The anatomy of hallux valgus. J. Bone Joint Surg., *36-B:*272, 1954.

220. Hardy, R. H., and Clapham, J. C. R.: Observations on hallux valgus. Based on controlled series. J. Bone Joint Surg., *33-B:*376, 1951.

221. Hardy, R. H., and Clapham, J. C. R.: Hallux valgus. Predisposing anatomic causes. Lancet, *1:*1180, 1952.

222. Jones, A. R.: Hallux valgus in the adolescent. Proc. Roy. Soc. Med. (Section of Orthopedics), *41:*392, 1948.

223. Keller, W. L.: Surgical treatment of bunion and hallux valgus. New York Med. J., *80:*741, 1904.

224. Keller, W. L.: Further observations on the surgical treatment of hallux valgus and bunions. New York Med. J., *95:*696, 1912.

225. Kelikian, H.: Hallux Valgus, Allied Deformities of the Forefoot and Metatarsalgia. Philadelphia, W. B. Saunders Co., 1965.

226. Lapidus, P. W.: Operative correction of the metatarsus varus primus in hallux valgus. Surg. Gynec. Obstet., *58:*183, 1934.

227. McBride, E. D.: A conservative operation for bunions. J. Bone Joint Surg., *10:*735, 1928.

228. McBride, E. D.: Hallux valgus, bunion deformity; its treatment in mild, moderate and severe stages. J. Int. Coll. Surg., *21:*99, 1954.

229. McBride, E. D.: The McBride bunion hallux valgus operation. Refinements in the successive surgical steps of the operation. J. Bone Joint Surg., *42-A:*965, 1960.

230. Mitchell, C. L., Fleming, J. L., Allen, R., Glenney, C., and Sanford, G. A.: Osteotomy-bunionectomy for hallux valgus. J. Bone Joint Surg., *40-A:*41, 1958.

231. Piggott, H.: The natural history of hallux valgus in adolescence and early adult life. J. Bone Joint Surg., *42-B:*749, 1960.

232. Silver, D.: The operative treatment of hallux valgus. J. Bone Joint Surg., *5:*225, 1923.

233. Simmonds, F. A., and Menelaus, M. B.: Hallux valgus in adolescents. J. Bone Joint Surg., *42-B:*761, 1960.

TARSAL COALITION

234. Anderson, R. J.: The presence of an astragalo-scaphoid bone in man. J. Anat. Physiol., *14:*452, 1880.

235. Anthonsen, W.: An oblique projection for roentgen examination of the talo-calcanean joint, particularly regarding intra-articular fracture of the calcaneus. Acta Radiol., *24:*306, 1943.

236. Austin, F. H.: Symphalangism and related fusions of tarsal bones. Radiology, *56:*882, 1951.

237. Badgley, C. E.: Coalition of the calcaneus and the navicular. Arch. Surg., *15:*75, 1927.

238. Bargellini, D.: Fusione calcaneo-cuboidea e piede piatoo. Arch. Ital. Chir., *21:*386, 1928.

239. Basu, S. S.: Naviculo-cuneo-metatarso-phalangeal synostoses. Indian J. Surg., *25:*750, 1963.

240. Bentzon, P. G. K.: Bilateral congenital deformity of the astragalocalcanean joint. Coalition calcaneonavicularis, mit besonderer Bezugnahme auf die operative Behandlung des durch diese Anomalie bedingten Plattfüsses. Verh. Deutsch. Orthop. Ges., *23:*269, 1929.

241. Bersani, F. A., and Samilson, R. L.: Massive familial tarsal synostosis. J. Bone Joint Surg., *39-A:*1187, 1957.

242. Blockey, N. J.: Peroneal spastic flat foot. J. Bone Joint Surg., *37-B:*191, 1955.

243. Boyd, H. B.: Congenital talonavicular synostosis. J. Bone Joint Surg., *26:*682, 1944.

244. Braddock, G. T. F.: A prolonged follow-up of peroneal spastic flat foot. J. Bone Joint Surg., *43-B:*734, 1961.

245. Brobeck, O.: Congenital bilateral synostosis of the calcaneus and cuboid and of the triquetral and hamate bones: Report of a case. Acta Orthop. Scand., *26:*217, 1957.

246. Bullitt, J. B.: Variations of the bones of the foot. Fusion of the talus and navicular, bilateral and congenital. Amer. J. Roentgen., *20:*548, 1928.

247. Chambers, C. H.: Congenital anomalies of the tarsal navicular with particular reference to calcaneo-navicular coalition. Brit. J. Radiol., *23:*580, 1950.

248. Conway, J. J., and Cowell, H. R.: Tarsal coalition: Clinical significance and roentgenographic demonstration. Radiology, *92:*799, 1969.

249. Cowell, H. R.: Extensor brevis arthroplasty. J. Bone Joint Surg., *52-A:*820, 1970, and personal communication.

250. Cruveilhier, J.: Anatomie Pathologique du Corps Humain. Tome I. 1829.

251. Del Sel, J. M., and Grand, N. E.: Cubonavicular synostosis: A rare tarsal synostosis. J. Bone Joint Surg., *41-B:*149, 1959.

252. Demarchi, E., Gambier, R., and Vespignani, L.: Les synostoses tarsiennes dans le pied plat valgus douloureux. J. Radiol., *36:*665, 1955.

253. Devoldere, J.: A case of familial congenital synostosis in the carpal and tarsal bones. Arch. Chir. Neerland., *12:*185, 1960.

254. Dwight, T.: A Clinical Atlas. Variations of the Bones of the Hands and Feet. Philadelphia, J. B. Lippincott Co., 1907.

255. Feist, J. H., and Mankin, H. J.: The tarsus. Radiology, *79:*250, 1962.

256. Gaynor, S. S.: Congenital astragalocalcaneal fusion. J. Bone Joint Surg., *18:*479, 1936.

257. Glessner, J. R., Jr., and Davis, G. L.: Bilateral calcaneonavicular coalition occurring in twin boys. A case report. Clin. Orthop., *47:*173, 1966.

258. Grashey, R.: Articulatio talo-calcanea (Os sustentaculi). Röntgenpraxis, *14:*139, 1942.

259. Hall, M. C.: The normal movement at the sub-talar joint. Canad. J. Surg., *2:*287, 1959.

260. Hark, F. W.: Congenital anomalies of the tarsal bones. Clin. Orthop., *16:*21, 1960.

261. Harle, T. S., and Stevenson, J. R.: Hereditary symphalangism associated with carpal and tarsal fusions. Radiology, *89:*91, 1967.

262. Harris, B. A.: Anomalous structures in the developing human foot (Abstract). Anat. Rec., *121*:399, 1955. (Original thesis in University of California library.)

263. Harris, R. I.: Rigid valgus foot due to talocalcaneal bridge. J. Bone Joint Surg., *37-A*:169, 1955.

264. Harris, R. I.: Peroneal spastic flat foot. A.A.O.S. Instructional Course Lectures. Vol. 15. Ann Arbor, J. W. Edwards, 1958, p. 116.

265. Harris, R. I.: Retrospect: Peroneal spastic flat foot (rigid valgus foot). J. Bone Joint Surg., *47-A*:1657, 1965.

266. Harris, R. I., and Beath, T.: Army foot survey. Ottawa. National Research Council of Canada, *44*, 1947.

267. Harris, R. I., and Beath, T.: Etiology of peroneal spastic flat foot. J. Bone Joint Surg., *30-B*:624, 1948.

268. Harris, R. I., and Beath, T.: John Hunter's specimen of talocalcaneal bridge. J. Bone Joint Surg., *32-B*:203, 1950.

269. Hayek, W.: Synostosis talonavicularis. Z. Orthop. Chir., *69*:231, 1934.

270. Heikel, H. V. A.: Coalition calcaneo-navicularis and calcaneus secundarius. A clinical and radiographic study of twenty-three patients. Acta Orthop. Scand., *32*:72, 1962.

271. Hodgson, F. G.: Talonavicular synostosis. Southern Med. J., *39*:940, 1946.

272. Holl, M.: Beiträge zur chirurgischen Osteologie des Füsses. Arch. Klin. Chir., *25*:211, 1880.

273. Isherwood, I.: A radiological approach to the subtalar joint. J. Bone Joint Surg., *43-B*:566, 1961.

274. Jack, E. A.: Bone anomalies of the tarsus in relation to "peroneal spastic flat foot." J. Bone Joint Surg., *36-B*:530, 1954.

275. Jaubert De Beaujeu, A., and Benmussa: Synostose, astragalo-scaphoïdienne congenitale, bilaterale et isolée. J. Radiol. Electrol., *23*:348, 1939.

276. Johansoon, S.: A case of congenital ankylosis of the ankle joints and other malformations. Acta Orthop. Scand., *5*:231, 1934.

277. Jones, R.: Peroneal spasm and its treatment. Report of meeting of Liverpool Medical Institution held 22nd April, 1897. Liverpool Med. Chir. J., *17*:442, 1897.

278. Jones, R.: The soldier's foot and the treatment of common deformities of the foot. Brit. Med. J., *1*:709, 1916.

279. Kadelbach, G.: Ein Beiträg zu den Fusswurzelsynostosen. Arch. Orthop. Unfallchir., *40*:363, 1940.

280. Kendrick, J. I.: Treatment of calcaneonavicular bar. J.A.M.A., *172*:1242, 1960.

281. Kirmisson, E.: Double pied bot varus par malformation osseuse primitive associé á des ankyloses congenitales des doigts et des orteils chez quatre membres d'une même famille. Rev. Orthop., *9*:392, 1898.

282. Korvin, K.: Coalition Talocalcanea. Z. Orthop. Chir., *60*:105, 1934.

283. Kozlowski, K.: Hypoplasie bilaterale congénitale du cubitus et synostose bilaterale calcaneocuboide chez une fillette. Ann. Radiol., *8*:389, 1965.

284. LaGrange, M.: Anomalie du pied. Soudure des os du tarse et du metatarse. Progr. Med., *10*:367, 1882.

285. Lapidus, P. W.: Bilateral congenital talonavicular fusion. Report of a case. J. Bone Joint Surg., *20*:775, 1938.

286. Lapidus, P. W.: Spastic flat foot. J. Bone Joint Surg., *28*:126, 1946.

287. Lissoos, I., and Soussi, J.: Tarsal synostosis with partial adactylia. Med. Proc., *11*:224, 1965.

288. Lusby, H. L. J.: Naviculo-cuneiform synostosis. J. Bone Joint Surg., *41-B*:150, 1959.

289. Mahaffey, H. W.: Bilateral congenital calcaneocuboid synostosis. Case report. J. Bone Joint Surg., *27*:164, 1945.

290. Maudsley, R. S.: Spastic pes varus. Proc. Roy. Soc. Med., *49*:181, 1956.

291. Miller, E. M.: Congenital ankylosis of joints of hands and feet. J. Bone Joint Surg., *4*:560, 1922.

292. Mitchell, G. P., and Gibson, J. M. C.: Excision of calcaneo-navicular bar for painful spasmodic flat foot. J. Bone Joint Surg., *49-B*:281, 1967.

293. Nievergelt, K.: Positiver Vaterschaftsnachweis auf Grund Erbicher mit Bildungen der Extremitaten., Arch. Julius Klaus Stift, *19*:157, 1944.

294. O'Donoghue, D. H., and Sell, L. S.: Congenital talonavicular synostosis. J. Bone Joint Surg., *25*:925, 1943.

295. O'Rahilly, R.: A survey of carpal and tarsal anomalies. J. Bone Joint Surg., *35-A*:626, 1953.

296. O'Rahilly, R.: Gardner, E., and Gray, D. J.: The skeletal development of the foot. Clin. Orthop., *16*:7, 1960.

297. Outland, T., and Murphy, I. D.: Relation of tarsal anomalies to spastic and rigid flat feet. Clin. Orthop., *1*:217, 1953.

298. Outland, T., and Murphy, I. D.: The pathomechanics of peroneal spastic flat foot. Clin. Orthop., *16*:64, 1960.

299. Pearlman, H. S., Edkin, R. E., and Warren, R. F.: Familial tarsal and carpal synostosis with radial head subluxation. J. Bone Joint Surg., *46-A*:585, 1964.

300. Pfitzner, W.: Die Variationen im Aufbar des Fussekelts. Bertrage zur Kenntniss des menschlichen Extremitatenskelets. VII. Morphol. Arbeit., *6*:245, 1896.

301. Rompe, G.: Ankylosen des Unteren Sprunggelenkes nach Offenem Unterschenkelbruch. Arch. Orthop. Unfallchir., *54*:339, 1962.

302. Rothberg, A. S., Feldman, J. W., and Schuster, O. F.: Congenital fusion of astragalus and scaphoid: Bilateral; Inherited. New York J. Med., *35*:29, 1935.

303. Rutt, A.: Zur Genese der Coalitio calcaneo naviculare. Z. Orthop., *96*:96, 1962.

304. Sanghi, J. K., and Roby, H. R.: Bilateral peroneal spastic flat feet associated with congenital fusion of the navicular and talus. A case report. J. Bone Joint Surg., *43-A*:1237, 1961.

305. Schreiber, R. R.: Talonavicular synostosis. J. Bone Joint Surg., *45-A*:170, 1963.

306. Seddon, H. J.: Calcaneo-scaphoid coalition. Proc. Roy. Soc. Med. (Section of Orthopedics), *26*:419, 1932.

307. Shands, A. R., and Wentz, I. J.: Congenital anomalies, accessory bones, and osteochondritis in the feet of 850 children. S. Clin. N. Amer., *33*:1643, 1953.

308. Simmons, E. H.: Spastic tibialis varus with tarsal coalition. J. Bone Joint Surg., *47-B*:533, 1965.

309. Sloane, M. W. M.: A case of anomalous skeletal development in the foot. Anat. Rec., *96*:23, 1946.

310. Slomann, H. C.: On coalitio calcaneo-navicularis. J. Orthop. Surg., *3*:586, 1921.

311. Slomann, H. C.: On the demonstration and analysis of calcaneo-navicular coalition by roentgen examination. Acta Radiol., *5*:304, 1926.

312. Solger, B.: Ueber abnorme Verschmelzung Knorpeliger Skelettheile Beim Fotus. Zbl. Allg. Path., *1*:124, 1890.

313. Sutro, C.: Anomalous talocalcaneal articulation. Cause for limited subtalar movements. Amer. J. Surg., *74*:64, 1947.

314. Trolle, D.: (Trans. by E. Aagesen): Accessory Bones of the Human Foot. Copenhagen, Munksgaard, 1948.

315. Vaughan, W. H., and Segal, G.: Tarsal coalition with special reference to roentgenographic interpretation. Radiology, *60*:855, 1953.

316. Veneruso, L. C.: Unilateral congenital calcaneocuboid synostosis with complete absence of a metatarsal and toe. Case report. J. Bone Joint Surg., *27*:718, 1945.

317. Wagoner, G. W.: A case of bilateral congenital fusion of the calcanei and cuboids. J. Bone Joint Surg., *10*:220, 1928.

318. Waugh, W.: Partial cubo-navicular coalition as a cause of peroneal spastic flat foot. J. Bone Joint Surg., *39-B*:520, 1957.

319. Webster, F. S., and Roberts, W. M.: Tarsal anomalies and peroneal spastic flat foot. J.A.M.A., *146*:1099, 1951.

320. Wray, J. B., and Herndon, C. N.: Hereditary transmission of congenital coalition of the calcaneus to the navicular. J. Bone Joint Surg., *45-A*:365, 1963.

321. Zock, E.: Ein Beiträg zu den Synostosen der Fusswurzel. Zbl. Chir., *78*:845, 1953.

322. Zuckerkandl, E.: Ueber einen Fall von Synostose zwischen Talus und Calcaneus. Allg. Wein. Med. Zeitung., *22*:293, 1877.

CONGENITAL CONVEX PES VALGUS

323. Armknecht, P.: Orthopädische Lieden bei Zwillingen. Verh. Deutsche. Orthop. Ges., *26*:62, 1931.

324. Aschner, B., and Engelmann, G.: Konstitutronspathologie in der Orthopädie. Erbbiologie des peripheren Bewegungsapparates. Vienna, Julius Springer, 1928.

325. Bender, G., and Horvath, F.: Uber eine seltene Entwicklungsanomalie des Talus und des Os haviculare pedis. Fortschr. Rontgenstr., *94*:281, 1961.

326. Berman, J. L., Rankin, J. K., Harrison, P. A., Donovan, D. J., Hogan, W. J., and Bearn, A. O.: Autosomal trisomy of a group 16–18 chromosome. J. Pediat., *60*:503, 1962.

327. Böhm, M.: Der Kongenitale Plattfuss. Zbl. Chir., pp. 2987–2990, 1932.

328. Camera, V.: A proposito del piedo piatoo valgo congenito. Arch. Ortop., *42*:432, 1926.

329. Coleman, S. S., Martin, A. F., and Jarrett, J.: Congenital vertical talus: Pathogenesis and treatment. J. Bone Joint Surg., *48-A*:1442, 1966.

330. Coleman, S., Stelling, F. H., and Jarrett, J.: Pathomechanics and treatment of congenital vertical talus. Clin. Orthop., *70*:62, 1970.

331. Drennan, J. C., and Sharrard, W. J. W.: The pathologic anatomy of convex pes valgus. J. Bone Joint Surg., *53-B*:455, 1971.

332. Eyre-Brook, A.: Congenital vertical talus. J. Bone Joint Surg., *49-B*:618, 1967.

333. Grice, D. S.: The role of subtalar fusion in the treatment of valgus deformities of the feet. A.A.O.S. Instructional Course Lectures. Vol. 16. St. Louis, C. V. Mosby Co., 1959, p. 127.

334. Gunz, E.: Die pathologische Anatomie der angeborenen Plattfusses. Z. Orthop., *69*:219, 1939.

335. Haliburton, R. A., Sullivan, C. R., Kelly, P., and Peterson, L. F. A.: The extra-osseous and intra-osseous blood supply of the talus. J. Bone Joint Surg., *40-A*:1115, 1958.

336. Hark, F. W.: Rocker-foot due to congenital subluxation of the talus. J. Bone Joint Surg., *32-A*:344, 1950.

337. Harrold, A. J.: Congenital vertical talus in infancy. J. Bone Joint Surg., *49-B*:634, 1967.

338. Haveson, S. B.: Congenital flatfoot due to talonavicular dislocation (vertical talus). Radiology, *72*:19, 1959.

339. Henken, R.: Contribution à l'etude des formes osseuses du pied plat valgus congénital. Thèse de Lyon, 1914.

340. Herndon, C. H., and Heyman, C. H.: Problems in the recognition and treatment of congenital convex pes valgus. J. Bone Joint Surg., *45-A*:413, 1963.

341. Heyman, C. H.: The diagnosis and treatment of congenital convex pes valgus or vertical talus. A.A.O.S. Instructional Course Lectures, Vol. 16. St. Louis, C. V. Mosby Co., 1959, p. 127.

342. Hohman, G.: Fuss und Bern. Munchen, I. F. Bergann, 1934, pp. 26–33.

343. Hughes, J. R.: Congenital vertical talus. J. Bone Joint Surg., *39-B*:580, 1957.

344. Hughes, J. R.: Pathologic anatomy and pathogenesis of congenital vertical talus and its practical significance. J. Bone Joint Surg., *52-B*:777, 1970.

345. Joachimsthal: Ueber pes valgus congenitus. Deutsch. Med. Wschr., *29*:(Vereins-Beilage):123, 1903.

346. Lamy, L., and Weissman, L.: Congenital convex pes valgus. J. Bone Joint Surg., *21*:79, 1939.

347. Lange, F.: Plattfusebeschwerben und Plattfussbehandlung. Munchen. Med. Wschr., *59*:300, 1912.

348. Lloyd-Roberts, G. C., and Spence, A. J.: Congenital vertical talus. J. Bone Joint Surg., *40-B*:33, 1958.

349. Mau, C.: Muskelbefunde und ihre Bedeutung beim angeborenen Klumpfussleiden. Arch. Orthop. Unfallchir., *28*:292, 1930.

350. Mead, N. C., and Anast, G.: Vertical talus. Clin. Orthop., *21*:198, 1961.

351. Nové-Josserand: Formes anatomiques du pied plat. Rev. Orthop., *10*:117, 1923.

352. Osmond-Clarke, H.: Congenital vertical talus. J. Bone Joint Surg., *38-B*:334, 1956.

353. Outland, T., and Hserk, H. H.: Congenital vertical talus. A.A.O.S. Instructional Course Lectures. Vol. 16. St. Louis, C. V. Mosby Co., 1959, p. 214.

354. Parrish, T. F.: Congenital convex pes valgus accompanied by previously undescribed anatomic derangements. Southern Med. J., *60*:983, 1967.

355. Patterson, W. R., Fitz, D. A., and Smith, W. S.: The pathologic anatomy of congenital convex pes valgus. J. Bone Joint Surg., *50-A*:458, 1968.

356. Rocher, H. L., and Pouyanne, L.: Pied plat congénital par subluxation sous-astragalienne congénitale et orientation verticale de l'astragale. Bordeaux Chir., *5*:249, 1934.

357. Sharrard, W. J. W., and Grosfield, I.: The management of deformity and paralysis of the foot in myelomeningocele. J. Bone Joint Surg., *50-B*:456, 1968.

358. Sonnenburg: Klumpfuss. *In* Eulenburg: Real-Encylopadie der gesamten Heilkunde, Aufl. 3. Bd 12, s. 368. Wein, Urban and Schwarzenberg, 1897.

359. Stone, K. H., and Lloyd-Roberts, G. C.: Congenital vertical talus: A new operation. Proc. Roy. Soc. Med., *56*:12, 1963.

360. Storen, H.: On the closed and open correction of congenital convex pes valgus with a vertical astragalus. Acta Orthop. Scand., *36*:352, 1965.

361. Storen, H.: Congenital convex pes valgus with vertical talus. Acta Orthop. Scand. Suppl., *94*:1, 1967.

362. Towns, P. L., Dettart, G. K., Hecht, F., and Manning, J A.: Trisomy 13-15 in a male infant. J. Pediat., *60*:528, 1962.

363. Uchida, I. A., Lewis, A. J., Bowman, J. M., and Wang, H. C.: A case of double trisomy No. 18 and Triple X. J. Pediat., *60*:498, 1962.

364. Wainwright, D.: The recognition and cure of congenital flat foot. Proc. Roy. Soc. Med., *57*:357, 1964.

CONGENITAL BALL-AND-SOCKET JOINT

365. Brahme, F.: Upper talar enarthrosis. Acta Radiol, *55*:221, 1961.

366. Jacobs, P.: Some uncommon deformities of the ankle and foot. Brit. J. Radiol., *35*:776, 1962.

367. Lamb, D.: The ball-and-socket ankle joint. J. Bone Joint Surg., *40-B*:240, 1958.

368. Robins, R. H. G.: The ankle joint in relation to arthrodesis of the foot in poliomyelitis. J. Bone Joint Surg., *41-B*:337, 1959.

369. Schreiber, R. R.: Congenital and acquired ball-and-socket ankle joint. Radiology, *84*:940, 1963.

370. Weston, W. J.: Congenital ball and socket ankle joint. Brit. J. Radiol., *35*:871, 1962.

METATARSUS PRIMUS ATAVICUS (CONGENITAL SHORT FIRST METATARSAL)

371. Harris, R. I., and Beath, T.: Report 1574, Army Foot Survey. Ottawa, National Research Council of Canada, 1947.

372. Harris, R. I., and Beath, T.: The short first metatarsal. J. Bone Joint Surg., *31-A*:553, 1949.

373. Morton, D.: The Human Foot. New York, Columbia University Press, 1935.

CONGENITAL HALLUX VARUS

374. Farmer, A. W.: Congenital hallux varus. Amer. J. Surg., *95*:274, 1958.

375. Kelikian, H., Clayton, L., and Loseff, H.: Surgical syndactylism of the toes. Clin. Orthop., *19:*208, 1961.
376. McElvenny, R. T.: Hallux varus. Quart. Bull. Northwest. Med. Sch., *15:*277, 1941.
377. Thomson, S. A.: Hallux varus and metatarsus varus. Clin. Orthop., *16:*109, 1960.

CONGENITAL SPLIT OR CLEFT FOOT (LOBSTER CLAW)

378. Barsky, A. J.: Cleft hand: Classification, incidence and treatment. J. Bone Joint Surg., *46-A:*1707, 1964.
379. Cowan, R. J.: Surgical problems associated with congenital malformations of the forefoot. Canad. J. Surg., *8:*29, 1965.
380. Lewis, T., and Embleton, D.: Split-hand and split-foot deformities, their types, origin and transmission. Biometrika, *6:*26, 1908.
381. McMullen, G., and Pearson, K.: On the inheritance of the deformity known as split foot or lobster claw. Biometrika, *9:*381, 1913.
382. Meyerding, H. W., and Upshaw, J. E.: Heredofamilial cleft foot deformity (lobster-claw or split foot). Amer. J. Surg., *74:*889, 1947.
383. Phillips, R. S.: Congenital split foot (lobster claw) and triphalangeal thumb. J. Bone Joint Surg., *53-B:*247, 1971.
384. Potter, E. L., and Nadelhoffer, L.: A familial lobster claw. J. Hered., *38:*331, 1947.
385. Stiles, K. A., and Pickard, I. S.: Hereditary malformations of the hands and feet. J. Hered., *34:*341, 1943.
386. Vogel, F.: Verzogerte Mutation Beim Mescchen. Einige Kritische Bemerkungen zu ch. Auberbachs Arbeit. Ann. Hum. Genet., *22:*132, 1958.
387. Walker, J. C., and Clodius, L.: The syndromes of cleft lip, cleft palate and lobster-claw deformities of hands and feet. Plast. Reconstr. Surg., *32:*627, 1963.

PES CAVUS

388. Alvik, I.: Operative treatment of pes cavus. Acta Orthop. Scand., *23:*137, 1953.
389. Barenfeld, P. A., Weseley, M. S., and Shea, J. M.: The congenital cavus foot. Clin. Orthop., *79:*119, 1971.
390. Barwell, R.: Pes planus and pes cavus: An anatomical and clinical study. Edinburgh Med. J., *3:*113, 1898.
391. Bentzon, P. G. K.: Pes cavus and the m. peroneus longus. Acta Orthop. Scand., *4:*50, 1933.
392. Bertrand, P.: Discussion. Symposium—Le Pied Creux Essentiel and Meary, P. Rev. Chir. Orthop., *53:*423, 1967.
393. Beykirch, A.: Ein Beitrag zur Atiologie und Therapie des Klanenhohlfusses. A. Orthop. Chir., *52:*41, 1929.
394. Brewerton, D. A., Sandifer, P. H., and Sweetman, D. R.: "Idiopathic" pes cavus, an investigation of its etiology. Brit. Med. J., *5358:*659, 1963.
395. Brockway, A.: Surgical correction of talipes cavus deformities. J. Bone Joint Surg., *22:*895, 1940.
396. Cole, W. H.: The treatment of claw-foot. J. Bone Joint Surg., *22:*895, 1940.
397. Coonrad, R. W., Irwin, C. E., Gucker, T., III, and Wray, J. B.: The importance of plantar muscles in paralytic varus feet; results of treatment by neurectomy and myoneurectomy. J. Bone Joint Surg., *38-A:*563, 1956.
398. Duchenne, G. B.: Physiology of Motion. (Translated and edited by E. B. Kaplan). Philadelphia, W. B. Saunders Co., 1959, p. 384.
399. Dwyer, F. C.: Osteotomy of the calcaneum for pes cavus. J. Bone Joint Surg., *41-B:*80, 1959.
400. Fowler, B., Brooks, A. L., and Parrish, T. F.: The cavovarus foot. *In* Proceedings of Amer. Acad. Orthop. Surg. J. Bone Joint Surg., *41-A:*757, 1959.
401. Frank, G. R., and Johnson, W. M.: The extensor shift procedure in the correction of clawtoe defromities in children. Southern Med. J., *59:*889, 1966.
402. Garceau, G. J., and Brahms, M. A.: A preliminary study of selective plantar-muscle denervation for pes cavus. J. Bone Joint Surg., *38-A:*553, 1956.

403. Hallgrimsson, S.: Pes cavus, seine Behandlung und einige Bennerkungen über seine Aetiologie. Acta Orthop. Scand., *10:*73, 1939.
404. Hammond, G.: Elevation of the first metatarsal bone with hallux equinus. Surgery, *13:*240, 1943.
405. Heyman, C. H.: The operative treatment of clawfoot. J. Bone Joint Surg., *14:*335, 1932.
406. Hibbs, R. A.: An operation for "claw-foot." J.A.M.A., *73:*1583, 1919.
407. Hughes, W. K.: Talipes cavus. Brit. Med. J., *2:*902, 1940.
408. Ingelrans, P.: Discussion-Symposium—Le Pied Creux Essentiel. Ed. Meary, R. Rev. Chir. Orthop., *53:*422, 1967.
409. Japas, L. M.: Surgical treatment of pes cavus by tarsal V-osteotomy. Preliminary report. J. Bone Joint Surg., *50-A:*927, 1968.
410. Jones, R.: The soldier's foot and the treatment of common deformities of the foot. Part II: Claw-foot. Brit. Med. J., *1:*749, 1916.
411. Kelikian, H.: Hallux Valgus, Allied Deformities of the Forefoot, and Metatarsalgia. Philadelphia, W. B. Saunders Co., 1965, p. 305.
412. Kleinberg, S., Horwitz, T., and Sobel, R.: Pes cavus. Bull. Hosp. Joint Dis., *10:*252, 1949.
413. Lambrinudi, C.: An operation for claw-toes. Proc. Roy. Soc. Med., *21:*239, 1927.
414. McElvenny, R. T., and Caldwell, G. D.: A new operation for correction of cavus foot. Fusion of first metatarsocuneiform-navicular joints. Clin. Orthop., *11:*85, 1958.
415. Meary, R.: Le pied creux essentiel. Symposium. Rev. Chir. Orthop., *53:*389–467, 1967.
416. Mills, G. P.: The etiology and treatment of claw foot. J. Bone Joint Surg., *6:*142, 1924.
417. Parkin, A.: Causation and mode of production of pes cavus. Brit. Med. J., *1:*1285, 1891.
418. Rütt, A.: Der Hohlfuss. *In* Handbuch der Orthopädie. Bd. IV/2. 1068–1095. Stuttgart, 1961.
419. Saunders, J. T.: Etiology and treatment of clawfoot. Arch. Surg., *30:*179, 1935.
420. Scheer, G. E., and Crego, C. H., Jr.: A two-stage stabilization procedure for correction of calcaneocavus. J. Bone Joint Surg., *38-A:*1247, 1956.
421. Schnepp, K. H.: Hammer-toe and claw-foot. Amer. J. Surg., *36:*351, 1937.
422. Sell, L. S.: Pes cavus. Spectator Correspondence Club Letter. Dec. 11, 1961.
423. Sherman, H. M.: The operative treatment of pes cavus. Amer. J. Orthop. Surg., *2:*374, 1904–1905.
424. Siffert, R. S., Forster, R. I., and Nachamie, B.: "Beak" triple arthrodesis for correction of severe cavus deformity. Clin. Orthop., *45:*101, 1966.
425. Steindler, A.: Stripping of the os calcis. J. Orthop. Surg., *2:*8, 1920.
426. Steindler, A.: The treatment of pes cavus. Arch. Surg., *2:*325, 1921.
427. Taylor, R. G.: The treatment of claw toes by multiple transfer of flexors into extensor tendons. J. Bone Joint Surg., *33-B:*539, 1951.

PRONATED FEET

428. Basmajian, J. V., and Stecko, G.: The role of muscles in arch support of the foot. An electromyographic study. J. Bone Joint Surg., *45-A:*1184, 1963.
429. Bettmann, E.: The treatment of flat-foot by means of exercise. J. Bone Joint Surg., *19:*821, 1937.
430. Butte, F. L.: Navicular-cuneiform arthrodesis for flatfoot. J. Bone Joint Surg., *19:*496, 1937.
431. Chambers, E. F. S.: An operation for correction of flexible flat feet of adolescents. Western J. Surg., *54:*77, 1946.
432. Chandler, F. A.: Children's feet, normal and presenting common abnormalities. Amer. J. Dis. Child., *63:*1136, 1942.
433. Clark, W. A.: A rebalancing operation for pronated feet. J. Bone Joint Surg., *13:*867, 1931.

434. Crego, C. H., Jr., and Ford, L. T.: An end-result study of various operative procedures for correcting flat feet in children. J. Bone Joint Surg., *34-A*:183, 1952.

435. Grice, D. S.: An extra-articular arthrodesis of the subastragalar joint for correction of paralytic flat-feet in children. J. Bone Joint Surg., *34-A*:927, 1952.

436. Haraldsson, S.: Pes plano-valgus staticus juvenilis and its operative treatment. Acta Orthop. Scand., *35*:234, 1965.

437. Harris, R. I., and Beath, T.: Hypermobile flat-foot with short tendo achillis. J. Bone Joint Surg., *30-A*:116, 1948.

438. Helfet, A. J.: A new way of treating flat feet in children. Lancet, *1*:262, 1956.

439. Hicks, J. H.: The function of the plantar aponeurosis. J. Anat., *85*:414, 1951.

440. Hicks, J. H.: The mechanics of the foot. I. The joints. J. Anat., *87*:343, 1953.

441. Hicks, J. H.: The mechanics of the foot. II. The plantar aponeurosis and the arch. J. Anat., *88*:25, 1954.

442. Hoke, M.: An operation for the correction of extremely relaxed flat feet. J. Bone Joint Surg., *13*:773, 1931.

443. Jack, E. A.: Naviculocuneiform fusion in the treatment of flat-foot. J. Bone Joint Surg., *35*:75, 1953.

444. Koutsogiannis, E.: Treatment of mobile flat foot by displacement of osteotomy of calcaneus. J. Bone Joint Surg., *53-B*:96, 1971.

445. Leavitt, D. G.: Subastragaloid arthrodesis for the os calcis type of flat-foot. Amer. J. Surg., *59*:501, 1943.

446. Leonard, M. H., Gonzolez, S., Beck, L. W., Basom, C., Palafox, M., and Kosick, Z. W.: Lateral transfer of posterior tibial tendon in certain selected cases of pes planovalgus. Clin. Orthop., *40*:139, 1965.

447. Lowman, C. L.: An operative method for correction of certain forms of flat foot. J.A.M.A., *81*:1500, 1923.

448. Lowman, C. L.: The treatment of flat foot. Orthopedic Correspondence Club Letter, 1941.

449. Miller, O. L.: A plastic flat foot operation. J. Bone Joint Surg., *9*:84, 1927.

450. Purvis, G. D.: Surgery of the relaxed flat foot. Clin. Orthop., *57*:221, 1968.

451. Rose, G. K.: Correction of the pronated foot. J. Bone Joint Surg., *40-B*:674, 1958.

452. Rose, G. K.: Correction of the pronated foot. J. Bone Joint Surg., *44-B*:642, 1962.

453. Rugtveit, A.: Extra-articular subtalar arthrodesis according to Green-Grice in flat feet. Acta Orthop. Scand., *34*:367, 1964.

454. Seymour, N.: The late results of naviculo-cuneiform fusion. J. Bone Joint Surg., *49-B*:558, 1967.

455. Seymour, N., and Evans, D. K.: A modification of the Grice subtalar arthrodesis. J. Bone Joint Surg., *50-B*:372, 1968.

456. Young, C. S.: Operative treatment of pes planus. Surg. Gynec. Obstet., *68*:1099, 1939.

457. Zadek, I.: Transverse wedge arthrodesis for the relief of pain in rigid flat-foot. J. Bone Joint Surg., *17*:453, 1935.

HALLUX RIGIDUS

458. Bingold, A. C., and Collins, D. H.: Hallux rigidus. J. Bone Joint Surg., *32-B*:214, 1950.

459. Bonney, G., and MacNab, I.: Hallux valgus and hallux rigidus. A critical survey of operative results. J. Bone Joint Surg., *34-B*:366, 1952.

460. Breitenfelder, G.: Hallux rigidus Jugendlicher. Verh. Deutsch. Orthop. Ges., *80*:313, 1951.

461. Cochrane, W. A.: An operation for hallux rigidus. Brit. Med. J., *1*:1095, 1927.

462. Cotterill, J. M.: On the condition of stiff great toe in adolescents. Edinburgh, Trans. Med. Chir. Soc., 1886–87, p. 277.

463. Davies-Colley, N.: On contraction of the metatarsophalangeal joint of the great toe (hallux flexus). Trans. Clin. Soc. London, *20*:165, 1887.

464. Glissan, D. J.: Hallux valgus and hallux rigidus. Med. J. Aust., *2*:585, 1946.

465. Harrison, M. H. M., and Harvey, F. J.: Arthrodesis of the first metatarsophalangeal joint for hallux valgus and rigidus. J. Bone Joint Surg., *45-A*:471, 1963.

466. Jack, E. A.: The aetiology of hallux rigidus. Brit. J. Surg., *27*:492, 1940.

467. Jansen, M.: Hallux valgus, rigidus and malleus. J. Orthop. Surg., *3*:27, 1921.

468. Kelikian, H.: Hallux Valgus, Allied Deformities of the Forefoot, and Metatarsalgia. Philadelphia, W. B. Saunders Co., 1965, p. 273.

469. Kessel, L., and Bonney, G.: Hallux rigidus in the adolescent. J. Bone Joint Surg., *40-B*:668, 1958.

470. Kingreen, O.: Zur Aetiologie des Hallux flexus. Zbl. Chir., *60*:2116, 1933.

471. Lambrinudi, C.: Metatarsus primus elevatus. Proc. Roy. Soc. Med. (Section of Orthopaedics), *31*:1273, 1938.

472. McMurray, T. P.: The treatment of hallux valgus and rigidus. Brit. Med. J., *2*:218, 1936.

473. Moynihan, F. J.: Arthrodesis of the metatarsophalangeal joint of the great toe. J. Bone Joint Surg., *49-B*:544, 1967.

474. Nilsonne, H.: Hallux rigidus and its treatment. Acta Orthop. Scand., *1*:295, 1930.

475. Severin, E.: Removal of the base of the proximal phalanx in hallux rigidus. Acta Orthop. Scand., *17*:77, 1947.

476. Steinhauser, W.: Osteochondrose der basalen epiphyse der Grundphalanx, Grosszehe und Hallus rigidus. Beitr. Ges. Orthop., *6*:177, 1959.

477. Walsham, W. J., and Hughes, W. K.: The deformities of the human foot. London, Bailliere, Tindall and Cox, 1895, pp. 512–514.

478. Watermann, H.: Die Arthritis deformans Grosszehengrundgelenkes. Z. Orthop. Chir., *48*:346, 1927.

479. Watson-Jones, R.: Treatment of hallux rigidus. Brit. Med. J., *1*:1165, 1927.

HAMMER TOE

480. Ely, L. W.: Hammertoe. Surg. Clin. N. Amer., *6*:433, 1926.

481. Glassman, F., Wallin, L., and Sideman, S.: Phalangectomy for toe deformities. Surg. Clin. N. Amer., *29*:275, 1949.

482. Jones, R.: Notes on Military Orthopaedics. New York, P. B. Hoeber, 1917, pp. 38–57.

483. Krenz, L.: Die Hammerzehen und ihre Operation nacht Bocht. Arch. Orthop. Unfallchir., *21*:459, 1923.

484. Lapidus, P. W.: Operation for correction of hammertoe. J. Bone Joint Surg., *21*:977, 1939.

485. Merrill, W. J.: Conservative operative treatment of hammertoe. Amer. J. Orthop. Surg., *10*:262, 1912.

486. Michele, A. A., and Krueger, F. J.: Operative correction for hammertoe. Mil. Surg., *103*:52, 1948.

487. Milgram, J. E.: Office measures for relief of painful foot. J. Bone Joint Surg., *46*:1095, 1964.

488. O'Neil, J.: An arthroplastic operation for hammertoe. J.A.M.A., *57*:1207, 1911.

489. Sehig, S.: Hammertoe: A new procedure for its correction. Surg. Gynec. Obstet., *72*:101, 1941.

490. Soule, R. E.: Operation for the cure of hammertoe. New York Med. J., *91*:649, March 26, 1910.

491. Taylor, R. G.: An operative procedure for the treatment of hammer toe and claw toe. J. Bone Joint Surg., *22*:608, 1940.

492. Trethowan, W. H.: The treatment of hammertoe. Lancet, *1*:1257–1312, 1925.

493. Young, C. S.: An operation for correction of hammertoe and claw toe. J. Bone Joint Surg., *20*:715, 1938.

CLAW TOES

494. Dickson, F. D., and Dively, R. L.: Operation for correction of mild claw foot, the result of infantile paralysis. J.A.M.A., *87*:1275, 1926.

495. Forrester-Brown, M. F.: Tendon transplantation for clawing of the great toe. J. Bone Joint Surg., 20:57, 1938.
496. Girdlestone, G. R.: Physiotherapy for hand and foot. Journal of Chartered Society of Physiotherapy, 32:176, 1947.
497. Lambrinudi, C.: An operation for claw-toes. Proc. Roy. Soc. Med., 21:239, 1927.
498. Pyper, J. B.: The flexor-extensor transplant operation for claw toes. J. Bone Joint Surg., 40-B:528, 1958.
499. Taylor, R. G.: The treatment of claw toes by multiple transfers of flexor into extensor tendons. J. Bone Joint Surg., 33-B:539, 1951.

CONGENITAL CURLY (OR VARUS) TOES

500. Kelikian, H.: Hallux Valgus, Allied Deformities of the Forefoot, and Metatarsalgia. Philadelphia, W. B. Saunders Co., 1965, p. 330.
501. Sharrard, W. J. W.: The surgery of deformed toes in children. Brit. J. Clin. Pract., 17:263, 1963.
502. Sweetnam, R.: Congenital curly toes. An investigation into the value of treatment. Lancet, 2:398, 1958.
503. Taylor, R. G.: The treatment of claw toes by multiple transfers of flexor with extensor tendons. J. Bone Joint Surg., 33-B:539, 1951.
504. Trethowan, W. H.: The treatment of hammertoe. Lancet, 1:1257 and 1312, 1925.

CONGENITAL DIGITUS MINIMUS VARUS (CONGENITAL DORSAL OVERRIDING OF FIFTH TOE)

505. Butler, R. W.: Personal communication to J. Cockin, 1964. (See Ref. No. 506.)
506. Cockin, J.: Butler's operation for an overriding fifth toe. J. Bone Joint Surg., 50-B:78, 1968.
507. DuVries, H. L.: Surgery of the Foot. St. Louis, C. V. Mosby Co., 1959, p. 347.
508. Gocht, H., and DeBrunner, H.: Orthopaedische Therapie. Leipzig, F. C. W. Vogel, 1925, p. 238.
509. Goodwin, F. C., and Swisher, F. M.: The treatment of congenital hyperextension of the great toe. J. Bone Joint Surg., 25:193, 1943.
510. Kelikian, H.: Hallux Valgus, Allied Deformities of the Forefoot, and Metatarsalgia. Philadelphia, W. B. Saunders Co., 1965.
511. Kelikian, H., Clayton, L., and Loseff, H.: Surgical syndactylia of the toes. Clin. Orthop., 19:208, 1961.
512. Lantzounis, L. A.: Congenital subluxation of the fifth toe and its correction by a periosteocapsuloplasty and tendon transplantation. J. Bone Joint Surg., 22:147, 1940.
513. Lapidus, P. C.: Transplantation of the extensor tendon for correction of the overlapping fifth toe. J. Bone Joint Surg., 24:555, 1942.
514. McFarland, B.: Congenital deformities of the spine and limbs. *In* Platt, H. (ed.): Modern Trends in Orthopedics. New York, P.B. Hoeber, Inc.; London, Butterworth & Co., 1950, p. 107.
515. Ruiz-Mora, J.: Personal communication to L. R. Straub, 1954. (See No. 518.)
516. Scrase, W. H.: The treatment of dorsal adduction deformities of the fifth toe. J. Bone Joint Surg., 36-B:146, 1954.
517. Stamm, T. T.: Surgery of the foot. *In* British Surgical Practice. Vol. IV. London, Butterworth & Co.; St. Louis, C. V. Mosby Co., 1948, p. 160.
518. Straub, L. R.: Orthopedic surgery. *In* Cecil, R. L. (ed.): The Specialties in General Practice. Philadelphia, W. B. Saunders Co., 1951, p. 60.
519. Thompson, C. T.: Surgical treatment of disorders of the fore part of the foot. J. Bone Joint Surg., 46-A:1117, 1964.
520. Wilson, J. N.: V-Y correction for varus deformity of the fifth toe. Brit. J. Surg., 41:133, 1953.

CONGENITAL CONTRACTURE OF TRICEPS SURAE MUSCLE

521. Hall, J. E., Salter, R. B., and Bhalla, S. K.: Congenital short tendo calcaneus. J. Bone Joint Surg., 49-B:695, 1967.

SKIN AND NAIL LESIONS

522. Branson, E. C., and Rhea, R. L., Jr.: Plantar warts. Cure by injection. New Eng. J. Med., 248:631, 1953.
523. Dickson, J. A.: Surgical treatment of intractable plantar warts. J. Bone Joint Surg., 30-A:757, 1948.
524. DuVries, H. L.: New approach to the treatment of intractable verruca plantaris (plantar wart). J.A.M.A., 152:1202, 1953.
525. Heifetz, C. J.: Ingrown toe-nail. Amer. J. Surg., 38:298, 1937.
526. Heifetz, C. J.: Operative management of ingrown toe-nail. J. Missouri Med. Ass., 42:213, 1945.
527. Kopell, H. P., Winokur, J., and Thompson, W. A. L.: Ingrown toe-nail. New concept. New York J. Med., 66:1215, 1966.
528. Lapidus, P. W.: Orthopedic skin lesions of the soles and the toes. Clin. Orthop., 45:87, 1966.
529. McElvenny, R. T.: Corns — their etiology and treatment. Amer. J. Surg., 50:761, 1940.
530. May, H.: The surgical treatment of intractable plantar warts. Surg. Clin. N. Amer., 31:607, 1951.
531. Robinson, D. W.: Treatment of complications of plantar warts. Arch. Surg., 66:434, 1953.

TORSIONAL DEFORMITIES OF THE LOWER LIMBS

532. Appleton, A. B.: Positional deformities and bone growth. An experimental study. Lancet, 1:451, 1934.
533. Arkin, A. M., and Katz, J. F.: Effects of pressure on epiphyseal growth. The mechanism of plasticity of growing bone. J. Bone Joint Surg., 38-A:1056, 1956.
534. Banks, S. W., and Evans, E. A.: Simple transverse osteotomy and threaded pin fixation for controlled correction of torsion deformities of the tibia. J. Bone Joint Surg., 37-A:193, 1955.
535. Bardeen, C. R., and Lewis, W. H.: Development of the limbs, body-wall and back in man. Amer. J. Anat., 1:1, 1901.
536. Bernbeck, R.: Zur pathologischen Anatomie und funktionellen Pathologie der Huftuerrenkung und des Luxationsbeckens. Arch. Orthop. Unfallchir., 45:268, 1952.
537. Blount, W. P.: Bow leg. Wisconsin Med. J., 40:484, 1941.
538. Blount, W. P., and Clarke, G. R.: Control of bone growth by epiphyseal stapling. A preliminary report. J. Bone Joint Surg., 31-A:464, 1949.
539. Blumel, J., Eggers, G. W. N., and Evans, B.: Eight cases of hereditary bilateral medial tibial torsion in four generations. J. Bone Joint Surg., 39-A:1198, 1957.
540. Böhm, M.: Infantile deformities of the knee and hip. J. Bone Joint Surg., 15:574, 1933.
541. Brookes, M., and Wardle, E. N.: Muscle action and the shape of the femur. J. Bone Joint Surg., 44-B:398, 1962.
542. Browne, D.: Congenital malformations. Practitioner, 131:20, 1933.
543. Crane, L.: Femoral torsion and its relation to toeing-in and toeing-out. J. Bone Joint Surg., 11-A:421, 1959.
544. Dega, W.: Ricerche anatomiche e meccaniche sull'anca fetale rivolte a chiarire l'etiologia e la patogenesi della lussazione congenita. Chir. Organi Mov., 18:425, 1933.
545. Delpech, J. M.: De l'orthomorphie, par rapport a l'espece humaine. Paris, Gabon, 1829, p. 301.
546. Dunlap, K., Shands, A. R., Jr., Hollister, L. C., Jr., Gaul, J. S., Jr., and Streit, H. A.: A new method for determination of torsion of the femur. J. Bone Joint Surg., 35-A:289, 1953.
547. Dunn, D. M.: Anteversion of the neck of the femur. J. Bone Joint Surg., 34-B:181, 1952.

548. Dupuis, P. V.: La Torsion Tibiale. Sa Mesure—Son Intérêt Clinique, Radiologique et Chirurgical. Paris, Masson & Cie, 1951.

549. Durham, H. A.: Anteversion of the femoral neck in the normal femur. J.A.M.A., 65:223, 1915.

550. Elftman, H.: Torsion of the lower extremity. Amer. J. Phys. Anthrop., 3:255, 1945.

551. Fitzhugh, M. L.: Faulty alignment of the feet and legs in infancy and childhood. Physioth. Rev., 21:239, 1941.

552. Haas, S. L.: Retardation of bone growth by a wire loop. J. Bone Joint Surg., 27:25, 1945.

553. Harris, N. H.: A method of measurement of femoral neck anteversion and a preliminary report on its practical application. J. Bone Joint Surg., 47-B:188, 1965.

554. Hueter, C.: Anatomische Studien an den Extremitätengelenken Neugeborener und Erwachsener. Virchow. Arch., 25:572, 1862.

555. Hutter, C. G., Jr., and Scott, W.: Tibial torsion. J. Bone Joint Surg., 31-A:511, 1949.

556. Khermosh, O., Lior, G., and Weissman, S. L.: Tibial torsion in children. Clin. Orthop.,79:25, 1971.

557. Kingsley, P. C., and Olmsted, K. L.: A study to determine the angle of anteversion of the neck of the femur. J. Bone Joint Surg., 30-A:745, 1948.

558. Kite, J. H.: Torsion of the lower extremities in small children. J. Bone Joint Surg., 36-A:511, 1954.

559. Kite, J. H.: Torsion of the legs in small children. J. Med. Ass. Georgia, 43:1035, 1954.

560. Kite, J. H.: Flat feet and lateral rotation of legs in young children. J. Int. Coll. Surg., 25:77, 1956.

561. Kite, J. H.: Torsion of the legs in young children. Clin. Orthop., 16:152, 1960.

562. Knight, R. A.: Developmental deformities of the lower extremities. J. Bone Joint Surg., 36-A:521, 1954.

563. Laage, H., Barnett, J. G., Brady, J. M., Dulligan, P. J., Fett, H C , Jr , Gallagher, T. F., and Schneider, B. A.: Horizontal lateral roentgenography of the hip in children. A preliminary report. J. Bone Joint Surg., 35-A:387, 1953.

564. LeDamany, P.: La torsion du tibia, normal, pathologique, expérimentale. J. Anat. Physiol., 45:598, 1909.

565. MacEwen, D.: Personal communication.

566. McSweeny, A.: A study of femoral torsion in children. J. Bone Joint Surg., 53-B:90, 1971.

567. Magilligan, D J : Calculation of the angle of anteversion by means of horizontal lateral roentgenography. J. Bone Joint Surg., 38-A:1231, 1956.

568. Nachlas, I. W.: Medial torsion of the leg. Arch. Surg., 28:909, 1934.

569. Nachlas, I. W.: Common defects of the lower extremity in infants. Southern Med. J., 41:302, 1948.

570. O'Donoghue, D. H.: Controlled rotation osteotomy of the tibia. Southern Med. J., 33:1115, 1940.

571. Pearson, K., and Bell, J.: A study of the long bones of the English skeleton. Draper's Company Research Memoirs. Biometric series X and XI. Part I. London, Cambridge University Press, 1919.

572. Pick, J. W., Stack, J. K., and Anson, B. J.: Measurements on the human femur. I. Length, diameters, and angles. Quart. Bull. Northwest. Med. Sch., 15:281, 1941.

573. Rogers, S. P.: A method for determining the angle of torsion of the neck of the femur. J. Bone Joint Surg., 13:821, 1931.

574. Rogers, S. P.: Observations on torsion of the femur. J. Bone Joint Surg., 16:284, 1934.

575. Rosen, H., and Sandick, H.: Measurement of tibiofibular torsion. J. Bone Joint Surg., 37-A:847, 1955.

576. Ryder, C. T., and Crane, L.: Measuring femoral anteversion: The problem and a method. J. Bone Joint Surg., 35-A:321, 1953.

577. Salter, A. R., Jr., Kostuik, J., and Schatzker, J.: Experimental dysplasia and its reversibility in newborn pigs. J. Bone Joint Surg., 45-A:1781, 1963.

578. Salter, R.: The present state of innominate osteotomy in congenital dislocation of the hip. J. Bone Joint Surg., 48-B:853, 1966.

579. Shands, A. R., Jr., and Steele, M. K.: Torsion of the femur. J. Bone Joint Surg., 40-A:803, 1958.

580. Somerville, E. W.: Persistent foetal alignment. J. Bone Joint Surg., 39-B:106, 1957.

581. Somerville, E. W.: Rotational abnormalities of the lower limbs. J. Bone Joint Surg., 45-B:627, 1963.

582. Soutter, R., and Bradford, E. H.: Twists in normal and in congenital dislocated femora. New York Med. J., 78:1071, 1903.

583. Stewart, S. F., and Karschner, R. G.: Congenital dislocation of the hip. A method of determining the degree of antetorsion of the femoral neck. Amer. J. Roentgen., 15:258, 1926.

584. Swanson, A. B., Greene, P. W., and Allis, H. D.: Rotational deformities of the lower extremity in children and their clinical significance. Clin. Orthop., 27:157, 1963.

585. Thelander, H. E., and Fitzhugh, M. L.: Posture habits in infancy affecting foot and leg alignments. J. Pediat., 21:306, 1942.

586. Volkmann, R.: Chirurgische Erfahrungen uber Knochenverbiegungen und Knochenwacsthum. Arch. Path. Anat., 24:512, 1862.

587. Weinmann, J. P., and Sicher, H.: Bone and Bones. Fundamentals of Bone Biology. St. Louis, C. V. Mosby Co., 1947.

588. Wilkinson, J. A.: Femoral anterversion in the rabbit. J. Bone Joint Surg., 44-B:386, 1962.

589. Wolff, J.: Ueber die inner Architektur der Knochen und ihre Bedeutung fur die Frage von Knochenwachsturm. Virchow. Arch. Path. Anat., 50:389, 1870.

590. Wynne-Davies, R.: Talipes equinovarus. A review of 84 cases after completion of treatment. J. Bone Joint Surg., 46-B:464, 1964.

ANGULAR DEFORMITIES OF THE LONG BONES OF THE LOWER LIMBS

591. Böhm, M.: Infantile deformities of the knee and hip. J. Bone Joint Surg., 15:574, 1933.

592. Brittain, H. A.: Treatment of genu valgum. Brit. Med. J., 2:385, 1948.

593. Caldwell, G. A., Shorkey, R. L., and Duncan, T. L.: Treatment of mild knock knees and pronated feet in childhood (results in 63 cases). N. Orleans Med. Surg. J., 104:304, 1952.

594. Girdlestone, G. R.: Night splint for knock knees. Lancet, 1:312, 1944.

595. Howorth, M. B.: Dynamic posture. J.A.M.A., 131:1938, 1946.

596. Howorth, M. B.: Textbook of Orthopedics. Philadelphia, W. B. Saunders Co., 1951. pp. 199, 301.

597. Howorth, M. B.: Knock knees: With special reference to the stapling operation. Clin. Orthop., 77:233, 1971.

598. Hueck, H.: Osteotomy for genu valgum adolescentium. Deutsch. Z. Chir., 160:245, 1920.

599. Junghans, H.: End results of supracondylar wedge osteotomy of femur for genu valgum. Deutsch. Z. Chir., 209:394, 1928.

600. Kellgren, H. A.: Treatment of postural abnormalities of legs in children. J. Roy. Inst. Public Health, 3:97, 1940.

601. Knight, R. A.: Developmental deformities of the lower extremities. J. Bone Joint Surg., 36-A:521, 1954.

602. Lloyd, E. I.: Night splint for knock knee in children. Brit. Med. J., 1:676, 1939.

603. Lloyd, E. I.: Knock knees and bowlegs. Practitioner, 150:238, 1943.

604. Morley, A. J. M.: Knock knee in children. Brit. Med. J., 2:976, 1957.

605. Morris, H. D.: Treatment of infantile bowlegs and knock knees with special consideration for the therapeutic use of large doses of activated ergosterol. Analysis of 58 cases. Southern Med. J., 44:435, 1951.

606. Parker, C. A.: Treatment of bowlegs and knock knees. Surg. Clin., 4:705, 1920.

607. Perthes, G.: Curvilinear osteotomy of tibia in genu valgum and genu varum. Zbl. Chir., *50*:891, 1923.
608. Seiger, H. W.: A night splint for correction of genu valgum. J. Bone Joint Surg., *28*:178, 1946.
609. Sherman, M.: Physiologic bowing of the legs. Southern Med. J., *53*:830, 1960.
610. Thelander, H. E., and Fitzhugh, M. L.: Posture habits in infancy affecting foot and leg alignments. J. Pediat., *21*:306, 1942.
611. Wynen, W.: Curvate osteotomy in angular ankylosis of hip and genu valgum. Deutsch. Z. Chir., *197*:420, 1926.

LEG LENGTH INEQUALITY

612. Abbott, L. C.: The operative lengthening of the tibia and fibula. J. Bone Joint Surg., *9*:128, 1927.
613. Abbott, L. C., and Grego, C. H.: Operative lengthening of the femur. Southern Med. J., *21*:823, 1928.
614. Abbott, L. C., and Gill, G. G.: Surgical approaches to the epiphyseal cartilages of the knee and ankle joint. Arch. Surg., *46*:591, 1943.
615. Abbott, L. C., and Saunders, J. B. de C. M.: The operative lengthening of the tibia and fibula. Preliminary report on further development of principles and technic. Ann. Surg., *110*:961, 1939.
616. Accinno, M. A., and Parker, M. V.: Leg length inequality treated by epiphyseal arrest and stimulation. A preliminary report. J. Med. Ass. Alabama, *24*:38, 1954.
617. Acheson, R. M.: The Oxford method of assessing skeletal maturity. Clin. Orthop., *10*:19, 1957.
618. Acheson, R. M.: The environment and the growth of children. Irish J. Med. Sci., *6*:397, 1959.
619. Agerholm, J.: The zig-zag osteotomy. Acta Orthop. Scand., *29*:63, 1959.
620. Aitken, A. P.: Overgrowth of the femoral shaft following fracture. Amer. J. Surg., *49*:147, 1940.
621. Aitken, A. P., Blackett, C. W., and Ciacotti, J. J.: Overgrowth of the femoral shaft following fractures in childhood. J. Bone Joint Surg., *21*:334, 1939.
622. Allan, P. G.: Bone lengthening. J. Bone Joint Surg., *30-B*:490, 1948.
623. Allan, P. G.: Leg lengthening. Brit. Med. J., *1*:218, 1951.
624. Allan, P. G.: Simultaneous femoral and tibial lengthening. J. Bone Joint Surg., *45-B*:206, 1963.
625. Amako, T., and Honda, K.: An experimental study of the epiphyseal stapling. Kyushu J. Med. Sci., *8*:131, 1957.
626. Anderson, M., and Green, W. T.: Length of femur and tibia: Norms derived from orthoroentgenogram of children from 5 years of age until epiphyseal closure. Amer. J. Dis. Child., *75*:279, 1948.
627. Anderson, M., Green, W. T., and Messner, M. B.: Growth and predictions of growth in the lower extremities. J. Bone Joint Surg., *45-A*:1, 1963.
628. Anderson, M., Messner, M. B., and Green, W. T.: Distribution of lengths of the normal femur and tibia in children from one to eighteen years of age. J. Bone Joint Surg., *46-A*:1197, 1964.
629. Anderson, M., Horton, B. G., and Green, W. T.: Orthoroentgenography for accurate long bone measurement. Modifications of technique possible with use of rectangular bone collimator. (Personal communication.)
630. Anderson, W. V.: Leg lengthening. J. Bone Joint Surg., *34-B*:150, 1952.
631. Anderson, W. V.: Lengthening of the lower limb: Its place in the problems of limb length discrepancy. *In* Graham, W. D. (ed.): Modern Trends in Orthopedics, Vol. V. London, Butterworth & Co., 1967.
632. Armstrong, W. D.: Bone growth in paralyzed limbs. Proc. Soc. Exp. Biol. Med., *61*:358, 1946.
633. Baldwin, B. T.: The physical growth of children from birth to maturity. University of Iowa Publication, *1*: 1921.
634. Barford, B., and Christensen, J.: Fractures of the femoral shaft in children with special reference to subsequent overgrowth. Acta Chir. Scand., *116*:235, 1958–1959.
635. Barr, J. S., and Ober, F. R.: Leg lengthening in adults. J. Bone Joint Surg., *15*:674, 1933.
636. Barr, J. S., Stindfield, A. J., and Reidy, J. A.: Sympathetic ganglionectomy and limb length in poliomyelitis. J. Bone Joint Surg., *32-A*:793, 1950.
637. Bayer, L. M., and Bayley, N.: Growth Diagnosis. Chicago, University of Chicago Press, 1959.
638. Bayley, N.: Table for predicting adult height and skeletal age and present height. J. Pediat., *28*:49, 1946.
639. Bayley, N.: Growth curves of height and weight by age for boys and girls. Scaled according to physical maturity. J. Pediat., *48*:187, 1956.
640. Bayley, N.: Individual patterns of development. Child. Develop., *27*:45, 1956.
641. Bayley, N., and Pinneau, S. R.: Tables for predicting adult height from skeletal age: Revised for use with the Greulich-Pyle Hand Standards. J. Pediat., *40*:423, 1952.
642. Belchier, J.: An account of the bones of animals being changed to a red color by aliment only. Phil. Trans. Roy. Soc., *39*:287, 1735–1736.
643. Belchier, J.: A further account of the bones of animals being made red by aliment only. Phil. Trans. Roy. Soc., *39*:299, 1735–1736.
644. Bell, J. S., and Thompson, W. A. L.: Modified spot scanography. Amer. J. Roentgen., *63*:915, 1950.
645. Bertrand, P.: Technique d'allongement du fémur dans les grands raccourcissements. Rev. Chir. Orthop., *37*:530, 1951.
646. Bertrand, P., and Trillat, A.: Le traitement des inégalités de longueur des membres inférieurs pendant la croissance. Rev. Orthop., *34*:264, 1948.
647. Bier, A.: Hyperemia as a therapeutic agent. Authorized translation. Ed. by Dr. G. M. Glech. Chicago, A. Robertson & Co., 1905.
648. Bisgard, J. D.: Effect of sympathetic ganglionectomy upon bone growth. Proc. Soc. Exp. Biol., *29*:229, 1931.
649. Bisgard, J. D.: Longitudinal bone growth, the influence of sympathetic deinnervation. Ann. Surg., *97*:374, 1933.
650. Bisgard, J. D.: Longitudinal overgrowth of long bones with special reference to fractures. Surg. Gynec. Obstet., *62*:823, 1936.
651. Bisgard, J. D., and Bisgard, M. E.: Longitudinal growth of long bones. Arch. Surg., *31*:568, 1935.
652. Blomqvist, E., and Rudström, P.: Über Femurfrakturen bei Kindern unter besonderer Berücksichtigung des gesteigerten Längenwachstums. Acta Chir. Scand., *88*:267, 1943.
653. Blount, W. P.: Blade-plate internal fixation for high femoral osteotomies. J. Bone Joint Surg., *25*:319, 1943.
654. Blount, W. P.: Unequal leg length in children. Surg., Clin. N. Amer., *38*:1107, 1958.
655. Blount, W. P.: Unequal leg length. A.A.O.S. Instructional Course Lectures, Vol. 17. St. Louis, C. V. Mosby Co., 1960.
656. Blount, W. P., and Clark, G. R.: Control of bone growth by epiphyseal stapling. Preliminary report. J. Bone Joint Surg., *31-A*:464, 1949.
657. Blount, W. P., and Zeier, E.: Control of bone length. J.A.M.A., *148*:451, 1952.
658. Bohlman, H. R.: Experiments with foreign materials in the region of the epiphyseal cartilage plate of growing bones to increase their longitudinal growth. J. Bone Joint Surg., *11*:365, 1929.
659. Bost, F. C.: Operative lengthening of the bones of the lower extremity. A.A.O.S. Instructional Course Lectures, Vol. 1. Ann Arbor, J. W. Edwards, 1944, p. 50.
660. Bost, F. C., and Larsen, L. J.: Experiences with lengthening of the femur over an intramedullary rod. J. Bone Joint Surg., *38-A*:567, 1956.
661. Bosworth, D. M.: Skeletal distraction of the tibia. Surg. Gynec. Obstet., *66*:912, 1938.

662. Boyd, R. J., and Ault, L. L.: An experimental study of vascular implantation with the femoral head. Surg. Gynec. Obstet., *121*:1009, 1965.

663. Brockway, A.: Clinical resume of 46 leg-lengthening operations. J. Bone Joint Surg., *17*:969, 1935.

664. Brockway, A., and Fowler, S. B.: Experiences with 105 leg lengthening operations. Surg. Gynec. Obstet., *75*:252, 1942.

665. Brockway, A., Craig, W. A., and Cockrell, B. R., Jr.: End result study of sixty-two stapling operations. J. Bone Joint Surg., *36-A*:1063, 1954.

666. Brodin, H.: Longitudinal bone growth. The nutrition of the epiphyseal cartilages and the local blood supply. Acta Orthop. Scand., Suppl. 20, 1955.

667. Broman, B., Dahlberg, G., and Lichtenstein, A.: Height and weight during growth. Acta Pediat., *30*:1, 1942.

668. Brooke, R.: Bone shortening for inequality of length in the lower limbs. Proc. Roy. Soc. Med., *30*:441, 1937.

669. Brooks, M.: Femoral growth after occlusion of the principal nutrient canal in day-old rabbits. J. Bone Joint Surg., *39-B*:563, 1957.

670. Burdick, C. G., and Siris, L. E.: Fractures of the femur in children. Ann. Surg., *77*:736, 1923.

671. Calvé, J., and Galland, M.: A new procedure for compensatory shortening of the unaffected femur in case of considerable asymmetry of the lower limbs, fractures of the femur, coxalgia. Amer. J. Orthop. Surg., *16*:211, 1918.

672. Camera, H.: 32 casi di accorciamento dell'arto inferiore sano a scopo ortopedico; indicazioni, tecnica, risultati. Chir. Organi Mov., *17*:569, 1933.

673. Cameron, B. M.: A technique for femoral-shaft shortening. A preliminary report. J. Bone Joint Surg., *39-A*:1309, 1957.

674. Carpenter, E. B., and Dalton, J. B., Jr.: A critical evaluation of epiphyseal stimulations. J. Bone Joint Surg., *38-A*:1089, 1956.

675. Carpenter, E. B., and Dalton, J. B., Jr.: A critical evaluation of a method of epiphyseal stimulation. Follow-up notes on article previously published in the Journal. J. Bone Joint Surg., *45-A*:642, 1963.

676. Cartwright, L. J.: Orthoroentgenography as applied to the lower extremities of children. Radiography, *15*:234, 1949.

677. Chapchal, G., and Zeldenrust, J.: Experimental research for promoting longitudinal growth of lower extremities by irritation of growth region of femur and tibia. Acta Orthop. Scand., *17*:371, 1948.

678. Codivilla, A.: On the means of lengthening in the lower limbs, the muscles and the tissues which are shortened through deformity. Amer. J. Orthop. Surg., *2*:353, 1905.

679. Cole, W. M.: Leg lengthening for shortening due to infantile paralysis. Minn. Med., *13*:901, 1930.

680. Coleman, S. S., and Noonan, T. D.: Anderson's method of tibial lengthening by percutaneous osteotomy and gradual distraction. Experiences with thirty-one cases. J. Bone Joint Surg., *49-A*:263, 1967.

681. Compere, E. L.: Indications for and against the leg lengthening operation. J. Bone Joint Surg., *18*:692, 1936.

682. Compere, E. L., and Adams, C. O.: Studies of longitudinal growth of long bones; the influence of trauma to the diaphysis. J. Bone Joint Surg., *19*:922, 1937.

683. Dalton, J. B., Jr., and Carpenter, E. B.: Clinical experiences with epiphyseal stapling. Southern Med. J., *47*:544, 1954.

684. David, V. C.: Shortening and compensatory overgrowth following fractures of the femur in children. Arch. Surg., *9*:438, 1924.

685. Dickerson, R. C., and Duthie, R. B.: The diversion of arterial blood flow to bone. A preliminary report. J. Bone Joint Surg., *45-A*:356, 1963.

686. Digby, K. H.: The measurement of diaphyseal growth in proximal and distal directions. J. Anat. Physiol., *50*:187, 1915–1916.

687. Duhamel, H. L.: Sur une racine qui a la faculté de teindre en ronge les os des animaux vivants. Mém. Acad. Roy. des Sci., 1–13, 1739.

688. Duhamel, H. L.: Sur le devéloppeme et la crué des os des animaux. Mém. Acad. Roy. des Sci., 354–370, 1742.

689. Duhamel, H. L.: Quatrième mémoire sur les os. Mém. Acad. Roy. des Sci., 87–111, 1743.

690. Duhamel, H. L.: Cinquième mémoire sur les os. Mém. Acad. Roy. des Sci., 111–146, 1743.

691. Duhamel, H. L.: Sixième mémoire sur les os. Mém. Acad. Roy. des Sci., 288–317, 1743.

692. Elo, J. O.: The effect of subperiosteally implanted autogenous whole-thickness skin graft on growing bone. An experimental study. Acta Orthop. Scand., Suppl. 45, 1960.

693. Eyre-Brook, A. L.: Bone shortening for inequality of leg lengths. Brit. Med. J., *1*:222, 1951.

694. Fahey, J. J.: The effect of lumbar sympathetic ganglionectomy on longitudinal bone growth as determined by the teleoroentgenographic method. J. Bone Joint Surg., *18*:1042, 1936.

695. Fassett, F. J.: On inquiry as to the practicability of equalizing unequal legs by operation. Amer. J. Orthop. Surg., *16*:277, 1918.

696. Ferguson, A. B.: Surgical stimulation of bone growth by a new procedure. J.A.M.A., *100*:26, 1933.

697. Flourens, P.: Recherches sur le développement des os et des dents. Archives du museum d'histoire naturelle, *2*:315, 1841.

698. Flourens, P.: Recherches sur le développement des os. C. R. Acad. Sci., Paris, *15*:875, 1842.

699. Flourens, P.: Théorie expérimentale de la formation des os. Paris, Ballière, 1847.

700. Flourens, P.: Note sur le développement des os en longueur. C. R. Acad. Sci., Paris, *52*:186, 1861.

701. Freiberg, A. H.: Codivilla's method of lengthening of the lower extremity. Surg. Gynec. Obstet., *14*:614, 1912.

702. Frejka, B., and Fait, M.: Clinical evaluation of linear growth stimulation. *In* Septième Congrès International de Chirurgie Orthopédique. Barcelone, 16–21, Septembre, 1957. Bruxelles, Imprimerie des Sciences, 1958, pp. 644–661.

703. Gay, W. I.: A method for surgical lengthening of the femur of the dog. Milit. Med., *123*:283, 1958.

704. Gelbke, H.: Influence of pressure and tension on growing bone in experiments with animals. J. Bone Joint Surg., *33-A*:947, 1951.

705. Gill, G. G.: Cause of discrepancy in length of the limbs following tuberculosis of the hip in children; arrest of growth from premature central closure of the epiphyseal cartilage about the knee. J. Bone Joint Surg., *26*:272, 1944.

706. Gill, G. G.: A simple roentgenographic method for the measurement of bone length: A modification of Millwee's method of slit scanography. J. Bone Joint Surg., *26*:767, 1944.

707. Gill, G. G., and Abbott, L. C.: Practical method of predicting growth of the femur and tibia in the child. Arch. Surg., *45*:286, 1942.

708. Goff, C. W.: Growth determinations. A.A.O.S. Instructional Course Lectures, Vol. 7, 1951, p. 160.

709. Goff, C. W.: Surgical Treatment of Unequal Extremities. Springfield, Ill., Charles C Thomas, 1960.

710. Goldstein, L. A., and Dreisinger, F.: Spot roentgenography—a method for measuring the length of the bones of the lower extremities. J. Bone Joint Surg., *32-A*:449, 1950.

711. Granieri, P.: Results with epiphysiodesis in the treatment of leg length discrepancy. Bull. Hosp. Special Surg., *1*:33, 1958.

712. Green, W. T., and Anderson, M.: Experiences with epiphyseal arrest in correcting discrepancies in length of the lower extremities in infantile paralysis. J. Bone Joint Surg., *29*:659, 1947.

713. Green, W. T., and Anderson, M.: Discrepancy in length of the lower extremities. A.A.O.S. Instructional Course

Lectures, Vol. 8. Ann Arbor, J. W. Edwards, 1951, p. 294.

714. Green, W. T., and Anderson, M.: The problem of unequal leg lengths. Pediat. Clin. N. Amer., 2:1137, 1955.

715. Green, W. T., and Anderson, M.: Epiphyseal arrest for the correction of discrepancies in length of the lower extremities. J. Bone Joint Surg., 39-A:353, 1957.

716. Green, W. T., and Anderson, M.: Skeletal age and the control of bone growth. A.A.O.S. Instructional Course Lectures, Vol. 17. St. Louis, C. V. Mosby Co., 1960, p. 199.

717. Green, W. T., Wyatt, G. M., and Anderson, M.: Orthoroentgenography as a method of measuring the bones of the lower extremity. J. Bone Joint Surg., 28:60, 1946.

718. Greulich, W. W., and Pyle, S. I.: Radiographic atlas of skeletal development of the hand and wrist. Stanford, Calif., Stanford University Press, 1950. 2nd Ed., 1959.

719. Gross, R. H.: An evaluation of tibial lengthening procedures. J. Bone Joint Surg., 53-A:693, 1971.

720. Gullickson, G., Jr., Olson, M., and Kottke, F. J.: Effect of paralysis of one lower extremity on bone growth; preliminary report. Arch. Phys. Med., 13:392, 1950.

721. Haas, S. L.: The relation of the blood supply to the longitudinal growth of bone. Amer. J. Orthop. Surg., 15:157, 305, 1917.

722. Haas, S. L.: The localization of the growing point in the epiphyseal cartilage plate of bones. Amer. J. Orthop. Surg., 15:563, 1917.

723. Haas, S. L.: Interstitial growth in growing long bones. Arch. Surg., 12:887, 1926.

724. Haas, S. L.: Retardation of bone growth by a wire loop. J. Bone Joint Surg., 27:25, 1945.

725. Haas, S. L.: Mechanical retardation of bone growth. J. Bone Joint Surg., 30-A:506, 1948.

726. Haas, S. L.: Restriction of bone growth by pins through the epiphyseal cartilaginous plate. J. Bone Joint Surg., 32-A:338, 350, 1950.

727. Haas, S. L.: Stimulation of bone growth. Amer. J. Surg., 95:125, 1958.

728. Hales, S.: Statistical essays: Containing vegetable staticks; or, an account of some statical experiments on the sap in vegetables. Vol. 1. 2nd Ed. London, Innys, Woodward and Peele, 1731.

729. Hansson, L. I.: Daily growth in length of diaphysis measured by oxytetracycline in rabbit normally and after medullary plugging. Acta Orthop. Scand., Suppl. 101, 1967.

730. Harmon, P. H., and Krigsten, W. M.: The surgical treatment of unequal leg length. Surg. Gynec. Obstet., 71:482, 1940.

731. Harris, H. A.: Bone Growth in Health and Disease: The Biological Principles Underlying the Clinical, Radiological and Histological Diagnosis of Perversions of Growth and Disease in the Skeleton. London, Oxford Univ. Press, 1933.

732. Harris, R. I., and McDonald, J. L.: The effect of lumbar sympathectomy upon the growth of legs paralyzed by anterior poliomyelitis. J. Bone Joint Surg., 18:35, 1936.

733. Hart, G. H.: Femoral shortening for equalization of leg lengths. Lancet, 78:1, 1958.

734. Hatcher, C. M.: Growth increment curve for the femur and tibia. *In* Campbell, W. C., Operative Orthopaedics. St. Louis, The C. V. Mosby Co., 1939. p. 954.

735. Hellstadius, A.: Investigation, by experiments on animals, of role played by epiphyseal cartilage in longitudinal growth. Acta Chir. Scand., 95:156, 1947.

736. Hellstadius, A.: On the importance of epiphyseal cartilage to growth in length. Acta Orthop. Scand., 20:84, 1950.

737. Hellstadius, A.: A reply in consideration of Walter Duben and Heinz Gelbke's article; animal experiments concerning the problem of epiphyseal or interstitial osseous growth in length, conclusions on the articles of A. Hellstadius and P. Macroix. Acta Orthop. Scand., 25:26, 1955.

738. Hendryson, I. E.: An evaluation of the estimated percentage of growth from the distal epiphyseal line. J. Bone Joint Surg., 27:208, 1945.

739. Herndon, C. H., and Spencer, G. E.: An experimental attempt to stimulate linear growth of long bones in rabbits. J. Bone Joint Surg., 35-A:758, 1953.

740. Hewitt, D.: Some familial correlations in height, weight and skeletal maturity. Ann. Hum. Genet., 22:26, 1957.

741. Hickey, P. M.: Teleoroentgenography as an aid in orthopedic measurements. Amer. J. Roentgenol., 11:232, 1924.

742. Hodgen, J. T., and Frantz, C. H.: Arrest of growth of epiphyses. Arch. Surg., 53:664, 1946.

743. Howorth, M. B.: Leg-shortening operation for equalizing leg length. Arch. Surg., 44:543, 1942.

744. Hunter, J.: Experiments and observations on the growth of bones, from the papers of the late Mr. Hunter. By Everard Home. Read October 4, 1798. Transactions of the society for improvement of medical and chirurgical knowledge, 2:277–286, 1800.

745. Hunter, J.: Experiments and observations on the growth of bones, from papers of the late Mr. Hunter. In The works of John Hunter with notes. Ed. by J. F. Palmer. Vol. IV, 315–318, 1835. Longman, Rees, Orme, Brown, Green and Longman, London.

746. Hutchinson, W. J., and Burdeaux, B. D., Jr.: The influence of stasis on bone growth. Surg. Gynec. Obstet., 99:413, 1954.

747. Ingalls, M. W.: Bone growth and pathology as seen in the femur (and tibia); studies on the femur. Arch. Surg., 26:787, 1933.

748. Janes, J. M., and Jennings, W. K.: Effect of induced arteriovenous fistula on leg length. 10 year observations. Proc. Mayo Clin., 36:1, 1961.

749. Janes, J. M., and Musgrove, J. E.: Effect of arteriovenous fistula on growth of bone. Preliminary report. Proc. Mayo Clin., 24:405, 1949.

750. Janes, J. M., and Musgrove, J. E.: Effect of arteriovenous fistula on growth of bone. Surg. Clin. N. Amer., 30:1191, 1950.

751. Johnson, R. W.: A physiological study of the blood supply of the diaphysis. J. Bone Joint Surg., 9:153, 1927.

752. Judy, W. S.: Attempt to correct asymmetry in leg length by roentgen irradiation; preliminary report. Amer. J. Roentgen., 46:237, 1941.

753. Kawamura, B., Mosono, S., Takahashi, T., Yano, T., Kobayashi, Y., Shibata, N., and Shinoda, Y.: Limb lengthening by means of subcutaneous osteotomy: Experimental and clinical studies. J. Bone Joint Surg., 50-A:851, 1968.

754. Keck, S. W., and Kelly, P. J.: The effect of venous stasis on intraosseous pressure and longitudinal bone growth in the dog. J. Bone Joint Surg., 47-A:539, 1965.

755. Kelly, P. J., Janes, J. M., and Peterson, L. P. A.: The effect of arteriovenous fistulae on the vascular pattern of the femora of immature dogs; microradiographic study. J. Bone Joint Surg., 41-A:1101, 1959.

756. Key, J. A.: Survival and growth of an epiphysis after removal and replacement. J. Bone Joint Surg., 31-A:150, 1949.

757. Khoury, S. C., Silberman, F. S., and Cabrini, R. L.: Stimulation of the longitudinal growth of long bones by periosteal stripping. J. Bone Joint Surg., 45-A:1679, 1963.

758. Kunkle, H. M., and Carpenter, E. B.: A simple technique for x-ray measurement of limb-length discrepancies. J. Bone Joint Surg., 36-A:152, 1954.

759. LaCroix, P.: Remarques sur le méchanisme de l'allongement des os. Paris, Arch. Biol., 56:185, 1945.

760. LaCroix, P.: Excitation de la croissance en longueur du tibia pas décollement de son périoste diaphysaire. Rev. Orthop. Paris, 33:3, 1947.

761. LaCroix, P.: The organization of bones. London, Churchill, 1951.

762. von Langenbeck, B.: Ueber Krankhaftes Längenwachsthum der Rohrenknochen und seine Verwerthung für

die chirurgische Praxis. Berlin. Klin. Wschr., *6*:265, 1869.

763. Langenskiöld, A.: Growth disturbance appearing 10 years after roentgen ray injury. Acta Chir. Scand., *105*:350, 1953.

764. Langenskiöld, A.: Inhibition and stimulation of growth. Acta Orthop. Scand., *26*:308, 1957.

765. Langenskiöld, A., and Edgren, W.: The growth mechanism of the epiphyseal cartilage in the light of experimental observation. Acta Orthop. Scand., *19*:19, 1949.

766. LeCoeur, P.: Égalisation des membres inférieurs par allongement avec fixation immédiate. Rev. Chir. Orthop., *49*:217, 1963.

767. Lewis, O. J.: The blood supply of developing long bones with special reference to the metaphyses. J. Bone Joint Surg., *38-B*:928, 1956.

768. McCarroll, H. R.: Trials and tribulations in attempted femoral lengthening. J. Bone Joint Surg., *32-A*:132, 1950.

769. McGibbon, K. C., Deacon, A. E., and Raisbeck, C. G.: Experiences in growth retardation with heavy Vitallium staples. J. Bone Joint Surg., *44-B*:86, 1962.

770. Macewen, W.: The Growth of Bone. Observations on Osteogenesis. An Experimental Inquiry into the Development and Reproduction of Diaphyseal Bone. Glasgow, Maclehose, 1912.

771. Magnuson, P. B.: Lengthening shortened bones of the leg by operation. Ivory screws with removable heads as a means of holding the two bone fragments. Univ. Pa. Med. Bull., *21*:103, 1908–1909.

772. Magnuson, P. B.: Lengthening of shortened bones of the leg by operation. Surg. Gynec. Obstet., *17*:63, 1913.

773. Maresh, M. M.: Growth of the major long bones in healthy children; a preliminary report on successive roentgenograms of the extremities from early infancy to 12 years of age. Amer. J. Dis. Child., *66*:227, 1943.

774. Maresh, M. M.: Linear growth of long bones of extremities from infancy through adolescence. *89*:725, 1955.

775. May, V. R., Jr., and Clemens, E. L.: Epiphyseal stapling: With special reference to complications. Southern Med. J., *58*:1203, 1965.

776. Merle D'Aubigné, R., and Dubousset, J.: Surgical correction of large length discrepancies in the lower extremities of children and adults. J. Bone Joint Surg., *53-A*:411, 1971.

777. Merrill, O. E.: A method for the roentgen measurement of the long bones. Amer. J. Roentgen., *48*:405, 1942.

778. Millwee, R. H.: Slit scanography. Radiology, *28*:483, 1937.

779. Mitchell, G. P.: L'élongation du tibia. Rev. Chir. Orthop., *49*:205, 1963.

780. Montgomery, W. S., and Ingram, A. J.: Experimental studies and clinical evaluation of linear growth stimulation. Southern Med. J., *49*:793, 1956.

781. Moore, B. H.: A bone lengthening apparatus. J. Bone Joint Surg., *13*:170, 1931.

782. Moore, B. H.: A critical appraisal of the leg lengthening operation. Amer. J. Surg., *52*:415, 1941.

783. Moore, J. R.: Tibial lengthening and femoral shortening. Pa. Med. J., *36*:751, 1933.

784. Moore, R. D.: Supracondylar shortening of the femur for leg length inequality. Surg., Gynec. Obstet., *84*:1087, 1947.

785. Mueller, W. K., and Higgason, J. M.: Spot scanography: Method of determining bone measurements. Amer. J. Roentgen., *61*:402, 1949.

786. Ollier, L.: Traité expérimental et clinique de la régénération des os et de la production artificielle du tissu osseux. Paris, V. Masson & fils, 1867.

787. Ombredanne: Allongement d'un fémur sur un membre trop court. Bull. Mém. Soc. Chir., *39*:1177, 1913.

788. Park, E. A.: Bone growth in health and disease. Arch. Dis. Child., *29*:269, 1954.

789. Park, E. A., and Richter, C. P.: Transverse lines in bone; mechanism of their development. Bull. Johns Hopk. Hosp., *93*:234, 1953.

790. Parker, S. G.: Regulation of longitudinal bone growth. Arch. Surg., *59*:1100, 1949.

791. Pearse, H. E., Jr., and Morton, J. J.: The stimulation of bone growth by venous stasis. J. Bone Joint Surg., *12*:97, 1930.

792. Pease, C. N.: Local stimulation of growth of long bones, a preliminary report. J. Bone Joint Surg., *34-A*:1, 1952.

793. Peck, M. E.: Obstructive anomalies of the iliac vein associated with growth shortening in the ipsilateral extremity. Ann. Surg., *146*:619, 1957.

794. Phalen, G. S., and Chatterton, C. C.: Equalizing the lower extremities; a clinical consideration of leg lengthening versus leg shortening. Surgery, *12*:678, 1942.

795. Phemister, D. B.: Operative arrestment of longitudinal growth of bones in the treatment of deformities. J. Bone Joint Surg., *15*:1, 1933.

796. Phemister, D. B.: Bone growth and repair. Ann. Surg., *102*:261, 1935.

797. Pilcher, M. F.: Epiphyseal stapling: 35 cases followed to maturity. J. Bone Joint Surg., *44-B*:82, 1962.

798. Poirier, H.: Epiphysial stapling and leg equalization. J. Bone Joint Surg., *50-B*:61, 1968.

799. Pugh, D. G., and Winkler, N. T.: Scanography for leg length measurement: An easy satisfactory method. Radiology, *87*:130, 1966.

800. Pujadas, G. M.: A method of measuring the length of the bones. J. Int. Coll. Surg., *22*:308, 1954.

801. Putti, V.: The operative lengthening of the femur. J.A.M.A., *77*:934, 1921.

802. Putti, V.: Operative lengthening of the femur. Surg. Gynec. Obstet., *58*:318, 1934.

803. Pyle, S. L., and Hoerr, N. L.: Radiographic Atlas of Skeletal Development of the Knee. Springfield, Ill., Charles C Thomas, 1955.

804. Pyle, S. L., Reed, R. B., and Stuart, H. C.: Patterns of skeletal development in the hand. Pediatrics., *24*:(Suppl.), 886, 1959.

805. Ratcliff, A. H. C.: The short leg in poliomyelitis. J. Bone Joint Surg., *41-B*:56, 1959.

806. Regan, J. M., and Chatterton, C. C.: Deformities following surgical epiphyseal arrest. J. Bone Joint Surg., *28*:265, 1946.

807. Reidy, J. A., Lingley, J. R., Gall, E. A., and Barr, J. S.: The effect of roentgen irradiation on epiphyseal growth. II. Experimental studies upon the dog. J. Bone Joint Surg., *29*:853; discussion, 873, 1947.

808. Richards, V., and Stofer, R.: The stimulation of bone growth by internal heating. Surgery, *46*:84, 1959.

809. Ring, P. A.: Shortening and paralysis in poliomyelitis. Lancet, *2*:980, 1957.

810. Ring, P. A.: Experimental bone lengthening by epiphysial distraction. Brit. J. Surg., *46*:169, 1958.

811. Ring, P. A.: Prognosis of limb inequality following paralytic poliomyelitis. Lancet, *2*:1306, 1958.

812. Ring, P. A.: Congenital short femur. J. Bone Joint Surg., *41-B*:73, 1959.

813. Ring, P. A., and Ward, B. C. H.: Paralytic bone lengthening following poliomyelitis. Lancet, *2*:551, 1958.

814. Rook, R. F.: Modified osteotomy of the tibia. Surg., Gynec. Obst., *109*:771, 1959.

815. Royle, N. D.: The treatment of inequality of length in the lower limbs. Med. J. Aust. *1*:716, 1923.

816. Rubin, P.: Dynamic Classification of Bone Dysplasias. Chicago, Year Book Medical Publishers, 1964.

817. Rush, W. A., and Steiner, H. A.: A study of lower extremity length inequality. Amer. J. Roentgen., *56*:616, 1946.

818. Sandaa, K.: Orthoroentgenographic measurement of long bones. Acta Orthop. Scand., *22*:76, 1952.

819. Selye, H.: On the mechanism controlling the growth in length of the long bones. J. Anat., *68*:289, 1934.

820. Sevastrikoglou, J.: A simple application of orthoroentgenography. Acta Orthop. Scand., *22*:80, 1952.

821. Shands, A. R.: Shortening of the long leg. Int. J. Surg., *30*:273, 1917.

822. Sofield, H. A.: Leg lengthening. Surg. Clin. N. Amer. *19*:69, 1939.

823. Sofield, H. A., Blair, S. J., and Millar, E. A.: Leg lengthening . A personal follow-up of 40 patients some years after the operation. J. Bone Joint Surg., *40-A*:311, 1958.

824. Speed, K.: Longitudinal overgrowth of long bones. Surg. Gynec. Obstet., *36*:787, 1923.

825. Stamp, W. G., and Lansche, W. E.: Treatment of discrepancy in leg length. Southern Med. J., *53*:764, 1960.

826. Stein, A. H., Morgan, H. C., and Porras, R.: The effect of an arteriovenous fistula on intramedullary bone pressure. Surg. Gynec. Obstet., *109*:287, 1959.

827. Stinchfield, A. J., Reidy, J. A., and Barr, J. S.: Prediction of unequal growth of the lower extremities in anterior poliomyelitis. J. Bone Joint Surg., *31-A*:478, 1949.

828. Stirling. R. I.: Equalisation of limb length. Presented at the meeting of the British Orthop. Assoc., Paris, May 5 – 7, 1955. J. Bone Joint Surg., *37-B*:511, 1955.

829. Straub, L. R., Thompson, T. C., and Wilson, P. D.: The results of epiphysiodesis and femoral shortening in relation to equalization of leg length. J. Bone Joint Surg., *27*:254, 1945.

830. Thompson, T. C., Straub, L. R., and Campbell, R. D.: An evaluation of femoral shortening with intramedullary nailing. J. Bone Joint Surg., *36-A*:43, 1954.

831. Thoms, H.: A new method for roentgen pelvimetry. J.A.M.A., *92*:1515, 1929.

832. Todd, T. W.: Atlas of skeletal maturation. St. Louis, C. V. Mosby Co., 1937.

833. Troupp, H.: Nervous and vascular influence on longitudinal growth of bone. An experimental study of rabbits. Acta Orthop. Scand., Suppl., *51*: 1961.

834. Truesdell, E. D.: Inequality of the lower extremities following fractures of the shaft of the femur in children. Ann. Surg., *74*:498, 1921.

835. Trueta, J.: The influence of the blood supply in controlling bone growth. Bull. Hosp. Joint Dis., *14*:147, 1953.

836. Trueta, J.: Trauma and bone growth. Septième Congrès International de Chirurgie Orthopédique. Barcelona, 1957, Bruxelles, Imprimerie des Sciences, 1958 pp. 329 – 353.

837. Tupman, G. S.: Treatment of inequality of the lower limbs. The results of operations for stimulation of growth. J. Bone Joint Surg., *42-B*:489, 1960.

838. Tupman, G. S.: A study of bone growth in normal children and its relationship to skeletal maturation. J. Bone Joint Surg., *44-B*:42, 1962.

839. Vanderhoeft, P. J., Kelly, P. J., Janes, J. M., and Peterson, L. F. A.: Growth and structure of bone distal to an arteriovenous fistula: Quantitative analysis of tetracycline-induced transverse growth patterns. J. Bone Joint Surg., *45-B*:582, 1963.

840. Vesely, D. G., and Mears, T. M.: Surgically induced arteriovenous fistula. Its effect upon· inequality of leg length. Southern Med. J., *57*:129, 1964.

841. Weinmann, D. T., Kelly, P. J., and Owen, C. A., Jr.: Blood flow in bone distal to a femoral arteriovenous fistula in dogs. J. Bone Joint Surg., *46-A*:1676, 1964.

842. Westin, G. W.: Femoral lengthening using a periosteal sleeve. Report of 26 cases. J. Bone Joint Surg., *49-A*:83, 1967.

843. White, J. W.: A simplified method for tibial lengthening. J. Bone Joint Surg., *12*:90, 1930.

844. White, J. W.: Femoral shortening for equalization of leg length. J. Bone Joint Surg., *17*:597, 1935.

845. White, J. W.: A practical graphic method of recording leg length discrepancies. Southern Med. J., *33*:946, 1940.

846. White, J. W.: Overlapping procedure for shortening bone defects. A. A. O. S. Instructional Course Lectures. Vol. 2. Ann Arbor, J. W. Edwards, 1944, p. 48.

847. White, J. W.: Leg length discrepancies. A. A. O. S. Instructional Course Lectures. Ann Arbor, J. W. Edwards, 1949, p. 201.

848. Wilk, L. H., and Badgley, C. E.: Hypertension, another complication of leg lengthening procedure. Report of a case. J. Bone Joint Surg., *45-A*:1263, 1963.

849. Wilson, P. D., and Thompson, T. C.: A clinical consideration of the methods of equalizing leg length. Ann. Surg., *110*:992, 1939.

850. Woodruff, H. J., and Lane, G.: A technique for slit scanography. Amer. J. Roentgen., *96*:907, 1966.

851. Wray, J., and Goodman, H. O.: Postfracture vascular phenomenon and long-bone overgrowth in the immature skeleton of the rat. J. Bone Joint Surg., *43-A*:1047, 1961.

852. Wu, Y. K., and Miltner, L. J.: A procedure for stimulation of longitudinal growth of bone. An experimental study. J. Bone Joint Surg., *19*:909, 1937.

853. Yabsley, R. H., and Harris, W. R.: The effect of shaft fractures and periosteal stripping on the vascular supply to epiphyseal plates. J. Bone Joint Surg., *47-A*:551, 1965.

854. Yosipovitch, Z. H., and Palti, Y.: Alterations in blood pressure during leg-lengthening. A clinical and experimental investigation. J. Bone Joint Surg., *49-A*:1352, 1967.

CONGENITAL HEMIHYPERTROPHY

855. Bryan, R. S., Lipscomb, P. R., and Chatterton, C. C.: Orthopedic aspects of congenital hypertrophy. Amer. J. Surg., *96*:654, 1958.

856. Campbell, W. C.: Congenital hypertrophy; report of a case with diffuse neurofibromatosis. Surg. Gynec. Obstet., *36*:699, 1923.

857. Carron, R.: L'hémihypertrophie congénitale. Pediatrie, *6*:969, 1951.

858. Carter, F. S., and Dockeray, M. C.: A case of congenital hemihypertrophy showing variations in bone age and development. Arch. Dis. Child., *28*:321, 1953.

859. Crosby, E. H.: Hemihypertrophy totalis: Case report. J. Bone Joint Surg., *17*:1025, 1935.

860. Fordyce, A. D.: Hemi-hypertrophie alterne. Arch. Dis. Child., *3*:300, 1928.

861. Friedberg, H.: Riesenwuchs des rechten Beines. Arch. Path. Anat., *40*:353, 1867.

862. Gesell, A.: Hemihypertrophy and mental defect. Arch. Neurol. Psychiat., *6*:400, 1921.

863. Gesell, A.: Hemihypertrophy and twinning. A further study of the nature of hemihypertrophy with report of a new case. Amer. J. Med. Sci., *173*:542, 1927.

864. Harwood, J., and O'Flynn, E.: Right sided hemihypertrophy associated with pubertas praecox. Proc. Roy. Soc. Med., *28*:857, 1935.

865. Kazanjian, V. H., and Sturgis, S. H.: Surgical treatment of hemiatrophy of the face. J.A.M.A., *115*:348, 1940.

866. MacEwen, D. G., and Case, J. L.: Congenital hemihypertrophy. Clin. Orthop., *50*:147, 1967.

867. McFarland, B. L.: Hemihypertrophy. Brit. Med. J., *1*:345, 1928.

868. Mayers, L. H.: Hemihypertrophy. Surg. Gynec. Obstet., *43*:746, 1926.

869. Morris, J. V., and MacGillivray, R. C.: Mental defect and hemihypertrophy. Amer. J. Ment. Defic. *59*:645, 1955.

870. Peabody, C. W.: Hemihypertrophy and hemiatrophy; congenital total unilateral somatic asymmetry. J. Bone Joint Surg., *18*:466, 1936.

871. Penfield, W., and Robertson, J. S. M.: Growth asymmetry due to lesions of the postcentral cerebral cortex. Arch. Neurol. Psychiat., *50*:405, 1943.

872. Peremans, G.: An unusual case of congenital asymmetry of the pelvis and lower extremities. J. Bone Joint Surg., *5*:331, 1923.

873. Roget, J., Beaudoing, A., and Guilhot, J.: Un cas d'hémihypertrophie congénitale avec aspect anormal des cisternes de la base du crâne. Pédiatrie, *10*:195, 1955.

874. Rugel, S. J.: Congenital hemihypertrophy. Report of a case with postmortem observations. Amer. J. Dis. Child., *71*:530, 1946.

875. Sabanas, A. O., and Chatterton, C. C.: Crossed congenital hemihypertrophy. J. Bone Joint Surg., *37-A*:871, 1955.

876. Schwartzman, J., Grossman, L., and Dragutsky, D.: True total hemihypertrophy. Case report. Arch. Pediat., *59*:637, 1942.

877. Scott, A. J.: Hemihypertrophy: Report of four cases. J. Pediat., *6*:650, 1935.

878. Silver, H. K., Kiyasu, W., George, J., and Deamer, W. C.: Syndrome of congenital hemihypertrophy, shortness of stature and elevated urinary gonadotropines. Pediatrics, *12*:368, 1953.

879. Stoesser, A. U.: Hyertrophies of infancy and childhood. Amer. J. Dis. Child., *35*:885, 1928.

880. Wagner, H.: Hypertrophie der rechten Brust und der rechten oberen Extremität besonders der Hand und der Finger. Med. Jahrb. d. K.K. Österreichischen Staates, *19*:378, 1839.

881. Wakefield, E. G., and Hines, E. A.: Congenital hemihypertrophy. Amer. J. Med. Sci., *185*:493, 1933.

882. Ward, C. E., and Horton, B. T.: Congenital arteriovenous fistulas in children. J. Pediat., *16*:763, 1940.

883. Ward, J., and Lerner, H.: A review of the subject of congenital hemihypertrophy and a complete case report. J. Pediat., *31*:403, 1947.

884. Williams, J. A.: Congenital hemihypertrophy with lymphangioma. Arch. Dis. Child., *26*:158, 1951.

885. Wisenberg, M.: Unusual case of hemigigantism. Canad. Med. Ass. J., *25*:591, 1931.

GENERAL

886. Dickson, F. D., and Diveley, R. L.: Functional Disorders of the Foot: Their Diagnosis and Treatment. 2nd Ed. Philadelphia, J. B. Lippincott & Co., 1944.

887. DuVries, H. L.: Surgery of the Foot. 2nd Ed. St. Louis, C. V. Mosby Co., 1965.

888. Gianestras, N. J.: Foot Disorders—Medical and Surgical Management. Philadelphia, Lea & Febiger, 1967.

889. Hauser, E. D. W.: Diseases of the Foot. 2nd Ed. Philadelphia, W. B. Saunders Co., 1950.

890. Hoerr, N. L., and Pyle, S. I.: Radiographic Atlas of the Skeletal Development of the Foot. Springfield, Ill., Charles C Thomas, 1957.

891. Jones, F. W.: Structure and Function as Seen in the Foot. 2nd Ed. London, Bailliére, Tindall and Cox, 1950.

892. Keith, A.: The history of the human foot and its bearing on orthopedic practice. J. Bone Joint Surg., *11*:10, 1929.

893. Kelikian, H.: Hallux Valgus, Allied Deformities of the Forefoot and Metatarsalgia. Philadelphia, W. B. Saunders Co., 1965.

894. Lake, N. C.: The Foot. 4th Ed. Baltimore, Williams & Wilkins Co., 1952.

895. Lapidus, P. W.: Subtalar joint. Its anatomy and mechanics. Bull. Hosp. Joint Dis., *16*:179, 1955.

896. Lewin, P.: The Foot and Ankle: Their injuries, Diseases, Deformities and Disabilities. 4th Ed. Philadelphia, Lea & Febiger, 1959.

897. Morton, D. J.: The Human Foot; Its Evolution, Physiology and Functional Disorders. New York, Columbia University Press, 1935.

8. *Fractures and Dislocations*

Fractures in children differ from those in adults in several ways: (1) Injuries may involve the physis and disturb growth. (2) The normal process of bone remodeling in the growing child will realign the malunited fragments and make accurate anatomic reduction of somewhat less importance than in the adult. Bone remodels in response to the stresses of body weight and the pull of muscles. In general, the younger the child and the closer the fracture site to the physis, the greater is the potential for spontaneous correction. Angular deformities in the plane of motion of an adjacent hinge joint, such as the knee, ankle, or elbow, are corrected readily, whereas spontaneous correction of angular deformities in other directions, such as cubitus varus following supracondylar fracture of the humerus, is minimal if it takes place at all. Rotational deformities do not correct themselves spontaneously. (3) Fractures stimulate growth by increasing the blood supply to the physis and epiphysis; thus, some degree of overriding with bayonet or side-to-side apposition is desirable in certain age groups, particularly in the long bones of the lower limb. (4) Bone healing is rapid in childhood because of the thickened periosteum and abundant blood supply. The younger the child, the more rapid is the union; for example, in the neonatal period, a fracture of the femoral shaft heals in two to three weeks; during early childhood, in four weeks; in the period from seven to ten years, in six weeks; whereas, in adolescence, in eight to ten weeks. Nonunion usually does not occur. With few exceptions, open surgical reduction of fractures is not indicated in children; such intervention merely delays normal healing and predisposes to nonunion. Among these biological differences, it is injury to the physis that warrants special detailed discussion, however, as it presents unique problems in the diagnosis and management of fractures in children.

The Normal Physis and Its Response to Trauma

The physis (also referred to in the literature as the epiphyseal plate, epiphyseal cartilage, and epiphyseal growth plate), is separated from the epiphysis by the *bone plate,* which is a rudimentary cortex formed by a variable number of lamellae, usually six to eight, its thickness being about one fifth that of the physis (Fig. 8–1A). The bone plate has openings through which vessels penetrate. It remains visible in the roentgenogram until late in life after epiphyseal closure.

The physis proper consists of four zones. The first, a zone of *undifferentiated* or *resting cartilage cells* is located immediately adjacent to the bone plate. The chondrocytes are arranged in irregular clusters separated from one another by abundant cartilage matrix (Fig. 8–1B). This is the germinal layer that supplies the developing cartilage cells. The source of its cells, in turn, is from the perichondral ring at its periphery, which grows by apposition. Injury to this zone of resting cells will result in cessation of growth.

The second, the *zone of proliferating cartilage,* is the site where length is provided to the tubular bone by active growth of carti-lage cells (Fig. 8–1C). The former concept of these cartilage cells being lined up in linear columns parallel to the long axis of the shaft is incorrect; they are best visualized as a stack of coins, i.e., flattened and largest at their transverse diameter. Each row of cartilage cells is separated from its neighboring abundant cartilage matrix containing bundles of collagen fibrils. The number of cells in the zone of proliferation reflects the activity of the growth plate; the greater their number, the greater is the productivity of the plate. The zone of resting cells and the zone of proliferation together constitute approximately half the physis.

The third, the *zone of vacuolization,* or *hypertrophic cell zone,* is the layer in which the chondrocytes become swollen and vacuolated in the process of maturation leading to cell death (Fig. 8–1D). There is no active growth in this zone; length is added to the bone passively by hypertrophy of the cells. As the chondrocytes swell, the intercellular cartilage matrix diminishes.

The fourth, the *zone of provisional calcification,* or *cell degeneration,* is the area where, with the death of chondrocytes and the

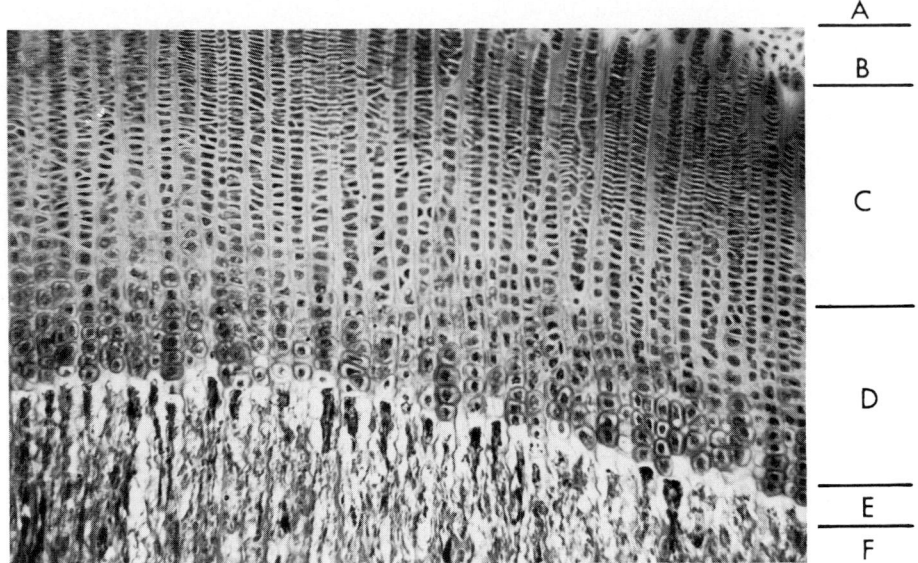

FIGURE 8–1.   The growth plate from the upper epiphyseal cartilage of a rabbit's tibia.

A. Bone plate. **B.** Zone of resting cartilage cells. **C.** Zone of proliferation. **D.** Zone of hypertrophic or giant cells. **E.** Zone of cell degeneration or provisional calcification. **F.** The layer of bone formation. (× 40) (Courtesy of J. Trueta.)

production of alkaline phosphatase, the longitudinal bars of cartilage matrix become calcified. Dead cells are soon absorbed by invasion of vascular mesenchyme.

Injury to the germinal cells of the epiphyseal plate by direct trauma, circulatory loss, or compression will arrest longitudinal bone growth.

Direct Trauma

Experimental investigations on the effects of injury to the physis are numerous: Ollier, in 1867, performed experiments in immature rabbits and cats by making linear incisions across the epiphyseal plate. Superficial cuts did not affect growth, whereas deep cuts arrested growth. He also found that growth was not disturbed as a result of multiple needle punctures of the plate.[22] Vogt was unable to produce any disturbance of growth by separating the epiphysis through the natural line of cleavage in the epiphyseal plates of goats and sheep.[34] The strength of the physis is provided by the intercellular cartilage matrix. In the first two zones of the physis, there is abundant cartilage matrix and the growth plate is strong; whereas, in

the third zone (hypertrophic cell zone), the chondrocytes enlarge to the detriment of their extracellular support, making this zone the weakest portion of the epiphyseal plate. This weakness is to shearing, bending, and tension stresses, not to compression. The fourth zone is reinforced by the addition of calcification. The region of trabecular formation in the metaphysis also contributes to the strength of the physis. The bone matrix laid about the spurs of calcified intercellular substance firmly unites the diaphyseal side of the fourth zone with the metaphysis (Fig. 8–1F).

The weakest part of the physis is the third layer (or the zone of cartilage cells). This was first demonstrated by Haas, who found that when the periosteum about the periphery of an epiphyseal plate was incised, the epiphysis could be easily detached from the metaphysis by gentle pressure. The plane of cleavage was constant, passing through the layer of hypertrophic cartilage cells.[15] Harris designed an apparatus to determine the shearing strength of the upper tibial epiphysis in the rat, and confirmed the finding of Haas that, when the epiphysis separates from the diaphysis, the plane of cleavage consistently passes through the third layer of the physis.[18] The clinical significance of these findings is that the growing cartilage cells in the physis remain adherent to the epiphysis.

From the circulatory point of view, epiphyses can be subdivided into two types: those that are entirely covered by articular cartilage, and those that are only partially covered. In the former (Type A), the artery enters the epiphysis by traversing the perichondrium at the periphery of the epiphyseal plate. Examples of this type are the proximal radial and upper femoral epiphyses. In the second type (Type B), those that are only partially covered, the nutrient vessels enter the bone by penetrating the cortex at the side of the epiphysis, like the blood supply of the diaphysis of a long bone. Frequently, more than one vessel enters the epiphysis or a single vessel may branch into many tributaries. The majority of the epiphyses in the body are classified as Type B (Fig. 8–2).[10]

Harris and Hobson studied the histologic changes in experimentally displaced upper femoral epiphyses in rabbits. As previously stated, this epiphysis is intra-articular and is entirely covered by articular cartilage; its nutrient vessels must enter it by being closely applied to the periphery of the epiphyseal plate. Their being so situated makes them vulnerable to injury and they inevitably become damaged in epiphyseal separation. In the study of Harris and Hobson,

complete displacement of the upper femoral epiphysis resulted in aseptic necrosis, which was slowly repaired by growth of callus and blood vessels from the stump of the femoral neck. As the bulk of the epiphyseal plate remains attached to the epiphysis, it acted as a barrier to successful revascularization. Deliberate removal of the epiphyseal cartilage permitted earlier revascularization.[19]

Dale and Harris demonstrated that when a Type B epiphysis (such as the proximal tibial epiphysis) is separated from the metaphysis, the nutrient vessels are not damaged and its capacity for growth is not disturbed. Enchondral ossification is temporarily interfered with, as evidenced by the increased thickness of the physis; however, healing takes place rapidly within three weeks and avascular necrosis does not occur. Thus, the prognosis of an epiphyseal separation is dependent upon the degree of damage to its blood supply rather than the mechanical disturbance of the epiphyseal plate.[10]

Brashear produced fractures through the distal femoral epiphysis of rats by applying a varus angulation force. This resulted in distraction on the lateral side of the epiphyseal plate. On the distraction side, the cleavage plane passed through the zone of hypertrophic cartilage cells; whereas on the compression side, the fracture line passed through the metaphyseal trabeculae. A

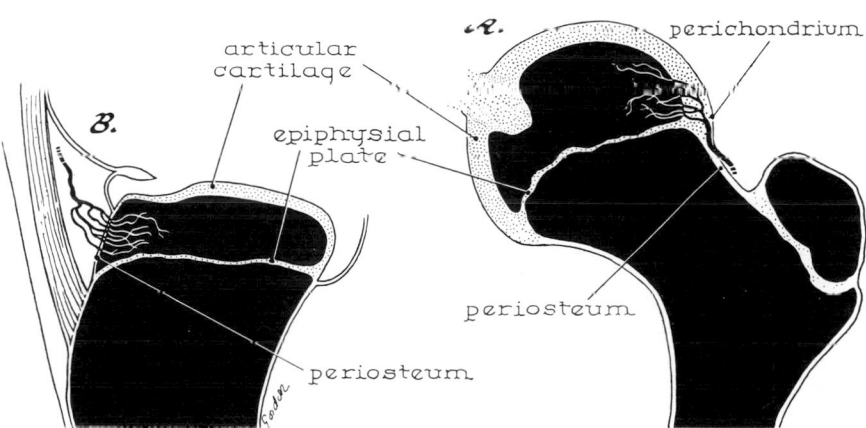

FIGURE 8–2. *Two basic patterns of blood supply to the epiphysis.*

A. *Epiphysis is entirely covered by articular cartilage* (the upper femoral epiphysis). The blood vessels enter the epiphysis by traversing the perichondrium at the periphery of the epiphyseal plate. During epiphyseal displacement these vessels are vulnerable to rupture. **B.** *Epiphysis is partly covered by articular cartilage.* The vessels enter bone by penetrating the cortex at the side of the epiphysis (proximal tibial epiphysis). In this type epiphyseal separation could occur without serious damage to vessels. (*From* Dale, G. G., and Harris, W. R.: Prognosis in epiphyseal separations. J. Bone Joint Surg., *40–B*:117, 1958.)

combination of shearing and compression stresses ground the metaphyseal bone into the epiphyseal plate, damaging all layers of cells.[7]

Depending upon the level of fracture within the epiphyseal plate, three types of healing are observed: (1) If the fracture is proximal in the hypertrophic zone, healing takes place by resorption of the proximal cartilage and fracture debris, a process that temporarily delays enchondral bone formation and causes moderate widening of the epiphyseal plate. After resorption of the proximal cartilage and debris, normal enchondral ossification is resumed. This healing process is usually completed by the end of the third week. (2) If the fracture is more distal or deeper in the hypertrophic zone, there is considerable delay in resorption of the proximal cartilage, with marked widening of the epiphyseal plate distal to the fracture. The cells in the middle of this wide plate mature and are invaded by avascular tissue. This results in a split epiphyseal line—a second healing process, which may not be completed until after the fifth week. (3) If the injury involves the entire depth of the growth plate, the healing process will be incomplete. It occurs either by hyperplasia of the few scattered remaining cartilage cells of the resting zone or by narrowing of the defect by encroachment of the normal epiphyseal cartilage on all sides. If the defect is very large, healing cannot take place and growth in that segment of the epiphysis ceases.[7]

Campbell, Grisolia and Zanconato studied the histologic effects and growth disturbances caused by surgical trauma to the epiphyseal plate of immature dogs (Table 8–1). Their conclusions are as follows:

1. After epiphyseal injury in an immature animal of specified age and growth potential, the amount of retardation of growth is roughly proportional to the amount of destruction of the region or zone of the epiphyseal plate which is responsible for replenishing the cells of the cartilage columns.
2. A defect in the cartilaginous epiphyseal plate caused by trauma which extends from the epiphysis to the metaphysis is not repaired by cartilage with the structural pattern of the normal epiphyseal plate. If there is nothing to obstruct the ingrowth of tissue, the defect is filled at first by an undifferentiated mesenchymal tissue which later forms a cancellous-bone bridge.
3. A bone may continue to grow in length normally if a relatively small cancellous-bone bridge connects the epiphysis to the metaphysis. When retardation occurs, the amount of retardation is usually proportional to the size and stability of the bone bridge. A cortical-bone graft, when placed across an epiphyseal plate, causes growth arrest if it unites to the bone of the epiphysis and metaphysis and does not break or is not absorbed.
4. Smooth metallic pins or nails of small gauge inserted from the epiphysis into the metaphysis at an angle perpendicular to the epiphyseal plate may cause less growth retardation than a cancellous-bone bridge of equal size. With growth, the epiphysis may glide over the pin if there is sufficient growth potential left in the epiphyseal plate.
5. Threaded pins or screws placed across the epiphyseal plate cause growth arrest if the threads are of sufficient gauge so that the epiphysis is mechanically fixed to the metaphysis until the epiphyseal plate is closed.*

Loss of Circulation

The normal vascular supply of the physis has been described by Trueta and Morgan.[32] There are two separate systems of circulation to the growth plate, one that supplies its epiphyseal surface (or E side), and the other, its metaphyseal surface (or M side).

Vascular Supply to the Epiphyseal Side of the Physis. Numerous branches of the epiphyseal artery reach to the bone plate, traverse it through canals, expand into terminal loops and tufts underneath the bone plate, and return to the epiphysis as large veins, not always through the same canal.

A former erroneous belief was that a rich blood supply existed *only* on the metaphyseal side of the growth plate. On the contrary, circulation underneath the bone plate is very rich, the vascular expansions forming a "ceiling" of blood with their endothelium in close contact with the "resting" chondrocytes, thus serving as an abundant vascular supply to the reproductive side of the growth plate (Figs. 8–3 to 8–5).

---

*From Campbell, C. J., Grisolia, A., and Zanconato, G.: The effects produced in the cartilaginous epiphyseal plate of immature dogs by experimental surgical traumata. J. Bone Joint Surg., *41-A:*1221, 1959. Reprinted with permission.

Table 8-1. *Operations on Immature Dogs**

Group	Operation	Line Drawing of Operation	No. of Operations	General Effect on Growth
1	Resection of the margin of the epiphyseal plate, epiphysis, and adjoining metaphysis		6	Minimum angulation
2	Longitudinal osteotomy through the distal radial and femoral epiphysis crossing the plate in a plane perpendicular to it			
	a. No internal fixation		5	Minimum retardation
	b. Internal fixation—one screw transversely across the metaphysis		15	Minimum retardation
	c. Detachment of all soft tissues from fragment, with replacement and fixation		5	Maximum retardation
	d. Detachment of soft tissues, insertion in 90 per cent alcohol for ten minutes, replacement, and fixation		3	Maximum retardation
3	Longitudinal osteotomy in the metaphysis of the radius extending distally to the epiphyseal plate with separation across the plate in the line of cleavage		15	Variable retardation (none to moderate)
4	Drilling of holes longitudinally across the distal epiphyseal plate of the radius and femur			
	a. One hole, one-quarter of an inch in diameter		2	Maximum retardation
	b. One hole, five-thirty-seconds of an inch in diameter		13	Minimum retardation
	c. One hole, five-thirty-seconds of an inch in diameter, with the insertion of beeswax		5	Minimum retardation
	d. Eight to ten holes, 0.45 millimeter in diameter		5	No retardation
5	Longitudinal insertion of cortical-bone graft (homogenous), five-thirty-seconds of an inch in thickness, through a drill hole across the distal epiphyseal plate of the femur		8	Arrest
6	Longitudinal insertion of smooth metallic pins extending from the articular surface of the epiphysis into the metaphysis of the distal part of the femur and radius			
	a. Steinmann pin, five-thirty-seconds of an inch		14	Minimum retardation
	b. Five Kirschner pins, 0.045 centimeter		4	Variable retardation (none to minimum)
7	Longitudinal insertion of threaded metallic pins (one-quarter of an inch and five-thirty-seconds of an inch) from the articular surface of the epiphysis into the metaphysis of the distal part of the femur		17	Arrest

*From Campbell, J. C., Grisolia, A., and Zanconato, G.: The effects produced in the cartilaginous epiphyseal plate of immature dogs by experimental surgical traumata. J. Bone Joint Surg., *41–A*:1221, 1959. Reprinted with permission.

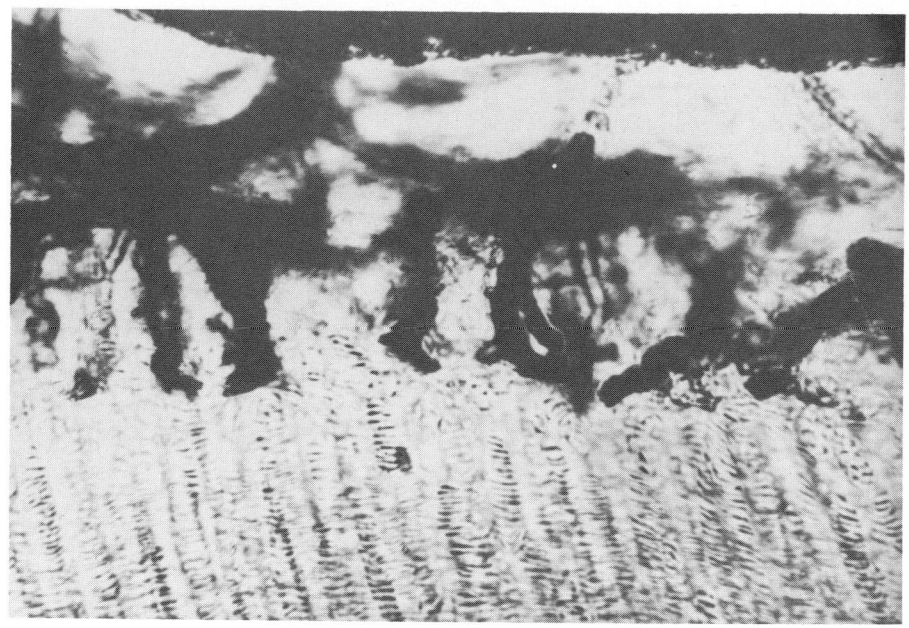

FIGURE 8–3.   Epiphyseal vessels.

After progressive branching and anastomosis, the epiphyseal arteries reach the bone plate, cross it, and expand into terminal loops or tufts underneath the bone plate, giving the appearance of a rake. These vessels supply the germinal layer or the zone of resting cells. The bone plate is seen as being white in this illustration and the injected vessels as black (× 35). (From Trueta, J., and Morgan, J. D.: The vascular contribution to osteogenesis. J. Bone Joint Surg., *42-B:*103, 1960.)

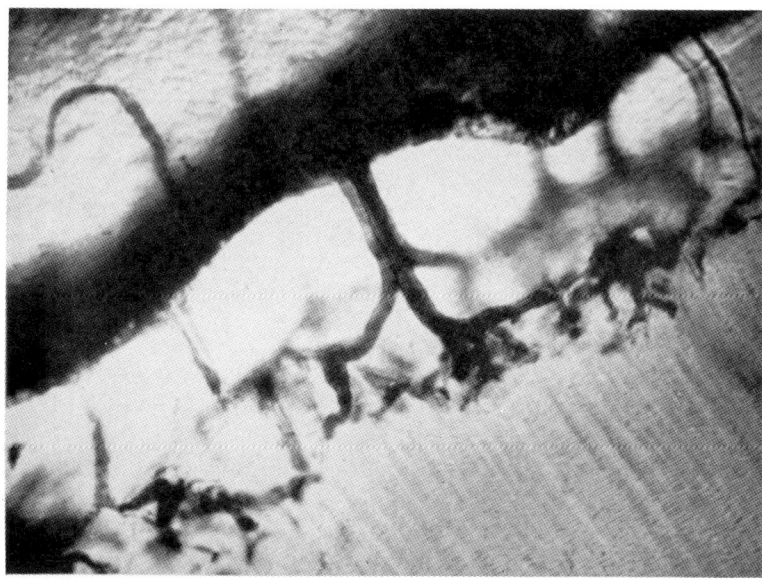

FIGURE 8–4.   The epiphyseal vessels traverse the bone plate through canals toward the zone of "resting" cartilage cells (× 40).

(From Trueta, J., and Morgan, J. D.: The vascular contribution to osteogenesis. J. Bone Joint Surg., *42-B:*102, 1960.)

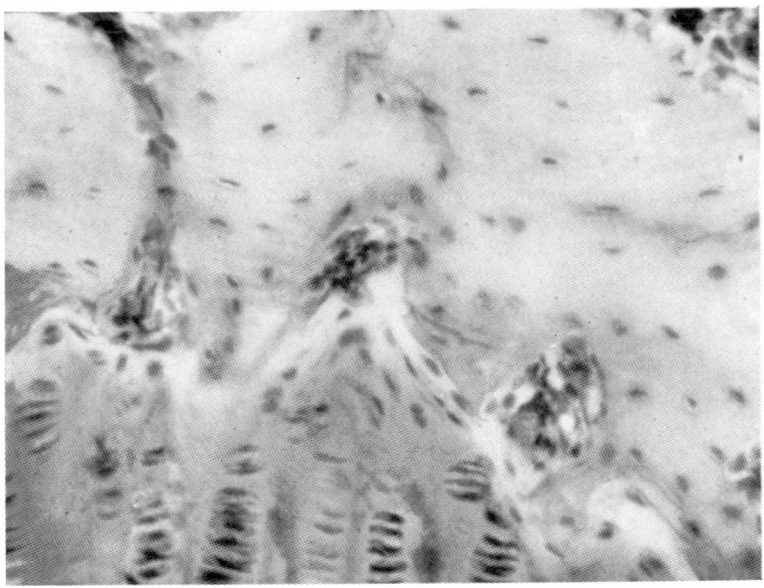

FIGURE 8–5. Epiphyseal vascular ends under the bone plate.

Each terminal bulging of a vessel covers the space corresponding to form four to ten cell columns. Note the close contact of the vascular endothelium to the "resting" cartilage cells (× 240). (From Trueta, J., and Morgan, J. D.: The vascular contribution to osteogenesis. J. Bone Joint Surg., *42–B:*102, 1960.)

Vascular Supply to the Metaphyseal Side of the Physis. The terminal ramifications of the nutrient artery constitute about four fifths of the vessels that reach the growth plate from the metaphyseal side; their branches are evenly distributed over the central three fourths or more of the growth plate. The periphery of the growth plate on its metaphyseal side is supplied from a system of large periosteal vessels known as the perforating vessels of the metaphysis (Fig. 8–6).

Effect of Ischemia on the Physis. This has been studied by Trueta and Amato on the tibiae of rabbits. Through a small drill hole (made with a fine dental drill on the medial

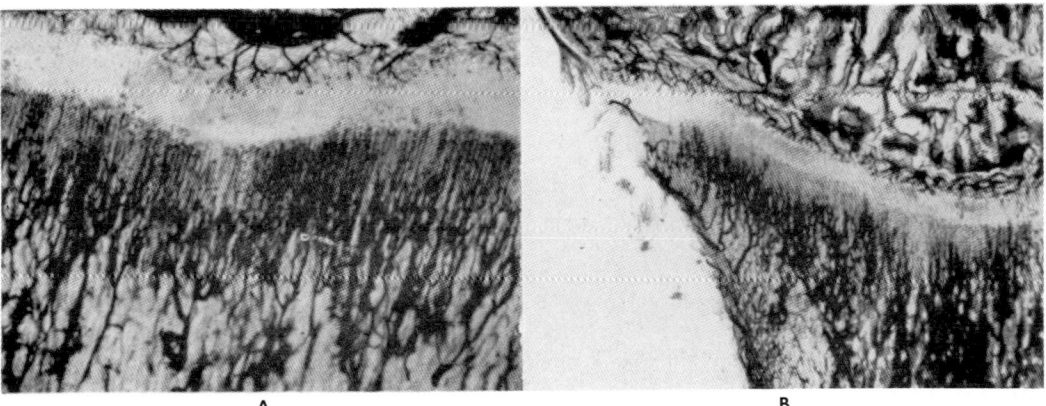

A   B

FIGURE 8–6. Metaphyseal vessels

The nutrient artery supplies about four fifths of the vessels reaching the growth plate from its metaphyseal side, and the loops of its branches cover the central three fourths or more of the physis (**A** × 8 and **B** × 15). (From Trueta, J., and Morgan, J. D.: The vascular contribution to osteogenesis. J. Bone Joint Surg., *42–B:*104, 1960.)

side of the proximal epiphysis of the right tibia and thus avoiding any direct injury to the physis), a flat spatula was introduced to the center of the epiphysis. A cavity was made parallel to the plane of the physis, and a strip of polyethylene film was placed in the cavity to prevent revascularization near the growth plate. The lateral side of the epiphysis was left intact to serve as a control. In the left tibia, using a similar technique, the polyethylene film was placed on the metaphyseal side of the physis and at a sufficient distance to prevent any direct damage. Groups of rabbits were sacrificed at varying intervals after operation to study the changes in the growth plate produced by ischemia. In other groups of rabbits, the polyethylene film was removed at varying intervals after the first operation, and then the rabbits were killed at 2 to 24 days after the second operation to study the revascularization that had occurred. The results of this investigation showed that the epiphyseal vessels are responsible for the nourishing blood supply of the reproductive cells of the physis; any extensive interruption of the epiphyseal vessels will result in irreparable damage to the growth plate. The principal role of the metaphyseal vessels—carrying calcium and vitamin D in the serum and phosphates in the erythrocytes—is calcification of the matrix, the removal of degenerate cells, and the deposition of lamellar bone along the inner side of the empty tubes. Thus, the metaphyseal vessels are of no nutritional importance to the proliferative chondrocytes of the physis. The absence of calcification will keep the cartilage cells alive.[31]

Compression

Trueta and Trias, in their studies of the effect of pressure on the epiphyseal cartilage of the rabbit, came to the following conclusions: (1) Persistent compression affects the growth plate by interference with the blood flow on one or both sides of the physis. (2) Despite exertion of the same pressure upon both sides of the growth plate, only the metaphyseal side is readily affected in the early stages; as long as no damage is caused to the epiphyseal side of the growth plate, the lesions are fully revers-

ible. (3) Interference with growth is directly proportionate to the damage caused by compression to the epiphyseal side of the growth plate, and, in general, to the duration of compression. (4) Severe continuous compression of the epiphyseal plate will affect its growth by interrupting its blood supply.[33] Trueta and Trias summarized their findings, designating the following four stages of compression injury:

Stage one: up to seven days of compression there is an inhibition of degeneration of the hypertrophic cells at the end of the growth columns. This allows the cells to survive for an, as yet, indefinite number of days: in some of our experiments, up to more than twelve days. During all this time cells from the proliferative section of the columns continue to develop into hypertrophic cells while the rate of cell division at the proliferative level of the columns remains apparently normal. In these circumstances the growth cartilage at the area of greatest pressure may develop to about four times its normal height.

Stage two: at approximately eight to ten days after the initiation of compression, the continuous accumulation of the new cartilage cells and their lack of subsequent removal at the metaphyseal end of the epiphyseal cartilage causes the compression to increase. This occurs despite the increase in the distance between the pins, because of compression of the springs of the clamp. In about ten days changes appear in the epiphyseal end of the growth cartilage. From then on, the suffering cartilage cells and their organization appears progressively greater until the next phase is reached.

Stage three: at about 14 days or more the disorganization is, in general, severe and mostly reversible. The bone plate covering the epiphyseal side of the cartilage has dead cells and appears broken into fragments. The new addition of cells by division of the proliferative section is interrupted and shortly after this, irregular vascular invasion occurs from both ends, despite the continuation of compression.

Stage four consists of fusion of the growth cartilage by bone formation following the vascular invasion of the previous phase, beginning by establishing a narrow bone bridge across the growth plate.*

Noteworthy, in the initial period, is the protection of the hypertrophic cells and the

---

*From Trueta, J., and Trias, A.: The vascular contribution to osteogenesis. J. Bone Joint Surg., *43-B:*800, 1961. Reprinted with permission.

lack of action on the proliferative segment of the physis.

Classification

Fractures involving the epiphyseal plate have been classified by several authors:

Foucher divided them into three classes: (1) pure separations of the epiphysis from the diaphysis (divulsion épiphysaire) without any osseous tissue adhering to it; (2) separation of the epiphysis with a thin, finely granular layer of osseous material attached to it (fracture épiphysaire); and (3) solution of continuity of the diaphysis in the midst of the osseous spongy tissue near the epiphysis (fracture pre-épiphysaire).[12]

Poland subdivided fractures involving the physis into the following types: *Type A*, pure and complete separation; *Type B*, partial separation with fracture of the diaphysis; *Type C*, partial separation with fracture of the epiphysis; and *Type D*, complete separation with fracture of the epiphysis (Fig. 8–7).[762]

Aitken designated the three types of fractures involving the epiphyseal cartilage plate as: *Type I*, an avulsion type of fracture due to shearing or twisting force in which

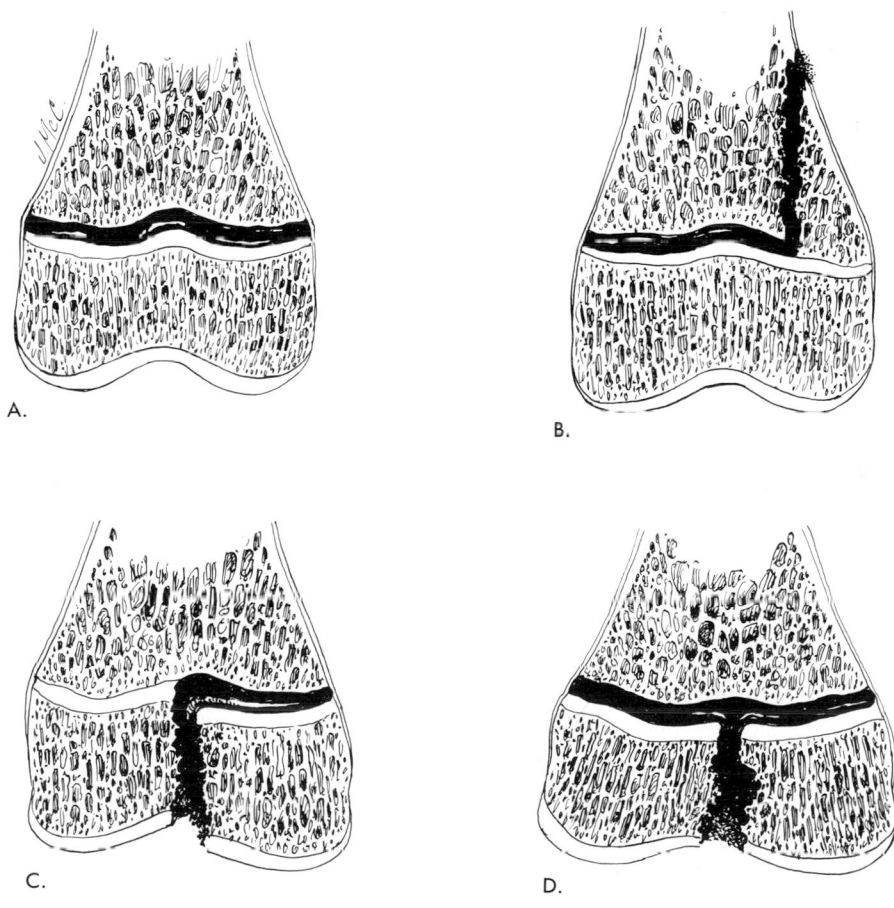

A.

B.

C.

D.

Partial

Complete

FIGURE 8–7. Poland's classification of epiphyseal separations.

A. Pure and complete separation. **B.** Partial separation with fracture of the diaphysis. **C.** Partial separation with fracture of the epiphysis. **D.** Complete separation with fracture of the epiphysis. (Redrawn after Poland, J.: Traumatic separation of the epiphysis. London, Smith, Elder & Co., 1898, p. 80.)

the fracture line passes through the zone of degenerating cartilage cells and emerges through a portion of the metaphyseal bone. Displacement in this type of fracture may be marked, but ultimate deformity due to displacement or growth disturbance is rare.

Type II, a compression type of fracture caused by a combination of crushing or shearing force, commonly involves the distal tibial epiphysis, but rarely the distal femoral epiphysis. The line of fracture originates in the joint and may emerge between the bony epiphysis and the zone of the degenerative cartilage cells of the physis; or the fracture line may cross the physis and emerge between it and the diaphysis. In the former, growth disturbance will not occur; whereas in the latter, premature arrest of growth and deformity will follow.

Type III is a compression type of injury in which the physis has been crushed between the bony epiphysis and the diaphysis. In this type, the fracture line may be so small as to be overlooked or may be considered of no clinical importance.[14]

Salter and Harris presented the following thorough and practical classification of physical injuries based on the mechanism of injury, the relationship of the fracture line to the germinal layer of the physis, and the prognosis concerning disturbance of growth.

Type I. This is produced by a shearing or avulsion force and is commonly encountered in infants whose physes are relatively thick. It may also occur in pathologic fractures such as those seen in rickets, scurvy, or osteomyelitis. The epiphysis separates from the metaphysis without any bony fragment, and the plane of cleavage is through the zone of the hypertrophying cells, with the germinal cells of the physis remaining with the epiphysis (Fig. 8–8A). Displacement of fragments is checked by the intact thick periosteal attachments. Reduction is usually unnecessary. Growth is not disturbed, unless there is associated aseptic necrosis and premature closure of the physis due to interruption of its blood supply; for example, in acute traumatic separation of the capital femoral epiphysis.

Type II. A shearing or avulsion force causes this fracture, which is the commonest type of physeal injury. It frequently occurs in children over ten years of age. The line of separation extends along the hypertrophic zone of the physis to a variable distance and then out through a portion of the metaphyseal bone (Fig. 8–8 B). In the roentgenogram, a triangular metaphyseal fragment is readily visible, which is referred to as "Thurston Holland's sign." The periosteum is intact on the concave side of the angulation (i.e., the side with the metaphyseal fragment), whereas on the convex side the periosteum is stripped and torn from the diaphysis, but still remains attached to the epiphysis. This is accounted for by the thickness, the great vascularity, and the loose connection of the periosteum with the diaphysis, but the intimate connection of the periosteum with the perichondrium of the epiphysis. In Type II physeal injury, reduction is ordinarily achieved and maintained with relative ease. The intact periosteal hinge on the concave side and the metaphyseal bone fragment prevent overreduction. Growth is not disturbed, as the germinal layer of chondrocytes remains attached to the epiphysis and circulation to the epiphysis is not interrupted.

Type III. This rare injury is caused by an intra-articular shearing force, which usually occurs in the proximal or distal tibial epiphysis. There is an intra-articular fracture of the epiphysis, with the plane of cleavage extending from the joint surface to the weak zone of hypertrophic cells of the physis and then extending parallel with the growth plate to its periphery (Fig. 8–8 C). Restoration of the congruous articular surface is essential in its treatment; in markedly displaced fractures, open surgery is often necessary to obtain accurate anatomic reduction. Prognosis for future growth is good, provided there is no impairment of circulation to the separated fragment of the epiphysis.

Type IV. This injury is most commonly seen at the lower end of the humerus in fractures of the lateral condyle. The fracture line begins at the articular surface and extends through the epiphysis, across the full thickness of the physis, and then through a segment of the metaphysis. There is a complete vertical split that involves the important germinal layer of the physis (Fig. 8–8 D). The fracture fragments may be undisplaced or separated to a varying extent. It is imperative to achieve per-

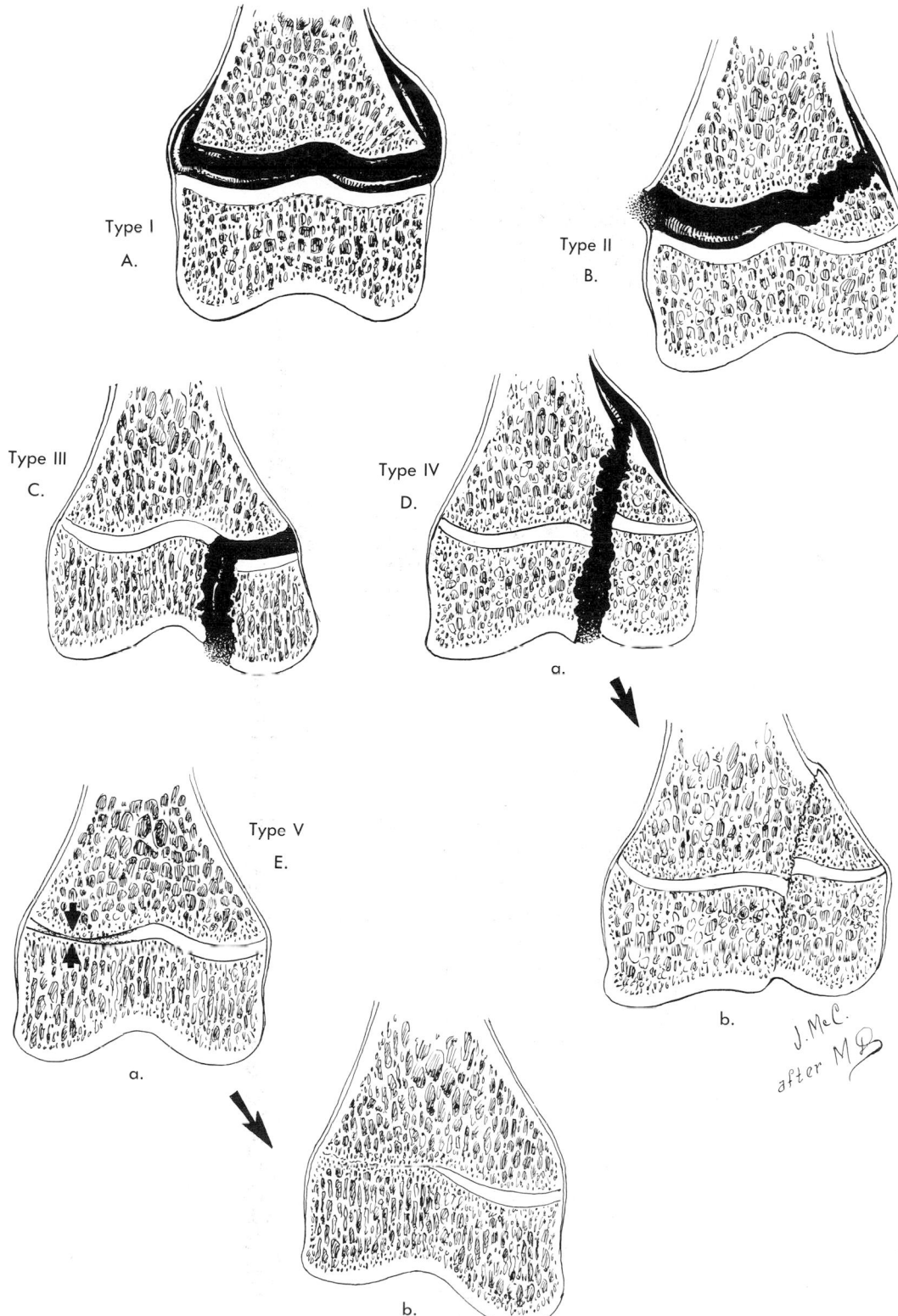

FIGURE 8–8. *Classification of epiphyseal plate injuries according to Salter and Harris.*

(Redrawn after Salter, R. B., and Harris, W. R.: Injuries involving the epiphyseal plate. J. Bone Joint Surg., *45-A*:587, 1963.)

fect anatomic reduction in order to restore a smooth articular surface and also to prevent osseous bridging across the physis with consequent local premature growth arrest. Only fine smooth Kirschner wires should be used for internal fixation; they should traverse the plate perpendicularly and be removed after four to six weeks.

Type V. This rare injury usually occurs in the knee or ankle—articulations that normally move only in one plane into flexion and extension. On the application of marked abduction or adduction strain, a severe compression force is transmitted through the epiphysis to a segment of the physis, crushing the germinal layer of the chondrocytes (Fig. 8–8 E). Displacement of the epiphysis is minimal in this type of physeal injury. Often the seriousness of the condition is not suspected and the injury is misdiagnosed as a simple sprain. In treatment, the part is supported in a cast, and weight-bearing is avoided for at least three weeks. The prognosis in Type V epiphyseal plate injury is poor, since premature arrest of growth almost always occurs.[27]

In this textbook, any physeal injury referred to by type will be according to the classification by Salter and Harris.

Incidence

Approximately 15 per cent of all fractures in children involve the physis.[27] The relative incidence of 2,500 consecutive epiphyseal injuries encountered at the New York Orthopedic Hospital is given in Table 8–2.

Principles of Management of Fractures Involving the Physis

These are well outlined by Salter and Harris:[27]

All reductions, whether closed or open, should be performed with the utmost gentleness in order to prevent damage to the delicate cartilage of the physis. Forceful manipulations are condemned. During open reduction, direct pressure on the physis by blunt instruments should be avoided.

Epiphyseal separations should be *reduced immediately*, as each day of delay will make it progressively more difficult. In fact, after ten days, Types I and II physeal injuries

Table 8–2. *Incidence—2,500 Epiphyseal Fractures**

Site	Per Cent
Lower radius	46
Lower humerus	14
Lower fibula	13
Lower tibia	11
Lower ulna	5
Upper radius	5
Upper humerus	3
Lower femur	1
Upper ulna	1
Upper tibia	0.8
Upper fibula	0.2

*From Neer, C. S. II, and Horwitz, B. S.: Fractures of the epiphysial plate. Clin. Orthop., *41*:24, 1965. Reprinted with permission.

cannot be reduced without exerting undue force and damaging the cartilaginous growth plate. When a Type I or Type II fracture is seen late (i.e., after seven to ten days), it is better to accept malunion than to cause growth arrest by forceful manipulation or open surgery. In Type III or IV physeal injuries, congruity of articular surfaces is essential; in such cases, delayed reduction is performed, if indicated.

As stated, reduction of Type I and Type II fractures involving the physis can be readily obtained and maintained. In Type III physeal injuries, open reduction may be indicated to restore a congruous articular surface, particularly in weight-bearing joints. Open reduction is required in almost all cases of Type IV fractures of the epiphyseal plate. Caution must be exercised in order to prevent injury to the circulation of the epiphysis. Only smooth Kirschner wires must be used for internal fixation, and under no circumstances should screws or threaded wires be inserted across the physis. The internal fixation device is removed when the fracture has healed.

Type III and Type IV physeal injuries require accurate anatomic reduction. In Type I and Type II fractures of the physis, perfect reduction is desirable, but not mandatory. Bone remodeling will correct moderate residual deformities. In general, one can accept a greater degree of deformity in multiplane joints (such as the shoulder) than in single plane joints (such as the knee and ankle).

Types, I, II, and III injuries consolidate

very rapidly, usually in about half the time required for a fracture through the metaphysis of the same bone. Type IV injuries require the same period for union as metaphyseal fractures.

Fractures involving the physis should be closely followed for possible development of growth disturbance. Parents should be warned of potential complications, but without causing much anxiety. As already indicated, the factors that determine the prognosis are: the type of epiphyseal plate injury, the age of the child at the time of fracture, the integrity of the blood supply to the epiphysis, the method of reduction, and whether the fracture is open or closed.

The Upper Limb

Injuries in the Region of the Shoulder

FRACTURES OF THE CLAVICLE

The clavicle (collar bone) is the most frequently broken bone in children. Extending from the acromion process of the scapula to the upper border of the manubrium sterni, it serves as the only connection between the arm and trunk, and is consequently subjected to all medially directed forces exerted upon the upper limb. This long bone has a double curve in the horizontal plane, being convex forward in its medial two thirds and concave forward in its lateral third. The shape of the clavicle is prismatic in its medial two thirds with anterior, posterior, and inferior surfaces; in its lateral third, it is flattened with superior and inferior surfaces. The lateral third of the clavicle provides attachment to the trapezius muscle posterosuperiorly and the deltoid muscle anteriorly. In its medial two thirds, the clavicular portion of the sternocleidomastoid muscle is inserted above and the pectoralis major muscle is attached in front and below. The superior surface of the clavicle is subcutaneous throughout its whole length. On its inferior surface, the costal tuberosity provides attachment for the strong costoclavicular ligaments medially; the conoid and trapezoid ligaments are inserted laterally, and the subclavius muscle originates in a groove in its middle two thirds. Because of the preceding anatomic features, the middle third of the clavicle is most vulnerable to injury.

The clavicle is the first bone in the body to ossify, doing so in membrane without going through a prior enchondral stage; cartilaginous growth areas develop later at both its ends, however. In adolescence, usually a single ossification center develops at the medial end of the clavicle, fusing with the shaft by 25 years of age. Occasionally an ossification center may develop at the acromion process, in which case it unites with the shaft immediately.[44] These ossification centers should not be mistaken for fractures.

Mechanism of Injury

The breaking force may arise from compression of the shoulders during a particularly difficult delivery at birth. The usual cause in a child is a fall, either from a high chair or out of bed onto the outstretched hand, elbow, or side of the shoulder. The fracture may occasionally be produced by direct violence applied from in front and above, the clavicle being forced against the upper ribs. An open fracture may occur following a direct blow, but this is extremely rare because of the mobility of the overlying skin and also because the fracture commonly results from indirect force.

Pathologic Anatomy

The most frequent site of the fracture is the junction of the middle and outer thirds of the bone. In the infant or young child, the break is often incomplete, being of the greenstick type. In older children and in adolescents, the fracture is frequently complete; the fragments may be undisplaced, but are bowed anteriorly, shortening the bone and increasing its normal anterior convexity. When there is overriding of the fragments, the affected shoulder drops downward, and inward, taking along the lateral fragment. This displacement is caused partially by the weight of the limb and partially by the pull of the pectoralis and trapezius muscles. The medial end of the lateral fragment is tilted posteriorly. The medial fragment is pulled upward and backward by the sternocleidomastoid muscle with the costoclavicular ligaments serving as a checkrein on the displacement (Fig. 8–9 A and B). The skin is then stretched over the lateral end of the medial fragment by the lowered shoulder.

If the breaking force is great, and particularly if it is direct, the fracture is comminuted. Occasionally, small, sharp fragments of bone may penetrate the skin or lacerate the subclavian vessels.

Fractures of the lateral third of the clavicle are infrequent and usually result from direct violence. The fracture is commonly transverse and may be comminuted. If the coracoclavicular ligaments are intact, displacement is minimal or negligible, the outer fragment being fixed to the acromion by the acromioclavicular ligaments and the inner fragment being bound to the coracoid process by the conoid and trapezoid ligaments. If the coracoclavicular ligaments are torn, the small lateral fragment is displaced with the acromion and the fracture acts like an acromioclavicular dislocation. The distal fragment, acromion, and shoulder are displaced downward and inward.

The medial third of the clavicle fractures vary rarely and then as a result of direct violence. The fragments are usually held together by the intact costoclavicular ligaments.

Diagnostic Features

BIRTH FRACTURES*

The clinical diagnosis of fractured clavicle in the newborn is made very occasionally, since the majority of these fractures are

---

*See References 37, 40, 47, 50–52, 54, 55, 57, 59.

asymptomatic. Farkas and Levine reported a roentgenographic survey of 300 consecutive living newborns; five were delivered with fractured clavicles (1.7 per cent). In none of the cases had the fracture been suspected following the routine pediatric examination in the delivery room and the nursery. On re-examination, however, Farkas and Levine were able to demonstrate crepitations at the fracture site. The break is usually complete, with overriding of the fragments. Involvement is usually unilateral, with no report of bilateral fractures. The injury occurs during delivery of the shoulders, with fracture of the anteriorly positioned clavicle predominating over that of the posterior clavicle.[43]

In clinically symptomatic cases, attention is drawn to the injury by the "pseudoparalysis"—i.e., lack of spontaneous movement of the upper limb on the affected side. This should be distinguished from obstetrical brachial plexus paralysis and from acute osteomyelitis of the humerus. Brachial plexus paralysis and fractured clavicle may coexist. On careful inspection and palpation, crepitation, local swelling, and tenderness will be found, suggesting the presence of a fractured clavicle. The diagnosis is confirmed by roentgenograms.

INFANCY AND CHILDHOOD

In infants and young children, a fractured clavicle of the greenstick type may escape notice until the appearance of the developing callus (Fig. 8–10). In such an instance, the condition should not be mistaken for congenital pseudarthrosis of the clavicle, which, likewise, is painless. The roentgenographic findings of congenital pseudarthrosis of the clavicle are characteristic: there is a definite wide zone of radiolucency with smooth margins at the site of the defect and no evidence of callus formation.

When the fracture is complete, with displacement, the clinical appearance is typical (Fig. 8–9 A). The shoulder on the affected side is lower than the opposite normal one, and it is drooped forward and inward. The patient rests the involved arm against his body and supports it at the elbow with the opposite hand. The tension on the sternocleidomastoid muscle tilts the head toward the affected side and rotates the chin

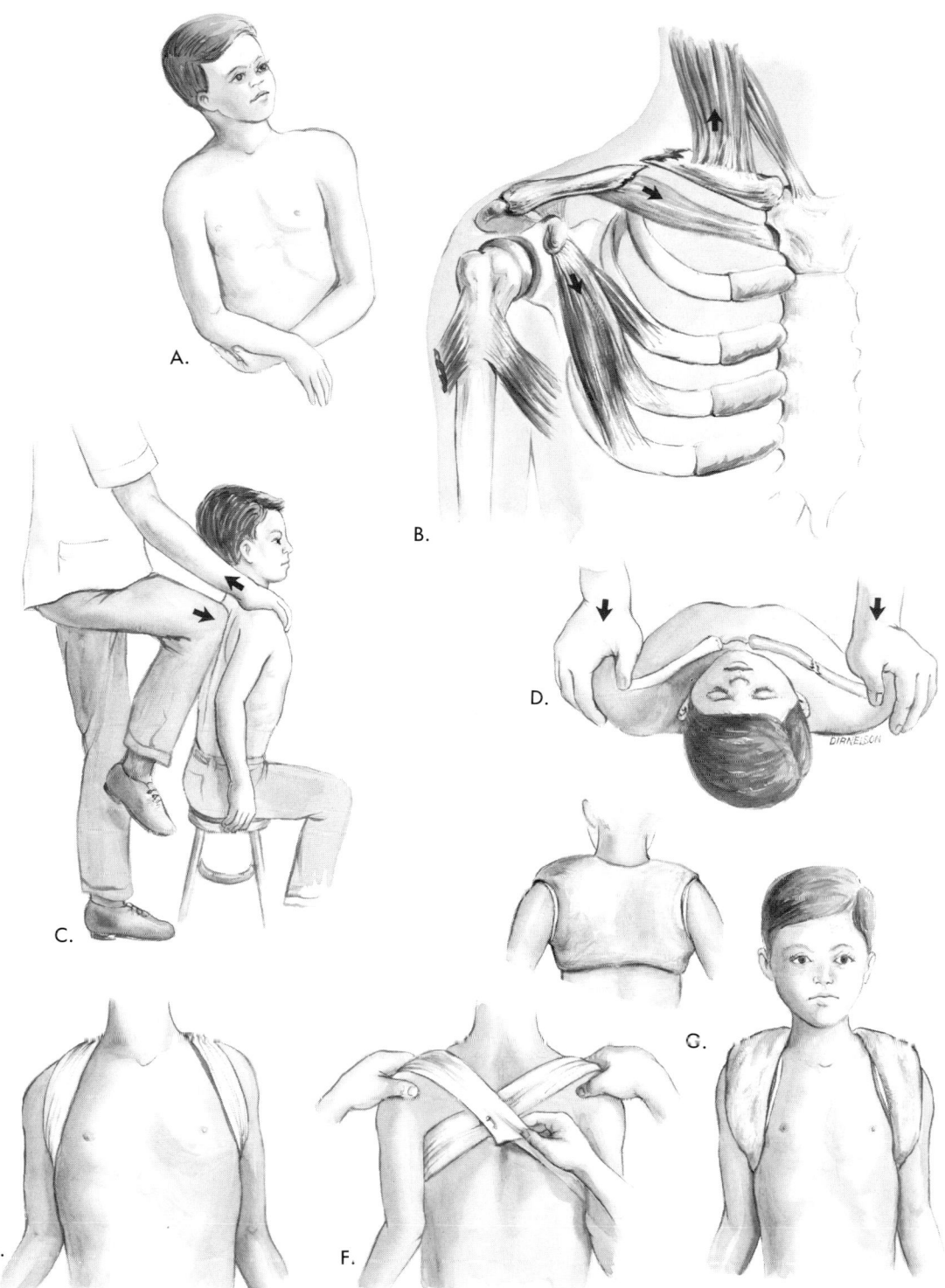

FIGURE 8–9. *Fracture of the clavicle.*

A and **B.** Deformity of fractured clavicle at the junction of its middle and outer thirds. Note the downward, forward, and inward drop of the affected shoulder because of the weight of the limb and the pull of the pectoral muscles. The medial fragment is pulled upward and backward by the pull of the sternocleidomastoid muscle. **C** and **D.** Method of reduction (see text for explanation). **E** and **F.** Figure-of-eight bandage used for immobilization. It is made of stockinette and orthopedic white felt. **G.** Figure-of-eight bandage made of plaster-of-Paris cast is used in children over six years of age.

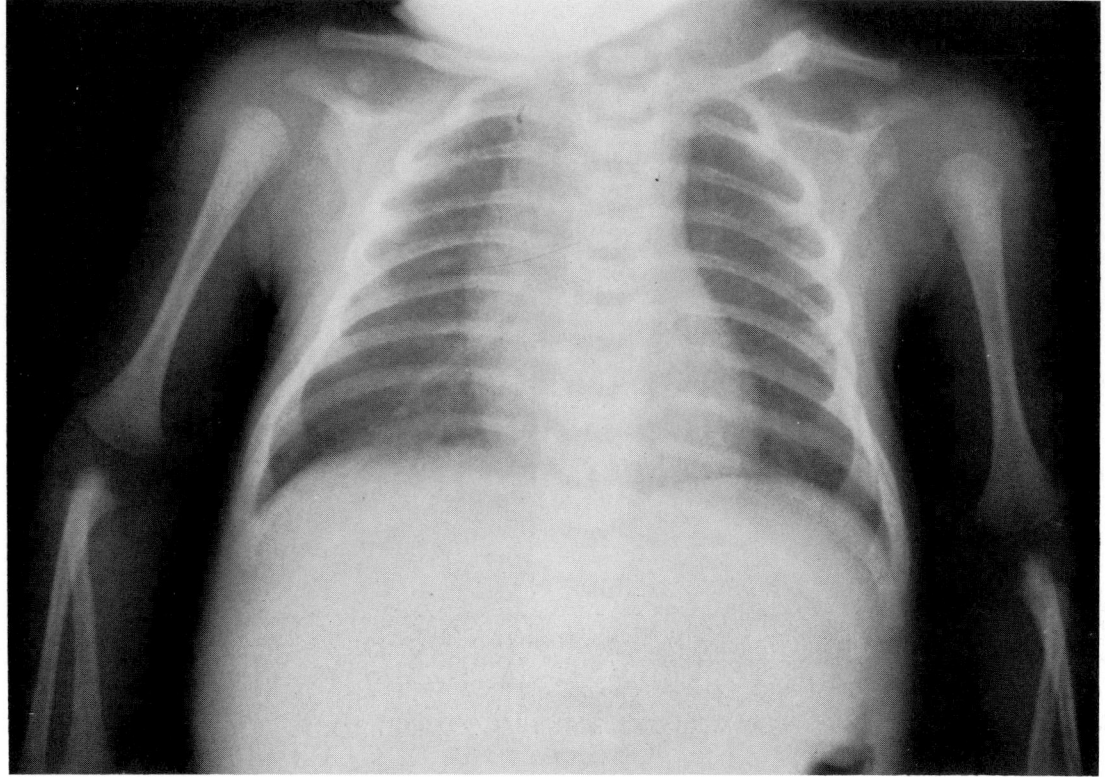

FIGURE 8–10. *Fracture of left clavicle in a newborn.*

This injury usually escapes notice until the development of callus.

toward the opposite side. Any change in position of the upper limb or of the cervical spine is painful. On palpation, there is local swelling, tenderness, and crepitation over the fracture site.

Fractures in the middle third of the clavicle will be clearly depicted in the anteroposterior roentgenogram (Fig. 8–11). To demonstrate fractures of the medial and lateral end of the clavicle, however, special oblique, lateral, or posteroanterior views may be required.

Treatment

BIRTH FRACTURES

An asymptomatic fracture in the neonate or young infant may be ignored. It will unite without external immobilization and any malalignment will correct itself with growth. The nurses and parents are instructed to

handle the infant gently, avoiding direct pressure over the broken clavicle. While the patient sleeps in prone position, soft padding may be placed under the affected shoulder to prevent it from drooping too far forward (this is done only when the fracture is grossly unstable and only for a few days).

When the fracture is painful and accompanied by "pseudoparalysis," it is best to protect it by splinting the arm for two weeks. A soft cotton pad is placed in the axilla, and with the elbow in acute flexion, the upper limb is loosely anchored across the front of the chest with two or three turns of elastic bandage. It is not necessary to encircle the elbow and clavicle with the bandage; and it is not advisable to apply a sling to hang from the opposite shoulder. The parents are instructed to reapply the bandage after each bath and skin care. Within 10 to 14 days, the pain will completely subside, the fracture will be united clinically, and the splint is removed. Muscle function in the upper limb is assessed by the reflex stimulation method to rule out associated obstetrical brachial plexus paralysis. Occasionally a birth fracture of the clavicle is accompanied by fracture of the upper humeral epiphysis involving the epiphyseal plate. In the initial roentgenograms, often this is not diagnosed; however, in the follow-up films, massive subperiosteal new bone formation will be seen and the condition may be mistaken for osteomyelitis. In the newborn with acute infection, there may be no systemic reaction. Osteomyelitis should be suspected if there is an area of rarefaction (bone destruction) in the metaphysis, if the pain is persistent, or if the swelling of the arm is marked and diffuse.

YOUNG CHILDREN

In children under six years of age, displaced fractures of the clavicle do not require reduction. Gross malalignment and the "bump" of the massive callus will remodel and disappear within six to nine months. The child is made comfortable by applying a figure-of-eight bandage (see Fig. 8–9 E and F). A 2- or 3-inch-wide stockinette is stuffed with orthopedic white felt. The patient is seated on a stool with the surgeon standing behind him. The bandage is applied in the following manner: Beginning posteriorly, the stockinette is passed in front of the normal clavicle, through the axilla, across the back, over the top of the fractured clavicle, through the axilla, and across the back, and then is anchored by two or three large safety pins to the other end of the stockinette. Tension is applied on the stockinette as it passes through the axilla of the involved side with the shoulder held upward and backward. It is imperative not to embarrass circulation. A circle of adhesive strapping on the back of the figure-of-eight bandage will maintain its tightness. Large pads of soft cotton may be placed over the superior and anterior aspects of the clavicle, reaching into the axilla; these are particularly indicated if the fracture fragments are overriding and unstable; the length and alignment of the clavicle are maintained by the weight of the arm over the axillary pads, which serve as fulcrums. If there is associated torticollis, the affected limb is supported with a sling suspended from the opposite shoulder.

The fracture is immobilized for three to four weeks. During this period tightness of the figure-of-eight bandage should be maintained. The parents are shown how to tighten the bandage by applying tension on the stockinette over the broken clavicle and securing it with an additional safety pin. They should be cautioned against excessive pressure on the axillary vessels and circulatory embarrassment, and they should check the skin for irritation and pressure sores. The surgeon should inspect, and if necessary, reapply the figure-of-eight bandage at weekly intervals.

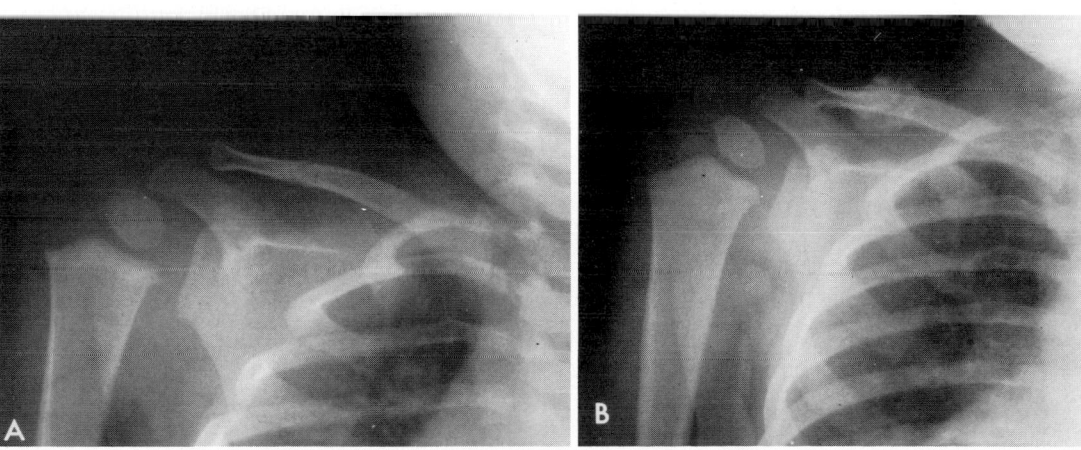

FIGURE 8–11. *Fracture of right clavicle in its middle third.*

A. Initial roentgenogram. **B.** Two weeks later, showing massive callus.

OLDER CHILDREN AND ADOLESCENTS

In children over six years of age and in adolescents, angulated greenstick fractures seldom, if ever, warrant reduction (Fig. 8–12). If the fracture is complete, however, or markedly displaced, or overridden, closed reduction is required. If anesthesia is indicated, under strict aseptic precautions, several milliliters of 1 per cent procaine is injected into the hematoma. General anesthesia is not required. Reduction is performed with the patient sitting on a stool. The operator places his knee between the scapulae and pulls the shoulders backward and upward. If the child is apprehensive, the fracture might be more comfortably reduced in the supine recumbent position. His lower limbs and pelvis are anchored on the table with sheets; a padded sandbag is placed posteriorly between the shoulders and the affected arm is allowed to hang in extended position at the side of the table. The weight of the arm alone will reduce the fracture, and this is less painful for the patient. If necessary, the operator can gently but firmly push the shoulders back to restore length and alignment to the fractured fragments. Roentgenograms are made to check reduction.

For the older child, immobilization is best provided by applying a plaster of Paris cast in a manner similar to the figure-of-eight bandage just described; with the child sitting on the table, felt padding and sheath wadding are applied in figure-eight fashion. Both the felt and sheath wadding should extend beyond the margins of the plaster cast. Then while an assistant pushes the shoulders upward and backward by pressure on the flexed elbows and the surgeon

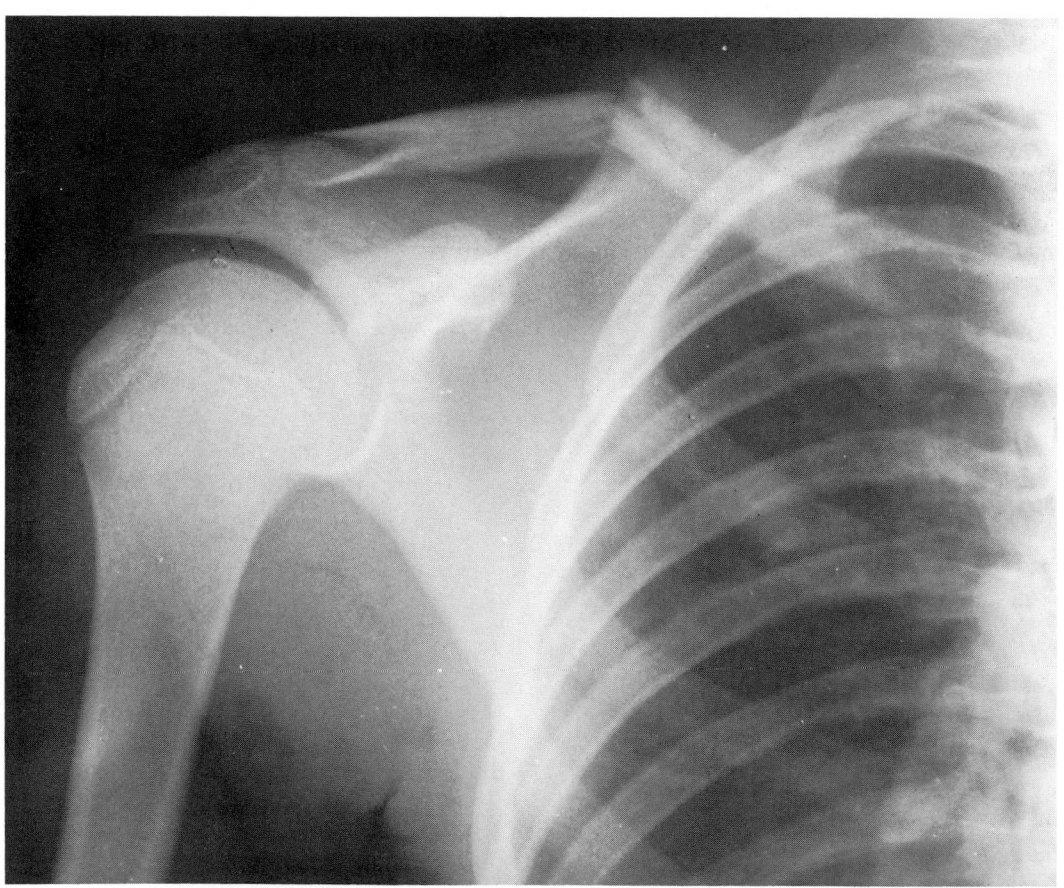

FIGURE 8–12. Angulated greenstick fracture of right clavicle.

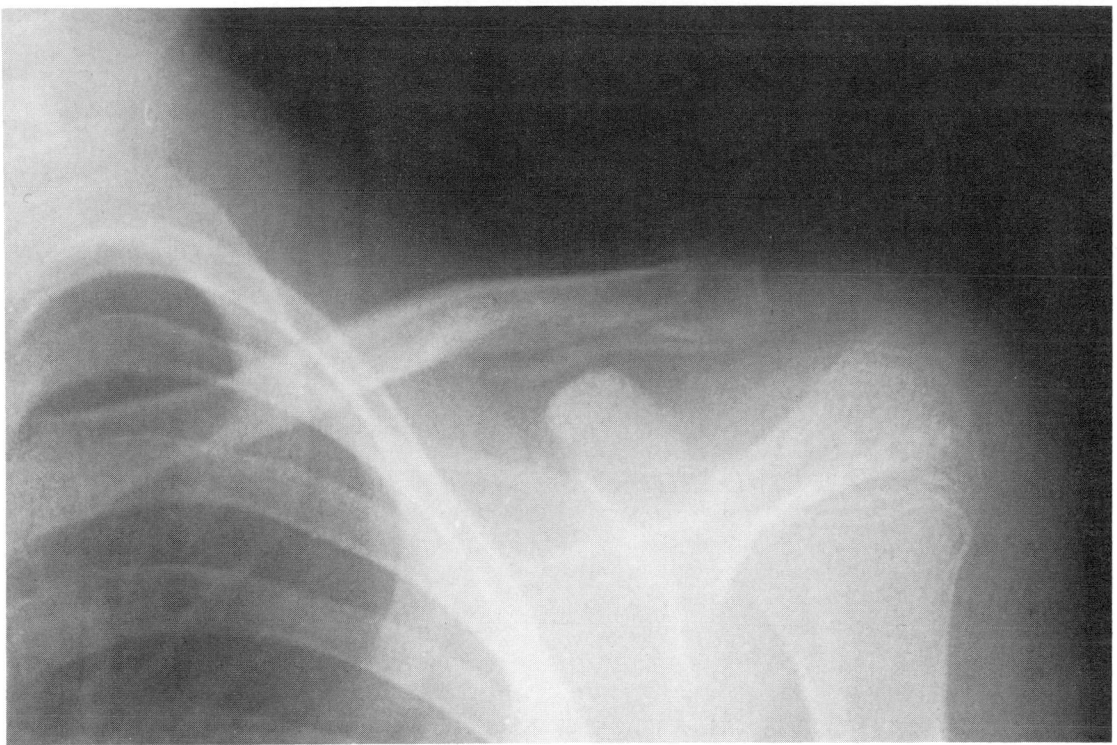

FIGURE 8-13. Fracture of lateral end of left clavicle.

applies posterior counterpressure with his knee on the upper dorsal spine, a 4-inch-wide plaster of Paris cast is applied. As soon as the plaster turns are completed, the patient is replaced in supine position and, using the sandbag as counterpressure, the operator pushes the shoulders posteriorly with the palms of his hands (see Fig. 8-9 G).

If the arm becomes swollen because of pressure of a tight splint against the axillary vessels, the cast is trimmed to relieve it. Five to six weeks of immobilization in the cast are required in the adolescent for osseous union to take place.

RECUMBENT TREATMENT

Fractures of the clavicle in the child with multiple injuries who is forced to rest in bed because of other major trauma (such as fractured femur, ruptured spleen, or subdural hematoma) are best managed by maintaining recumbent supine posture on a firm mattress. A small but firm pillow is placed between the scapulae, and the weight of the upper limb will gradually reduce the frac-

ture. For comfort, a stockinette and felt figure-of-eight bandage can be applied if necessary. In an adolescent girl, the cosmetic end-result of a displaced and overriding fracture may be improved by lateral arm skin traction, similar to modified Dunlop, with the shoulder in 90 degrees of abduction and 90 degrees of external rotation. Care is taken not to stretch the brachial plexus in a semicomatose or agitated patient. Bony union ordinarily occurs within three to four weeks.

Open reduction of a fractured clavicle is contraindicated in children. The only justification for open surgery is the repair of subclavian vessels that have been lacerated by the sharp bone fragments of a comminuted fracture. The presence of this rare complication is suggested by the large, rapidly increasing hematoma. Surgical intervention should be immediate, as the patient may die of extravasation or shock.[41]

Fractures of the lateral end of the clavicle are usually undisplaced (Fig. 8-13). The upper limb is supported in a triangular sling and immobilized across the chest with several circular turns of the elastic bandage. If the coracoclavicular ligaments are ruptured and the fracture fragments are displaced, treatment is similar to that of acromioclavicular dislocation, except that with the capsule and ligaments of the acromioclavicular joint intact, the fracture can be reduced and alignment maintained by closed methods. A downward force is exerted on the medial fragment of the clavicle, and the distal fragment and acromion are pushed upward by vertical pressure on the flexed elbow. After adequate padding with orthopedic felt, adhesive strapping is applied, encircling the elbow and clavicle. The strapping may become loose and should be changed as necessary at weekly intervals. In about a month, the fracture will be consolidated enough to discontinue the strapping. A simple triangular sling may be worn for an additional week to support the weight of the upper limb.

Fractures of the medial end of the clavicle are usually undisplaced and are adequately treated by support in a sling for three to four weeks.

EPIPHYSEAL SEPARATION OF MEDIAL END OF CLAVICLE

The epiphysis at the medial end of the clavicle does not begin to ossify until the eighteenth year; it fuses with the shaft between the twenty-second and twenty-fifth years. The acromial end of the clavicle has no epiphysis.

Traumatic separation of the epiphysis of the sternal end of the clavicle is a rare injury. Poland could collect only six cases; three of them were separations of an ossified epiphysis (ages 20, 18, and 17 years) and there were separations of cartilaginous epiphysis (14, 11, and 3 years).[762] Karlèn, in 1943, reported a case in a boy 12 years of age; Denham and Dingley reported four cases, all under 18 years of age (three 14 and one 16 years old).[60, 61]

The medial end of the clavicle is attached to the sternum and first rib by a heavy sheath of fibrous tissue. The injury is commonly caused by indirect violence, such as a fall or blow upon the point of the shoulder, causing the clavicle to be driven inward and forward. It may occasionally be produced by direct violence, as in the second case of Denham and Dingley, in which a wagon loaded with wood ran over the patient's chest.[60]

Roentgenograms will show the displacement of the sternal end of the clavicle, and on clinical examination, prominence of the sternal end of the clavicle may be sharp and palpable immediately beneath the skin. The clavicular part of the sternocleidomastoid muscle is pulled anteriorly with the bone and is in spasm, causing the patient's head to tilt toward the affected side. If the injury occurs before ossification has taken place in the medial epiphysis, the condition is often mistaken for common dislocation of the sternoclavicular joint.

Treatment consists of closed manipulative reduction and immobilization in a Velpeau dressing. Its reduction usually proves more stable than that of a sternal dislocation. Open reduction is indicated when manipulation under general anesthesia fails to replace the medial end of the clavicle; in such cases, it is best to drill a Kirschner wire obliquely through the anterior cortex of the clavicle, across the epiphyseal line, and into the epiphysis to stabilize the fragments. The lateral end of the wire is bent to prevent its migration. A Velpeau dressing is applied. The wire is removed in six weeks.

ACROMIOCLAVICULAR DISLOCATION

Injury to the acromioclavicular joint is very rare in children because the force of direct violence or a direct blow will instead fracture the clavicle. In adolescents, however, dislocation of the acromioclavicular joint is a quite common occurrence in sports. Three grades of injury are recognized: sprain of the acromioclavicular ligament; rupture of the acromioclavicular ligament; and rupture of the acromioclavicular, conoid, and trapezoid ligaments.

Clinical findings depend on the severity of the lesion. Immediately following injury, the patient will complain of pain on all motions of the shoulder, particularly forward rotation. There is definite local tenderness over the acromioclavicular joint. When the joint is dislocated, the upriding prominent lateral end of the clavicle can be palpated.

Roentgenograms should be made with the patient standing and holding weight in each hand and the central beam passing anteroposteriorly through the joint. In subluxation the acromion process is depressed in relation to the lateral end of the clavicle, whereas in dislocation there will be complete discontinuity of the articular ends. An associated fracture of the lateral end of the clavicle should be ruled out.

Treatment depends upon the degree of injury to the joint. In a *sprain* of the acromioclavicular ligament, simple strapping and a sling are all that is necessary. In *subluxation*, strapping and a plaster jacket are applied—the clavicle is depressed by a padded strap across the clavicle and the acromion is elevated by pushing the humerus upward with strapping. The acromioclavicular joint is immobilized for three weeks. *Dislocations* of the acromioclavicular joint require open reduction, capsular repair, and internal fixation with a threaded wire. For details of operative technique and other methods of treatment, the reader is referred to the cited literature.[62-66]

FRACTURES OF THE SCAPULA

The scapula is a flat triangular bone located between pads of muscles in the posterior upper thorax. Its borders are thickened and it is freely mobile on the chest wall. These anatomic features make injuries to the scapula very rare. Almost any part of the bone may be broken.

The scapula is ossified from seven or more centers: one for the body, two for the acromion, two for the coracoid process, one for the vertebral border, and one for the inferior angle.

At birth, the scapula is composed of a large osseous plate (consisting of its body and spine) and a cartilaginous mass comprising the coracoid process, the acromion, the glenoid, and the edge of the scapular spine. Between 15 and 18 months of age, the ossification center for the *middle of the coracoid process* appears. The base of the coracoid process that rests on the glenoid fossa begins to ossify between the seventh and tenth years; it is sometimes called the subcoracoid bone. When fully ossified, it is pyramidal in shape. Shortly following its appearance, the subcoracoid bone first joins posteriorly with the body of the scapula, and later (between the fourteenth and sixteenth years) with the middle of the ossified portion of the coracoid process. Frequently, a scalelike ossification nucleus appears on the tip of the coracoid process at about the fourteenth year, and joins on at the eighteenth year. Occasionally, an additional point of ossification in the form of a cap appears at the apex of the coracoid process at the seventeenth year, joining the body of the process between the twentieth and twenty-fifth years. This cap-shaped apophysis does not unite with the scalelike apophysis.

Ossification of the *acromion process* originates from two centers, one being at its base, and the other at its apex. These begin to ossify between the fourteenth and sixteenth years, and coalesce to form one apophysis at about the nineteenth year, connecting with the scapular spine from the twenty-second to the twenty-fifth year. Sometimes bony union may fail to take place between the acromion and the spine of the scapula, the junction created consisting only of fibrous tissue. Such tardy union or failure of osseous union should not be mistaken for fracture.

The *glenoid fossa* is composed of four segments: the subcoracoid bone on its upper third; a portion of the coracoid process internally; a part from the body of the scapula; and a cartilaginous plate in the lower part of the glenoid, which joins the body of the scapula between the twentieth and twenty-fifth years. In its early stages of development, the glenoid fossa is convex, but later becomes flat and then concave.

The ossification center for the inferior angle of the scapula appears at the fifteenth year and fuses by the twentieth year; and that of the vertebral border of the scapula appears by the seventeenth year, fusing by the twenty-fifth year.

Fractures of the Body of the Scapula

These are the result of direct violence such as a crushing injury in an automobile accident or a fall from a height. The blade of the scapula is often comminuted, the fracture lines running in various directions, but at times, the bone may split throughout its length in a transverse or oblique line. The spine of the scapula may be fractured with the body of the scapula. The intraspinous portion is more frequently fractured than the supraspinous one. Usually there is little if any displacement of the fractured fragments, as they are held together by the surrounding muscles. The fracture is rarely open, but the direct trauma may cause severe damage to the overlying soft parts. Frequently there are extensive crushing injuries of the thorax with multiple fractures of the ribs or the spinal column, pneumothorax, and subcutaneous emphysema. Because of the gravity of the accompanying conditions, the scapular fracture is often missed. In order to demonstrate the fracture, it is necessary to obtain oblique tangential views in addition to the routine anteroposterior roentgenograms.

The primary objective of treatment is to make the patient comfortable. It is not necessary to reduce the fracture or to immobilize the entire arm and shoulder. If the soft-tissue condition permits, the scapula is fixed against the chest wall by crisscross moleskin adhesive strapping across the shoulder and down over the patient's back to the level of his waist. If the patient is ambulatory, he can be made more comfortable by suspending his arm in a sling. The fracture will heal within four weeks and any resultant irregularity of bony contour will be remodeled and will disappear with growth. Shoulder stiffness is not a problem in children.

Fractures of the Scapular Neck

These are usually caused by a direct blow to the front or back of the shoulder. The fracture line usually begins in the suprascapular notch and runs downward and laterally to the axillary border of the scapular neck inferior to the glenoid. The capsular attachments of the glenohumeral joint and the articular surface of the glenoid remain intact. Depending upon the force of injury, the fracture may be undisplaced, minimally displaced, markedly displaced, or comminuted. If the coracoclavicular and acro-

mioclavicular ligaments are intact, there is little, if any, displacement of the articular fragment; however, if these ligaments are torn, or if the fracture line is lateral to the coracoid process, the articular fragment is displaced downward and inward by the weight of the limb and the muscle pull. In severe crushing injuries, the fracture line may include the acromion, scapular spine, and glenoid.

Treatment consists of support of the shoulder and arm in a triangular sling for a period of three to four weeks. Circumduction and pendulum exercises for the shoulder can be performed 14 days after injury when the patient is more comfortable.

Markedly displaced fractures of the scapular neck are treated by skeletal traction with a pin through the base of the olecranon; the shoulder is abducted to 90 degrees and the forearm is flexed to right angles. Gradually the glenoid fragment will be repositioned in normal anatomic alignment. After two to three weeks the traction is removed and the shoulder is immobilized in a triangular sling and swathe for an additional two weeks. Several times a day, the swathe is removed and circumduction shoulder exercises are performed to maintain range of motion of the shoulder.

Fractures of the Glenoid Cavity of the Scapula

These are produced either by direct or indirect force. Direct violence, such as a fall on the lateral side of the shoulder, will usually produce a stellate fracture, which may be minimally displaced or comminuted with separation of the fragments. In indirect injuries, such as a fall on the flexed elbow, the breaking force is transmitted up the shaft of the humerus, shearing off a fragment of the glenoid. When the shoulder is in extended and abducted position during the fall, the anterior part of the glenoid is fractured; whereas when the shoulder is in flexion and abduction, a fragment from the posterior part of the glenoid is detached. The humeral head may subluxate if the fracture fragment is large and markedly displaced. Avulsed fracture of the glenoid bone may result from acute traumatic dislocation of the shoulder. Sudden severe contraction of the long head of the triceps may cause avulsion fracture of the inferior brim of the glenoid cavity.

Fractures of the glenoid should be managed conservatively. The shoulder joint is immobilized in a triangular sling and swathe. After two to three weeks, pendulum and circumduction exercises are performed within tolerance of pain. Immobilization is discontinued after four weeks. Stellate fractures with marked displacement are treated with lateral arm skeletal traction with a Kirschner wire through the base of the olecranon. After two weeks, traction is removed and a triangular sling is applied for an additional two weeks. Open reduction of a fracture of the glenoid cavity is difficult and its results disappointing. Functional results of conservative treatment are good, despite gross irregularity of the joint. If avulsed fragments become symptomatic, they are excised at a later date.

When a large fragment of the anterior or posterior portion of the glenoid fossa is fractured and widely separated and causes the humeral head to subluxate, open reduction and internal fixation with a screw are indicated. Any tears of the capsule are repaired to stabilize the joint.

Fractures of the Acromion

The acromion process breaks occasionally from direct violence or from indirect force transmitted vertically by the humeral head. The line of fracture is usually lateral to the acromioclavicular joint, though occasionally it occurs at its base adjacent to the spine of the scapula. The shoulder is flattened, and there is localized pain, swelling, and tenderness. Abduction of the shoulder is very painful and restricted. The diagnosis is made on roentgen examination. Treatment consists of immobilization in a circular strapping (pushing the flexed elbow upward and the lateral part of the clavicle downward) and a sling for a period of three to four weeks. If, later, abduction of the shoulder is limited by a downward projecting malunited acromion, partial acromionectomy is performed to improve range of shoulder motion.

Fracture of the Coracoid Process

This isolated injury is a rare lesion. It may be caused by sudden muscular action of the short head of the biceps and the coracobrachialis muscles or by direct violence. Treatment consists of a triangular sling and swathe across the chest for a period of three weeks. Results are excellent, even in the presence of nonunion of the coracoid process.

Fracture-Separation of Epiphyses of Acromion and Coracoid Process

These occasionally occur in adolescents and young adults. Their treatment is the same as that of a fracture of a bone. Traumatic dislocation of the scapulocostal joint is a very rare injury.

FRACTURES INVOLVING THE PROXIMAL HUMERAL PHYSIS (Fracture-Separation of Upper Epiphysis of Humerus)

The proximal epiphysis of the humerus develops from three centers of ossification: one major central one for the head, which usually appears between the ages of four and six months (sometimes before birth); one for the greater tuberosity, which ossifies by three years; and one for the lesser tuberosity, which is visible on the roentgenogram by the age of five years. These ossification nuclei coalesce into a single center by the age of seven years. The epiphyseal plate is concave inferiorly; in its medial half, it follows the line of the anatomic neck and then passes laterally and downward to the distal border of the greater tuberosity. Fusion of the upper humeral epiphysis with the shaft takes place between 20 and 22 years of age. About 80 per cent of the longitudinal growth of the humerus is contributed by its proximal epiphyseal plate.

The supraspinatus, infraspinatus, and teres minor muscles are inserted on three flat impressions on the greater tuberosity, whereas the subscapularis muscle is inserted on an impression on the lesser tuberosity. In the metaphyseal and proximal diaphyseal regions, the pectoralis major tendon inserts to the crest of the greater tuberosity; the teres major is attached to the crest of the lesser tubercle of the humerus; and the floor of the intertubercular groove gives insertion to the latissimus dorsi muscle.

Fracture-separations of the upper humeral epiphysis may take place at any age while the epiphyseal plate is open, the period of greatest frequency being between the ages of 11 and 15 years. It can occur at birth, and the oldest patient reported in the literature is a 23-year-old man with pituitary gigantism, in whom epiphyseal closure was delayed secondarily to the endocrine lesion. It is three times more frequent in boys than in girls in the series of Smith, of Neer and Horwitz, and of Dameron and Reibel.[73, 77, 82] Bourdillon, however, reports four male patients to one female patient in his series.[71]

Mechanism of Injury

Fractures that involve the proximal humeral epiphyseal plate usually result from indirect violence, the force being exerted up through the humeral shaft with the arm in an adducted, extended, and externally rotated position. A common accident is a fall backward in which the person extends his elbow in an attempt to break the fall with his hand and gets the hand caught under his buttock. A direct blow or a fall on the lateral aspect of the shoulder may also cause a fracture. Neer and Horwitz reported a direct blow to the shoulder as the etiologic agent in 59 of their 89 cases; they believed the fracture is characteristically produced by a posterolateral shearing force that adducts the humeral shaft and displaces it forward.[77]

Pathologic Anatomy

Dameron and Reibel performed experimental studies on 12 anatomic specimens of the proximal ends of the humeri from stillborn infants. They could not fracture the humerus through the epiphyseal plate without displacing the metaphysis posteriorly or laterally; the fracture fragments were maintained in position by the thick periosteal envelope. By forceful manipulation it was extremely difficult to displace the metaphysis posteriorly at the epiphyseal plate; however, when the arm was extended and adducted, the metaphysis could be displaced anteriorly with relative ease. The upper end of the metaphysis ruptured the periosteum immediately lateral to the tendon of the long head of the biceps. (The anterior rather than the posterior displacement of the metaphysis is partly due to asymmetric configuration of the dome of the metaphysis, with its apex posterior and medial to its center, and partly due to firmer attachment of the periosteum along the posterior surface of the periphery of the epiphysis.) Once the periosteum was torn and began to strip distally, the fracture became progressively less stable. In all stillborn specimens, the fracture occurred at the epiphyseal plate without any metaphyseal bone fragment.[73]

This Type I epiphyseal injury is typical of that encountered in infants and young children. In older children and adolescents, a fragment of metaphysis usually remains attached to the posterior medial epiphysis (Type II epiphyseal injury). Thus, the cartilage cells contributing to the longitudinal growth of the humerus are spared. Types III, IV, or V epiphyseal injuries are not encountered in the upper end of the humerus; this is accounted for by the fact that the glenohumeral joint is the most mobile and multiplane joint in the body, and for mechanical reasons, crushing or splitting injuries of this plate are very unlikely.

The degree of displacement depends upon the force causing the injury and upon the muscular pull. There may be simple loosening of the epiphysis with practically no displacement, or the displacement may be partial or complete. Neer and Horwitz have graded the degree of displacement as: *Grade I*, less than 5 mm.; *Grade II*, to one third of the shaft; *Grade III*, to two thirds of the shaft; and *Grade IV*, greater than two thirds of the shaft, including total displacement.[77]

In grades III and IV displacement there is always a varying degree of angulation.

Partial displacement occurs more frequently than complete. The epiphysis remains in the glenoid fossa, but is rotated into abduction and external rotation by the pull of attached muscles, so that its articular surface is tilted inferiorly. The upper end of the humeral shaft is drawn upward, forward, and inward by the combined action of the pectoralis major, latissimus dorsi, and teres major muscles. The arm is abducted to a varying degree by the pull of the deltoid muscle. The periosteum is stripped off the lateral aspect of the humeral diaphysis to a varying extent. The intact portion of the periosteum on the posteromedial aspect holds the fragments together, making closed reduction difficult; it also forms a mold for the callus and later for the new bone produced by the epiphyseal plate. Occasionally the fracture is impacted with the upper end of the metaphysis driven into the epiphysis.

Diagnosis

This should be the first lesion to be thought of in injuries to the shoulder region in children between 9 and 15 years. Disability is great, with marked swelling and local tenderness.

With complete displacement of the fracture fragments, the presenting deformity is characteristic. The arm is shortened and is held in a varying degree of abduction and extension. There is a prominence in the front of the axilla near the coracoid process caused by the upper end of the distal fragment, which can be palpated and even seen. The anterior axillary fold is distorted, with a characteristic puckering of the skin caused by the lower fragment hooking into it. The humeral head is palpable in its normal position. On grasping the head of the humerus between the fingers and thumb of one hand while holding the flexed elbow with the other hand, the surgeon may be able to demonstrate false motion and crepitus between the fracture fragments. When the displacement is slight, most of these physical findings will be absent, the diagnosis being confirmed by roentgenograms in both the anteroposterior and lateral views (Fig. 8–14).

Treatment

In infants and young children (up to five years of age), the usual epiphyseal injury is Type I (Salter and Harris). It is difficult to delineate the position of the upper humeral epiphysis since it is mostly cartilaginous. If the arm is shortened and abducted, an attempt is made to restore length and alignment by applying longitudinal traction with the arm in 90 degrees of abduction, 90 degrees of flexion, and 15 to 25 degrees of external rotation. Exact apposition of the fragment is not necessary and administration of a general anesthetic is not justified. The shoulder and upper limb are immobilized in a modified Velpeau bandage. Within three to four weeks, solid union will take place. Any malalignment and angular deformity will correct itself with growth and remodeling.

In children over six years of age and in adolescents the usual fracture is a Type II epiphyseal injury. When there is no displacement, a modified Velpeau bandage is applied for four weeks, by which time the fracture will be firmly consolidated.

When there is minimal displacement with the degree of angulation less than 20 degrees, a gentle closed reduction is attempted without general anesthesia. Again, it is not necessary to reduce the fracture into normal anatomic alignment. Remodeling will correct any deformity and will have excellent functional and cosmetic results.

When the fracture is moderately angulated (more than 20 degrees) or completely displaced, it should be manipulated into an acceptable position. This is best carried out under general anesthesia. In a cooperative patient, local anesthesia with supplemental analgesia may be adequate, however. The longer its duration following injury, the more difficult this fracture is to reduce. The first few hours after trauma are the easiest time for manipulative reduction. The prime difficulty of reduction is the position assumed by the upper humeral epiphysis, which is small, mobile, and difficult to grasp and stabilize during manipulation. The proximal fragment is abducted and externally rotated; to permit reduction it is essential to place the distal fragment in line with the proximal fragment. Thus, traction is exerted with the arm in 90 degrees of abduction, 90 degrees of flexion, and slight external rotation. During the maneuver, an assistant grasps and stabilizes the humeral head between his thumb and fingers. The metaphysis is forced back through the defect in the anterior periosteum and im-

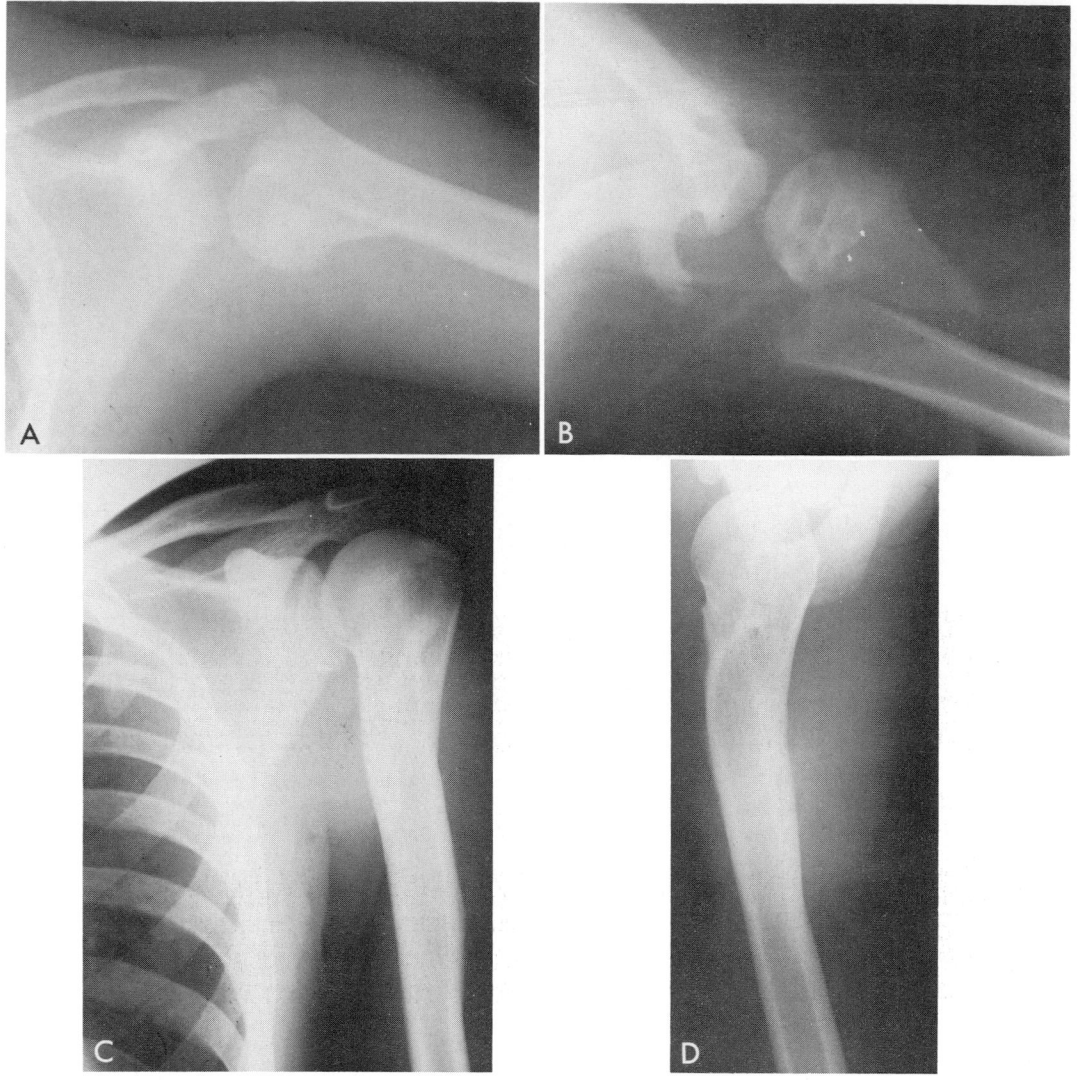

FIGURE 8-14. *Fracture involving the proximal humeral physis.*
A and **B.** Initial roentgenograms. **C** and **D.** Roentgenograms taken six years later, showing remodeling of malunion. (Courtesy of Dr. John J. Fahey.)

pacted into the epiphysis. Roentgenograms are made in anteroposterior and lateral views to check anatomic alignment. If reduction is stable, a modified Velpeau bandage is applied; if unstable, a shoulder spica cast is applied with the arm in 90 degrees of abduction, 60 degrees of forward flexion, and neutral rotation.

Closed reduction may be difficult or, at times, impossible. If the preceding manipulation fails, a heavy smooth Kirschner wire is inserted (under strict aseptic conditions and roentgenographic control) in a superoin-

ferior direction from the acromion into the upper humeral epiphysis, transfixing the two. The pin should not engage the metaphysis, however. The shoulder is positioned in abduction and flexion prior to fixing the humeral head to the acromion. The manipulative reduction is repeated. If it is successful and the fracture is stable, a modified Velpeau bandage is again applied; if it is successful but unstable, a shoulder spica cast is applied in the degree of abduction and flexion that affords the greatest stability. Osseous union will occur in four to six weeks. Alignment of fracture fragments is checked by periodic roentgenograms since it may be lost, even in a shoulder spica cast. A hanging cast, so commonly used in adults, is not effective in children, as the fragments become displaced when the arm is returned to the side.

Perfect anatomic reduction is not essential since gross malalignment is compatible with excellent functional result. This is because the shoulder is the most mobile articulation in the human skeleton and is not a weight-bearing joint. The greater the growth potential of the proximal humerus, the more

acceptable the malalignment. In general, in boys under 15 years of age and in girls under 13 years of age, 50 per cent bayonet apposition of the fragments will be corrected with growth and remodeling; however, one should be cautious in accepting angulation of more than 20 degrees (Fig. 8–15).

Only very occasionally is open reduction indicated in an older adolescent in whom conservative measures have failed to achieve adequate reduction. The tendon of the long head of the biceps may be caught between the fragments, or more frequently, a patient

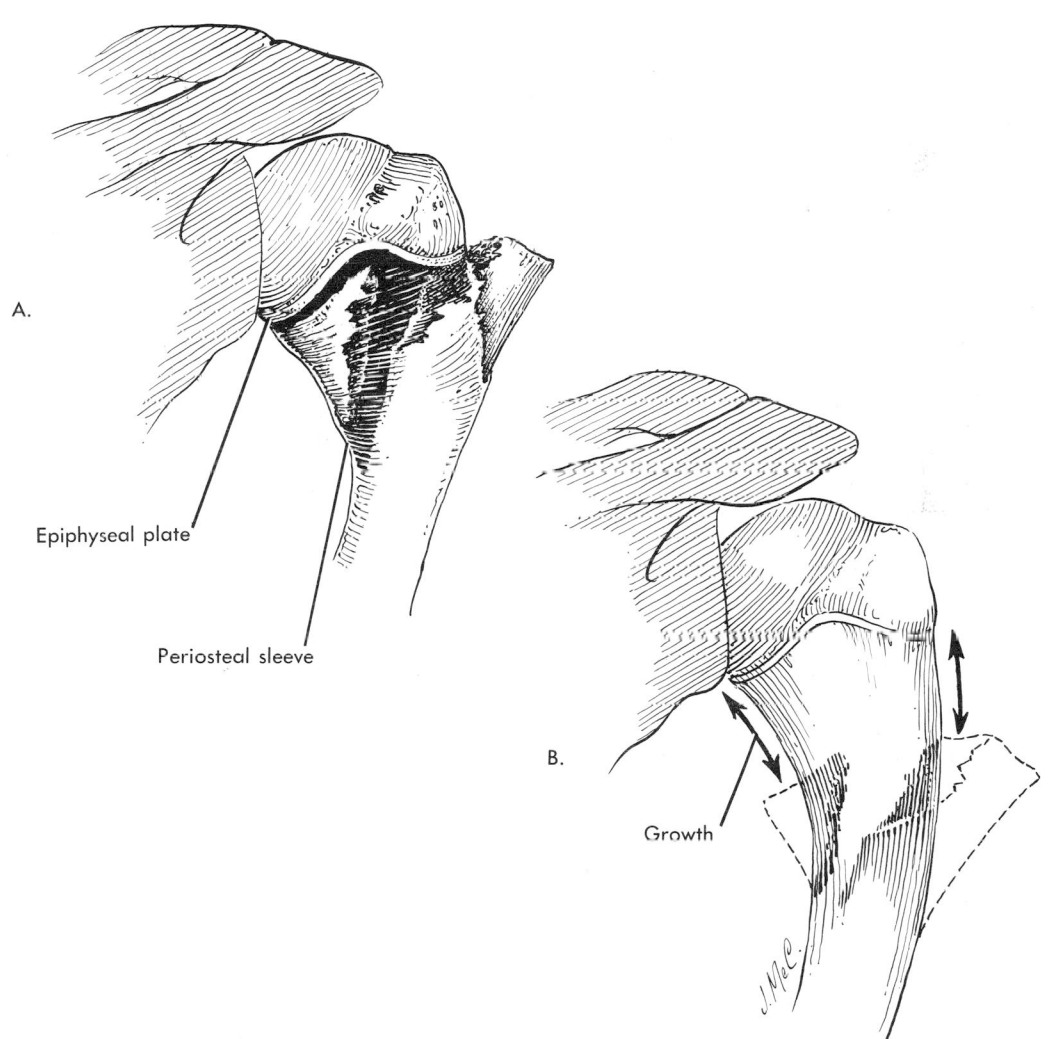

Epiphyseal plate

Periosteal sleeve

Growth

FIGURE 8–15. *Diagram showing remodeling process of a malunited fracture involving the proximal humeral physis.*

is seen several days after injury and the fragments are bound firmly together by the thickened reactive periosteum. Before embarking on open surgery, the consequences of the blemish of an unsightly scar should be weighed. In the author's experience, angulation can ordinarily be corrected if it is less than 20 degrees, and the marked overriding and shortening are acceptable. The protruding bony prominence of the upper end of the humeral shaft may restrict internal rotation and adduction to a varying degree; however, over a period of several years, the bony block will be absorbed by remodeling with excellent functional range of shoulder motion.

Side arm or overhead arm traction with a pin in the olecranon may be attempted, but usually fails. Instead of disengaging the fragments, it stretches the capsule and subluxates the humeral head.

Nilsson and Svartholm reported excellent results in 43 of 44 cases of fractures of the upper end of the humerus. They found considerable displacement does not in itself necessarily lead to any significant disability and advised open reduction only in those cases of serious displacement that cannot be treated with closed methods; i.e., dislocation of the upper humeral epiphysis or serious rotational displacement.[78] Dameron and Reibel, in an end-result study of 69 patients (46 of whom returned for end-result evaluation) with an average follow-up of seven years, concluded that more than the usual displacement and angulation can be accepted in the treatment of this epiphyseal injury, and believed open reduction is not indicated.[73] Neer and Horwitz, in a study of 89 fractures of the proximal humeral epiphyseal plate, presented the end-results in 62 patients with a minimum follow-up of 4.8 years. Shortening of the humerus of from 1 to 3 cm. occurred in 9 per cent of the patients with fractures of Grade I and Grade II displacement and in 33 per cent of those with Grade IV displacement. In children under 11 years of age, permanent shortening was not noted. In children 11 years of age and over, length and axis deformities of moderate degree were not infrequent; however, the functional results in all these cases were very satisfactory because of the compensation provided by the great mobility of the glenohumeral joint and because discrepancies in length are clinically less significant in the upper limb than in the lower limb. They concluded that the remodeling powers of the epiphysis of the proximal humerus are so great that the hazards of operative reduction are rarely, if ever, justified. It is advisable, however, to warn the parents of children over 11 years of age that growth and remodeling may not fully correct the inequality, and some permanent shortening and angulation may occur. This is especially true in cases with marked displacement.[77]

Injuries to the Arm

FRACTURES OF THE SHAFT OF THE HUMERUS

Fractures of the humeral shaft in children are uncommon in comparison to the frequency with which they occur in the adult. The shaft of the humerus is roughly cylindrical in its upper half, becoming gradually broadened and flattened below. Surgically, it may be considered as extending from the upper border of the insertion of the pectoralis major muscle proximally to the supracondylar ridges distally.

Its numerous muscle attachments must be considered in the analysis of humeral shaft fractures. The deltoid, biceps brachii, and brachialis anticus muscles cover it anteriorly. The coracobrachialis muscle inserts beneath the upper half of the biceps brachii muscle. The pectoralis major inserts into the lateral lip of the bicipital groove of the humerus. The posterior surface is covered by the deltoid and triceps brachii muscles. On the lateral and medial aspects of the humerus, intermuscular septa dip down between the muscles to be attached to the bone, dividing the arm into anterior and posterior compartments. The neurovascular bundle courses along the medial aspect of the humerus in the anterior compartment, consisting of the brachial vessels, the median, musculocutaneous, and ulnar nerves. The radial nerve lies in the posterior compartment in a shallow groove in the posterior and lateral surfaces of the middle and upper thirds of the shaft of the humerus between the origins of the medial and lateral heads of the triceps brachii muscle. The radial nerve traverses obliquely downward and laterally as it passes from the axilla to the anterolateral epicondylar region.

Mechanism of Injury

The majority of the fractures of the shaft of the humerus are caused by direct violence, such as falls on the side of the arm; these tend to be transverse or comminuted and not infrequently are open. The more severe the injury, the greater is the possibility of comminution or of open fracture (Fig. 8–16). Segmental fractures occasionally occur.

Indirect violence, such as a fall on the hand or elbow, will produce an oblique spiral fracture. A forceful muscular action, such as throwing a baseball, may also result in an oblique or spiral fracture; however, when a minor injury causes the humeral shaft to fracture, the possibility of a pathologic fracture, such as through a unicameral bone cyst or metastatic lesion, should be ruled out.

Pathologic Anatomy

The direction of displacement of the fracture fragments depends on whether the level of fracture is proximal or distal to the insertion of the deltoid muscle. When the fracture occurs in the lower third or at a level of the lower and middle thirds of the humerus below the deltoid insertion, the action of the supraspinatus, deltoid, and coracobrachialis muscles will tend to pull the proximal fragment laterally and anteriorly, whereas the distal fragment is drawn upward by contraction of the biceps and brachialis muscles (Fig. 8–17 A).

If the fracture occurs in the upper and middle thirds of the humeral shaft, i.e., above the insertion of the deltoid but distal

to that of the pectoralis major, the pull of the deltoid muscle will tend to displace the distal fragment laterally and upward, while the pectoralis major, latissimus dorsi, and teres major muscles will adduct and internally rotate the proximal fragment (Fig. 8–16 G).

The displacement of the fracture fragments is also influenced by gravity, the position in which the upper limb is held, and the forces causing the fracture. The distal fragment is usually internally rotated, as the arm is held across the chest while the proximal fragment remains in mid-position.

Diagnosis

The deformity, local swelling, and pain caused by humeral shaft fractures make the clinical diagnosis very obvious and simple; however, the pitfall is failure to detect associated neurovascular injury. The intimate relation of the radial nerve to the humerus in the musculospiral groove makes it especially vulnerable. Injury to nerves may result secondarily by their being stretched over the displaced fragments or primarily at the time of initial trauma by being torn or crushed between the fragments. With radial nerve paralysis, there is anesthesia over the dorsum of the hand between the first and second metacarpals and loss of motor strength of extensors of the wrist, fingers and thumb, and supinators of the forearm. The median and ulnar nerves are rarely injured. Vascular injury to brachial vessels is extremely rare.

Treatment

The preferred treatment of humeral shaft fractures in adults is a hanging cast. In children, this method of treatment is not effective, as it requires the cooperation of the patient in sleeping and staying in a semirecumbent or sitting posture without support beneath the elbow and also in the added responsibility for performing the proper exercises. A hanging cast is also not practical for the irrational or unconscious patient or for the patient who must remain recumbent in bed because of associated injuries.

Wherever there is marked displacement of the fragments, the initial step is to reduce

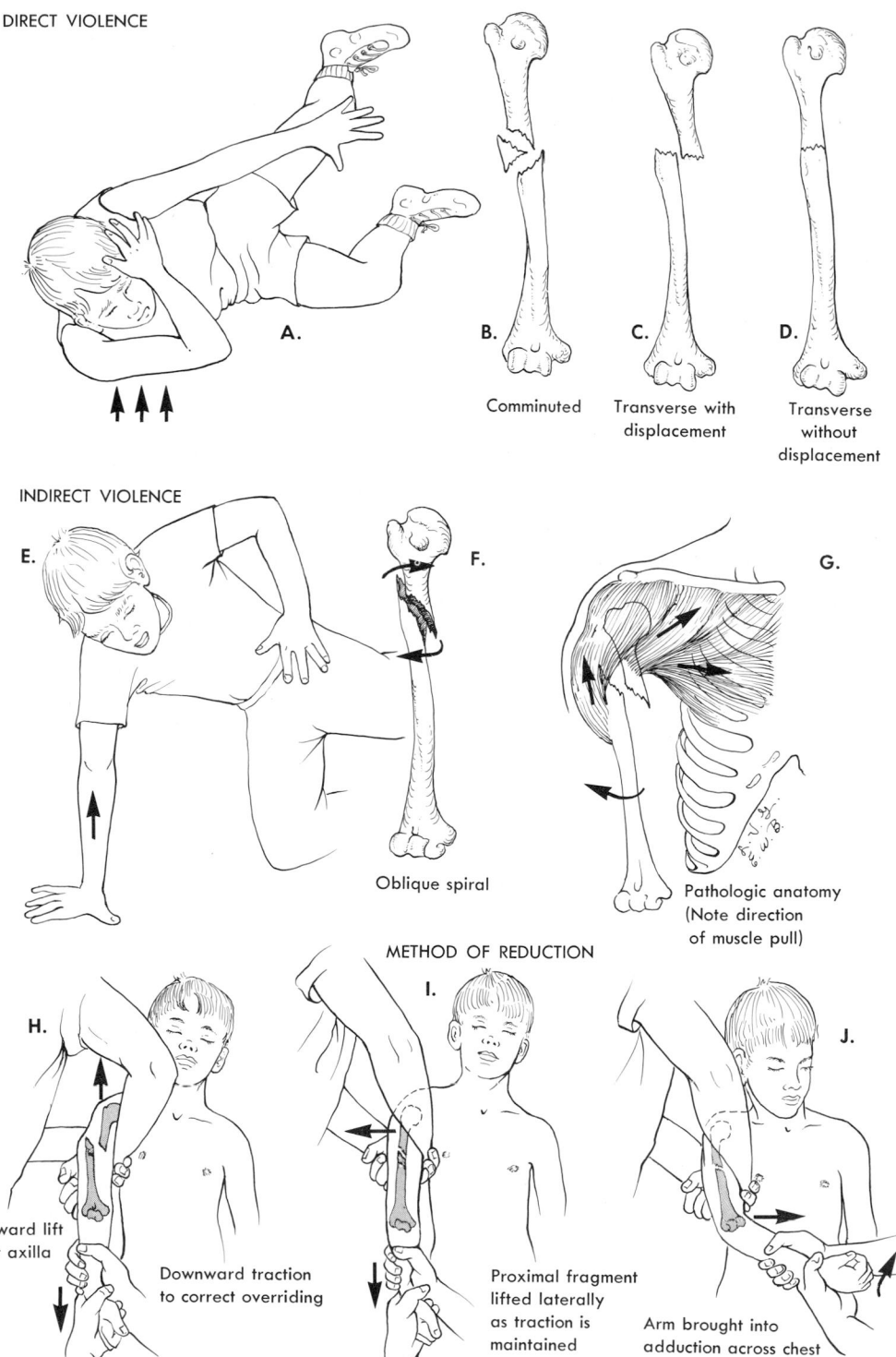

DIRECT VIOLENCE

A.

B.
Comminuted

C.
Transverse with displacement

D.
Transverse without displacement

INDIRECT VIOLENCE

E.

F.
Oblique spiral

G.
Pathologic anatomy
(Note direction of muscle pull)

METHOD OF REDUCTION

H.
Upward lift at axilla
Downward traction to correct overriding

I.
Proximal fragment lifted laterally as traction is maintained

J.
Arm brought into adduction across chest

FIGURE 8–16. *Fractures of the humeral shaft above insertion of deltoid and distal to attachment of pectoralis major muscles.* See opposite page for legend.

the fracture. When the level of the fracture is between the sites of insertion of the pectoralis major and deltoid muscles with adduction and internal rotation of the upper fragment, reduction is carried out by first applying downward traction to correct overriding and to disengage the fracture fragments, and then, while maintaining distal traction and with the surgeon's forearm in the patient's axilla, lifting the proximal fragment laterally into abduction. The reduction is completed by bringing the distal fragment into adduction and internal rotation by adducting the upper limb across the patient's chest (Fig. 8–16 H to J and Fig. 8–18).

When the level of the fracture is distal to the deltoid insertion with abduction and external rotation of the upper fragment, again downward traction is initially applied with the arm in abduction and external rotation to correct overriding of fracture fragments; then, while the assistant maintains distal traction, the surgeon lifts the upper end of the lower fragment into abduction with one hand and with his other, pushes the proximal fragment into adduction, reducing the fracture (Fig. 8–17 B and C).

Roentgenograms of the humerus, in both anteroposterior and lateral views, are taken to confirm the reduction, and its stability is checked clinically. It is not essential in children to obtain end-to-end anatomic alignment. Overriding of 1 to 1.5 cm. can be easily accepted, as overgrowth is common in a displaced shaft fracture of the humerus; however, angulation of more than 15 to 20 degrees is not desirable, and one should pay attention to rotational alignment.

In infants and young children, the fracture is immobilized for a period of four to six weeks by bandaging the arm to the side of the thorax in a modified Velpeau bandage or a sling and swathe (Fig. 8–17 E). If the fracture is unstable or oblique, with much overriding of the fragments, lateral adhesive skin traction is applied to maintain acceptable position of the fracture fragments for a period of two to three weeks until callus is demonstrable in the roentgenograms, and then it is immobilized as just described until healing is completed (Fig. 8–17 D).

In the older child or adolescent with an unstable fracture, following reduction, a shoulder spica cast is used for immobilization. This should extend distally to include the pelvis and should be well molded above the iliac crests (Fig. 8–17 E).

Skeletal traction with a Kirschner wire through the olecranon and suspension of the forearm and hand are indicated either when the local skin and soft-tissue conditions do not permit adhesive skin traction, when the fracture is open, or when there is marked comminution and displacement of the fracture fragments in a patient who must remain in bed because of associated trauma.

In the older adolescent who is cooperative, the hanging cast is the best method of treatment, as it permits him to be ambulatory and active. A long arm cast is applied from the metacarpal heads to the axilla with the elbow in 90 degrees of flexion and the forearm in neutral rotation. In fractures in the distal third of the humeral shaft, the forearm is placed in full pronation, however. Supinating force of the biceps brachii muscle is lost by a break in continuity of the humerus at this level, and the elbow joint is held in pronation by the unopposed action of the pronators. Since the joint is fixed in pronation, attempts to place the forearm in supination will result in varus deformity at the fracture site.[85] A collar and cuff is attached to a plaster loop at the wrist and

---

FIGURE 8–16. *Fractures of the humeral shaft above insertion of deltoid and distal to attachment of pectoralis major muscles.*

A to **F.** *Mechanism of injury.* Direct violence, such as falls on the side of the arm, will cause comminuted or transverse fractures (**A** to **D**). Indirect violence, such as falls on the hand, will cause oblique spiral fractures (**E** and **F**).

G. *Pathologic anatomy* when fracture site is at junction of upper and middle thirds. Note the pull of the deltoid muscle tends to displace the distal fragment laterally and upward, while the pectoralis major, latissimus dorsi, and teres major muscles will adduct and internally rotate the proximal fragment.

I and **J.** *Method of reduction* when the level of fracture is between the insertions of the pectoralis major and deltoid muscles.

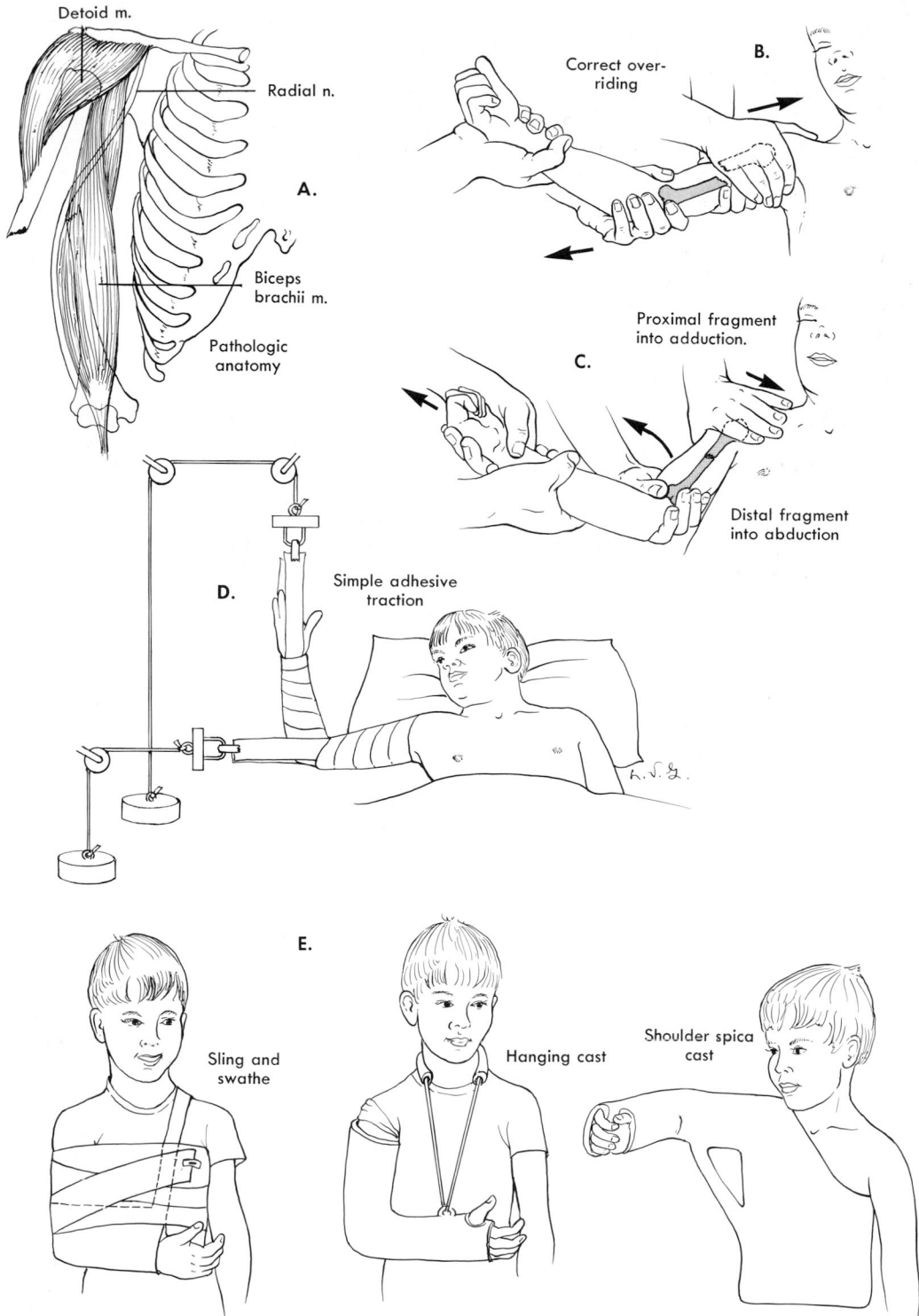

FIGURE 8–17. *Fractures of humeral shaft distal to insertion of deltoid muscle. See opposite page for legend.*

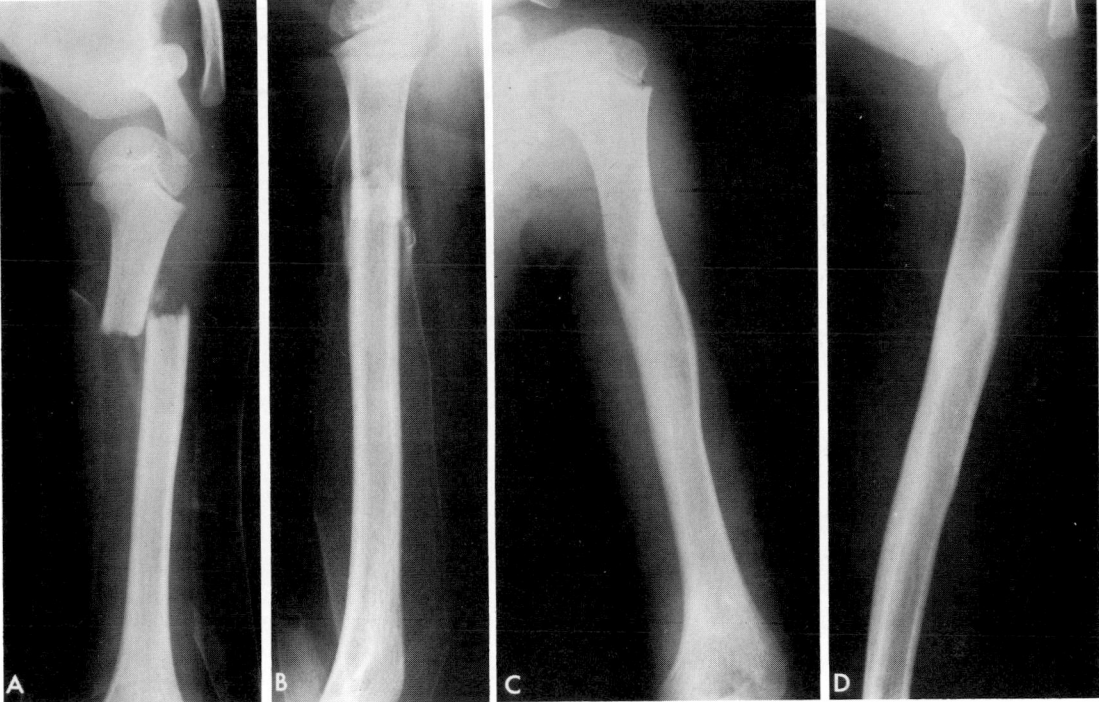

FIGURE 8–18. *Fracture of humeral shaft between the sites of insertion of the pectoralis major and deltoid muscles.*

Note the overriding and adduction of proximal fragment. Treated by closed reduction and plaster of Paris reinforced modified Velpeau bandage. **A** and **B.** Initial roentgenograms. **C** and **D.** Four months later, showing healing.

passed around the patient's neck. The weight of the cast should be slight; if it is excessive, the bone fragments will be distracted.

Improper length of the collar and cuff is a common error. If it is too long and the wrist drops below the horizontal plane, the distal fragment of the humerus will tilt posteriorly and anterior angulation of the fracture will result. Conversely, a short collar and cuff will cause posterior bowing. A pad of rolled sponge is attached to the medial aspect of the cast to serve as a fulcrum for the arm as it presses against the chest wall.

The patient sleeps in semirecumbent position. Erect position is maintained during the day as much as possible. There should be no support under the elbow. Pressure from clothing, as from a buttoned coat over the cast, or anything that might compress the arm against the body must be avoided, as it interferes with traction.

FIGURE 8–17. *Fractures of humeral shaft distal to insertion of deltoid muscle.*

A. *Pathologic anatomy* when site of fracture is at junction of the lower and middle thirds. Note the proximal fragment is displaced laterally by the pull of the deltoid muscle and anteriorly by the coracobrachialis muscle. The distal fragment is pulled upward by the action of the biceps and brachialis muscles.

B and **C.** *Method of reduction.* With the arm in abduction and external rotation, distal traction is applied to correct overriding; then, while an assistant maintains traction, the distal fragment is pulled into abduction with one hand and the proximal fragment is pushed into abduction with the other.

D. Traction when fracture is unstable or oblique with much overriding.

E. Methods of immobilization after reduction.

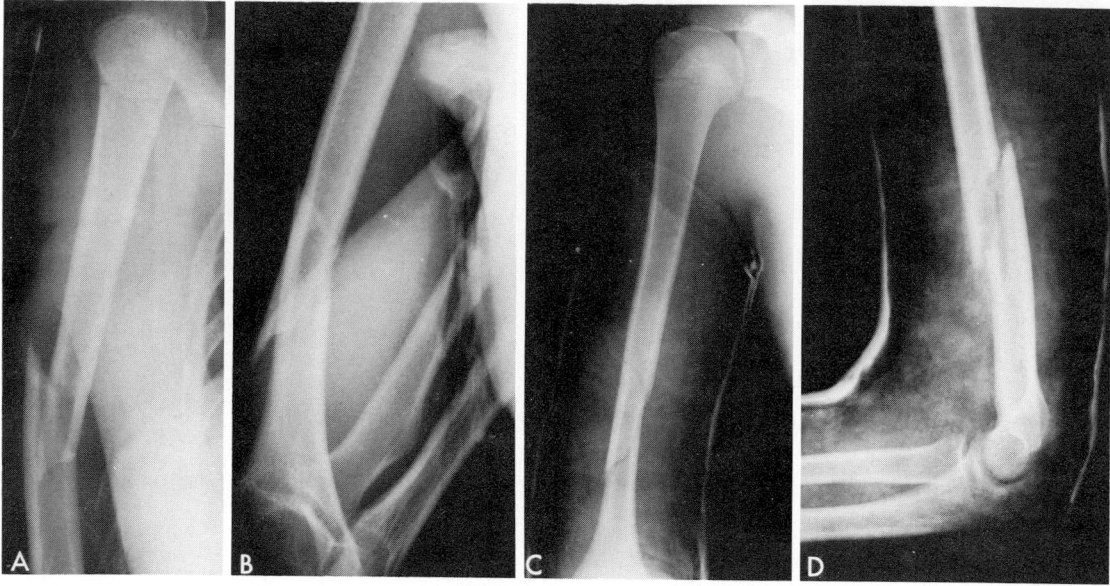

FIGURE 8–19. *Long spiral fracture of lower third of right humerus.*

Hanging cast is best method of treatment in the cooperative adolescent patient. **A** and **B.** Initial roentgenograms. **C** and **D.** Roentgenograms in cast, showing the satisfactory anatomic alignment.

Circumduction and pendulum exercises for the shoulder are demonstrated and begun early. The patient assumes a forward and laterally inclined position; he is then asked to swing the arm in increasingly larger circles through all motions of the shoulder to the limit of tolerance. The arm with the cast should hang free vertically, the wrist still supported by the collar and cuff.

The hanging cast method of treatment is ideal, particularly for long spiral oblique fractures and in comminuted fractures of the lower two thirds of the humeral shaft (Fig. 8–19).

Radial nerve paralysis, which is not un-common in adults, is rare in children. Complete severance of the nerve in closed fractures is very unlikely, and nerve function almost always recovers if the fracture is managed by conservative methods. Primary open reduction of a closed fracture of the humeral shaft is not indicated. The wrist and hand are splinted in functional position, and passive exercises are performed to maintain full range of motion of the joint. Electromyographic studies are helpful in following the return of nerve function. If, after three to four months, there is no evidence of nerve regeneration, the nerve is explored.

Injuries in the Region of the Elbow

SUPRACONDYLAR FRACTURE OF THE HUMERUS

This is the commonest type of elbow fracture in children and adolescents. According to most series, it accounts for between 50 and 60 per cent of elbow fractures, and is seen most frequently in children between the ages of three and ten years. Males predominate and the left arm is involved about twice as frequently as the right arm.[130]

The high incidence of deformities in the

elbow and the potential neurovascular complications that result make this a serious injury.

Mechanism of Injury and Classification

Two types of supracondylar fracture are designated according to the position of the forearm in relation to the arm at the time of injury, and the displacement of the distal fragment.

The more common *extension type* accounts for approximately 95 per cent of cases. It is caused by a fall on the outstretched hand with hyperextension of the elbow. The distal fragment is posteriorly displaced (Fig. 8–20)

The *flexion type* is rare and occurs in only 5 per cent of cases, usually following a fall with the elbow flexed and resulting in anterior displacement of the distal fragment (Fig. 8–21).

Clinically, according to the degree of displacement of the fragments, three grades of supracondylar fractures of the humerus are recognized: (1) fracture with no displacement, (2) fracture with minimal or moderate displacement, and (3) fracture with severe displacement.

It is important that in supracondylar fractures the exact type and the severity of the displacement be delineated, since the method of treatment varies accordingly.

Pathologic Anatomy

EXTENSION TYPE

In the sagittal plane, the fracture line traverses obliquely upward and backward, and in the frontal plane, it is frequently transverse. The older the patient, the more oblique the fracture line tends to be in the frontal plane. As a rule, transverse fractures are more stable than oblique ones. The fracture is usually complete, though occasionally greenstick fractures do occur.

The distal fragment is displaced proximally and posteriorly by the fracturing force transmitted upward through the bones of the forearm and because of the pull of the triceps muscle. It is often tilted laterally or medially and rotated medially.

The lower end of the proximal fragment projects anteriorly, pierces the periosteum, and forces its way into the brachialis anticus and biceps brachii. The periosteum is stripped from both the anterior surface of the lower fragment and the posterior surface of the upper fragment. The degree of displacement of the fracture fragments is limited by the extent of periosteal stripping. There is a considerable amount of local bleeding and swelling. The nerves and blood vessels are thus contused, compressed, or lacerated by the bone fragments or by the blood that infiltrates the antecubital fossa.

FLEXION TYPE

In the sagittal plane, the fracture line courses from below upward and forward. The proximal fragment is displaced posteriorly, whereas the distal fragment is displaced anteriorly and upward. There may be a varying degree of medial or lateral tilting and rotation. The periosteum is stripped from the posterior surface of the distal fragment and from the anterior surface of the proximal fragment. Soft-tissue swelling and damage are usually much less than in the extension type and neurovascular complications are rare.

Diagnosis

Supracondylar fracture of the humerus is diagnosed by the history, by clinical findings, and by roentgenographic studies.

In the simple undisplaced supracondylar fracture seen soon following injury, swelling may be minimal, and the most characteristic finding will be tenderness over the lower end of the humerus. When a supracondylar fracture is suspected, a true lateral projection of the distal humerus should be obtained in the roentgenogram; often a false diagnosis of fracture is made by the finding, in an oblique view, of anterior tilting of the distal humeral epiphysis (Fig. 8–22). When in doubt, one should make roentgenograms of both elbows for comparison.

(*Text continued on page 1572.*)

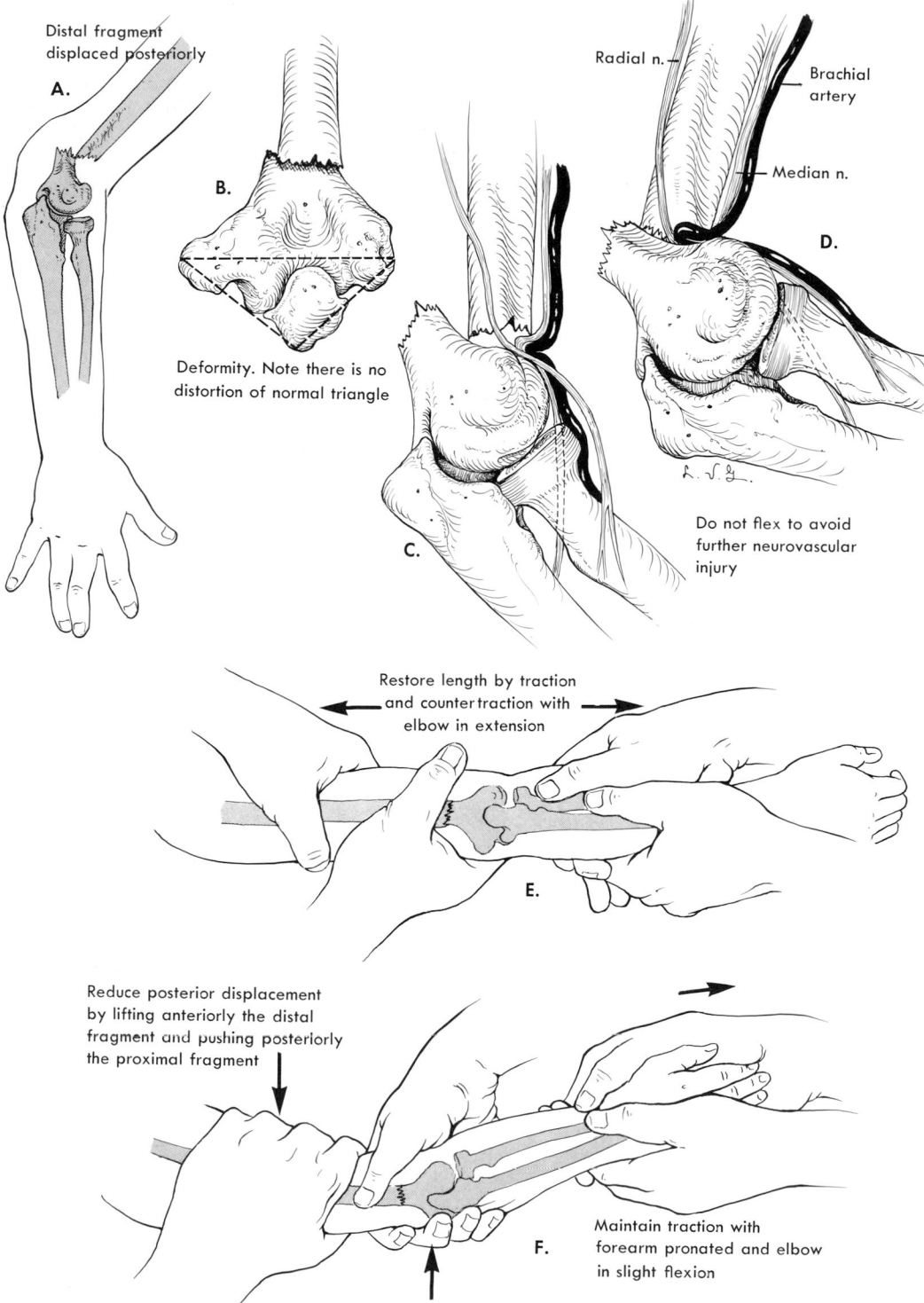

A. Distal fragment displaced posteriorly

B. Deformity. Note there is no distortion of normal triangle

C.

D. Radial n. — Brachial artery — Median n.

Do not flex to avoid further neurovascular injury

E. Restore length by traction and countertraction with elbow in extension

F. Reduce posterior displacement by lifting anteriorly the distal fragment and pushing posteriorly the proximal fragment

Maintain traction with forearm pronated and elbow in slight flexion

FIGURE 8–20.   Supracondylar fracture of the humerus—extension type (see text for explanation).

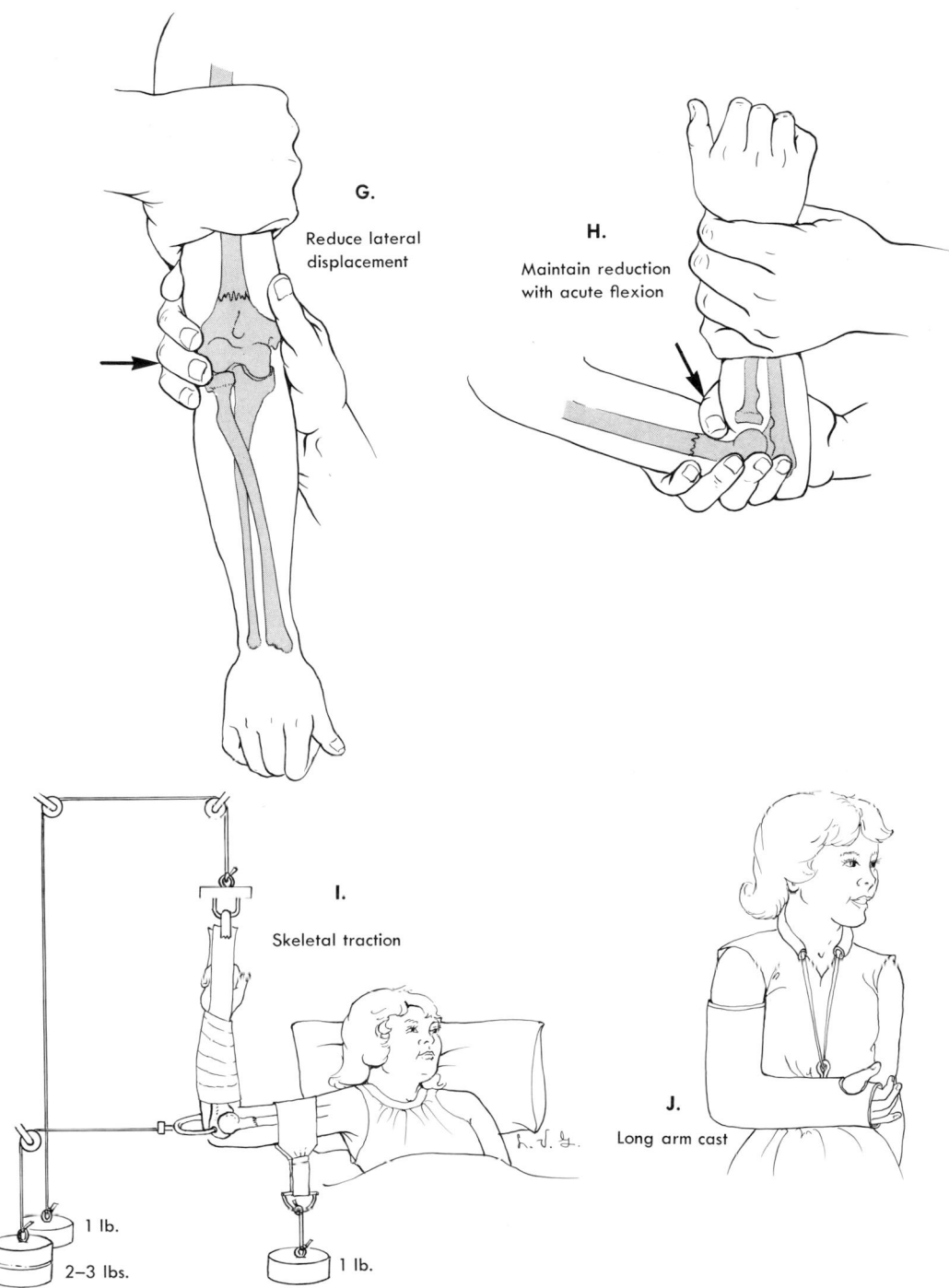

G.

Reduce lateral displacement

H.

Maintain reduction with acute flexion

I.

Skeletal traction

1 lb.

2–3 lbs.

1 lb.

J.

Long arm cast

FIGURE 8–20 Continued.   Supracondylar fracture of the humerus—extension type (see text for explanation).

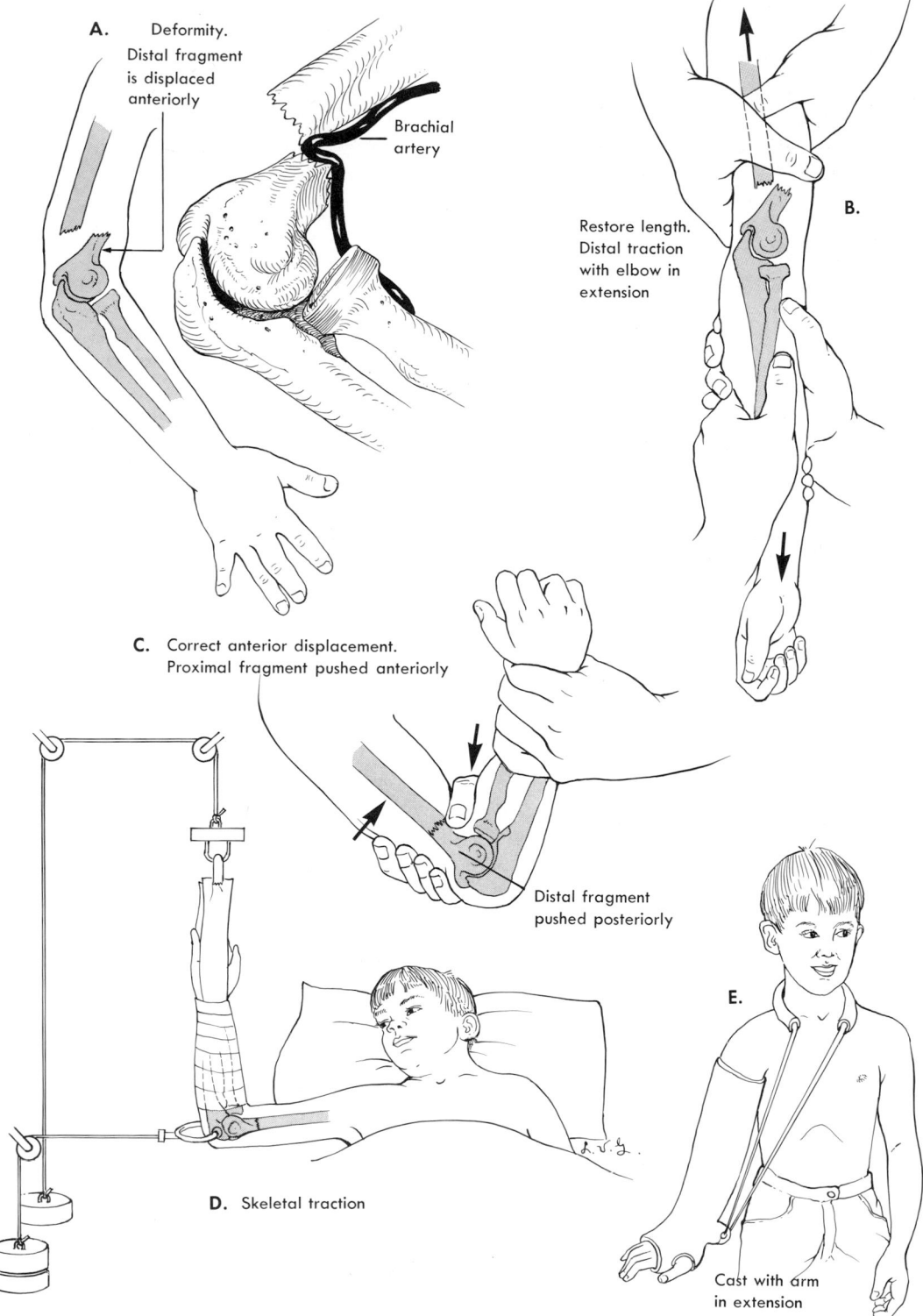

A. Deformity. Distal fragment is displaced anteriorly

Brachial artery

B. Restore length. Distal traction with elbow in extension

C. Correct anterior displacement. Proximal fragment pushed anteriorly

Distal fragment pushed posteriorly

D. Skeletal traction

E. Cast with arm in extension

FIGURE 8–21.   Supracondylar fracture of the humerus—flexion type (see text for explanation).

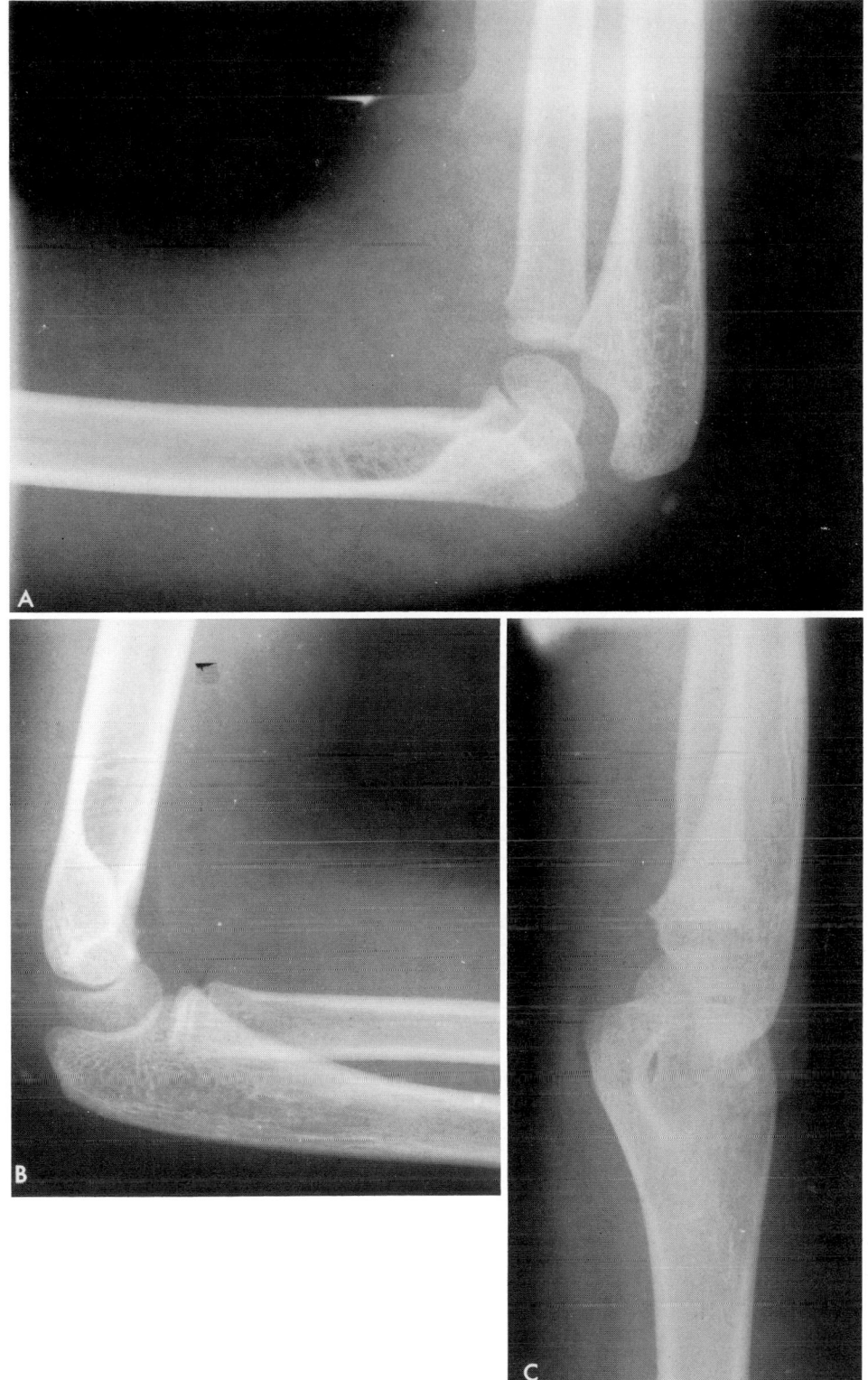

FIGURE 8–22. The importance of a true lateral view in suspected supracondylar fracture of humerus.

A. An oblique view of distal humerus suggesting supracondylar fracture and anterior tilting of distal fragment. **B** and **C.** A true lateral roentgenogram of the distal humerus and a semioblique view show that there is no fracture. These roentgenograms emphasize the importance of a true lateral view of the distal humerus; when in doubt, one should make comparative views of the opposite uninjured elbow.

In the presence of more violent injury with displacement of the fragments, swelling and deformity of the elbow become more characteristic. The amount of swelling in general depends on the severity of the fracture and the time that has elapsed between the occurrence of the injury and the examination of the patient; in a patient seen several hours following trauma, tension develops in the antecubital area owing to the extravasation of blood, and skin changes in the forms of blebs may occur. There is usually severe pain, and examination of the posterior aspect of the lower humerus will reveal a discontinuity of the bone. The anteriorly displaced proximal fragment is often palpable beneath the skin. In the presence of overriding, there will be shortening of the involved arm.

Most important in the physical examination is the careful assessment of the vascular and neural function in the injured limb. Any neurovascular deficit should be recorded. Failure to detect vascular injuries will be disastrous, resulting in permanent deformity and disability.

The treating physician should be constantly alert for any signs of pain, pallor, cyanosis, absence of pulse, coldness, or paralysis, any of which may indicate the possibility of impending Volkmann's ischemia.

Roentgenographic examination will confirm the diagnosis. Instructions on the x-ray requisition should specifically indicate that anteroposterior and true lateral projections of the distal humerus and including the elbow joint be taken. An anteroposterior view of the elbow will reveal whether the fracture line is transverse or oblique, and whether the distal fragment is medially or laterally angulated. A lateral view of the elbow will show whether the distal fragment is displaced posteriorly or anteriorly.

Treatment

EMERGENCY SPLINTING

Proper splinting of the limb before sending the patient to the x-ray department and while awaiting definitive treatment is very important. In extension type fractures, flexion of the elbow should be avoided, as it may cause further damage to neurovascular structures (see Fig. 8–20 D). The limb is immobilized in a simple splint (aluminum or padded board with loosely applied bandage) in the deformed position that it lies in, preferably with the elbow in extension and the forearm in pronation. Circulation should always be checked prior to and following application of the splint. The radial pulse should be assessed to determine whether it is normal and capillary return is good. Sensation is also carefully checked.

The method of treatment is dependent upon the degree of displacement of the fracture fragments, the amount of soft-tissue swelling, and whether there is any disturbance of neurovascular function.

Supracondylar fractures in children should be managed as acute emergencies. The most effective method of preventing local swelling (or decreasing it if the elbow is already swollen) is to achieve immediate reduction and restore normal alignment.

MINIMALLY DISPLACED FRACTURES

Treatment of undisplaced or minimally displaced supracondylar fractures of the humerus consists of application of a posterior plaster splint with the elbow flexed at 90 degrees and the forearm in pronation (Fig. 8–23). The plaster splint is kept on for four weeks. Follow-up x-rays are taken after a week and again at the time the posterior splint is removed. It is important that the status of circulation be assessed in the first 24 hours and the family of the patient be educated to recognize the signs and symptoms of circulatory embarrassment. In a mildly displaced fracture with moderate swelling, it is advised that the child be admitted to the hospital for a period of one or two days for observation.

The average time required for bony union to take place is three weeks; full range of movement in the elbow usually returns in about eight weeks.

Cubitus varus can occur following minimally displaced fractures treated by simple plaster immobilization. Two such cases were reported by Fahey, who cautioned that one must be on the alert for the possibility of such an unfavorable outcome, even in instances when the displacement does not appear to be of such magnitude that reduction is required.[88] If there is compression on the

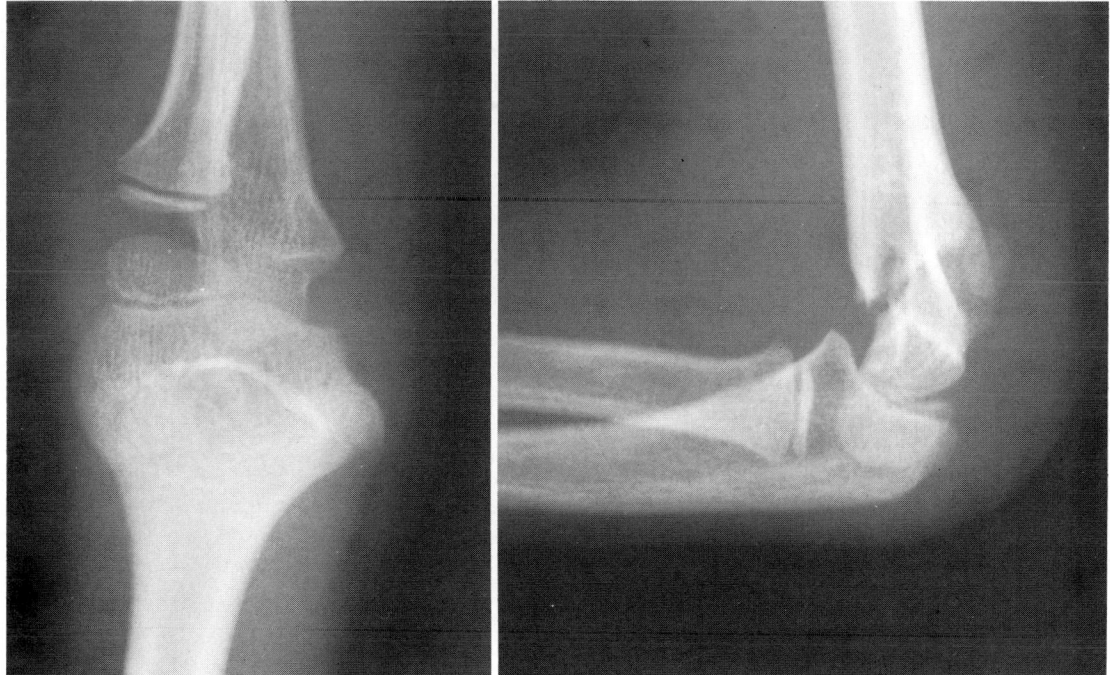

FIGURE 8-23.   Roentgenograms showing undisplaced supracondylar fracture of the humerus.

medial side, the fracture should be manipulated and medial tilting of the distal fragment corrected. The carrying angle of the elbow should always be matched with the normal side.

MODERATELY DISPLACED FRACTURES

The moderately displaced extension type supracondylar fracture with some bony contact, when local swelling is minimal and neurovascular function normal, is treated by closed reduction performed under general anesthesia. The technique is as follows: (1) Length should first be restored by traction and countertraction with the elbow in extension but *not hyperextension* to prevent pulling and injury of the brachial vessels (see Fig. 8-20 E). (2) Next, while maintaining traction (with the forearm pronated and the elbow in slight flexion), reduce posterior displacement of the distal fragment by lifting it anteriorly and by pushing the proximal fragment posteriorly (Fig. 8-20 F). (3) Then reduce lateral displacement by pushing the distal fragment medially; any rota-

tional deformity is also corrected at this time (Fig. 8-20 G). (4) The elbow is hyperflexed to 90 degrees to tighten the posterior hinge of the periosteum and to maintain the reduction.

In supracondylar fractures, the biceps brachii muscle loses its supinating action because of the break in continuity of the humerus. The unopposed action of the strong pronator teres muscle swings the proximal radioulnar joint into pronation Since the joint is fixed by the pronators, varus deformity at the fracture site will result. The direction of original displacement of the distal fragment is another consideration in deciding the position of the forearm when immobilized in the cast; if it was displaced medially, the forearm is *pronated* in order to tighten the medial hinge and to close the fracture line on the lateral side, thus preventing any cubitus varus deformity; but if the distal fragment was displaced *laterally, supination* of the forearm will tighten the lateral periosteal hinge and close the fracture line on the medial side, thus preventing cubitus valgus.

Next, roentgenograms are made in the

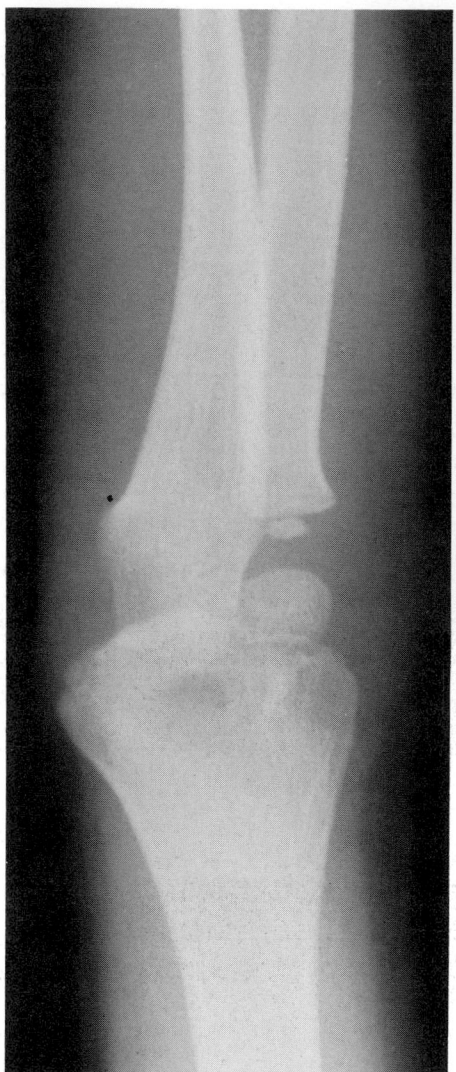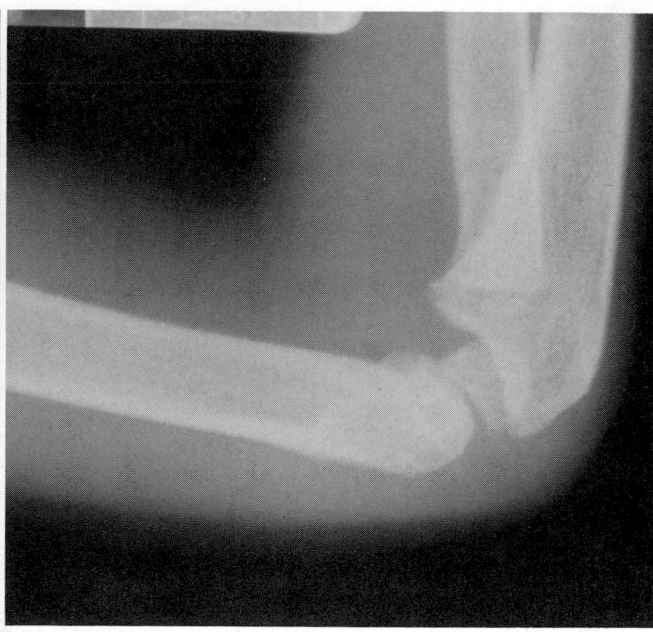

FIGURE 8–24.   Supracondylar fracture—extension type.

The fracture is minimally displaced and is treated by simple immobilization in a posterior plaster of Paris mold.

anteroposterior and lateral projections to determine the adequacy of reduction (Fig. 8–26). *Any lateral tilting must be completely corrected.* Appositional malalignments are inconsequential, as they will correct themselves spontaneously by extensive remodeling and have no effect on the carrying angle or final range of motion of the elbow. Rotation of the distal fragment is not corrected by remodeling and may look bizarre in the roentgenogram, but it is well compensated clinically by rotation at the shoulder. Posterior angulation of the distal fragment will result in hyperextension at the elbow, and anterior angulation in flex-

ion deformity; however, these deformities are in the plane of motion of the elbow and spontaneously correct themselves.[94, 161]

Vigorous manipulations and remanipulations should be avoided, as they may cause further damage to vessels and nerves.

Following achievement of satisfactory reduction, peripheral circulation is again assessed. If it is normal, a long arm cast is applied for immobilization. The cast should not constrict the soft tissues in the antecubital area. A window is cut out in the region of the radial artery at the wrist to check circulation.

In the presence of marked swelling,

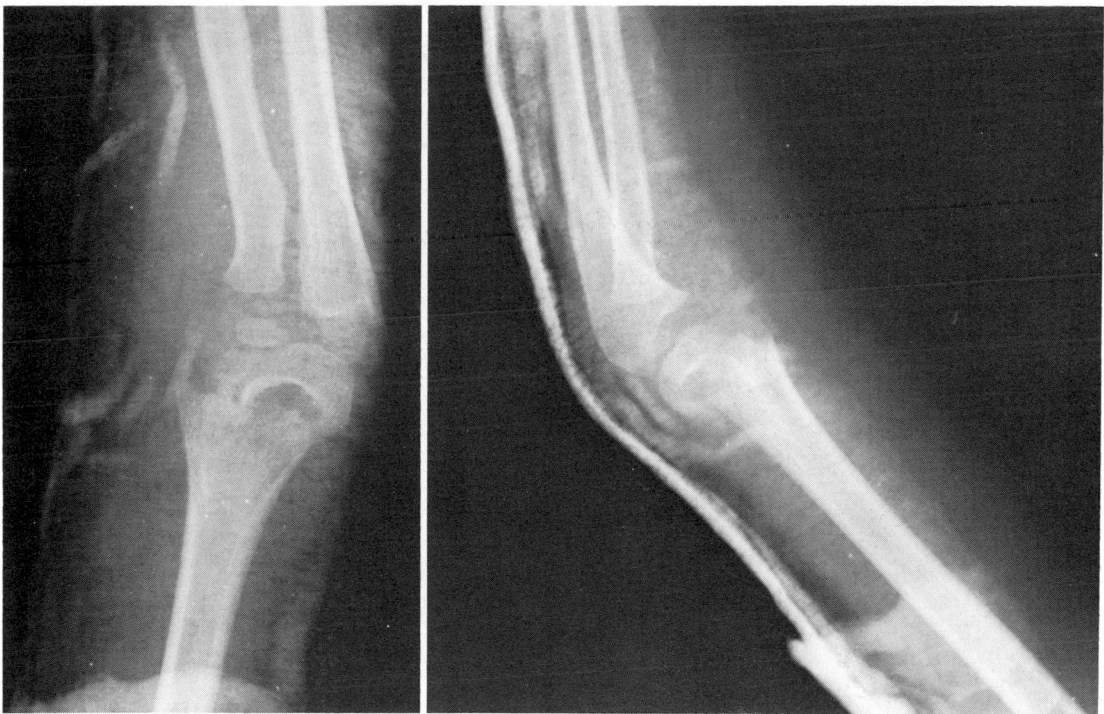

FIGURE 8-25. *Moderately displaced extension type of supracondylar fracture of the humerus with some bony contact.*

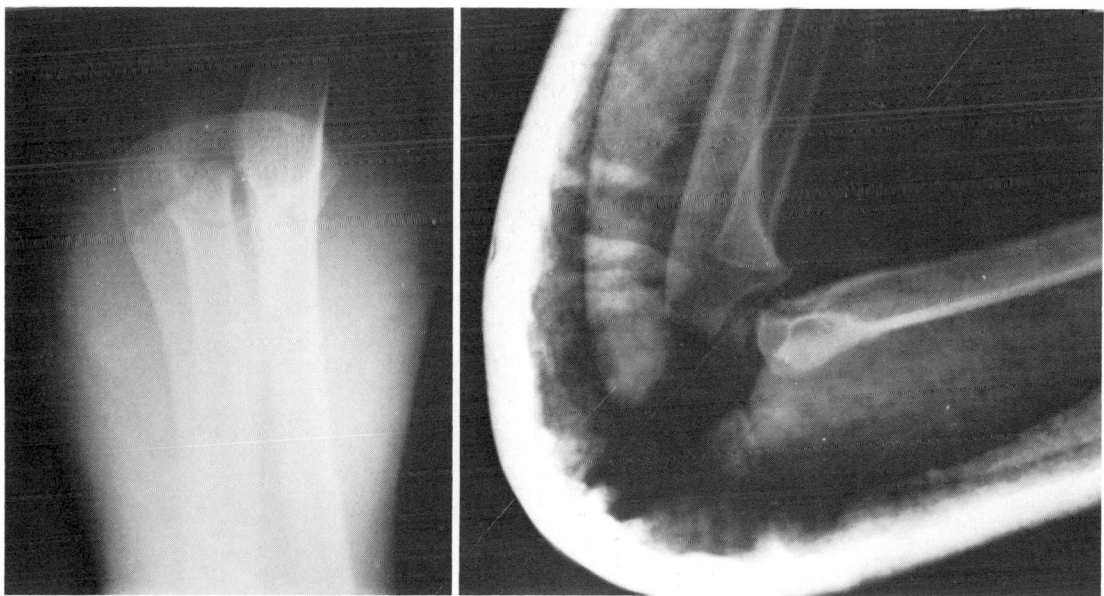

FIGURE 8-26. *Supracondylar fracture of humerus.*

Roentgenographic views immediately following reduction show accurate anatomic alignment.

closed reduction is carried out as just out-lined, but instead of immobilization in the cast, Dunlop skin traction is applied to the injured limb for five to seven days until the swelling subsides. Peripheral circulation is also closely observed. It is not necessary to apply skeletal traction when the original fracture was only moderately displaced with bony contact and when anatomic stable re-duction has been achieved. After the swell-ing subsides, the elbow is immobilized in a long arm cast, as previously described. Some surgeons prefer to elevate the injured arm in traction prior to attempting closed reduc-tion, but, as already stated, early reduction of the fracture will promote decrease of the swelling.

Roentgenograms are made at four and ten days following injury to check mainte-nance of reduction and then again, at four weeks.

The *flexion type of supracondylar fracture of the humerus* (the reverse type with the distal fragment displaced forward) is a simpler in-jury to treat (cf. Fig. 8–121) Closed reduc-tion is carried out by traction in flexion, followed by correction of lateral tilting and displacement by manual pressure. The elbow is immobilized in extension. Oc-casionally the fragments are severely dis-placed and the fracture may require treat-ment by skeletal traction as described next.

SEVERELY DISPLACED FRACTURES

A completely displaced supracondylar fracture of the humerus is best treated by closed manipulative reduction followed by skeletal traction (Figs. 8–27 and 8–28). The technique is as follows:

Under general anesthesia, the child's arm is suspended by an assistant, while the surgeon inserts a threaded Kirschner wire ($^3/_{32}$ inch in diameter) through the crest of the ulna about 3 cm. distal to the tip of the olecranon process. Bony landmarks about the elbow are carefully identified and the wire is drilled from the medial to the lateral side so as to avoid injury to the ulnar nerve. The assistant should not acutely flex the elbow in an attempt to increase the promi-nence of the olecranon. A threaded Kirschner wire is used to prevent it from becoming loose and causing pin tract infec-

tion. A traction bow is fastened to the wire and the fracture is manipulated as pre-viously described. The relationship of the bony prominence on the posterior aspect of the elbow is determined. As stated, any lat-eral or medial tilting of the distal fragment is unacceptable. The circulation is checked. Roentgenograms are made to determine the accuracy of reduction.

Lateral skeletal traction is applied with the shoulder abducted 60 degrees and the arm elevated 20 degrees above the horizon-tal (Fig. 8–20). This position provides max-imum venous drainage of the upper limb. Also, it curtails the patient's movements in bed, thus obviating the possibility of vascu-lar damage by inadvertent increase in the degree of elbow flexion. A hyperactive child is placed on a Bradford frame. The poste-rior aspect of the elbow is not obscured; all the surgeon has to do is to kneel down to inspect the bony prominences; the author finds with lateral traction, it is very simple to use the visual method of treatment, as ad-vocated by Lyman Smith (Fig. 8–29). The disadvantage of overhead traction is that it does not provide adequate control over the proximal fragment if the patient moves about in bed; thus, it is possible for him to force the elbow into acute flexion and cause circulatory embarrassment. Such an in-stance was reported by Staples.[163]

Fahey prefers the use of a screw through both cortices of the ulna for skeletal traction because of difficulties encountered in in-troducing a Kirschner wire in the presence of a swollen elbow and the possibility of damaging the ulnar nerve.[88] This has not been a problem in the experience of the author.

A 3- to 5-lb. weight is applied on the lat-eral traction bow and the forearm is sus-pended by adhesive strapping traction with 1 or 2 lb. of weight. In extension type supra-condylar fracture, in which the proximal fragment is anteriorly displaced, a sling with a 1-lb. weight is applied on the upper arm, pulling it posteriorly. Circulation and neural function are closely checked and recorded. The maintenance of reduction is determined by periodic roentgenograms. In two or three weeks, the fracture is stable enough to remove the Kirschner wire and continue immobilization in a long arm cast for an additional two to three weeks. Then the cast is removed and active exercises are instituted to restore range of motion of the elbow joint (Fig. 8–30). Passive stretching exercises are never performed, and weights should not be used to stretch the elbow into full extension.

Severely displaced supracondylar fractures of the humerus should not be treated by open reduction and internal fixation with Kirschner wires because of the possibility of growth disturbance and complications of persistent contractural deformity of the elbow.

Complications

MALUNION AND CHANGES IN CARRYING ANGLE

The carrying angle is the lateral angle that the longitudinal axis of the fully supinated forearm makes with the longitudinal axis of the upper arm when the elbow is completely extended. The carrying angle tends to disappear with pronation of the forearm and with flexion of the elbow. With progressive flexion of the elbow from complete extension, the carrying angle becomes less and less evident until complete flexion is reached, at which time the arm is covered by the forearm and there is no apparent deviation. Changes in the carrying angle cannot be detected when one examines the flexed elbow from the front. However, if the flexed elbow is examined posteriorly and compared with the opposite normal elbow, changes in the carrying angle will become quite apparent. The bony relations of the medial and lateral epicondyles and the olecranon process are palpated. The examiner grasps the child's left wrist with his left hand and places his right thumb upon the tip of the lateral condyle, the long finger on the tip of the medial epicondyle and the index finger on the olecranon process. When examining the right elbow, the surgeon reverses his hand positions for convenience.

With the elbow flexed to a right angle, the three points make a fairly symmetrical equilateral triangle and tend to lie in a plane parallel with the plane of the posterior surface of the upper arm. In some children, the capitellum becomes quite prominent in 90 degrees of flexion and disturbs the symmetry of the lateral segment of the triangle. When the elbow is in complete extension, three bony points are almost in a straight line.

It is important to remember that the carrying angle is subject to considerable normal individual variation. Lyman Smith studied the carrying angle of 150 normal children, 80 girls and 70 boys, aged 3 to 11 years (the age when supracondylar fracture is most common). He found the average carrying angle to be 6.1 degrees in the girls, with a range of 0 to 12 degrees, and 5.4 degrees in boys, with a range of 0 to 11 degrees. Some of the children (9 per cent) had no carrying angle or cubitus rectus, and 48 per cent had a carrying angle of 5 degrees or less.[161]

In measurements of the carrying angle of 100 subjects, Aebi found the average value for men to be 6.5 degrees, with a range of 0 to 14 degrees; in women, the average was 13 degrees, with a range from 4 to 20 degrees.[91]

The effect on the carrying angle caused by various types of displacement of the distal fragment in supracondylar fractures was experimentally studied by Smith. He simulated a transverse supracondylar fracture in an articulated upper extremity by an osteotomy through the supracondylar region, the fragments being held together by spring wiring. Medial and lateral displacement of the distal fragment did not change the carrying angle (Fig. 8–31 B and C). Internal rotation of the distal fragment also had no effect on the degree of the carrying angle (Fig. 8–31 D). Only medial or lateral tilt of the distal fragment changed the carrying angle (Fig. 8–31 E and F).

The compressional forces of normal muscle tone and of the elasticity of soft tissues surrounding the fracture fragments will tilt the distal fragment in the presence of medial and lateral displacement and instability of the fracture. This can be best prevented by traction on the distal fragment in the direction of the longitudinal axis of the distal part of the humerus.

Cubitus varus or valgus deformity results from malunion; it is not caused by epiphyseal growth disturbance (Figs. 8–32 and 8–33). If the varus or valgus deformity of the elbow is severe, its correction is indicated by supracondylar osteotomy of the humerus. The operative technique of osteotomy of

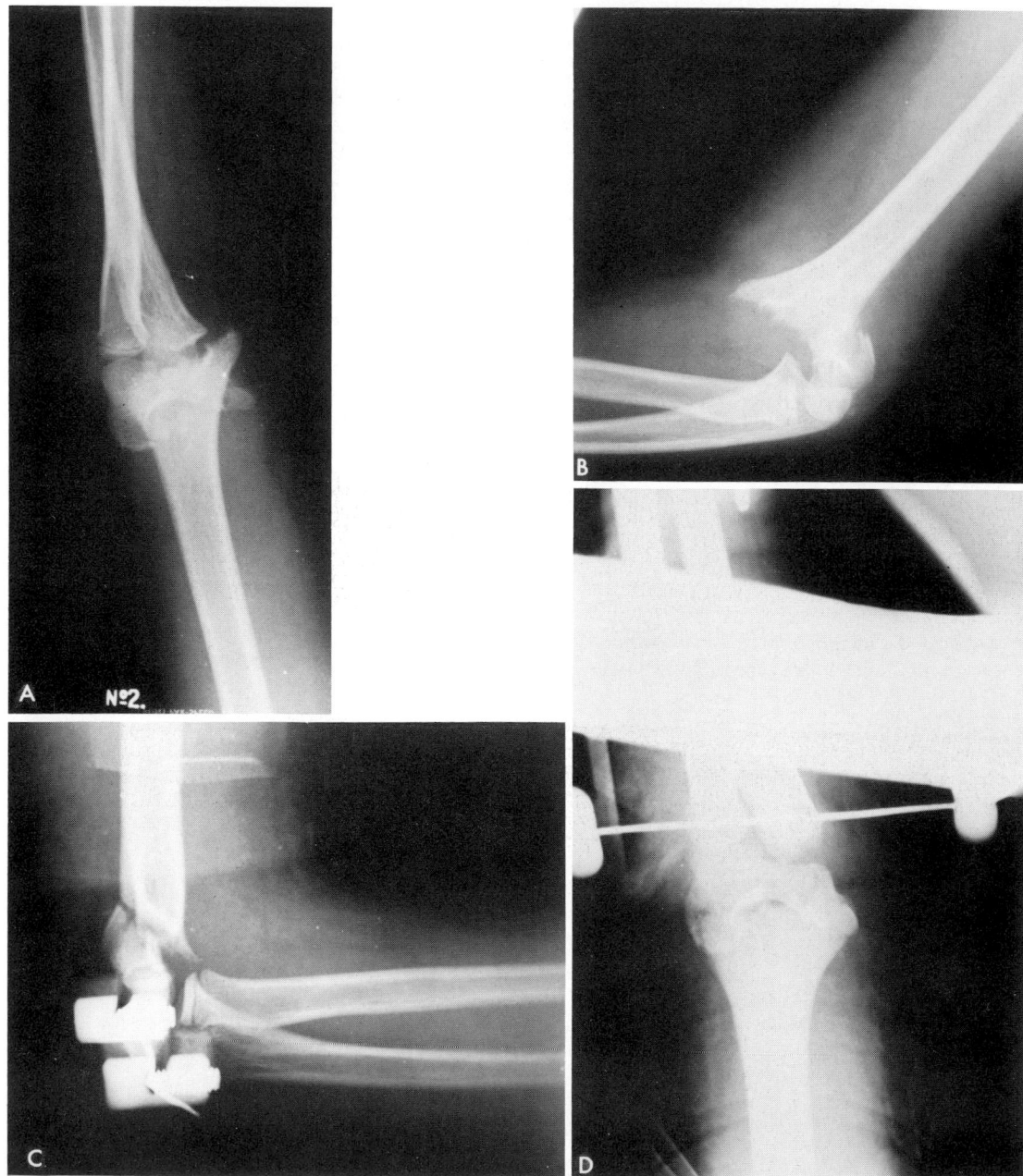

FIGURE 8–27.   *Supracondylar fracture of the humerus—markedly displaced.*

The fracture was treated by insertion of threaded Kirschner wire through olecranon, closed manipulative reduction, and skeletal traction for 18 days followed by immobilization in plaster of Paris cast for two more weeks. **A** and **B**. Initial roentgenograms. **C** and **D**. Roentgenograms while in traction, showing satisfactory alignment.

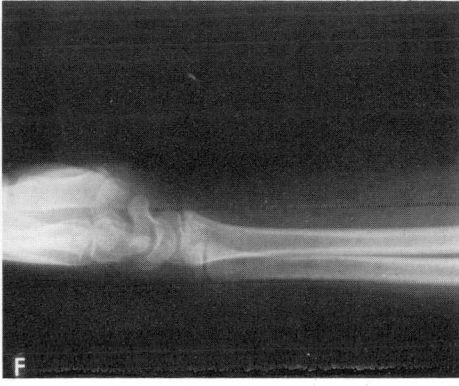

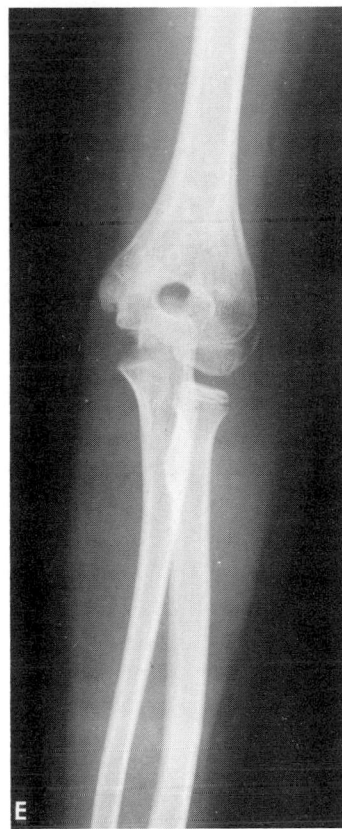

FIGURE 8–27 Continued.   Supracondylar fracture of the humerus — markedly displaced.

E and **F.** Roentgenograms three months later, showing healing in good position.

the distal humeral shaft to correct cubitus varus is described and illustrated in Plate 64.

VASCULAR COMPLICATIONS — VOLKMANN'S ISCHEMIA

In 1881, Richard von Volkmann described an ischemic paralysis and contracture of the muscles of the forearm and hand and less frequently of the leg, which followed the application of taut bandages in the treatment of injuries in the region of the elbow and knee. He suggested that the pathologic changes primarily resulted from obstruction of arterial blood flow, which, if unrelieved, after six hours, would result in death of the muscle.[229]

Initially supracondylar fractures of the humerus were the commonest cause of Volkmann's ischemia. With improved management of the elbow fractures in children, the incidence and type of predisposing injury is changing. For example, at the Mayo Clinic, Meyerding reported the incidence of

Volkmann's ischemic contracture as 0.18 per thousand new registrants prior to 1935.[210] This incidence decreased to 0.03 per thousand new registrants at the Mayo Clinic between 1955 and 1965. Eichler and Lipscomb found 35 per cent of the cases of Volkmann's ischemia were caused by supracondylar and elbow fractures, 20 per cent by fractures of both bones of the forearm, 20 per cent by soft-tissue or crush injuries without associated fractures. Other new causes noted by them were perfusion of the upper limb for treatment of malignant neoplasms, massive blood transfusion under pressure during cardiac surgery, and excision of congenital radioulnar synostosis in which it occurred as a complication. In the series of Eichler and Lipscomb, 70 per cent of the patients were males.[184]

In the past, there were two contending theories about the mechanism of Volkmann's ischemic contracture: one, that it resulted from arterial insufficiency and the other, that it developed secondarily to venous occlusion and stasis. In 1940, Griffiths

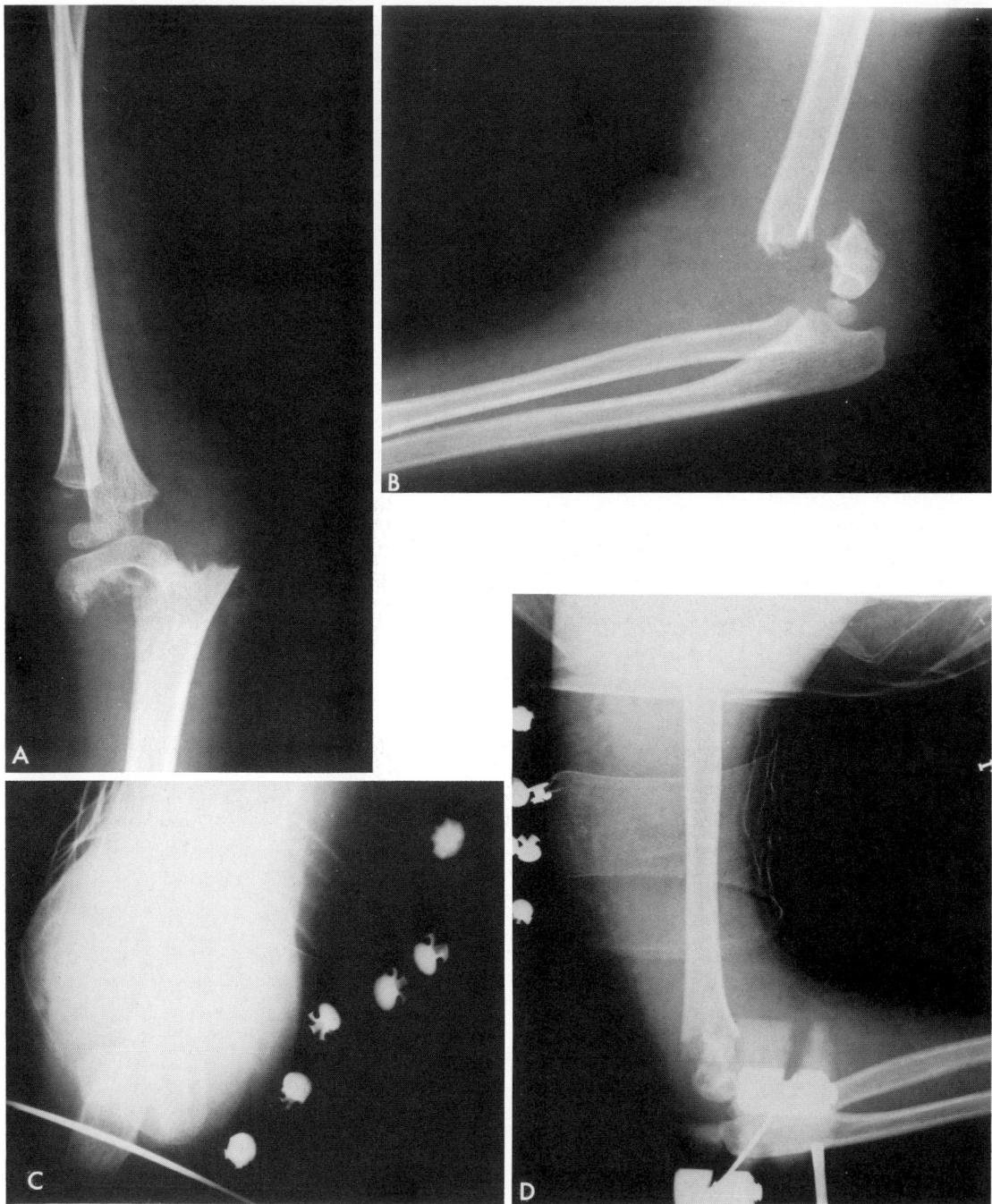

FIGURE 8-28.   *Supracondylar fracture of humerus — markedly displaced.*

Note the anterior displacement of lower end of the proximal fragment. This patient had impending Volkmann's contracture with absence of radial pulse, pain on extension of the digits, and pallor of fingertips. Immediate reduction was carried out. Ten minutes later, the radial pulse returned. **A** and **B.** Initial roentgenograms. **C** and **D.** Roentgenograms in traction, showing satisfactory alignment.

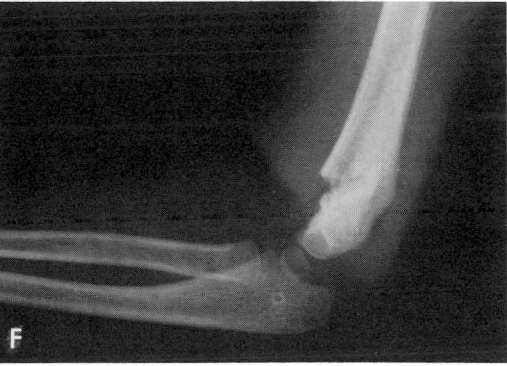

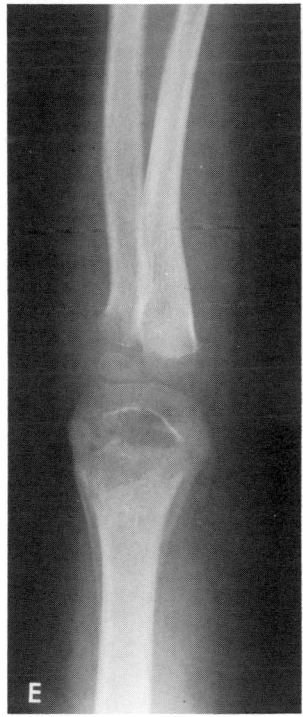

*FIGURE 8–28 Continued. Supracondylar
fracture of humerus — markedly displaced.*

E and **F**. Roentgenograms two months later,
showing the healed fracture.

firmly established that the process is caused
by arterial occlusion.[188]

Pathophysiology. The pathophysiology
of Volkmann's ischemia as outlined by
Eaton and Green is as follows:[182]

Ischemia produces anoxia in muscles,
which in turn causes formation of his-
tamine-like substances; consequently capillary permeability increases and conspicuous
intramuscular edema develops. This increasing intramuscular edema causes progressive increase in the intrinsic tissue pressure of the muscles. Circular unyielding
dressings on the limb and limited expansion
in a taut fascial envelope increase the venous compression, which causes further increase in intrinsic tissue pressure. Pressor
receptors within the compartment and
within the muscle itself stimulate a reflex
vasospasm affecting all vessels in this general area. This vasospasm aggravates and
perpetuates the initial vascular compromise,
and a destructive ischemia-edema cycle develops. Eaton et al. were able, experimentally, to produce transient yet complete
spasmodic shutdown of the brachial artery
by injecting a small bolus of autogenous
blood beneath the volar carpal ligaments of
rabbits.

The pathologic process is one of necrosis
of muscle with secondary fibrosis that may
develop calcification in its terminal phase.
The infarct has an ellipsoid shape with its
axis along the anterior interosseous artery
and its central point slightly above the middle of the forearm. The flexor digitorum
profundus, the flexor pollicis longus, and
the median nerve are the most commonly
and severely affected. During the acute
stage, when the volar compartment of the
forearm is surgically exposed, the deep fascia will be very taut and will spread widely
when split. The muscles, which are either
pale or blue-black from extravasation, will
protrude through the wound. The veins are
always engorged.

Circulatory embarrassment in supracondylar fractures of the humerus may
result from the brachial artery being caught
and kinked at the fracture site, from contusion and spasm of the artery at the moment of fracture, from compression of the
brachial vessels by a tight encircling cast, or
from rapidly progressive swelling in a taut
fascial compartment.

Distal to the lacertus fibrosus the brachial
artery branches into the radial and ulnar arteries. The radial artery is superficially lo-

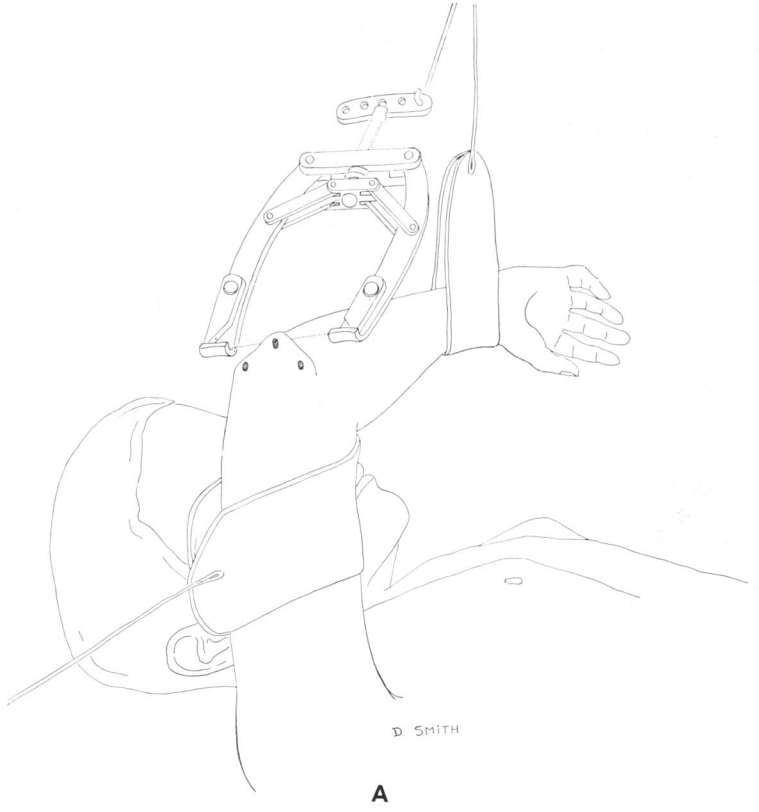

A

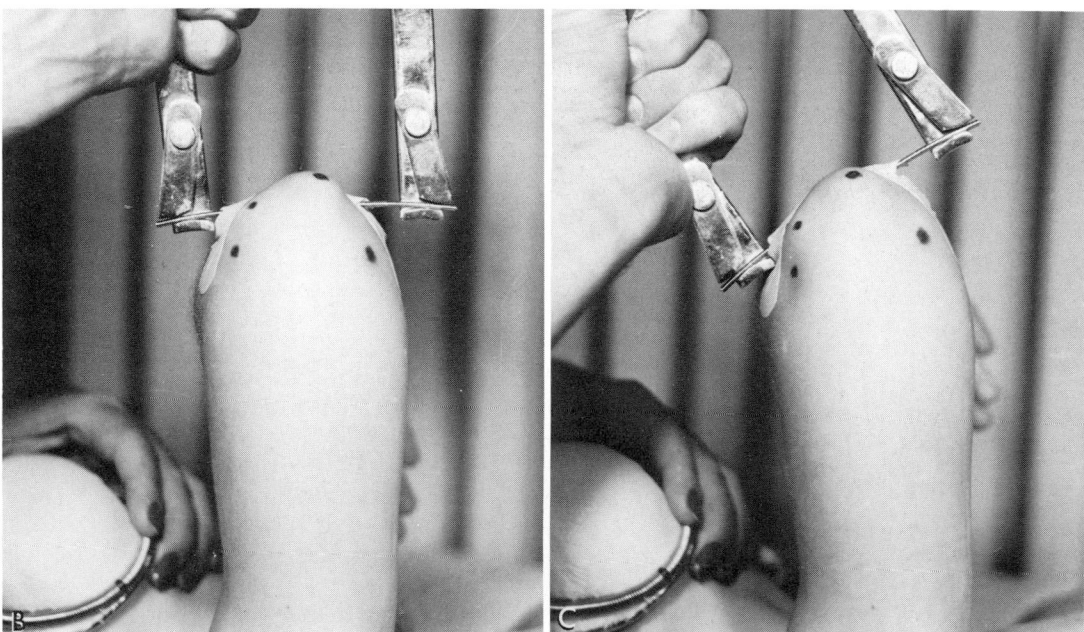

FIGURE 8–29.   *Overhead skeletal traction through a pin in the olecranon for treatment of markedly displaced supracondylar fractures of the humerus.*

A. Traction arrangement. **B.** Bony prominences are aligned like those of the contralateral normal elbow. **C.** The distal fragment has, for demonstration purposes, been tilted into valgus deformity. (From Smith, L.: Deformity following supracondylar fractures of the humerus. J. Bone Joint Surg., *42–A*:244 and 246, 1960.)

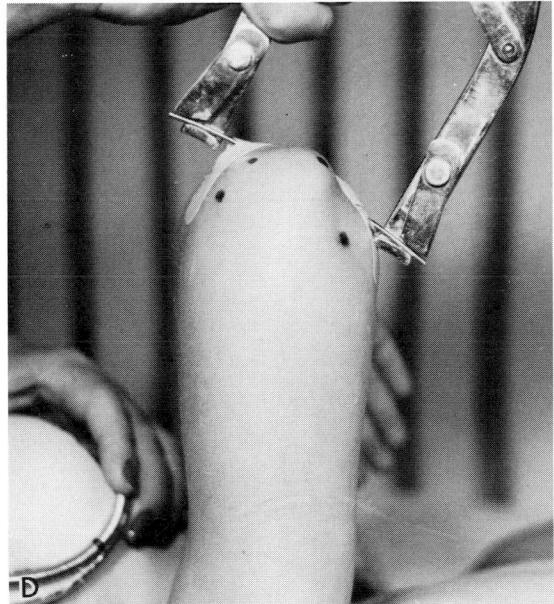
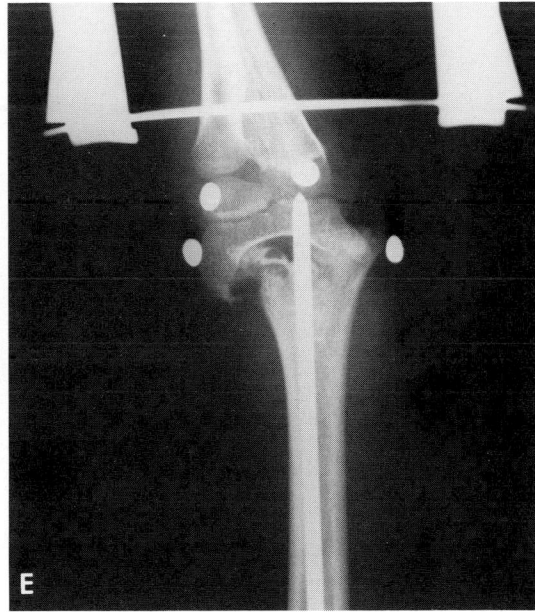

FIGURE 8-29 Continued. Overhead skeletal traction through a pin in the olecranon for treatment of markedly displaced supracondylar fractures of the humerus.

D. The distal fragment has been tilted into varus position. **E.** Roentgenographic appearance of the elbow as it is in **B.** Lead dots are placed on the ink markings and a wire taped along the long axis of the humerus. The lateral displacement of the distal fragment will have no effect on the carrying angle or function. (*From* Smith, L.: Deformity following supracondylar fractures of the humerus. J. Bone Joint Surg., *42-A*:244 and 246, 1960.)

cated, whereas the ulnar artery is deeply situated, traversing deep to the pronator teres muscles. The ulnar artery gives origin to the common interosseous artery, which divides immediately into anterior and posterior in terosseous branches. The flexor digitorum profundus and flexor pollicis longus muscles receive their blood supply through the anterior interosseous artery. The median nerve is particularly vulnerable to damage because of its course deep to the lacertus fibrosus and through the substance of the pronator teres muscle.

Diagnosis. The warning signs of Volkmann's ischemia are pain, pallor (or cyanosis), pulselessness, paresthesia, and paralysis. Of the five p's, the most important hallmark is pain. The possibility of Volkmann's ischemia should always be ruled out when increasing pain develops in the forearm following injury in the region of the elbow or forearm. A characteristic physical finding is exaggeration of the pain upon passive extension of the fingers. Within 6 to 12 hours, progressive swelling and firmness develops in the volar compartment of the forearm. The radial pulse may be present or absent. The presence of a normal radial pulse does not rule out Volkmann's ischemia, since the radial artery may not be compressed because of its superficial location and its pulsation may not disappear until the entire vascular system is in spasm. Paleness or cyanosis is best detected in the nailbed with delay of vascular return following compression. There is always a varying degree of sensory loss—the median nerve is almost always involved and the ulnar nerve is paralyzed in most cases.

The destructive process of Volkmann's ischemia is progressive, and within 12 to 24 hours, it becomes fully developed.

Within five to ten days, the swelling and sensitivity gradually subside and the muscles of the flexor compartment become hard and inelastic. Gradually fibrosis of the involved muscles produces fixed contractural deformity—the elbow is flexed, the forearm pronated, the wrist flexed, the metacarpophalangeal joints hyperextended, and the interphalangeal joints flexed.

Treatment. In the acute ischemic stage, treatment should be immediate. If signs of impending Volkmann's ischemia cannot be

(*Text continued on page 1587.*)

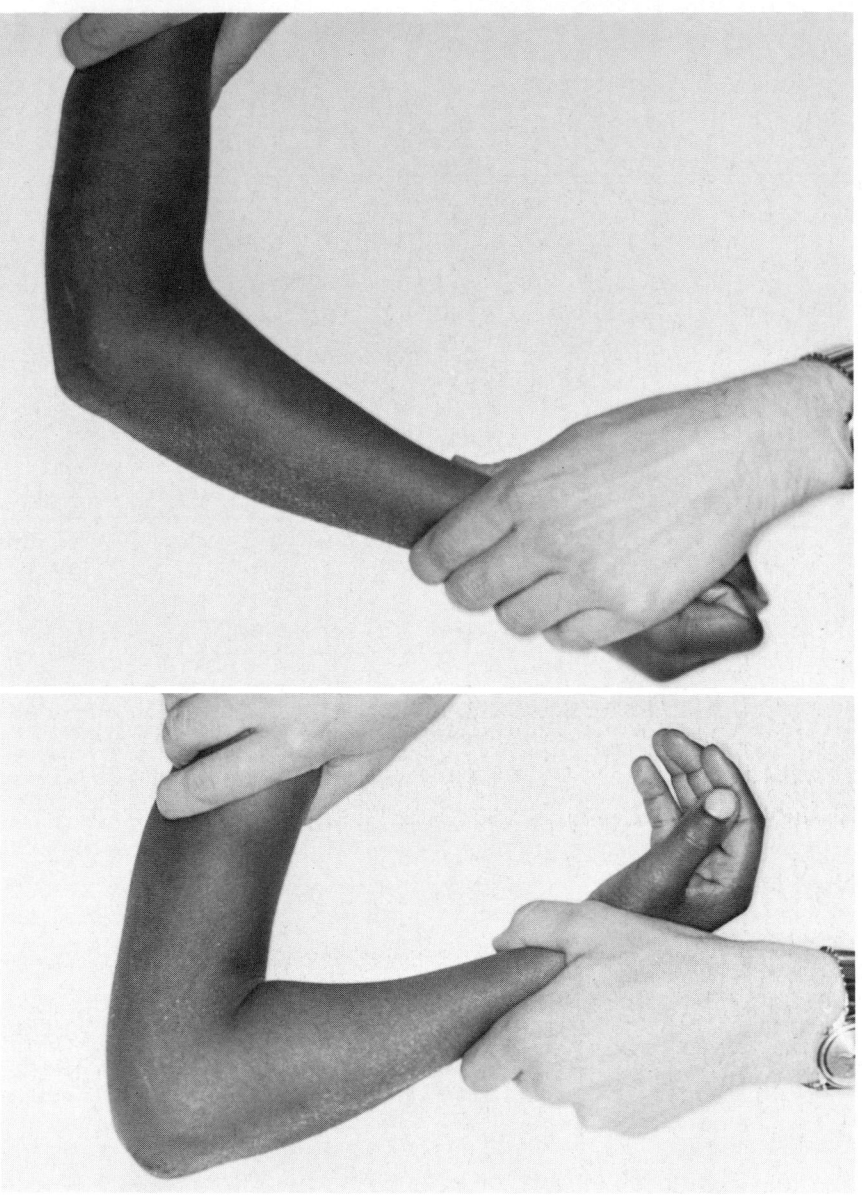

FIGURE 8–30.   Active exercises to develop range of motion of elbow joint.

The left hand of the therapist is used to guide the forearm into extension and flexion, motion is performed actively by the patient. Passive exercises and lifting of weights should not be performed.

FIGURE 8–31.   The effect on the carrying angle of various types of displacement of the distal fragment in supracondylar fractures of the humerus.

A. The carrying angle of the elbow—12 degrees. **B.** Following medial displacement of the distal fragment, the carrying angle did not change from its 12 degrees. **C.** Upon lateral displacement, the carrying angle again did not change. **D.** Fifteen-degree medial rotation of distal fragment did not change the carrying angle. **E.** Upon 32-degree medial tilting of the distal fragment, the carrying angle changed to 20 degrees varus. **F.** The distal fragment was tilted laterally 18 degrees, and the carrying angle increased to 30 degrees valgus. (From Smith, L.: Deformity following supracondylar fractures of the humerus. J. Bone Joint Surg., *42–A*:238, 239, 1960.)

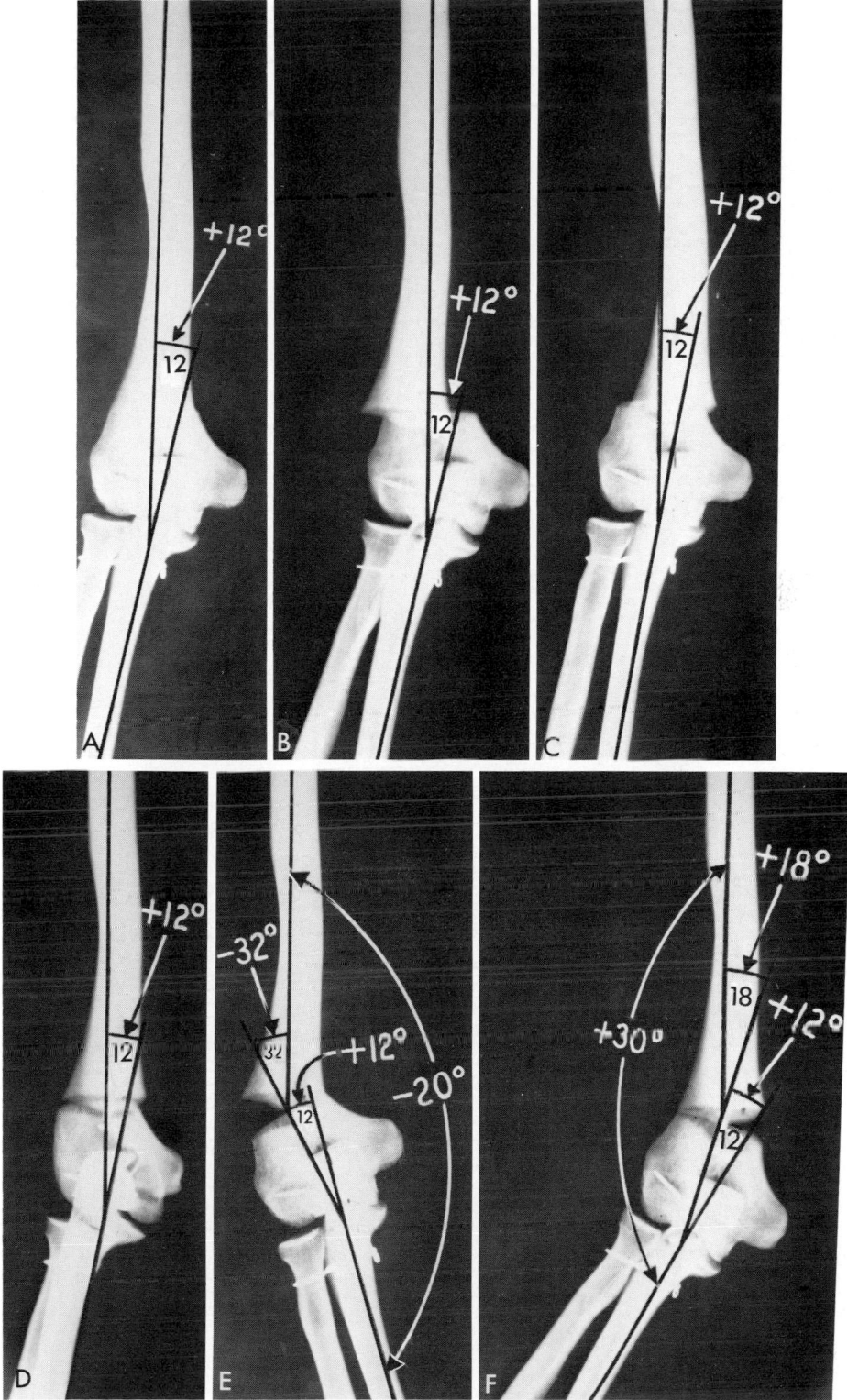

FIGURE 8-31. *The effect on the carrying angle of various types of displacement of the distal fragment in supracondylar fractures of the humerus.* See opposite page for legend.

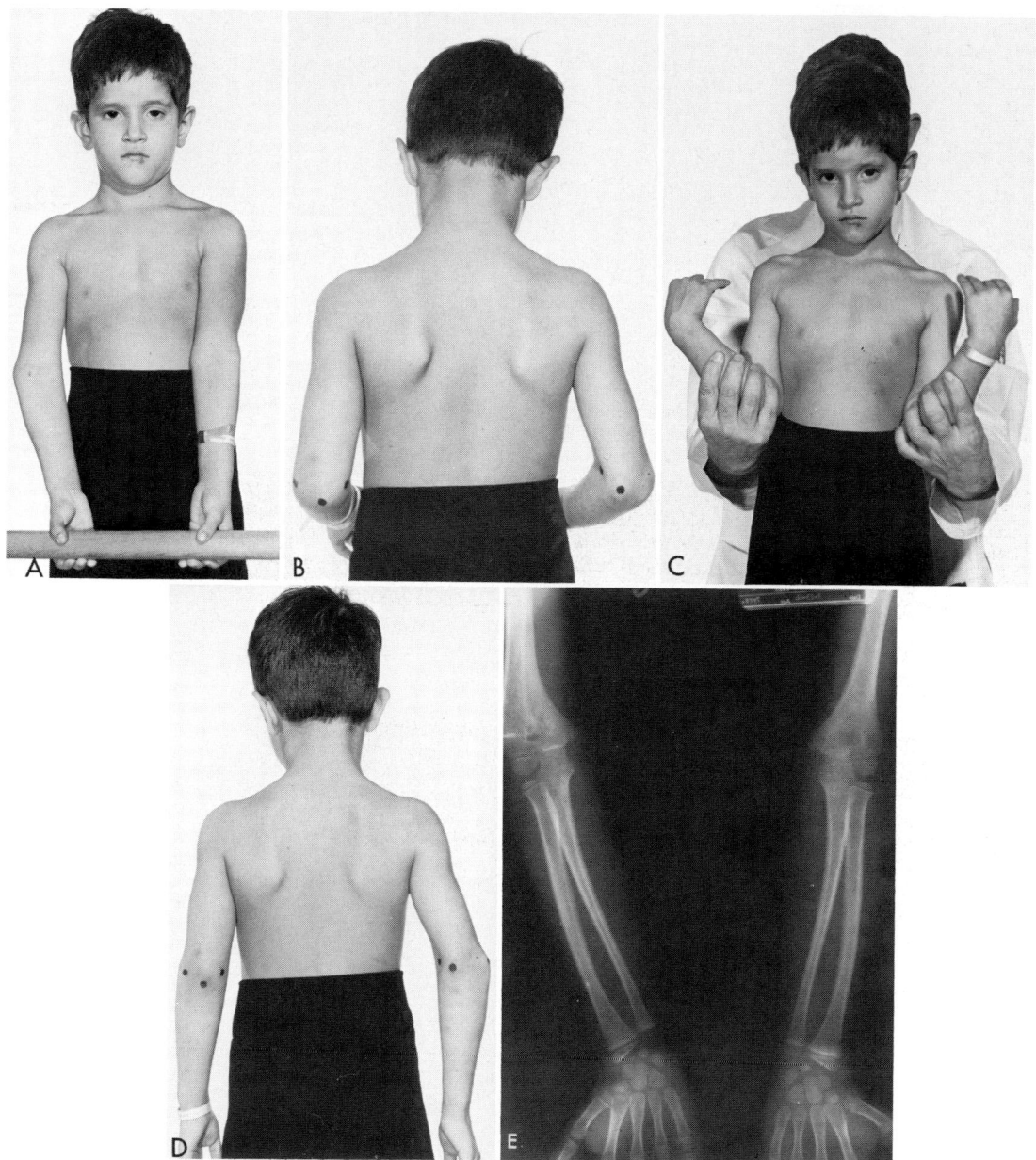

FIGURE 8–32. *Cubitus varus caused by malunion of supracondylar fracture of the humerus.*

Deformity on the right is due to medial tilting of the distal fragment. **A** to **D.** Clinical appearance. **E.** Anteroposterior roentgenogram with the elbows in extension.

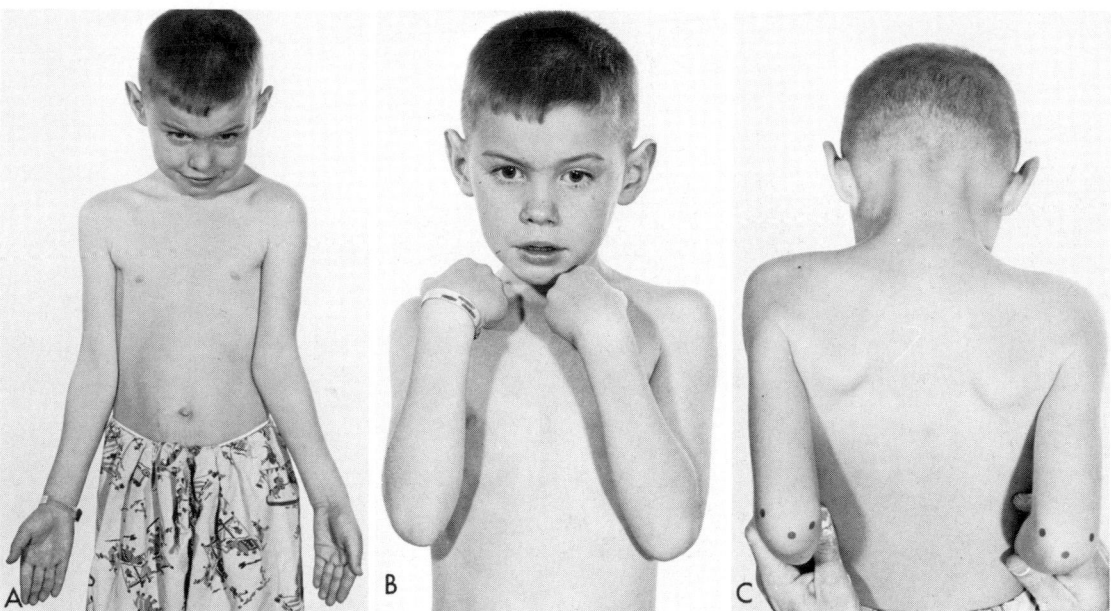

FIGURE 8–33. *Cubitus valgus due to malunion of supracondylar fracture of left humerus.*

Deformity on the left is caused by lateral tilting of the distal fragment. **A** to **C.** Clinical appearance.

relieved within 6 to 12 hours by extension of the elbow, removal of all tight encircling bandages, and reduction of the fracture, arteriography is performed. If a vascular surgeon is available, he should be called in consultation. If the brachial artery is in spasm only, a stellate ganglion block is performed. If, within 30 minutes, circulation does not improve, fasciotomy and epimysiotomy of the forearm and exploration of the brachial artery are indicated. The technique of epimysiotomy and fasciotomy is described by Eaton and Green as follows:[182]

A longitudinal incision is made at the flexor crease of the elbow medial to the biceps tendon and is extended along the middle of the volar surface of the forearm to the flexor crease of the wrist. Proximally the incision may be extended to expose the brachial artery without crossing the flexor crease. The subcutaneous tissue is divided and the antebrachial fascia is sectioned longitudinally throughout its entire length. The fascial sheath of each muscle (the epimysium or perimysium) is carefully divided from its lower to upper margin. Muscle fibers should not be sectioned and meticulous attention should be paid to avoiding inadvertent injury to any nerve branches that penetrate the epimysium.

Following decompression by fasciotomy and epimysiotomy there will be a dramatic return of circulation unless the muscles have become grossly gangrenous. If indicated, the brachial artery is explored. The major nerves are decompressed; particularly important is decompression of the median nerve as it passes beneath the humeral and ulnar heads of the flexor carpi ulnaris muscle.

The fascia is not closed. Often muscle edema prevents approximation of the skin edges. In such an instance, the wound is left open and covered with nonadherent dressing. Skeletal traction is applied with a pin through the olecranon. A delayed closure is performed in two to three days when the edema has subsided. Relaxing incisions and skin grafts may be utilized to cover the bulging muscle bellies.

In the postoperative period, proper splinting and active and passive exercises are essential to obtain good function.

Treatment of *established* Volkmann's ischemic contracture is dependent upon the severity of the deformity and the period following injury. Eaton and Green recommend that fasciotomy and epimysiotomy be performed weeks or even months following onset, as long as induration of the volar compartment is present. Two to three months postinjury, the author fractionally

(*Text continued on page 1592.*)

Osteotomy of Distal Humerus for Correction of Cubitus Varus

THE PROCEDURE

A. A longitudinal incision is made over the anterolateral aspect of the distal third of the arm, with the anterior margin of the brachioradialis muscle serving as an anatomic landmark. It begins 1 cm. proximal and anterior to the lateral epicondyle of the humerus and extends proximally for a distance of approximately 7 cm.

B. The subcutaneous tissue and fascia are divided in line with the skin incision. The skin flaps are mobilized and retracted. The anterior margin of the brachioradialis muscle laterally and the lateral margin of the biceps muscle medially are identified, and by blunt dissection in the loose areolar tissue between these two muscles, the radial nerve is located. A moist hernia tape is passed around the radial nerve for gentle handling and traction.

The biceps muscle is retracted medially, exposing the lateral half of the brachialis muscle beneath it. By blunt dissection with a periosteal elevator, the lateral one third to one half of the muscle fibers of the brachialis are raised, exposing the periosteum on the front of the lower end of the humerus. The periosteum is incised longitudinally as shown in the illustration, its distal end stopping 1 cm. proximal to the capsule of the elbow joint.

C. The periosteum is reflected with a periosteal elevator and the lower end of the shaft of the humerus is exposed. It is essential not to disturb the growth of the epiphyseal plates and to keep out of the elbow joint.

Plate 64. Osteotomy of Distal Humerus for Correction of Cubitus Varus

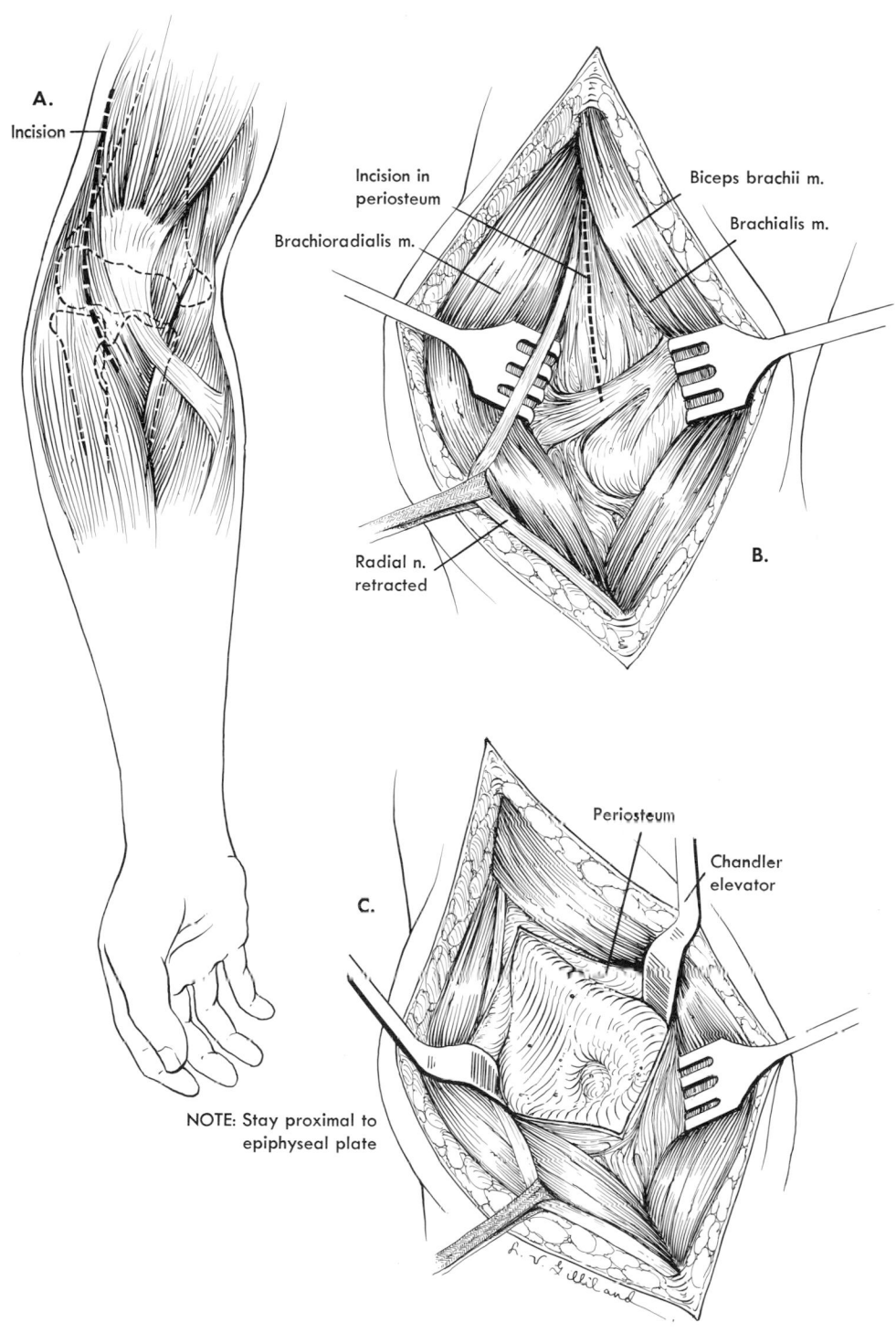

A.
Incision

Incision in periosteum

Brachioradialis m.

Biceps brachii m.

Brachialis m.

Radial n. retracted

B.

C.

Periosteum

Chandler elevator

NOTE: Stay proximal to epiphyseal plate

L. V. Gilliland

Osteotomy of Distal Humerus for
Correction of Cubitus Varus (Continued)

D. With a starter and drill, the line of a dome-shaped osteotomy is outlined with drill holes through both anterior and posterior cortices. The medial arch of the dome should be deeper and 1 to 1.5 cm. longer than the lateral arch, which is almost transverse.

Next, through stab wounds separate from the skin incision, two ⅛-inch Crow pins are drilled transversely across the distal portion of the proximal fragment. The pins should be perpendicular to the shaft of the humerus, 3 cm. apart, and should engage the medial cortex of the humerus. It is essential to drill the pins across the humerus under direct vision and lift the radial nerve anteriorly to protect it from injury. Then a third Crow pin is placed into the distal fragment at a predetermined angle so that when the varus deformity is corrected, the distal pin should be parallel to the proximal pins. The distal pin should not cross the osteotomy line and it should engage the medial cortex of the distal fragment. A Roger Anderson apparatus is applied to the Crow pins and the bolts are loosely fitted. With sharp thin osteotomes, the osteotomy is completed, great care being taken not to split the medial cortex of the dome of the proximal fragment.

E. The bone fragments are manipulated and the angular and rotational deformities are corrected. If necessary, a wedge of bone may be removed from the lateral side of the distal fragment with a rongeur. The osteotomy fragments are anchored together by fixing the Roger Anderson apparatus firmly. Roentgenograms are taken with the elbow in extension to check the correction of the deformity and the position of the Crow pins. The periosteum and the wound are closed in the usual manner.

F. Abundant sheath wadding and petrolatum gauze are placed over the Roger Anderson apparatus, and a long arm cast is applied with the elbow in 90 degrees of flexion.

POSTOPERATIVE CARE

Roentgenograms are made after five days and again at two weeks to check maintenance of anatomic alignment of the fracture fragments. The osteotomy usually heals in six weeks. The cast and pins are removed and *active* exercises are begun to restore range of motion of the elbow. Passive exercises are *not* performed. Weights should not be lifted for two months.

Plate 64. Osteotomy of Distal Humerus for Correction of Cubitus Varus

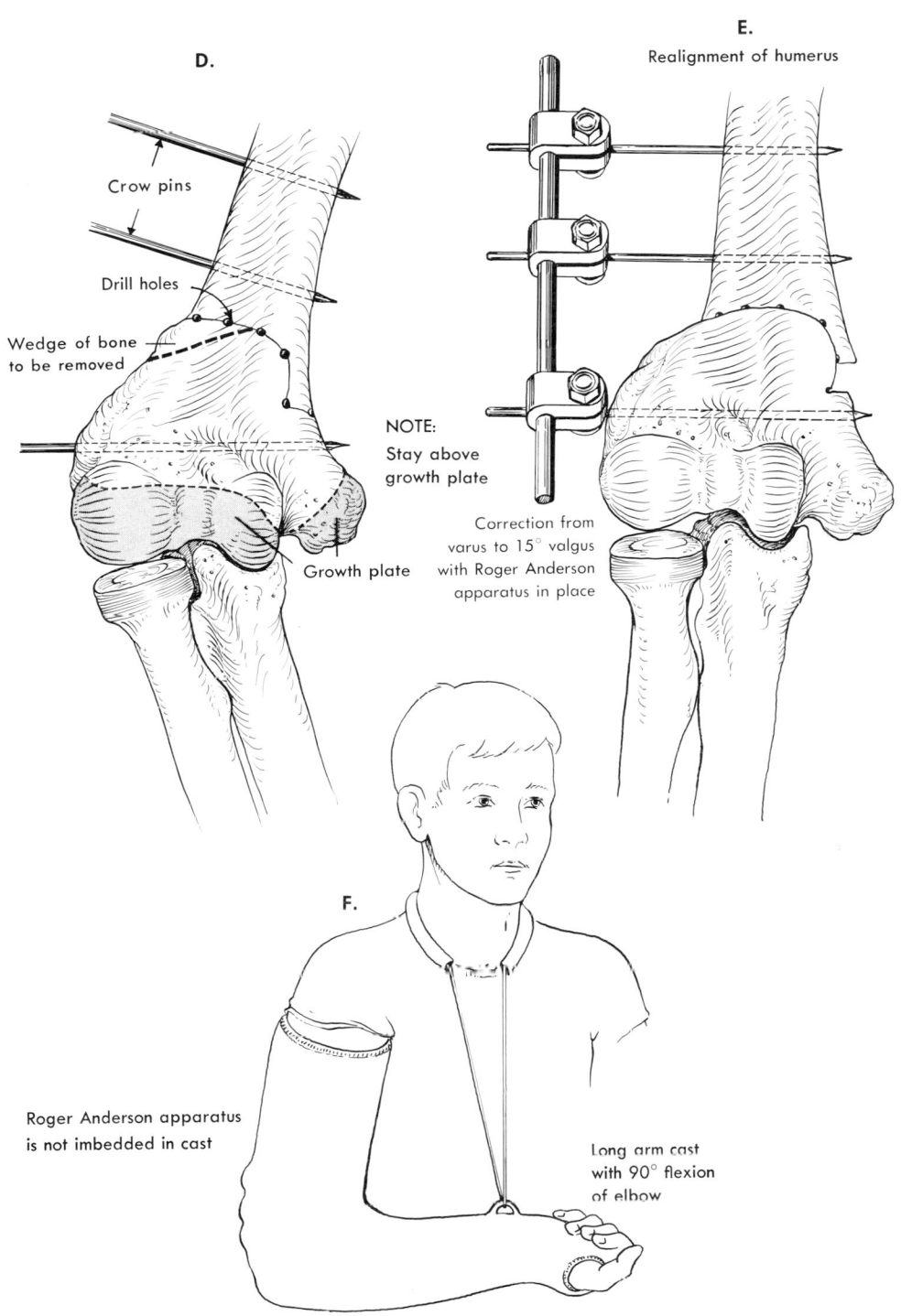

D.

Crow pins

Drill holes

Wedge of bone to be removed

NOTE:
Stay above growth plate

Growth plate

E.
Realignment of humerus

Correction from varus to 15° valgus with Roger Anderson apparatus in place

F.

Roger Anderson apparatus is not imbedded in cast

Long arm cast with 90° flexion of elbow

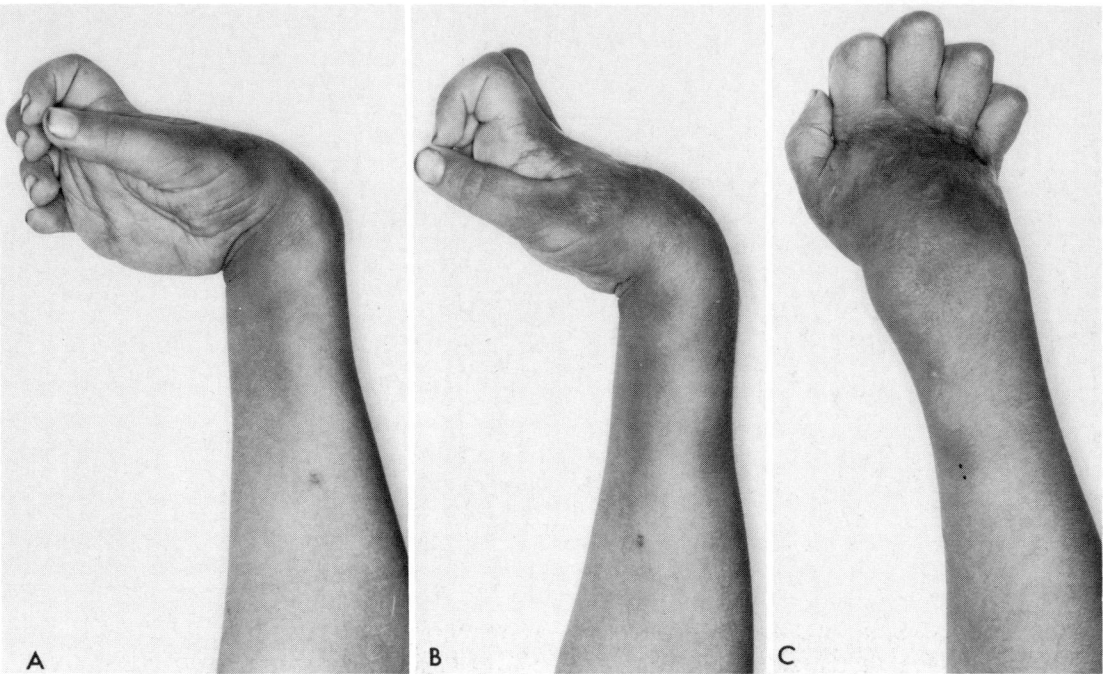

FIGURE 8–34.   *Volkmann's ischemic contracture caused by supracondylar fracture of the humerus.*

A to **C.** Clinical appearance.

lengthens the contracted flexor muscles of the forearm at their muscle junction. This is combined with neurolysis of the median and ulnar nerves.

In severe late cases, both bones of the forearm may be shortened to gain relative length of the contracted muscles.

NEURAL COMPLICATIONS

The radial, ulnar, and median nerves may be injured at the time of fracture, during attempts at reduction, or by compression during Volkmann's ischemia. Siris, in 1939, reported a series of 330 supracondylar fractures of the humerus, with 11 cases of nerve paralysis (7 of the radial nerve, 4 of the ulnar nerve).[159] Sorrel and Sorrel-Déjerine found an incidence of 7 per cent (16 of 207 supracondylar fractures) — 7 ulnar, 4 radial, 4 median, and 1 combined median and ulnar nerve paralysis.[162] Both Siris and Sorrel recommended exploration if there are no signs of improvement in 15 days.[159, 162]

Bailey reviewed 71 cases of supracondylar fractures of the humerus in children and found six cases of nerve injury (8 per cent);

four had radial nerve involvement only, one of the median nerve alone, and one of all three nerves — the radial, median, and ulnar. In two of the cases, paralysis was present prior to attempts at reduction, and in the remaining four cases, the nerves were injured during attempted reduction of the fracture. In all six cases the nerves were compressed or contused, and partial return of function in the paralyzed muscle took place before the end of two months and complete recovery before the end of 14 weeks.[173]

Lipscomb and Burleson reported a 16 per cent incidence of nerve injury in supracondylar fractures (in 17 of the 108 patients). Trauma to the radial nerve was most common. Five of the seventeen patients were treated expectantly; partial return or full return of function occurred in two to three weeks. In four patients, the nerve injury accompanied trauma to the brachial artery and surgical exploration was performed because of the vascular lesion. In one patient with radial nerve palsy, open reduction of the fracture was performed early, and tension on the nerve was released. Four pa-

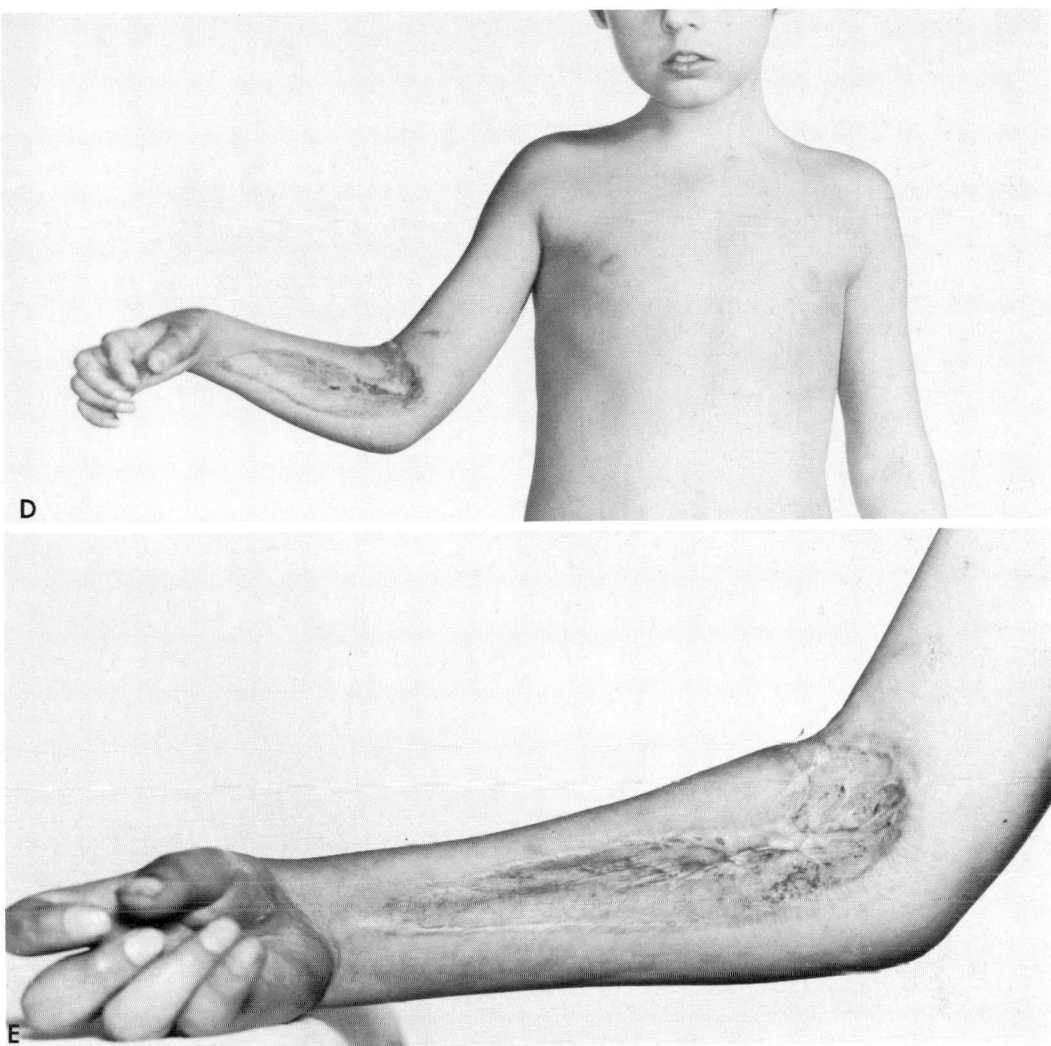

FIGURE 8-34 Continued. *Volkmann's ischemic contracture caused by supracondylar fracture of the humerus.*

D and **E.** This patient had decompression by fasciotomy.

tients with nerve palsy were observed for a period of three to four weeks. Because there was no recovery of nerve function, exploration was then performed. In no patient was a nerve found to be divided, but they were either compressed by old hemorrhage, bound down by fibrous tissue, or stretched over a bone fragment. Complete recovery was obtained by neurolysis. In one patient with palsy of all three nerves, partial return of function was obtained by neurolysis. Lipscomb and Burleson advised observation of nerve palsies for a few weeks after adequate reduction of the fracture. If no improvement occurred after this period, they advised surgical exploration.[205]

Spinner and Schreiber reported six cases of anterior interosseous nerve paralysis as a complication of supracondylar fractures of the humerus in children. They proposed traction as the mechanism of the paralysis, the distracting elements being the proximal fragment of the humerus and a tethering structure in the forearm. They believed the paralysis is caused by contusion of the nerve by the anteriorly displaced proximal fragment of the humerus at the level of the fracture. The characteristic physical finding of anterior interosseous nerve paralysis is loss of flexion power of the distal phalanx of the thumb and of the index finger with all other median nerve functions intact. In all six of their patients, spontaneous recovery occurred in six to eight weeks. They recommended exploration of the median nerve from the distal part of the humerus through the pronator teres, should clinical or electromyographic recovery not take place in six to eight weeks following surgery.[224]

A complete evaluation of radial, ulnar, and median nerve function should be performed before and after reduction of supracondylar fracture of the humerus. As stated, manipulation should be gentle to avoid injury to the nerves. If there is paralysis, passive exercises are performed to maintain range of motion of the digits, and the hand is splinted in functional position. Nerve function is periodically determined. If, within six to eight weeks, function has not returned, the nerves are explored and neurolysis is performed. It is best to transpose the ulnar nerve anteriorly. If the nerve palsy is associated with Volkmann's ischemia, neurolysis is performed along with fasciotomy and epimysiotomy.

FRACTURE-SEPARATION OF THE DISTAL HUMERAL EPIPHYSIS

This injury is extremely rare and is often misdiagnosed because of difficulties in interpreting the roentgenogram. One of the earliest case reports of a 12-year-old child was given by R. W. Smith, who emphasized the importance of the differential diagnosis between supracondylar fractures, dislocations, and epiphyseal separations of the elbow.[234] A critical review of six previously published cases in the literature was given by Poland, in 1898.[762] Ashhurst reported seven cases in his monograph.[86] Marmor and Bechtol described a Type I physeal injury (Salter-Harris) in a two-year-old child; Kaplan and Reckling reported a Type II physeal injury with medial displacement of the lower humeral epiphysis in an eight-year-old boy.[232, 233]

The entire lower epiphysis of the hu-

merus is displaced posteriorly, laterally, or forward, depending on the mechanism of injury. The violence may be indirect (a fall on the outstretched hand) or direct (a fall on the olecranon). The condition is easily confused with dislocation of the elbow. The salient distinguishing feature of fracture-separation of the lower humeral epiphysis is the normal relationship of the ossification center of the capitellum with the radius. A longitudinal line drawn up the shaft of the radius normally passes through the capitellum; in dislocation, however, it does not, indicating a disruption of the joint. A Type II physeal injury (Salter-Harris) should be differentiated from a fracture of the lateral condyle of the humerus; the latter is a Type IV physeal injury, in which the fracture fragment is often displaced by the pull of the common extensor muscles of the forearm with subsequent loss of its normal relationship to the radial head.[232]

Treatment consists of closed reduction and immobilization in a long arm cast for three weeks.

FRACTURES OF THE LATERAL CONDYLE OF THE HUMERUS

The ossification center of the lateral condyle appears between 18 months and two years of age. It extends medially to form the principal part of the lower articular end of the humerus. The ossific center for the medial part of the trochlea appears at 12 years of age. The lateral epicondyle ossifies at the age of 13 years and fuses with the capitellum at 16 or 17 years. The radial collateral ligament, the tendon of the supinator longus, and the common tendon of the extensor muscles of the forearm are attached to the lateral epicondyle.

Fractures of the lateral condyle of the humerus are rather common, constituting 13 to 18 per cent of all fractures in the region of the elbow in children.

The injury is a Type IV physeal injury (Salter-Harris), i.e., it is an intra-articular transepiphyseal fracture. It is mostly encountered in children between the ages of 3 and 14 years, the peak incidence being from 6 to 10 years of age. It is three to four times more common in boys than in girls.

Mechanism of Injury and Pathology

Fracture of the lateral condyle of the humerus usually results from indirect violence in a fall on the outstretched hand with the forearm in abduction and the elbow in extension. The force is transmitted up the radius; the lesion may also be produced by a traction force that thrusts the elbow into varus position.

The fracture line begins at the lateral side of the distal metaphysis of the humerus and extends obliquely downward and medially, traverses the physis, and enters the joint in the lateral portion of the trochlea. Thus, the distal fragment contains the epiphysis of the capitellum, a part of the trochlea, the lateral epicondyle, and a part of the metaphysis with the radial collateral ligament and the common tendon of the extensor muscles of the forearm attached to it.

The fractured fragment may be undisplaced, as shown in Figure 8–35, minimally displaced, or markedly displaced and rotated by the pull of the extensors of the wrist and the fingers. The degree of rotation of the fragment varies; when it is 90 degrees, the articular surface faces inward

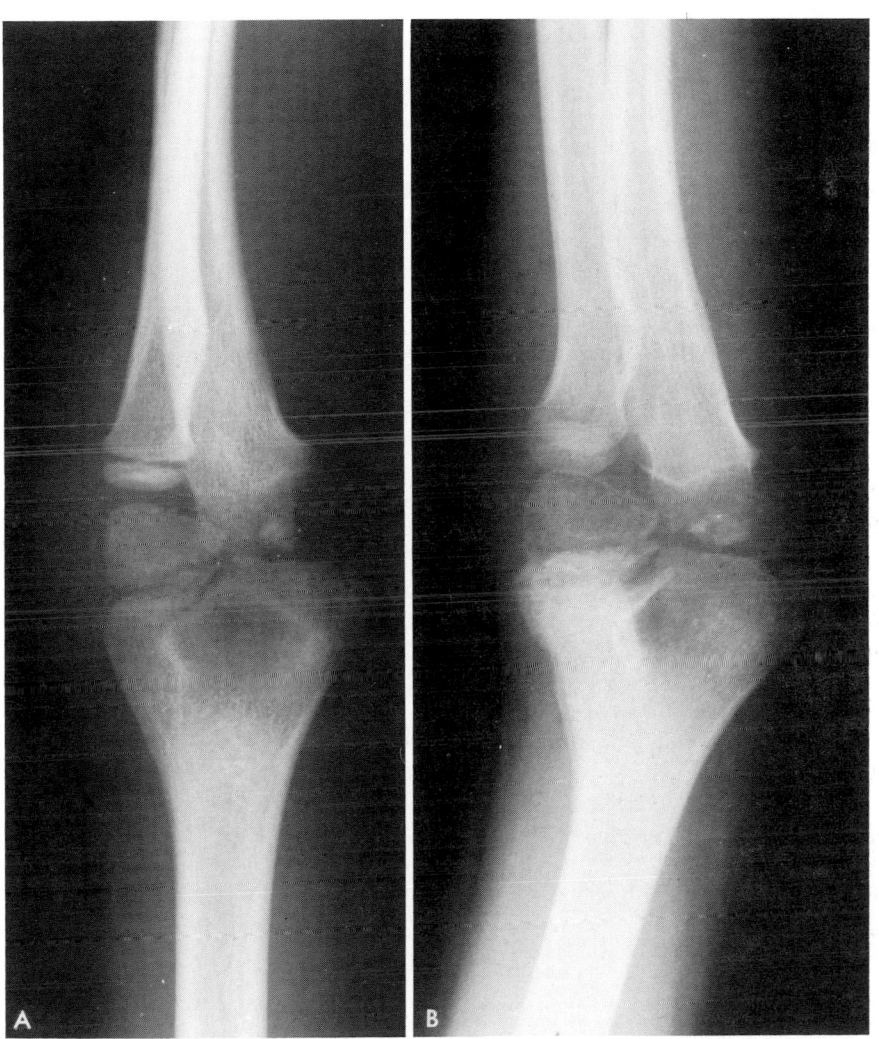

FIGURE 8–35.   *Undisplaced fracture of lateral condyle of humerus.*

Fracture was treated by simple immobilization in long arm cast. **A.** Initial roentgenogram. **B.** Roentgenogram taken after two months, showing healing.

and the fractured surface, laterally; in its extreme form of 180-degree rotation around both the horizontal and vertical axes, the distal articular surface faces cephalad toward the fracture site, the inner trochlear surface faces outward, and the lateral surfaces faces inward. Fracture of the lateral condyle of the humerus may be associated with medial dislocation of the elbow (cf. Fig. 8–41).

Diagnosis

Following injury, these patients complain of severe pain. There is marked swelling, ecchymosis, and local tenderness over the lateral aspect of the elbow. In the absence of soft-tissue swelling, one may be able to palpate the detached fragment. Ordinarily rotation of the forearm is not restricted.

The diagnosis is made by the roentgenographic findings. Anteroposterior, lateral, and oblique projections are obtained. Sometimes only the oblique view will disclose displacement. Undisplaced fractures may not be diagnosed unless comparative roentgenograms of the opposite elbow are obtained.

Treatment

Fractures of the lateral condyle of the humerus are unstable; they tend to become displaced even when immobilized because of the pull of the common extensors. As the fracture line crosses the physis, accurate anatomic repositioning is imperative to decrease the likelihood of growth damage. Congruity of the joint must be restored. This fracture is intra-articular and synovial fluid bathes the fracture line, predisposing to delayed union and nonunion.

The *undisplaced fracture* is treated by simple immobilization in a long arm cast with the elbow in 90 degrees of flexion and the forearm in full supination to minimize the pull of the extensor muscles. Even undisplaced fractures of the lateral condyle are unstable and may become displaced while immobilized in the cast. Repeated roentgenograms are made during the first 10 to 14 days to detect further displacement. If such a complication occurs, immediate open reduction and internal fixation are carried out.

In the *displaced fracture,* primary open reduction and internal fixation constitute the treatment of choice. The operative technique is described and illustrated in Plate 65.

In the literature some authors recommend conservative closed treatment of minimally displaced fractures of the lateral condylar epiphysis. The author recommends that such fractures be internally fixed with two smooth Kirschner wires (sometimes this is easily done subcutaneously under image intensifier control). Nonunion and growth arrest more commonly result from minimally displaced fractures than from markedly displaced and rotated fractures because the severe fractures are treated more adequately.[240]

Complications

Nonunion will result in progressive cubitus valgus due to retardation or arrest of growth of the lateral condyle and continued normal growth of the medial condyle. The ulnar nerve is repeatedly stretched by motion of the elbow over the apex of the deformity, and may become inflamed in its course behind the medial epicondyle. At the earliest signs of neuritis, the ulnar nerve is transferred anteriorly to the medial epicondyle in order to prevent permanent neural deficit.

Bone grafting to obtain union before completion of growth is not recommended because functional disability is unsignificant in the presence of nonunion.

Malunion and premature growth arrest of the lateral condyle will also cause progressive cubitus valgus and tardy ulnar nerve palsy. The deformity of the elbow is corrected by open-up osteotomy of the distal humerus with a graft wedge and the ulnar nerve is transposed anteriorly (Fig. 8–36).

Wadsworth studied 28 children with fracture of the capitulum (8 undisplaced and 20 displaced), and found six cases of premature epiphyseal fusion. He distinguished two types of premature fusion; in the first, the capitular epiphysis fused to the metaphysis, and in the second, the capitular and trochlear epiphyses fused together and then to the metaphysis. Either type of premature fusion resulted in valgus deformity.

Delayed union will result in prolonged hyperemia and stimulation of growth on the lateral side of the elbow, producing cubitus varus.

Avascular necrosis of the capitellum will cause growth disturbance and deformity of the capitellum and adjacent radial head.

FRACTURES OF THE MEDIAL EPICONDYLE OF THE HUMERUS*

The ossification center of the medial epicondyle of the humerus appears at about five years of age and unites with the humeral diaphysis between 18 and 20 years of age. The common tendon of the flexor muscles of the forearm (flexor carpi radialis, flexor carpi ulnaris, flexor digitorum sublimis, palmaris longus, and part of the pronator teres) takes its origin from the anterior aspect of the medial epicondyle, which also gives attachment to the ulnar collateral ligament of the elbow joint. The ulnar nerve runs in a groove in the posterior aspect of this epicondyle—an anatomic relation responsible for the frequent occurrence of the ulnar nerve injury in this fracture. The medial epicondyle is an apophysis and does not contribute to longitudinal growth of the humerus.

Fractures of the epicondyle usually occur between 7 and 15 years of age. They constitute about 10 per cent of all fractures in the region of the elbow joint in children.

The mechanism of injury is a valgus strain of the joint, producing traction on the medial epicondyle through the flexor muscles. The epicondyle may be minimally displaced, moderately displaced to the level of the joint, markedly displaced and incarcerated into the elbow joint, or severely displaced in association with posterolateral dislocation of the elbow (Fig. 8–37). About half of the cases of fractures of the medial epicondyle are associated with dislocation of the elbow (cf. Fig. 8–40 C).

Incarceration of the fragment into the joint usually occurs at the time of reduction of the dislocation; or it may be pulled into the joint by the abduction force when the elbow is temporarily opened on its medial side, or while the joint is momentarily dislocated.

*See References 261 to 265.

Diagnosis

Physical findings depend upon the degree of displacement of the medial epicondyle. The elbow is held in partial flexion and any motion is painful. There is local tenderness over the medial aspect of the joint. When valgus strain is exerted at the elbow joint, the pain is aggravated.

Roentgenograms will disclose the absence of the medial epicondyle from its normal position. The displaced fragment may be seen in the lateral, anteroposterior, or oblique projections of the elbow. If the diagnosis is in doubt, roentgenograms of the opposite elbow are made for comparison. When the medial epicondyle is incarcerated into the joint, the articular cartilage space is widened on its medial aspect and the bony fragment is best visualized in the lateral views. When the elbow is dislocated posterolaterally, the medial epicondyle is usually located posterior to the trochlea. Ulnar nerve paresis is a common complication of this injury.

Treatment

If the medial epicondyle is *minimally displaced,* the joint is immobilized in a long arm cast with the elbow in moderate flexion and the forearm in pronation for three weeks.

If the epicondyle is *moderately displaced* but the elbow is *stable* on valgus strain, treatment again consists of simple immobilization in a long arm cast for three weeks. The functional result will be excellent despite the fact that healing is by fibrous union. Occasionally the fragment may fail to heal and produces symptoms due to irritation by local pressure, such as rubbing on a table while writing; in such an instance, complete relief of symptoms is obtained by excision of the loose fragment.

If the medial epicondyle is *markedly displaced* and the elbow joint is *unstable* on application of valgus strain, open reduction and internal fixation are indicated.

The medial longitudinal skin incision starts at the fractured medial epicondyle and extends proximally for a distance of 5 to 7 cm. parallel with the epicondylar ridge of the humerus. The subcutaneous tissue and deep fascia are divided in line with the skin incision. The ulnar nerve is identified,

(*Text continued on page 1604.*)

Open Reduction and Internal Fixation of Fracture of Lateral Condyle of Humerus

THE PROCEDURE

A. The incision begins 5 to 7 cm. proximal to the lateral epicondyle of the humerus and extends distally over the epicondylar ridge of the lateral epicondyle and then continues distally and posteriorly over the interval between the anconeus and the extensor carpi ulnaris muscles for a distance of 2.5 cm.

B. The deep fascia is opened in line with the skin incision. Working distally to proximally, the plane between the triceps muscle posteriorly and the brachioradialis muscle anteriorly is developed. One should avoid the radial nerve in the proximal end of the wound where it enters in the interval between the brachialis and brachioradialis muscles. The dissection is carried distally between the anconeus and the extensor carpi ulnaris muscles, exposing the joint capsule.

C. The periosteum is incised along the lateral epicondylar ridge and adjacent humerus, and the joint capsule is opened.

D. On exposure of the fracture site, the wound is irrigated with normal saline to remove small pieces of loose bone. The lateral condylar fracture segment is usually larger than it appears on the roentgenogram, and it is rotated distally.

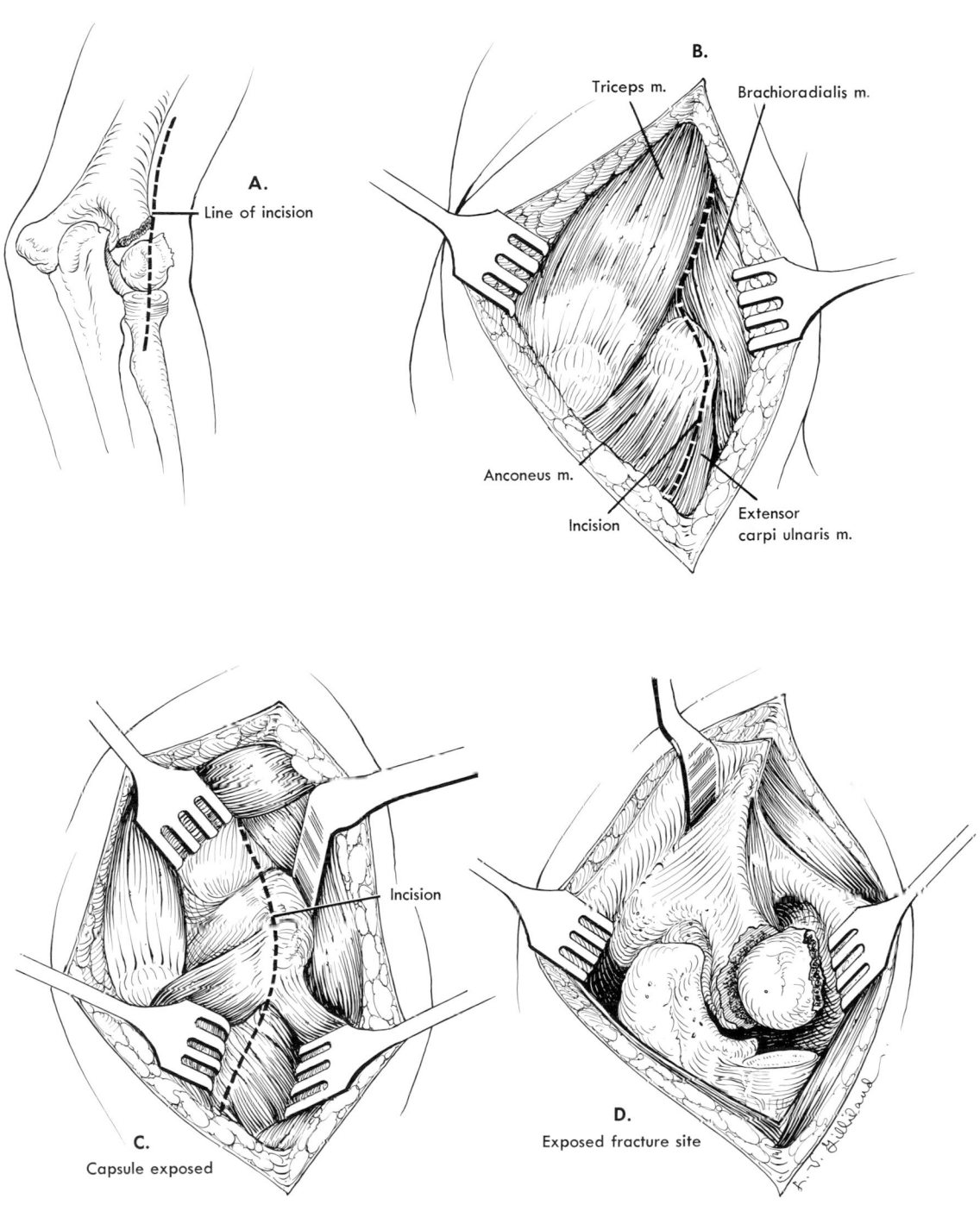

A.
Line of incision

B.
Triceps m.

Brachioradialis m.

Anconeus m.

Incision

Extensor carpi ulnaris m.

C.
Incision

Capsule exposed

D.
Exposed fracture site

Open Reduction and Internal Fixation of Fracture of Lateral Condyle of Humerus (Continued)

E. Holding the lateral condyle fracture fragment with a bone tenaculum or a towel clip, the surgeon reduces the fracture. It is not necessary to detach the soft tissues from the lateral epicondyle. Two smooth Kirschner wires are drilled across the fracture site, through stab wounds separate from the skin incision. The wires should engage the medial cortex of the humerus. The reduction and position of the wires are checked by roentgenograms. The distal ends of the wires are cut off, but left protruding slightly from the skin, and their ends are bent to prevent migration.

F and **G.** The periosteum and the capsule of the joint are closed by interrupted sutures. The wound is closed and the upper extremity is immobilized in a long arm cast, with the elbow in 90 degrees of flexion and the forearm in neutral position.

POSTOPERATIVE CARE

In about four to six weeks, the wires are removed and immobilization is discontinued. Gentle active exercises are performed to restore range of motion of the elbow joint. It is imperative to follow the patient for possible premature closure of the lateral portion of the distal humeral physis, cubitus valgus, and tardy ulnar nerve palsy.

Plate 65. Open Reduction and Internal Fixation of Fracture of Lateral Condyle of Humerus

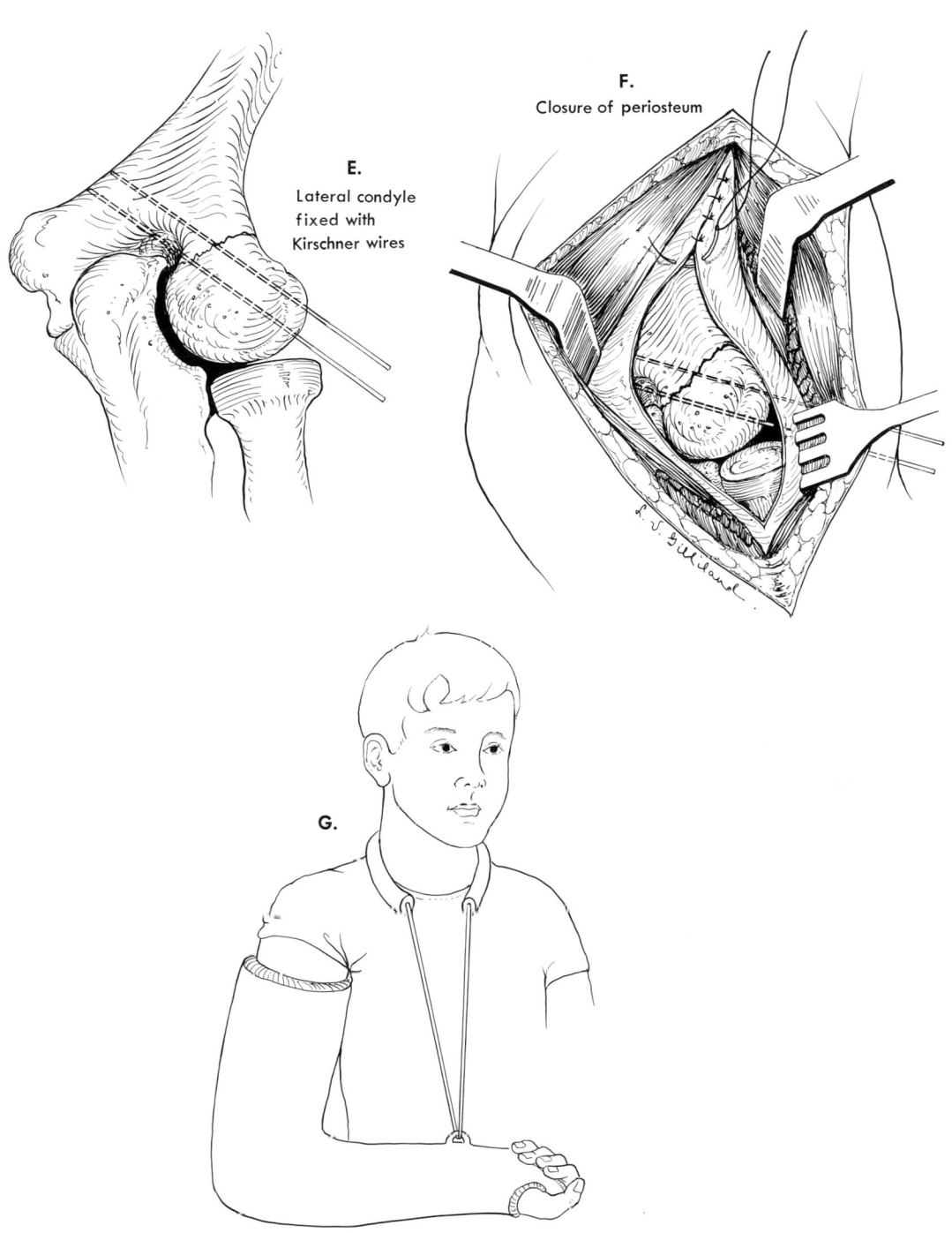

E.
Lateral condyle
fixed with
Kirschner wires

F.
Closure of periosteum

G.

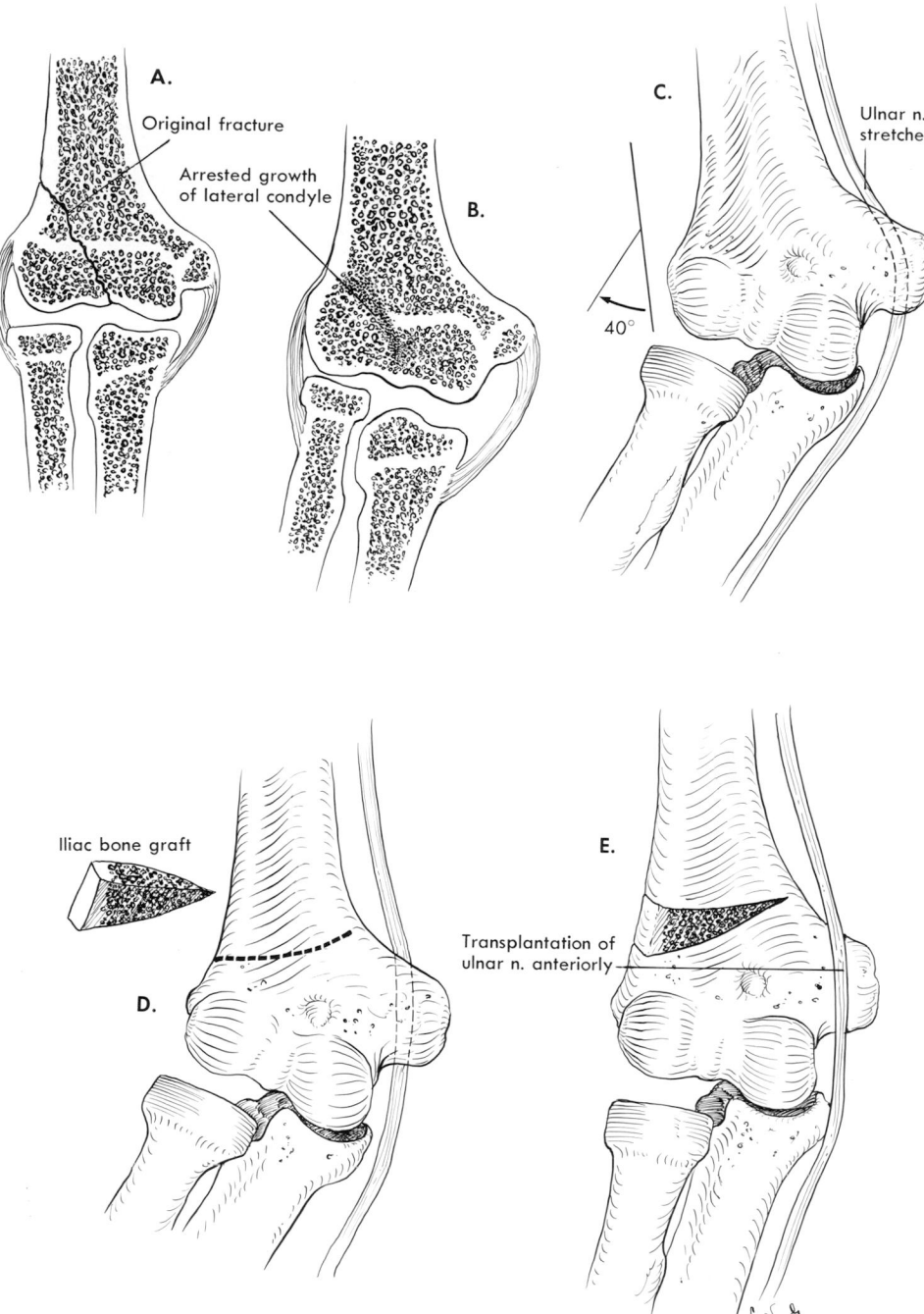

FIGURE 8–36. *Cubitus valgus and tardy ulnar nerve palsy caused by fracture of lateral condyle of the humerus.*

A. Original fracture is Type IV epiphyseal plate injury. **B.** Premature closure of the physis of distal humerus on the lateral side. **C.** Progressive increasing cubitus valgus deformity will stretch the ulnar nerve and cause paresis. **D** and **E.** Correction of cubitus varus deformity by open-up osteotomy with bone graft wedge. The ulnar nerve is transposed anteriorly.

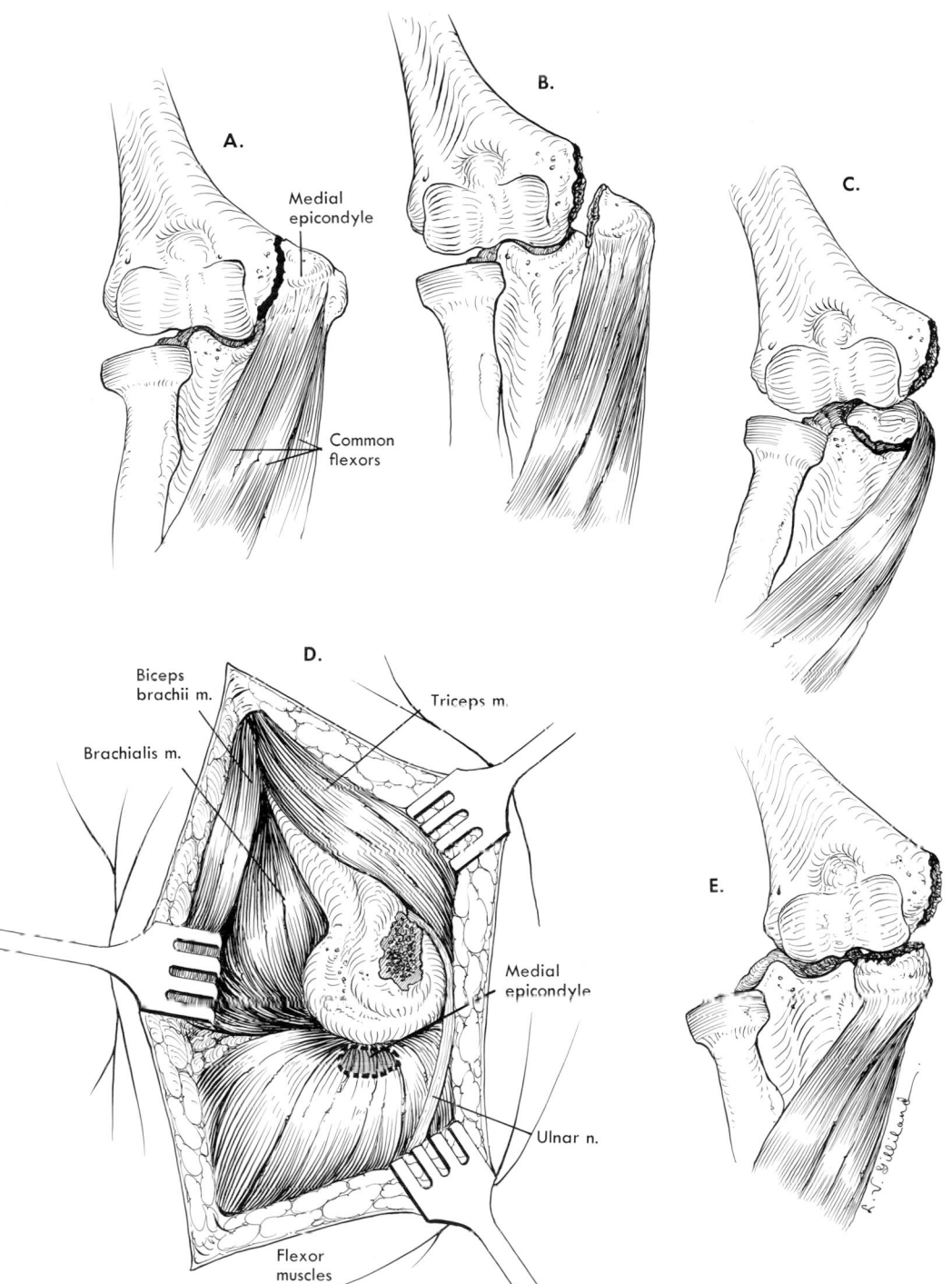

FIGURE 8–37. *Fracture and displacement of medial epicondyle of the humerus.*

A. Minimal displacement. **B.** Moderate displacement. **C** and **D.** Marked displacement and incarceration into the elbow joint. **E.** Fracture and displacement associated with posterolateral dislocation of the elbow joint.

dissected free, and retracted posteriorly with a moist hernia tape. The fractured medial epicondyle is identified, and with a sharp towel clip on the common tendon of the flexor muscles, it is anatomically repositioned. Next, through two small stab wounds in the skin, separate from the incision, two smooth medium sized Kirschner wires are drilled across the fracture site in a proximal and lateral direction. The pins should engage the lateral cortex. The position of the wires and the accuracy of reduction are verified by making roentgenograms of the elbow in the anteroposterior and lateral projections. The distal parts of the wire are bent to prevent migration and then are cut off with a wire cutter, leaving the ends protruding slightly through the skin. The periosteum and capsule are repaired with interrupted sutures, giving further stability to the reduction of the fracture fragments. After closure of the wound, a long arm cast is applied, immobilizing the elbow in 90 degrees of flexion and the forearm in full pronation.

In about four weeks, the cast and pins are removed and active exercises are instituted to restore range of motion of the elbow.

The author does not recommend closed reduction of markedly displaced medial epicondyle fractures. Immobilization in a long arm cast with the elbow in acute flexion and the forearm in full pronation for six weeks (in order to maintain reduction by relieving the pull of the flexor muscle) will result in fixed flexion deformity of the elbow.

When the epicondyle is incarcerated in the joint, manipulation to dislodge the fragment should not be performed, because frequently this method is unsuccessful, and there is a definite danger of injury to the ulnar nerve, which is often incarcerated with the fragment. It is best to dislodge the trapped epicondyle by open surgery. Whether the epicondyle should be reattached or not depends upon the age of the patient and the extent of damage to the epicondyle. In children under ten years of age, the epicondyle, if normal and not crushed, is reattached to its bed of origin to avoid any underdevelopment of the medial aspect of the elbow. In the older child or in a case in which the bone fragment is damaged, it is excised. Ordinarily if the fracture is associated with dislocation, rehabilitation is prolonged, and often some fixed flexion deformity remains.

DISLOCATION OF THE ELBOW

Dislocation of the elbow is a common injury in children, usually occurring between 11 and 15 years of age. It is more frequently encountered in boys, with the left elbow being more often affected than the right.

The direction of displacement varies according to the direction of the force. The most common type of dislocation is, by far, posterior, usually accompanied by some lateral displacement. Rotatory luxation with total displacement of one bone and part of the other bone may occur in the posterior type when only one collateral ligament is torn. Other rare forms are anterior, lateral, and medial dislocations. Divergent dislocation of the radius and ulna is extremely rare.

Mechanism of Injury and Pathologic Anatomy

Posterior dislocation usually results from a fall on the outstretched hand with the forearm supinated and the elbow extended or partially flexed (Fig. 8–38 A). The coronoid process, which normally resists posterior displacement of the ulna, is relatively small in children. The anterior capsule of the elbow joint is torn by the force of the impact transmitted upward through the ulna and radius; and the momentum of the body applied to the lower end of the humerus tears the joint capsule anteriorly. The collateral ligaments are stretched or ruptured. The radius and ulna, being firmly bound by the annular ligament and the interosseous membrane, are displaced upward and posteriorly together; the coronoid process of the ulna becomes locked in the olecranon fossa of the humerus. The periosteum is stripped from the posterior surface of the humerus and the brachialis muscle becomes stretched.

As already stated, with posterior luxations, there is often a varying degree of lateral displacement of the forearm bones (Fig. 8–39). With the ulnar collateral ligament, a portion of the medial epicondyle may be avulsed and displaced posteriorly (Fig. 8–40). On reduction, the medial epicondyle may be incarcerated in the joint. With posteromedial dislocation, fracture of the lateral condyle of the humerus may occur (Fig. 8–41). Fracture-separation of the upper epiphysis of the radius is another complication. Injury to brachial vessels or ulnar and median nerves may occur.

Anterior dislocation is a rare injury caused by a direct blow or fall on the olecranon process; the latter, with the proximal end of the radius, is displaced anteriorly to the lower end of the humerus. Medial or lateral luxations usually result from direct trauma, violent twisting of the forearm, or falls upon the hand.

Diagnosis

Immediately following the injury, the patient presents with a painful and swollen elbow, which is held in partial flexion and supported at the forearm by the opposite hand. Any attempted motion of the elbow is very painful and restricted, with marked muscle spasm. When a normal elbow is extended, the olecranon process and the medial and lateral epicondyles form three points on a straight line; and when the normal elbow is flexed to 90 degrees in the lateral view, the olecranon is aligned vertically with the epicondyles; the tip of the olecranon is, however, definitely posterior to the plane of the epicondyles (Fig. 8–38 B). In posterior dislocation, the olecranon process is displaced backward from its normal position in relation to the humerus, and one can palpate the concavity of the semilunar notch (Fig. 8–38 C and D) increasing the degree of elbow flexion exaggerates the prominence of the olecranon process. The radial head can be usually palpated behind the lateral condyle of the humerus and lateral to the olecranon. In the antecubital fossa, there is definite fullness due to prominence of the humerus. From the anterior view, the forearm appears to be shortened, whereas from the posterior view, the upper arm appears to be decreased in length. The foregoing physical findings, however, are soon obscured by the development of marked soft-tissue swelling in the region of the elbow.

It is imperative to assess and record neuromuscular function in the upper limb, particularly of the ulnar and median nerves.[293] The brachial artery may be torn.

Roentgenograms should always be made prior to treatment; they should be meticulously scrutinized to rule out the presence of associated fractures of the medial epicondyle, coronoid process, proximal radius, or lateral condyle.

Treatment

Reduction of recent *posterior dislocation* is easily accomplished. General anesthesia is usually not necessary. There are several methods available.[268]

In children, a gentle and effective method is as follows: Place the patient in prone position with the injured limb hanging over the edge of the table. The weight of the arm provides distal traction. The surgeon encircles the patient's arm with his fingers (to give countertraction), and, with his thumbs, pushes the olecranon downward and forward (Fig. 8–38 F). Following reduction, the elbow is acutely flexed as much as swelling will permit and without causing circulatory embarrassment.

An alternate method of reduction is by hyperextension, downward traction, and flexion: (1) Hold the upper arm with one hand to apply steady countertraction (an assistant, if available, can do it). With the other hand, grasp the forearm and, with the elbow in some hyperextension, exert moderate traction to disengage the tip of the coronoid process from the olecranon fossa (Fig. 8–38 G). Marked hyperextension of the elbow should be avoided in order to avoid unnecessary strain on the already torn capsule and other soft tissues on the anterior aspect of the joint. (2) Then apply downward traction with the elbow in neutral extension to restore length. While traction is maintained, any lateral displacement and increase in the carrying angle is corrected. (3) Next, the elbow is gently flexed. Often, as the olecranon engages the articular surface of the humerus, a "click" can be palpated and heard. Postreduction roentgeno-

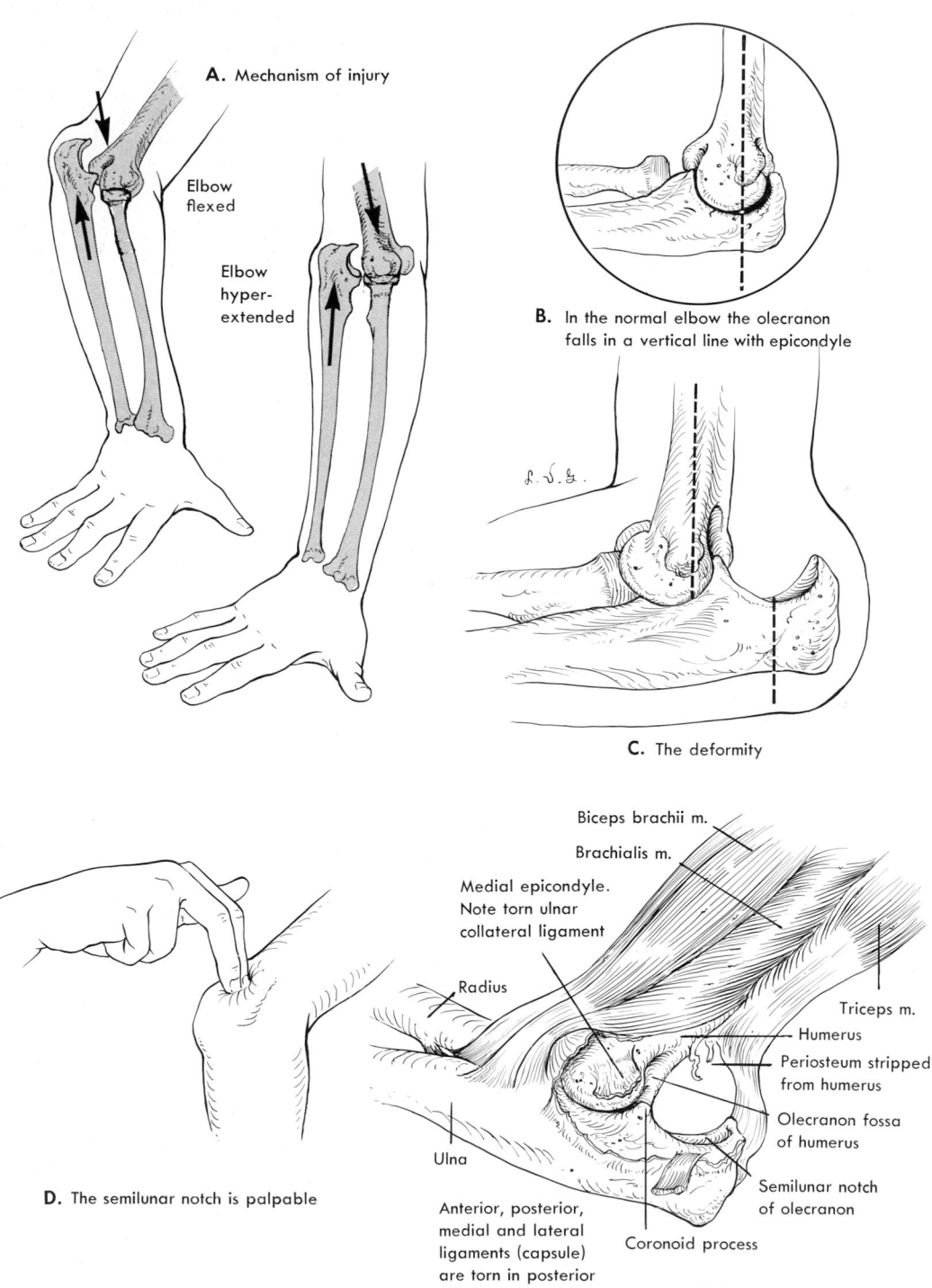

A. Mechanism of injury

Elbow flexed

Elbow hyper-extended

B. In the normal elbow the olecranon falls in a vertical line with epicondyle

C. The deformity

D. The semilunar notch is palpable

Biceps brachii m.

Brachialis m.

Medial epicondyle. Note torn ulnar collateral ligament

Radius

Triceps m.

Humerus

Periosteum stripped from humerus

Olecranon fossa of humerus

Semilunar notch of olecranon

Ulna

Coronoid process

Anterior, posterior, medial and lateral ligaments (capsule) are torn in posterior displacement of ulna

E. Pathology

FIGURE 8–38. Posterior dislocation of the elbow (see text for explanation).

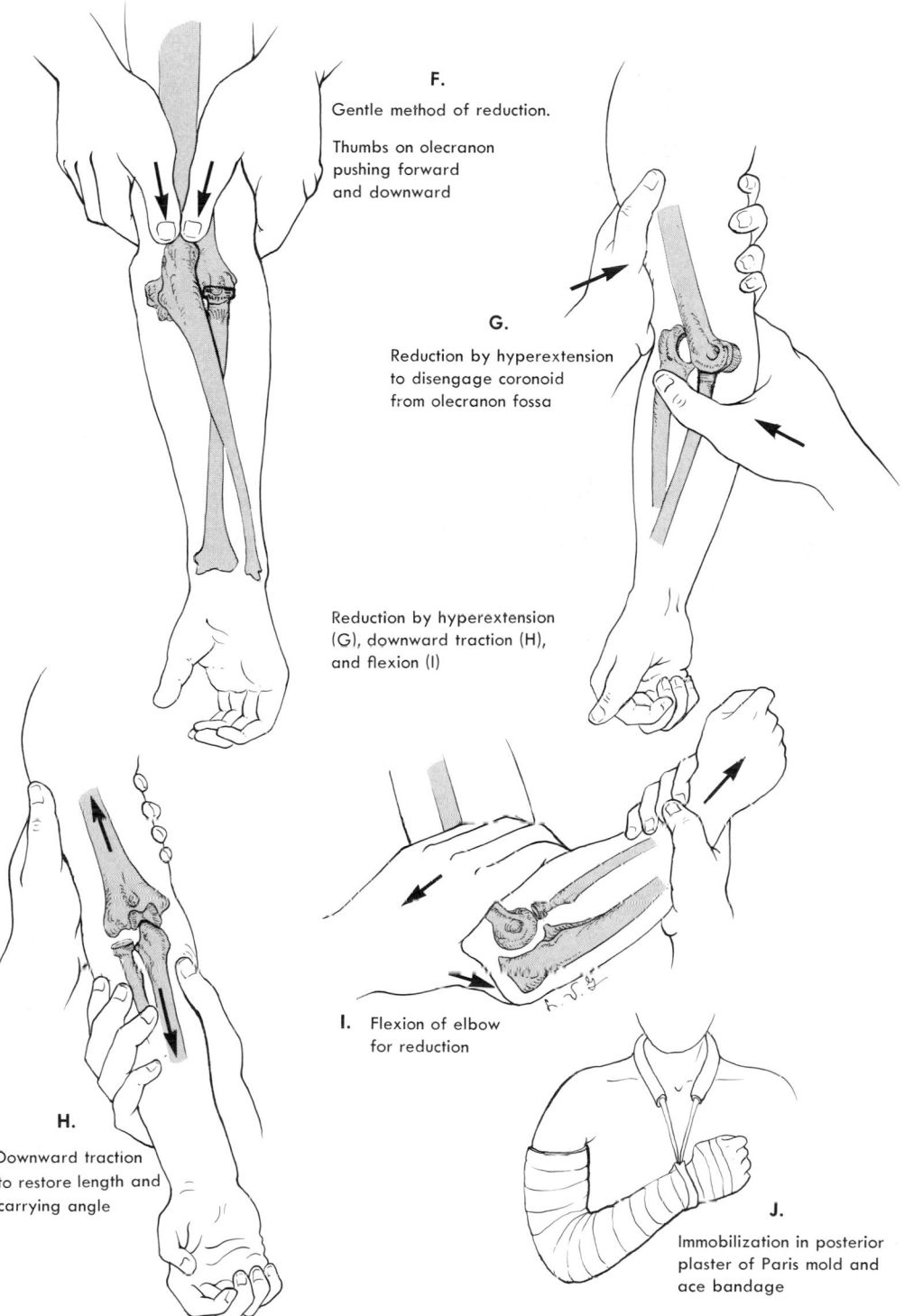

F.

Gentle method of reduction.

Thumbs on olecranon
pushing forward
and downward

G.

Reduction by hyperextension
to disengage coronoid
from olecranon fossa

Reduction by hyperextension
(G), downward traction (H),
and flexion (I)

I. Flexion of elbow
for reduction

H.

Downward traction
to restore length and
carrying angle

J.

Immobilization in posterior
plaster of Paris mold and
ace bandage

FIGURE 8–38 Continued.   Posterior dislocation of the elbow (see text for explanation).

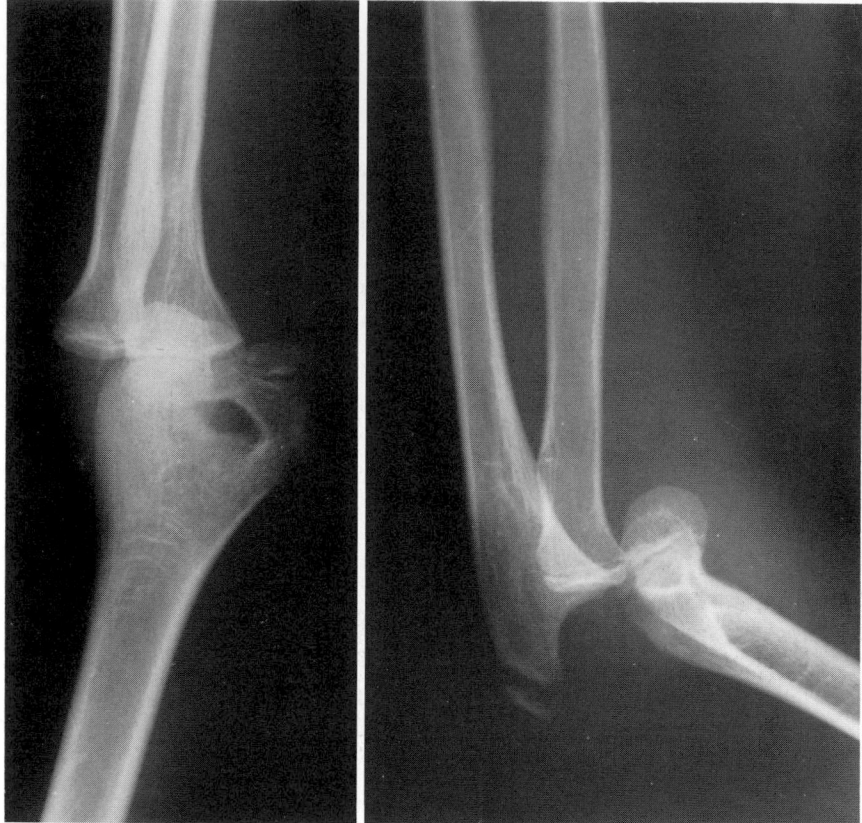

FIGURE 8–39. Roentgenograms of posterolateral dislocation of elbow.

grams are obtained to check the accuracy of reduction and, most important, to rule out the presence of associated fractures. The elbow is flexed to the degree that swelling will permit without interfering with circulation and immobilized in a posterior plaster of Paris splint and ace bandage.

Three weeks after closed reduction, the plaster splint is removed and active exercises are instituted to restore normal range of motion of the elbow. A triangular sling may be worn for seven days for comfort. Passive exercises should *not* be performed, as they promote the development of myositis ossificans. Any lifting strain or forced hyperextension should be avoided for two months following the injury.

Anterior dislocation is a very rare injury. Cohn, in a review of the early literature, found only 23 cases.[267] Linscheid and Wheeler reported two cases of anterior dislocation out of 110 elbow dislocations and stated that there are less than 50 reported cases in the literature.[278] In anterior disloca-

tion of the elbow, there is extensive soft-tissue damage, and often associated fractures of the olecranon or of the proximal shaft of the ulna. Reduction is accomplished as follows: (1) Apply longitudinal traction with the elbow in flexion to distract the articular surfaces; (2) then, while maintaining traction, exert firm steady pressure distally and posteriorly on the upper part of the forearm as the elbow is gradually extended. A click will indicate the achievement of reduction.

Reduction of the extremely rare medial, lateral, or divergent dislocations of the elbow follows the principles outlined for treatment of posterior dislocation, i.e., first, traction in the line of deformity to disengage the articular ends of both bones of the forearm; then, while traction is maintained, correction of any lateral or medial displacement; next, as reduction is achieved, flexion of the elbow.

When a dislocated elbow is associated with fracture, first reduce the dislocation. In the

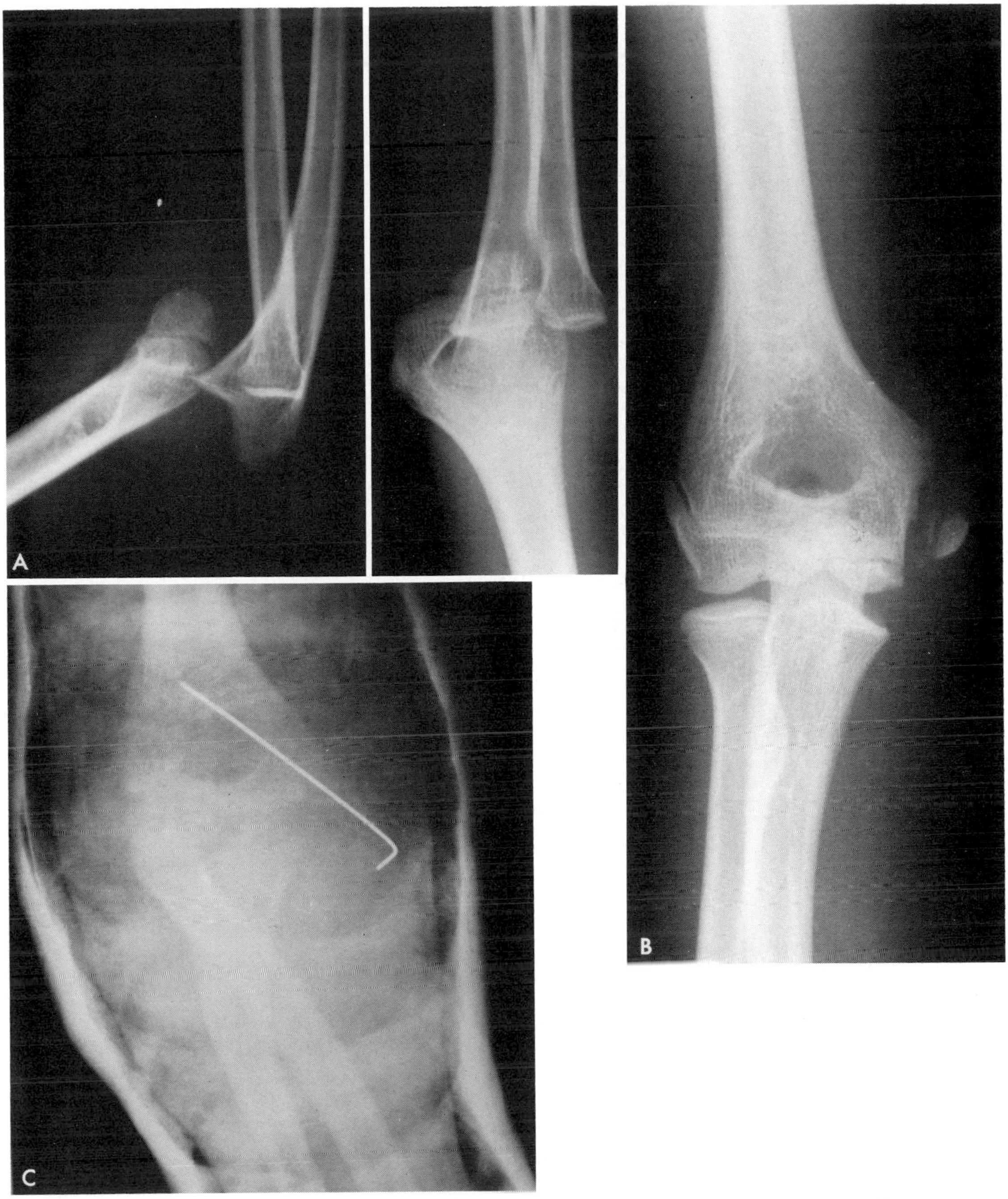

FIGURE 8-40.   *Posterolateral dislocation of the elbow with fracture of the medial epicondyle.*

A. Initial roentgenograms. **B.** Immediate postreduction roentgenogram showing the displaced fracture of the medial epicondyle. This patient had persistent ulnar nerve paralysis. The bony fragment was excised and the ulnar nerve transposed anteriorly. **C.** An alternate method is pinning of the medial epicondyle with a Kirschner wire, as shown in this roentgenogram of another patient.

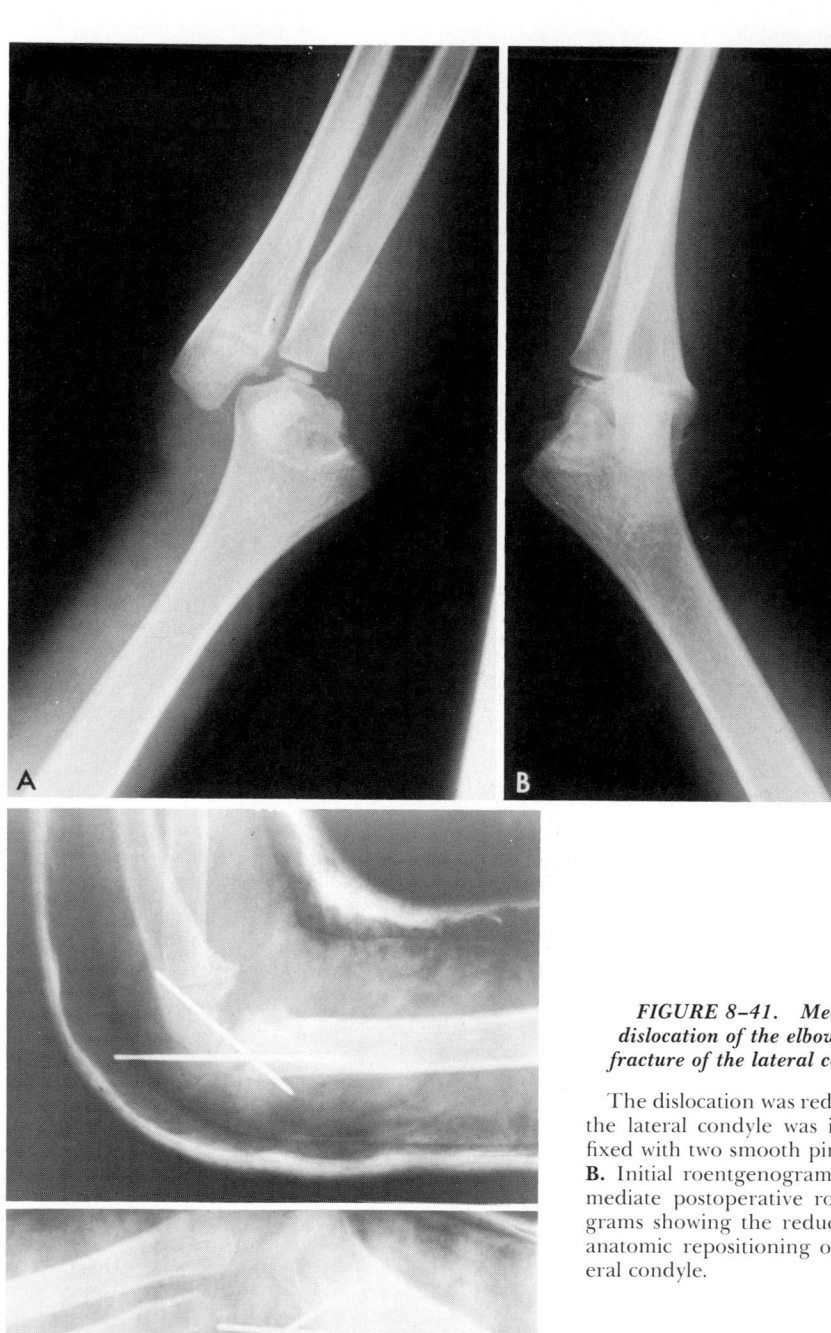

FIGURE 8–41. *Medial dislocation of the elbow with fracture of the lateral condyle.*

The dislocation was reduced and the lateral condyle was internally fixed with two smooth pins. **A** and **B.** Initial roentgenograms. **C.** Immediate postoperative roentgenograms showing the reduction and anatomic repositioning of the lateral condyle.

immediate postreduction roentgenograms, assess the fracture and treat it as if the dislocation had not occurred.

Old dislocations of the elbow usually require open reduction.

Complications

VASCULAR INJURIES

These are associated with more violent injuries, and in general, are more common in cases of open dislocation than in closed dislocations. The severity of trauma to the brachial artery varies from simple contusion to laceration or rupture.

Linscheid and Wheeler reported vascular complications in 8 of the 110 elbow dislocations seen during a 15-year period at the Mayo Clinic. In two of these patients, circulatory embarrassment consisted of loss of radial pulse until reduction was accomplished. In the remaining six patients, injury to the brachial artery was more serious. Three patients sustained lacerations of the brachial artery; ligations were performed in two, and arterial repair was attempted in one. The latter patient developed a hematoma during anticoagulant therapy, and redislocation occurred with failure of the anastomosis. Three of the six patients sustained stretching injuries of the brachial artery. In one patient this was associated with severe skin abrasions and contusions; the second patient, despite rather prompt reduction, had thrombosis of the radial artery; the third had sensory loss, and the radial pulse was absent when the cast was removed after five weeks.[278]

The author has encountered two children with Volkmann's ischemic contracture of the forearm following posterior dislocation of the elbow. Both were treated by reduction in the emergency room and were sent home after application of a solid cast. One cannot overemphasize the importance of assessing the status of circulation in the limb prior to reduction of dislocation. Following reduction, adequacy of circulation is again determined. *It is best to admit these children to the hospital for close supervision of circulation,* particularly if there is marked swelling of the elbow. If the child is sent home from the emergency room, the parents should be instructed how to check the circulation in the hand, and the physician himself should examine the child at close intervals. One should realize that Volkmann's ischemic contracture occurs as frequently with elbow dislocations as with supracondylar fractures of the humerus. In cases with laceration of the brachial artery, immediate exploration of the antecubital area is indicated for ligation of the artery or anastomosis. In stretching vascular injuries, the stretching force should be relieved.

NEURAL INJURIES

Injury to the nerves occurs more frequently than injury to the vessels. The ulnar nerve is rather firmly anchored down in the groove behind the medial epicondyle, and may be easily damaged in dislocations, particularly if there is an associated avulsion of the medial epicondyle, which, when trapped in the joint, compresses the ulnar nerve by holding taut the band of fibrous tissue that crosses the nerve.

Linscheid and Wheeler reported neural complications in 24 of 110 elbow dislocations. The ulnar nerve only was involved in 16 patients; the involvement consisted of transient paresthesia and anesthesia in 11 of these patients (in 7, it disappeared in less than one day, and the others had full return of ulnar sensation within two months of reduction). Of the remaining five patients, one had a persistent ulnar nerve palsy but received no further treatment. The other four patients had anterior translocation of the ulnar nerve from three weeks to two years after dislocation, with fair to good return of function in all. The dislocation was associated with avulsion of the medial epicondyle in three patients. Three patients had median nerve hypesthesia only, and four patients had both ulnar and median nerve involvement. The remaining patient with neural damage sustained a brachial plexus stretch injury.[278]

Treatment of neural complications should be conservative in the beginning, as most cases will recover spontaneously. If ulnar nerve paralysis persists, the nerve probably is entangled in dense scar tissue in the region of the medial epicondyle. Two months after reduction of the joint, it is advisable to free the nerve and transpose it anteriorly into a normal tissue bed free of scar. If ulnar nerve palsy is associated with displaced fracture of the medial epicondyle, it is best to translocate the nerve anteriorly when excising the detached medial epicondyle. When confronted with persistent median nerve palsy, one should rule out the possible presence of Volkmann's ischemic contracture.

HETEROTOPIC BONE FORMATION

This disabling complication may restrict elbow motion permanently. Linscheid and Wheeler reported heterotopic bone formation in 32 of 110 elbow dislocations. The heterotopic bone is most commonly located below the medial or lateral epicondyle along the course of the collateral ligaments. In these areas, it is usually of small size, extending only a short distance. In five of their patients, the heterotopic bone developed in the region of the anterior capsule; in four of these patients, the large deposits of heterotopic bone interfered significantly with the degree of functional return. In two cases, they believed the heterotopic bone was partially caused by excessive passive manipulation and the use of heavy weights in an attempt to straighten the elbow. One patient was treated with capsulotomy and partial excision of the heterotopic mass seven months after dislocation, with improvement in extension amounting to 40 degrees.[278]

The possible complication of heterotopic new bone formation should be suspected if, following removal of the cast, the elbow joint is unusually tender and remains so for a long time, and if the elbow joint is stiff with very slow restoration of motion. The diagnostic features and treatment of heterotopic new bone formation (myositis ossificans conscripta) are described on pages 1102 to 1103.

RECURRENT DISLOCATION OF THE ELBOW

This is a rare but disabling complication. The first case was reported by Albert in 1881.[266] It usually occurs in boys who first sustained dislocation when younger than 15 years of age (about 80 per cent of cases). Osborne and Cotterill discovered 18 cases in a three-year period and found reports of 30 other cases.[281] Except for two patients, all re-

current dislocations have been posterior or posterolateral. Three cases of recurrent bilateral dislocation of the elbow have been described in the literature.[273, 280, 283]

Osborne and Cotterill proposed that the basic pathologic defect causing recurrent dislocation of the elbow is laxity of the posterolateral ligamentous and capsular structures due to failure of reattachment following a tear at the time of simple traumatic dislocation. A pocket of capsule is formed into which the radial head becomes displaced as it slides off its articulation with the capitellum.[281] An osteochondral fracture may take place with the detached bone fragment lying in the posterolateral capsule. A permanent defect or crater develops in the posterolateral margin of the capitellum, and the radial head also becomes damaged, sometimes with a crater or a "shovel-like" defect. Roentgenograms will often demonstrate the abnormal shape of the capitellum and of the radial head, but the roentgenographic changes will not be detected unless the lesions are confined to the cartilaginous surfaces.

A defect in the trochlea, possibly due to osteochondritis dissecans, has been described by Reichenheim and by King.[274, 283] Spring has reported loose bodies in the joint.[291]

Treatment. In childhood, if recurrence of dislocation is infrequent, one should refrain from operative treatment, since the normal process of growth may cause tightening of the capsule and ligaments with consequent decrease of frequency and eventual cessation of dislocations. Also, occasional dislocations at intervals of once a year or so are not an indication for surgery.

Operative treatment is indicated if dislocations occur following minimal injury in the older adolescent. Several methods of surgical correction have been described in the literature, namely:

1. Transfer of the biceps tendon to the coronoid process of the ulna, reinforcing the joint anteriorly by an active tenodesis.[274, 283]

2. Increase in the depth of the coronoid process by an intra-articular bone graft.[280, 294]

3. Repair or reinforcement of soft tissues about the elbow joint, using either fascial strips or tendinous straps to reinforce the collateral ligaments.[276, 291] Kapel constructed an intra-articular ligament by using

portions of the biceps and triceps tendons passed through a hole in the distal humerus between the olecranon and coronoid fossa.[273] Osborne and Cotterill repaired the capsular and ligamentous laxity.[281]

The soft-tissue repair described by Osborne and Cotterill is recommended by the author, as it is simple and effective. They reported successful results with no recurrence in eight patients. The author's experience is limited to only two cases, in both of which there was no recurrence and the range of motion was normal.

The operative technique of Osborne and Cotterill is as follows (Figure 8-42):

Technique. An incision is made on the lateral side of the elbow from the lateral epicondylar ridge to the annular ligament. The elbow is opened behind the lateral ligament and any fragments of bone are removed from the postero-lateral part of the capsule. The bone of the lateral epicondyle and of the lateral side of the capitulum is cleared of soft tissue and scarified. . . . One or two transverse holes are drilled with an awl, and catgut is passed through the bone and through the postero-lateral capsule in order to tie the capsule down tightly so that it will adhere to the bone of the lower end of the humerus as close to the articular margin as possible. A similar repair of the medial ligament is done if it is necessary. A plaster cylinder is applied with the elbow at about 40 degrees for four weeks, after which the patient is allowed to recover movements gradually.*

---

*From Osborne, G., and Cotterill, P.: Recurrent dislocation of the elbow. J. Bone Joint Surg., 48-B:340, 1966.

FRACTURES INVOLVING THE PROXIMAL RADIAL PHYSIS AND RADIAL NECK

The disc-shaped head of the radius is of greater diameter than its neck. The shallow, cuplike, and slightly concave upper surface of the radial head that articulates with the capitellum of the humerus is covered by hyaline cartilage. The smooth radial head rotates within the annular ligament and articulates medially with the radial notch of the ulna. On the posterior aspect of the radial neck, there is a small ridge for insertion of a part of the upper fibers of the supinator muscle. The radial tuberosity for the insertion of the biceps brachii muscle is immediately distal to the neck.

The shape of the radial head in the child is identical to that in the adult, with the same eccentric concavity and sharp anterolateral rim; however, they differ in size and in the amount of cartilage. The ossification center of the upper epiphysis of the radius appears at the fifth year and fuses with the body between the ages of 16 and 18 years. In children, the proximal radial epiphysis is cartilaginous and resilient; thus, a fracture through the articular surface of the radial head is extremely rare. The site of fracture in childhood is either through the physis with a metaphyseal fragment (Type II physeal injury, according to the classification of Salter and Harris), or through the neck proper (3 to 4 mm. distal to the epiphyseal plate). In the report of 34 cases by Jones and

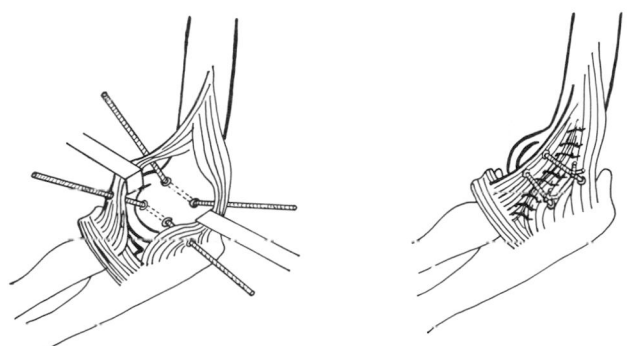

FIGURE 8–42. *Osborne and Cotterill operation for repair of the lateral capsular damage in recurrent dislocation of the elbow.*

(From Osborne, G., and Cotterill, P.: Recurrent dislocation of the elbow. J. Bone Joint Surg., *48–B*:344, 1966.)

Esah, 50 per cent were through the radial neck proper and 50 per cent were Type II fractures involving the proximal radial physis.[303]

It occurs on the average at the age of 10 years, with the upper age limit being 13 years and the lower, 5 years (i.e., after the appearance of the ossification center of the proximal radial epiphysis). Approximately three fourths of cases occur in children aged nine years or older. There is no sex predilection.[303]

Injuries involving the proximal radial epiphyseal plate constitute five per cent of all physeal injuries, and account for 4.5 to 10 per cent of fractures about the elbow in children under 16 years of age.

Mechanism of Injury

The fracture is caused by a fall on the outstretched hand with the elbow in extension and the forearm usually supinated. The force is transmitted through the shaft of the radius, and the momentum of the body drives the capitellum against the lateral half of the radial head, tilting and displacing it laterally (Fig. 8–43). At the moment of impact, there is a valgus strain on the medial aspect of the elbow; the distraction force may rupture the medial collateral ligament, avulse the medial epicondyle, or cause fracture of the olecranon or upper shaft of the ulna. The compression force may also fracture the lateral epicondyle or condyle of the humerus. The displacement of the fragments in those associated with fracture is usually minimal. In the series of 30 cases of Reidy and Van Gorder, there were 11 associated injuries in nine of the patients.[370]

The direction of tilting of the displaced head relative to the shaft of the radius depends upon the rotational attitude of the radius at the time of injury; if the forearm is fully supinated, the displacement is lateral; if the forearm is in neutral mid-position, it is posterior.[302]

Another mechanism of injury according to Jeffery is as follows: The patient first falls on the hand and sustains a temporary posterior dislocation or subluxation of the elbow joint. The resultant upward force on the flexed elbow displaces the radial head posteriorly almost 90 degrees by the impact

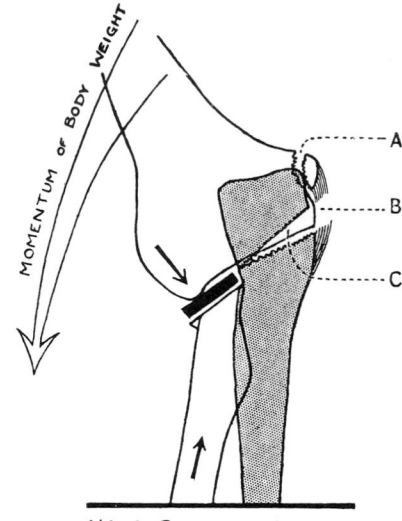

HAND FIXED TO GROUND

FIGURE 8–43. *Diagram to illustrate the mechanism of fractures involving the proximal radial physis.*

The compression force on the radial side as the capitellum of the humerus is driven against the outer side of the radial head as indicated. The distraction force in the ulnar side of the joint may produce the following lesions. A, Avulsion of the medial epicondylar apophysis; B, rupture of the medial collateral ligament; C, fracture of the olecranon or upper ulna of abduction type. (From Jeffery, C. C.: Fractures of the head of the radius in children. J. Bone Joint Surg., 32–B:314, 1950.)

against the inferior aspect of the capitellum. Spontaneous reduction of elbow dislocation leaves the separated radial head beneath the capitellum (Fig. 8–44). This second form of injury is rare. Jeffery reported 2 such cases in his series of 24; Reidy and Van Gorder, 1 of 30 cases; and Wood, 2 similar cases from the Royal Hospital for Sick Children, Glasgow, Scotland.[302, 310, 314]

O'Brien found two cases of posterior displacement of the proximal radial epiphysis (Fig. 8–45). He proposed a double mechanism of injury in its causation. First, a fall on the outstretched hand produces a posterior dislocation with displacement of the proximal end of the radius beneath the capitellum; second, a further blow on the forearm or the elbow spontaneously reduces the posterior dislocation, but displaces the radial epiphysis posteriorly.[308] Both mechanisms are likely to occur in different cases; i.e., the radial epiphysis may fracture and become displaced either at the

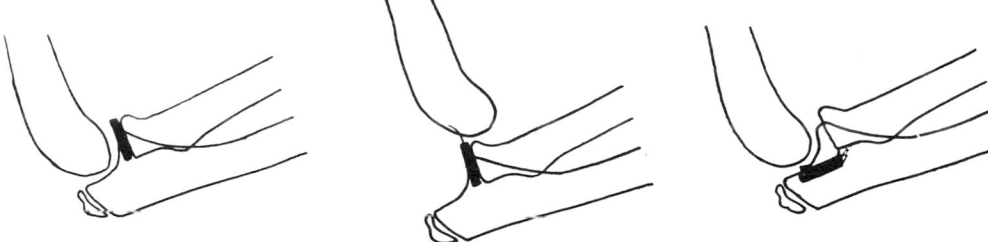

FIGURE 8–44. *Diagrams to show the mechanism of 90-degree posterior displacement of the radial head.*

(From Jeffery, C. C.: Injuries of the head of the radius in children. J. Bone Joint Surg., *32–B*:3, 1950.)

time of posterior dislocation or at the time of spontaneous reduction.

Direct crushing of the radial head by the convex lateral condyle of the humerus will cause an intra-articular fracture of the proximal radial epiphysis (Fig. 8–46).

Displacement of the radial head may be subdivided into the three categories shown in Figure 8–47: *Minimal* — when the degree of downward tilting of the superior surface of the head from the horizontal is from zero

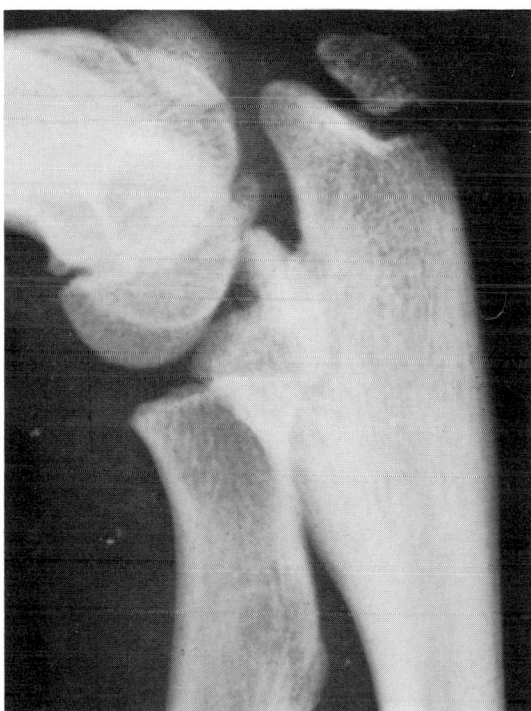

FIGURE 8–45. *Posterior displacement of proximal radial epiphysis in a 12-year-old girl.*

(From O'Brien, P. I.: Injuries involving the proximal radial epiphysis. Clin. Orthop., *41*:57, 1965.)

to 30 degrees; *moderate* — when it is from 31 to 60 degrees; *marked* — 61 to 90 degrees. This gradation serves as a guide in both treatment and prognosis.[308, 310]

Diagnosis

The affected elbow is held in moderate flexion, with the opposite hand supporting the forearm, which is held in neutral rotation. There will be local swelling and ecchymosis over the lateral aspect of the elbow. When pressure is applied with the tip of the index finger, the radial head and neck are exquisitely tender; the pain may be referred to the radial side of the wrist.[311]

Gentle passive flexion and extension of the elbow are restricted in range, but are relatively less painful than pronation and supination of the forearm, which are accompanied by severe pain. Radial deviation of the forearm at the elbow is also very painful. Ordinarily, crepitation is absent.

Roentgenograms should be made of the *proximal end of the radius* in the anteroposterior and lateromedial views. When the clinical findings are suggestive but the x-rays are inconclusive, it is best to make roentgenograms of the normal proximal forearm held in the same degree of flexion and supination as the affected side.

It is also advisable to take several views with the proximal radius in various degrees of rotation. The degree of the tilting of the radial head is measured in the films that most clearly depict the profile of the radius at the fracture site. The surgeon should always look for associated fractures, particularly of the medial epicondyle and olecranon or proximal ulna.

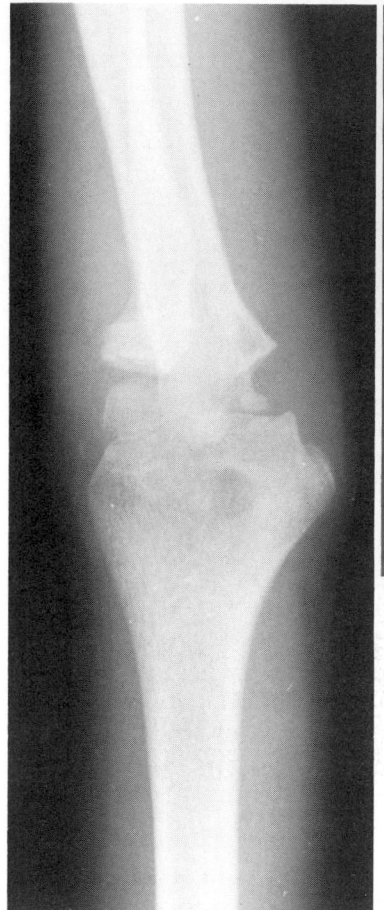
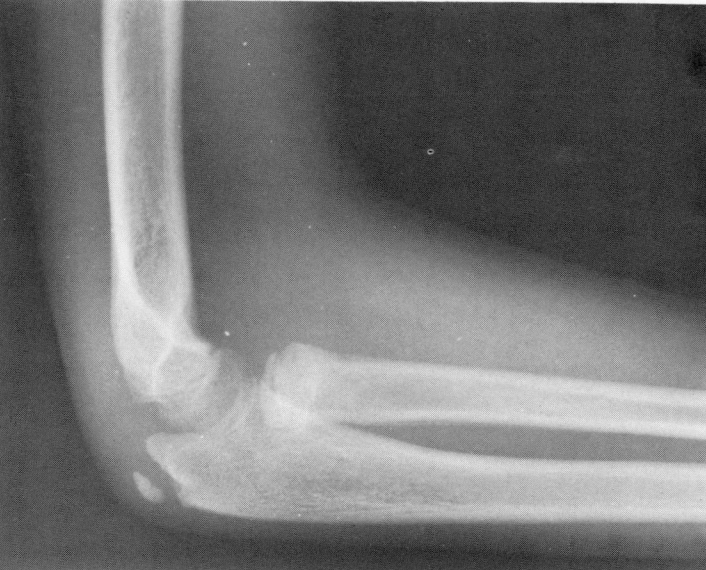

FIGURE 8–46. *Intra-articular fracture of the proximal radial eiphysis caused by a direct crushing injury by the lateral condyle of the humerus.*

Treatment

In *undisplaced or minimally displaced* fractures, treatment consists of simple immobilization of the elbow (in 90 degrees of flexion and neutral rotation of the forearm) in a posterior plaster splint for two weeks. Then the elbow and forearm are gradually mobilized and partially supported in a sling. With such early use of the limb, an excellent result can be obtained. When a child is over ten years of age, it is preferable to correct the tilting of the radial head to less than 15 degrees by closed reduction. When the child is younger than ten years of age, lateral tilting of up to 30 degrees can be accepted, as it

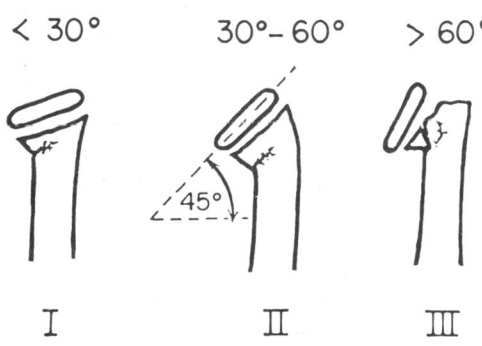

FIGURE 8–47. *Degrees of displacement of proximal radial epiphyses.*

I. Minimal displacement. II. Moderate displacement. III. Marked displacement. (From O'Brien, P. I.: Injuries involving the proximal radial epiphysis. Clin. Orthop., *41*:52, 1965.)

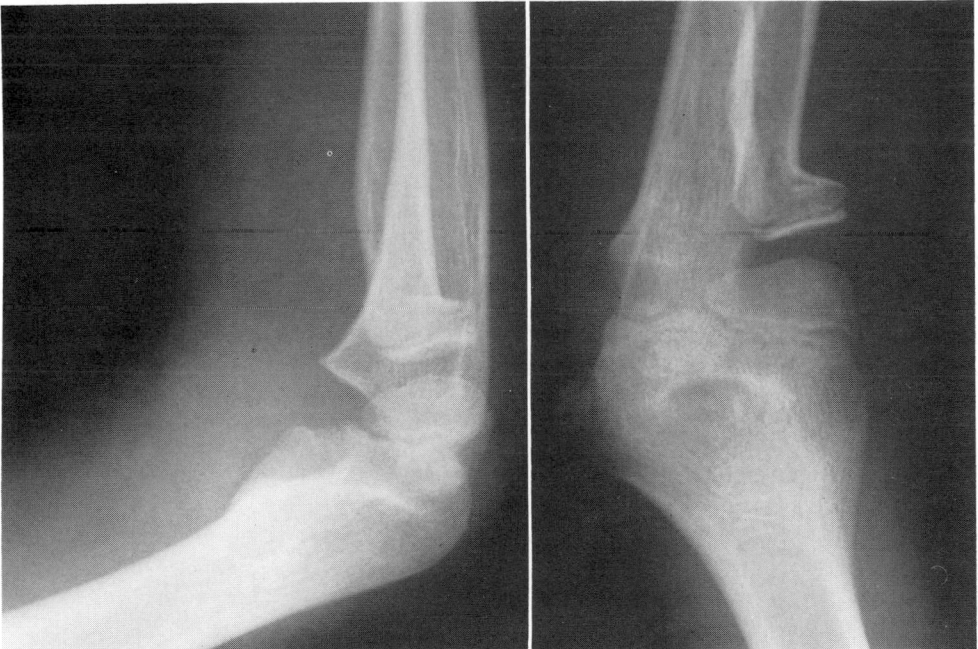

FIGURE 8-48. *Fracture involving the proximal radial physis — minimal displacement.*

will be spontaneously corrected with re-modeling.

In *moderately displaced* fractures (31 to 60 degrees of lateral tilting of the radial head), a closed reduction under general anesthesia should be attempted. The technique is as follows:

First, the elbow is completely extended to provide some fixation of the ulna in relation to the humerus. The forearm is then fully supinated to bring the most prominent part of the displaced radial head into a superficial location in the lateral aspect of the elbow between the common extensor muscle mass and the anconeus muscle. As emphasized by Jeffery, it is important to determine the direction of displacement of the radial head by studying anteroposterior roentgenograms centered upon the head of the radius and taken in various recorded positions of rotation.[302] The manipulative reduction is then carried out with the forearm in the degree of rotation that brings the most prominent part of the displaced head farthest laterally. The forearm is forcibly deviated ulnarward to widen the lateral aspect of the radiohumeral articulation; this maneuver provides space into which the tilted radial head can be moved. Firm digital pressure is applied in an upward and inward di-rection upon the displaced radial head to complete the reduction.

Roentgenograms are made to check restoration of normal anatomic relationship of the fracture fragments. If satisfactory reduction is achieved, i.e., the degree of tilting of the radial head is corrected to less than 30 degrees, a long arm cast is applied with the elbow joint held in right angle flexion and neutral mid-rotation. In three to four weeks, bony union is usually adequate for the cast to be removed and gradual active mobilization of the elbow begun. Repeated roentgenograms are taken to ensure maintenance of reduction. Certain of these fractures are unstable, and the initial satisfactory reduction may be lost while in the cast; this occurred in 2 of the 7 cases of Dougall and 3 of the 34 cases of Jones and Esah.[299, 303] If the position is lost while in the cast, closed reduction is repeated; often the second time, it can be maintained with a snug cast; however, if it is lost again, internal fixation with a Kirschner wire is required.

Markedly displaced fractures often require open reduction. A very gentle closed manipulative reduction is attempted under general anesthesia; if unsuccessful, open reduction is immediately performed. O'Brien warns that a closed manipulation of a head tilted more than 60 degrees can cause further damage to the cartilaginous epiphysis and he recommends early gentle open reduction, as it will minimize such damage and achieve stable repositioning of the radial head on the neck.[308]

A posterolateral approach is used for surgical exposure. The capsule is divided and the elbow joint is entered. Care is taken that the posterior interosseous nerve is not damaged. Jones and Esah recommend that the posterior interosseous nerve be exposed by separating the fibers of the supinator muscle with a blunt dissector; they also recommend retracting the soft tissues away from the nerve rather than pulling on both the tissues and the nerve. This wide exposure prevents neuropraxia of the posterior interosseous nerve and facilitates repositioning of the radial head on its neck.[303] Sectioning of the orbicularis ligament is not performed unless it is necessary to achieve reduction. The forearm is fully pronated and supinated to test the stability of reduction. The author recommends internal fixation with one smooth Kirschner wire (of adequate diameter), which is inserted through the capitellum of the humerus into the center of the radial head and along half the length of the radial shaft. As the wire traverses the radiohumeral joint, the elbow is flexed to 90 degrees and the forearm is placed in mid-rotation prior to transfixion of the joint. The proximal end of the wire is bent and cut but allowed to extend percutaneously in order to prevent migration and permit later removal. The orbicularis ligament is repaired, if it is simple to do so. The wound is closed and a long arm cast applied. Breakage of the wire across the joint is not a problem as long as the elbow is immobilized in the cast. The Kirschner wire is removed in three weeks and a new snug cast is applied for an additional one or two weeks.

There is variance of opinion in the literature concerning the necessity of internal fixation following open reduction. Key placed one or two sutures of fine catgut in the periosteum of the neck and then sutured the annular ligament about it. He suggested that the elbow and forearm be manipulated and placed in a position in which the head is fairly stable before any sutures are placed.[304] Reidy and Van Gorder do not use internal fixation except for an occasional suture.[310] O'Brien occasionally finds that he has to use a Kirschner wire to hold the head in place.[308] Jones and Esah recommend internal fixation, particularly if the radial head is found to be detached and unstable following reduction. They introduce two Kirschner wires behind and lateral to the lateral condyle of the humerus, crossing the radial head obliquely from the margin of its articular surface into the radial shaft. The wires are removed between three and eight weeks later. They used Kirschner wires in six elbows, with functional results rated good in four and satisfactory in two.[303]

In children, unlike adults, the radial head should not be excised because of consequent growth disturbance and deformity of the wrist and elbow. When the fracture is diagnosed late the deformity of radial head tilting can be corrected by open-up wedge osteotomy with a bone graft.

Complications

Malunion results from failure either to achieve adequate reduction or to maintain reduction.

Premature fusion of the upper radial epiphysis occurs quite often in moderately and markedly displaced fractures. This will cause shortening of the radius and increased cubitus valgus, depending upon the age of the child at the time of injury and the severity of the cartilaginous damage. This occurred in about one third of the cases of O'Brien, but in none was the cubitus valgus severe enough to require osteotomy.[308] Premature fusion occurred in 11 of 30 cases reported by Reidy and Van Gorder.[310]

Avascular necrosis of the radial head occurred in 10 per cent of the cases of Jones and Esah; they were unable to relate it to the degree of initial displacement or to the age at the time of injury. The results were poor in all three cases.[303]

New bone formation and deformity of the radial head with enlargement results in some cases, restricting elbow motion. A notch on the radial neck was found in 6 of 125 cases by O'Brien, who believed it to be caused by a taut scarred orbicular ligament.[308]

Synostosis between the proximal radius and ulna has been reported by Fielding, Dougall, and O'Brien.[299, 300, 308] Fibrous adhesions between the radius and ulna were noted in one case by Jones and Esah.[303] These will block rotation of the forearm.

Two factors seem to have a definite influence on the prognosis: the degree of displacement of the upper radial epiphysis (the more severe it is, the worse the prognosis), and the patient's age at the time of injury. After open operation, the children under ten years of age have a higher percentage of good and excellent results than those in the older age group. Reidy and Van Gorder correlated the results in the 24 patients with maximum displacement (60 degrees or more) with age and type of treatment. Twenty had open reductions; four, closed reduction. Of the 20 with open reduction, 8 were 6 to 9 years of age and 12 were 10 to 13 years old. Seven of the eight younger patients had good or excellent results; one, a poor result. Only 4 of the 12 older patients had excellent or good results, however, and eight, fair or poor.[310]

FRACTURES OF THE OLECRANON

These result either from direct violence (such as a fall on the point of the elbow) or from indirect violence (as when the elbow is suddenly flexed against the opposing triceps muscle). Fractures of the olecranon also occur in association with various injuries about the elbow produced by an abduction force—such as fractures of the capitellum, radial neck, or medial epicondyle. Secondary centers of ossification of the olecranon (bipartite olecranon or patella cubiti) should not be misdiagnosed as fractures.

If the fracture is undisplaced or minimally displaced, treatment consists of simple immobilization of the elbow in a long arm cast for three or four weeks (Figs. 8–49 and 8–50). Flexion of the elbow is rapidly restored in children following removal of the cast, and extension contracture is not a problem. Markedly displaced fractures require open reduction, soft-tissue repair, and internal fixation with a wire (Fig. 8–51).

PULLED ELBOW

The term *pulled elbow* is used to denote a clinical entity in young children in whom traumatic subluxation of the radial head is produced by sudden traction on the hand with the elbow extended and the forearm pronated. This common injury was known in historic times; Van Arsdale states that Hippocrates was the first to recognize the

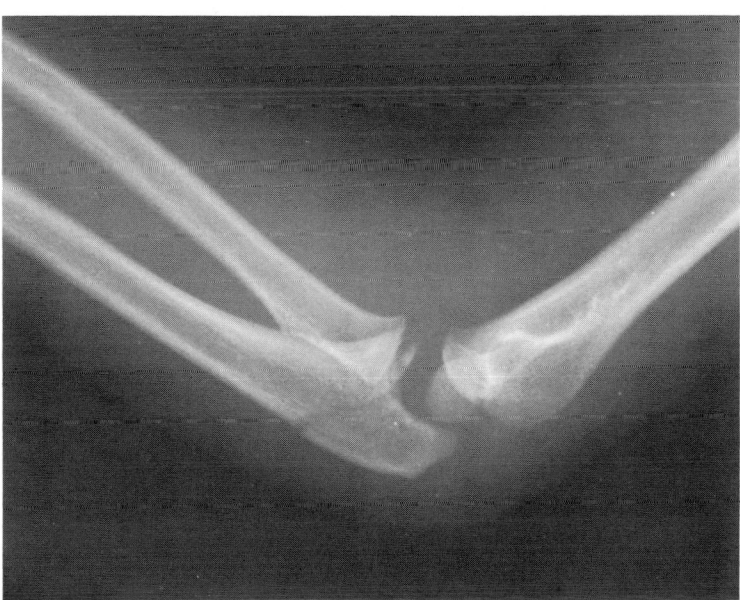

FIGURE 8–49. *Undisplaced fracture of olecranon.*

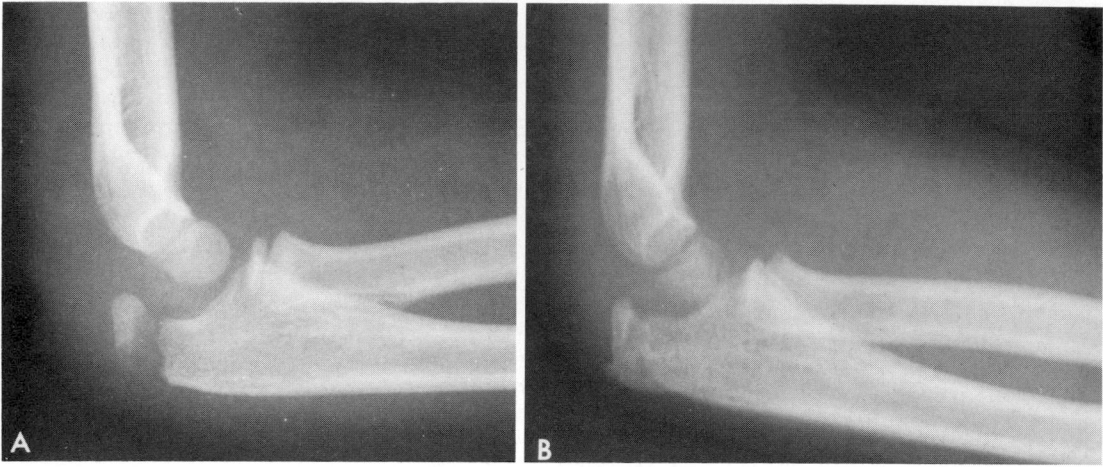

FIGURE 8-50.   *Moderately displaced fracture of olecranon treated by long arm cast with the elbow in extended position.*

A. Initial roentgenogram. **B.** Roentgenogram taken after five weeks, showing healing.

condition, though Fournier is usually given credit for first accurately describing the injury in 1671.[328, 350]

Various eponyms and synonyms have been used to denote this traumatic lesion, some of which are subluxation of the head of the radius, subluxation of the radius by elongation, subluxation of the annular ligament at the proximal radioulnar joint, "nursemaid's elbow," "temper tantrum elbow," and Malgaigne's injury or luxation.[315–351]

Pulled elbow is one of the most common musculoskeletal injuries in children under four years of age, and is rarely, if ever, found in children over five. The peak incidence is between the ages of one and three years. It is more frequent in boys than in girls, and the left side is more commonly subluxated than the right. In the emergency department of the Hospital for Sick Children, Toronto, 112 children with pulled elbow were seen in a period of one year, according to Salter and Zaltz.[343] This average incidence of two per week is also reported by Griffin and by Snellman.[331, 347]

Mechanism of Injury and Pathologic Anatomy

The lesion is caused by sudden longitudinal traction on the wrist of a young child whose elbow is extended and forearm is pronated. Common circumstances that precipitate this injury are pulling a child as he stumbles in an attempt to keep him from falling, lifting him by the hand up a curb, pulling the hand through the sleeve of a dress or sweater, swinging the child around while holding him by the hand, or forcefully pulling a child away from something by his hand. Occasionally, the injury may be sustained in a fall.

In the literature, there has been much speculation about the exact etiology. One of the theories offered has been that in young children the head of the radius is not fully developed and that the perimeter of the cartilaginous head is smaller than the neck; hence, it is not firmly held in place by the annular ligament.[338] This is an error probably based on a misinterpretation of a statement by Pierseol.[343]

Ryan examined the upper end of the radius in 15 fetal specimens and found that the radial head is definitely larger than the radial neck, and that the ratio of the two does not differ greatly from that of the adult, the average of the fetal radii being 1.53, and that of the adult radii, 1.50. The smallest ratio among the fetal radii was 1.10; the smallest ratio in the adult radii was 1.25. The largest ratio in fetal radii was 1.79; the largest in the adult, 1.80.[342] This investigation was supported by Salter and Zaltz, who

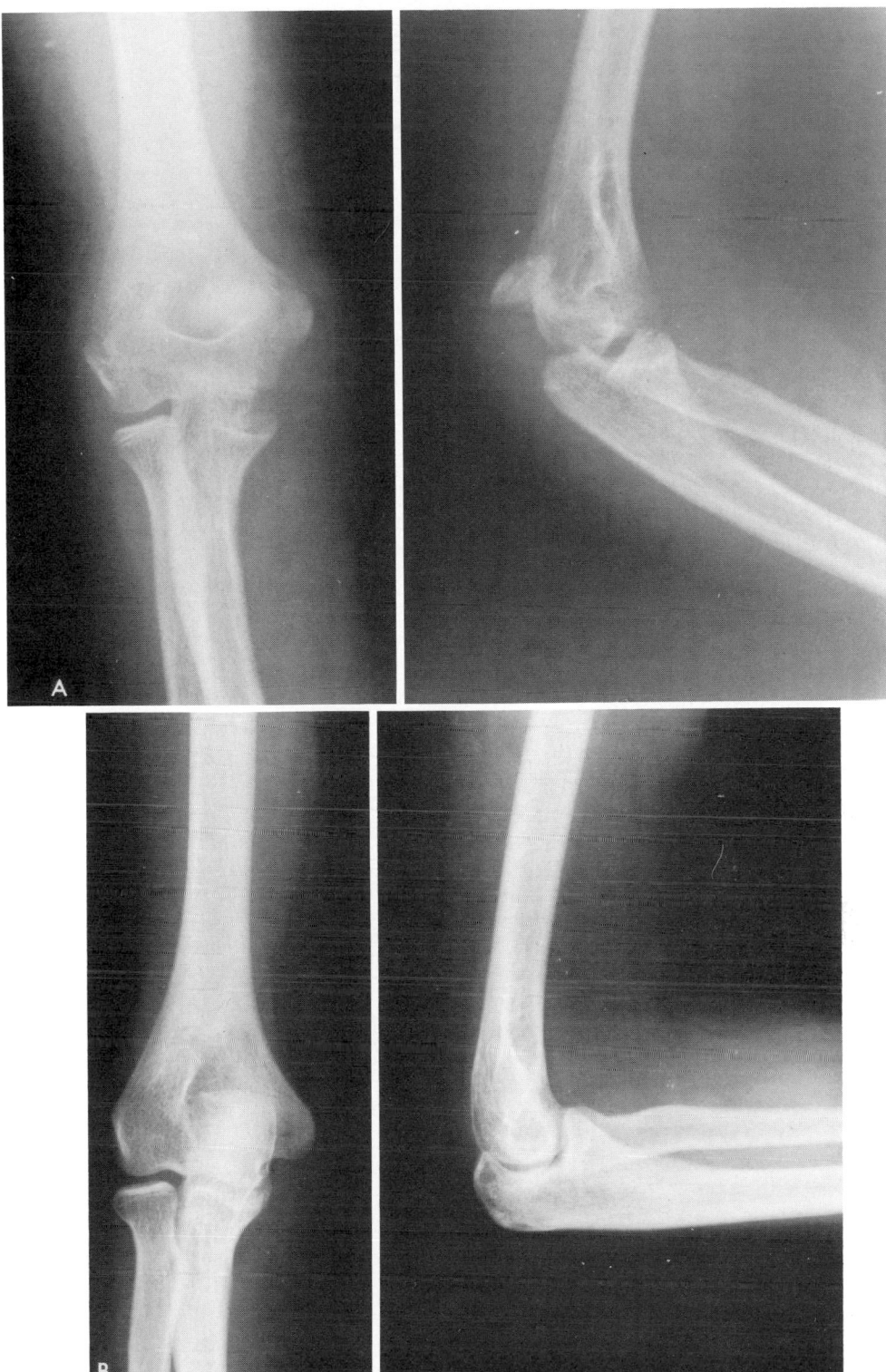

FIGURE 8–51. *Markedly displaced fracture of olecranon.*

Fracture was treated by open reduction, soft-tissue repair, and internal fixation with wire. **A.** Initial roentgenograms. **B.** Three years later, roentgenograms show healing and remodeling.

examined the proximal end of the radius in 12 child cadavers ranging in age from two days to nine years; in each and every specimen they found the diameter of the radial head to be larger than that of the neck by 30 to 60 per cent, the ratio varying from 1.3:1 to 1.6:1.[343] Thus, the former concept that the radial head is easily pulled through the annular ligament because it is smaller than the radial neck is erroneous and should be discarded.

Stone studied the mechanism of injury in 12 anatomic specimens, and was able to produce the lesion in six of the elbows, observing that the annular ligament slipped over the radial head only when the forearm was pronated. He also noted that the radial head is oval in outline rather than circular, and that when the forearm is supinated, the anterior aspect of the radial head is elevated sharply from the neck; when traction was applied with the forearm in supination, the annular ligament was pulled against this sharp bony elevation. Laterally and posteriorly, the radial head rises rather gradually, so that when traction is applied with the forearm in pronation, the annular ligament lies over this part and becomes stretched until it slips over the head.[348]

In their investigations of the elbows of 25 stillborn infants, McRae and Freeman concluded that pulled elbow is caused by the annular ligament slipping over the radial head.[336]

Salter and Zaltz also observed that the superior surface of the radial head (viewed axially from above) is slightly oval rather than circular, and that with the forearm supinated, the sagittal diameter of the radial head is consistently greater (less than 1 mm.) than the coronal diameter. These findings were similar to the measurements of Stone.[343, 348]

Salter and Zaltz studied the pathologic anatomy in the 12 aforementioned anatomic specimens. The proximal radiohumeral and radioulnar joints were exposed, leaving the joint capsule and annular ligament intact. Sudden firm and steady traction was exerted on the extended elbow by pulling on the hand, first with the forearm in supination, and then in pronation. They could not subluxate the radial head in any of the 12 specimens when traction was applied to the extended elbow with the forearm in *supination;* but in the child

cadavers under five years of age, when traction was applied on the extended elbow with the forearm in *pronation*, a transverse tear in the thin distal attachment of the annular ligament to the periosteum of the radial neck could be produced. When the forearm is pronated, the narrowest diameter of the radial head is in the anteroposterior plane. Once a transverse tear in the orbicularis ligament has occurred, the anterior portion of the radial head escapes from under the anterior part of the annular ligament, which, in turn, becomes interposed and is caught between the articular surfaces of the radial head and the capitellum when traction is discontinued (Fig. 8–52). When the interposed part of the annular ligament extended beyond the equator of the radial head, its reduction could not be achieved by passive supination of the forearm (Fig. 8–53 A); but when the proximal edge of the annular ligament did not extend beyond the

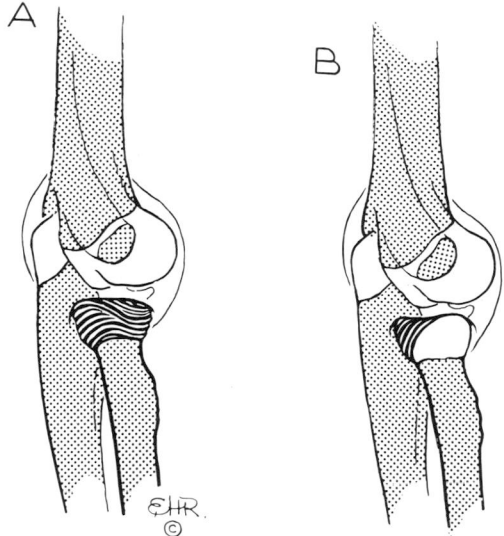

FIGURE 8–52. *Diagram illustrating pathologic anatomy of pulled elbow in a young child.*

A. Normal arrangement of the annular ligament, as seen from the lateral view. **B.** Lateral view of the pulled elbow. Note the tear in the distal attachment of the annular ligament through which the radial head has protruded slightly; the detached portion of the annular ligament has slipped into the radiohumeral joint where it has become trapped when traction was discontinued. (From Salter, R. B.: Disorders and Injuries of the Musculoskeletal System. Baltimore, Williams & Wilkins Co., 1970, p. 430.)

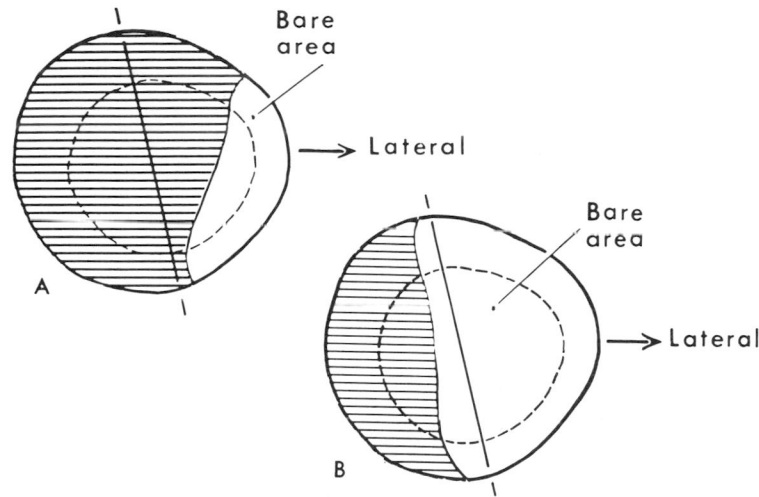

FIGURE 8-53. *Diagram showing pathologic anatomy of two degrees of pulled elbow (superior axial view of radial heads).*

A. The detached margin of the annular ligament has slid beyond the equator or widest part of the head. This severe degree results when the tear in the attachment of the annular ligament extends over more than half of its length. It occurs very rarely, and reduction cannot be achieved by closed manipulation. **B.** The detached margin of the annular ligament has not slid beyond the equator of the radial head. This is the common form of pulled elbow. The interposed annular ligament is readily freed from the radiohumeral joint by simply supinating the forearm with the elbow in slight flexion. (From Salter, R. B., and Zalta, C.: Anatomic investigations of the mechanism of injury and pathologic anatomy of "pulled elbow" in young children. Clin. Orthop., 77:141, 1971.)

equator of the radial head, the interposed annular ligament could be repositioned in its normal site by simple supination of the forearm with the elbow in slight flexion (Fig. 8-53 B).

In the anatomic specimens of children five years of age or older, a tear in the annular ligament could not be produced by firm traction with the elbow in extension and the forearm in pronation. This is because of the thicker and stronger distal attachment of the annular ligament to the periosteum of the radial neck in the older child; with continued traction, the entire elbow was dislocated.

The foregoing anatomic findings of Salter and Zaltz correlate well with the many characteristic clinical features of pulled elbow in living children.

The child will hold the injured elbow by his side, supporting the forearm with his opposite hand. The forearm is *always pronated* and the elbow partially flexed. On gentle palpation, one can elicit local tenderness over the anterolateral aspect of the radial head. There is no restriction to flexion and extension of the elbow, but supination of the forearm is markedly limited and voluntarily resisted.

Roentgenograms of the elbow are normal. There is no distal displacement of the proximal radius from the capitellum; it is the relationship of the radius and ulna that indicates the pronated posture of the forearm. The diagnosis of subluxation of the radial head is made by the typical clinical findings.

Diagnosis

The clinical picture is characteristic. Immediately following the injury, the child cries with pain and refuses to use the affected limb. A "click" may have been heard or felt in the child's elbow by the person who pulled it.

Treatment

Often reduction of the pulled elbow is unknowingly carried out by the x-ray technician, who passively forces the forearm into full supination in an attempt to obtain a true anteroposterior projection of the elbow. If the child escapes such "treatment,"

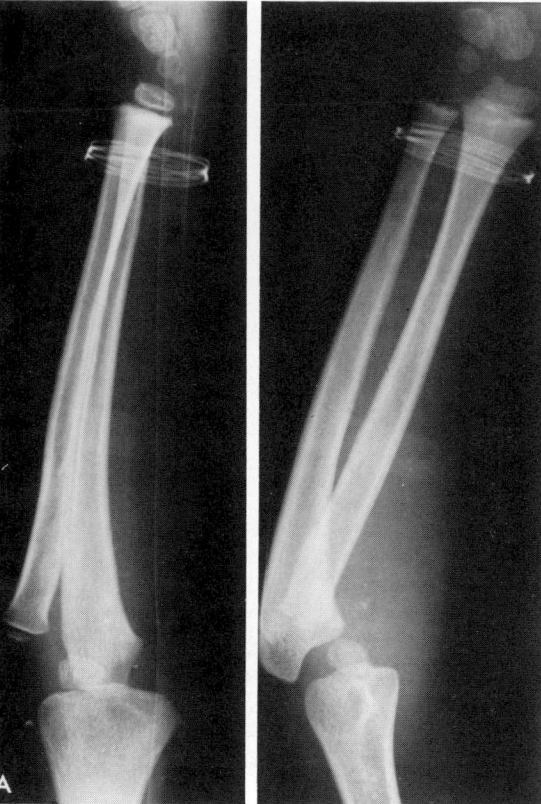

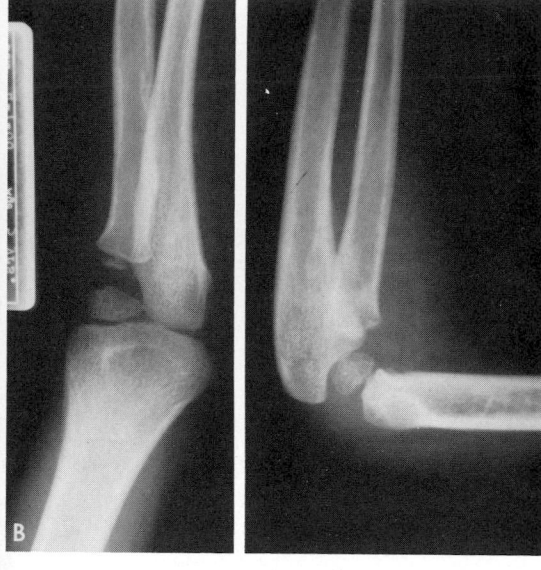

FIGURE 8–54. *Traumatic posterolateral dislocation of the radial head.*

A. Initial roentgenograms. **B.** Roentgenograms taken after reduction. Note the absence of associated fractures.

the pediatrician or orthopedic surgeon performs the reduction of radial head subluxation as follows: The elbow is gently flexed to 90 degrees by holding the child's forearm above the wrist with one hand while, with the other hand, the lower end of the humerus and elbow are firmly held to prevent rotation at the shoulder; the thumb is placed in the region of the radial head for palpation and the exertion of mild pressure if necessary. Then the child's forearm is rapidly and firmly rotated into full supination. As reduction is achieved, a palpable and sometimes audible click can be felt in the region of the radial head. Another signal of reduction is the spectacular and instantaneous relief of pain. The child stops crying and begins to use the arm in a normal manner almost immediately. Should treatment have been delayed and subluxation persist following reduction, the child will still be in some discomfort and will not be anxious to use the limb for several hours or days.

Immobilization is not necessary if it is the first time that subluxation has occurred. A simple sling may be used for a week to keep the elbow out of harm's way. It is important to educate the parents to the potential danger of pulling the child by his hands.

If treatment of subluxation is delayed for more than 12 hours following reduction, the upper limb is immobilized for 10 days in a long arm posterior splint with the elbow in 90 degrees of flexion and the forearm in full supination.

Recurrence of subluxation as a result of a subsequent pull on the hand occurs in about 5 per cent of cases. Following manipulative reduction of a recurrent case, it is best to immobilize the upper limb in a long arm cast for at least two to three weeks.

In a very few children over four years of age, the subluxated radial head may be irreducible by closed manipulation, particularly if it is recurrent, necessitating open operation. In one such case, Salter and Zaltz had to divide the annular ligament, withdraw its ends from the radiohumeral joint, and repair it.

MONTEGGIA FRACTURE-DISLOCATION

In 1814, Giovanni Monteggia first described two cases of fracture of the proximal third of the ulna in association with anterior dislocation of the radial head.[363] Almost 100 years later, Perrin suggested that the condition be called *Monteggia fracture*.[366] The eponym "Monteggia lesion" is used by some authors as a more general term to designate various types of dislocation of the radial head in association with fracture of the ulnar shaft.

The Monteggia fracture is a rare injury, constituting about 2 per cent of fractures involving the elbow in children. Despite its rarity, this lesion has been the subject of great interest because of its inherent serious complications as a result of having been inadequately treated or having gone unrecognized. An entire monograph has been devoted to this injury.[352]

There are three types of Monteggia fracture: *Type I* or *extension type* in which the head of the radius is dislocated anteriorly with volar angulation of the fractured shaft of the ulna (Figs. 8–55 and 8–56); *Type II* or *flexion type*, in which the radial head is dislocated posteriorly, with dorsal angulation of the fractured shaft of the ulna (Figs. 8–57 and 8–58); *Type III*, in which the radial head is dislocated laterally with the fractured shaft of the ulna (Fig. 8–59). Type I is the most common form, accounting for about 85 per cent of cases. Type II accounts for approximately 10 per cent of cases, and Type III, 5 per cent.[358, 370]

The level of the fracture varies. In approximately two thirds of the cases, it is located at the junction of the proximal and middle thirds of the shaft; in one sixth of the cases, in the middle third; in the remainder, it is equally distributed between the distal third of the ulnar shaft and the olecranon process. Fractures of both bones of the forearm at the same level with anterior dislocation of the radial head is sometimes referred to as Type IV Monteggia fracture.

Mechanism of Injury

Three theories have been proposed to explain the pathogenesis of the anterior or extension type of Monteggia fracture. The *direct blow* was proposed as the cause by Speed and Boyd, and subsequently by Smith.[368, 370] The radius and ulna are firmly bound to each other at their upper and lower ends by strong ligaments and throughout their extent by a strong interosseous membrane; as the ulna fractures and shortens, it puts stress on the radial head, which becomes dislocated following rupture of the annular ligament. The torn ligament may be loose or may fold in behind the radial head. In certain instances, the radial head may be pulled out from beneath the annular ligament, coming to lie anterior to an intact ligament.

The *hyperpronation theory* was proposed by Evans, who noted that in extension type Monteggia fractures, the skin over the subcutaneous border of the ulna was always intact. He believed Type I Monteggia fracture resulted from hyperpronation during a fall on the outstretched hand, with the body rotating around the fixed and pronated forearm. In a series of experiments on cadavers, he was able to produce fracture of the middle third of the ulna with anterior dislocation of the radial head by subjecting the specimens to hyperpronation. However, Evans stripped the forearm and arm of all soft tissues, save for the capsule and ligaments of the elbow and the interosseous membrane.[360] Bado, in his monograph, supported the theory that Type I Monteggia fracture is a hyperpronation injury.[352]

Tompkins objected to both the direct blow and hyperpronation theories, proposing that this fracture is a *hyperextension injury* sustained when the child falls on his outstretched hand with his forearm in any degree of rotation. At the moment of impact, the elbow is in the position of hyperextension. The radial head is dislocated anteriorly by strong contraction of the biceps muscle. When this occurs, all the body weight is borne by the ulna, which fractures and is deflected anteriorly as the result of longitudinal compressive force coupled with the pull of the intact interosseous membrane and the simultaneously contracting brachialis muscle.[372]

(*Text continued on page 1630.*)

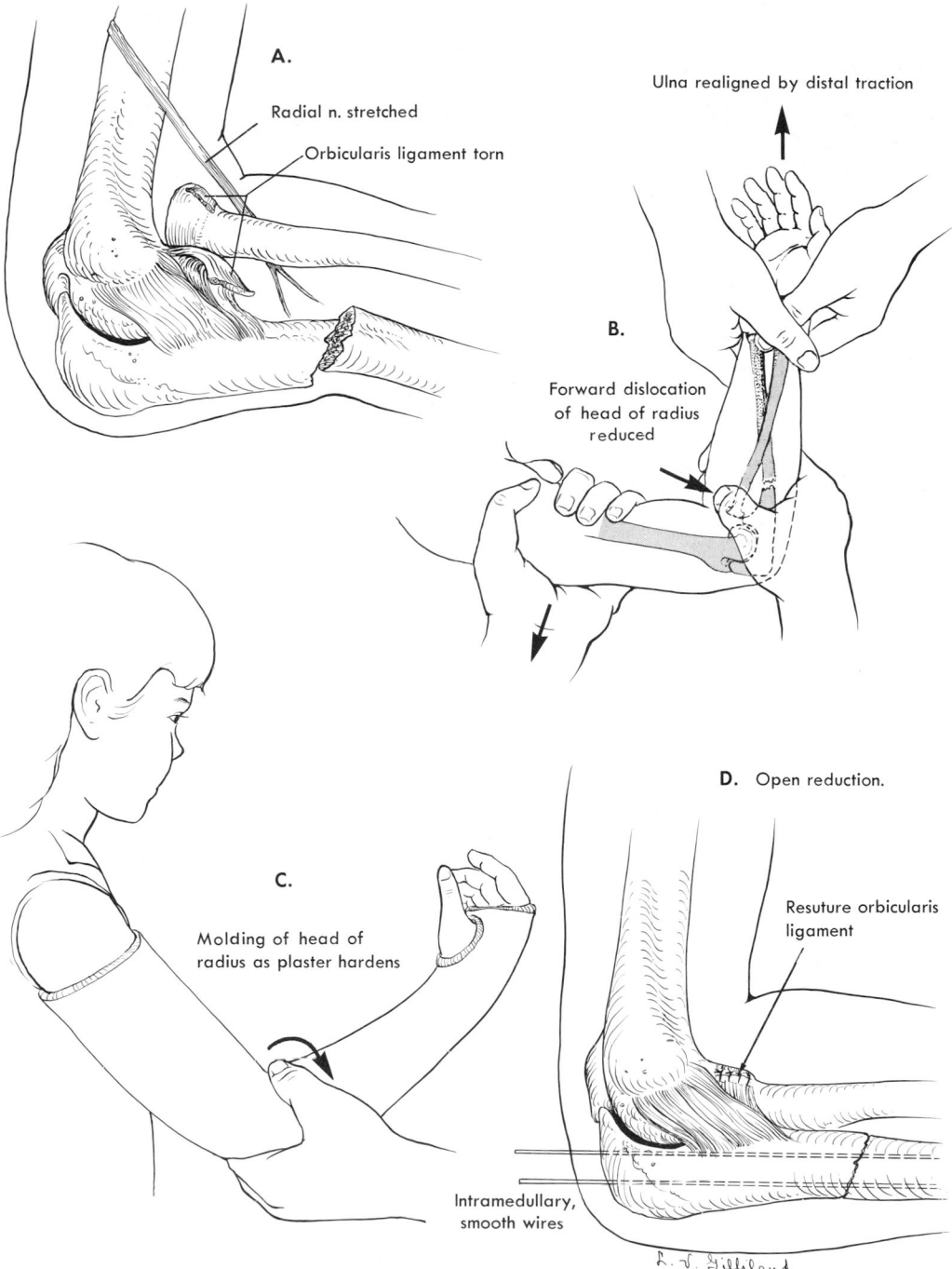

FIGURE 8–55. *Monteggia fracture-dislocation—anterior type (see text for explanation).*

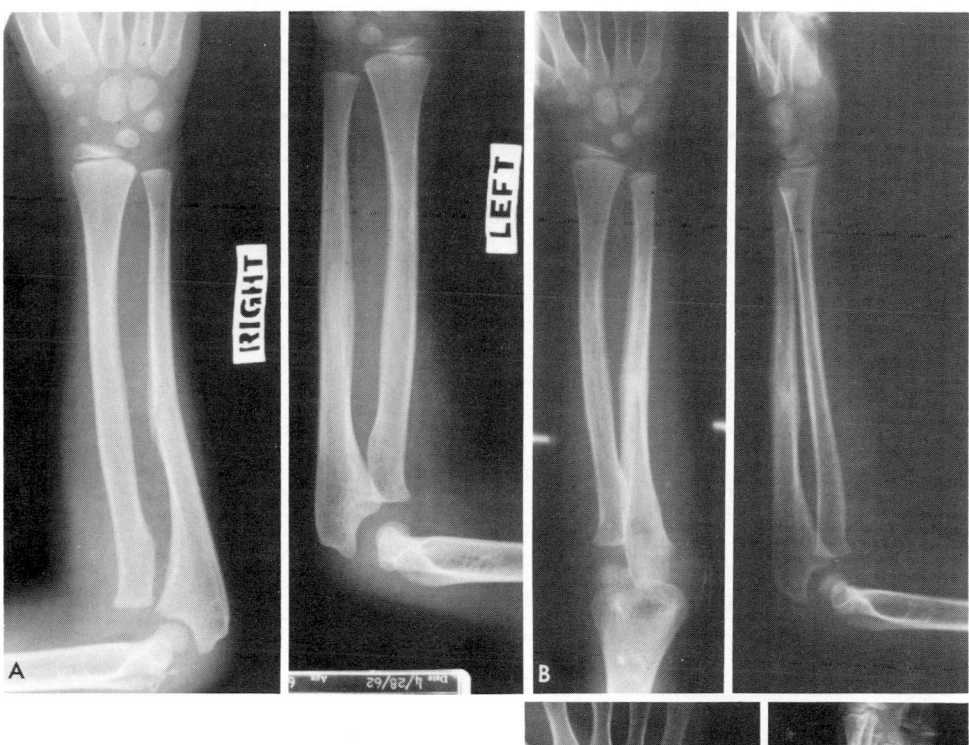

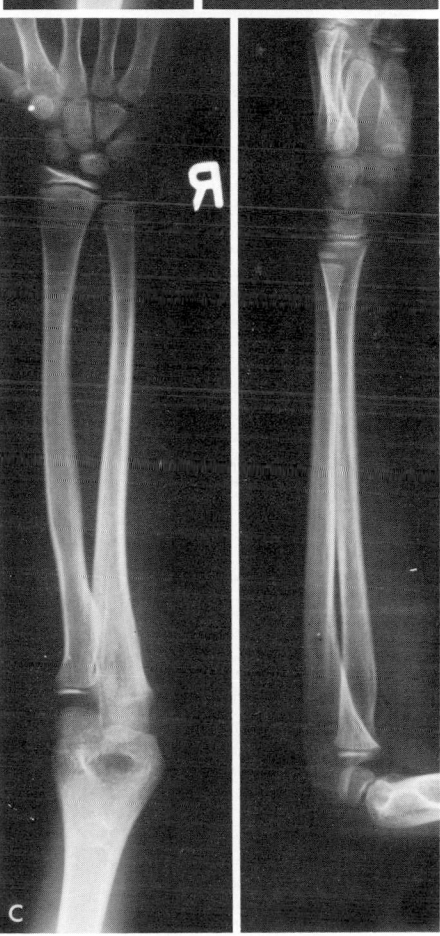

FIGURE 8-56. *Monteggia fracture-dislocation—*
anterior type on the right.

A. Initial roentgenogram of both forearms including wrists and elbows (the normal left one is for comparison). Note the anterior dislocation of the radial head and anterior angulation of the green stick fracture of the ulna in its middle third. **B.** Roentgenograms of right forearm three months following closed reduction. The fracture has healed and the reduction of the radial head has been maintained. **C.** Two years later, roentgenograms show remodeling and complete healing.

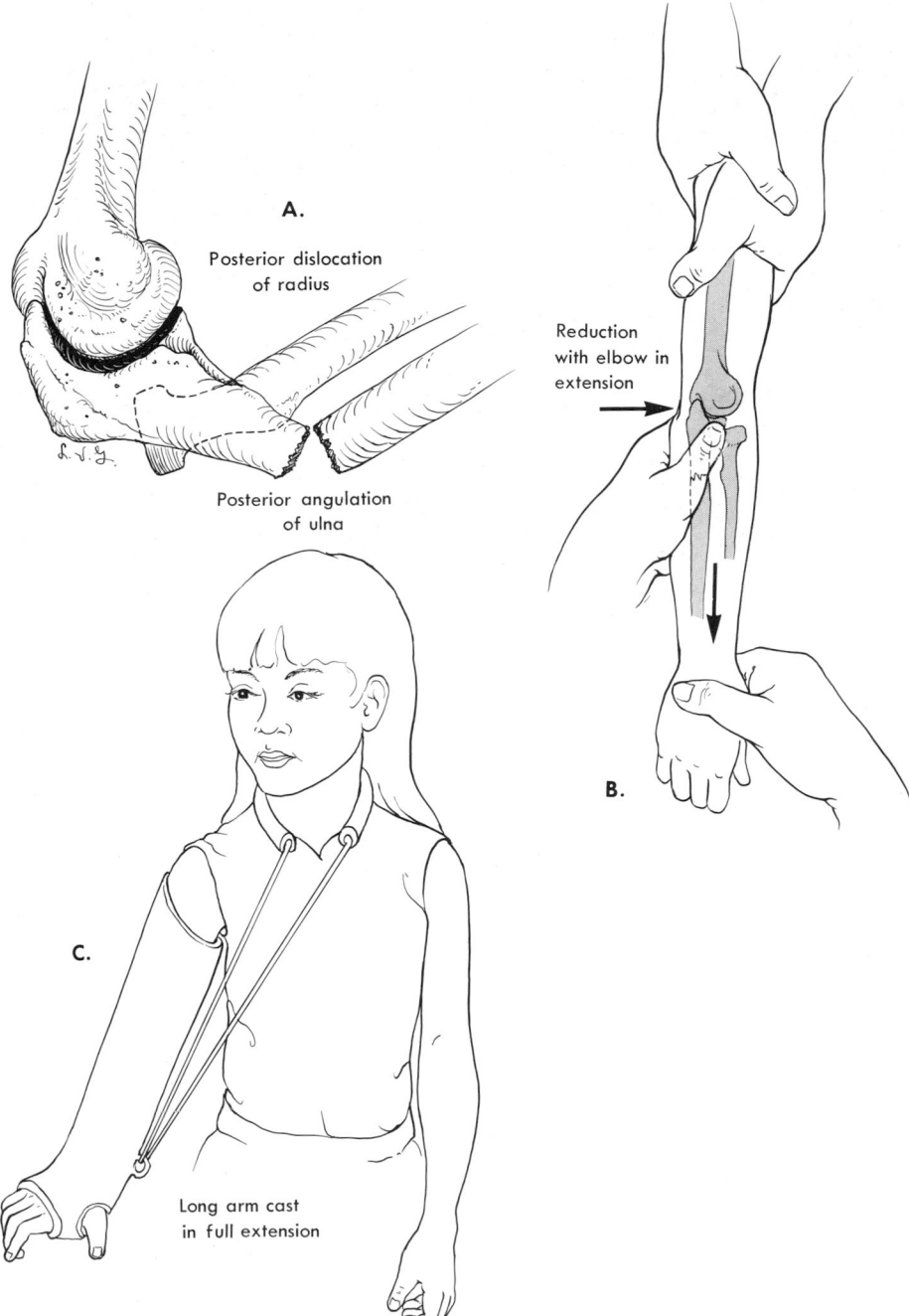

A.

Posterior dislocation
of radius

Posterior angulation
of ulna

Reduction
with elbow in
extension

B.

C.

Long arm cast
in full extension

FIGURE 8–57. *Monteggia fracture-dislocation—posterior type (see text for explanation).*

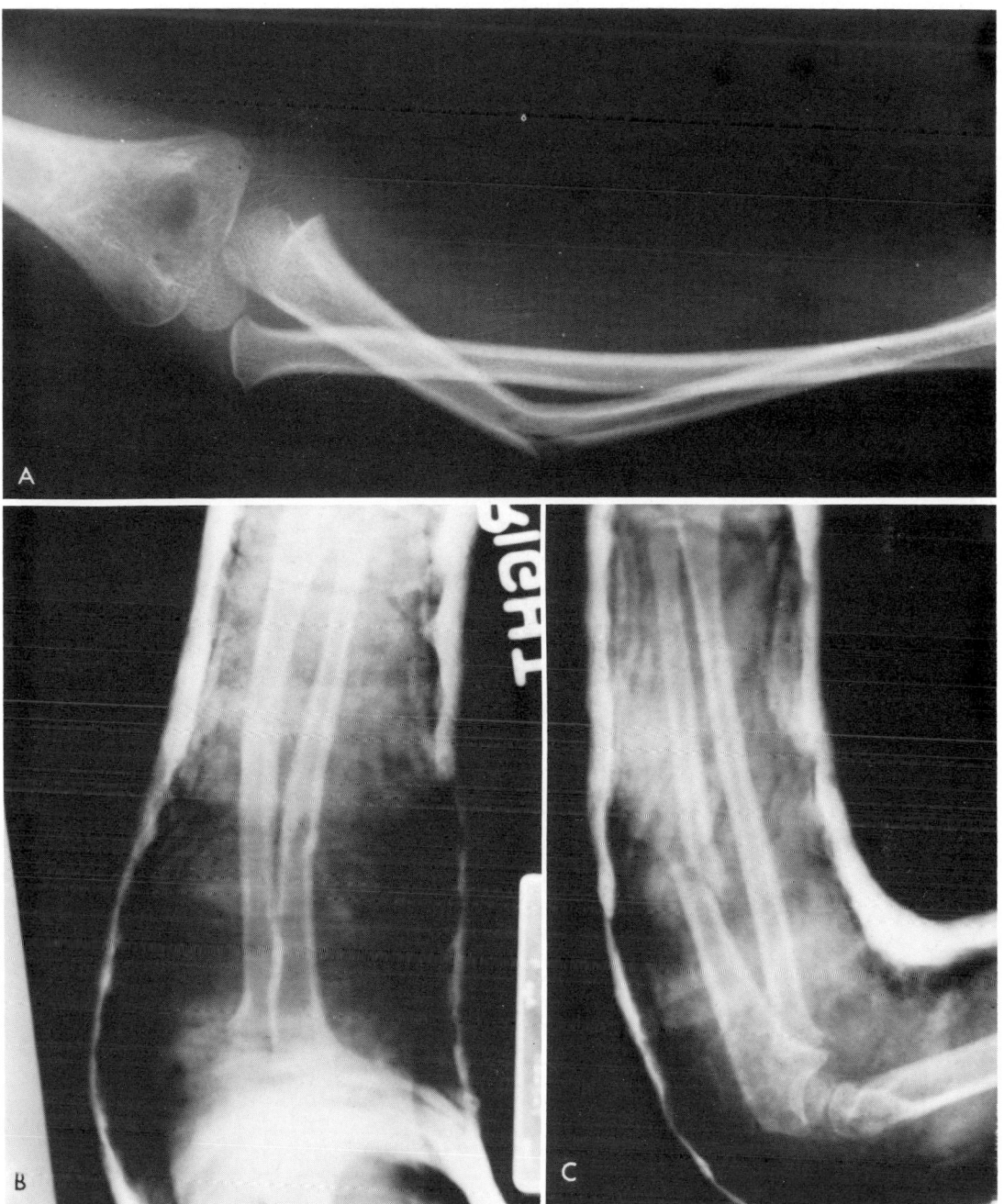

FIGURE 8–58. Monteggia fracture-dislocation — posterior type.

A. Initial roentgenogram. Note the posterior dislocation of the radial head and fracture of the ulna in its middle third. **B** and **C.** Postreduction views.

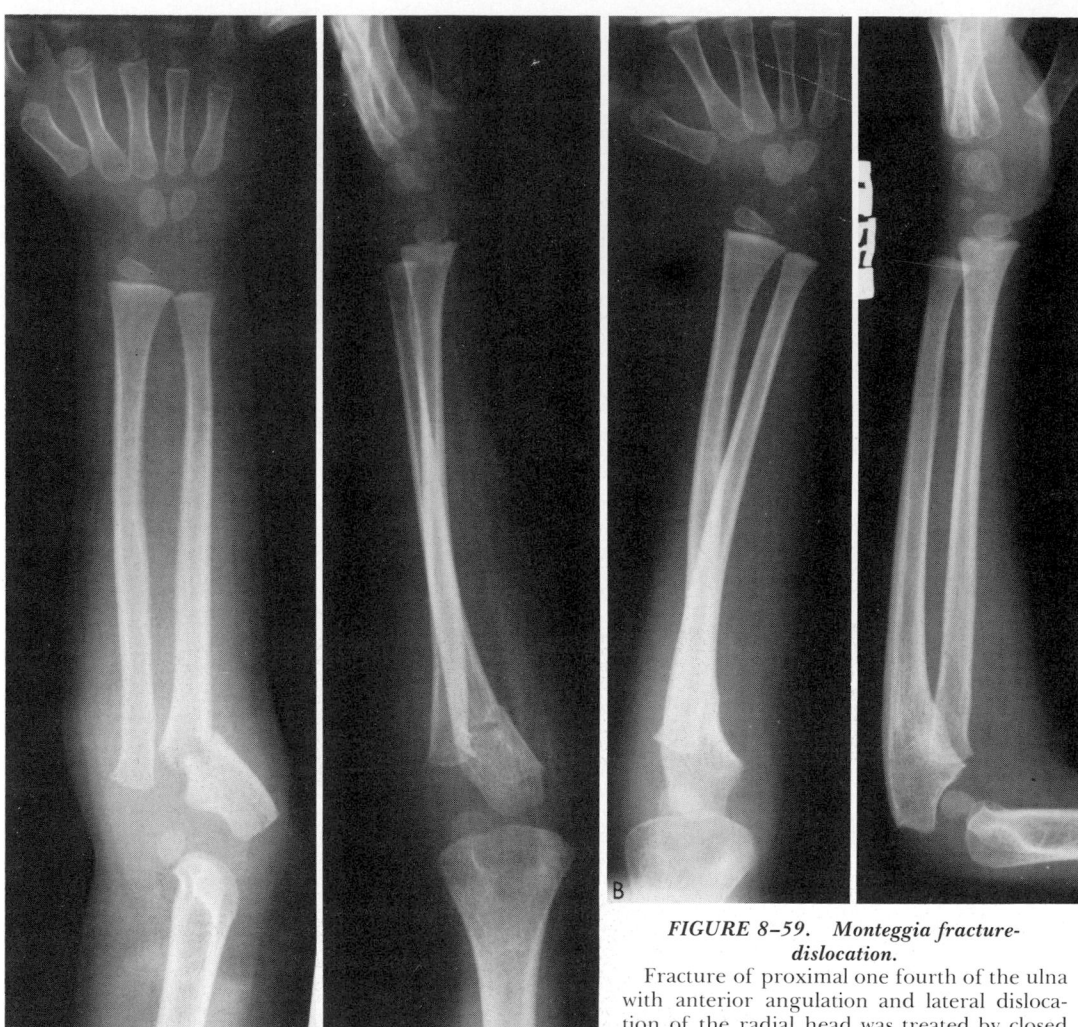

FIGURE 8–59. *Monteggia fracture-dislocation.*
Fracture of proximal one fourth of the ulna with anterior angulation and lateral dislocation of the radial head was treated by closed reduction. **A.** Initial roentgenograms. **B.** Roentgenograms six months later, showing healing and remodeling.

Diagnosis

The patient with a Monteggia fracture usually holds his elbow partially flexed and his forearm in pronation. Any rotation of the forearm or flexion-extension of the elbow is painful and restricted. The elbow is swollen, ecchymotic, and tender. Depending upon the type of Monteggia fracture, the radial head is palpable anterior, posterior, or lateral to its normal location. Palpation of the ulnar diaphysis will reveal the deformity of the angulated fracture.

In order to recognize this injury, it is imperative to obtain roentgenograms of the forearm that include both the elbow and wrist. Particular attention should be paid to detecting luxation of the radial head. Normally, the longitudinal axis of the radius should pass through the ossification center of the capitellum of the humerus; if it does not, then the radial head is dislocated. Possible associated fractures of the wrist should always be ruled out.

Treatment

Early closed reduction is usually successful in children. The anterior Monteggia fracture is reduced as follows: With the forearm in full supination, longitudinal traction is applied first; then the elbow is gently flexed to beyond 90 degrees to relax the biceps muscle. The radial head is gently repositioned by direct manual pressure anteriorly on the bone. The angulated ulnar shaft is reduced by firm manual pressure; this is rarely difficult, once the radial head has been repositioned. Following reduction, the radial head will be quite stable as long as the elbow is kept in acute flexion.

Tompkins has pointed out that, subsequent to reduction during immobilization, the ulnar fracture has a tendency to develop an increasing radial bow; this is caused by the normal slight bowing of the ulna, the contraction of the flexor muscles in the forearm, and perhaps by the anconeus muscle. Tompkins recommends immobilization of the forearm in neutral rotation in only slight supination, with the cast carefully molded over the lateral side of the ulna at the level of the fracture. As long as the elbow is in acute flexion (110 degrees), and the biceps is relaxed, it will not be necessary to keep the forearm in full supination to maintain the reduction.[372]

Posterior Monteggia fracture is reduced by applying traction to the forearm with the elbow in full extension. The radial head is reduced manually. The posteriorly angulated ulnar fracture is anatomically aligned, and a long arm cast is applied with the elbow in full extension.

Immobilization is maintained until there is union of the ulna; this ordinarily requires six to ten weeks, depending upon the age of the patient.

Occasionally open reduction is indicated when one is unable to replace the radial head into normal position by closed methods. The obstacles to closed reduction are: interposition of torn portions of the ruptured orbicular ligament, interposition of an intact orbicular ligament that may have slipped over the radial head without rupturing, or interpositioning of a cartilaginous or osteochondral fragment in the radial notch of the ulna. Open reduction of the radial head and repair of the annular ligament always carry the risk of traumatic ossification.

In instances when the diagnosis of Monteggia fracture is delayed, open surgery is required to reduce the radial head. In the event that three months or more have elapsed from the time of injury, it is wise to leave unreduced Monteggia fractures untreated because ankylosis of the elbow following surgery will be more disabling than the joint instability consequent to persistent dislocation of the radial head. In a child, a dislocated radial head should not be resected, as it will cause cubitus valgus, prominence of the distal end of the ulna, and radial deviation of the head. Removal of the radial head should be deferred until completion of skeletal growth.

Complications that one may encounter following Monteggia fracture are: posterior interosseous or radial nerve palsy from anterior displacement of the radial head, nonunion of fracture of the ulnar shaft, radiohumeral ankylosis, radioulnar synostosis, recurrence of radial head dislocation, and myositis ossificans.

Injuries to the Forearm and Hand

FRACTURES OF THE SHAFT OF RADIUS AND ULNA

The upper end of the ulna articulates with the trochlea of the humerus and provides flexion-extension of the elbow; in its lower portion the ulna splints the radius and provides stability to the forearm. The radius articulates with the carpus and through its rotatory motions of pronation and supination it provides dexterity to the hand.

In the forearm the radius and ulna are firmly bound together by the interosseous membrane, which provides a hinge mechanism for rotatory movements. The annular ligament holds together the proximal radioulnar joint; the distal radioulnar and radiocarpal joints are firmly connected by the dorsal and volar radiocarpal ligaments, and the medial ulnocarpal and lateral radiocarpal ligaments.

Fractures of the shaft of the radius and

ulna may occur in their distal third, middle third, or upper third. One or both bones may be broken. The fracture may be of the greenstick type or complete; the latter may be undisplaced, minimally displaced, or markedly displaced with overriding. The fracture may be greenstick or complete in both radius and ulna, or it may be complete in one bone and greenstick in the other. Angulation may be volar, dorsal, or toward or away from the interosseous space. When only one bone of the forearm is broken, the integrity of the proximal and distal radioulnar joints should always be determined by obtaining roentgenograms that include the elbow and wrist joints with the entire forearm. *Monteggia fracture* — dislocation of the radial head with fracture of the ulna — has been discussed. *Galeazzi fracture* is dislocation of the inferior radioulnar joint with a fracture of the lower third of the radius.

According to Blount, 75 per cent of the fractures of the shaft of the radius and ulna are in the distal third, 18 per cent in the middle third, and 7 per cent in the proximal third.[376-378]

Mechanism of Injury and Pathologic Anatomy

In children, the common injury is by indirect violence sustained in a fall on the outstretched hand. The breaking force is transmitted to the radius. With the hand fixed on the ground, the momentum of the body rotates the humerus and ulna externally and a fracture of the ulna results. Direct violence occasionally is the cause of "both-bone" fractures in children; often these are associated with severe soft-tissue trauma and the fracture may be open.

Once the bones break, the direction and extent of displacement of the fractured fragments is dependent upon the level of the fracture, muscle action, and the direction of breaking force. In the reduction and immobilization of these fractures, the origin, insertion, and action of the forearm muscles must be considered. The biceps brachii and supinator brevis muscles insert into the proximal third of the radius; these muscles are the powerful supinators of the forearm. The pronator teres, originating

above the elbow medially, inserts into the middle third of the radius. The pronator quadratus, located on the anterior aspect of the lower forearm, inserts into the distal third of the radius. The brachioradialis muscle originates from the lower end of the lateral aspect of the humerus and inserts into the lateral surface of the distal radius, immediately above the styloid process; the brachioradialis muscle assists in elbow flexion and is also a semipronator and semisupinator of the forearm, bringing it from supine or prone position to neutral rotation. The extensors of the wrist and digits have no deforming influence on the fracture fragments, but act as a dynamic posterior splint when under tension, as when the elbow is flexed. The extensors and abductors of the thumb act with the brachioradialis muscle in fractures of the distal third of the radius and pull the distal fragment of the radius proximally. The powerful flexor muscles of the forearm tend to pull the distal fragments anteriorly and produce dorsal bowing of the radius and ulna during healing.

In fractures of the *upper third* of the forearm and above the insertion of the pronator teres muscle, the *proximal fragment* of the radius is supinated and flexed because of the unopposed action of the biceps brachii and supinator brevis muscles, and the distal fragment is pronated by the action of the pronator teres and pronator quadratus muscles. Therefore to obtain alignment of the fracture, the distal fragment should be supinated.

In fractures of the *middle third* of the forearm (below the insertion of the pronator teres), the *proximal fragment* of the radius is held in neutral rotation, as the action of the supinator muscles is counteracted by the pronator teres. The proximal fragment is drawn into flexion by the action of the biceps muscle. The *distal fragment* is pronated and drawn toward the ulna by the pronator quadratus muscle. To achieve anatomic reduction, the distal fragment is brought into neutral rotation — midway between full supination and full pronation.

In fractures of the *lower third* of the forearm, the distal fragment of the pulled radius is pronated and pulled inward by the pronator quadratus muscle. Overriding and shortening are caused by the obliquity of the fracture and the pull of the muscles.

The preservation and restoration of the interosseous space are important factors to consider in forearm fractures. Any deviation of the radius and ulna toward each other will encroach on the interosseous membrane; the result is narrowing or obliteration of the interosseous space and marked restriction or loss of rotation of the forearm. Functional handicap will be great, as the dexterity of the hand is contingent on the power of supination and pronation of the forearm.

Diagnosis

The history of injury, the clinical signs of local swelling and tenderness, angular deformity, pain on motion of the forearm, and the roentgenographic findings make the diagnosis obvious.

Treatment

Fractures of both bones of the forearm are difficult to treat, and often they are mismanaged. There are certain pitfalls that should be avoided.

The Loose Cast. In order to maintain reduction, fixation should be secure. As the swelling about a fracture site subsides and muscle atrophies, the cast becomes loose and the fracture fragments are displaced. This loss of position can occur as late as the third week following reduction. A loose cast can be detected in the roentgenogram. The author prefers a circular solid cast; at seven to ten days after reduction, the cast is removed if its is loose, the alignment of fracture fragments is determined, and a new snug cast is applied. Others may prefer bandaged sugar-tong plaster splints for immobilization because they are easily adjusted and tightened as the swelling subsides. One cannot overemphasize the importance of a *snug cast* in preventing loss of alignment.

Inadequate Fixation. Displaced fractures of the radius and ulna should always be immobilized in a sturdy long arm cast, extending from the axilla to the metacarpal heads, with the elbow in 90 degrees of flexion. In children, stiffness of joints from prolonged immobilization is not a problem. In unstable fractures of the distal third of the radius,

the plaster cast should include the proximal phalanges to immobilize the metacarpophalangeal joints; secure fixation of the proximal phalanx of the thumb is particularly important. Blount recommends the use of finger traction on a banjo splint;[376, 377] the author does not believe it is effective in preventing or correcting loss of position of fragments.

Failure to Detect and Correct Loss of Position. In unstable fractures of both bones of the forearm, the position of the fragments should be determined by roentgenograms at three days, seven days, and then at weekly intervals for four weeks. If satisfactory position is lost, the fracture should be remanipulated promptly. Between 10 and 14 days postfracture, the repeated reduction is apt to be more stable because of the "stickiness" of the fragments consequent to the healing process. A common error is to accept inadequate roentgenograms. The x-ray projections should be "true" anteroposterior and "true" lateral. Oblique views are misleading. If necessary, the surgeon himself should assist the x-ray technician in proper positioning of the forearm.

Failure of Adequate Initial Reduction. The more accurate the fracture reduction, the less is the potential for loss of alignment. Reduction of displaced overriding fractures of the distal forearm is difficult in the presence of marked local swelling. There is no emergency in the treatment of these fractures. Often such a child has a full stomach at the time of injury. Compression with a plaster splint is applied, and the child is admitted to the hospital and put to bed with the limb elevated. Within a day or two, the swelling will have receded and, under general anesthesia, the fracture can be manipulated under optimal conditions.

Failure to Immobilize Forearm in Position of Stability. The degree of rotation of the forearm in which fractures of the radius and ulna should be immobilized has been the subject of some controversy. The *forearm is immobilized in the position of rotation in which reduction is most stable.* The standard routine has been full supination in fractures of the upper third, neutral rotation in those of the middle third, and full pronation in the lower-third fractures. Once stable and adequate reduction is achieved, the preservation and restoration of the interosseous space is the important consideration. If reduction is stable, the author recommends the position of full supination in all fractures. As stated before, in full supination of the forearm, the radius and ulna are parallel to each other; and, if a snug cast is maintained during the healing period, the pull of the muscles will not cause malalignment of a satisfactorily reduced stable fracture. However, if fractures of the middle third of the radius and ulna are stable in neutral rotation, the position of the forearm in the cast should be neutral rotation. Stability of reduction is determined clinically and by roentgenographic examination.

Failure to Break the Cortex Competely. In angulated greenstick fractures, this is another common pitfall. The strong advice of Blount should be followed.[376, 377] To merely straighten the bone is not adequate; the intact cortex must be broken through as described in the following section.

Circulatory Embarrassment and Volkmann's Ischemia. These can be caused by frac-tures of both bones of the forearm. When the forearm is swollen or when a displaced fracture is reduced by manipulation, it is wise to admit the child to the hospital, elevate the limb, and closely observe the circulation for one to three days.

Open Reduction. Rarely, if ever, should this be performed in fractures of both bones of the forearm in a child because of the definite risk of delayed union and nonunion. Radioulnar synostosis and infection are other serious complications.

Keeping the foregoing principles in mind, one treats "both-bone" fractures of the forearm as follows:

GREENSTICK FRACTURES OF MIDDLE THIRD OF RADIUS AND ULNA

The usual deformity is dorsal angulation of the distal fragment with the apex of the

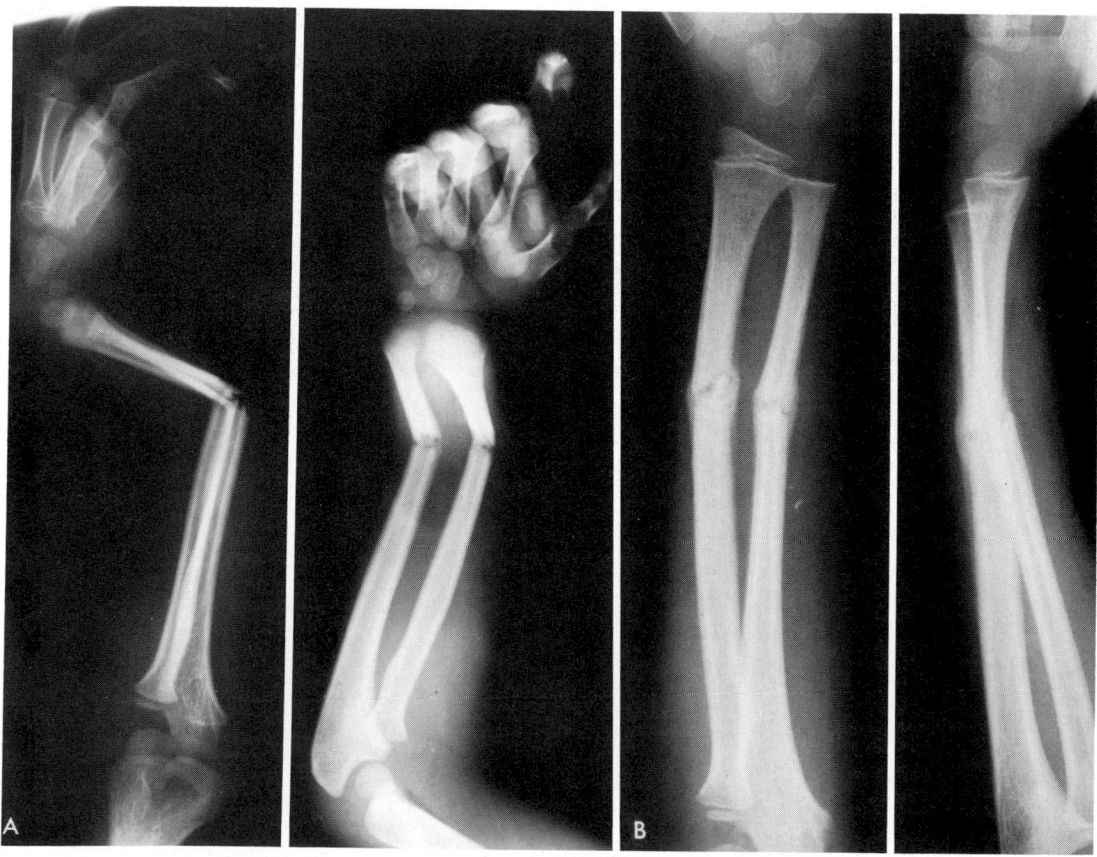

FIGURE 8–60. *Fracture of both bones of forearm with marked dorsal angulation of distal fragments.*

A. Initial roentgenogram. **B.** Four weeks after closed reduction.

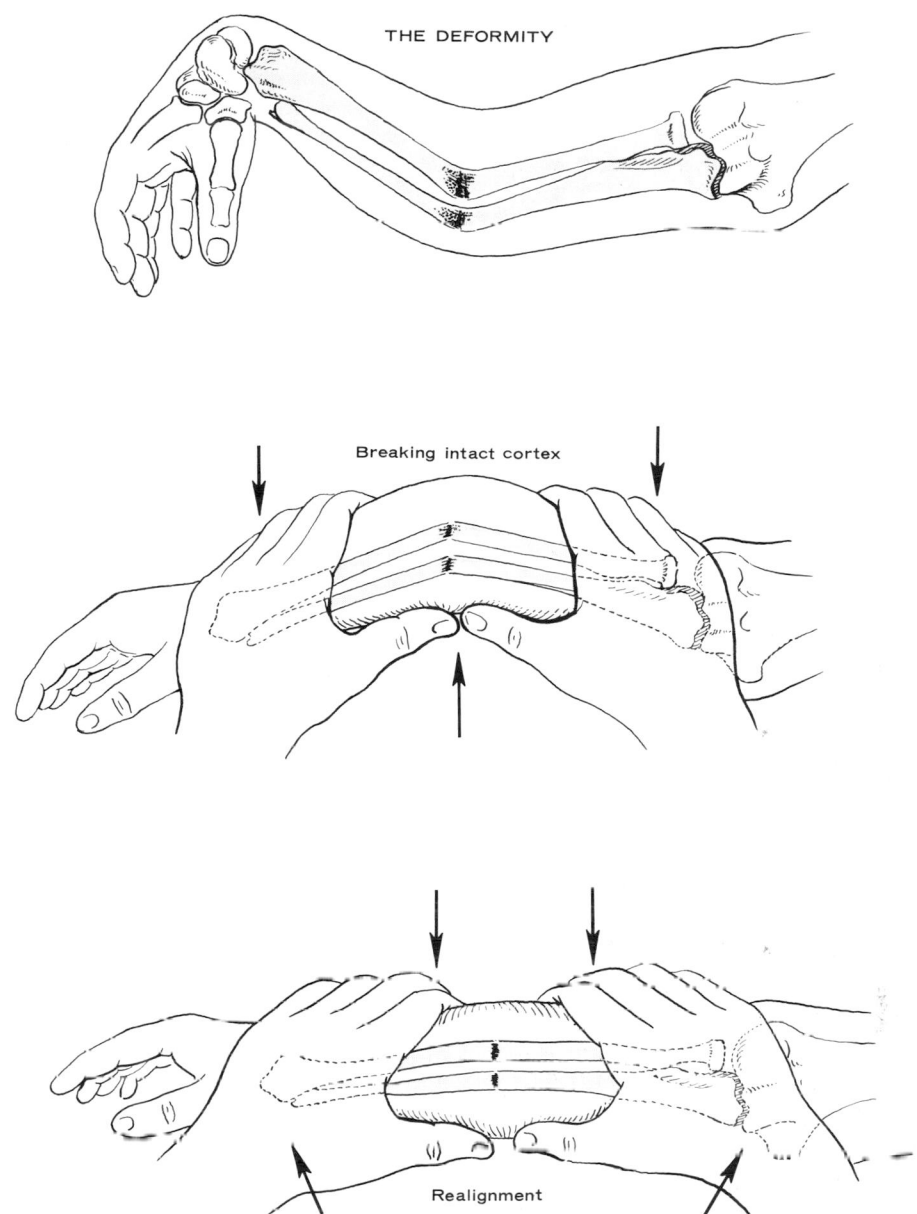

THE DEFORMITY

Breaking intact cortex

Realignment

FIGURE 8-61.   Method of closed reduction of greenstick fracture of middle third of radius and ulna.

fracture toward the volar aspect. Simple straightening of the bones and immobilization in the cast is not adequate, as the deformity will recur. The intact cortex should be completely broken through. Ordinarily in a recent fracture, general anesthesia is not required. The technique of manipulative reduction is as follows: (1) Grasp the forearm with one hand above and one hand below the fracture site. (2) Place the volar aspect of the apex of the forearm deformity over your knee; then suddenly reverse it and break the intact cortex on the dorsal aspect. The periosteal tube remains intact and holds the fragments together in normal alignment. A long arm cast is applied with the elbow in 90 degrees of flexion and the forearm in full supination or midway between pronation and supination. The fracture will consolidate in four to six weeks (Figs. 8–60 and 8–61).

DISPLACED FRACTURES OF MIDDLE THIRD OF BOTH BONES OF FOREARM

These require correction of angular and rotational deformities. If normal alignment is not restored, there will be restriction of pronation and supination of the forearm. Bayonet (side-to-side) apposition with some overriding is acceptable, provided there is no deviation of the radius and ulna toward each other and no encroachment on the interosseus space. In the determination of the degree of angulation and rotation, the injured and normal forearm should be compared, both clinically by inspection and by roentgenograms made in symmetrical positions and several projections. The technique of manipulative reduction is as follows: (1) With the patient in supine position, the elbow is flexed to right angles and the forearm is supinated. One assistant applies longitudinal traction by grasping the distal ends of the radius and ulna at the wrist, while another assistant applies countertraction at the elbow. (2) The surgeon repositions the fragments into anatomic alignment with his thumbs. The width of the interosseous space is restored by digital pressure on the soft tissues between the bones. (3) While traction is maintained, a long arm cast is applied with the elbow in 90 degrees of flexion and the forearm fully supinated. The cast should be well molded over the volar aspect of the radius.

Displaced fractures in the middle third of the radius and ulna require six to eight weeks to heal. Postreduction care follows the principles outlined previously — namely, a snug cast, frequent x-rays to detect loss of position, and prompt remanipulation if such loss occurs.

If closed manipulation fails to correct angular deformity, open surgical reduction should not be performed. A well-padded cast is applied for immobilization and to act as a compression dressing to reduce the local swelling. After five to seven days, the fracture is remanipulated. Often this second attempt will be successful in obtaining anatomic alignment. If unsuccessful, reduction is achieved with skeletal traction through the shafts of the metacarpals. *Rarely, if ever, is open reduction of "both-bone" fractures warranted in children.*

FRACTURES OF THE DISTAL THIRD OF THE RADIUS AND ULNA

"Torus" or buckle fracture of the distal metaphysis of the radius and ulna is the commonest fracture in the lower forearm in young children. (The word *torus* is derived from the Latin *tori* meaning a swelling or protuberance.) The impact of the indirect violence of a fall on the outstretched hand crumples the dorsal cortex, but the volar cortex remains intact. The distal fragment is angulated dorsally. Treatment consists of a below-elbow cast or volar splint for a period of three weeks.

Greenstick Fractures of the Distal Radius and Ulna

These do not require reduction if the dorsal angulation is insignificant; however, if it exceeds 30 degrees in infants and 15 degrees in children, closed reduction is required. During manipulation the deformity is reversed, i.e., the distal fragment is angulated toward the volar aspect until the intact dorsal cortex is broken through completely. Then a long arm cast is applied for a period of four to six weeks. In greenstick fractures, if the intact cortex is not completely broken through, the deformity will recur.

Complete Fractures of the Distal Third of the Radius and Ulna

The distal fragments are displaced dorsally and radially with varying degrees of overriding (Fig. 8–62). The fracture of the radius may be complete and that of the ulna, greenstick. They should be reduced, preferably under general anesthesia or 1 per cent lidocaine local anesthesia. The technique of reduction is as follows: (1) With the patient supine, an assistant grasps the fingers

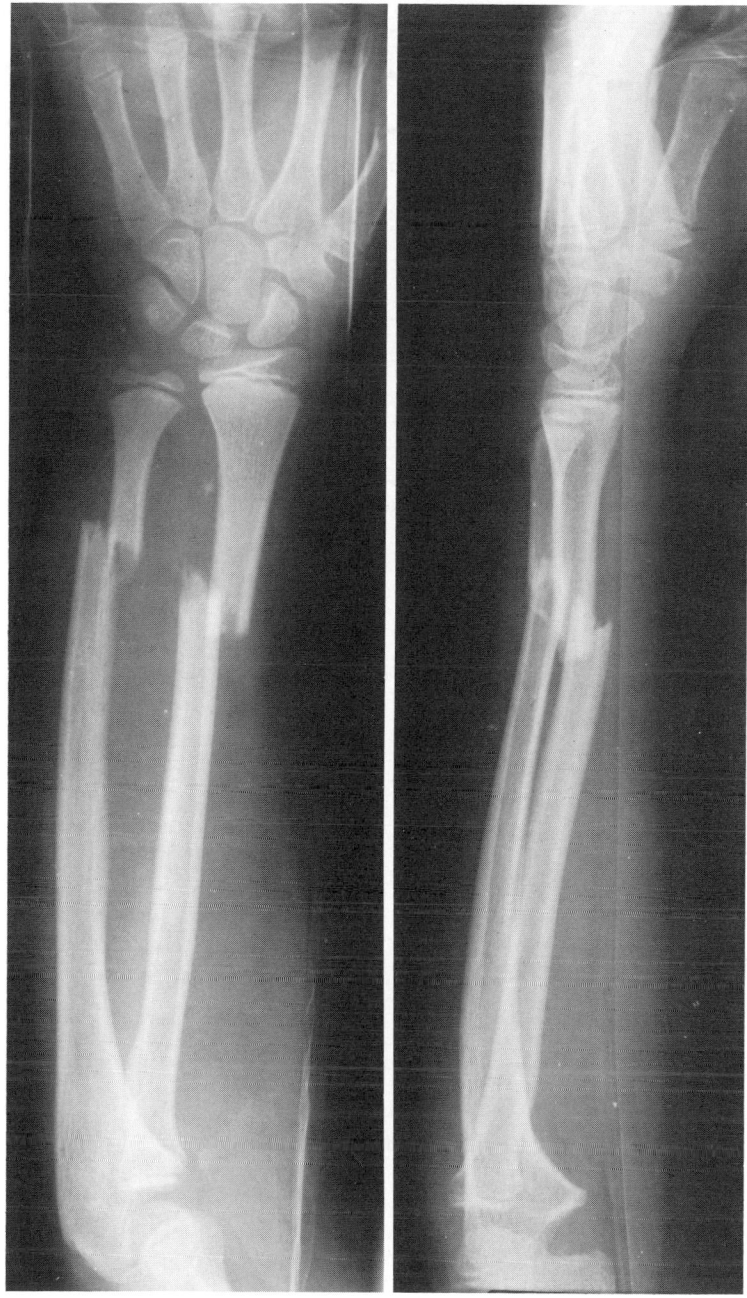

FIGURE 8–62. Fracture of radius and ulna in its distal fourth.

in one hand and the thumb in the other hand, and applies strong longitudinal traction *in the line of deformity*; another assistant applies countertraction at the elbow. (2) The surgeon pushes the fragments into normal position with his thumb and fingers. The soft tissues between the distal radius and ulna are pressed to restore the width of the interosseous space. It is desirable to achieve perfect anatomic alignment; however, side-to-side bayonet apposition in good alignment is acceptable. Encroachment on the interosseous space by the fragments should be corrected, as it will restrict rotation of the forearm (Figs. 8–63, 8–64, and 8–65). Minimal overriding will be remodeled.

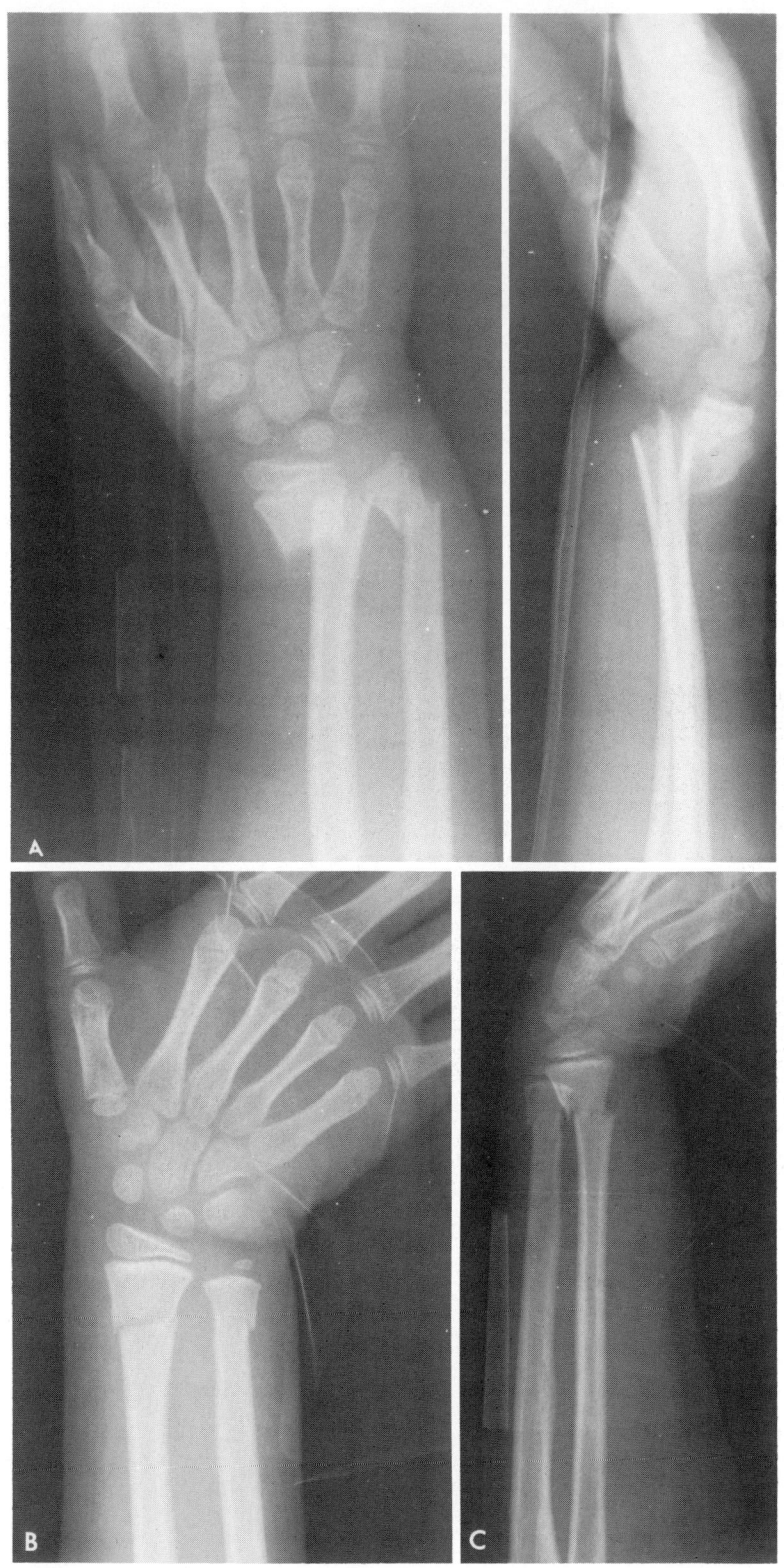

FIGURE 8–63. *Fracture of the right radius and ulna at the junction of the distal metaphyses with the diaphyses.*

A. Initial roentgenogram. **B** and **C.** Following closed reduction.

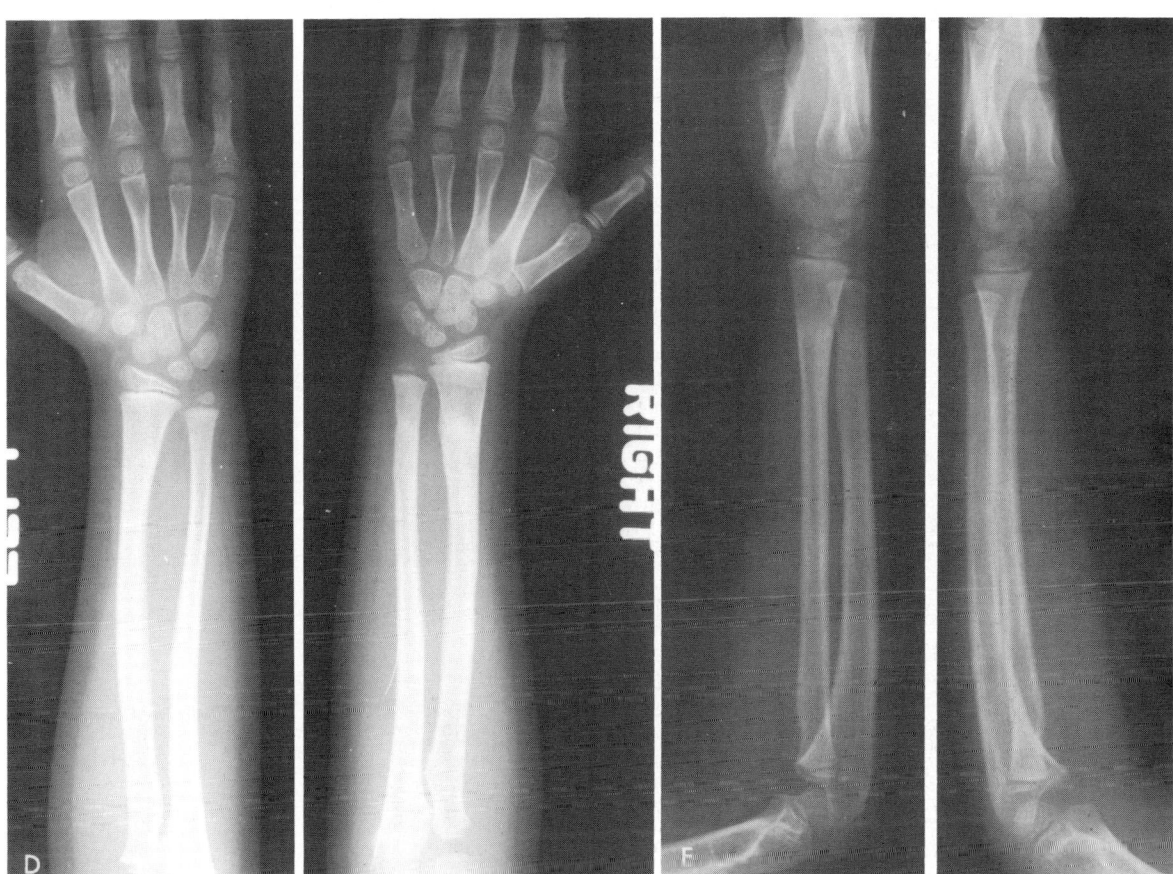

FIGURE 8–63 Continued. *Fracture of the right radius and ulna at the junction of the distal metaphysis with the diaphysis.*

D and **E.** Anteroposterior and lateral roentgenograms made eight months later, showing healing and remodeling.

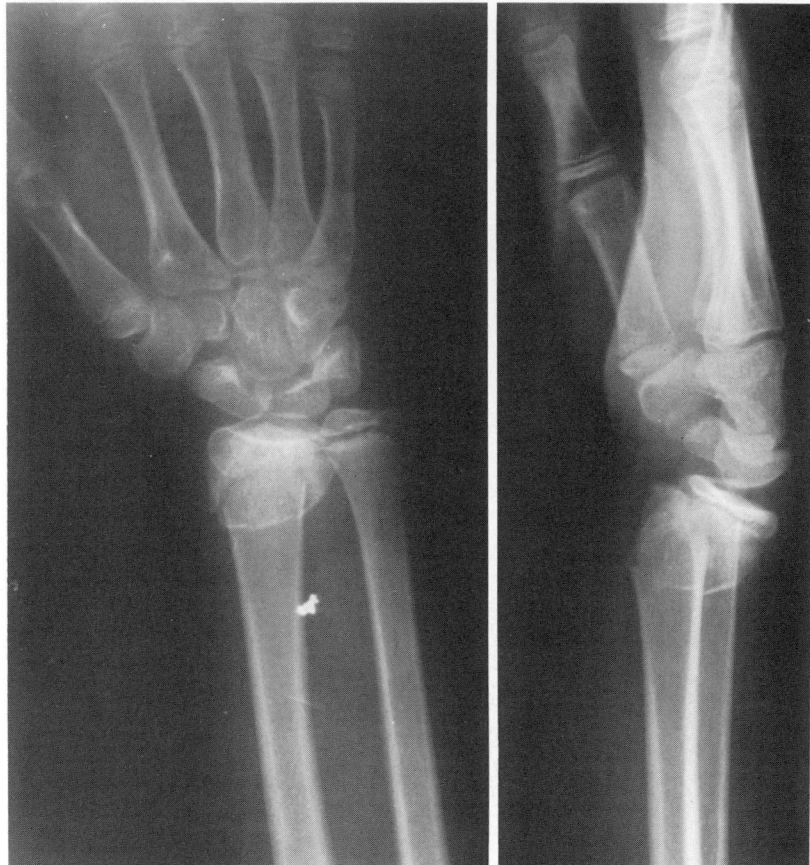

FIGURE 8–64.   *Fracture of lower end of diaphysis of radius.*

Note marked dorsal angulation and displacement.

Marked overriding may occasionally require skeletal traction through the metacarpals for correction.

An above-elbow cast is applied for immobilization, which is maintained for six weeks. When both bones are fractured, neutral rotation of the forearm may provide more stability, whereas if only the radius is broken, the reduction may be more stable in pronation.

Fractures of the Proximal Third of the Shaft of the Radius and Ulna

These relatively rare injuries are often caused by direct trauma. Frequently one bone is fractured. As in all fractures of the forearm, the elbow and wrist should be included in the roentgenogram to rule out dislocation of the radial head or of the inferior radioulnar joint (Fig. 8–66).

Isolated fracture of the proximal third of the radial shaft is reduced and immobilized with the forearm in full supination.

Remodeling of Malunion of Fractures of Both Bones of the Forearm

The degree of spontaneous correction of residual deformities by remodeling depends upon the age of the child, the distance of the fracture site from the physis, the amount of deformity, and the direction of angulation.[376] To reiterate, narrowing of the interosseous space by angulation of the radius and ulna toward each other is not acceptable

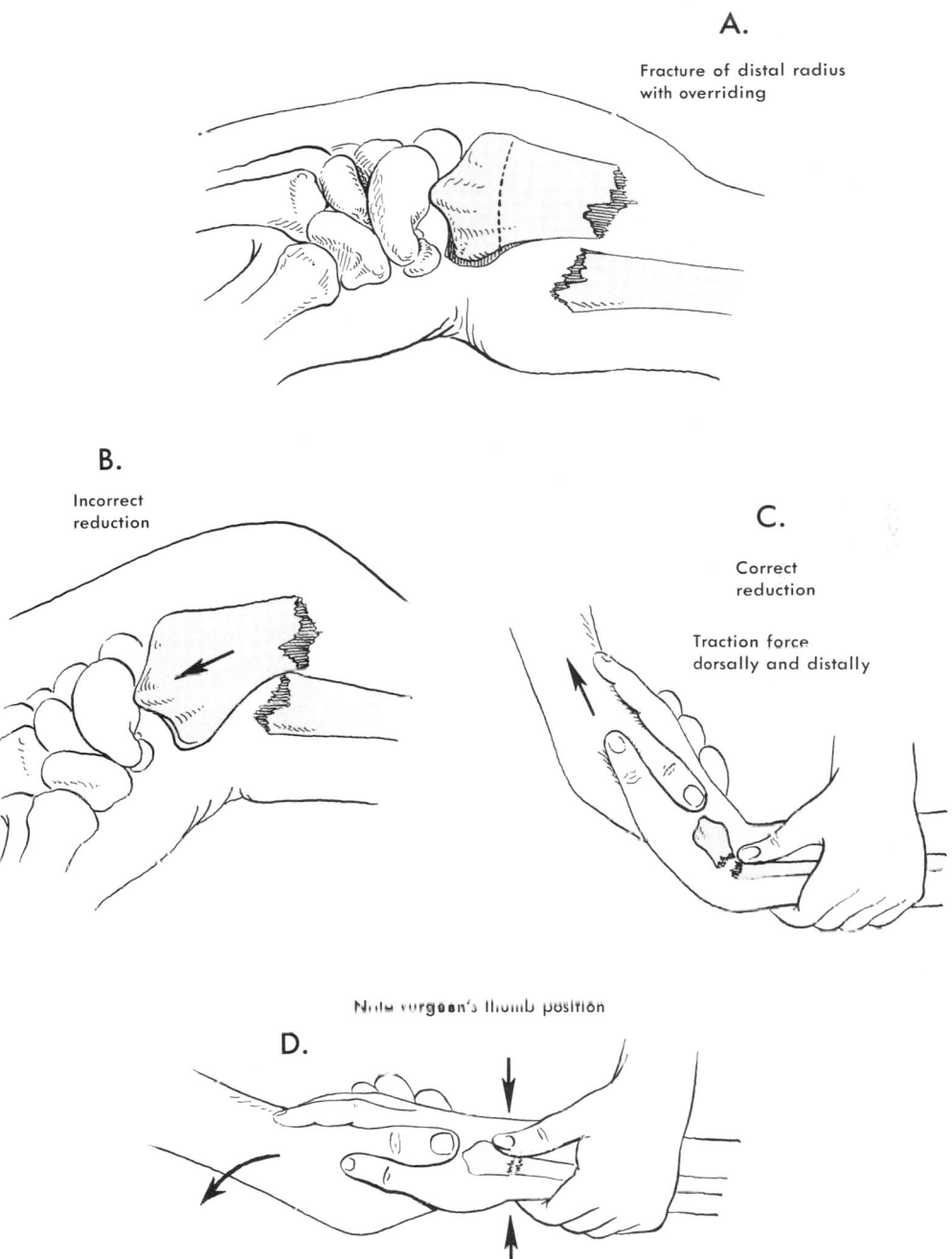

A.

Fracture of distal radius
with overriding

B.

Incorrect
reduction

C.

Correct
reduction

Traction force
dorsally and distally

Note surgeon's thumb position

D.

FIGURE 8–65. *Technique of closed reduction of fracture of lower end of radial shaft (see text for explanation).*

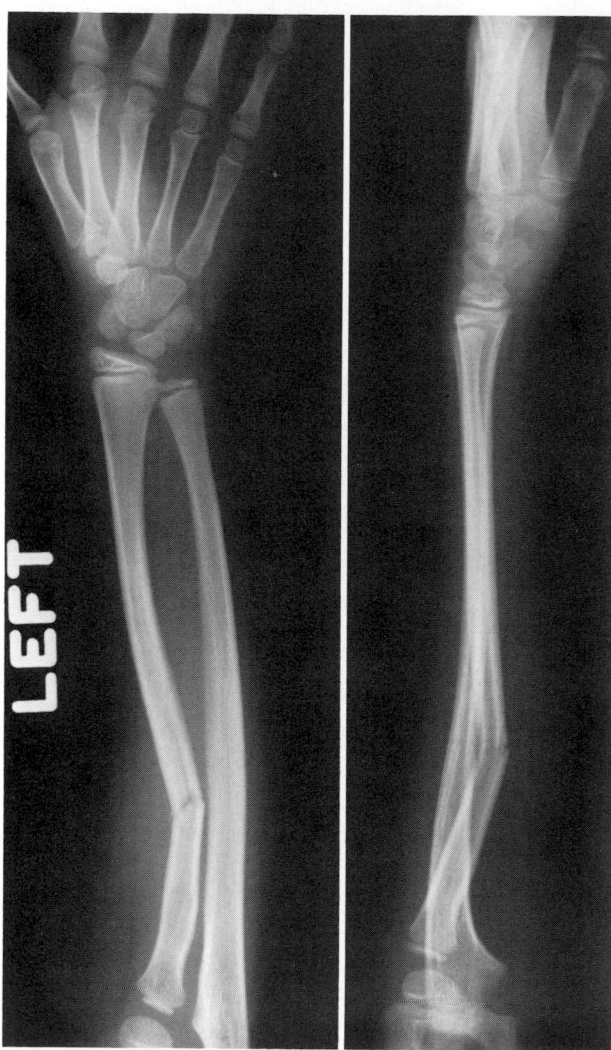

FIGURE 8–66.   *Greenstick fracture of the shaft of the radius at the junction of its proximal and middle thirds.*

The ulna is not fractured, but the inferior radioulnar joint was subluxated. Always roentgenograms of the entire forearm, including the elbow and wrist joints, should be made.

because invariably it will result in some degree of restriction of pronation-supination of the forearm. Dorsal angulation of the distal fragment (apex volar) will be remodeled rapidly. Figs. 8–67 to 8–69 illustrate spontaneous correction of malunion of fractures of both bones of the forearm.

FRACTURES INVOLVING THE DISTAL RADIAL PHYSIS

This fracture is the most common physeal injury, constituting about 50 per cent of the total. It usually occurs in children between the ages of six and ten years who sustain injury by falling on an outstretched hand. The shearing forces of hyperextension and supination displace the distal radial epiphysis dorsally. The physeal injury is Type II (Salter-Harris), with a small metaphyseal bone fragment attached to the dorsal or dorsoradial aspect of the epiphysis. The distal radial epiphysis may be displaced alone, or it may be associated with a greenstick fracture of the metaphysis of the ulna, separation of the distal ulnar epiphysis, or fracture of the tip of the ulnar styloid process.

Clinically, there is local pain, swelling, and "silver fork" deformity. Roentgenograms will establish the diagnosis by revealing posterior displacement of the epiphysis, which is best visualized in the lateral projection (Fig. 8–70). The dorsal metaphyseal bone fragment is usually small, requiring close scrutiny for detection.

Treatment consists of closed reduction and immobilization in a long arm cast for a period of three to four weeks. Repeated forceful manipulations should be avoided, as they cause damage to the physis. That malposition does not persist has been well demonstrated by Aitken.[386, 387] Within a maximum period of two to three years (usually five to eight months), the distal radial epiphysis will assume its normal relation to the radial metaphysis. Remodeling takes place by new bone formation on the dorsum of the distal radius so that the diaphysis is elevated to the epiphysis. The volar portion of the radius is gradually absorbed. If one or two attempts at gentle closed reduction fail, it is wise to leave the epiphysis displaced; open reduction of the markedly displaced epiphysis should not be performed.

The prognosis for a Type II physeal injury is good. Occasionally, the longitudinal forces of the impact may crush the germinal cells of the physis, producing a Type V physeal injury. This crushing of the physis cannot be detected in the early roentgenograms; but within 6 to 12 months, the follow-up roentgenograms will disclose growth arrest by the gradual narrowing and obliteration of the radiolucent line of the physis and overgrowth of the ulna in relation to the radius.

FRACTURES OF THE PHALANGES AND METACARPALS IN THE HAND

Fractures of the bones in the hand are rare injuries in children, but if encountered, they are treated as in the adult.

Comminuted fracture of the distal phalanx caused by direct crushing force is frequently seen in children. The nail is trephined to release the hematoma and to relieve the intense pain due to the distended pulp. A padded aluminum finger splint is applied to protect the fingertip.

When the level of fracture is proximal to the insertion of the flexor digitorum sublimis, the angulation is dorsal (Fig. 8–71 C and D). It is reduced and immobilized with the interphalangeal joints in extension. A displaced T-fracture of the distal end of the proximal phalanx requires open reduction and internal fixation with a Kirshner wire.

Fractures of the *middle phalanx* may be undisplaced or angulated. If the site of the fracture is distal to the insertion of the flexor digitorum sublimis tendon, the proximal fragment is angulated toward the palm; this is treated by manual traction and flexion of the distal fragment. It is immobilized in a below-elbow plaster cast with a volar padded aluminum splint. The interphalangeal joints are completely flexed; the metacarpophalangeal joint is partially flexed, whereas the wrist is in neutral position (Fig. 8–71 E and F).

In fractures of the mid-shaft of the proximal phalanx, the apex of the angulation is

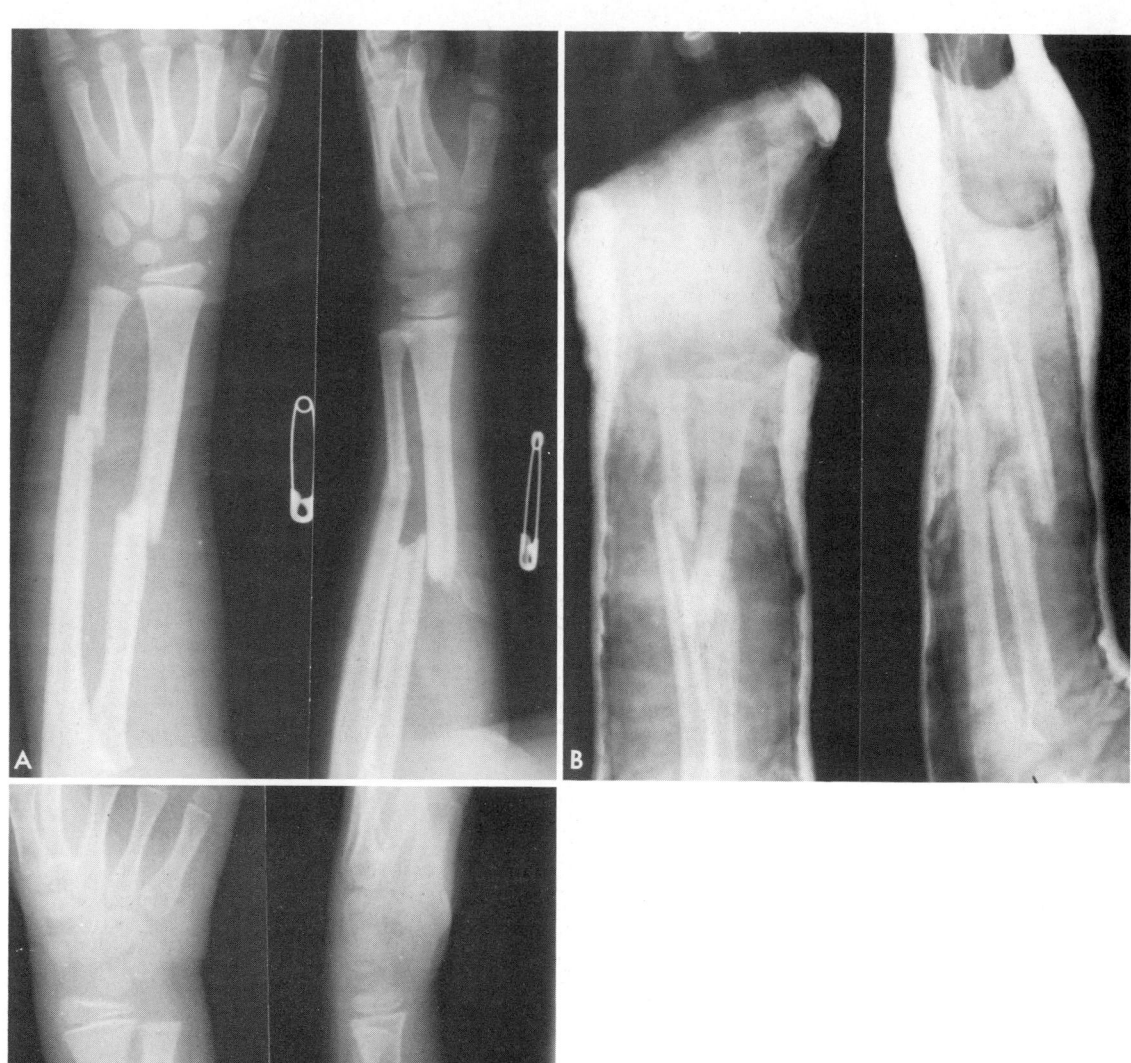

FIGURE 8–67. *Remodeling of fracture of both
bones of the forearm.*

A. Initial roentgenograms. **B.** In cast, showing the
marked displacement of the fragments. **C.** Four weeks
later, showing the malunion.

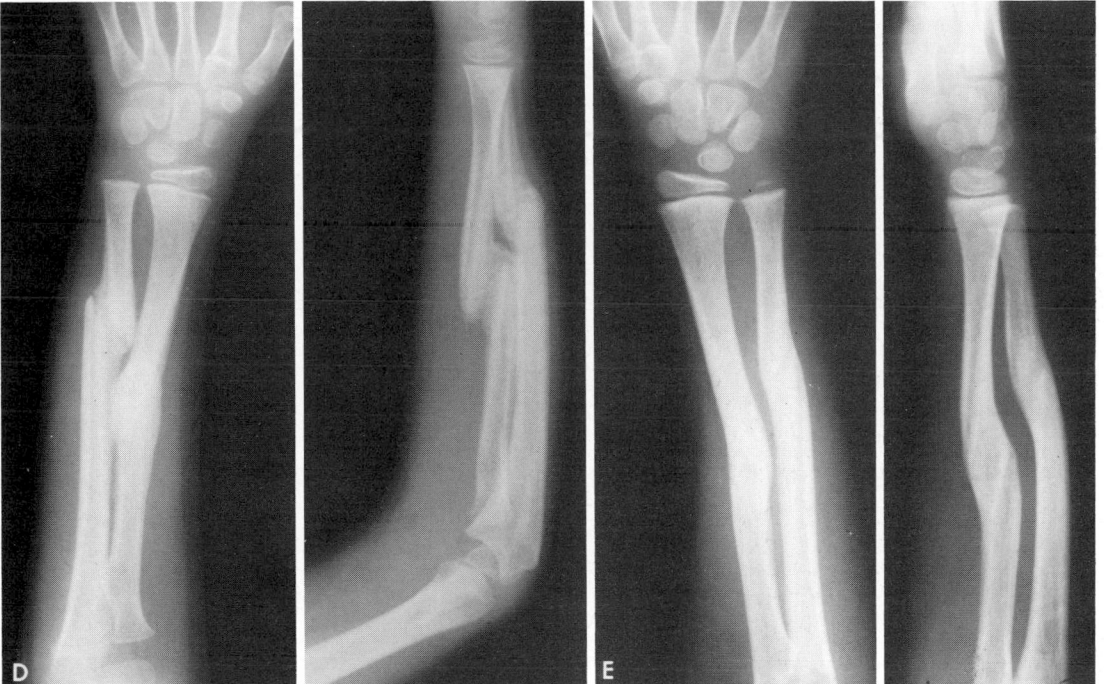

FIGURE 8–67 Continued.   Remodeling of fracture of both bones of the forearm.

D. After one month there is solid bony union. Parents were unhappy and desired surgery to correct the deformity. They were assured it would be spontaneously corrected by remodeling. **E.** Six months later, alignment was good, child had normal looking arm with excellent function.

volar owing to the action of the intrinsic muscles (Fig. 8–71 A and B). The fracture line may be transverse or oblique. Reduction is achieved and maintained in flexion; it should never be immobilized in extension. Those fingers adjacent to the injured ones are splinted as well. Unstable fractures may require skeletal traction with a pin through the distal phalanx. Attention should be given to maintaining correct rotational alignment. Fractures involving the physis of the phalanges require accurate reduction.

Metacarpal fractures usually occur in adolescents who get into fist fights. The dorsally angulated fracture of the shaft of a metacarpal is easily reduced by elevation of the distal fragment (Fig. 8–72). The displaced fracture of the metacarpal neck is reduced by acute flexion of the metacarpophalangeal joint and by pushing the distal fragment dorsally along the longitudinal axis of the proximal phalanx. These fractures are immobilized in a below-elbow cast for four weeks with the finger of the affected metacarpal in moderate flexion.

Bennett's fracture may require open reduction and internal fixation with smooth Kirschner wire. Metacarpophalangeal dislocation of the thumb usually results from a hyperextension force; the metacarpal head may be trapped through a buttonhole in the capsule and require open reduction.

WRINGER INJURY TO THE UPPER LIMB*

Wringer injuries of the upper limb are sustained by a child whose hand is drawn into the power-driven rollers of a washing machine. If the elbow is flexed as the forearm is drawn into the roller, the maximum damage to the soft tissues is sustained in the antecubital fossa; whereas if the elbow is extended, the maximum trauma is to the axilla. The extent of injury is increased by applying countertraction to the extremity or

(*Text continued on page 1650.*)

*See References 396 to 408.

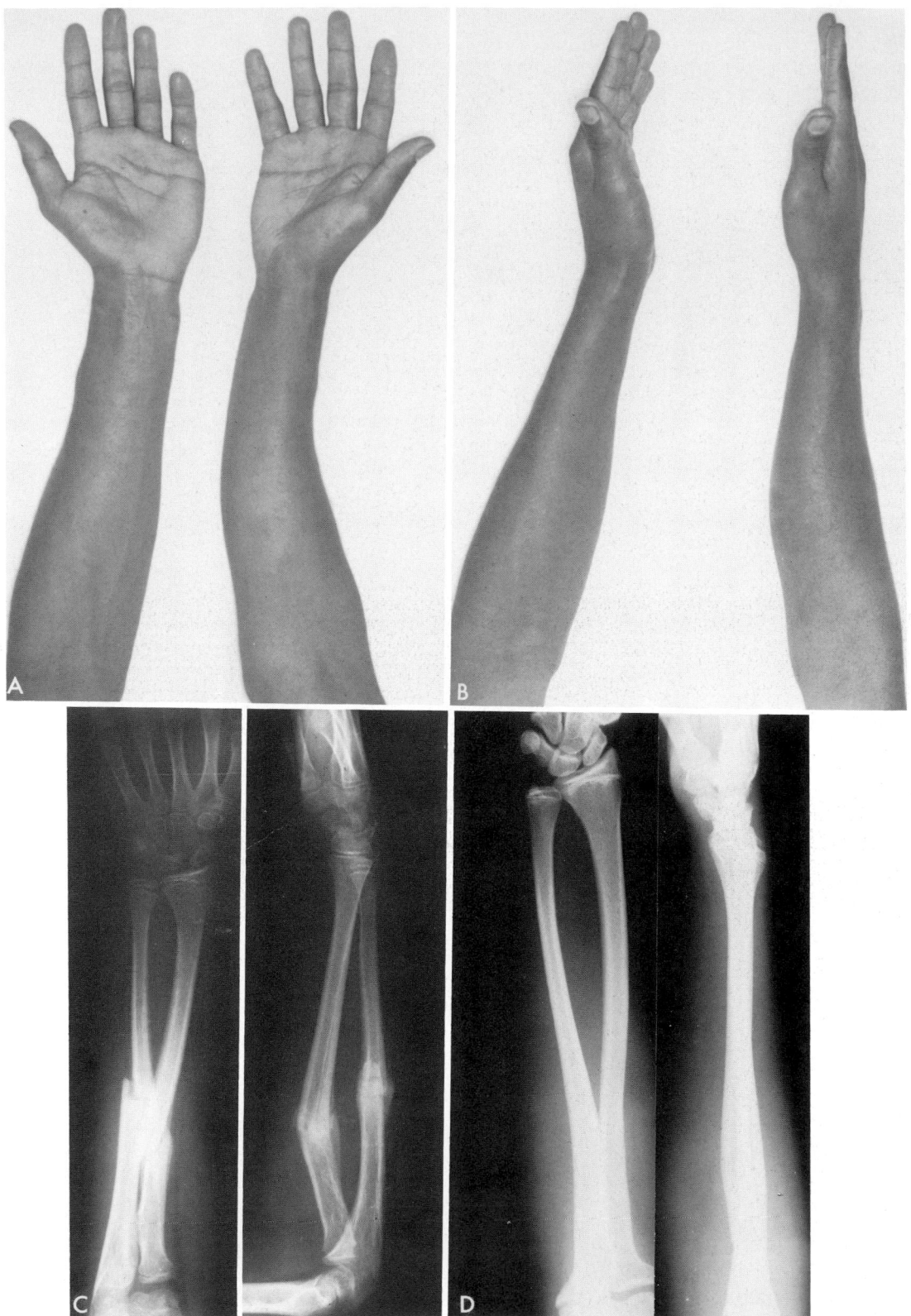

FIGURE 8–68. *Malunited fracture of both bones of the forearm at junction of middle and proximal thirds.*

A and **B.** Clinical appearance of the deformity. The distal fragment is angulated dorsally and radially. **C.** Roentgenograms showing the malalignment. **D.** Four years later. Note the spontaneous correction by remodeling.

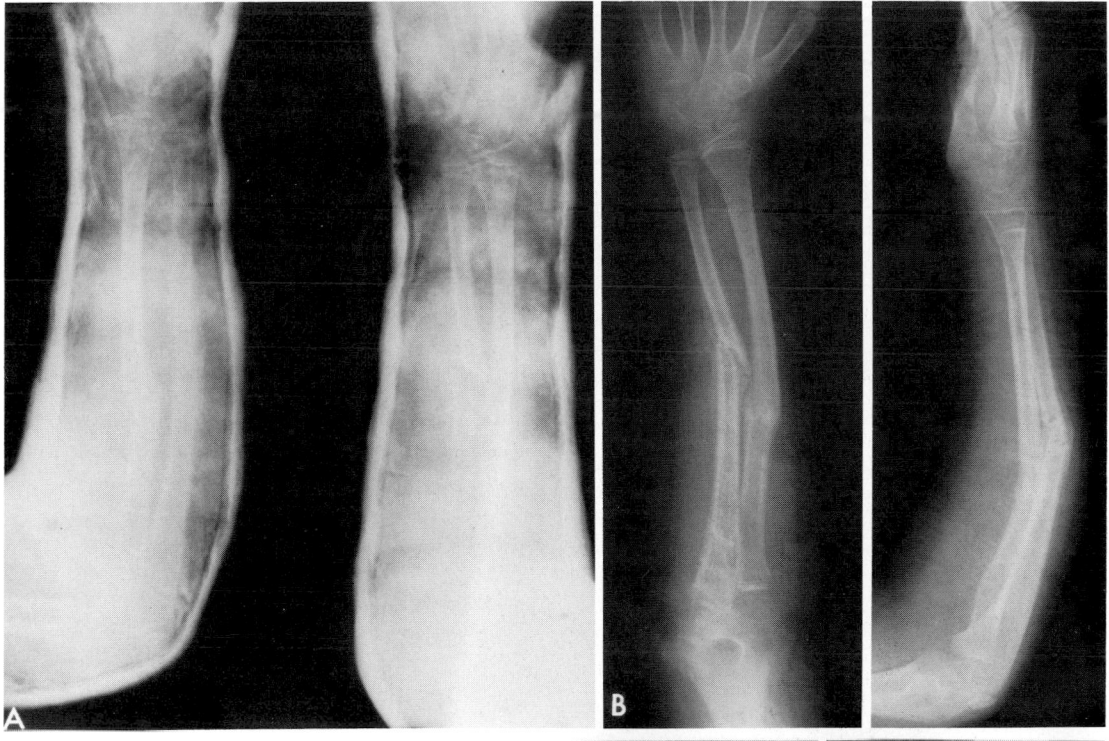

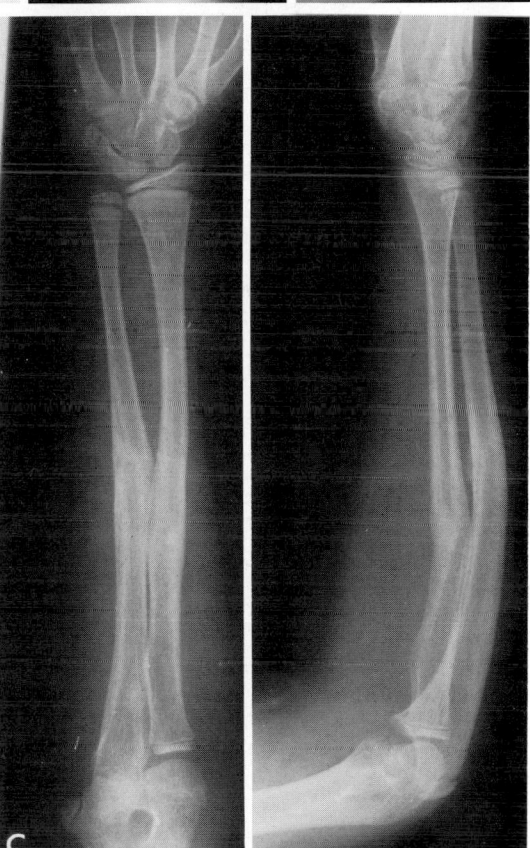

FIGURE 8–69. *"Both-bone" fractures of forearm.*

These views illustrate the importance of changing the cast when it becomes loose and obtaining a true lateral view. **A.** Roentgenograms following reduction. Alignment was interpreted to be satisfactory. Note this is an oblique and not a true lateral view. The patient was told to return in a month. **B.** On removal of the cast, the dorsal angulation of fracture fragments was noted. **C.** Six months later, remodeling has taken place.

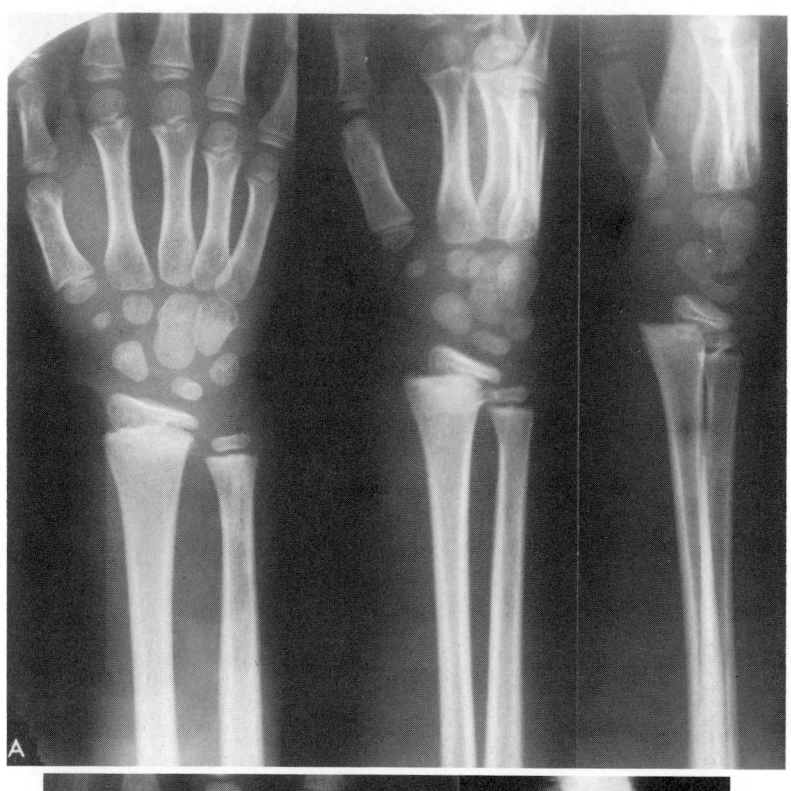

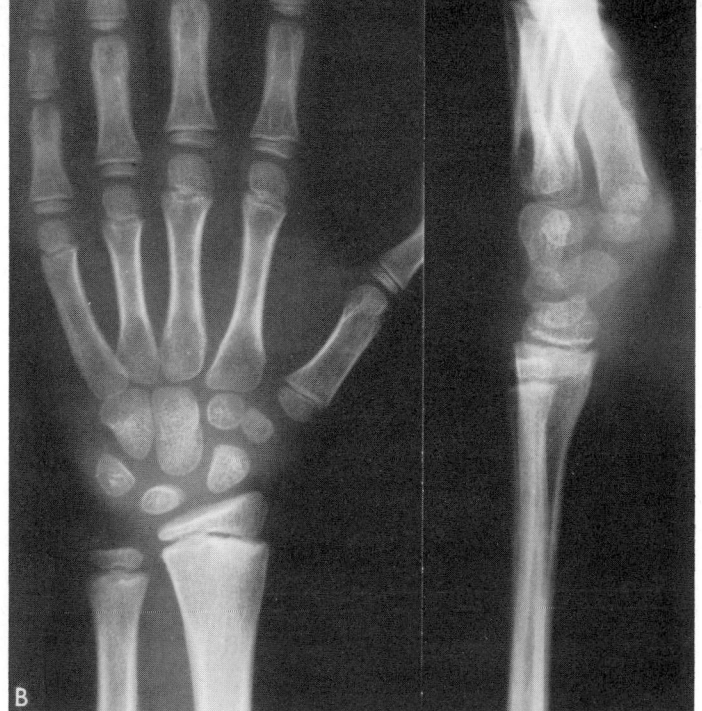

FIGURE 8–70.   *Fracture involving the distal radial physis.*

   A. Initial roentgenogram showing dorsal displacement of distal radial epiphysis. It was treated by closed reduction. **B.** Roentgenogram of same wrist a year later.

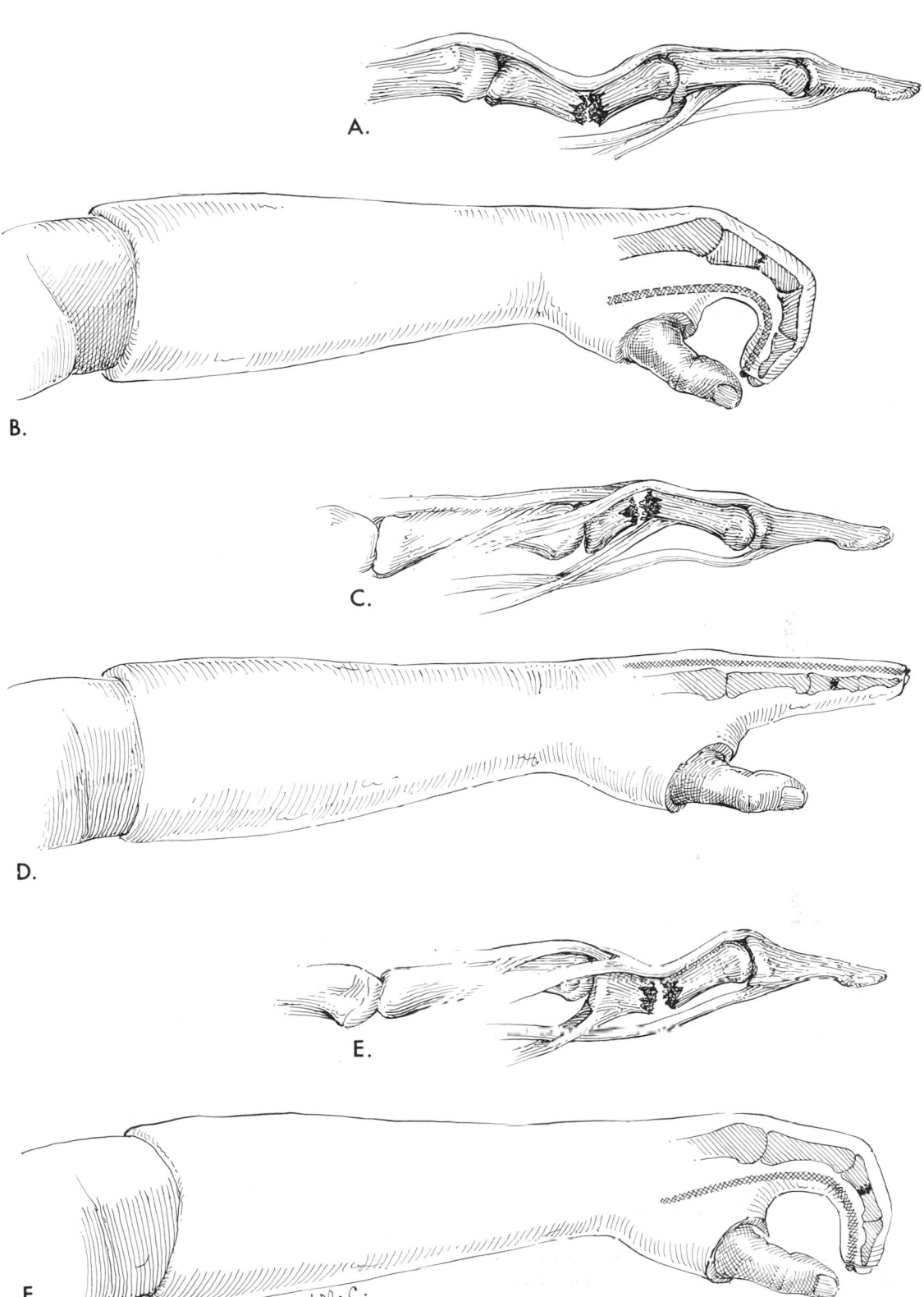

FIGURE 8–71. *Fracture of middle and proximal phalanges.*

A and **B.** Fracture of proximal phalanx. **C** and **D.** Fracture of middle phalanx proximal to insertion of flexor digitorum sublimis tendon. **E** and **F.** Fracture of middle phalanx distal to insertion of flexor digitorum sublimis tendon.

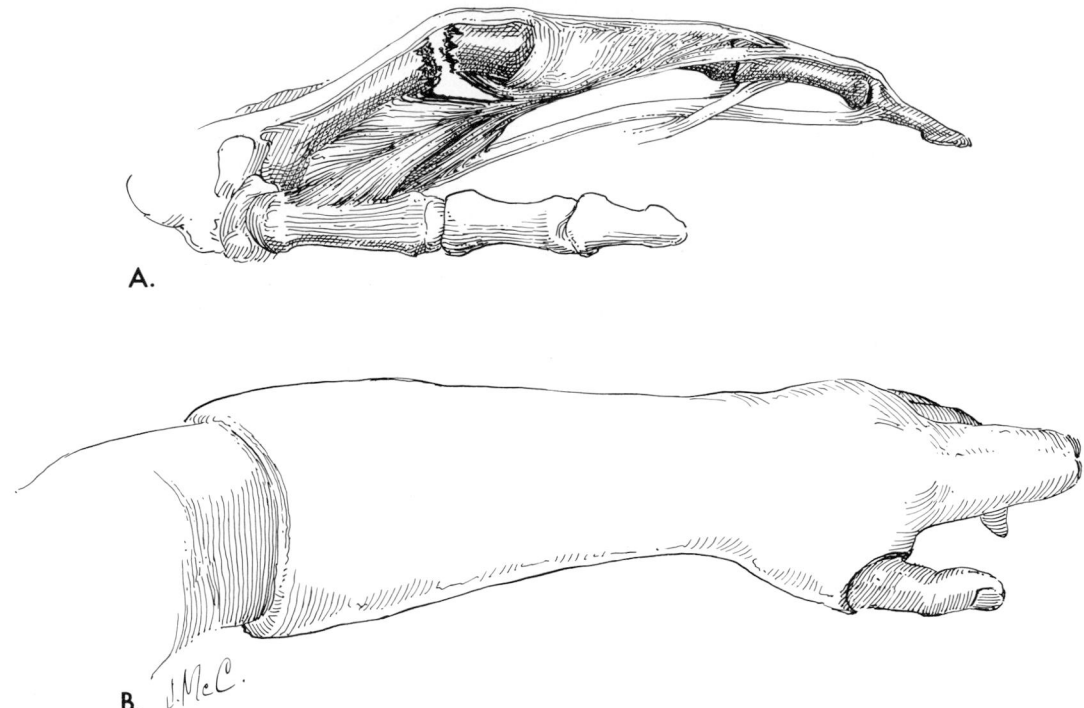

A.

B.

FIGURE 8-72. *Fracture of metacarpal (see text for explanation).*

by reversing the direction of the rollers, thus subjecting it to a second crushing. Other factors determining the severity of the damage are the length of time during which the limb was caught between the rollers, the size of the limb, the tension of the rollers, and the rapidity of their revolution.

The crushing injury is primarily to the soft tissues, i.e., the skin, subcutaneous tissue, muscles, tendons, and nerves. The bones are rarely fractured, but it is important to take roentgenograms to detect any possible damage.

Clinically, the limb may be found diffusely swollen and ecchymotic in some areas, especially in the antecubital fossa, and in the axilla. Minor abrasions are common. Occasionally there is avulsion of the skin.

Nerve and muscle function in the crushed limb is determined. There may be disruption of nerves and tearing of tendons or muscles without a break in the skin. In the beginning, it is difficult to assess the extent of the injury, and it is wise to make a guarded prognosis. Within a day or two, what appears to be a minor injury may

progress to sloughing of the regional skin and devitalization of the muscles.

Treatment

Regardless how benign the appearance of the injury, it is best to hospitalize the patient for at least two or three days to observe the progression of the damage. After proper sedation, the limb is washed with a mild antiseptic soap, a sterile compression bandage is applied, and the limb is elevated to minimize edema and further swelling.

Once a day, under aseptic precautions, the sterile compression bandage is changed and the limb is inspected for progression of injury. If there are subcutaneous collections of transudate or blood, they should be decompressed by aspiration to allow the skin to fall back into a nutritive bed. If there is sloughing of skin, the area is allowed to granulate for seven to ten days, and is then covered with a split-thickness graft. A pedicle type of graft is indicated where tendons, nerves, and bone are exposed. The joints are splinted in functional position.

The Lower Limb

TRAUMATIC DISLOCATION OF THE HIP

Seldom does a child sustain traumatic dislocation of the hip. Maffei, in a review of 1,842 cases at the Rizzoli Institute of Bologna, could find only three in children.[454] Choyce, in 1924, collected from the literature 58 cases of children with traumatic dislocation of the hip and added 6 cases of his own.[421] Mason covered the period between 1922 and 1954, studying 88 reported cases.[456] Pineschi, in 1956, presented a careful study of 150 reported cases in the world literature.[429] In 1968, the Scientific Research Committee of the Pennsylvania Orthopedic Society gave a final report based on 51 cases collected from the membership of the Society between 1959 and 1966. Earlier, they had presented the initial findings in 32 children.[407] In addition to these comprehensive reviews, the literature also contains reports of scattered cases in children, as well as general studies of traumatic dislocation of the hip in which cases in children are included.

Types

Traumatic disolocation of the hip is classified according to the position of the displaced femoral head in relation to the acetabulum (Fig. 8–73).

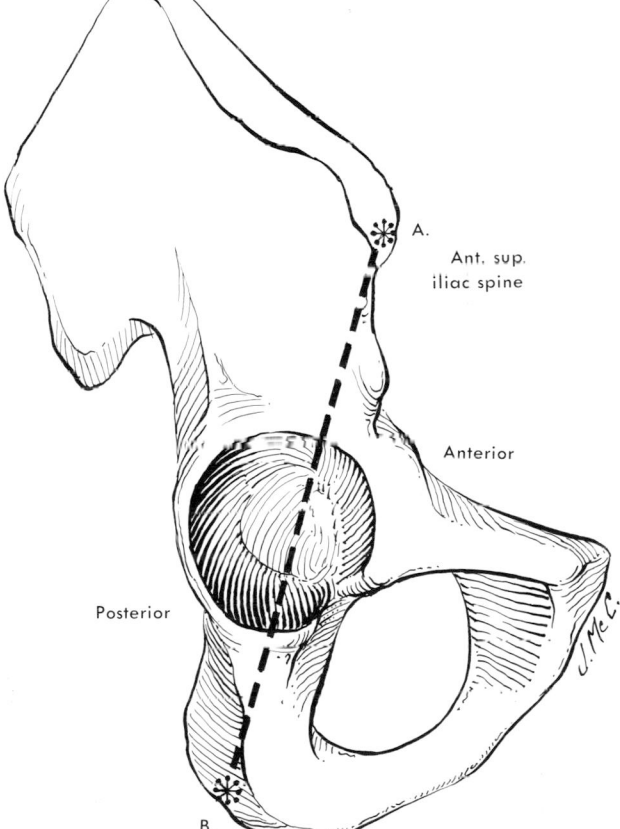

FIGURE 8–73. A line drawn from the anterior-superior iliac spine to the ischial tuberosity bisects the acetabulum, dividing anterior from posterior luxation. When the femoral head is displaced anterior to this line the dislocation is called anterior and vice versa.

A. Post. iliac
dislocation

B. Post. ischial
dislocation

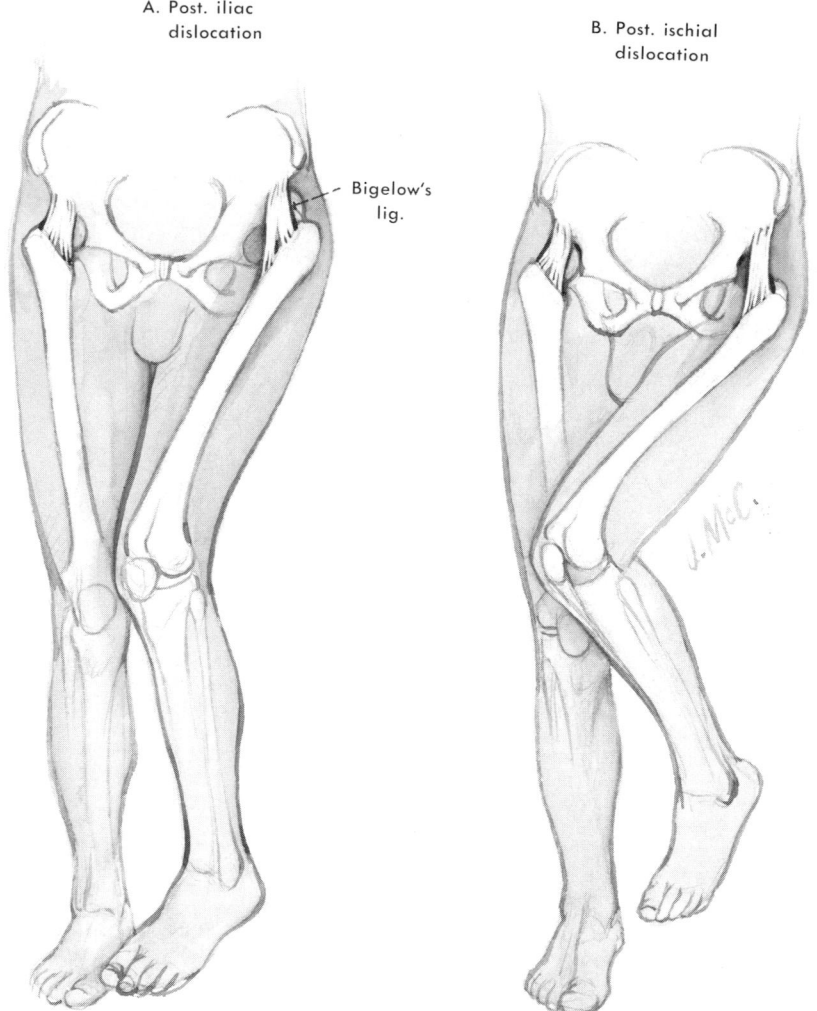

Bigelow's
lig.

FIGURE 8–74. *Types of traumatic hip dislocation.*

Posterior

Iliac—femoral head lies posteriorly and superiorly along the lateral aspect of the ilium (Fig. 8–74 A).

Ischial—femoral head is displaced posteroinferiorly and lies adjacent to the greater sciatic notch (Fig. 8–74 B).

Anterior

Obturator—femoral head lies in the region of the obturator membrane (Fig. 8–74 D). Perineal type is the extremely inferiorly displaced form of anterior dislocation.

Pubic—femoral head is displaced anterosuperiorly along the superior ramus of the pubic bone. Suprapubic type is the extremely superiorly dis-

placed form of pubic dislocation (Fig. 8–74 C).

Central—there is a comminuted fracture of the central portion of the acetabulum with displacement of the femoral head and acetabular fragments into the pelvis.

Central dislocations of the hip are actually fractures of the pelvis; however, as the associated hip-joint injury presents the greater disability, they are discussed with hip dislocation.

Stewart and Milford have further subdivided fracture-dislocations of the hip according to the severity of the associated fracture of the acetabulum or the femoral head:

Grade I: simple dislocation without frac-

C. Ant. pubic
dislocation

D. Ant. obturator
dislocation

Bigelow's
lig.

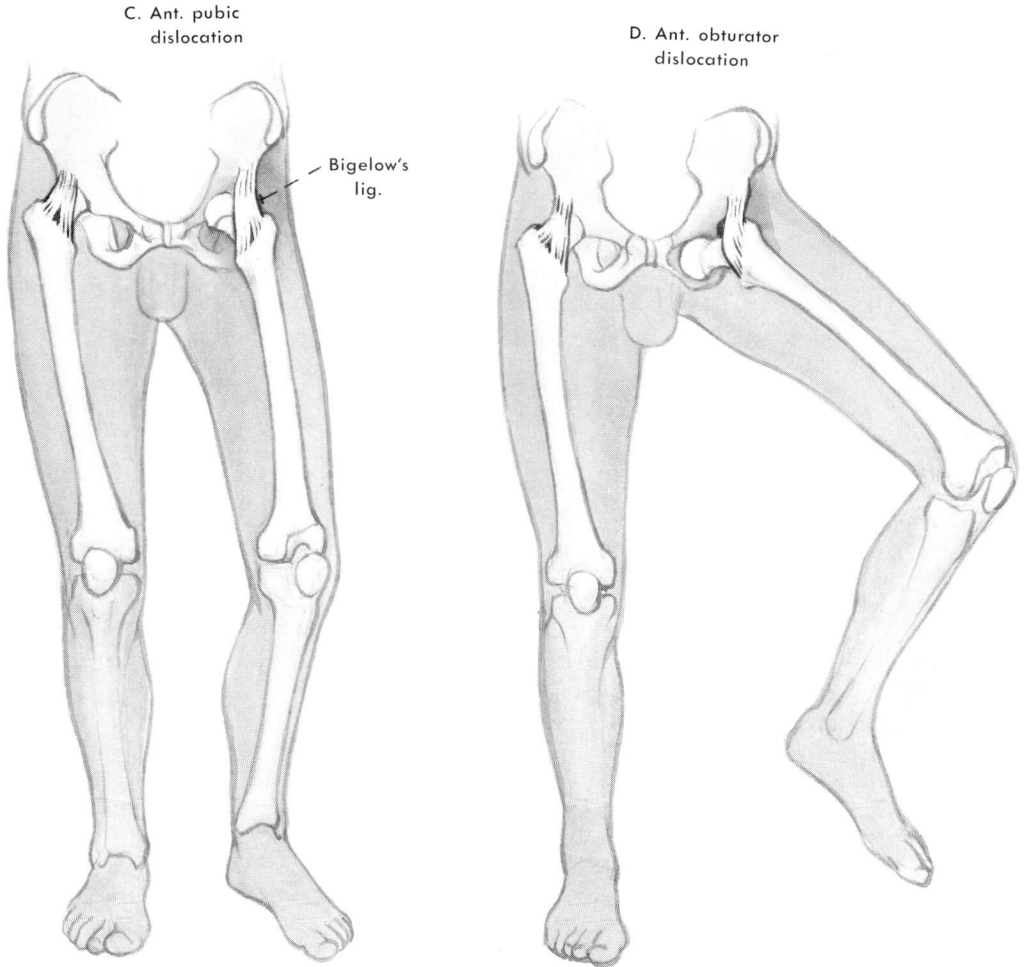

FIGURE 8-74 Continued. Types of traumatic hip dislocation.

ture or with a chip from the acetabulum so small as to be of no consequence

Grade II: dislocation with one or more large rim fragments, but with sufficient socket remaining to ensure stability after reduction

Grade III: explosive or blast fracture with disintegration of the rim of the acetabulum that produces gross instability

Grade IV: dislocation with a fracture of the head or neck of the femur

Dislocation with fracture of the femoral shaft presents a unique problem of management, and for this reason, the author recommends it be added, as a fifth grade, to the four just given.[473]

Central dislocations of the hip were classified as follows by Stewart and Milford:

Grade I Central: linear or stellate fracture through the floor of the acetabulum but without appreciable dislocation

Grade II Central: comminuted fracture with mild to moderate central displacement of the femoral head and acetabular fragments

Grade III Central: marked displacement of the fragments and protrusion of the head of the femur into the pelvis, with or without comminution of the superior portion of the acetabulum

Grade IV Central: dislocation with an associated fracture of the head or neck of the femur[473]

In children, the majority of traumatic dislocations of the hip are of the posterior type. In the 1968 study of 51 patients by the

Pennsylvania Orthopedic Society, 80 per cent of the dislocations were of the posterior type, 16 per cent anterior, and 4 per cent central.[466]

There is a definite predilection for males, the injury being four times more common in boys than in girls. It may occur in any age group, but there are two peak periods of incidence—between 4 and 7 years, and between 11 and 15 years. The right and left hips are involved equally. Very rarely are both hips dislocated.

Mechanism of Injury

Because the femoral head may become displaced out of the acetabular socket only as a result of very extreme force, its dislocation is found in persons who have been subjected to severe trauma, as in a serious automobile collision. Posterior dislocation is produced when the flexed knee strikes against the dashboard with the hip flexed and adducted. The driver of the car is more likely to sustain an associated fracture of the posterior wall of the acetabulum, because on applying the brakes, his hip is in semi-flexed position and the femoral head is displaced posterosuperiorly by the impact (Fig. 8–75 A); whereas the passenger's hip is more often in hyperflexion at the moment of the impact and the femoral head is driven downward and backward, with the acetabulum sustaining less damage (Fig. 8–75 B). In this type of injury, often there may be associated fracture of the patella, the upper end of the tibia, the femoral shaft, or the head and neck of the femur.

Anterior dislocation is usually sustained in a fall from a height, whose impact inflicts a direct blow on the posterior aspect of the abducted and externally rotated thigh (Fig. 8–76 A). The femoral head is displaced forward, commonly lying external to the obturator foramen; greater force will displace the femoral head forward and upward in the region of the pubic crest.

Central dislocations with fractures of the acetabulum are frequently caused by a direct blow to the greater trochanter, such as that which results from the impact of a falling object or a fall from a height (Fig. 8–76 B). It may also be produced in "dashboard injuries," when the hip is in an extended and abducted position at the time of the direct blow on the flexed knee.

Pathologic Anatomy

In posterior dislocation, the ligamentum teres is ruptured and the capsule is torn in its posterior aspect. The tear in the capsule may be at its pelvic attachment or femoral insertion, or may run irregularly between the two. Upon departing from the acetabular socket, the femoral head migrates and enlarges the rent in the capsule. The iliofemoral ligament (the Y-ligament of Bigelow) is usually taut, with the hip in extended position, or it may be torn (Fig. 8–77 D and E). The short external rotator muscles—obturator internus, pyriformis, obturator externus, and quadratus muscles—are either partially or completely torn with the posterior part of the capsule. Occasionally, the femoral head may push its way between the short external rotators without causing them to tear. The gluteus maximus, medius, and minimus muscles are stretched and pushed backward by the femoral head, which lies deep to or within the fibers of these muscles. The hip adductors are stretched or partially torn by the indirect force and pull of the displaced femoral head.

In anterior dislocations, the anterior part of the capsule and the ligamentum teres are ruptured. The iliofemoral ligament is usually intact (Fig. 8–77 C). Muscles in the direct path of the femoral head are stretched or may be partially torn. In the pubic type of luxation the femoral nerve may be damaged. Very occasionally femoral vessels may be injured, particularly when the femoral head is dislocated anteriorly by hyperextension of the hip.

In central dislocations, the femoral head splits the acetabulum and lies inside the pelvis. The pelvic fascia is strong, but injury to viscera in the pelvis or to the obturator nerve may occur.

Diagnostic Features

In *posterior dislocations* the deformity has a typical appearance (see Fig. 8–74 A and B). The involved lower limb is held in flexion, adduction, and internal rotation at the hip

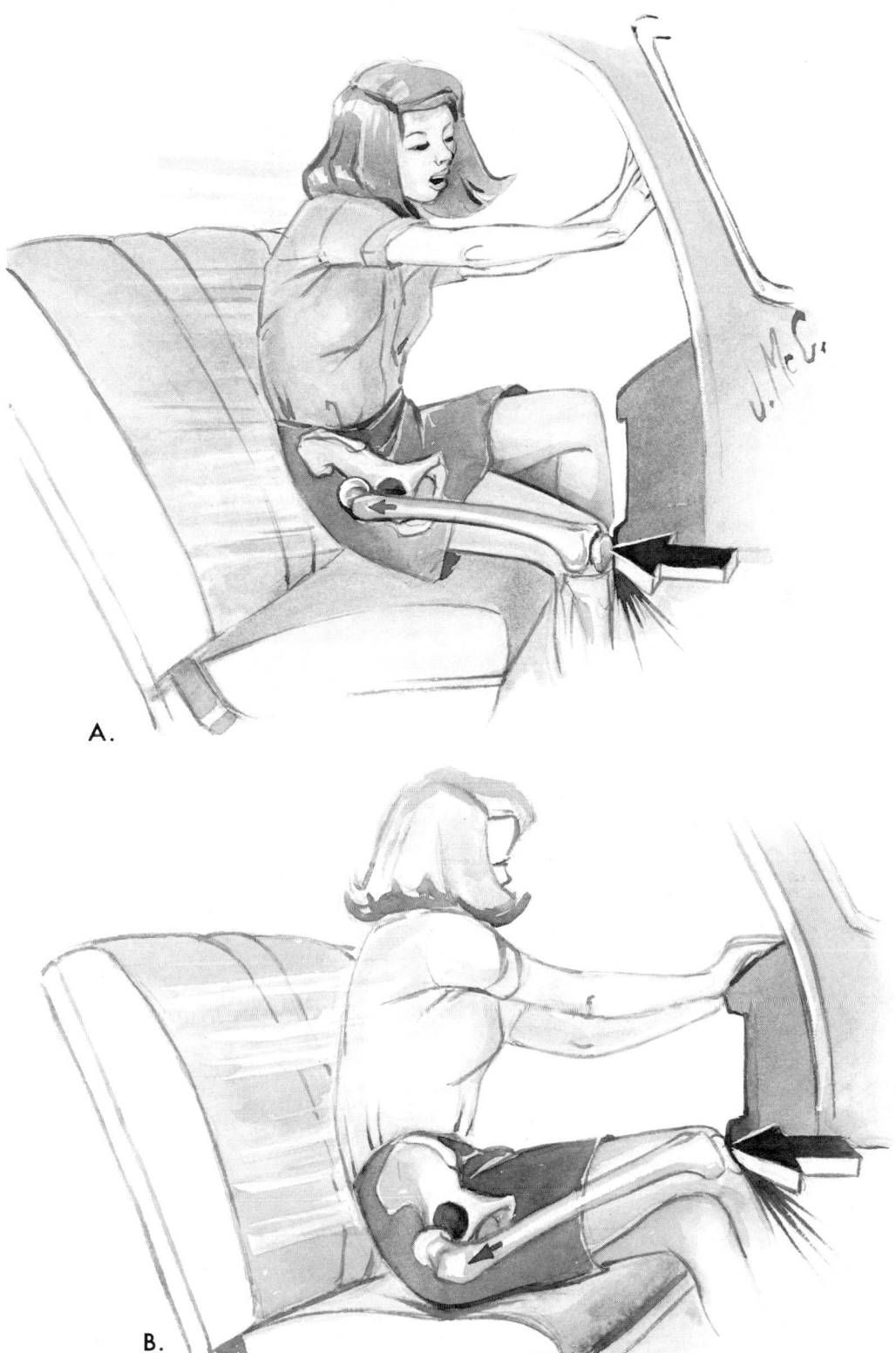

FIGURE 8–75. *Mechanism of injury in posterior dislocation of the hip (see text for explanation).*

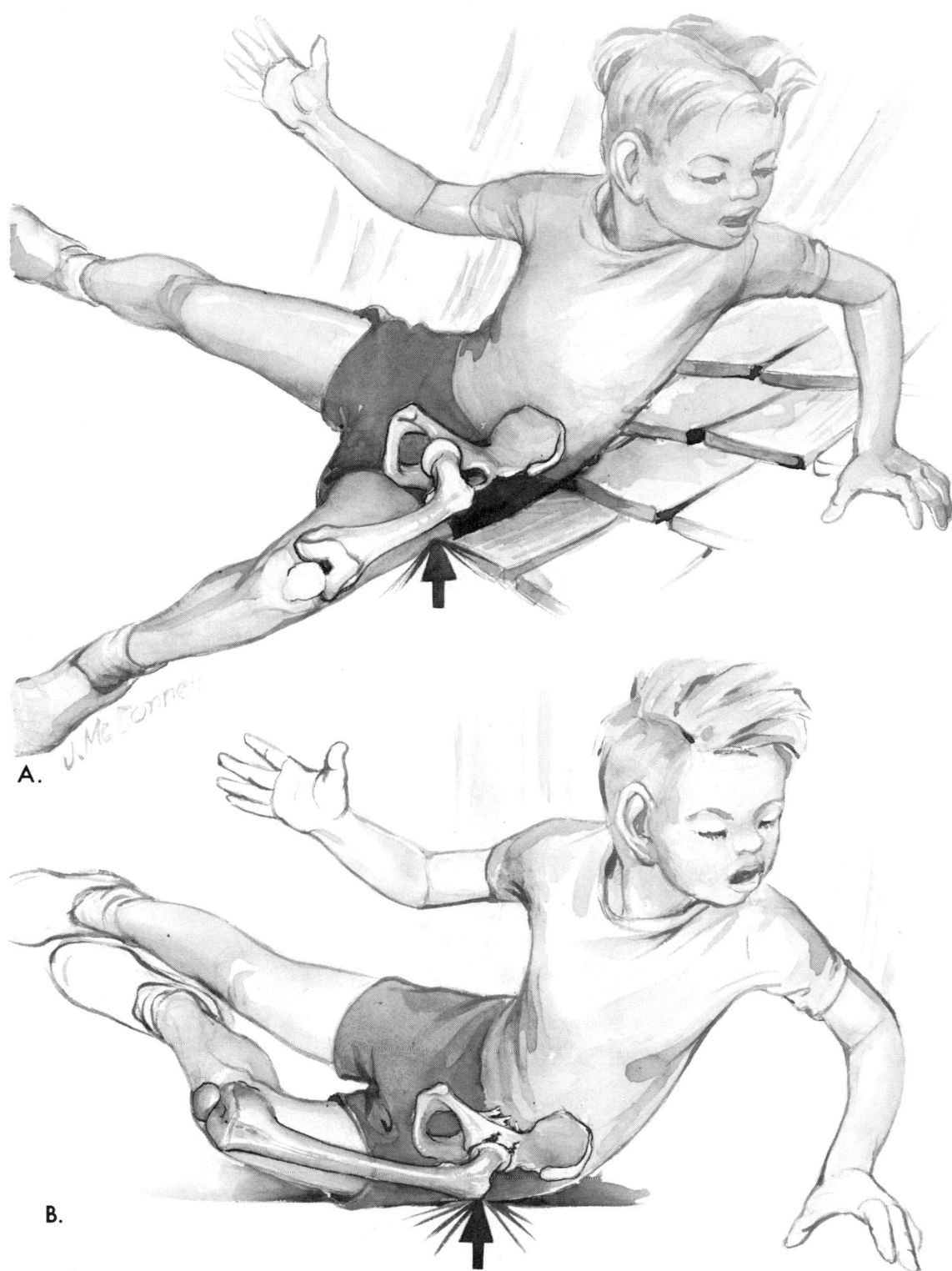

FIGURE 8–76.   *Mechanism of injury in dislocation of the hip.*
A. Anterior dislocation. **B.** Central dislocation (see text for explanation).

with the knee or foot resting on the normal leg. There is both apparent and actual shortening of the limb. The femoral head cannot be palpated in its normal location deep to the femoral vessels below the inguinal ligament; occasionally, it may be palpable posteriorly in the gluteal region. The patient is in excruciating pain and is unable to stand or walk on the affected limb. Any motion of the hip is painful and guarded by muscle spasm. Extension, abduction, and external rotation of the hip are markedly restricted. Flexion and internal rotation contracture of the hip are primarily produced by tension on the Y-ligament of Bigelow; they are directly proportionate to the amount the femoral head is displaced out of the acetabular socket. When the Y-ligament is torn (referred to as the "irregular type of hip dislocation" by Bigelow), the limb lies in external rotation, with no restriction of hip extension and external rotation (Fig. 8–77 E).

Posterior dislocations are commonly of the iliac type, with the femoral head lying between the sciatic notch and the acetabulum. High iliac luxations with the femoral head up, behind, and definitely on the lateral surface of the ilium are rare. Ischial posterior luxations are also uncommon.

In *anterior dislocations*, the hip is held in abduction, external rotation, and some flexion. There is fullness in the region of the obturator foramen, where the femoral head may be palpable. Because of its abducted position, there is apparent lengthening of the limb. Motion of the hip is markedly restricted, with almost no adduction and external rotation. In pubic luxations, the femoral head is displaced upward and forward, lying inferior to the pubic ramus or riding on it, in which case, it can be easily palpated. There is loss of prominence of the greater trochanter (Fig. 8–74 C and D).

In *central dislocations* with fractures of the acetabulum, all motions of the hip are markedly restricted by muscle spasm. The limb is not maintained in any characteristic deformed posture. Shortening is minimal. The lateral aspect of the hip is flattened because of inward displacement of the greater trochanter. Intrapelvic hemorrhage is common, as evidenced by the finding of suprapubic dullness on percussion of the abdomen. On rectal examination, a tender mass may be palpated deep to the fractured acetabulum, and the femoral head may be felt.

Roentgenograms will disclose the specific type of dislocation (Figs. 8–78 and 8–79). It is imperative that adequate films be made and associated fractures be ruled out.

In the badly injured patient, failure to examine and x-ray the hip joint adequately is a common pitfall, and fracture-dislocations of the hip have often been overlooked.

Treatment

Reduction of traumatic dislocation of the hip should be immediate; the longer it is delayed, the more difficult is the reduction and the poorer the prognosis.

Forceful manipulations must be avoided. It is best to administer a general anesthetic to obtain complete muscle relaxation.

The chief obstacle to reduction in posterior hip dislocation is the iliofemoral ligament, which is perhaps the strongest ligament in the body. Its somewhat triangular shape resembles an inverted Y, and it is often referred to as the Y-ligament of Bigelow. The apex of the ligament is in the markedly thickened fibers of the longitudinal fibers of the capsule, originating in the anteroinferior iliac spine and extending downward across the anterior aspect of the hip joint to be attached to the anterior intertrochanteric line. As it passes distally, it becomes broad and tends to separate into two bands; for this reason, its base may be considered to have a bifid attachment (Fig. 8–77).

Normally, the iliofemoral ligament limits hyperextension and lateral rotation of the hip joint—an important function, because in stance the weight of the body tends to rotate the pelvis posteriorly upon the two femoral heads.

CLOSED REDUCTION OF POSTERIOR DISLOCATION

The three methods of closed reduction of posterior dislocation are those of Bigelow, Allis, and Stimson, all of which utilize the principle of hip flexion, causing the Y-ligament to relax, and bringing the femoral

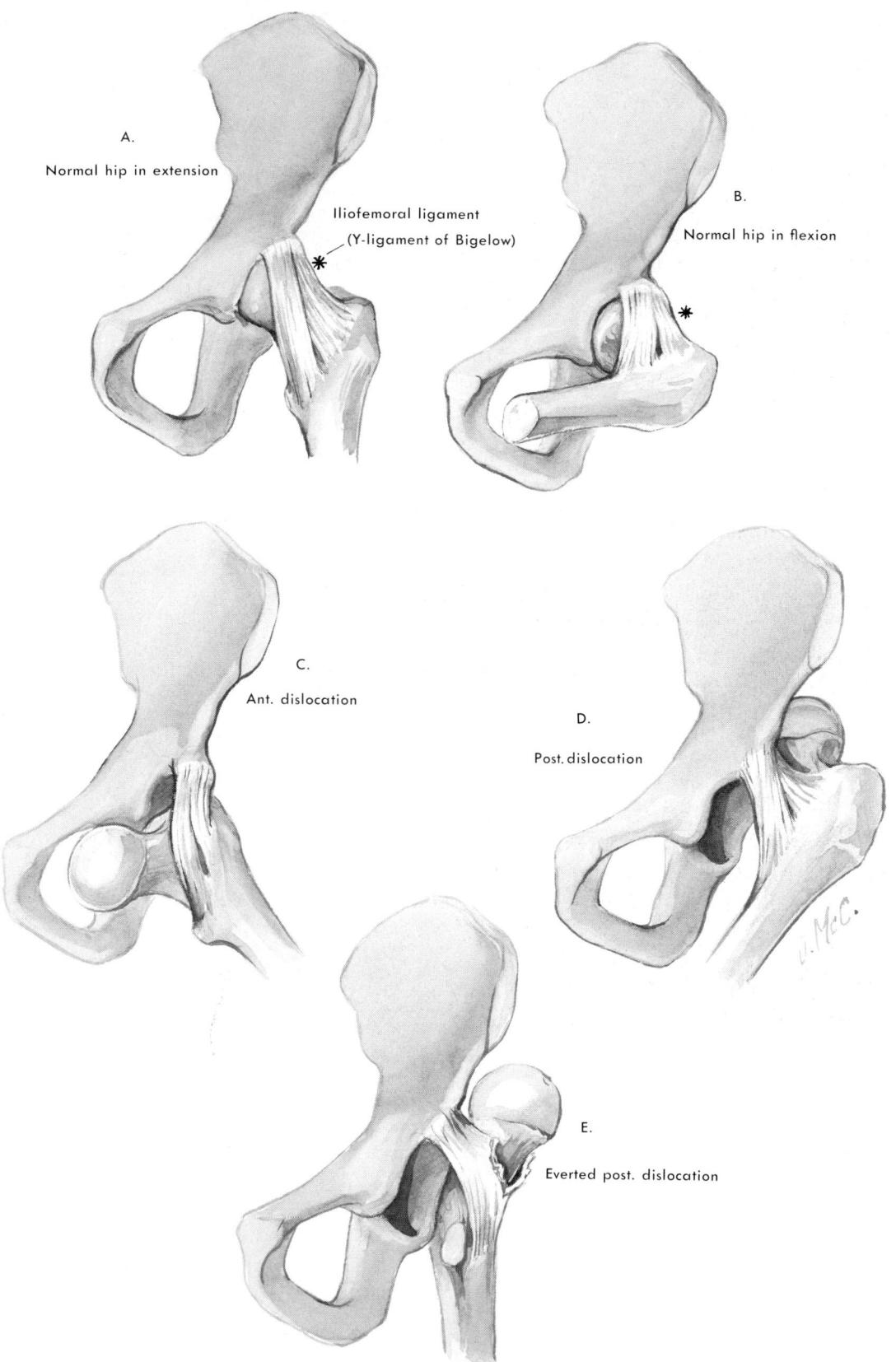

FIGURE 8–77. *The iliofemoral ligament (or Y-ligament of Bigelow).* *See opposite page for legend.*

1658

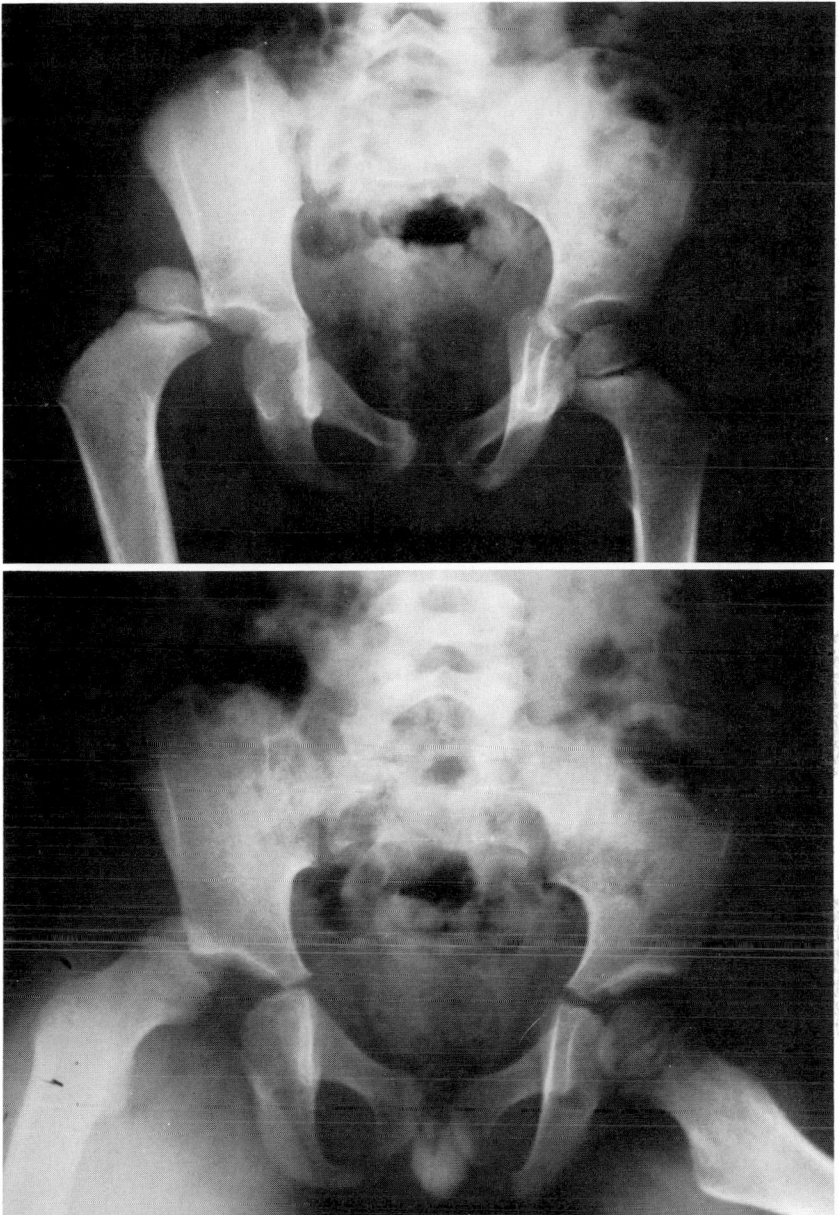

FIGURE 8-78. Traumatic posterior dislocation of right hip—iliac type.

FIGURE 8-77. The iliofemoral ligament (or Y-ligament of Bigelow).

A. Normal ligament with the hip in extension. **B.** With hip in flexion it is relaxed. **C.** Anterior dislocation. **D.** Posterior dislocation. **E.** In everted posterior dislocation it is partially torn.

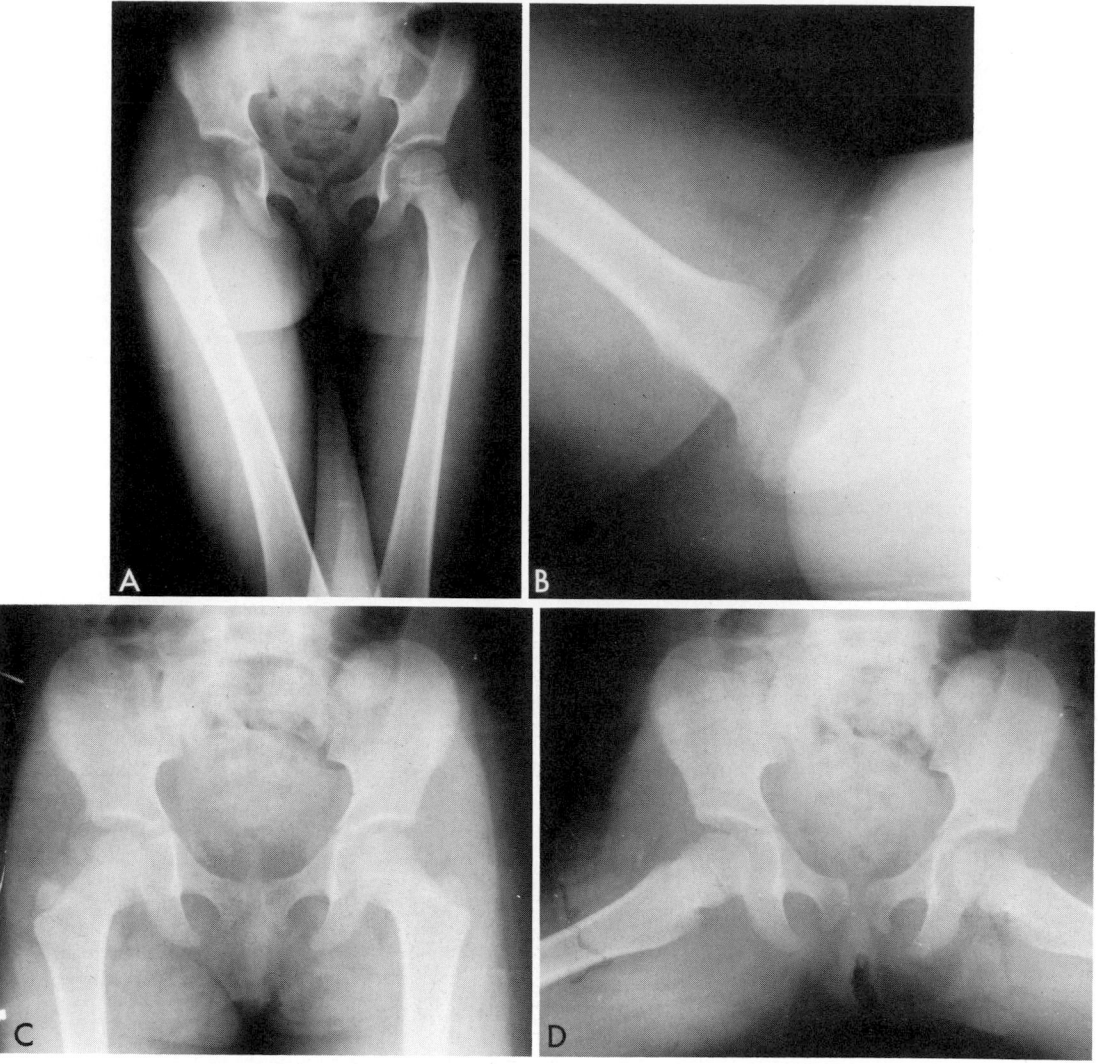

FIGURE 8–79.   Traumatic posterior dislocation of right hip—ischial type.

A and **B.** Initial roentgenograms. **C** and **D.** Postreduction views. It is imperative that adequate films be obtained to rule out the presence of associated fractures.

head adjacent to the acetabular margin near the rent in the capsule.

Gravity Method of Stimson (Fig. 8–80). The patient is placed in prone position with his lower limbs hanging free from the end of the table. His pelvis is immobilized by an assistant who presses down on the sacrum. With his left hand, the surgeon holds the ankle and flexes the knee of the injured limb to 90 degrees, and with his right hand, applies downward pressure to the leg just below the bent knee. Gentle rocking or rotatory motions of the limb and direct pressure

over the femoral head may assist in the reduction. This method is the least forcible and most desirable, as it utilizes the weight of the limb to help the reduction. If necessary, a sandbag may be strapped to the leg to relax the tight muscles.

"Direct Method" of Allis (Fig. 8–81).   The patient is placed in supine position on the floor and his pelvis is immobilized by an assistant or by the surgeon's foot pressing on the anterior superior iliac spine. The hip and knee of the affected hip are flexed to 90 degrees, with the thigh in slight adduction and medial rotation. Then, with his forearm behind the knee, the surgeon applies vertical traction, and the femoral head is lifted over the posterior rim of the acetabulum, through the hole in the capsule, into the acetabular socket. The hip and knee are then gently extended. Occasionally one encounters soft-tissue resistance when lifting the femoral head; in such an instance, the capsule is first relaxed by increasing the degree of hip adduction and medial rotation, and reduction is again attempted by lifting the femoral head anteriorly and extending the hip. If this is unsuccessful, excessive force should be avoided because the femoral head may be caught by the short rotator muscles or by the sciatic nerve. Reduction is again initiated from the first step; however, this time, after the hip is flexed, it is gently rotated laterally to disengage the

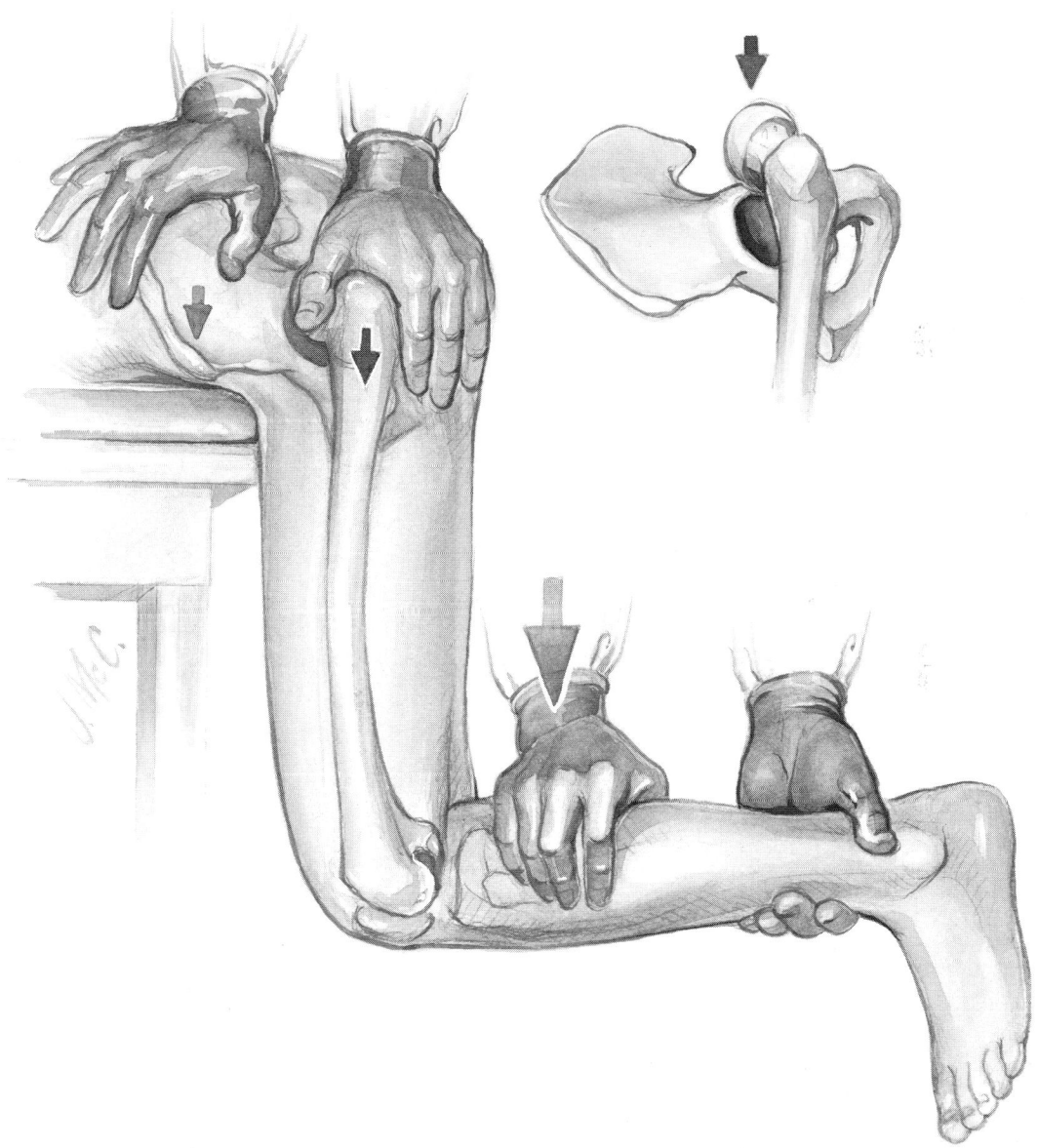

FIGURE 8–80. *Gravity method of reduction (Stimson) of traumatic posterior dislocation of the hip (see text for explanation).*

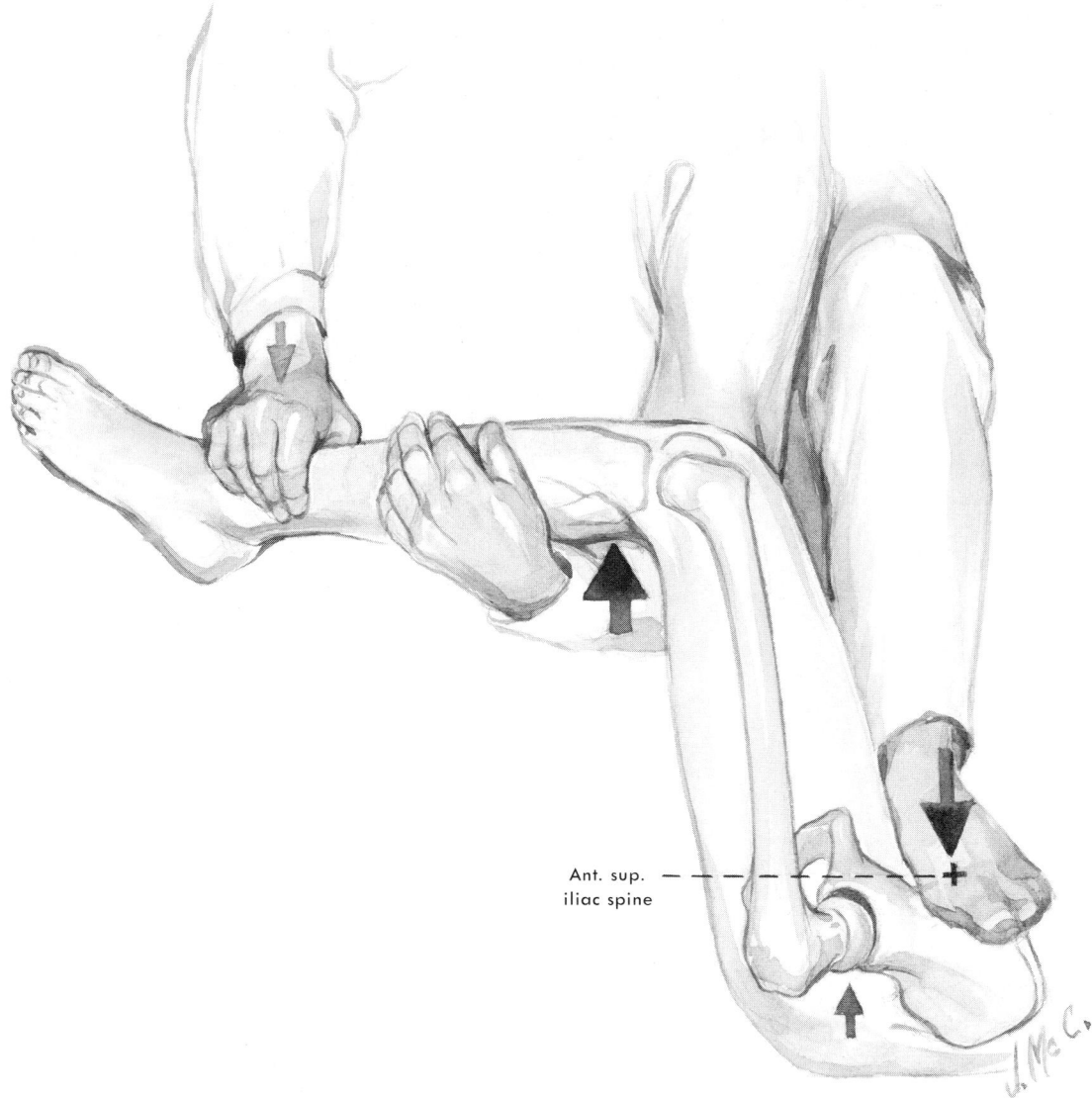

Ant. sup.
iliac spine

FIGURE 8–81. *"Direct" method (Allis) of reduction of posterior dislocation of the hip (see text for explanation).*

femoral head from the soft tissues. Direct pressure may be applied over the femoral head to assist it to slip back into place.

Circumduction Method of Bigelow (Fig. 8–82). The fully anesthetized patient is placed supine on the floor. An assistant applies countertraction by pressing downward on the anterior superior iliac spines and the ilia. If an assistant is not available, an alternate method is for the surgeon to apply pressure with his foot over the anterior superior iliac spine. The surgeon then grasps the affected limb at the ankle with one hand and places his opposite forearm behind the knee. First, the adducted and internally rotated thigh is flexed 90 degrees or more on the abdomen and longitudinal traction is applied in the line of the deformity. This maneuver will relax the Y-ligament and bring the femoral head near the posterior rim of the acetabulum. The femoral head is then freed from the rotator muscles by gently rotating and "rocking" the thigh forward and backward. Next, while traction is maintained, the femoral head is levered into the acetabulum by gentle abduction, ex-

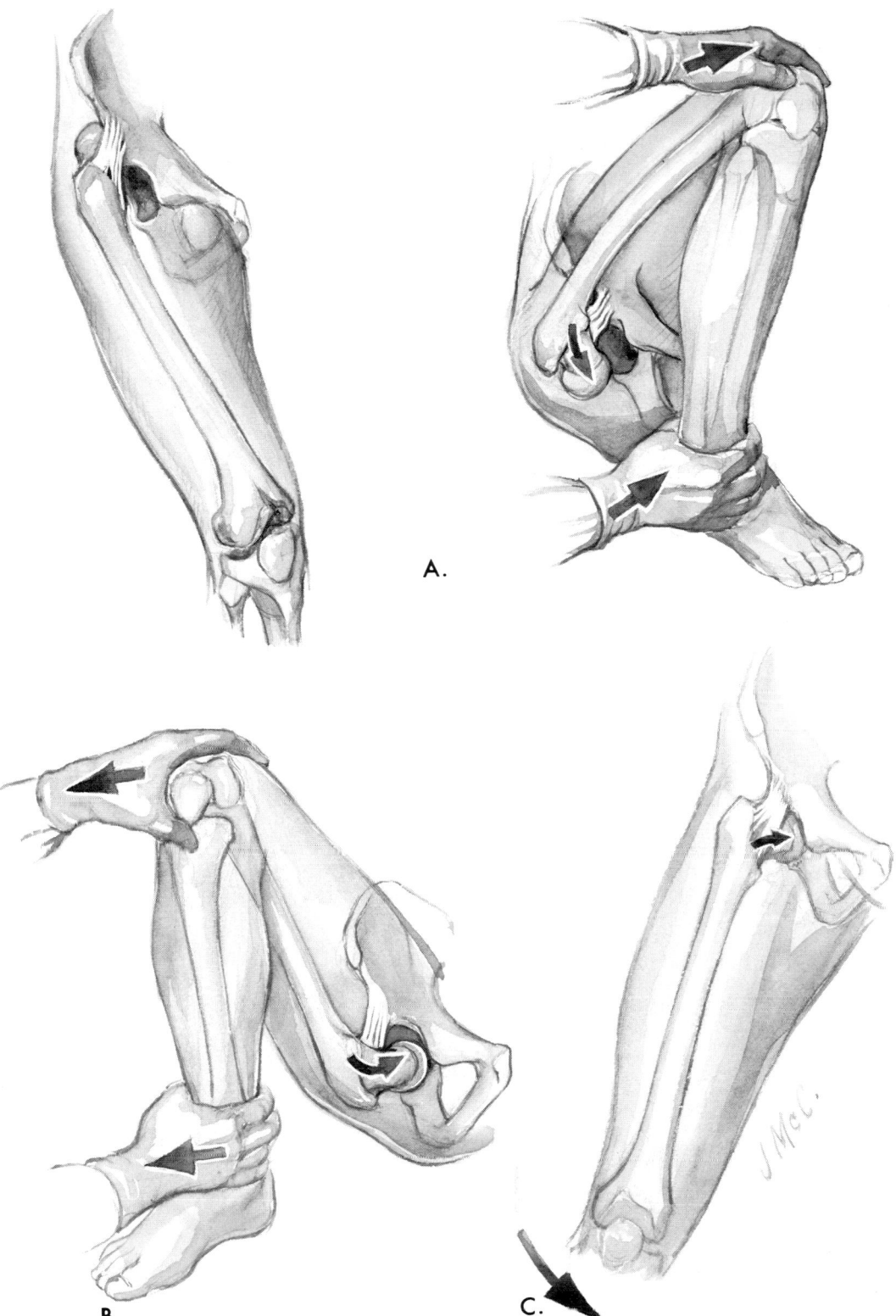

FIGURE 8–82. *Circumduction method (Bigelow) of reduction of posterior dislocation of the hip (see text for explanation).*

ternal rotation, and extension of the hip. During extension, the iliofemoral ligament is used as a fulcrum to force the femoral head into the acetabular socket. One must avoid excessive force in order to prevent rupture of the Y-ligament or damage to the sciatic nerve.

CLOSED REDUCTION OF ANTERIOR DISLOCATION

With anterior and medial displacement of the femoral head, no bony fulcrum is available to be used for reduction. The iliofemoral ligament lies across the femoral neck. During manipulation the femoral head is dislodged and brought opposite the tear in the capsule through which it is levered into the acetabular socket. The simplest and safest method is that of *Allis' reduction*. With the anesthetized patient in supine position on the floor, the following maneuver is carried out: (1) Flex the knee to relax the hamstrings. (2) Fully abduct the hip and bring it into flexion, the exact degree depending upon whether the femoral head is in the obturator or pubic location (Fig. 8–83 A). (3) Apply longitudinal traction in line with the longitudinal axis of the femur. (4) An assistant should fix the femoral head with the palm of his hand. Then, using the patient's thigh as the lever and the assistant's hand as the fulcrum while maintaining moderate traction, the surgeon gently adducts the hip and replaces the femoral head in the acetabulum (Fig. 8–83 B and C). The hip may be medially rotated as it is adducted to achieve reduction. Occasionally it is necessary to utilize a reverse Bigelow maneuver in which the hip is partially flexed and abducted; then, with moderate traction applied in line with the longitudinal axis of the femur, the hip is adducted in flexion, sharply internally rotated, and extended. Circumduction is in a clockwise direction.

Postoperative Care

Following reduction, roentgenograms are made to confirm its completeness. Again, x-rays are carefully scrutinized to rule out the possibility of any associated fractures. Reduction is maintained in a one and one half

hip spica cast with the affected hip in neutral extension and some abduction. In simple dislocations, the period of immobilization is four weeks in young children and six weeks in adolescents—this period should be sufficient for healing of capsular and soft-tissue structures. Following removal of the cast, the hip is partially protected with a three-point crutch gait. As soon as pain-free full range of motion of the hip is obtained, the patient is allowed to bear full weight with no protection, as the general consensus of various authors is that a prolonged period without weight-bearing neither prevents aseptic necrosis nor does it affect the prognosis.

Fracture-Dislocations of the Hip

The method of treatment depends upon the severity of associated fracture of the acetabulum or the femoral head. Grade I and Grade II fracture-dislocations are treated by closed reduction and immobilization in a hip spica cast for six weeks.[473] Grades III and IV fracture-dislocations always require open reduction and internal fixation of the acetabular fragments with screws. These injuries are very rare in children; the reader is referred to King and Richards for a description of operative technique.[447]

Central Dislocations of the Hip

These are essentially comminuted fractures of the central portion of the acetabulum with displacement of the fragments and the femoral head into the pelvis. Associated injury to the pelvic viscera should be ruled out.

Reduction is achieved by skeletal traction applied through a Kirschner wire inserted into the distal femoral metaphysis. In moderate inward displacements, it is best to also apply direct lateral traction through a large screw or Kirschner wire (inserted in an anteroposterior plane) through the greater trochanter. After two or three weeks, the lateral traction is discontinued and distal traction is increased to correct upward displacement and to maintain the reduction. Active exercises are performed while the

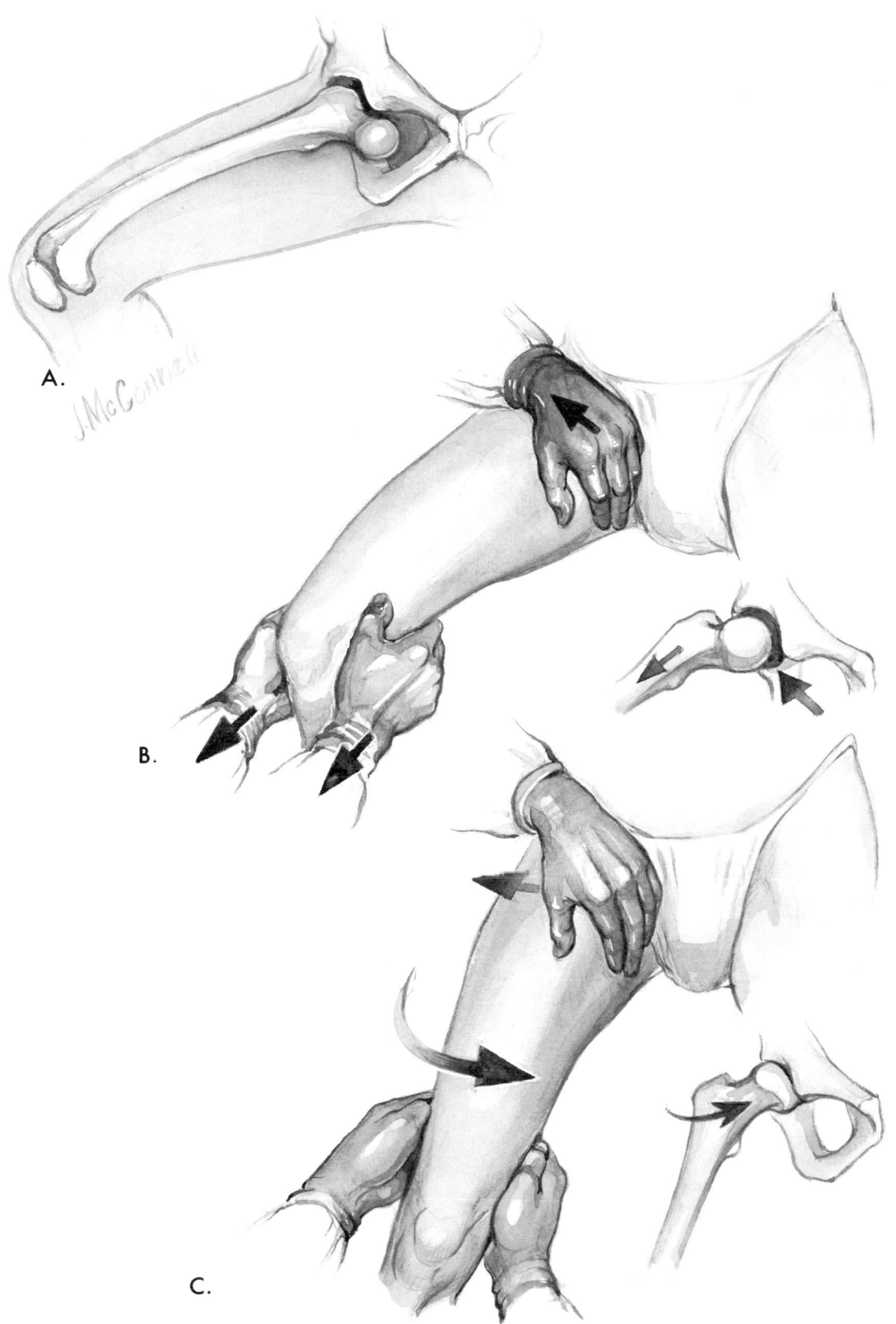

A.

B.

C.

FIGURE 8–83. *Closed reduction of anterior dislocation of the hip by the method of Allis (see text for explanation).*

patient is in traction to mold the acetabulum.

Complications

These may be aseptic necrosis, sciatic nerve palsy, degenerative arthritis of the hip, myositis ossificans, and recurrence of hip dislocation.

ASEPTIC NECROSIS

This complication occurs in 10 per cent of the cases. Factors that influence the incidence of avascular necrosis are a delay in reduction over 24 hours, and severe trauma to the hip joint. In the very young patient, there appears to be some protection against aseptic necrosis. According to the Pennsylvania Orthopedic Society study, the zero to five year age group had the lowest incidence of this complication.[467] Treatment of avascular necrosis of the femoral head follows the same principles as those described for treatment of Legg-Perthes disease.

Sciatic nerve palsy is rare in children because of the low incidence of associated fracture. When sciatic nerve palsy fails to show evidence of improvement in four to eight weeks, exploration is warranted. *Degenerative arthritis* in a child develops much less frequently than in an adult following traumatic dislocation of the hip.

RECURRENT POST-TRAUMATIC DISLOCATION OF THE HIP

Recurrent dislocation of the hip due to marked ligamentous laxity is not uncommon in children, particularly in those with Down's syndrome. Recurrent post-traumatic dislocation of the hip is rare, however. Sullivan, Bickel and Lipscomb reported one such case and traced several others of recurrent dislocation of the hip unassociated with fracture, acetabular dysplasia, sepsis, or paralysis.[474] Brav reported four cases of redislocation in 264 traumatic dislocations of the hip (1.5 per cent); however, only one of his cases was not associated with fracture of the acetabulum or the femoral head.[417] Eleven cases of recurrent post-traumatic dislocation of the hip have been reported in children—five cases found

by Choyce in a review of the literature;[421] and one each by Freeman, Funk, Aufranc et al., Hohmann, and Townsend et al.[411, 430, 431, 444, 476] In the majority of these cases, there were aseptic necrotic changes in the femoral head.

An important etiologic factor is inadequate immobilization of the hip following reduction, with consequent incomplete healing of the capsule. Liebenberg and Dommisse, in their report of two cases of recurrent post-traumatic dislocation in adults, noted that the initial dislocation was caused by major trauma; often there was a significant delay in reduction. Subsequent dislocations followed slight injury. At operation, they found a large synovium-lined pouch or false joint cavity communicating with the true joint cavity through a broad defect in the posterior capsule. The ligamentum teres was ruptured and could not be found at operation. The hips could not be dislocated by applying moderate force unless intra-articular levers were used. On the basis of these anatomic findings, Liebenberg and Dommisse proposed the following theory:

The synovial fluid flows freely through the capsular defect between the hip joint space and the pseudocavity. During normal locomotion and movement of the lower limb, changes of volume within the two cavities occur, and the flow of fluid from one cavity to the other represents a normal adjustment of unequal hydrostatic pressures. Under certain circumstances consequent to temporary closure of the valvelike posterior defect, an increase of hydrostatic pressure of the fluid within the true cavity of the hip joint could develop. This pressure differential could be of such magnitude that it could force the femoral head across the acetabular rim, through the capsular defect, and into the pseudocavity. They believe the most important factor in development of the pseudocavity is probably a delay in reduction of the dislocation.[450]

Treatment consists of excision of the posterior pouch and repair of the capsular defect. If there is a defect or erosion of the fibrocartilaginous labrum, it is reinforced by bone blocks.[443, 450, 462, 474]

Failure to detect associated fractures of the femoral shaft, the patella, or the tibial plateau is a common pitfall. Conversely, in femoral shaft fractures, traumatic dislocation of the hip should always be ruled out.

FRACTURES OF THE NECK OF THE FEMUR

Fractures of the femoral neck are rare in children and indeed were hardly known to exist until the latter part of the nineteenth century. The initial case reports in the English literature were those of Barber, in 1871, and Cromwell, in 1885.[483, 491] Whitman, in 1891, described a fracture of the femoral neck in a child, and subsequently, in a series of papers (the last of which appeared in 1909), reported a total of 31 cases.[518-522] Most of Whitman's cases were encountered prior to the discovery of x-rays, and were recognized late because of the presence of coxa vara. Russell, in 1898, in his report of two femoral neck fractures in children, stressed the importance of distinguishing this rare injury from various diseases of the hip joint.[508] In 1917, Taylor reported six cases;[512] and Bland-Sutton, in 1918, described the pathologic features of an anatomic specimen, dated 1893, of an intracapsular fracture of the neck of a child's femur found in the museum of Middlesex Hospital.[485]

The rarity of this injury is indicated by the scanty literature with few case reports on the subject; 12 cases by Colonna, 10 cases by Wilson, 10 cases by Carrell and Carrell, 8 cases by Allende and Lezama, and 24 cases by McDougall.[482, 487, 489, 490, 501, 523]

Detailed studies of a large series of cases were recently reported. Ratliff, in 1962, described 71 cases (19 of his own and 52 those of other local surgeons) and later, in 1966, he added 49, a total of 120 cases.[506, 507] Lam's study in 1971 comprised 75 fractures of the femoral neck; he was personally responsible for the care of 57 of them.[500]

At the Manchester Royal Infirmary, in 12 consecutive years (1947–1959), seven children with femoral neck fractures were admitted, as opposed to 900 adults with the same injury. In an eight-year period (beginning of 1962 to end of 1969), of 260 fractures admitted to the Children's Memorial Hospital, Chicago, only 8 involved the femoral neck, a relative incidence of about 3 per cent.

The injury is more common in boys, with the male to female ratio being approximately 3:2. Lam, however, reports 57 of the 75 fractures in boys, or approximately 75 per cent.[500] The fracture may occur at any age, with the highest incidence between 11 and 12 years.

Classification

Fractures of the hip in children are classified according to anatomic location into four types (originally developed by Delbet and subsequently popularized by Colonna).[492]

Type I, or *transepiphyseal*—an acute traumatic separation of a previously normal epiphysis. It should not be confused with an acute slip of the upper femoral epiphysis. Anatomically, it is similar to the Type I epiphyseal injury of Salter and Harris.

Type II or *transcervical*—the mid-portion of the femoral neck.

Type III or *cervicotrochanteric*—the base of the femoral neck.

Type IV or *pertrochanteric*—between the base of the femoral neck and the lesser trochanter. The incidence of various types of fractures is shown in Table 8–3.

In the newborn there is another type of injury to the hip, namely, birth fracture of the metaphysis of the femoral neck (Fig. 8–84). As the capital femoral and greater trochanteric epiphyses are not yet ossified, these fractures are often mistaken for dislocation of the hip. Metaphyseal birth fractures and pathologic fractures of the femoral neck are considered elsewhere.

Mechanism of Injury

In children the femoral neck and head are hard and the force required to break them is considerable—such as that of a fall from a height, an automobile accident, or a fall off a bicycle. (In the latter the saddle of the bicycle is wedged against the perineum and acts as a fulcrum over which the femoral neck fractures.) This is in contrast to the fractures of the femoral neck in the elderly adult, in whom the osteoporotic bone breaks because of such minimal trauma as tripping over a carpet.

Because of the nature of severe violence producing the hip injury, in children there is often associated major trauma such as fractures of the skull, pelvis, and femoral shaft; visceral rupture; and soft-tissue loss over the affected limb. It is imperative to rule out multiple injury; conversely, when the fracture is caused by trivial injury, it is necessary to eliminate the possibility of pathologic fracture.

Diagnosis

The diagnosis is not difficult. There is a history of severe injury following which the patient complains of sudden pain in the hip. He is usually unable to stand or walk; however, if the fracture is of the greenstick or impacted type, he may be able to bear weight on the affected limb.

On physical examination, the injured limb is held rigidly in a varying degree of external rotation and slight adduction. In displaced fractures, the patient is unable to move the injured hip actively. Actual shortening of 1 to 2 cm. is present. On palpation, local tenderness is elicited, and is most marked posteriorly where the femoral neck is superficially located. Some swelling in Scarpa's triangle may be noted. There is marked restriction of passive motions of the hip, particularly those of flexion, abduction, and internal rotation.

The diagnosis is confirmed by the use of roentgenograms, which should be made in the anteroposterior and lateral views. The direction of the fracture line and the degree of coxa vara are noted. The femoral head is retained in the acetabulum in its normal location, but the distal fragment of the femoral neck is displaced upward, anteriorly, and into slight external rotation.

Treatment

In the literature, various methods of treatment of femoral neck fractures in children have been advocated, and because this is a particularly difficult fracture, they are briefly reviewed here.

Traction was the method chosen by Barber, in 1871.[483] Forced manipulative reduction and immobilization in a hip spica cast were advocated by Whitman, who felt that it is imperative to restore normal anatomic alignment to prevent future deformity. He achieved forced reduction as follows: (1) The anesthetized patient is placed on the fracture table with the pelvis resting on a sacral support and the extended lower limbs held by assistants (or secured on a foot plate of the fracture table in the older child). (2) The normal hip is fully abducted to determine its range and to fix the pelvis. (3) Then, under longitudinal traction, the fractured hip is slowly abducted to its full limit. (4) With his hands, the surgeon presses the greater trochanter downward, utilizing the upper border of the acetabular rim as a fulcrum, to restore the normal relationship between the head-neck and shaft of the femur (Fig. 8–85). The extended hip is rotated medially to 20 degrees beyond neutral position, and the hip is then immobilized in this position in a one and one half hip spica cast.[518-522]

Table 8–3. *Incidence of Various Types of Femoral Neck Fractures in Children*

Author	Total No. of Cases	Transepiphyseal	Transcervical	Cervicotrochanteric (or Basal neck)	Petrochanteric
Lam (1971)	75	2	37 (9 seen late)	23 (5 seen late)	13 (1 seen late)
Ratliff (1962)	70	2	38	26	4
McDougall (1961)	24	2	11	8	3
Ingram and Bachynski (1953)	24	6	11	5	2
Allende and Lezama (1951)	8	1	5	1	1
Carrell and Carrell (1941)	12	—	4	8	—
Total	213	13 (6%)	106 (50%)	71 (33%)	23 (11%)

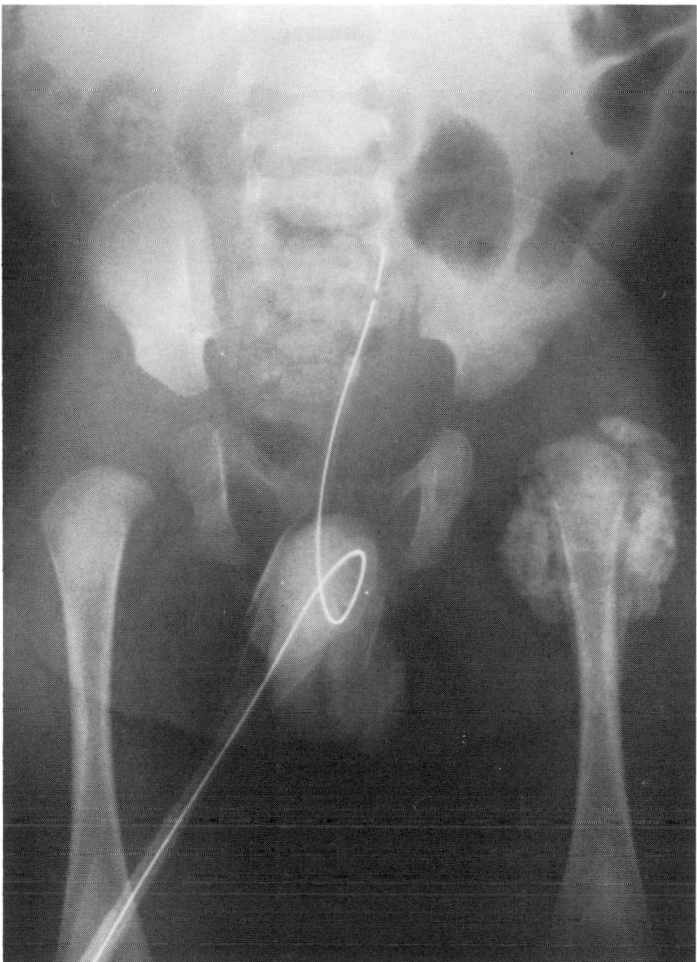

FIGURE 8–81. *Metaphyseal fracture of the left femoral neck in a newborn infant.*

Russell recommended traction for a period of three weeks to allow "soft union" to occur prior to forced abduction and immobilization in a hip spica cast.[508] Taylor and Colonna followed Whitman's method of early forced manipulative reduction.[489, 490, 512] Böhler advocated continuous traction for three months, stating that femoral neck fractures in children should be treated like any other fracture of the femur in a child.[486]

Mitchell, in 1936, reported a series of ten fractures of the hip in children, of which only three were seen within two weeks of the initial trauma and were, therefore, classified as recent. Of these three, two were treated by the Whitman forced abduction method, the result being good in one and poor in the other. The third fracture was treated by manipulative reduction, followed by continuous well-leg traction with the hip immobilized in abduction in a plaster of Paris cast; the latter method showed a good result. Thus, Mitchell concluded that the method of choice in treatment of recent fractures of the femoral neck is continuous well-leg traction combined with immobilization in abduction in a hip spica cast.[503]

Wilson analyzed eight of his own cases of femoral neck fractures, four of which were treated initially by the Whitman method, with good results in some. He pointed out the difficulties involved in maintaining reduction by the Whitman method and recommended internal fixation with a nail, provided the epiphyseal plate is not damaged.[523]

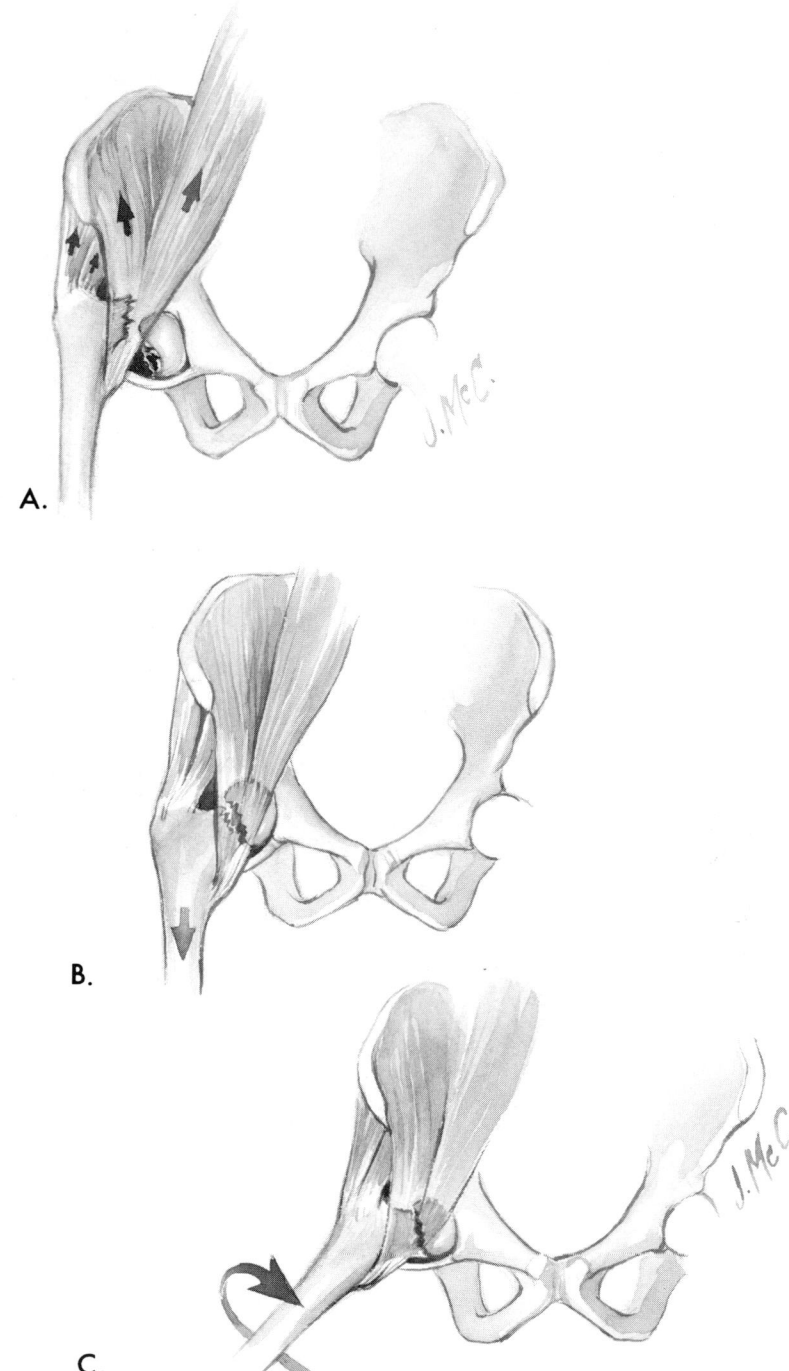

FIGURE 8–85. *Diagram illustrating Whitman's method of reduction of femoral neck fractures.*

  A. The deformity is increased by the pull of the iliopsoas and gluteal muscles. **B.** Longitudinal traction is applied to pull the lower fragment distally. **C.** Gradual abduction of the hip and utilization of the upper border of the acetabular rim as a fulcrum reduce the fracture. The extended and abducted hip is rotated medially to 20 degrees beyond neutral position.

Carrell and Carrell found it difficult to maintain reduction with the Whitman method, as alignment was retained in only one of their five patients treated in this manner. Three of their patients with four fractures were treated by closed reduction and immobilization in a Hoke type plaster cast with leg countertraction. As reduction was maintained in all three cases, they concluded that this is the best method of immobilization, particularly in the cervicotrochanteric type of fracture. Adductor myotomy was performed as necessary.[487]

The importance of the plane or the angle of the fracture line was pointed out by Allende and Lezama. When Pauwel's angle is less than 50 degrees, the fracture is considered stable and reduction can be maintained by the Whitman method; if the angle is greater than 50 degrees, the fracture is unstable and cannot be held by the Whitman method. In such cases, they recommended an intertrochanteric osteotomy to modify the angle of the fracture, and also advised a fibular bone graft at the time of osteotomy to promote union.[482]

Ingram and Bachynski recommended routine use of internal fixation preceded by closed reduction in all femoral neck fractures in children, except in the undisplaced cervicotrochanteric type. Knowles pins were used for internal fixation. They cautioned against the use of the Smith-Peterson nail because of its tendency to distract the fracture fragments. In cases of intertrochanteric fractures, treatment by closed manipulative reduction and immobilization in a Hoke-Martin traction cast was advised.[496] Green, in discussing the foregoing paper, cautioned against the use of threaded pins or screws of wood type for internal fixation, as they firmly hold the femoral head and arrest growth by compression of the epiphysis. On the other hand, a smooth nail or pin of a reasonable size will not do this. Green recommended the use of one or two pins or nails of small caliber in most fractures, with accessory protection as needed. In fractures of the distal portion of the femoral neck, he advised that the pins be stopped short of the physis, thereby decreasing the possibility of growth arrest. This is feasible because of the dense nature of the cancellous bone in the proximal portion of the child's femoral neck.[494] Sullivan, in his discussion of Ingram

and Bachynski's paper, emphasized the difficulties in the technique of nailing because of the smaller target in the neck of the child's femur, the firm and springy cancellous bone, and the tendency of the fragments to separate as the nail is driven across the fracture line. He also agreed that use of a cast without internal fixation is not adequate to maintain reduction. Sullivan recommended immediate open reduction, drilling with a large-sized drill into the neck under roentgenographic visualization, and insertion of a graft of cancellous bone. He had done this in one case, in which x-rays subsequently showed healing of the fracture and solid union.[511]

In 1955, Blount advocated accurate reduction and internal fixation with $\frac{1}{8}$-inch adjustable nails for treatment of displaced femoral neck fractures. McDougall, in 1961, in his end-result study of 24 femoral neck fractures, observed equally good or bad results from either conservative or operative methods.[501] It should be noted, however, that all his cervicotrochanteric fractures were treated conservatively by plaster cast, splint, or traction; whereas the transcervical fractures were, for the most part, treated by internal fixation. The duration of follow-up was 14 months to 16 years. In the cervicotrochanteric fractures, excellent or good results were obtained in only three of the eight cases (37.5 per cent), with the remainder (62.5 per cent — five patients) requiring secondary operative procedures. Excellent or good results were obtained in five of the eight transcervical fractures treated with internal fixation (62.5 per cent). Of the three transcervical fractures treated conservatively, the one treated by a plaster cast did poorly; however, the two treated by traction and a splint did well. It would seem that the evidence is in favor of internal fixation.

Ratliff, in his review of 71 cases, stressed the importance of the distinction between displaced and undisplaced fractures. The management of an undisplaced fracture presented no great problem and the results were good with immobilization in a hip spica cast. Occasionally avascular necrosis developed. Treatment of displaced fractures (49 cases), however, was fraught with complications.[506]

Manipulative reduction and immobilization in

a plaster hip spica cast was employed in 19 patients. The fracture was either not reduced or it became displaced following reduction in 15 out of 19 patients (79 per cent). In two patients, good position was maintained, but avascular necrosis developed, with consequent poor results, and in only two patients was the result good. *Manipulative reduction and internal fixation* was employed in 19 patients (transcervical fractures in 15 cases and basal neck fractures in 4 cases). Only one patient was under 11 years of age at the time of injury. Various types of internal fixation were used. The results were good in nine (about 50 per cent), fair in five, and poor in five. *Manipulative reduction and Thomas splint* were used in three patients, with poor results in two, and good in one. He did not recommend this method, as the Thomas splint is not designed to maintain the reduction of a femoral neck fracture. *Primary subtrochanteric osteotomy* was performed in four patients, in three because of failure of manipulative reduction; the results were good in two, and fair in the remaining two. Ratliff gave two indications for primary osteotomy: first, in a displaced fracture in a child under ten years of age (because of the great difficulty of internal fixation in this age group without disturbing the growth plate); and second, in a displaced fracture of the femoral neck in an older child in whom adequate manipulative reduction cannot be achieved.[506]

Lam reached the following conclusions in his study of 75 fractures of the femoral neck: (1) Undisplaced transcervical and cervicotrochanteric fractures can be adequately treated by simple immobilization in a plaster of Paris cast. (2) All pertrochanteric fractures can be satisfactorily treated by conservative means. (3) Minimally displaced transcervical and cervicotrochanteric fractures with considerable bony contact are best treated by closed reduction and immobilization in a plaster of Paris cast. (4) Displaced transcervical and cervicotrochanteric fractures with loss of all bony contact present a difficult problem. Lam could not give any firm advice based on his experience. Closed reduction should be attempted, and if successful, the hip immobilized in a one and one half plaster spica cast or well-leg traction in a younger child, or by the insertion of two or more threaded pins reinforced by

a plaster spica in the older child. If closed reduction fails, open reduction is performed. In Lam's series, primary subtrochanteric osteotomy was not employed.[500] The various methods of treatment of femoral neck fractures in children are summarized in Table 8–4.

A categorical statement cannot be made as to the best method of treatment. Factors to consider are the type of fracture, the plane or angle of the fracture line, the degree of displacement, and the age of the patient. It is imperative to preserve the blood supply to the femoral head and neck. The vessels are most vulnerable to injury at the cervicotrochanteric area and at the epiphyseal plate when they are in close proximity to bone and are quite rigidly fixed. Ordinarily circulation is disturbed as a result of the original trauma; however, the surgeon must take all precautions that his treatment does not aggravate the original injury. *Closed reductions must be performed very gently.*

Another important factor to consider is that growth of the capital femoral epiphysis should not be disturbed. In children, the cancellous bone of the femoral neck is dense, and whenever possible, the pins should stop short of the physis. Added protection and immobilization are provided by the hip spica cast. If the fracture is trans-

Table 8–4. *Methods of Primary Treatment of Femoral Neck Fractures in Children*

Traction (Barber, Böhler)

Manipulative closed reduction and plaster hip spica cast (Whitman)

Manipulative closed reduction and immobilization in bilateral hip spica cast with well-leg countertraction

Manipulative closed reduction and Thomas splint

Gradual reduction by skeletal or skin traction and later plaster of Paris hip spica cast

Manipulative closed reduction, primary subtrochanteric osteotomy, internal fixation, and hip spica cast

Open reduction and internal fixation

Open reduction, bone grafting, and internal fixation

epiphyseal or high cervical in location, and it is necessary to penetrate the capital epiphysis, only one or two smooth sharp pins of adequate size should be used. Wood screws or threaded pins that firmly hold the head will stop growth by compression of the epiphysis. Under no circumstances should the Smith-Peterson nail or any other type of three-flanged nail be used because it will distract the fracture fragments.

The author recommends the following plan of treatment, based upon his experience with 32 femoral neck fractures in children at the Children's Memorial Hospital, Chicago, and at the Children's Hospital Medical Center, Boston. First, all children with fractured hips are placed *immediately* in bilateral split Russell traction with medial rotation straps on both the thigh and leg of the affected limb. This measure will relieve muscle spasm, prevent further displacement, and may achieve gentle reduction. Rough handling of the limb should be avoided during examination.

TRANSEPIPHYSEAL FRACTURES

If the fracture is undisplaced or minimally displaced (less than one fourth) immobilize the hip in a one and one half hip spica cast with the affected hip in moderate abduction, neutral extension, and ten degrees of medial rotation. If displaced (more than one fourth), perform gentle closed manipulative reduction under general anesthesia; fix internally with two sharp smooth pins, which should penetrate the epiphysis; and immobilize in a one and one half hip spica cast. Ordinarily, eight to ten weeks are required to achieve bony union. Prognosis is poor. The patient should be carefully followed by periodic roentgenograms for possible development of the complications of avascular necrosis, coxa vara, or premature fusion of the physis. Early treatment of these complications by appropriate measures will salvage the hip.

UNDISPLACED TRANSCERVICAL OR CERVICOTROCHANTERIC FRACTURES

There is a great temptation to treat these conservatively by immobilization in a one and one half hip spica cast; however, anatomical alignment may be lost, leading to

displacement and greater incidence of complications. As a general rule, if Pauwel's angle is less than 40 degrees, these fractures can be adequately treated by a one and one half hip spica cast. Absolutely no weightbearing should be permitted. In an especially active child, a double hip spica cast is preferable. Frequent roentgenograms are made. If loss of position occurs, the fracture is internally fixed. If Pauwel's angle is more than 40 degrees, anatomic alignment is maintained by internal fixation with two small threaded pins, which should stop short of the epiphyseal plate (Fig. 8–86). Again, a one and one half hip spica cast is applied to provide adequate immobilization. One cannot overemphasize the importance of internal fixation in maintaining reduction when Pauwel's angle is greater than 40 degrees. In personal experience with five such cases, the author lost position in four treated by simple immobilization in a hip spica cast. Some surgeons may prefer to treat these by a double hip spica cast with well-leg countertraction. The author recommends this only when a transcervical fracture is too close to the epiphyseal plate.

DISPLACED TRANSCERVICAL AND CERVICOTROCHANTERIC FRACTURES

These should be treated by gentle closed reduction and internal fixation with two or three threaded pins (preferably of the Moore type). Age is not a factor. With modern image intensifier roentgenographic control, the author finds it is feasible to pin the femoral neck accurately in a child under ten years of age. Again, the pins should stop short of the physis and a one and one half hip spica cast should be applied for added protection (Fig. 8–87). If adequate reduction cannot be achieved, or if, following reduction (particularly in transcervical fractures), Pauwel's angle is greater than 50 to 60 degrees with consequent high shearing stress, a primary subtrochanteric valgus osteotomy is recommended.

If closed reduction cannot be achieved, open reduction is performed; it is combined with a primary subtrochanteric abduction osteotomy if Pauwel's angle is greater than 50 to 60 degrees. One cannot overemphasize the importance of *not* using a Smith-

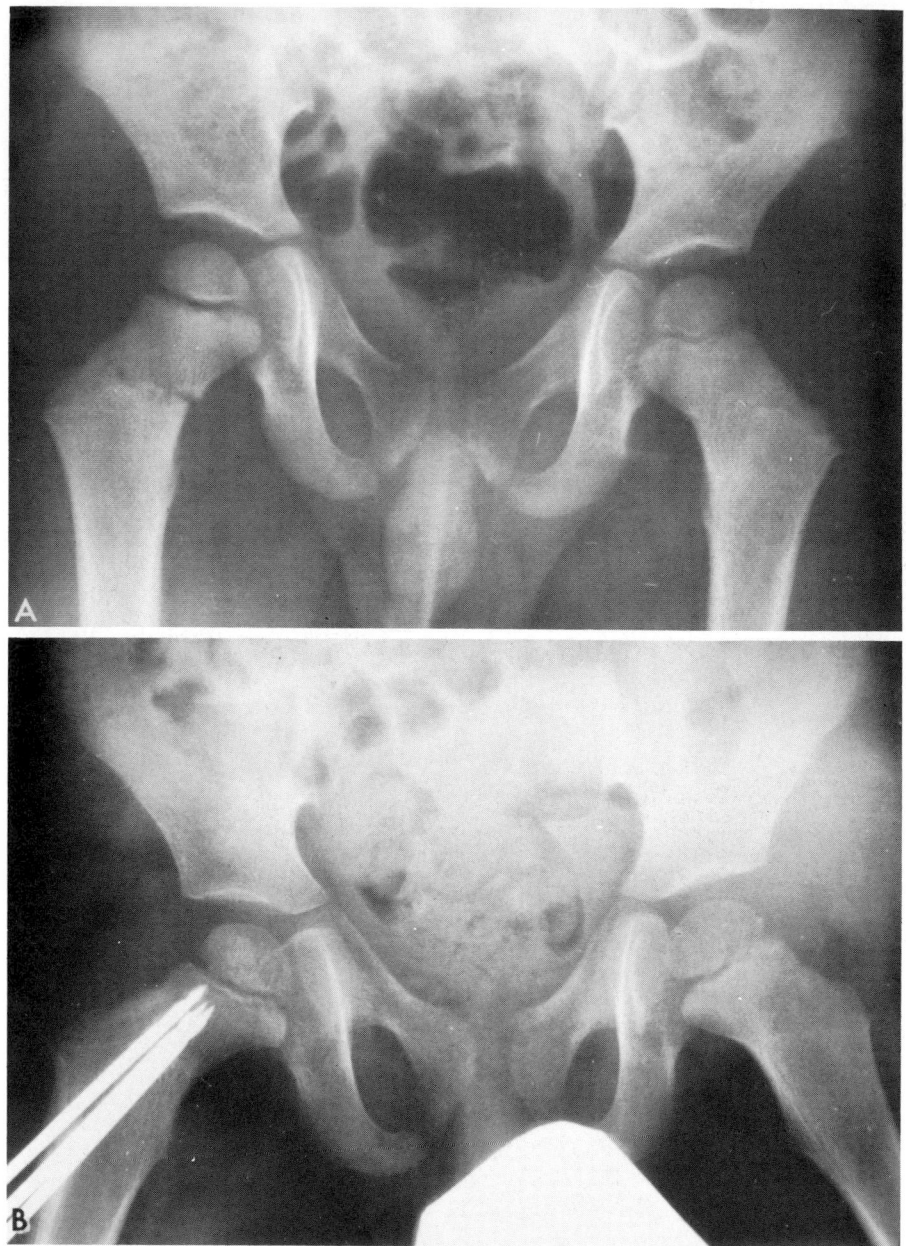

FIGURE 8–86. *Minimally displaced cervicotrochanteric fracture of the left hip treated by percutaneous pinning and hip spica cast.*

A. Preoperative roentgenogram. **B.** Postoperative roentgenogram showing that the pins have stopped short of the growth plate.

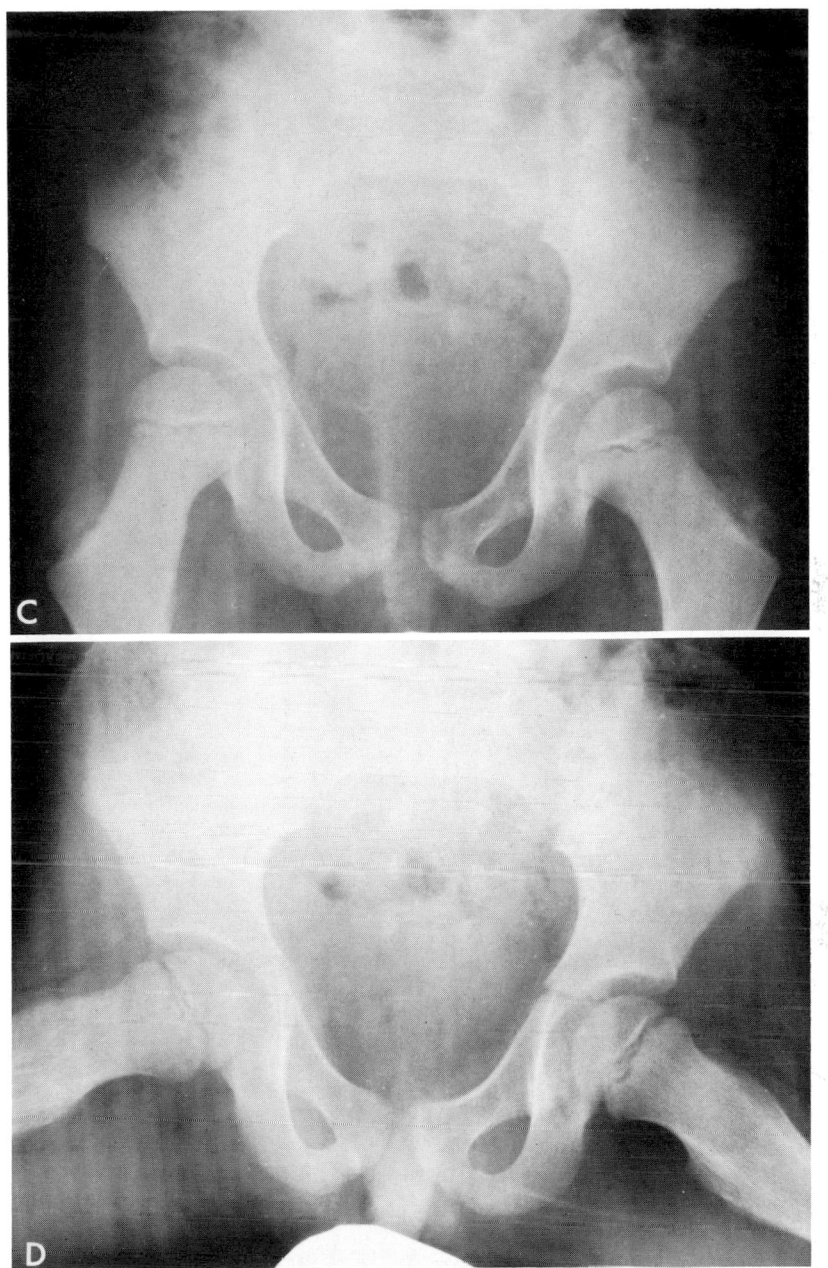

FIGURE 8–86 Continued. ***Minimally displaced cervicotrochanteric fracture of the left hip treated by percutaneous pinning and hip spica cast.***

C and **D.** Roentgenograms two and one half years later, showing the healed fracture.

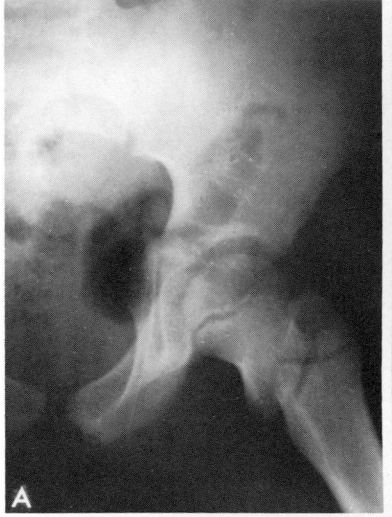
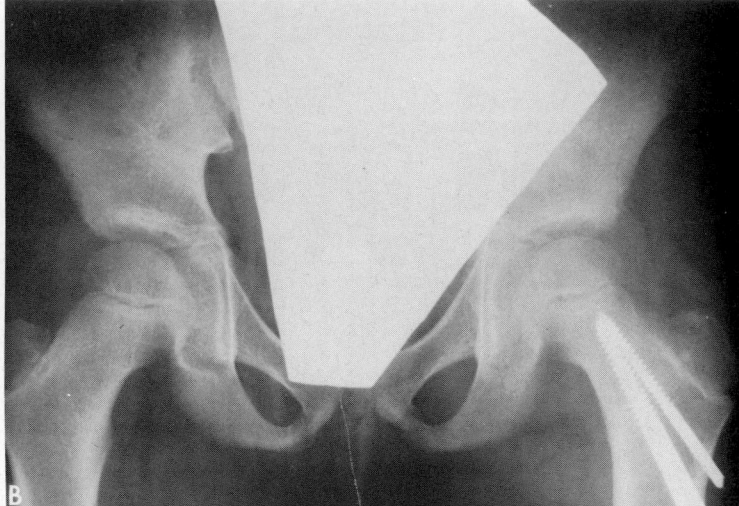

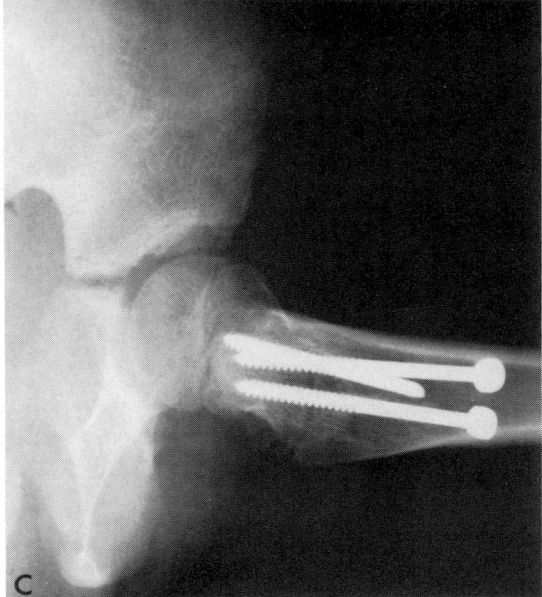

FIGURE 8–87. *Displaced cervicotrochanteric fracture in a ten-year-old girl treated by closed reduction, internal fixation, and hip spica cast.*

A. Preoperative roentgenogram. **B** and **C.** Postoperative roentgenograms eight months later. Note the healed fracture. Thin threaded pins have stopped short of the capital femoral physis.

Peterson or a trifin nail or a nail plate for internal fixation as it is difficult for the nail to penetrate the hard femoral head and neck; when it is being driven in the fracture fragments will become distracted.

Intertrochanteric fractures of the hip can be effectively treated by traction followed by immobilization in a hip spica cast (Fig. 8–88).

Complications

Treatment of fractures of the femoral neck is fraught with complications. Even with the most masterful reduction and ade-quate fixation, a normal hip cannot be assured; avascular necrosis, coxa vara, premature closure of the epiphyseal plate, and nonunion may occur. Of the 189 cases reported in five large series in the literature, 110 (60 per cent) developed one or more of these complications. The displaced fracture of the femoral neck in children still remains an unsolved problem and a challenge to the orthopedic surgeon.

ASEPTIC NECROSIS

The great hazard of femoral neck fractures in children is aseptic necrosis. The

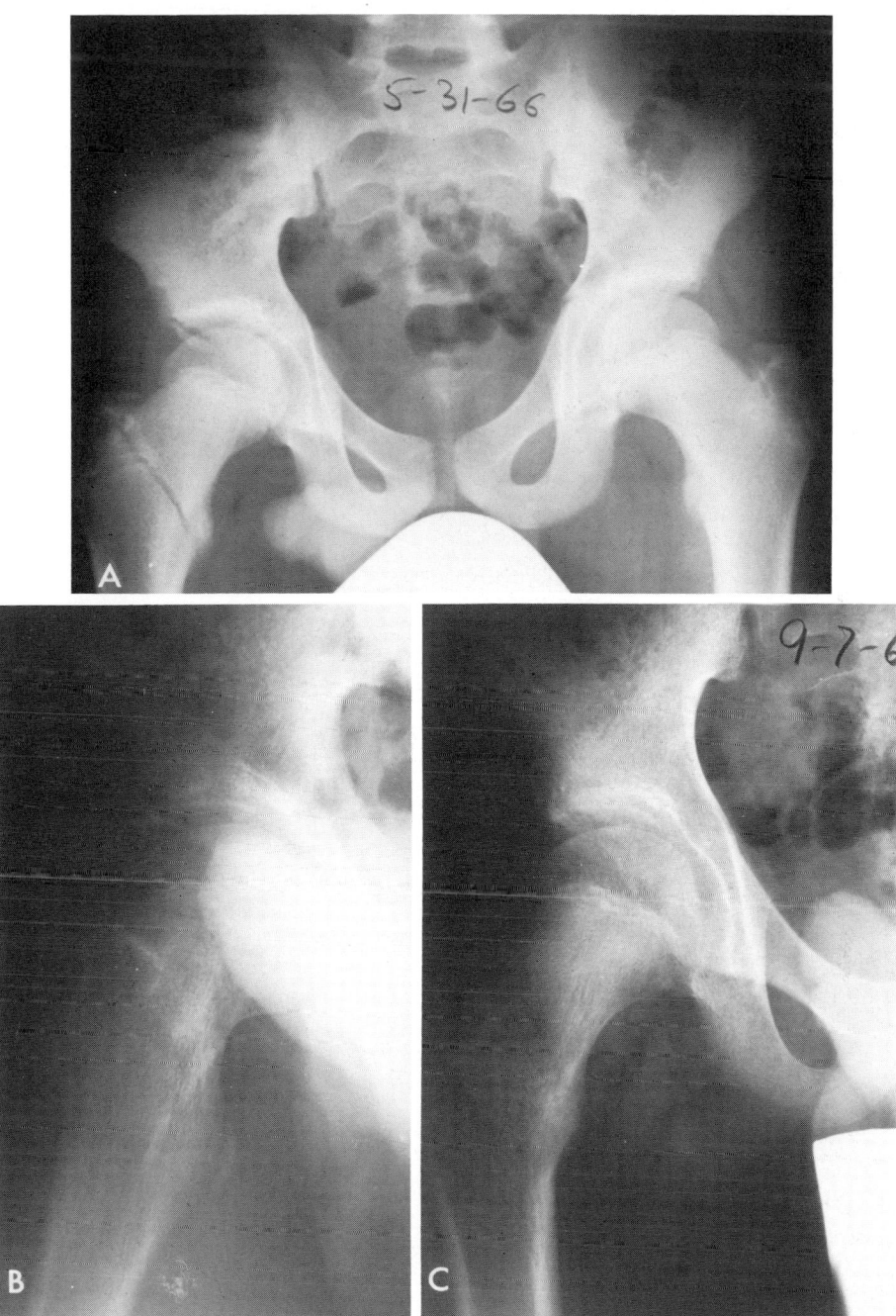

FIGURE 8–88. *Intertrochanteric fracture of right hip in a 15-year-old boy.*

Fracture was treated by traction for three weeks, followed by immobilization in a hip spica cast for five more weeks. **A.** Preoperative roentgenogram. **B** and **C.** Four months later. Note the healed fracture.

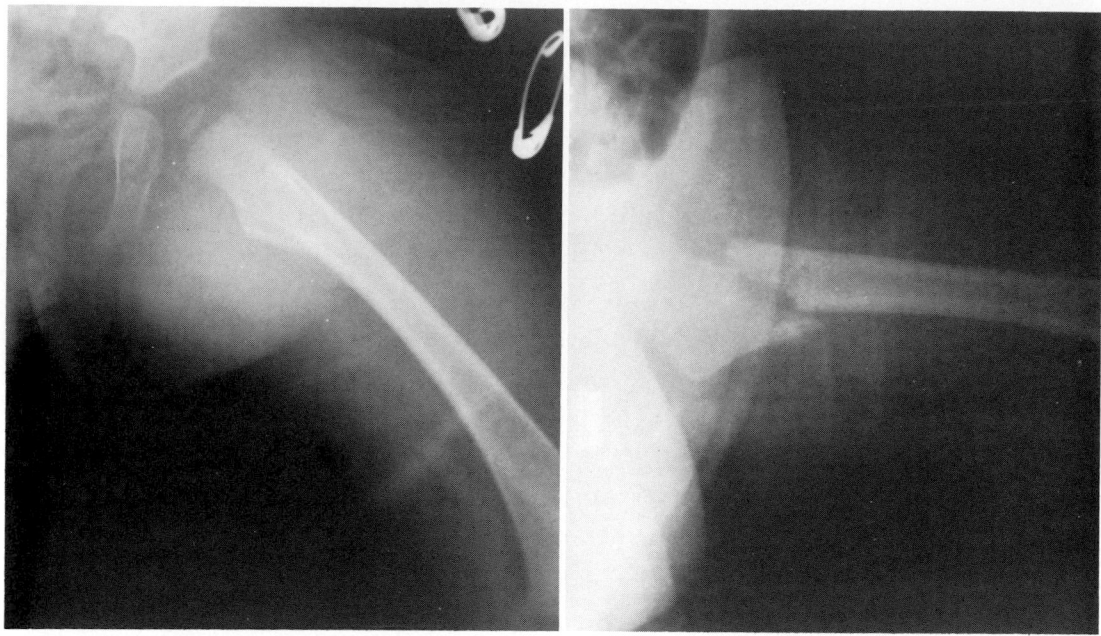

FIGURE 8-89. *Pertrochanteric fracture in a one-year-old girl.*

blood supply to the femoral head and neck has been studied by Wolcott, Tucker, and Trueta.[513-515, 524] The artery of the ligamentum teres from the acetabular branch of the obturator artery contributes little to the growing capital femoral epiphysis until about eight or nine years of age. The principal source of blood supply is through the lateral epiphyseal and superior and inferior metaphyseal vessels—all branches of the medial femoral circumflex artery. These vessles enter the capsule at its distal attachment posteriorly at the distal third of the femoral neck and traverse proximally in close proximity to the bone within the synovium. The epiphyseal plate in children acts as a barrier, precluding any significant anastomosis between those blood vessels that supply the epiphysis and those that supply the metaphysis. A fracture divides the vascular supply from the intraosseous nutrient vessels; it also produces a tear of the synovium, and therefore readily lacerates the posterior circumflex artery or its metaphyseal and lateral epiphyseal branches.

Ratliff has described three patterns of avascular necrosis following fractures of the femoral neck in children (Fig. 8–90). In *Type I* there is severe diffuse necrosis of the femoral head and of the proximal fragment of the femoral neck, produced by interruption of the blood supply to the lateral epiphyseal vessels, metaphyseal vessels, and nutrient vessels (Fig. 8–90 A). This is the most common pattern, and occurs in approximately 50 per cent of those with necrosis; also, it has the poorest prognosis, with total collapse of the femoral head; none of the patients has attained a good end-result. In *Type II*, the necrotic changes are more localized (usually in the anterosuperior half of the femoral head), and are accompanied by minimal collapse of the bony epiphysis. It is caused by damage to only the lateral epiphyseal vessels before they enter the epiphysis (Fig. 8–90 C). Collapse occurs in 25 per cent of cases with this type of necrosis, but it has a good prognosis. In *Type III* the area of necrosis is confined to the femoral neck, delimited proximally by the fracture line. This occurred in the remaining 25 per cent of cases of avascular necrosis (Fig. 8–90 B). Ratliff proposes the cause of isolated necrosis of the femoral neck to be damage to only the superior metaphyseal vessels, with the lateral epiphyseal vessels remaining intact. It is noteworthy that almost all patients with Type III avascular necrosis were under 12 years of age, and that in 85 per cent of the cases, premature fusion of the upper femoral epiphyseal plate took place. In Type III avascular necrosis, the prognosis is fair, as the femoral head does not fragment or collapse.[506]

Approximately one third of children with femoral neck fractures develop avascular necrosis. On critical analysis of the cases reported in the literature, including the author's, it is obvious that transcervical fractures are somewhat more likely to undergo necrosis than are cervicotrochanteric fractures (34 per cent versus 27 per cent, respectively). Displaced transepiphyseal fractures have the poorest prognosis, with

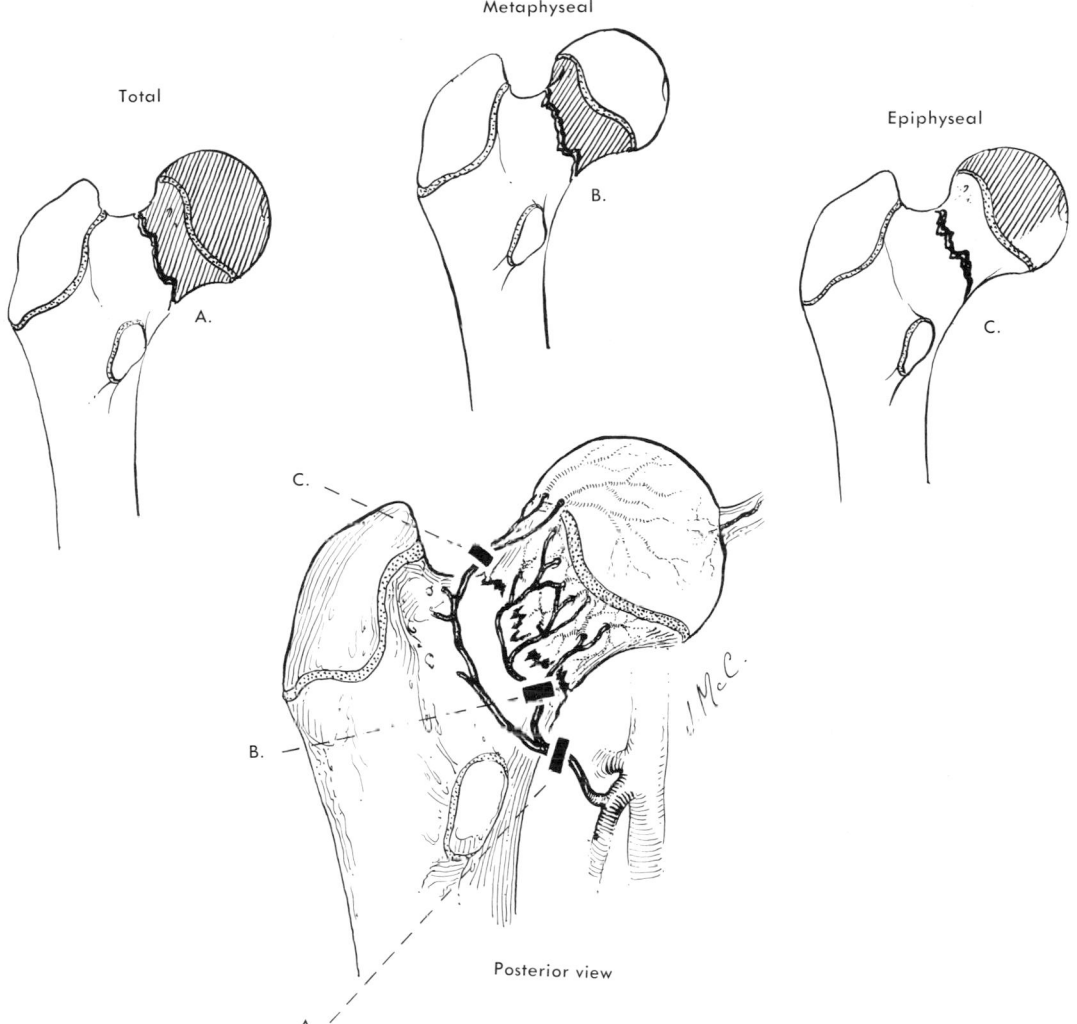

FIGURE 8–90. Patterns of aseptic necrosis following fractures of the femoral neck in children.

Type A or *total.* There is severe diffuse necrosis of the entire capital epiphysis and proximal fragment of the femoral neck. It is produced by interruption of blood supply from the lateral epiphyseal, metaphyseal, and nutrient vessels. (Contribution to circulation of the femoral head from the vessels along the ligamentum teres is minimal. The epiphyseal plate acts as a barrier to anastomosis between vessels supplying the epiphysis and those supplying the metaphysis.)

Type B or *metaphyseal.* The avascular necrosis is confined to the femoral neck, being outlined proximally by the epiphyseal plate and distally by the fracture line. The femoral head does not collapse or fragment. Necrosis is caused by interruption of blood supply from superior metaphyseal vessels with the lateral epiphyseal vessels remaining intact.

Type C or *partial epiphyseal.* The avascular necrotic changes are confined to the femoral head, usually in its superior half. This type is produced by interruption of lateral epiphyseal vessels before they enter the capital epiphysis. (Redrawn after Ratliff.)

development of aseptic necrosis in 80 per cent of cases. The incidence of aseptic necrosis in those who are ten years of age or younger is 21 per cent, whereas in those over ten years of age it is 47 per cent.

The method of treatment seems to be a factor in the development of aseptic necrosis; 35 per cent of those fractures treated conservatively were complicated by necrosis, as opposed to only 27 per cent of those treated by internal fixation. That extreme abduction of the hip in the treatment of congenital dislocation of the hip decreases circulation to the femoral head has been well demonstrated and the practice is condemned. It is noteworthy that in Whitman's conservative method of treatment the fractured hip is *forced into extreme abduction* to reduce the fracture and then is immobilized in that position. The principle of reduction by Whitman's method is mechanically sound; however, following reduction, the affected hip should be brought into 30 to 40 degrees of abduction and moderate flexion, and then immobilized in that position. Likewise, following internal fixation, the hip should not be immobilized in extreme abduction. One cannot overemphasize the importance of not further decreasing an already precarious circulation to the femoral head. Durbin has pointed out that aseptic necrosis may occur following undisplaced as well as displaced fractures of the femoral neck in children.[493]

Radiologic evidence of aseptic necrosis is usually apparent within one year after injury. Occasionally it is heralded by premature closure of the epiphyseal plate.

Treatment follows the same principles as those outlined in the section on management of Legg-Perthes disease. Congruity of the femoral head in the acetabulum is achieved and maintained by the trilateral socket ischial weight-bearing hip abduction orthosis until the necrotic bone is reconstituted by normal bone.

COXA VARA

This is a common complication. Lam reported 23 instances of this deformity in 75 femoral neck fractures in children (32 per cent); it developed in 18 fresh fractures (30 per cent), and in five of the 15 late fractures.[500]

Coxa vara may be caused by several factors: (1) failure to reduce the fracture; (2) loss of alignment in a hip spica cast, either because of inadequate immobilization or delayed union: or (3) aseptic necrosis and premature fusion of the capital femoral epiphyseal plate, in which instance, relative discrepancy of growth between the capital femoral epiphysis and the greater trochanteric apophysis will result in progressive decrease of the neck-shaft angle.

In the series of Lam, 3 of the 18 cases of coxa vara in fresh fractures were associated with avascular necrosis of the proximal fragment in whole or in part with premature epiphyseal fusion: two with avascular necrosis alone; and two with premature fusion of the epiphyseal plate in the absence of avascular necrosis. In the remaining 11 cases, coxa vara occurred alone.[500]

Ratliff noted that coxa vara was associated with delayed union in 14 of his 71 cases.[506] Undoubtedly, this is an important predisposing factor.

Allende and Lezama, to reiterate, emphasized the importance of the obliquity of the fracture line. Fractures with a Pauwel's angle of less than 50 degrees responded well to treatment with a plaster cast; whereas those with an angle greater than 50 degrees did poorly, with coxa vara being the end-result. Mitchell, Wilson, and Ingram and Bachynski stressed the importance of internal fixation in prevention of coxa vara.[496, 503, 523] Of the 11 patients in whom Ingram and Bachynski used internal fixation, not one developed coxa vara.[496] McDougall, however, reported four cases of coxa vara in the seven transcervical fractures treated by internal fixation that went on to union. It is of interest to note, also, that all eight of his cervicotrochanteric fractures were treated conservatively and that five of them developed coxa vara. McDougall proposed that "in these fractures there is a degree of plasticity at the fracture site for a long time after union appears adequate, with a tendency to bending of the neck of the femur."[501]

The clinical signs of coxa vara—prominence and elevation of the greater trochanter, shortening of the limb, decreased hip abduction, and a gluteus medius limp are well known. Treatment consists of subtrochanteric abduction osteotomy. If the capital femoral epiphyseal plate has prematurely fused, the varus deformity will recur with growth, necessitating repeat osteotomy after several years.

Epiphyseodesis of the greater trochanter will prevent recurrence of coxa vara; however, the resultant leg length discrepancy will require arrest of the distal femoral epiphysis at the appropriate age.

PREMATURE EPIPHYSEAL FUSION

This will result in total shortening of the lower limb and in coxa vara. In the literature, attention was drawn to this complication by Ratliff, who reported 11 patients with premature fusion of the upper femoral epiphyseal plate; in 6 of these, it followed avascular necrosis of the femoral head.[506] In the series of Lam, premature fusion of the upper femoral physis occurred in nine fresh and in six late fractures. He postulated long continued trauma to the capital femoral physis because of lack of immobilization to be the cause in the late cases.[500]

DELAYED UNION AND NONUNION

This complication usually develops in transcervical fractures (about 85 per cent of cases) with a Pauwel's angle greater than 60 degrees that are treated conservatively by plaster cast immobilization (about 70 per cent of cases). In those treated by internal fixation, the fracture fragments may be separated during insertion of trifin nails or held apart by the threaded portion of a large pin such as the Knowles pin. Aseptic necrosis is another important etiologic factor in delayed union.

Nonunion is treated by bone grafting and subtrochanteric abduction osteotomy aimed at converting the fracture angle from one of shearing stress to one of compression. In delayed union, abduction osteotomy alone is adequate; it is not necessary to bone graft.

AVULSION FRACTURES OF THE GREATER AND LESSER TROCHANTERS

These injuries occur as a result of muscular violence. The ossification center of the greater trochanter appears during the fourth year and that of the lesser trochanter, between the thirteenth and fourteenth years. They fuse with the femoral shaft between 18 and 19 years of age.

The *greater trochanter* is avulsed by sudden contraction of the gluteus medius and minimus muscles against resistance. The bone fragment is retracted proximally. Treatment consists of immobilization of the hip in a spica cast with the hip in wide abduction, bringing the greater trochanter into apposition with the upper end of the femoral shaft. The fracture will be healed in about six weeks.

The *lesser trochanter* is avulsed by the powerful contraction of the iliopsoas muscle against resistance, such as that which occurs during a football tackle or in an attempt to stop suddenly while running (Fig. 8–91). The displaced fracture heals, with little or no disability. Open reduction is not indicated. The patient is kept in bed with the hips in flexion until he is comfortable and then he is allowed to ambulate with crutches —three-point partial weight-bearing gait. Immobilization in a hip spica cast is not necessary.

FRACTURES OF THE FEMORAL SHAFT

Fractures of the shaft of the femur are relatively frequent in children and should be considered serious injuries because of the blood loss and potential shock that may accompany the primary trauma.

The largest bone in the body, the femur is a long cylinder of heavy compact bone that is bowed anteriorly and laterally. The linea aspera, a sturdy elevated ridge extending along the middle of the posterior surface of the femoral shaft, acts as a thickened buttress, providing strength and serving as an attachment for muscles.

In normal stance, the femoral shaft inclines medially at an angle varying from 3 to 15 degrees with an average of 9.56 degrees. This tends to partially overcome the effect of the angle of inclination of the femoral neck by bringing the weight-bearing articular surfaces of the knee closer to the center of gravity.[582]

The femoral shaft can be broken only by tremendous force. The majority of these

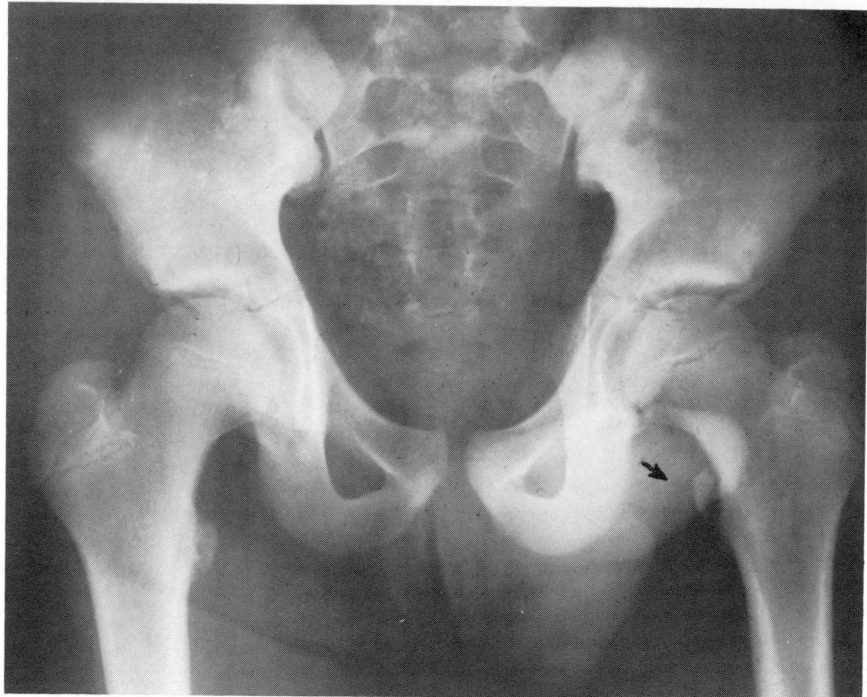

FIGURE 8–91.   *Avulsion of lesser trochanter on the left.*

fractures occur as a result of major violence, either direct or indirect, such as that sustained in automobile accidents and falls from a height.

Pathologic Anatomy

The commonest site of fracture of the femoral shaft is in its middle third, where the normal anterolateral bowing of the diaphysis is at its maximum; this is also the area most commonly subjected to severe direct violence. Of 250 cases of fracture of the femoral shaft admitted to the Children's Memorial Hospital, Chicago, 66 per cent were in the middle third, 17 per cent in the proximal third, 12 per cent in the distal third, and 5 per cent in the subtrochanteric region. Griffin, Green, and Anderson reported 70 per cent of the fractures in the middle third, 22 per cent in the proximal third, and 8 per cent in the distal third.[555] A similar distribution is reported by Blount, LeMesurier, Neer and Cadman, and Staheli.[535, 566, 575, 589]

The torsional force produced by indirect violence results in a long spiral or oblique fracture, whereas a transverse fracture is caused by direct trauma (Figs. 8–92 and 8–93). When the direct force is very severe, there may be comminution, or the fracture may be segmental, or both. Greenstick fractures may occur and are more common in the distal third.

Birth fractures, resulting from obstetrical trauma, usually occur in the middle third of the shaft and are transverse. Occasionally, however, they are metaphyseal in location (Fig. 8–95).

The displacement of the fragments in fracture of the femur depends upon the breaking force, the pull of the attached muscles, and the force of gravity acting upon the limb. As a rule, the distal fragment is laterally rotated consequent to outward rotation of the leg by the force of gravity. The severity of violence and the strong pull of the muscles will cause the fracture fragments to be completely displaced with variable amounts of overriding.

In fractures of the upper third of the femoral shaft, the proximal fragment is pulled into flexion by the iliopsoas muscle, into abduction by the gluteus medius and minimus, and into external rotation by the short external rotators and gluteus maximus. The shorter the proximal fragment, the greater is the degree of displacement. The distal fragment is drawn proximally by the hamstrings and quadriceps femoris muscles and into adduction by the adductors of the thigh. The distal fragment also falls posteriorly because of the force of gravity. Thus, the upper end of the distal fragment tends to lie posterior and medial to the proximal fragment, which is in flexion, abduction, and external rotation (Fig. 8–96).

Displacement of the fragments in the middle third does not follow any regular pattern. The tendency is for the proximal fragment to be in flexion and the distal fragment to be displaced backward; when the fracture level is in the upper half of the middle third, the proximal half is abducted; when the break is in the lower half, it is adducted. However, displacements are not necessarily constant.

In fractures of the lower third, the fracture line may be transverse or oblique, or the break may be of the greenstick type. The gastrocnemius muscle is a chief deforming force. It arises from the posterior surface of the lower femur and pulls the distal fragment posteriorly into the popliteal space where it may cause damage to vessels and nerves. The lower end of the proximal fragment is driven forward and distally into the quadriceps femoris muscle.

Soft-tissue injury inevitably accompanies

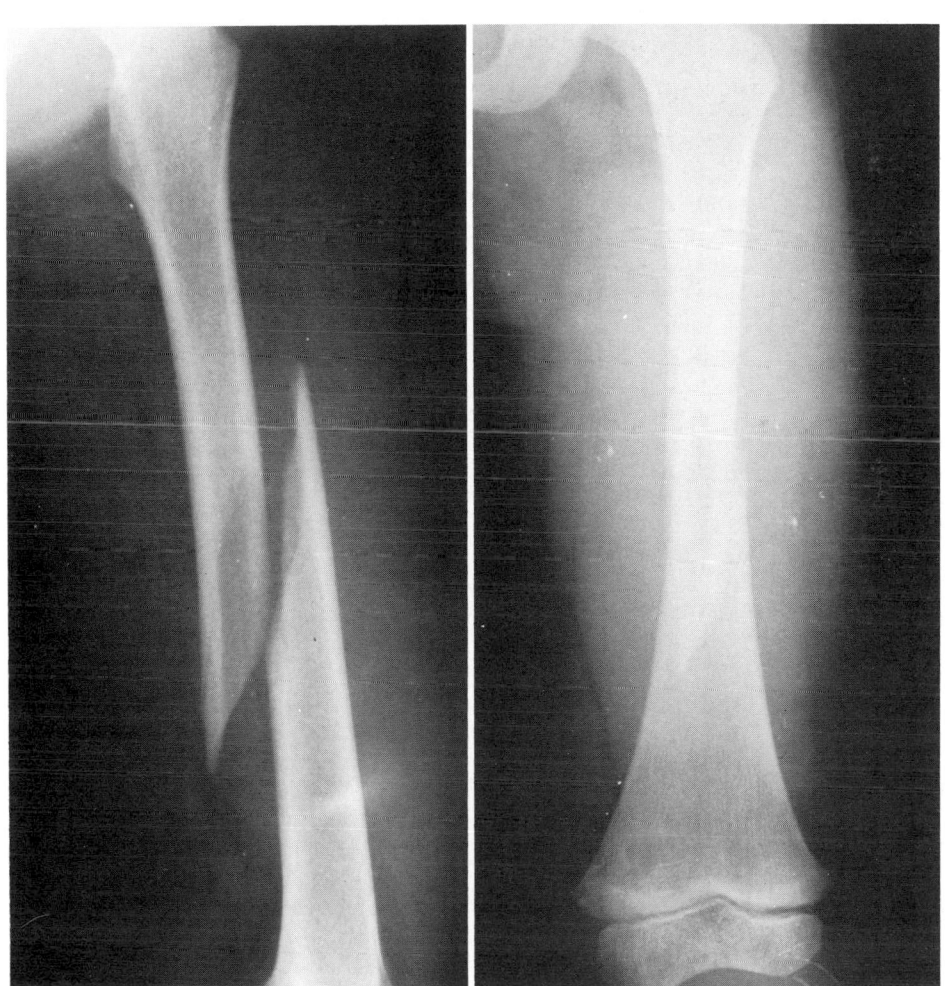

FIGURE 8–92. *Long spiral fracture of the femoral shaft produced by torsional force of indirect violence.*

The commonest site of fracture of the femoral shaft is in its middle third.

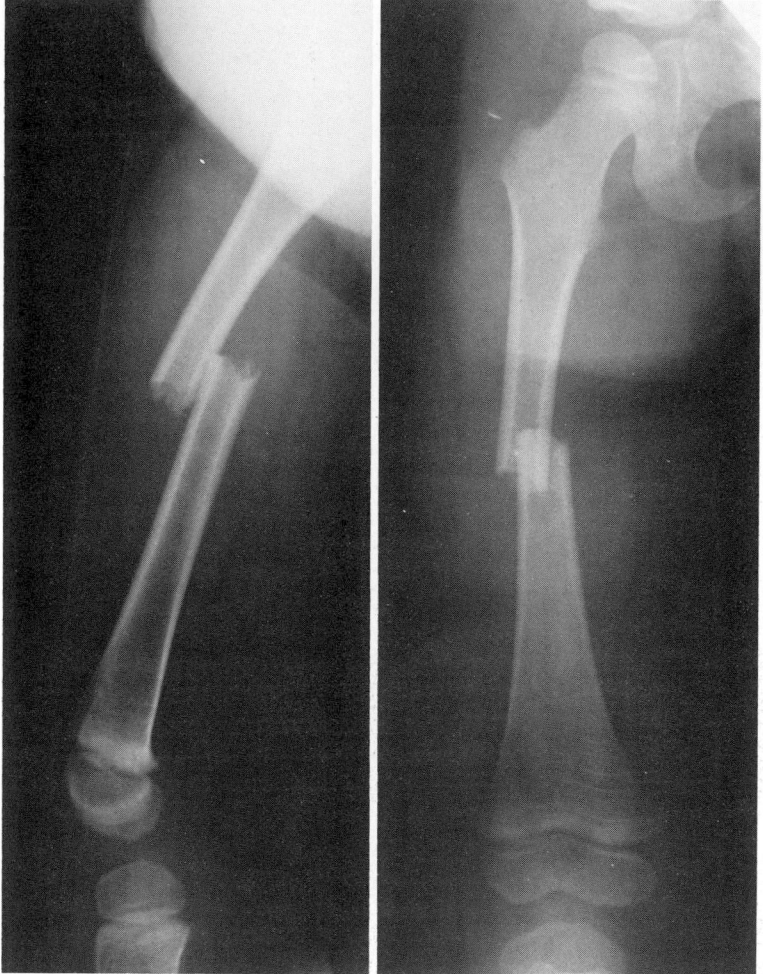

FIGURE 8–93. *Transverse fracture of the femoral shaft—it is usually caused by direct trauma.*

a femoral shaft fracture. Excessive hemorrhage with blood loss of 500 ml. or more is not uncommon. The source of bleeding may be either one or several branches of the profunda femoris artery (which courses around the posterior and lateral surfaces of the femoral shaft), the vessels of the richly vascular muscles that envelop the femur, or the vessels in the bone itself. Occasionally, the femoral artery itself may be torn.

Diagnosis

A history of injury, with the resultant local pain, tenderness, and swelling, inability to move the affected limb, deformity, shortening, abnormal mobility, lateral roll-ing of the limb distal to the level of the fracture, and crepitus render the diagnosis self-evident.

Examination of the patient should be very gentle, with great care exercised not to inflict unnecessary pain that might add to the possibly already present shock. The soft parts should not be damaged further. The fracture is distinguished as being either open or closed. Neurovascular status in the lower limb should be carefully assessed and recorded because injury to the femoral or popliteal vessels or to the sciatic nerve, or both, may occur, especially from posterior displacement of the distal fragment in fractures of the lower third of the shaft.

Because femoral shaft fractures usually result from major violence, it is imperative

(Text continued on page 1689.)

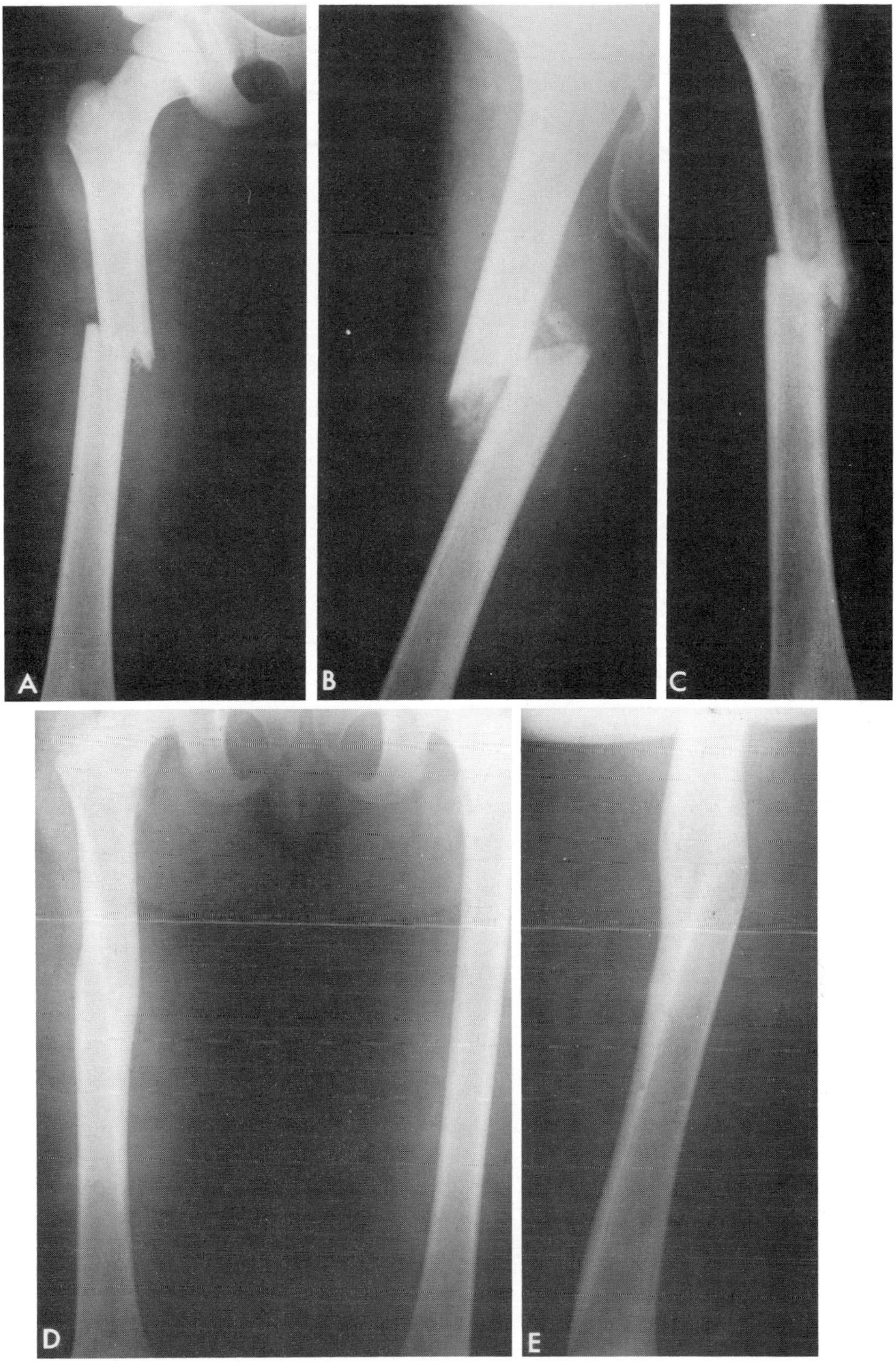

FIGURE 8–94. *Short oblique fracture of the femoral shaft at the junction of its middle and proximal thirds in a six-year-old child.*

A and **B.** Initial roentgenograms. Treated by 90°–90° skeletal traction followed by immobilization in a one and one half hip spica cast. **C.** Anteroposterior roentgenogram made when traction was discontinued. Note the 1 cm. overriding of the fragments, which is desirable in this age group. **D** and **E.** Ten months later—note the remodeling.

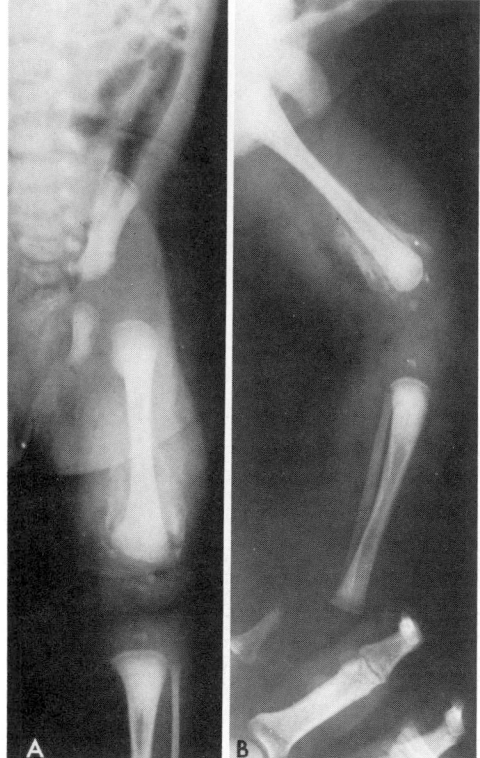

FIGURE 8–95.   *Birth fracture through metaphyseal region of distal left femur.*

A and **B.** Initial roentgenograms showing excessive subperiosteal calcification. A diagnostic feature is the extension of new bone formation distal to the area of bone density of the diaphysis. The condition should not be mistaken for osteomyelitis. There is no area of radiolucency in the metaphysis. Syphilis, tuberculosis, and scurvy are other entities to consider in the differential diagnosis. No treatment is necessary. **C** and **D.** These are roentgenograms made three months later. Note the remodeling of the callus. **E.** An anteroposterior roentgenogram taken a year later.

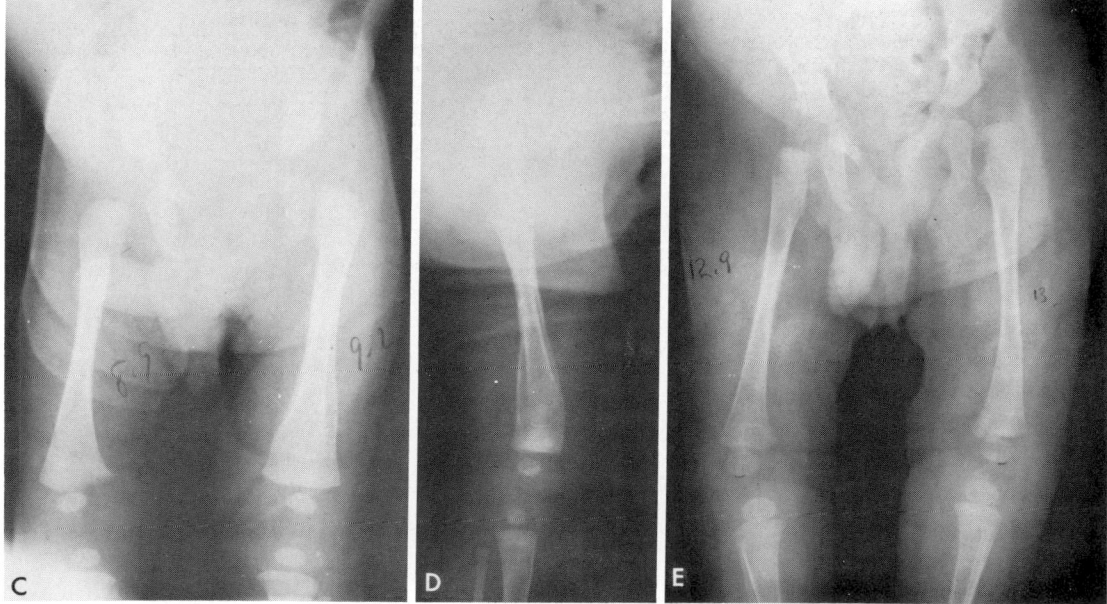

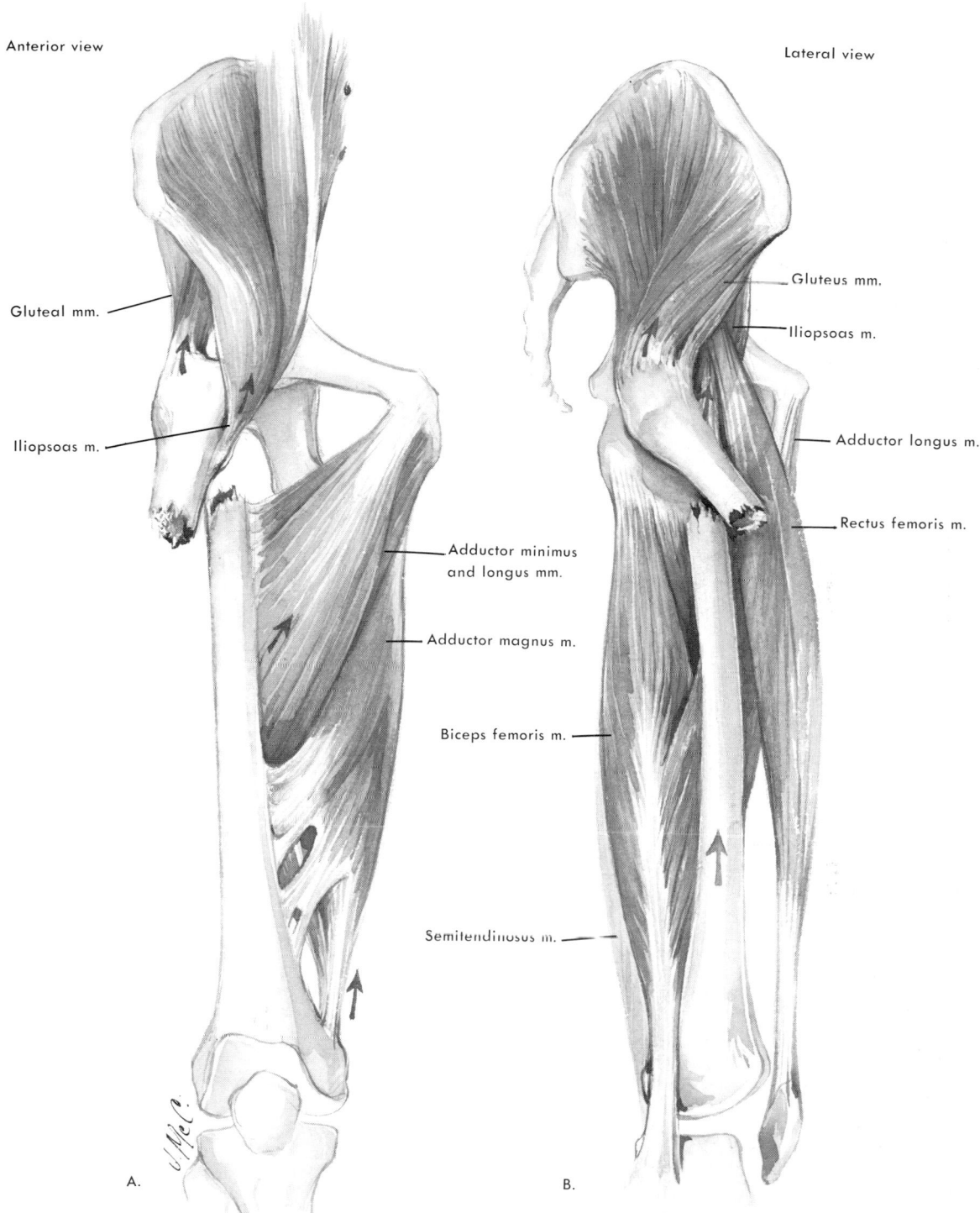

Anterior view

Gluteal mm.

Iliopsoas m.

Adductor minimus and longus mm.

Adductor magnus m.

Biceps femoris m.

Semitendinosus m.

A.

Lateral view

Gluteus mm.

Iliopsoas m.

Adductor longus m.

Rectus femoris m.

B.

FIGURE 8–96.   *Displacement of fragments in fractures of the upper third of the femoral shaft.*

Note the upper end of the distal fragment tends to lie posterior and medial to the proximal fragment, which is displaced into flexion, abduction, and external rotation by the pull of the iliopsoas, gluteal muscles, and short external rotators.

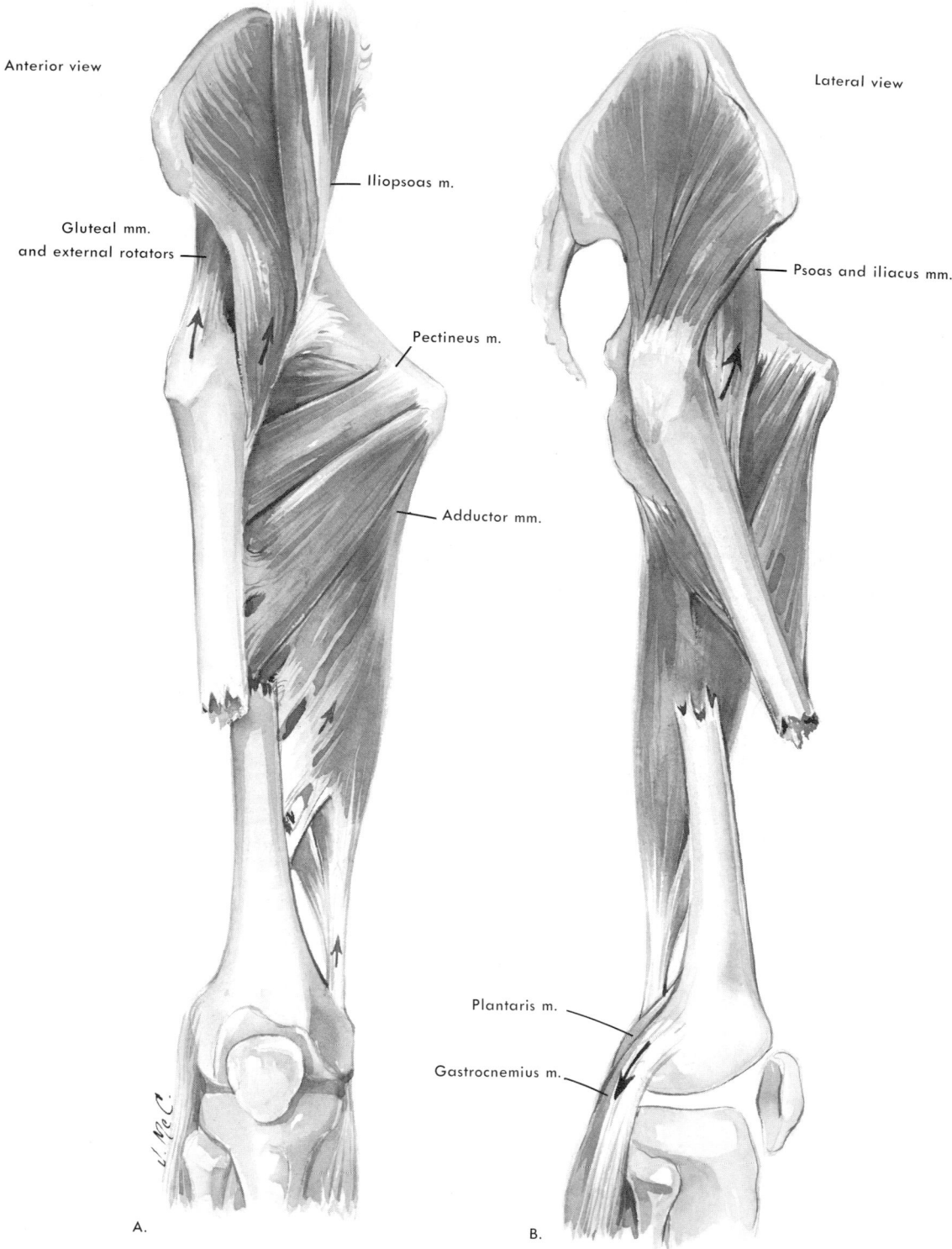

FIGURE 8–97.   Displacement of fragments in fractures of the middle third of the femoral shaft.

to evaluate the general condition of the patient meticulously. The sensorium, blood pressure, and pulse should be observed, and careful examination performed to detect any visceral damage in the intra-abdominal and genitourinary areas, cranial injury, other fractures, or hip dislocation.

Roentgenograms are taken to determine the exact level and nature of the fracture; however, this should not be done prior to proper splinting of the limb.

Treatment

Proper emergency care, i.e., initial gentle handling and adequate splinting of the fracture, is extremely important to prevent shock and further injury to the soft parts. Any movement of the injured limb will be quite painful, and one should *not* attempt to remove the patient's clothing or shoes.

An efficient means of immobilization is the Thomas splint or the Blake modification, in which there is only half of the ring. The size of the splint should be suitable for the child. The person applying the splint places his arm through the ring of the splint, grasps the patient's foot, and applies gentle and steady traction. Then, without releasing the traction on the foot, the splint is pushed proximally against the ischial tuberosity and traction is applied by a twisted rope or a strap sling that extends from the well-padded ankle to the end of the splint. The thigh and leg are supported on slings tightened under them or by encircling strips of cloth.

If a Thomas splint is not available, a splint may be improvised by using long boards or sticks, which should be padded to prevent pressure over bony prominences. The lateral splint extends from near the axilla to below the foot, and the medial one extends distally from the groin. Both splints are secured to the limb and the lateral one also to the trunk by means of an elastic bandage.

Another fairly satisfactory method of immobilization is to bandage the two lower limbs together. It is best to place some form of padding such as a folded blanket or clothing between the legs, and bind the feet together in order to control rotation. A pressure dressing over the fracture site will minimize bleeding into the soft tissues of the

thigh. The author does not recommend the use of airsplints when transporting children with femoral shaft fractures, because of potential circulatory embarrassment.

In the definitive care of femoral shaft fractures in children, various factors determine the method chosen, namely: (1) the age of the patient; (2) the preference of the surgeon, based on past experience; (3) the condition of the skin and soft tissues; and (4) the level and degree of displacement or comminution of the fracture.

INFANTS AND CHILDREN UP TO TWO YEARS OF AGE

In infants and children in this age group, Bryant's traction is most efficient and satisfactory, provided there is no spasticity and contracture of the hamstrings and, with the knees in extension, the hips can be flexed to 90 degrees (Fig. 8–98).

Bryant's Traction. An overhead frame is placed over the crib—the type used varies in different hospitals. The child is placed on a Bradford frame to facilitate nursing care and to maintain the hip joint in a position directly underneath the overhead pulleys. A chest restraint is used to secure the patient on the frame (Figs. 8–99 and 8–100). Bryant originally put only the fractured femur in direct overhead vertical traction. Some surgeons still prefer to apply traction to the involved legs only, claiming that more traction force can be achieved in this way. The author, however, believes that traction on both legs both provides more effective control of the pelvis and also prevents rotatory movements. Pressure on the malleoli is precluded by placing padding over them—a rolled short piece of stockinette or sheath wadding. Adhesive traction strips of proper length are smoothly applied, beginning proximally at the upper third of the thighs, and attached distally by straps to a spreader foot piece. Elastic bandages encircle the traction strips, beginning above the ankle and extending proximally; these should not be tight. The ropes extend from the foot piece and pass through pulleys located directly over the hip joints. The same amount of weight is applied on each leg and should be sufficient to lift the infant's pelvis by suspension until no weight is borne on the back of the sacrum. One should be cautious not

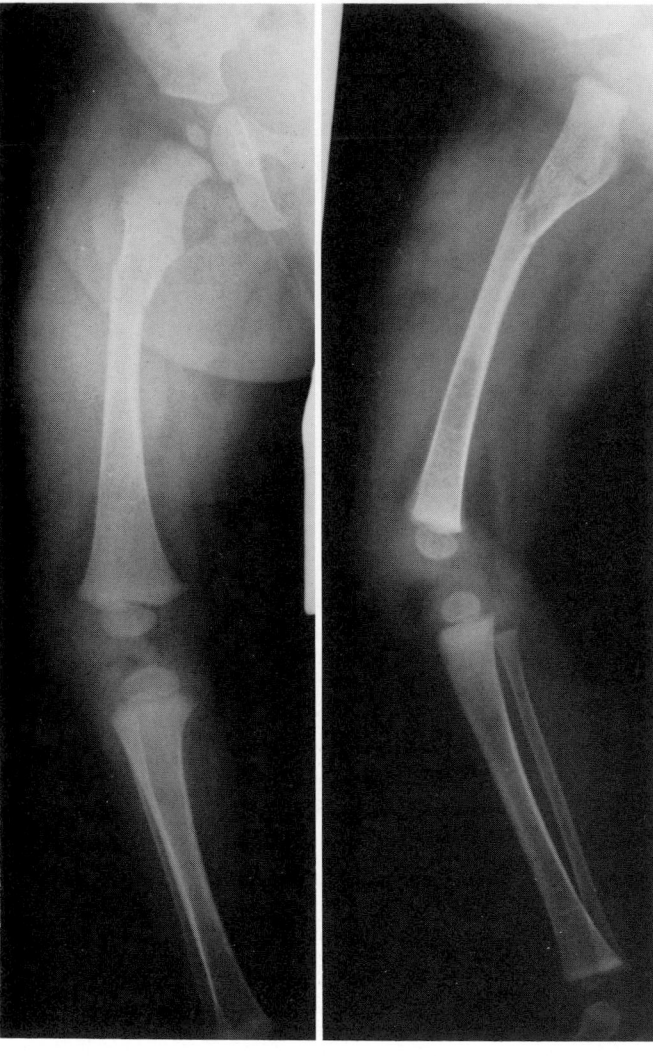

FIGURE 8–98. Fracture of the femoral shaft at its proximal third in a nine-month-old infant.

This fracture is best treated by Bryant's traction.

to overpull the small infant and suspend him in the air. Adhesive tape applied between the foot pieces will control rotational alignment of the lower limbs.

The position of the fracture is checked by periodic roentgenograms. Distraction of the fragments should be avoided. Medial bowing caused by excessive pull of the hip adductors is corrected by decreasing the amount of weight on the affected limb and increasing traction on the contralateral normal limb. By tilting the pelvis distally on the contralateral side, the pull of the hip adductors will be released (Fig. 8–101).

The expectation that a bony deformity in childhood will correct itself spontaneously with growth and remodeling is not an ex-

cuse for ignoring it, if correction can be obtained by simple means. At the same time, a child should not be subjected to too frequent manipulations or unjustified trauma to correct mere minor displacements.

Callus forms rapidly in infants. Two to three weeks from the time of trauma, the tenderness of the callus will have disappeared and the fracture will usually be stable enough to remove the traction and continue immobilization in a one and one half hip spica cast without the risk of losing the position of the fragments. The normal hip and thigh are included in the cast to stabilize the pelvis. The patient can then be discharged from the hospital. Immobilization in the hip spica cast is continued at home until there is solid union of the fracture. In birth fractures, this usually occurs in three weeks, and in infants and young children, from four to six weeks from the day of original injury. The immobile joints spontaneously regain their full range of motion within a few weeks.

Complications of Overhead Traction. Bryant's traction does have its drawbacks, nevertheless, and its apparent simplicity should not lull the surgeon into a false sense of security. It should *not* be used in children over two years of age or in those weighing over 25 pounds. Constant vigil should be kept for the possible development of any vascular, neurologic, or skin complications. Of these, circulatory embarrassment is the most serious and one that may assume tragic proportions.

Treatment of fractured femora by direct overhead traction may result in three degrees of circulatory insufficiency. The first is ischemic fibrosis of the muscles of the lower leg, with patches of sensory loss. There is almost complete paralysis of the muscles distal to the knee, except in the short toe flexors. The foot and ankle are usually deformed in rigid equinovarus position. The second degree of involvement is characterized both by the changes described in the first degree and by the presence of circumferential

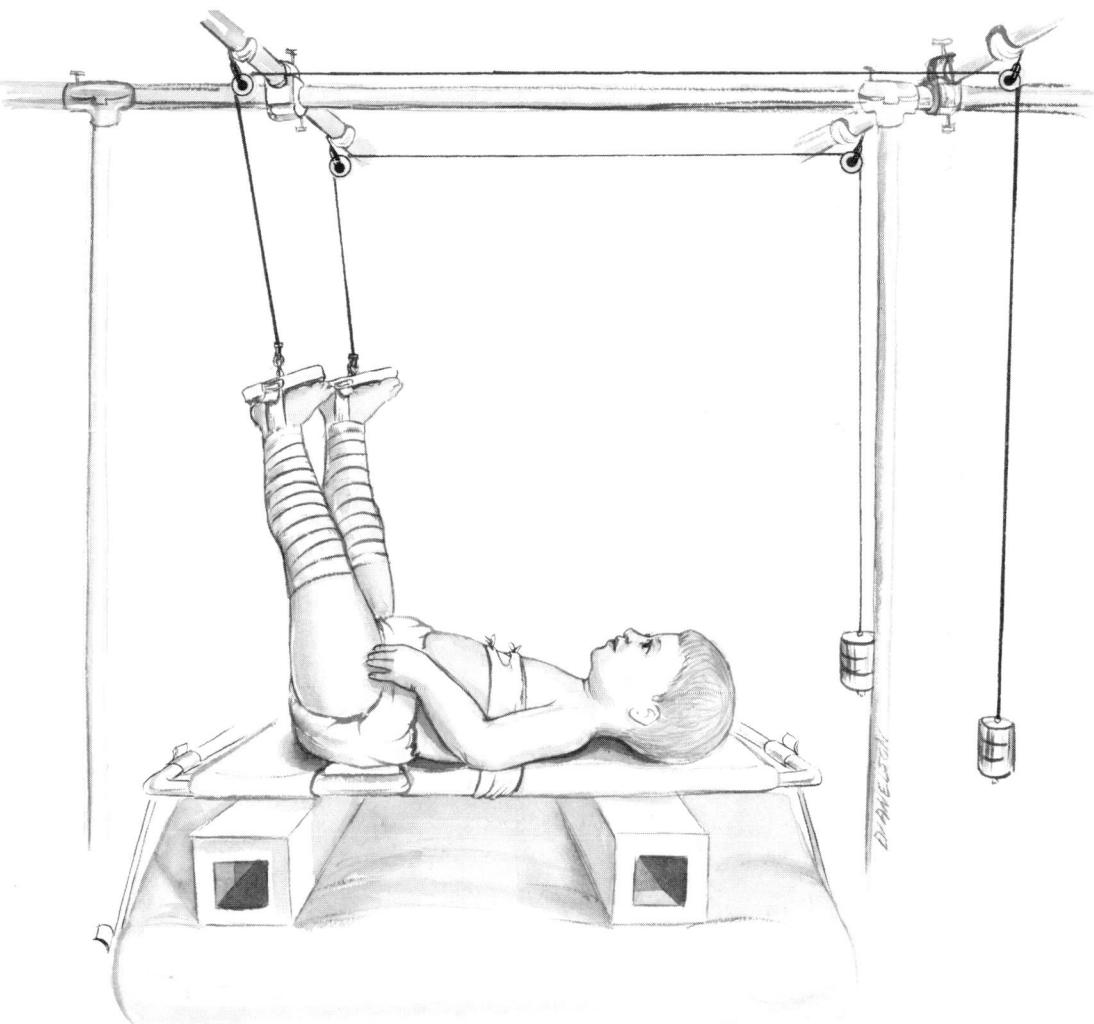

FIGURE 8–99. Bryant's direct overhead traction (see text for explanation).

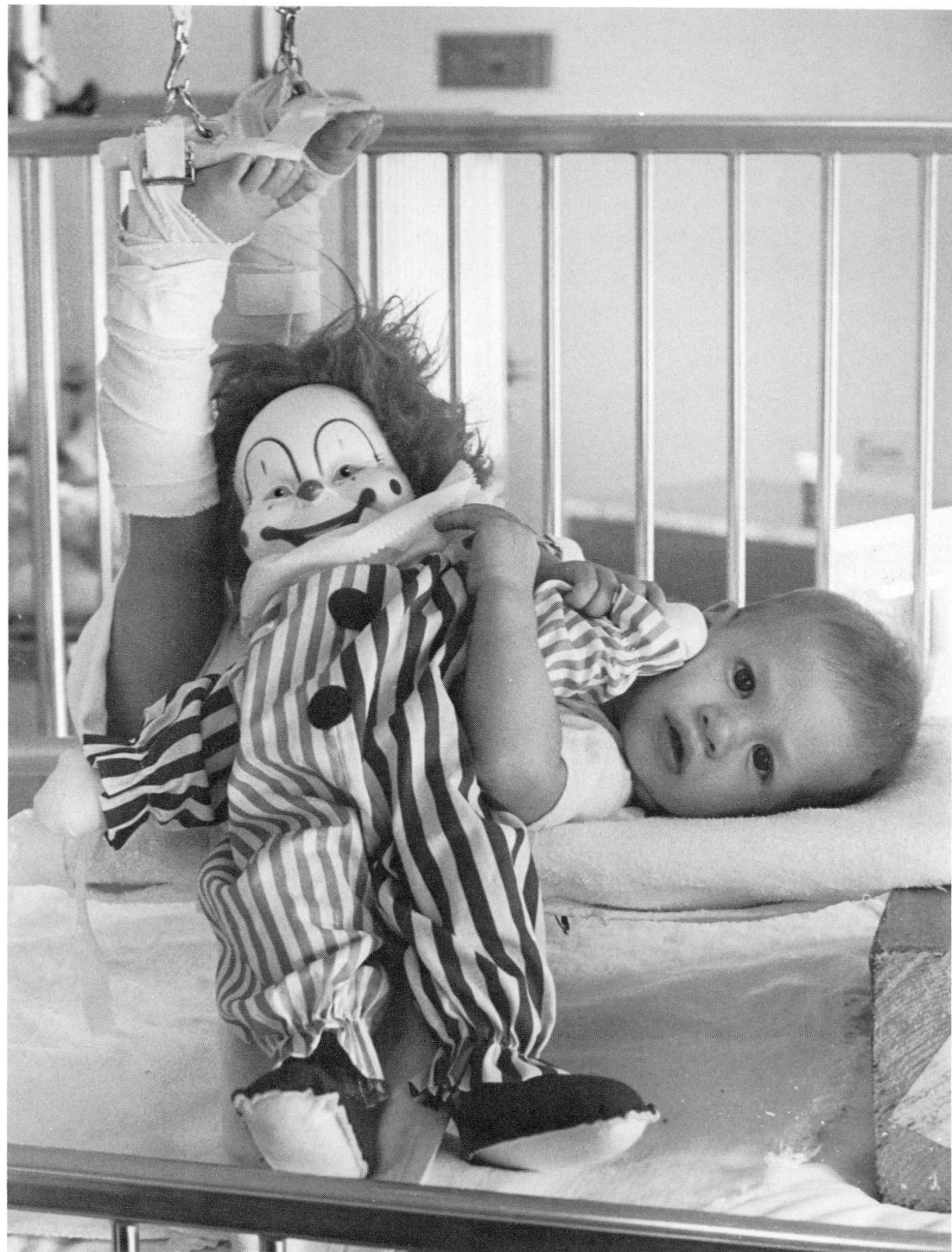

FIGURE 8–100.   *An infant with fractured femoral shaft treated in Bryant's traction.*

A.

Incorrect

B.

Correct

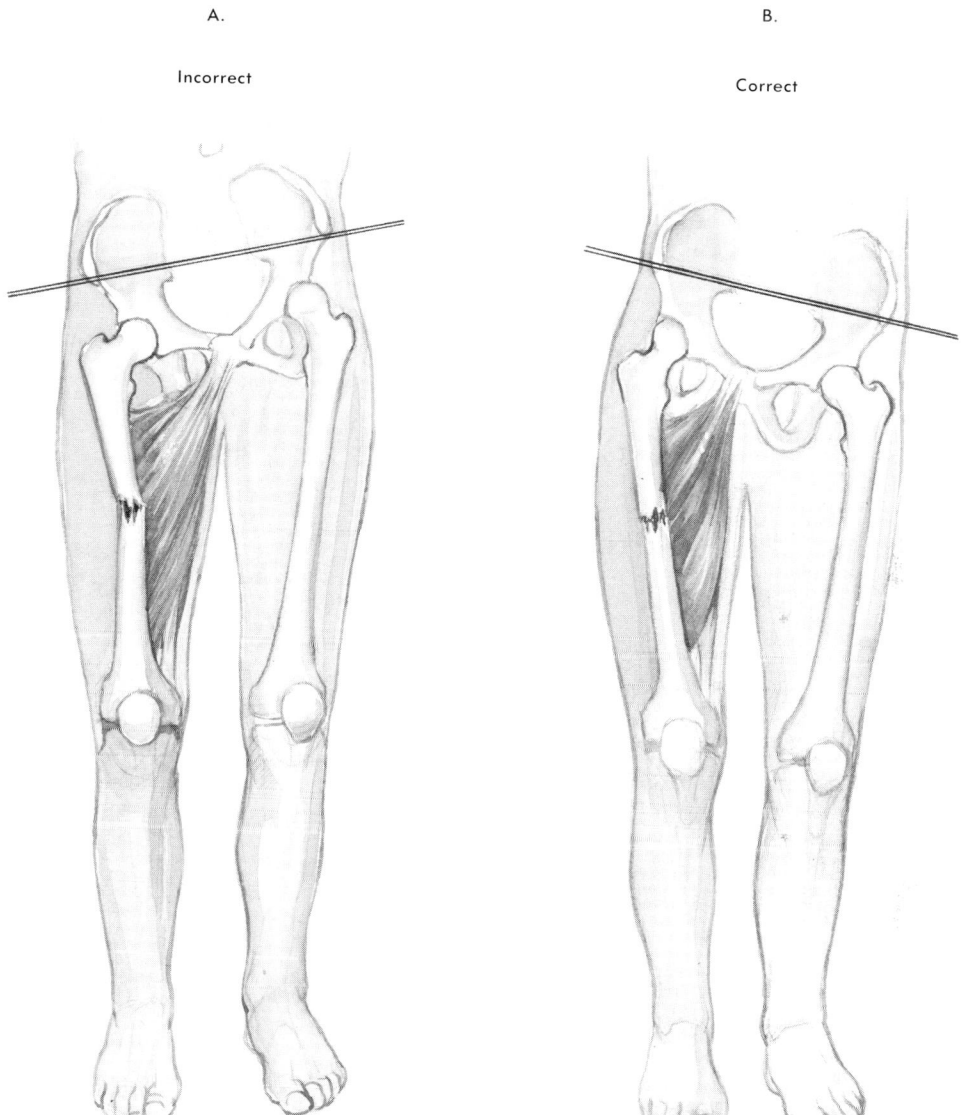

FIGURE 8-101. *The wrong and right ways of correcting medial bowing of fracture of the femoral shaft caused by pull of the hip adductors.*

A. *Wrong way.* Increasing weight on the fractured limb will tilt the pelvis distally, exaggerate functionally the degree of hip abduction, and increase the pull of the hip adductors; thus, the deformity is aggravated.

B. *Right way.* Increase the weights on the contralateral normal hip and tilt the pelvis distally on the normal side. Thus, the hip on the affected side is functionally in adducted position and the medial bowing is corrected by relaxing the pull of the hip adductors. (Redrawn after Blount.)

necrosis of the skin and underlying muscles in the calf. The third degree is the most severe form of circulatory insufficiency in which, in addition to the circumferential necrosis in the calf, the foot and ankle have become gangrenous.[576]

The first report of ischemic contracture in the lower limb in children was given in 1951 by Thompson and Mahoney, who described its occurrence following fractures of the femur in 13 children, one of whom had been treated by Bryant's traction.[592] Previously, Jones and Cotton had reported Volkmann's ischemia in the lower limb in two adults who had sustained crush injuries in the popliteal area.[561] Miller, Markin, and Grossman, in 1952, reported ischemic fibrosis of the lower limbs of seven children being treated for fractured femur, with six of the seven being treated in Bryant's traction. In all six, the ischemia manifested itself within the first two days. In three of the seven children, ischemia developed in the normal leg.[570] Nicholson, Foster, and Heath, in 1955, reported circulatory insufficiency in the legs of six children treated with Bryant's traction for simple fracture of the femur. In five of the six children, circulatory impairment developed in the uninjured leg.[576]

Impairment of circulation may be caused by several factors: (1) *The reduced hydrostatic pressure in the lower limbs* when they are held in vertical position makes it difficult for the blood to reach the foot and maintain adequate circulation. Nicholson, Foster, and Heath found an inversely proportionate ratio between the blood pressure of the ankle and the height of the ankle above the heart. When the leg was dependent over the side of the bed, blood pressure at the ankle was raised; when the leg was in horizontal position, it returned to normal; and with the leg in the elevated, or Bryant's position, the blood pressure was lowered. They further demonstrated, by making repeated oscillometric readings over a period of time, that with the leg maintained in Bryant's traction, the lowered blood pressure at the ankle remained constant and was not compensated.[576] (2) *Tautly applied circular bandages on the leg* can alter the level of blood pressure at the ankle. The pressure did not alter when the bandages were loosely applied; but when the bandages were tightly wrapped, particularly in children over two years of age, it could be reduced to zero.[576]

(3) *Shock* is an important factor. The lowered systemic blood pressure may produce ischemia in legs held by Bryant's traction. (4) *Traction* and stretching of the vascular tree from its normal resting state in one lower limb produce a variable degree of spasm in both main and collateral arteries in both limbs. This was shown experimentally in dogs by Mustard and Simmons.[574] Allowing a fractured femur to maintain the vessels in a shortened state for 24 hours and then distracting them will result in diffuse arterial spasm. (5) *Hyperextension of the knee* can impair circulation. Nicholson et al. investigated the effect of knee position on the vascular supply to the lower leg. They made oscillometric readings at the ankle with the traction and bandages on the leg, with the knee held in hyperextension, both with the limb in the horizontal and in the vertical position. In children under two years of age, reasonable snugness and extent of the bandage made no appreciable difference; whereas in children over four years of age, the oscillometric readings at the ankle with the limb vertical and the knee hyperextended were invariably zero. Nicholson et al. demonstrated that one significant factor that interferes with circulation in the vertically held leg, with or without the use of traction, is knee hyperextension. Its effect is apparent in patients more than two years of age and is constant in patients more than four years old. They emphasized the dangers of using Bryant's traction in patients over two years of age. Elevation of the leg to a vertical position with the knee hyperextended or fully extended may result in circulatory impairment.[576]

Peroneal nerve paralysis can occur. It is important that circulation, the degree of sensation in both feet, and the ability to move the toes be checked at frequent intervals. The circular turns of the elastic bandage may be displaced distally and cause as in children over four years of age, pressure sores on the heel. Careful inspection of the skin and rewrapping of the elastic bandages will prevent pressure necrosis of the skin.

Modification of Bryant's Traction. Ferry and Edgar modified Bryant's traction by utilizing the principles of Russell's traction (Fig. 8–102). This method is as follows: (1) The skin is painted with tincture of benzoin from the ankle to the midthigh. The

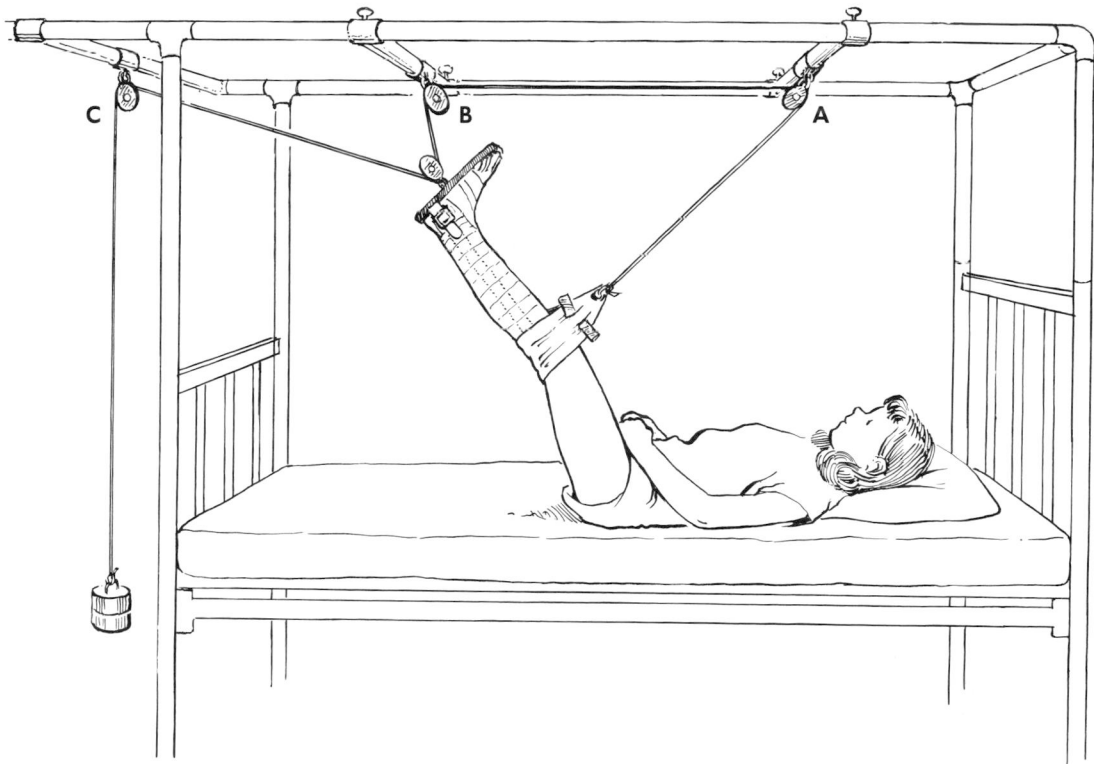

FIGURE 8–102. *Ferry and Edgar modification of Bryant's traction utilizing the principle of Russell (see text for explanation).*

painted area is then covered with stockinette that is smooth and not wrinkled. The malleoli are padded with a cotton-roll bandage. Traction strips are applied longitudinally on the medial and lateral aspects of the prepared area and are held in place by elastic bandage wrapped from the toes to the upper margin of the traction straps. The traction straps are then connected to a footplate that has a pulley on its bottom surface; it should be of adequate size to prevent pressure on the malleoli. A well-padded sling is secured on the back of the proximal part of the calf and distal to the popliteal fossa; the traction rope connected to the anterior end of the sling is passed to an overhead pulley A, through overhead pulley B, then through the pulley on the foot piece, and finally through overhead pulley C. Traction is applied on both lower limbs with sufficient weight on each limb to raise the buttocks slightly off the bed. Ordinarily 2 to 4 lb. of weight is sufficient. With this method, longitudinal traction force is applied in the direction of the long axis of the femur, raising the buttocks from the bed, but also maintaining the knees in a partially

flexed position. In this position, the hydrostatic force working against the pulse pressure is less because the heart-to-toe height is less than in the vertical position maintained in Bryant's traction. It is not necessary to wrap the circular bandages tightly, as part of the traction force is exerted through the calf sling. With the knees maintained in flexion, the likelihood of vascular and neurologic complications is minimized.[550]

The author recommends the use of the Ferry and Edgar modification of Bryant's traction for children over two years of age in whom insertion of a pin through the distal femur for skeletal traction is undesirable, such as in pathologic fractures in osteogenesis imperfecta or in cases of children with myelomeningocele who have markedly osteoporotic bones.

CHILDREN OVER TWO YEARS OF AGE AND ADOLESCENTS

If the fracture is undisplaced it is treated only with immobilization in a hip spica cast. If it is displaced, several choices of treatment are available: immediate reduction and immobilization in a plaster of Paris cast, with or without traction being incorporated into the cast; or reduction and some type of traction until callus is formed and then immobilization in a spica cast until bony union is firm. In children, open reduction and internal fixation of femoral shaft fractures should not be performed.

Regardless of the type of treatment used, if the fracture is displaced, it is best to perform a closed manipulative reduction initially.

The author prefers to employ traction to maintain alignment until there is adequate callus for stability (i.e., the callus is no longer tender and the femur moves as a unit on manipulation) and then immobilize in a one and one half hip spica cast. There are several types of traction available, namely: (1) skin traction—Russell or split Russell, (2) suspension skeletal or skin traction with a Thomas splint and Pearson attachment, and (3) "90°–90°" skeletal traction with a pin through the distal femur or the proximal tibia.

90°–90° Skeletal Traction. The author prefers 90°–90° skeletal traction with a pin through the distal femur because of its effectiveness and simplicity. Alignment of the fracture is easily achieved and maintained, as there is one line of traction and the pin through the distal femur provides good control of the fracture fragments. The gastrocnemius, hamstring, and iliopsoas muscles are relaxed by the flexed position of the hip and knee, making alignment of the fracture fragments relatively easy. Other advantages of 90°–90° traction are that it promotes dependent drainage; the thigh is readily accessible for clinical inspection of alignment without the use of portable x-ray equipment, and it facilitates change of dressings and wound inspection in infected open fractures. Preferably under general anesthesia, a heavy threaded Steinmann pin or a large Kirschner wire is inserted 2 cm proximal to the adductor tubercle at the junction of the posterior third and anterior two thirds of the femoral shaft; using this site, one avoids injuring the epiphyseal plate and puncturing the suprapatellar pouch and knee joint. Small stab incisions in the skin are desirable. The pin is introduced at right angles to the longitudinal axis of the thigh. Pushing the skin slightly upward while drilling the wire through it will prevent undue pressure on the skin while traction is applied. Sterile dressings are placed over the skin wounds and a traction bow of correct size is applied with the pin under tension. A light below-knee cast is applied with the ankle in neutral position. This should be well padded in the popliteal area and the dorsum of the foot and ankle to prevent pressure sores. Through two metal rings or plaster of Paris cast loops, one distal, the other proximal in position, traction ropes are extended to pulleys on the overhead frame to suspend the lower leg in horizontal position with the knee in 90 degrees of flexion. The weights are adjusted to counterbalance the weight of the leg plus that of the plaster boot, thus merely suspending the lower leg. A closed reduction of the fracture is performed next. Weights are placed via a rope on the traction bow with the hip in 90 degrees of flexion, the traction forces acting vertically in line with the longitudinal axis of the femoral shaft. The pelvis should be slightly lifted from the bed (Figs. 8–103 and 8–104).

Angulation and rotation can be easily corrected by shifting the overhead traction in the appropriate direction. If additional external support is necessary in an unstable fracture, coaptation splints may be employed; these are made of strips of balsa wood 2.5 cm. in width cut to the desired lengths and laid side-by-side between two pieces of moleskin. The splint is applied circumferentially around the thigh and held in place with buckled webbing straps over thin felt. Slings with 1 or 2 lb. of weight can be applied over the fracture site to control lateral or anteroposterior angulation. Small children are usually placed on a Bradford frame with split Russell traction on the normal leg for immobilization. A chest restraint is advisable if the child is very active.

The position and alignment of the fracture fragments are checked by periodic roentgenograms. Under no circumstances should one allow distraction of the fragments to take place. In children between two and ten years of age, side-to-side apposition with 0.5 to 1 cm. overriding is the ideal position (but it should not exceed 1.5 cm.). In infants and adolescents, however, end-to-end apposition is desirable.

Traction is continued for two to four

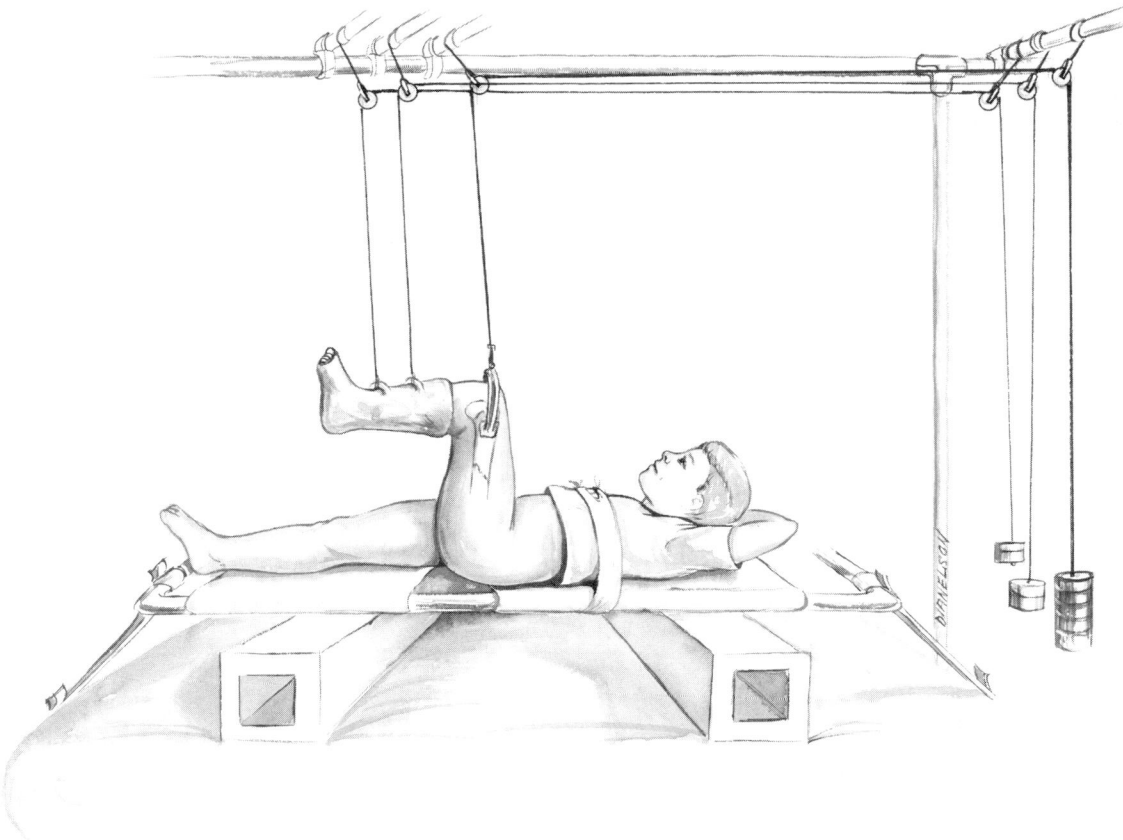

FIGURE 8–103. *Ninety-ninety skeletal traction with wire through the distal femur.*

It is used in children over two years of age for treatment of fractures of the femoral shaft.

weeks, until the callus is no longer tender on palpation and the femur moves in one piece. Adequate callus should also be visible on the roentgenograms. The patient is then placed in a one and one half hip spica cast. The affected thigh should be in 10 degrees of abduction or in neutral position with the opposite hip in moderate abduction to facilitate perineal hygiene. A common pitfall is to place the fractured thigh in marked abduction with resultant lateral bowing due to the pull of the strong adductors. It is always wise to extend the hip and knee gradually to 45 degrees of flexion before applying the hip spica cast. The pin in the femur is removed and is not incorporated in the cast.

Complications of this method of 90°–90° skeletal traction have been negligible in 280 fractures of the femoral shaft treated at the Children's Memorial Hospital, Chicago.

Humberger and Eyring have described a method of 90°–90° skeletal traction with the Kirschner wire inserted through the proximal tibia.[558] The author does not recommend their method because the Kirschner wire may injure the apophysis of the proximal tibial tubercle, either at the time of insertion or if it should migrate. Also, the wire in the proximal tibia does not provide direct control over the femur as does a wire through the distal femur. The only instance in which the author uses a wire through the proximal tibia is when the fracture is open and local skin lacerations preclude the use of a wire through the distal femur.

Suspension Traction. This method is preferred by many orthopedic surgeons for use in older children and adolescents. Skin traction is often unsatisfactory in the heavy child, and skeletal traction is applied with a Kirschner wire inserted through the distal femur.

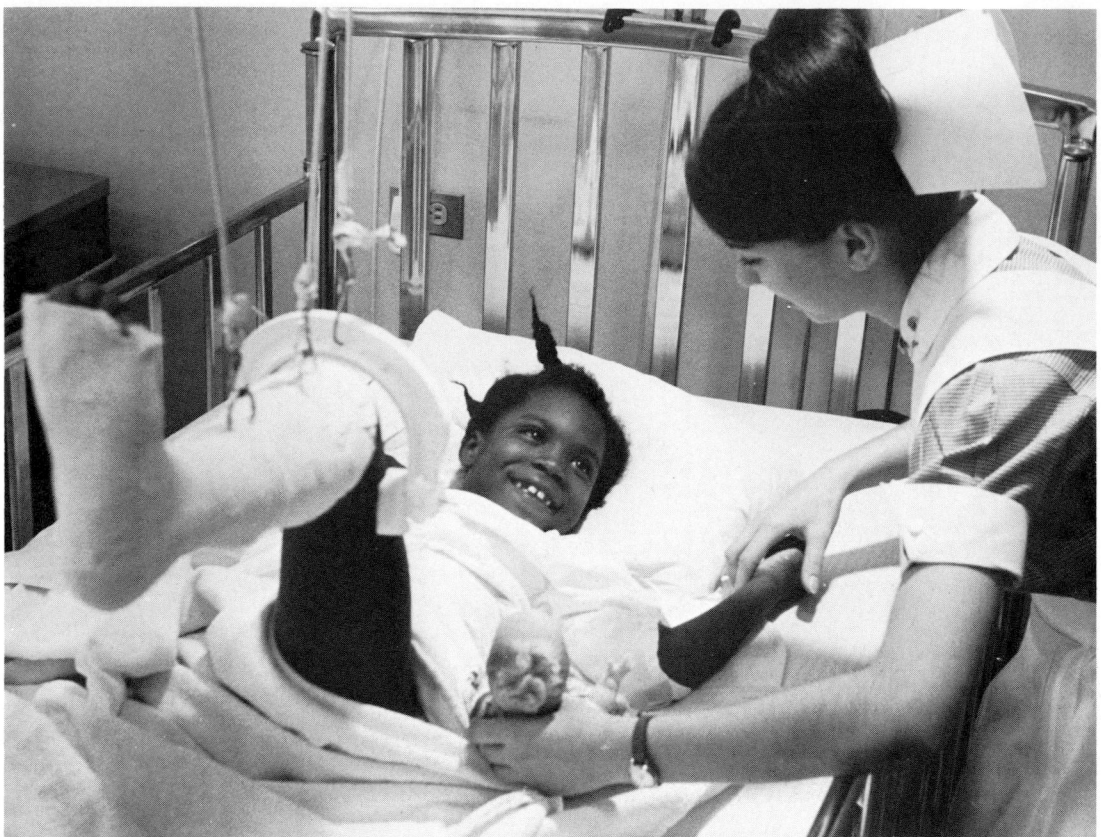

FIGURE 8–104. *A seven-year-old girl with fracture of the femoral shaft is being treated by 90°–90° skeletal traction with a wire through the distal femur.*

This is a very effective and simple method. The child is pain-free while in traction.

The thigh and leg are supported on a felt pad covered with stockinette and placed on webbing slings attached to the Thomas splint and Pearson attachment with safety pins or clips. There should be no wrinkles in the stockinette that encloses the felt pad. With the hip in 35 to 40 degrees of flexion, the Thomas splint (full or half-ring) is pushed up firmly against the ischial tuberosity and supported at both ends by sufficient weight to balance the limb. The traction ropes on the Thomas ring should pull in a somewhat cephalad direction to prevent the splint from sliding off the leg. The level of the Pearson attachment should be just above the knee joint level so that the knee can be flexed 30 degrees to relax the hamstrings. A traction rope with sufficient weight on the distal end of the Pearson attachment supports the weight of the leg. By careful ad-

justments of the weights, the limb can be so counterbalanced that it moves up and down with the patient without discomfort during nursing care. The foot of the bed is elevated, so that the weight of the patient's body acts as countertraction (Fig. 8–105).

In midshaft fractures, the tendency is toward posterior angulation due to the pull of gravity. To prevent this and to restore the normal anterior bowing of the femur, the slings under the thigh should be taut and the knee should be in flexion to relax the gastrocnemius muscle. If there is persistent posterior angulation, a thick pad may be placed beneath the thigh at the fracture site, or a sling with direct overhead vertical pull at the appropriate level may be employed. Medial or lateral angulation may be corrected by aligning the distal fragment with the proximal one by shifting the position of the outer or inner upper ends of the Pearson attachment, either proximally or distally on the Thomas splint, or by changing the direction of the pull, or both. Rotation is controlled by adjusting the suspension.

In about three to four weeks, good callus will usually be depicted in the roentgenogram. Traction is removed and the fracture is immobilized in a one and one half hip spica cast for an additional three to five weeks, at which time it will be solidly healed.

The author does not use suspension traction because of the advantages listed previously for 90°–90° traction in which there are no shifting splints with multiple suspension ropes to be adjusted.

Russell Skin Traction.[584] This is preferred by some as an ideal method for treatment of femoral shaft fractures in older children. The medial and lateral adhesive traction strips extend from the ankle to a point just below the knee and are attached

with straps to a footplate with a pulley on its inferior surface. There should be two pulleys at the foot of the bed and one overhead. A well-padded sling is placed beneath the knee. The traction rope extends from the sling to the overhead pulley, which is distal to the knee joint, so that the rope is directed upward and distally at an angle of 25 degrees, passing over the superior pulley attached to the end of the bed to which the skin traction straps are fixed and back again over the inferior pulley at the foot of the bed, where 5 to 8 lb. of weight is suspended. The lower limb rests on two pillows arranged so that the knee is in 30 degrees of flexion, the thigh is supported, and the foot just clears the mattress. The foot of the bed is raised 10 to 20 cm. to provide countertraction. The vertical traction force is roughly equal to the amount of weight used; whereas the horizontal traction force, because of the double pull from the footplate

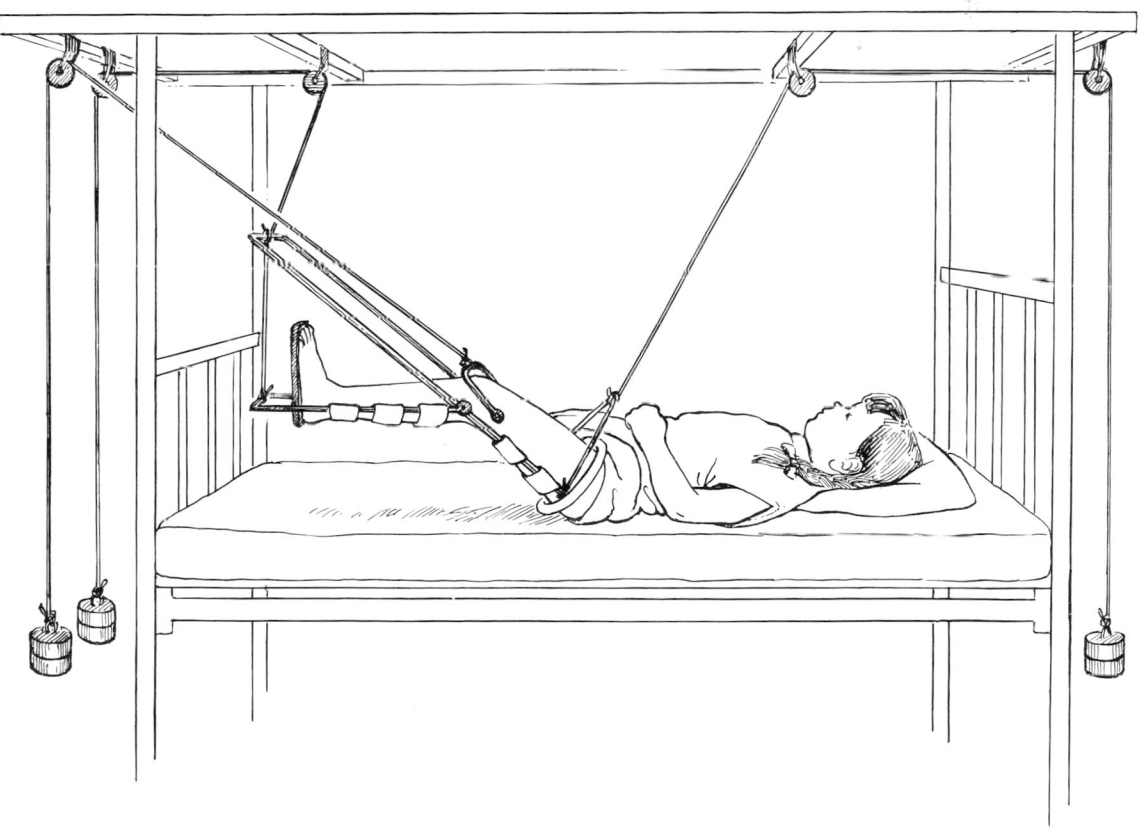

FIGURE 8–105. *Suspension traction with wire through the distal femur with Thomas splint and Pearson attachment (see text for explanation).*

to the foot of the bed, is equal to approximately twice the amount of weight. The vertical and horizontal forces create a parallelogram of forces, with the resultant force in line with the long axis of the shaft of the femur (Fig. 8–106 A).

Advocates of Russell traction prefer it because of the ease with which it may be applied. The muscles are kept in balance, relatively less traction weight is required to overcome shortening and deformity, and the need for skeletal traction with its possible complications is eliminated. The disadvantages of this technique are: (1) the possible serious complication of peroneal nerve palsy with the resultant foot drop due to pressure by the knee sling in the region of the common peroneal nerve; (2) the potential for development of posterior bowing at the fracture site due to lack of effective external support under the thigh (often it is necessary to apply an additional sling beneath the thigh with vertical traction to restore the normal anterior bowing of the femur); (3) the difficulty of nursing care and the necessity for careful vigil to ensure that correction traction is maintained; and (4) the child is initially in more pain than in 90°–90° traction.

The author employs split Russell traction instead of the original Russell traction with its 2:1 ratio of forces. In split Russell traction, skin traction is applied in the longitudinal axis of the limb and a balanced sling with a vertical force is placed under the distal femur or knee and suspended by weights to support the part and supply the necessary resolution of forces (Fig. 8–106 B). External rotation of the leg is controlled with medial rotation traction straps.

As stated previously, open reduction is not justified in femoral shaft fractures in children. Perfect anatomic reduction of fracture fragments is of less importance in the child than in the adult, as with growth and remodeling, malunion will correct itself.

When there is an open fracture of the femur, the wound is thoroughly debrided of all foreign material, and any contused dead tissue is excised. After copious irrigation with normal saline solution, suction catheters are inserted through separate stab wounds in the skin and the wound is primarily closed. The limb is placed in 90°–90° skeletal traction, as already described. Ap-

propriate antibiotics and tetanus antitoxin are administered. There is no justification for immediate internal fixation because the fracture is open and the bone ends are exposed. The suction catheters connected to the Hemovac are removed in two to three days. An open fracture ordinarily requires a longer period of time to consolidate.

Treatment by Closed Reduction and Immediate Immobilization in Double Hip Spica Cast. The chief advantage of this method is that it decreases the duration of the hospital stay, which has obvious financial advantages. However, to maintain reduction is difficult, requiring close supervision by repeated roentgenograms and wedging of the cast to correct angulation, should it occur.

Dameron and Thompson, in 1959, presented the end-results in 53 patients treated by closed reduction and immobilization in a hip spica cast. The average duration of follow-up was 6.9 years. In no patient could they find any deformity, abnormality of gait, or limitation of hip and knee motion. At the follow-up examination, the fractured limb was, on the average, 1/16 inch longer than the opposite normal limb. In only a few patients was the broken limb more than 1/4 inch shorter than the normal limb, and in five patients, the affected limb was more than 1/4 inch longer. Complications of malunion, delayed union, nonunion and Volkmann's contracture and gangrene were not encountered in any of their patients. They recommended it as a safe, certain, comfortable, and economical method of treatment of femoral shaft fractures.[544]

The method advocated by Dameron and Thompson is as follows:

Under general anesthesia and aseptic conditions, a Kirschner wire is inserted immediately distal to the proximal tibial epiphysis on the affected side; a sterile Kirschner wire bow is attached and, while longitudinal traction is applied, the patient is gently transferred to the fracture table. The foot on the normal side is secured by strapping it to the foot piece of the fracture table. Traction is applied on the fractured thigh and normal leg, while an assistant steadies the pelvis manually against the well-padded perineal post. The pull on the distal fragment should be in line with the proximal fragment. Ordinarily this is adequate to

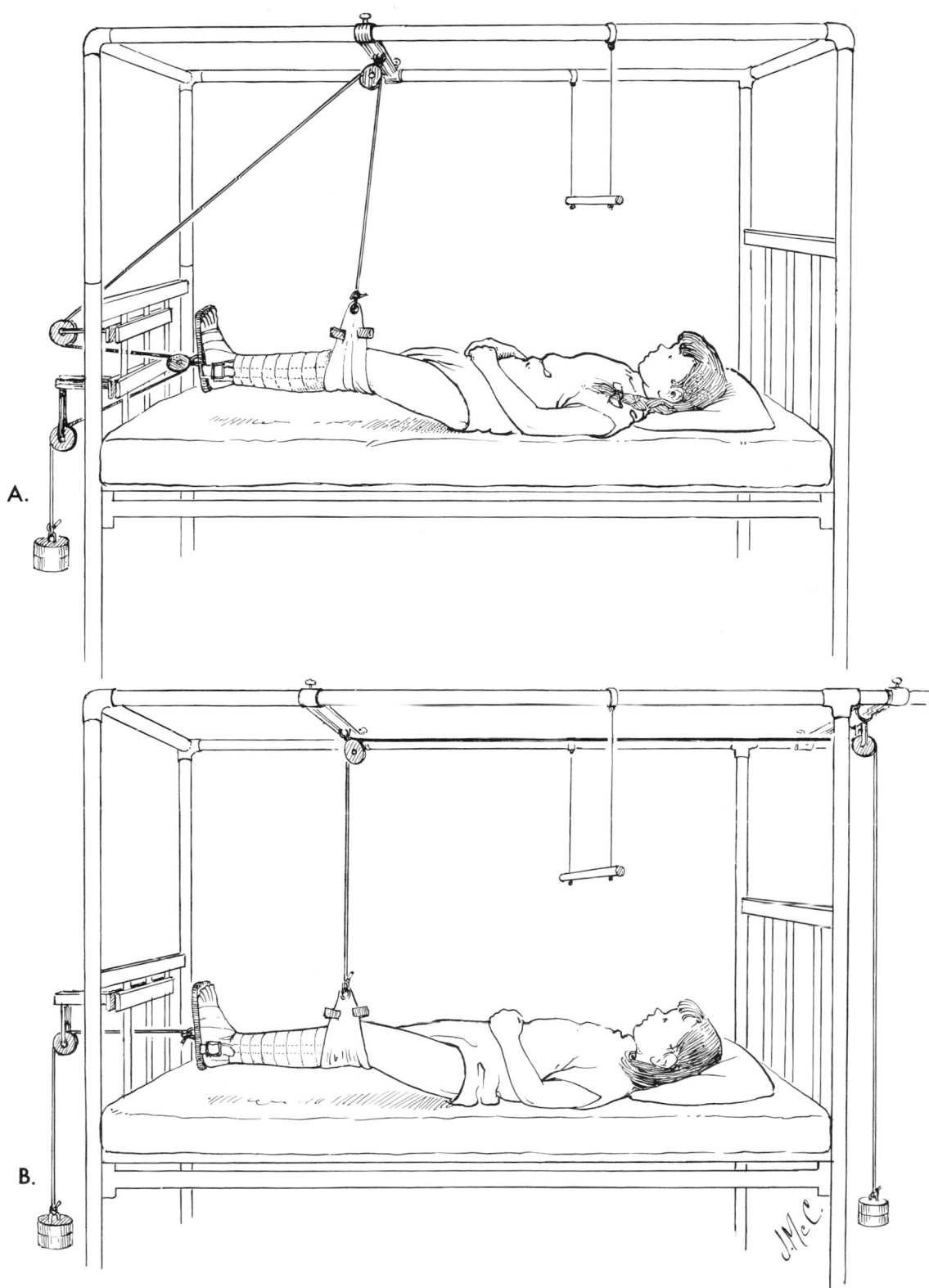

FIGURE 8–106.   *Russell skin traction (A) and split Russell traction (B). (See text for explanation.)*

achieve reduction of oblique fractures. Roentgenograms are made to determine alignment of fracture fragments. If any angulation is present, it is corrected by altering the direction of the traction forces.

A well-moulded double hip spica cast is applied from the nipple line to include both feet, incorporating the Kirschner wire bow in the plaster. The patient is discharged on the following day. Immobilization in the cast is continued for eight weeks; adolescents require an additional two to four weeks for solid bony union to take place.[20, 544]

Judet, Judet, and LeGrange immobilize the fractured femur in a hip spica cast, with the knee and hip on the affected side in 90 degrees of flexion.[758]

Complications

DISCREPANCY IN LIMB LENGTH

Inequality in limb length following femoral shaft fractures in children may result from excessive overriding or distraction of the fragments or from stimulation of linear growth. In the literature there are several "late follow-up" observations.* Aitken, in a study of the end-results in 71 cases of femoral shaft fractures in children, concluded that in children under 13 years of age, one should expect an average overgrowth of 1 cm. from the position at the time of discharge regardless of the method of treatment.[527] In a meticulous analysis of femoral shaft fractures in children, Greville and Ivins observed that, between the ages of four and eight years, an average overgrowth of 0.6 cm. can be expected in midshaft fractures; they also noted some added growth in the unbroken tibia on the same side as the fractured femur.[554]

Anderson, Griffin, and Green arrived at the following conclusions based upon serial data collected from the Growth Study of Children's Hospital Medical Center in Boston. A total of 107 patients were included in their study. (1) Between two and ten years of age, it is desirable for the fracture to heal with some overriding, but this should not exceed 1.5 cm. All children in this age group with displaced femoral fractures showed some stimulation of growth of the affected limb as compared with that of the normal side. (2) In children under two years of age and in adolescents, a similar degree of growth stimulation was not noted. This might be explained by the fact that in infants the fracture heals rapidly and there is a shorter period of hyperemia, and that in adolescents there are only a few years of growth remaining with a shorter period for relative acceleration of growth to operate on epiphyses that are less responsive to growth. Thus, in children under two years of age and in adolescents, they recommend end-to-end reduction and no overriding, since the degree of stimulation in these two age groups is usually small.[529]

Leg lengths should be carefully checked at periodic intervals following femoral shaft fractures to detect any significant discrepancy.

ANGULAR DEFORMITIES OF FEMORAL SHAFT

Linear growth of long bones takes place at the epiphysis with the addition of new bone. Growth displaces angulation away from the end of the bone, instead of decreasing the angle. The remodeling of angular deformity is primarily a response to functional stresses on the femur by muscle pull and the force of gravity. Remodeling and changes in alignment occur slowly; this is in contrast to stimulation in rate of growth of the fractured femur, which occurs mostly during the first two years after injury.

Angular deformities occur more frequently in fractures of the proximal third of the femoral shaft, often with medial angulation, and correct themselves more slowly in the proximal third than in the distal two thirds.

Anderson, Griffin, and Green noted the rate of reduction of an angular deformity to be dependent upon the direction of angulation. In their series of cases within a five-year period, the average reduction of anterior bowing was 26 per cent, medial bowing 30 per cent, lateral bowing 46 per cent; and in 8 of the 11 who showed zero to 6 degrees of posterior bowing, it was more

---

See References 527, 528, 532, 533, 542, 545, 554, 567, 585, 589, 593.

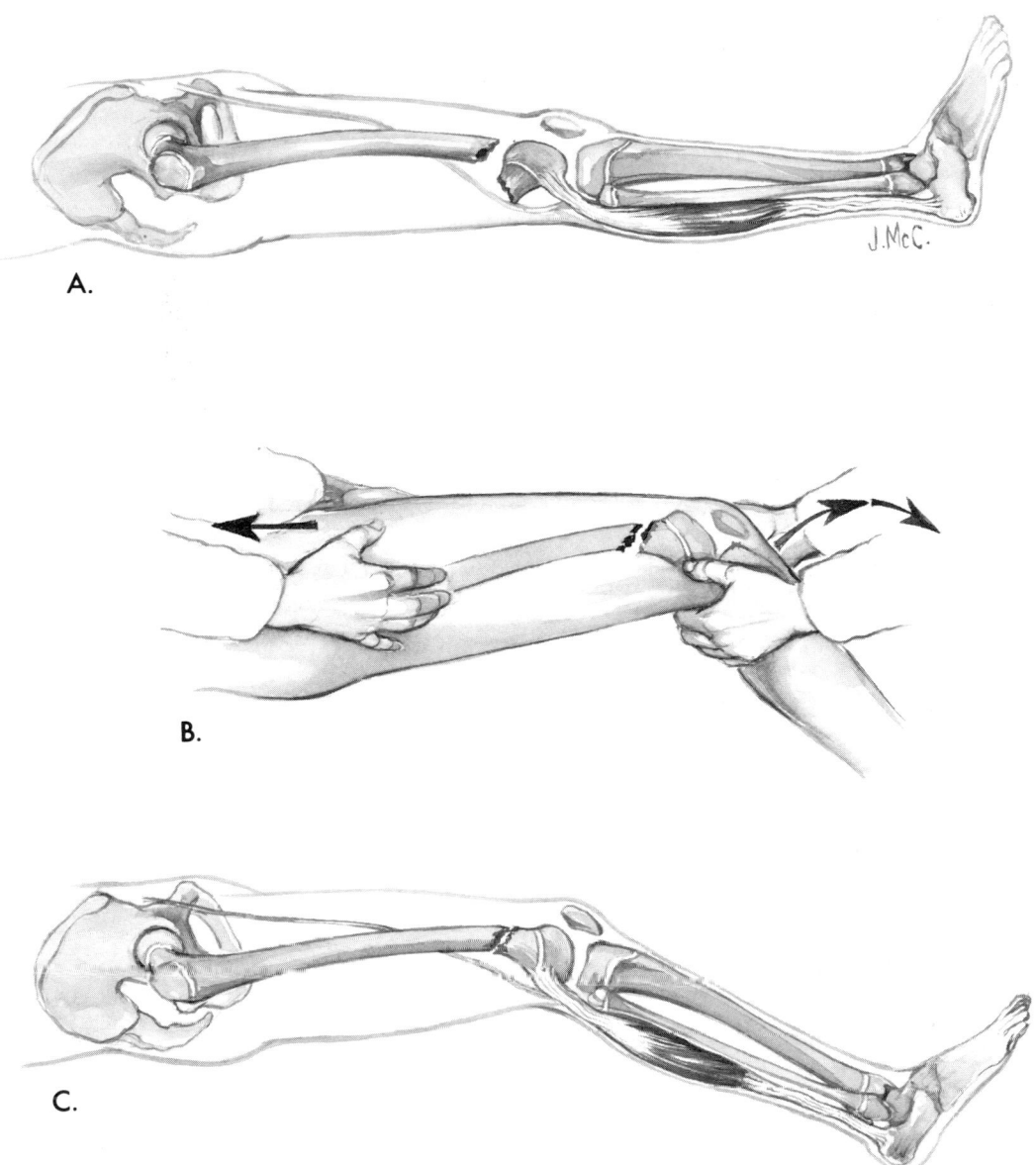

A.

B.

C.

FIGURE 8–107. Technique of reduction of supracondylar fracture of distal femur.

resistant to diminution through remodeling. They were unable to delineate the extremes of malalignment that will spontaneously correct themselves, as the patients in their series did not have severe angular deformities after reduction.[529]

Barford and Christiansen, in a follow-up study of 114 children with femoral shaft fractures 2 to 12 years following the original trauma, concluded that angulation of 25 degrees or less in the diaphyses of the femora can be expected to undergo sufficient correction with remodeling and growth so that a residual deformity is not apparent clinically, but may still be beyond normal limits when measured on the roentgenogram.[532]

It is recommended that fracture fragments be aligned in as near normal a relationship as is possible and that angles that exceed the normal range by more than 5 degrees not be accepted. The surgeon

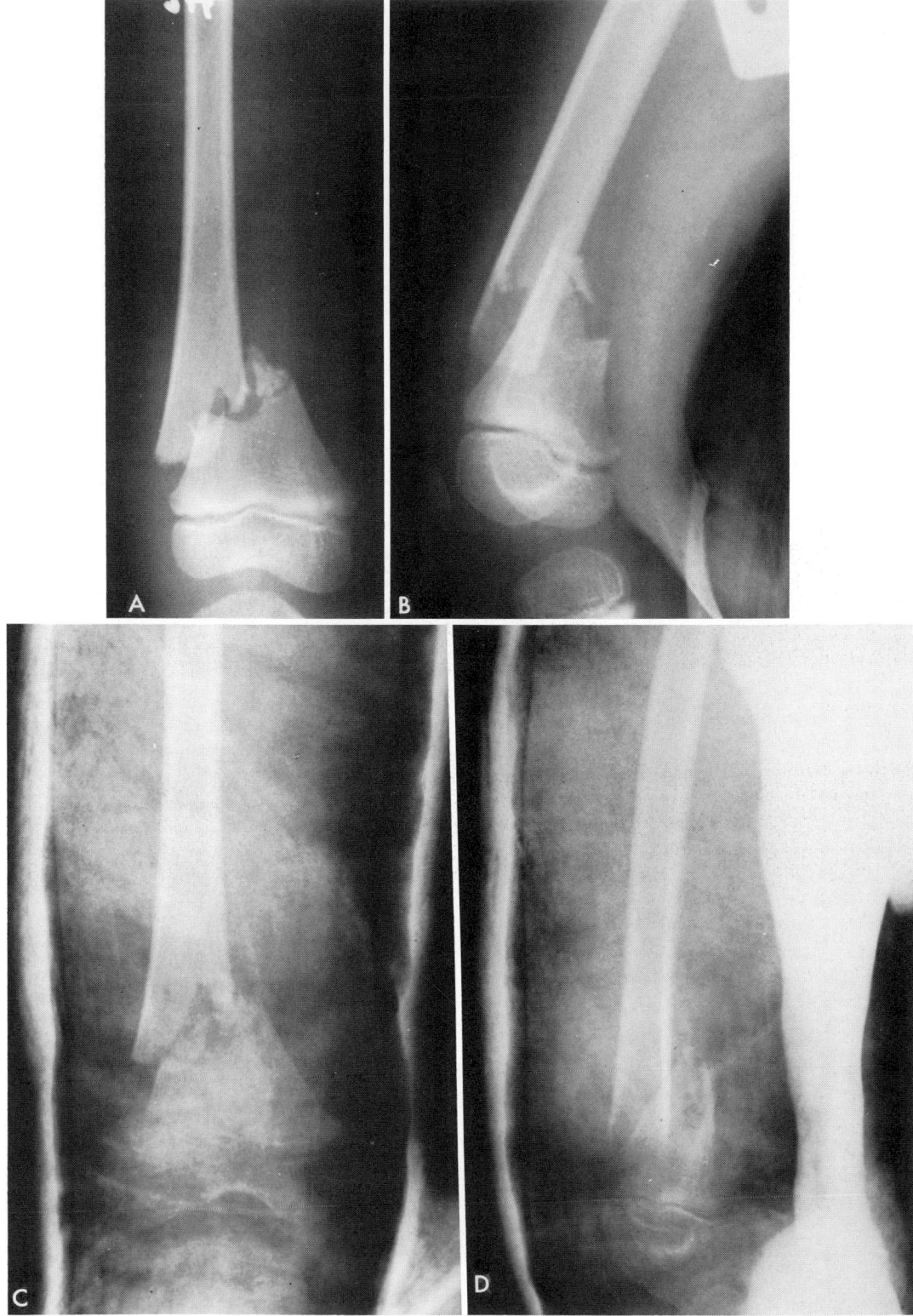

FIGURE 8–108.   *Remodeling of supracondylar fracture of distal femur.*

A and B. Initial roentgenograms. C and D. In cast. Note posterior angulation of distal fragment.

Figure continued on following page.

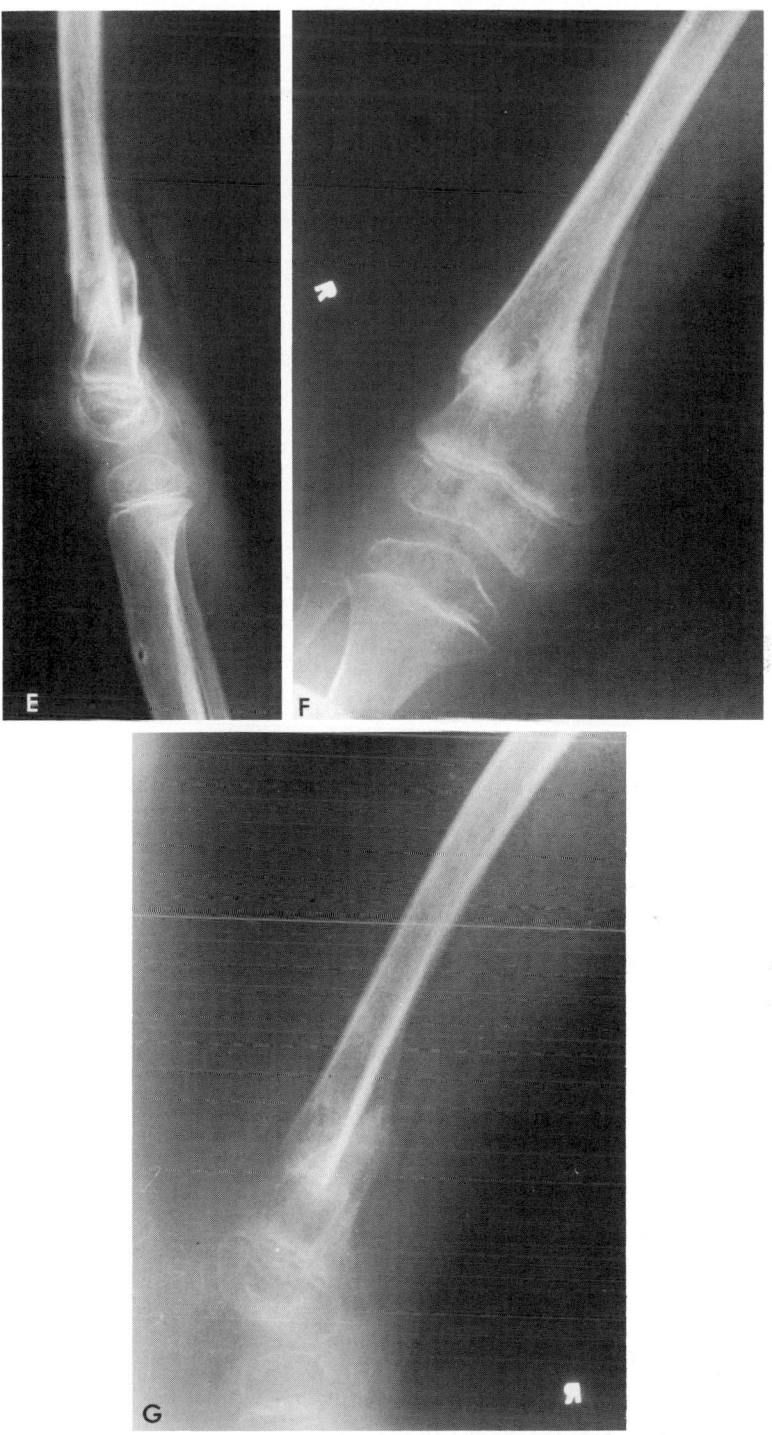

FIGURE 8–108 Continued.   Remodeling of supracondylar fracture of distal femur.

E to **G.** Remodeling of angular deformity in the plane of knee motion.

should aim at complete absence of rotational deformity, and should strive to achieve angular deformities that do not exceed 9 degrees in the mediolateral direction, 15 degrees anteriorly, and 5 degrees posteriorly. These borderlines are easily obtainable with adequate supervised traction.

FRACTURES INVOLVING THE DISTAL FEMORAL EPIPHYSIS

The ossification center of the distal femoral epiphysis is present at birth and becomes fused with the diaphysis between the eighteenth and nineteenth years. The largest and most actively growing epiphysis in the body, it contributes to 70 per cent of the length of the femur and 40 per cent of that of the entire lower limb.

The distal femoral epiphysis includes the entire articular surface of the lower end of the femur. The points of origin of the two heads of the gastrocnemius muscle and of the plantaris muscle are from the posterior surface of the distal diaphysis; the ligaments are attached to the medial and lateral femoral condyles. The bony configuration of the knee joint is such that in no position are the bones in more than partial contact. Thus, the strength of the knee joint is derived from the ligaments that surround it and not from the contour of the bones. An excessive force applied on the knee joint will put tension on the ligaments; when this strain is of sufficient degree, the epiphysis will separate from the diaphysis.

Fractures involving the distal femoral physis are rare, constituting 1 per cent of all physeal injuries. They may occur at any age before 17 years, the greatest incidence being between 11 and 15 years.

In the pre-automobile era when horse-drawn vehicles were the means of transportation, this injury was of common occurrence and was known as the "cartwheel" fracture. Boys stealing rides, while trying to board moving wagons from the rear, would get a leg or foot caught in the spokes of the rear wheel. Forced hyperextension of the knee was produced by the traction imparted by the rotatory force of the revolving rear wheel. The distal femoral epiphysis was displaced anteriorly, while the distal end of the diaphysis was forced into the popliteal space, lacerating or contusing the popliteal vessels or tibial nerve. These fractures were often open and were later complicated by gas-bacillus or tetanus infection. The extremely serious nature of this injury at that time is reflected by the report of Hutchinson, in 1894, who presented the end-results of 58 cases; among the 30 patients with open fractures, there were ten deaths; and of the remaining 20, 17 required amputation. Of the 28 closed fractures, reduction could not be obtained in 12 cases, 6 of which developed sloughs, necessitating amputation in 4. Only 16 of the 28 closed fractures could be reduced with good end-results.[607] Fortunately, this gloomy picture has altered today; however, trauma to the distal femoral epiphyseal plate is still a serious problem and may be the source of troublesome complications. For a critical review of the early literature, which is particularly voluminous in the latter part of the nineteenth century, the reader is referred to Poland.[762]

Mechanism of Injury and Pathologic Anatomy

Separation of the distal femoral epiphysis is caused by a sudden severe force applied in the region of the knee joint. With changes in the means of transportation, the scene of injury has moved to the highway, the football field, and the farm. About 50 per cent of the cases are caused by automobile accidents, 20 per cent by football injuries, 15 per cent by falls from a height, and the remaining 15 per cent by miscellaneous accidents such as stepping in a hole, catching the foot in a moving wheel, or being dragged by a horse. Fractures involving the distal femoral physis can be divided into the following types according to the direction of the force causing the injury:

Abduction Type. This is caused by a blow to the lateral side of the distal femur, usually occurring on the high school football field (the adult who receives the same kind of trauma will sustain tears of the medial collateral ligament, medial meniscus, and cruciate ligament). The result is a Type II (Salter-Harris) physeal injury. The periosteum is ruptured on the medial side and the distal femoral epiphysis is displaced laterally with a lateral fragment of the metaphysis. It is usually associated with some rotation. This fracture may reduce itself spontaneously and may be missed if the triangular piece of metaphyseal bone is small. One should carefully scrutinize the roentgenogram and take special abduction strain views to detect the lesion, if indicated.

Hyperextension Type. This was the common variety in the wagon wheel injury of old times. The distal femoral epiphysis is displaced anteriorly by the hyperextension force and by the pull of the contraction of the quadriceps muscle. The periosteum on the posterior aspect is torn and the fibers of the gastrocnemius muscle are stretched or partially torn. The triangular metaphyseal bone fragment and the intact periosteal hinge are anterior in location. The distal end of the femoral shaft is driven posteriorly into the soft tissues of the popliteal fossa, where it may injure the popliteal vessels as well as the common peroneal or posterior tibial nerves.

Hyperflexion Type. Posterior displacement of the distal femoral epiphysis is extremely rare. It results from a forceful flexion injury caused by a direct blow on the distal femur.

Type IV (Salter-Harris) Physeal Injury. In a fourth variety, the fracture line traverses the joint surface as well as the physis. It is usually sustained as a result of an automobile accident or a fall from a height, and results from longitudinal thrust and lateral compressional forces. The fracture may be comminuted. In this injury, the prognosis for subsequent growth is very poor.

Diagnosis

The child is presented in the emergency room with a history of violent injury to the lower limb. He is in severe pain and unable to bear weight on the affected leg. The knee is markedly swollen, tense, and held in partial flexion. Any attempt at passive extension of the joint is restricted and guarded by muscle spasm. There may be obvious deformity, with genu valgum in lateral displacements. In anterior displacements the femoral condyles may be palpable anterior to the distal diaphysis. The lower end of the femoral shaft or a large hematoma may be

felt in the popliteal fossa. The pulsations of the posterior tibial and dorsalis pedis arteries may be absent, and the leg and foot may be cold and cyanotic.

Roentgenograms will disclose the fracture (Fig. 8–109). As stated previously, in abduction fractures the roentgenograms may be misinterpreted as normal unless one meticulously looks for the triangular piece of metaphyseal bone or takes special abduction strain views.

Treatment

The method of reduction depends upon the type of fracture. Ordinarily a general anesthetic is required to obtain adequate relaxation of the limb and the patient. The markedly swollen joint is aspirated to facilitate reduction.

ABDUCTION TYPE FRACTURES

These are simple to treat. There are no special problems of vascular injury or growth disturbance. The technique of reduction is as follows: The anesthetized patient is placed on the fracture table with both feet strapped on the footplates. Longitudinal traction is applied on the extended knee. Reduction is accomplished by direct manual pressure, pushing the laterally displaced distal epiphysis medially and the lower end of the femoral shaft laterally. The fracture is held in a single hip spica cast. The knee is immobilized in extension. The three points of fixation—laterally at the ankle and the greater trochanter, and medially at the knee—are well padded. If only a long leg cast is applied, the fracture will become displaced. Plaster immobilization is maintained for from four to six months.

HYPEREXTENSION TYPE FRACTURES

The hyperextension type of fracture presents several problems of management: first, the potential injury to the popliteal vessels, and second, the difficulty of achieving and maintaining reduction. Since the plane of displacement and the plane of the knee joint motion are in the same direction, there is lack of an adequate lever arm to grasp the

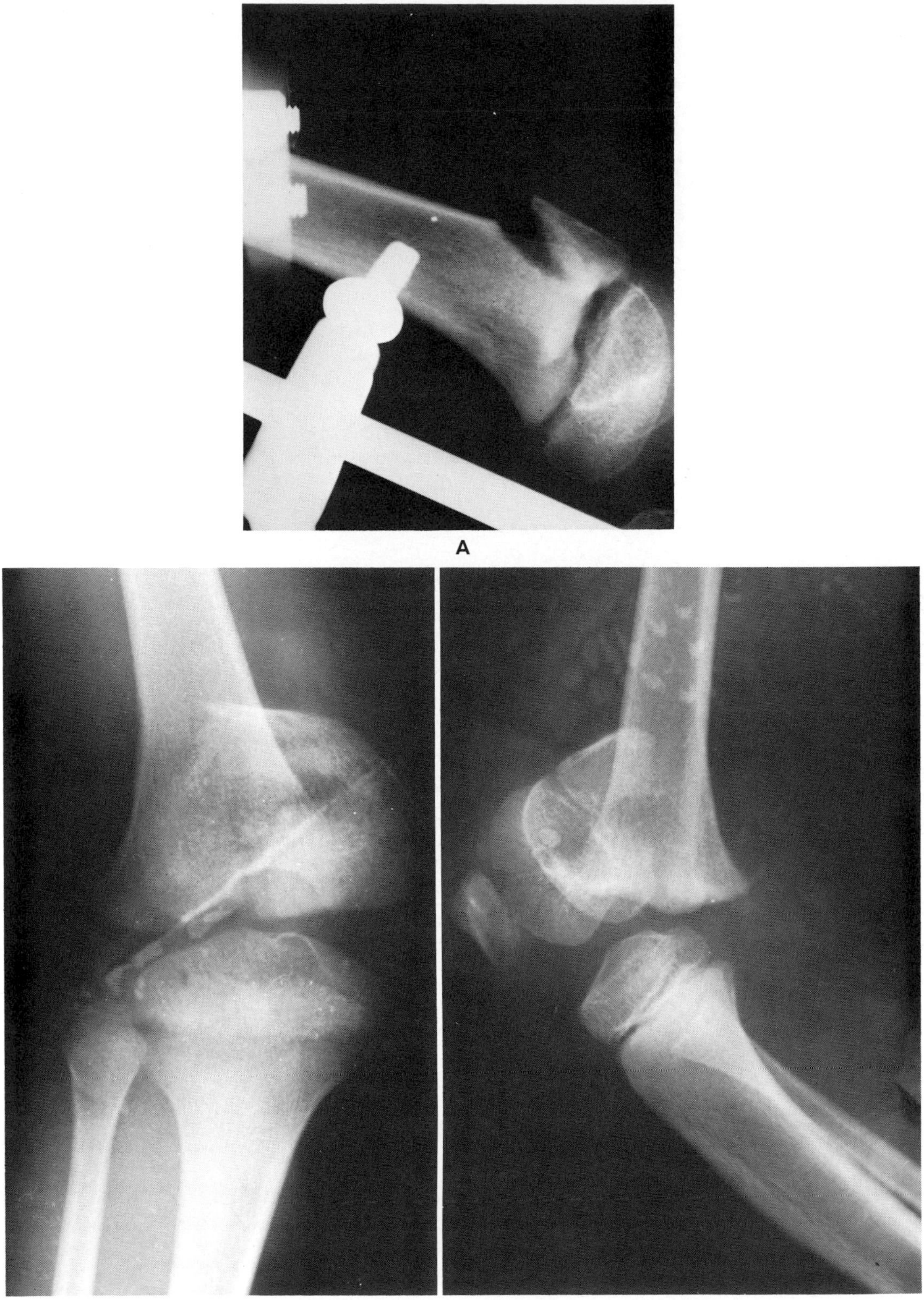

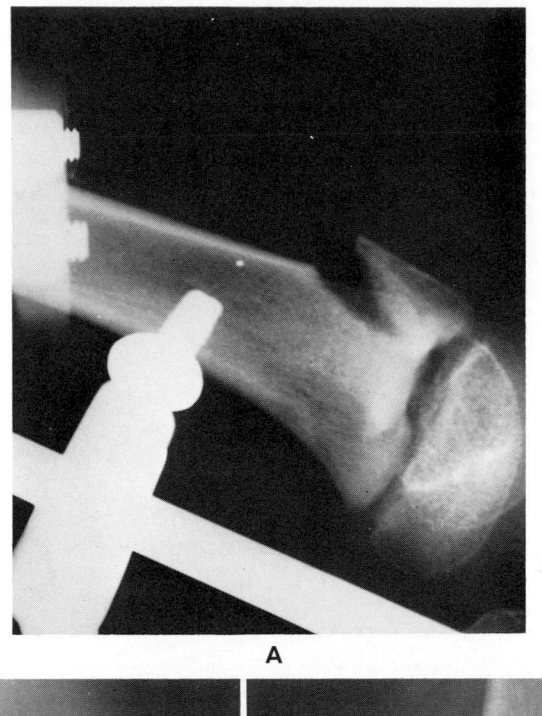

A

B

FIGURE 8–109.   Type II (Salter and Harris) fracture involving the distal femoral physis.

A. Minimally displaced. **B.** Markedly displaced.

distal fragment effectively. A closed reduction should be attempted first. The technique is as follows: The anesthetized patient is placed on the fracture table and the foot on the normal side is fastened to the footplate. The hip is flexed to relax the quadriceps muscle and the knee is flexed to relax the gastrocnemius and hamstring muscles. An assistant applies longitudinal traction on the lower leg, gradually increasing flexion of the knee; with his thumbs, the surgeon exerts direct pressure on the femoral epiphyses, pushing it first distally and then downward and posteriorly, while, with his other fingers, he pulls the lower femoral shaft anteriorly. Reduction is completed by acute flexion of the knee. Postreduction roentgenograms are made to check restoration of the epiphysis to its normal anatomic position. If reduction is successful, a single hip spica cast is applied, holding the knee in 60 to 90 degrees of flexion. The angle at which the knee is immobilized is of great importance in maintaining anatomic reduction. As pointed out by Aitken and Magill, recurrence of anterior displacement usually is caused by immobilization of the knee in insufficient flexion.[597]

In complete anterior displacements, a position of acute knee flexion may be necessary to maintain reduction; however, immobilization of the knee in such a position may cause marked difficulty in regaining extension. In complete anterior displacements, it is best to insert heavy threaded Steinmann pins transversely in the distal femoral shaft well above the fracture site, and another pin in the proximal third of the tibia well distal to the physis and avoiding the apophysis of the proximal tibial tubercle. Assistants apply gentle skeletal traction to disengage the bone fragments as the surgeon reduces anterior displacement by manual pressure on the epiphysis. The Steinmann pins are incorporated in the hip spica cast to secure maintenance of anatomic reduction (the author does not recommend immobilization of the knee in acute flexion by circular adhesive strapping around the thigh and leg, or by anterior plaster slab and circular plaster bandages to the thigh and calf). The position of the knee in the hip spica cast is 45 to 60 degrees of flexion. In three to four weeks, the cast and pins are removed and a long leg cast is applied

with the knee in 30 degrees of flexion. After two to three weeks, the second cast is removed, and active flexion-extension exercises are instituted to restore motor strength of the quadriceps muscle and joint motion. During this period the affected limb is protected by a three-point crutch gait. When the quadriceps muscle is of fair motor strength and the knee joint has attained complete extension, the crutches are discarded and full weight-bearing is allowed.

The use of Kirschner wires across the physis for internal fixation is not recommended. Open reduction of Type II (Salter-Harris) fractures is not indicated. In anterior displacements of distal femoral epiphyses, angulation is in the plane of motion of the knee, and any deformity will be spontaneously corrected by remodeling.

If the patient is seen late and the interval between the injury and the initial manipulation is such that some healing has occurred, it is best to reduce the fracture by 90°–90° skeletal traction with a pin through the proximal tibia (cf. Fig. 8–103).

HYPERFLEXION TYPE FRACTURES

The posteriorly displaced distal femoral epiphysis is reduced as follows: The patient is placed on a fracture table with the normal limb fastened on the footplate. An assistant applies straight longitudinal traction on the injured side by pulling on the lower leg with the knee in complete extension. As the fragments are disengaged, the surgeon pulls the distal epiphyses anteriorly with one hand while pushing posteriorly on the lower end of the femoral shaft with the other. The reduced fracture is immobilized in a single hip spica cast with the knee in *complete extension*. To re-emphasize: At no time should the knee be immobilized in a position of semiflexion. Supracondylar fracture of the femur requires a position of knee flexion to relax the pull of the gastrocnemius muscle; since the fracture site is proximal to the origin of the heads of the gastrocnemius, the unopposed pull of this muscle results in a posterior displacement of the femoral condyle in relation to the diaphysis, and also flexion of the condyles in relation to the tibia (Fig. 8–107). Aitken and Magill have pointed out that in fractures involving the distal femoral physis, the fracture line is distal to the origin of the medial head of the gastrocnemius. Consequently, the distal femoral epiphysis may be posteriorly displaced, but does not become flexed on the tibia. With the knee fully extended, the medial head of the gastrocnemius is taut and provides a posterior dynamic splint, preventing posterior displacement of the reduced lower femoral epiphysis. When the knee joint is immobilized in flexion, the medial head of the gastrocnemius is relaxed and enhances posterior displacement of the femoral epiphysis.[597]

Type IV (Salter-Harris) fractures involving the distal femoral epiphysis often require open reduction and internal fixation with smooth Kirschner wires. During surgery, care should be taken that the blood supply to the epiphysis is preserved.

TRAUMATIC DISLOCATION OF THE PATELLA AND OSTEOCHONDRAL FRACTURES OF THE KNEE

In children, dislocation of the patella in a normal knee is a rather uncommon injury. It is usually a lateral dislocation caused by a direct blow in the inner side of the patella; occasionally it may result from violent muscle contraction when the knee is in adduction and flexion. Dislocation may be complete, especially when the quadriceps muscle is relaxed, the patella slipping over the lateral edge of the femoral condyle and resting on its lateral surface; or it may be incomplete, the patella riding on the lateral edge of the condyle.

The patellar displacement is accompanied by a variable degree of injury and tearing of the soft tissues on the inner side of the knee, namely the patellar retinaculum, the vastus medialis, the capsule, and the synovial membrane. Usually there is also hemorrhage into the joint. In incomplete dislocations the soft-tissue injury may be minimal, but in complete dislocations, there may be wide longitudinal tears.

When lateral dislocation of the patella is produced by muscle action only, and especially when it recurs, genu valgum, deficient development of the lateral femoral condyle, and contracture of the iliotibial band or a high-riding patella are additional pathogenetic factors.

In rare instances, the patella is displaced medially, or it may be rotated upon its longitudinal axis so that its articular surface faces forward.

Diagnosis

Often the patella reduces itself spontaneously on extension of the knee, or a bystander may push it back into its normal position. Only rarely does the orthopedic surgeon see the patella in a dislocated state in which the injured limb is completely useless, with pain and swelling in the knee. The knee is maintained in flexion, with definite limitation of further flexion. Active extension of the knee is impossible; it can, however, be extended passively in its abnormal position. The smooth anterior surface of the femoral condyles can be easily identified beneath the skin and subcutaneous tissues. Occasionally one may be able to palpate a longitudinal tear on the medial side of the joint capsule and patellar retinaculum. The knee joint is distended with fluid.

Diagnosis of a recently reduced dislocation of the patella is difficult. It is based on the history and clinical findings of hemarthrosis and tenderness on the medial aspect of the patella, which has abnormal lateral mobility.

Treatment

Ordinarily reduction is very easy. The hip is flexed to relax the rectus femoris, the knee is extended, and the patella is pushed forward and medially into its normal position. Occasionally, in a hypersensitive adolescent patient, general anesthesia may be necessary to perform the reduction. After reduction there is, of course, some effusion in the knee joint, but as a rule, aspiration of the joint is not necessary. The limb is immobilized in an above-knee walking cylinder cast with the knee in full extension for a period of three weeks. This provides adequate time for the torn soft tissues to heal.

Surgical intervention is indicated in the very rare case in which a definite wide rent in the medial capsule can be palpated

A medial parapatellar incision is employed for the exposure. The capsule is repaired and imbricated by sutures to prevent recurrence, and the limb is immobilized in a cast, as just described. After removal of the cast, muscle power is restored by progressive quadriceps exercises.

Treatment of the rare medial and rotatory dislocations is similar to that described for lateral dislocations, except that reduction is accomplished by pushing outward in a medial dislocation and derotating in rotatory dislocation.

Osteochondral fractures of the lateral femoral condyle or of the posterior articular surface of the patella may be caused by rapid lateral dislocation and spontaneous reduction of the patella. Sporadic cases have been reported in the literature; Rosenberg reported 15 such fractures and Ahstrom, 18 cases.[615, 624]

The injury usually occurs in an adolescent patient who twists his flexed knee into a valgus position; he then falls down, his knee giving way because of the severe pain. On examination, the knee is markedly distended with effusion; there is loss of full active knee extension, local tenderness over the lateral femoral condyle, and over the medial capsule and patellar retinaculum.

On pressing the patella against the femur, local pain is elicited. The fracture fragment may be seen as a loose body; however, it is often very thin and difficult to visualize in the initial x-ray films. If clinical findings suggest the knee should be aspirated, the joint fluid is usually found to be bloody; the presence of fat globules indicates an intraarticular fracture. An arthrogram will assist in making the diagnosis.

Treatment consists of arthrotomy, removal of the loose fragment, and shaving down of the sites of origin. Medial capsular tissues are imbricated and the knee is immobilized in a long leg cast for three weeks.

FRACTURES OF THE PATELLA

The patella, embedded in the quadriceps tendon, is the largest sesamoid bone in the body. It usually has one center of ossification, which appears at two or three years of age but may, at times, be delayed until the sixth year. In approximately 2 to 3 per cent of patellae, a separate center of ossification is present in the upper lateral angle, where it may be unfused or incompletely fused to the main patella. These bipartite patellae are usually bilateral and should not be confused with fractures.[626, 627]

Fractures of the patella are rare in children. A direct blow will crush the patella against the femoral condyles and result in a stellate, comminuted fracture. Lateral marginal fracture is produced when the direct blow is applied to the periphery rather than to the center of the bone. A sudden powerful contraction of the quadriceps muscle with the knee flexed will cause a transverse avulsion type of fracture of the patella and a transverse tear in the quadriceps expansion.

Clinically, there is local pain, swelling, and effusion into the knee joint. If there is discontinuity of the quadriceps mechanism, the patient will be unable to extend the knee against gravity. The gap between the separated fragments may be palpable.

Roentgenograms will best disclose the fracture in the lateral projection (Fig. 8–110). If there is doubt, roentgenograms of the normal knee should be made for comparison.

Treatment of the fractured patella in a child follows the same principles as its treatment in an adult. Undisplaced or minimally displaced fractures are treated by immobilization of the knee in extension in a long-leg cylinder walking cast. Avulsion fractures with separation of the fragments require open reduction and repair of the torn medial and lateral quadriceps expansions. Undisplaced crush fractures are treated by immobilization in a long-leg cylinder walking cast; the hemarthrosis is aspirated if the joint is markedly swollen. Displaced comminuted fractures are treated by excision of all bone fragments and repair of the quadriceps expansion.

FRACTURES OF THE INTERCONDYLAR EMINENCE OF THE TIBIA

The intercondylar eminence (tibial spine) is located between the medial and lateral articular facets on the superior surface of the upper end of the tibia. In front of and behind the intercondylar eminence are rough

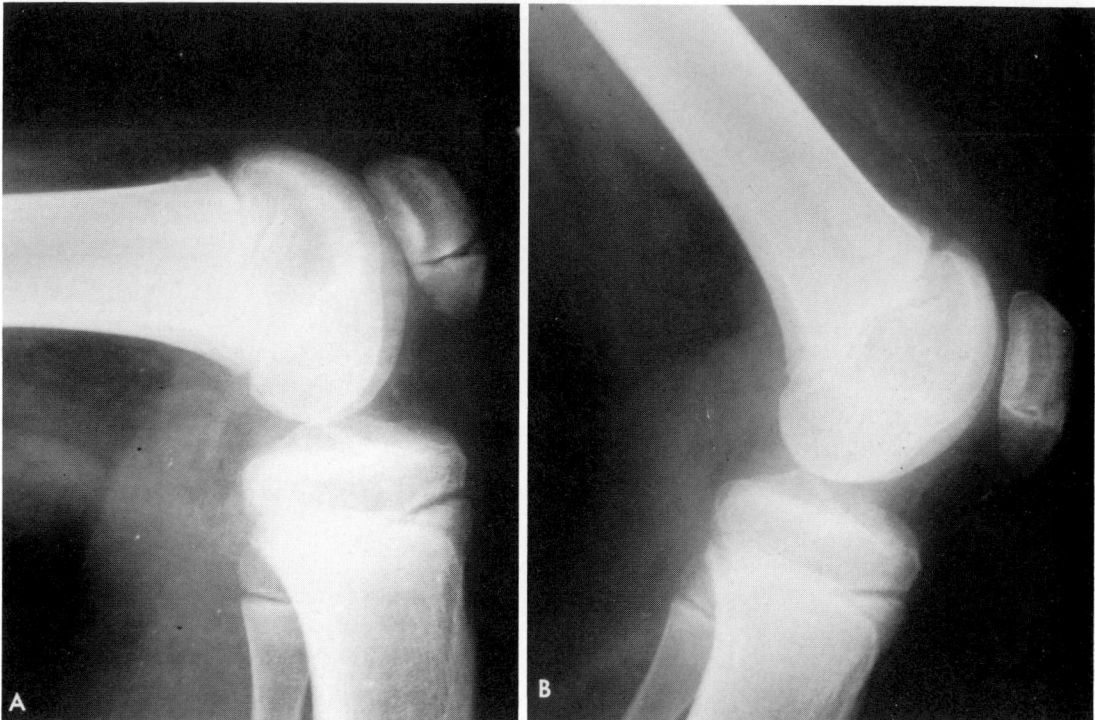

FIGURE 8–110. *Fracture of the patella—transverse, minimally displaced.*

Fracture was treated by immobilization in a long leg cast with the knee in extension. **A.** Initial lateral roentgenogram. **B.** Six weeks later.

depressions for the attachments of the menisci and the anterior and posterior cruciate ligaments. The intercondylar eminence is located directly beneath the hollow of the intercondyloid fossa of the femur, and does not articulate with the gliding articular surface of either femoral condyle.

Fractures of the intercondylar eminence of the tibia occur most frequently between the ages of 8 and 13 years; they are not found in children before the age of 7 years.

Mechanism of Injury

Fractures of the intercondylar eminence are essentially avulsions of either the anterior or posterior cruciate ligaments with an attached piece of bone. In children, the ligamentous tissues are resilient and seldom are avulsions of the tibial spine associated with tears of the menisci or of the ligaments. A blow to the front of the flexed knee will drive the femur posteriorly on the fixed

tibia and result in avulsion of the anterior part of the tibial spine; a common incident is a bicycle injury in which a child falls and lands on the front of the flexed knee. In Meyers and McKeever's series of 35 fractures of the intercondylar eminence of the tibia in children, 17 patients sustained the injury in a fall from a bicycle. Meyers and McKeever pointed out that the anterior cruciate ligament serves as a deterrent to excessive internal rotation of the tibia on the femoral condyles; they proposed that during the fall on the bent knee there is a violently forced internal rotation of the tibia on the femur, which places a severe strain on the anterior cruciate ligament.[628]

Avulsion of the posterior part of the tibial spine is very rare; it is caused by a direct force that strikes the proximal part of the flexed tibia and drives it posteriorly. Occasionally the same injury results from hyperextension injury of the knee joint; in such an instance, an associated tear of the posterior part of the capsule will almost invariably occur.

Classification

Meyers and McKeever subdivided fractures of the intercondylar eminence of the tibia into three types (Fig. 8–111).

In *Type I*, the avulsed fragment of bone is minimally displaced, with only slight elevation of its anterior margin. In *Type II*, there is greater displacement, with the anterior third to half of the avulsed fragment being elevated from its bone bed. This produces a beaklike deformity in the lateral roentgenogram. In a *Type III* fracture, the avulsed fragment is completely elevated from its bed on the tibia. There is total lack of bone apposition. In some instances, the avulsed fragment is rotated so that its cartilaginous surface faces the bare bone of the intercondylar eminence, making union impossible.

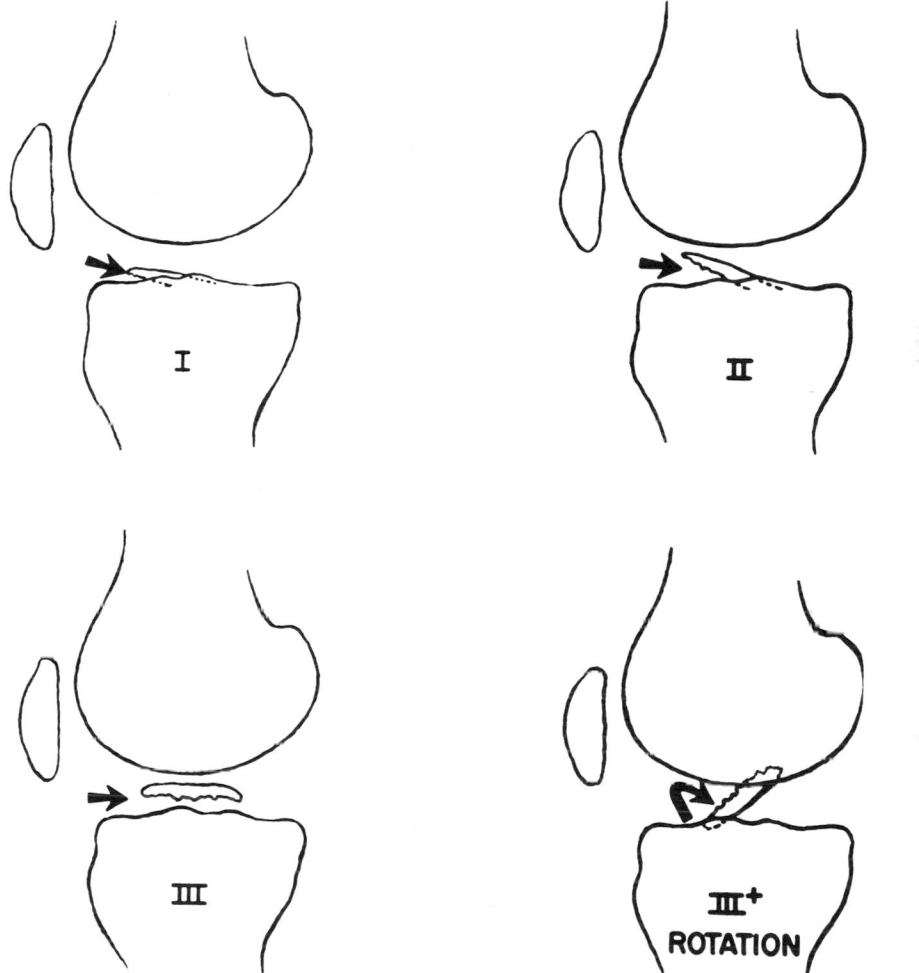

FIGURE 8–111. *Classification of fractures of the intercondylar eminence in children (according to Meyers and McKeever).*

Type I. No dislodgement of the fragment from its bed. There is minimal displacement and slight elevation of its anterior margin. *Type II.* Anterior third to half of the avulsed fragment is elevated from its bone bed. It has a beaklike appearance in the lateral roentgenogram. *Type III.* The avulsed fragment is completely dislodged from its bone bed. It may be rotated so that its cartilaginous surface faces the raw bone of the bone bed, making union impossible.

Type I and Type II fractures are treated by simple immobilization in a long leg cast with the knee in comfortable flexion. (The anterior cruciate ligament is taut in extension or hyperextension of the knee; it is relaxed in the first arc of flexion.) Type III fractures require open reduction, internal fixation (with simple catgut suturing to the adjacent meniscus) and immobilization. (From Meyers, M. H., and McKeever, F. M.: Fracture of the intercondylar eminence of the tibia. J. Bone Joint Surg., *41–A:*214, 1959.)

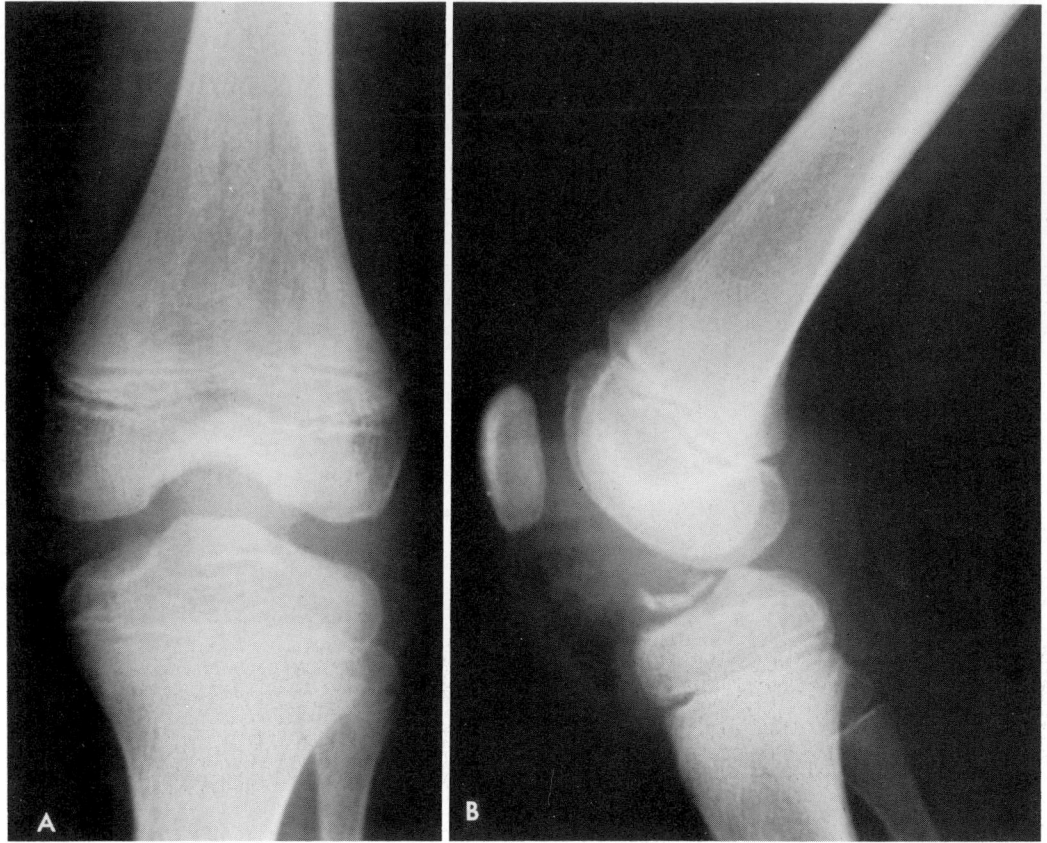

FIGURE 8–112. *Fractures of the anterior tibial spine.*

A and **B.** Minimally displaced fracture of anterior tibial spine was treated conservatively by a long leg cast with the knee in extension.

Diagnosis

Rapid development of hemarthrosis of the knee following an injury is a sign suggestive of fracture of the intercondylar eminence. The knee is held in partial flexion, and any attempt at passive extension of the knee is painful. From the position of fixed flexion deformity of 10 to 30 degrees, the knee can be further flexed to 60 to 100 degrees. Restriction of joint motion is caused by muscle spasm and not by the avulsed fragment; the latter lies below the hollow of the intercondylar notch of the femur and does not lock the knee by being trapped between the femur and the tibia. On palpation, the local tenderness is in the central region of the anterior aspect of the joint line, and not on the medial or lateral sides. Anteroposterior instability (drawer sign) is usually absent; when present, it is minimal. In children, even under the relaxation of a general anesthetic, lateral instability of the knee cannot be demonstrated.

Roentgenograms will disclose the avulsed bone fragment, which can best be visualized in the lateral projection (Fig. 8–112). When displacement is minor, the fracture may be completely overlooked in the anteroposterior film. It is extremely important to obtain adequate roentgenograms and to determine the type of fracture. In the differential diagnosis, one should consider osteochondral fractures of the femoral condyles and osteochondritis dissecans.

Treatment

This depends upon the type of fracture. When the joint is markedly swollen and tense, the hemarthrosis is aspirated first.

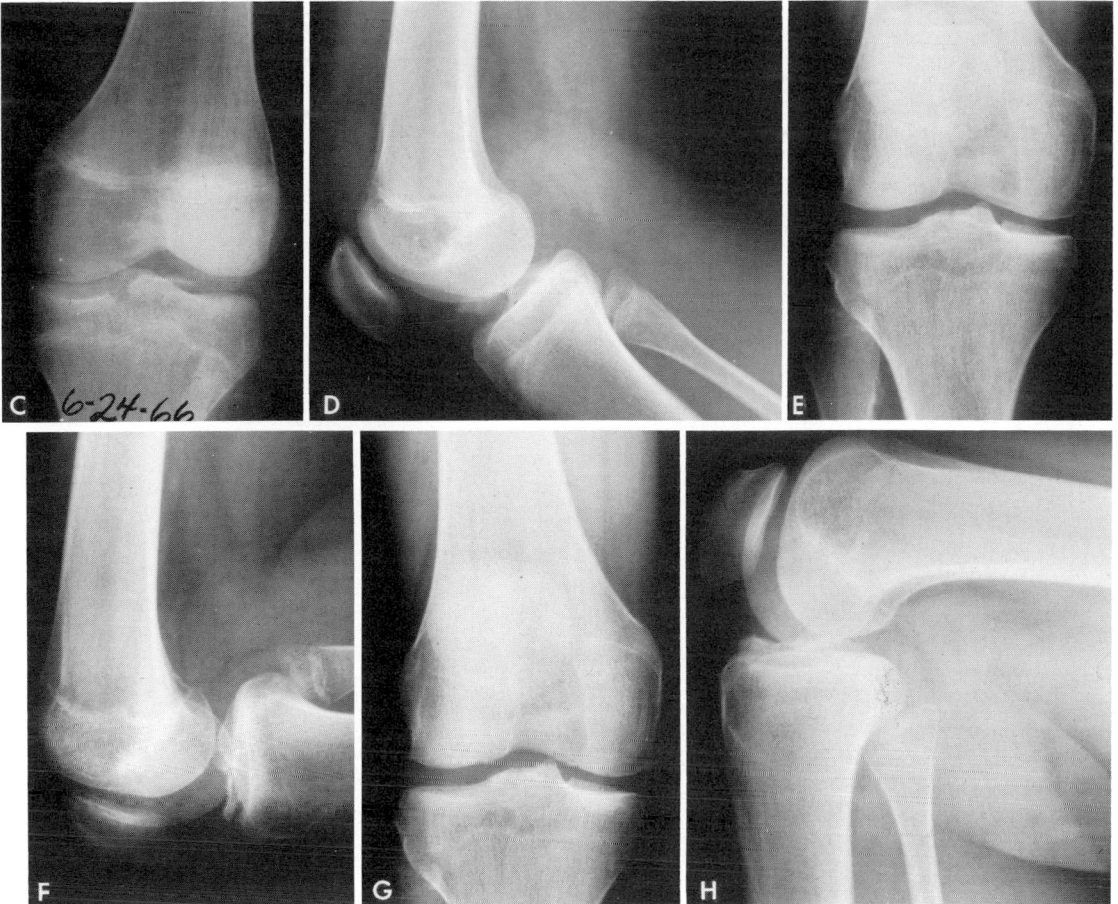

FIGURE 8-112 Continued. *Fractures of the anterior tibial spine.*

C to **H.** Markedly displaced fracture of the anterior tibial spine. This is treated by arthrotomy, open reduction, and internal fixation with simple catgut suture to the meniscus. **C** and **D.** Initial roentgenograms. **E** and **F.** Three months later. Note the slight separation of anterior tibial spine. **G** and **H.** Six months later; the fractured spine is well incorporated into the tibial plateau.

Type I and *Type II* fractures require simple immobilization in a long leg cast, as there is still some apposition between the avulsed fragment and its bed of origin. The position of the knee is 20 to 30 degrees of flexion; this is because the anterior cruciate ligament is taut when the knee is in extension and hyperextension, relaxed in the first portion of the arc of flexion, and becomes taut again as complete flexion is reached. General anesthesia is not necessary during application of the cast. Manipulating the knee into hyperextension with the patient anesthetized serves no useful purpose and may, in fact, further displace the avulsed fragment attached to the distal end of the anterior

cruciate ligament. Immobilization is maintained for 8 to 12 weeks or until union of the bone fragment to its bed on the tibia is demonstrated in the roentgenogram. After removal of the cast, active knee exercises and gradual weight-bearing are instituted. In a child, two to three months are usually required to restore normal motion and strength of the knee.

Type III fractures require open reduction. Meyers and McKeever have demonstrated that it is not necessary to transfix the fragment with a screw or nail, nor to drill a hole through the upper end of the tibia and pass removable retention sutures around the avulsed fragment. They recommend internal fixation with a simple absorbable catgut suture passed, with a cutting needle, through the thin edge of the avulsed fragment and through the meniscus near its sharp margin. They report excellent results in six patients treated by open reduction and suturing done in this fashion. Following open reduction, the knee is immobilized in a long leg cast in partially flexed position. Immobilization is continued until there is roentgenographic evidence of healing—usually about 12 weeks.[628]

FRACTURES INVOLVING THE PROXIMAL TIBIAL PHYSIS AND THE APOPHYSIS OF THE TIBIAL TUBERCLE

Injuries to the proximal tibial physis are rare, constituting only 0.8 per cent of all physeal injuries. This immunity from fractures is due to the relative lack of ligamentous attachments to the proximal tibial epiphysis; the lateral collateral ligament inserts to the fibular head, and the principal part of the medial collateral ligament is attached to the metaphyseal region, well distal to the physis. Thus, abduction or adduction strain is transmitted to the distal femur instead of to the proximal tibial epiphysis.

As stated, normally only a small part of the medial collateral ligament is inserted into the epiphysis. Occasionally this attachment is large, and upon exertion of a valgus strain, Type II (Salter-Harris) physeal injury is produced. This is the most common type of physeal injury involving the proximal tibial epiphysis (9 of 14 cases in the series of Aitken).[629] The distal fragment is usually displaced posterolaterally; circulatory embarrassment may result if the sharp upper end of the distal fragment impinges on the popliteal vessels (Fig. 8–113). A Type II (Salter-Harris) fracture with anteromedial displacement of the distal fragment has been reported by Aitken and Ingersoll.[630]

Type III (Salter-Harris) physeal injury can occur (2 of Aitken's 14 cases).[629] The detached epiphyseal fragment is usually unstable and becomes displaced either medially, anteriorly, posteriorly, or proximally.

Direct crushing injury may cause Type IV (Salter-Harris) fracture; this is usually associated with crushing of the physis and avulsion fracture of the tibial spine.

Treatment

Closed reduction is performed in all Type II fractures and the lower limb is immobilized in an above-knee cast for a period of four to six weeks. In Aitken's series of nine patients, despite some persistent displacement, complete spontaneous correction occurred without deformity or clinical shortening in all cases.

Type III fractures (Salter-Harris) require open reduction and internal fixation with bolt and screw. Open surgery is indicated also in Type IV fractures when fragments are displaced and cannot be anatomically reduced by closed methods. Premature growth arrest with resultant varus, valgus, or recurvatus deformity almost always occurs with Type IV fractures; these require osteotomy for correction.

AVULSION FRACTURES OF APOPHYSIS OF TIBIAL TUBERCLE

These avulsion fractures of the tibial tubercle commonly occur in boys between the ages of 14 and 16 years. The distal ligamentous expansion of the insertion of the quadriceps mechanism spreads out like a fan as it attaches to the proximal tibial surface. The apophysis of the tibial tubercle is located in the middle of this tendinous expansion. Because of the diffuse insertion of the quadriceps mechanism, it is rare for the tibial tubercle to be completely avulsed; however, partial avulsion is a frequent occurrence.

The tibial tubercle may develop in two different forms, according to Smillie: as a tongue-shaped downward protrusion of the proximal tibial epiphysis on the anterior proximal tibial surface, which fuses with the proximal tibia at the age of 18 years; or in the second form, as a separate center of ossification that fuses with the main body of the epiphysis at the age of 16 and, together with the main body of the epiphysis, fuses to the tibial diaphysis at the age of 18. In both complete and partial avulsions of the epiphysis of the tibial tubercle, injury occurs before the epiphysis fuses to the tibia at the age of 18.[633]

Mechanism of Injury. When complete

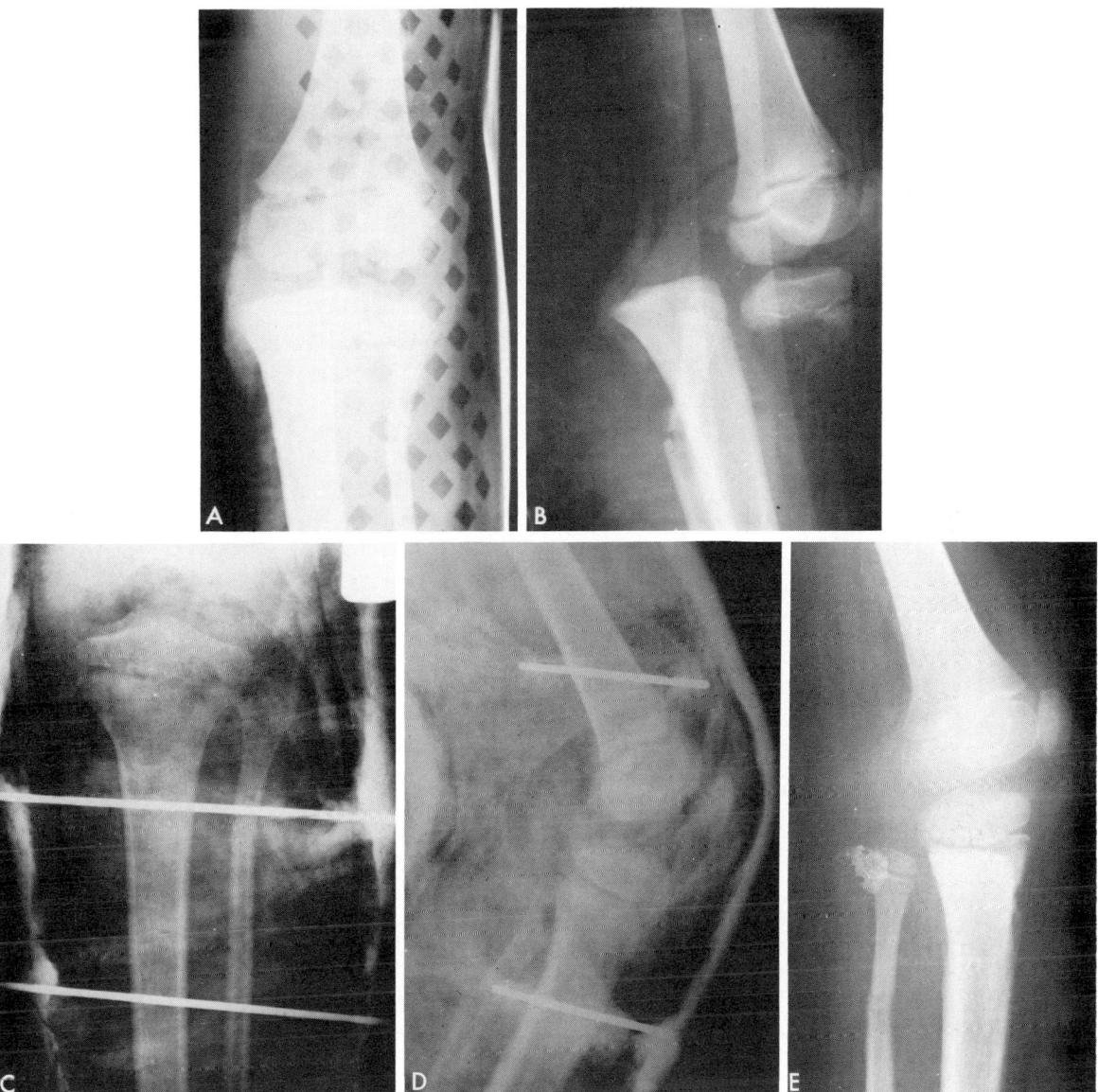

FIGURE 8–113. *Fracture involving the proximal tibial physis, Type II according to Salter-Harris.*

A and **B.** Initial roentgenograms. Note the complete separation with posterior and superior displacement of distal fragment. Anterior metaphyseal fragment is small; there is associated fracture of the proximal fibula. Posterior tibial and dorsalis pedis pulsations were absent and the foot and leg were cold. Immediate closed reduction was carried out with two pins in the tibia and one pin in the distal femur to secure maintenance of reduction. A long leg cast was applied. **C** and **D.** Immediate postreduction roentgenograms. Note the anatomic alignment **E.** Oblique-lateral roentgenogram four months later, showing healing.

avulsion occurs, it is usually the result of the knee being forcibly flexed against the resistance of the strongly contracting quadriceps muscle. These injuries are usually sustained in athletic activities, such as high jumping or football.

If the first of Smillie's two types of tibial tubercle apophysis is present, a projecting tongue-like flap may either be raised from the anterior tibial surface and not detached from the main body of the epiphysis, or it may be raised from the tibial surface and fractured from the main body of the epiphysis at its base. In the second of Smillie's two types, in which the injury occurs in a knee in which the tibial tubercle is developing as a separate center of ossification, this small fragment is avulsed from its bed.

Watson-Jones has classified these fractures into three types (Fig. 8–114): *Type I*

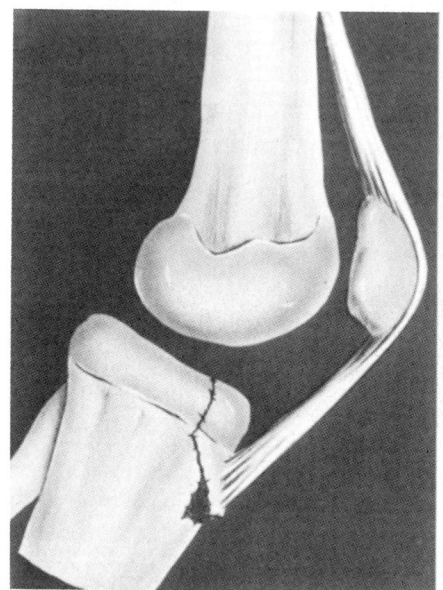
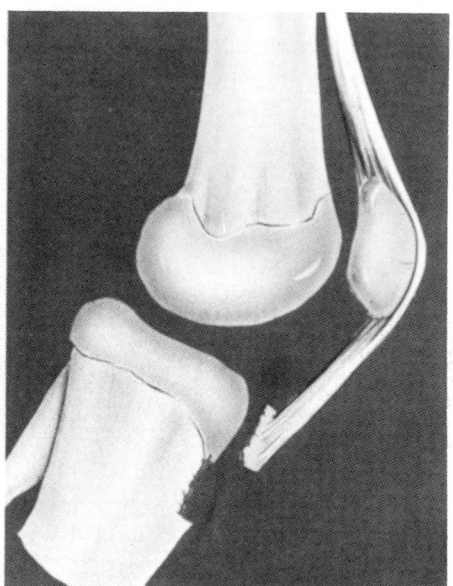

FIGURE 8–114.   Three types of fracture of the proximal tibial tubercle (according to Watson-Jones).

A. *Type I injury*—The tubercle is hinged upward without displacement at its proximal base. **B.** *Type II injury*—A small portion of the tubercle is avulsed and retracted proximally. **C.** *Type III injury*—This is the more severe form of Type I with fracture line extending across the articular surface. (From Hand, W. L.; Hand, C. R.; and Dunn, A. W., Avulsion fractures of the tibial tubercle. J. Bone Joint Surg., *53–A:*1550, 1971.)

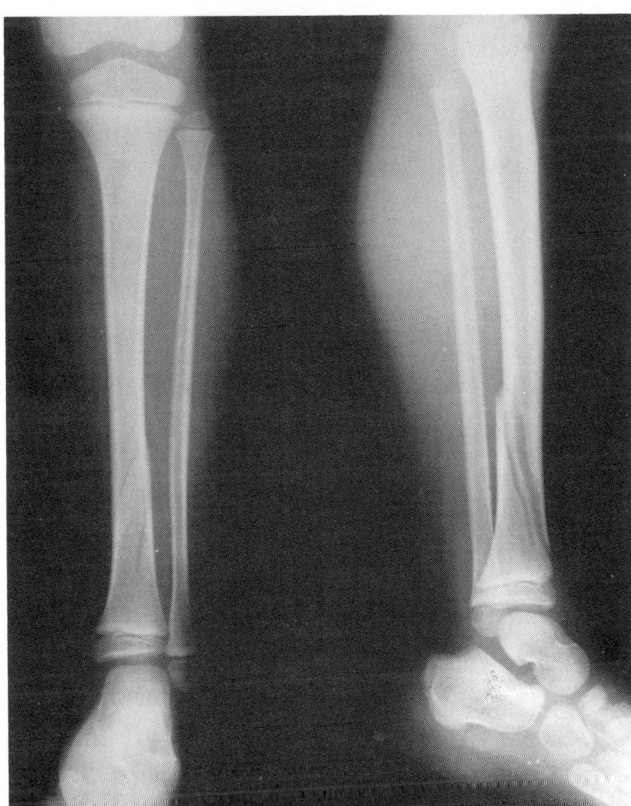

FIGURE 8-115. *Spiral fracture of distal third of tibia with the fibula intact results from torsional stress on the leg.*

fractures are those in which the tonguelike projection of the epiphysis has been lifted upward without displacement at its proximal base. *Type II* fractures correspond to injuries of the second of Smillie's two forms of epiphysis, in which the separate center of ossification, not having fused with the main body of the epiphysis, has been completely avulsed from its bed. *Type III* is the most severe injury and is actually an extension of the Type I fracture with extension across the articular surface.[634]

Treatment of the complete avulsion depends upon whether or not the tongue-shaped epiphysis has been completely detached from the main body of the epiphysis. If it is still attached, it may often be replaced by manipulative reduction and held by a long leg cast with the knee in extension. However, if it has fractured from the main body of the epiphysis, or if a separate center of ossification (Type II) has been avulsed, open reduction is indicated. The best means of maintaining anatomic repositioning is by suturing the epiphysis to the surrounding fibrous attachments of the quadriceps mechanism and immobilizing it in a long leg cast with the knee in extension.

FRACTURES OF THE SHAFT OF THE TIBIA AND FIBULA

The type of fracture sustained by the tibia varies with the age of the child and is dependent upon the nature of the violence – whether it is an indirect rotational twisting force or a direct blow.

In infants and young children, the typical injury is a spiral fracture of the tibia with an intact fibula. Between three and six years of age, a torsional stress applied on the medial aspect of the leg will result in a greenstick fracture of the proximal metaphysis or upper diaphysis of the tibia with an intact fibula, or it will cause a spiral fracture of the tibia, with or without a break of the fibula (Figs. 8–115 and 8–116). In the five- to ten-year age group, the common injury is a simple transverse fracture with or without

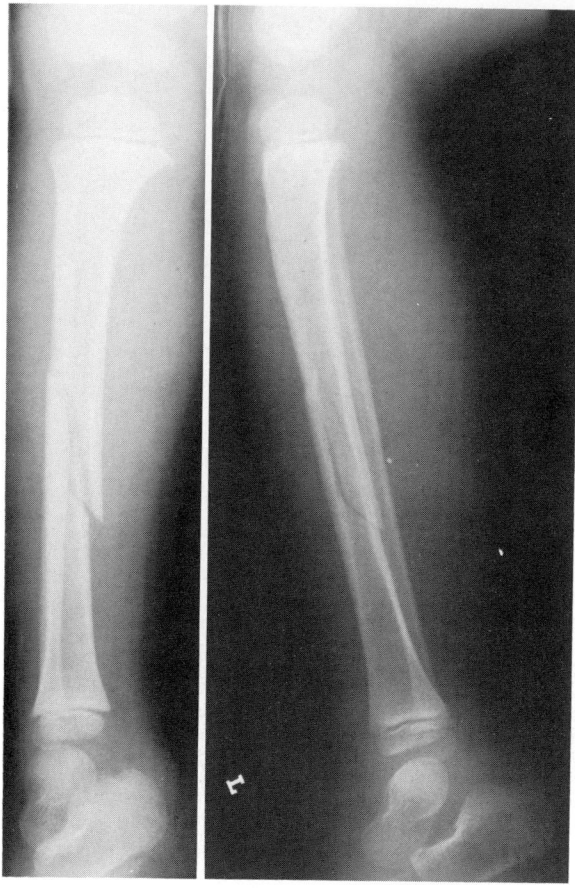

FIGURE 8–116.   *Long spiral fracture of the middle third of the tibia is due to lateral twisting injury applied on the foot.*

The fibula is intact. Note the lateral rotation of the distal fragment.

displacement due to direct trauma (Fig. 8–117). In adolescents, athletic injuries cause comminuted fracture of the middle third of the tibia and fibula with a butterfly fragment (Fig. 8–118).

Ordinarily, fracture fragments are held together by a thick periosteal sleeve and displacement of the fragments is minimal. Consequently, they are stable and can be adequately managed by closed methods; open surgical reduction is contraindicated in the treatment of closed fractures in infants and children. In automobile accidents, open fractures of the tibia and fibula with marked displacement of the fragments can occur.

Spiral Fracture of Tibia with Intact Fibula in Infancy and Early Childhood

This is produced by a torsional force on the leg when a child falls from his crib or twists his leg and falls down when attempting to pry his foot loose from the playpen. Because of its resiliency in infants, the fibula is usually not broken.

The child refuses to walk or bear weight on the affected lower limb, or he walks with an antalgic limp. He is unusually irritable and is constantly crying with pain. On examination, there is no obvious deformity; however, by careful palpation and by paying attention to the intensity of the cry, one should be able to localize the area of tenderness on the tibia. A common error is to suspect an injured foot, and on obtaining roentgenograms, to find that it is normal. Frequently spiral fractures of the tibia in an infant remain undiagnosed at the time of injury.

Then, a week or ten days later, because of persistence of the limp and irritability, the parents bring the child for another consultation. At this time, a tender thickening on the subcutaneous surface of the tibia is palpable. Roentgenograms will disclose subperiosteal new bone formation. A hairline fracture may or may not be visualized—the fracture line may not be demonstrated because the fracture has consolidated, leaving only the periosteal reaction as evidence of the healing fracture. This may be mistaken for osteomyelitis, eosinophilic granuloma, acute leukemia, or some other neoplastic lesion. However, the true diagnosis will be established by repeating the roentgenograms of the tibia in six to eight weeks, when, in a fracture, they will be normal and all periosteal reaction will have disappeared.

When the diagnosis is made at the time of initial injury, treatment consists of immobilization of the limb in a long leg cast for a period of three weeks.

Greenstick Fracture of Proximal Metaphysis or Upper Shaft of Tibia

An undisplaced or greenstick fracture of the proximal metaphysis or upper part of the diaphysis of the tibia is not uncommon in children. They usually occur between the ages of three and six years, although they may be encountered in the older child.

The mechanism of injury is usually a torsional stress applied from the medial aspect of the leg or, occasionally, direct violence. The distal fragment is angulated laterally, but there is no loss of apposition and the fragments do not override. The fibula ordinarily escapes injury, though occasionally it may sustain a greenstick fracture.

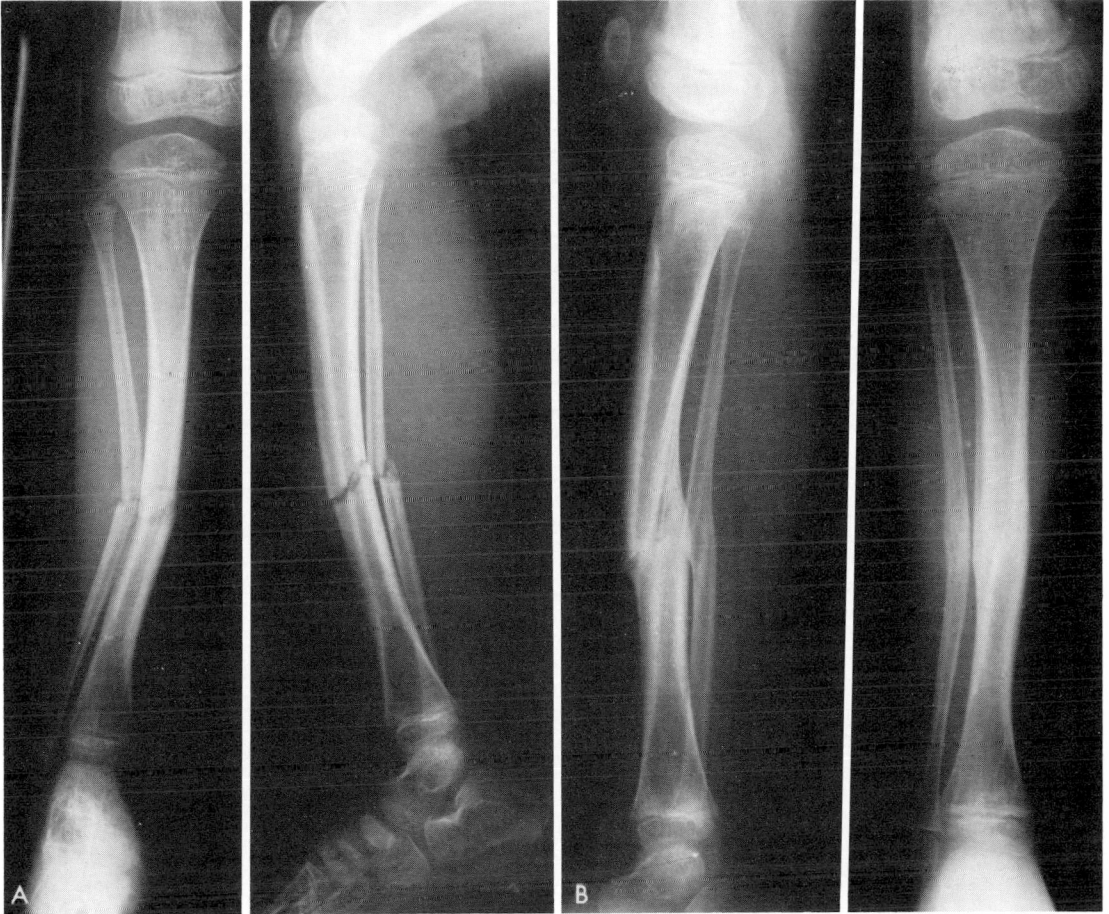

FIGURE 8–117. *Fracture of tibia and fibula in its middle third resulting from direct injury.*

A. Initial roentgenogram. **B.** Six weeks following closed manipulative reduction and immobilization in a long leg cast.

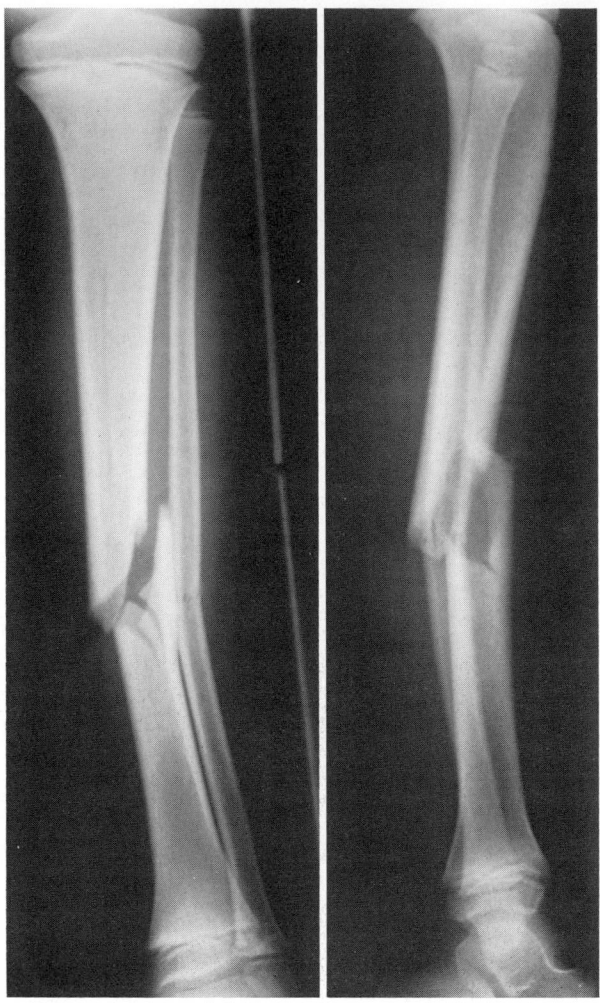

FIGURE 8–118. Comminuted fracture of middle third of tibia and fibula with butterfly fragment.

Treatment consists of correction of lateral angulation by manipulative reduction and immobilization in a long leg cast for a period of four to six weeks. An angulated greenstick fracture of the proximal tibia should be broken through by bending the leg toward the angulation, then slightly overcorrecting the deformity and applying a long leg cast. A common pitfall is failure to complete the fracture. The deformity will recur if the fracture is reduced by simple straightening of the leg prior to application of the cast.

The proximal metaphyseal fracture of the tibia is considered to be an innocuous injury. However, a common potential complication is asymmetrical tibial overgrowth and genu valgum. Orthoroentgenograms will disclose the increased length of the tibia, which is longer on its medial than on its lateral aspect. Another factor to consider is a discrepancy of growth between the tibia and fibula, with the fibula exerting a tethering effect.[637, 638]

Treatment consists of supportive shoes with a 1/8- to 3/16-inch medial wedge on the heel and longitudinal arch support. If the tibial valgus deformity exceeds 20 degrees, a knock-knee long leg orthosis may be given to accelerate correction. If the valgus deformity is severe and does not respond to the foregoing conservative methods, corrective osteotomy may be necessary. An osteotomy of the fibula is performed simultaneously to prevent recurrence of deformity.

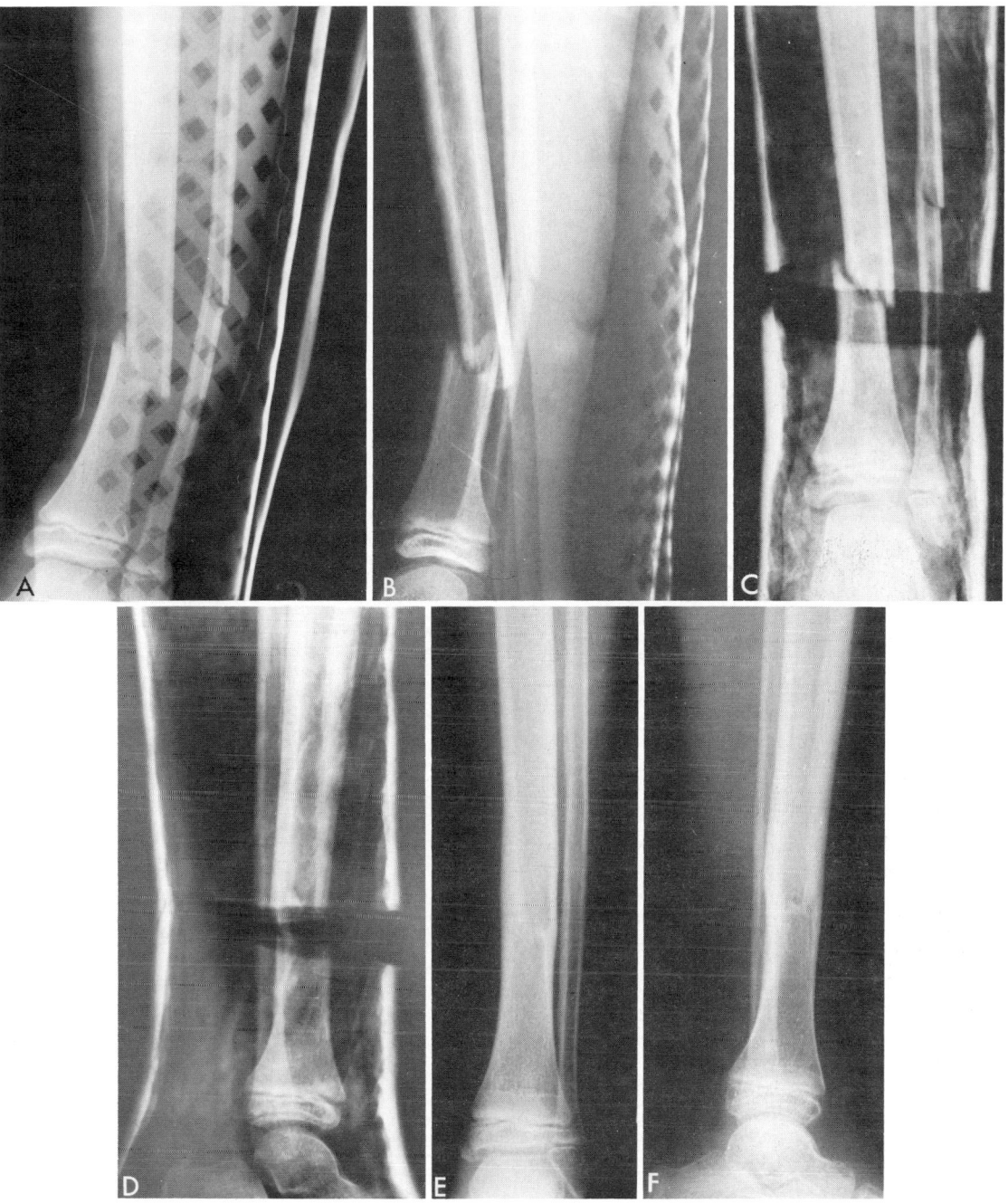

FIGURE 8–119.   Fracture of tibia and fibula at the junction of middle and distal thirds.

A and B. Initial roentgenograms. C and D. Following closed reduction and wedging of the cast, accurate alignment was obtained. E and F. Four months later, roentgenograms show excellent alignment and healing.

Fractures of Tibia and Fibula in Older Children and Adolescents

These are treated by closed reduction, correcting both angular and rotational malalignment. The limb is immobilized in a long leg cast, with the knee flexed to 90 degrees in order to control rotation and to prevent the child from bearing weight. In children, bayonet apposition of the fracture fragments and 1 cm. of overriding can be accepted. Immobilization is maintained for six weeks; during the last two weeks, the fracture may be sufficiently healed to permit partial weight-bearing in a walking cast.

In adolescents, comminuted unstable fractures of the tibia may be difficult to hold in a cast; in such an instance, pins are inserted above and below the fracture site and are incorporated in the cast to maintain reduction. Open reduction and internal fixation are not warranted.

FRACTURES INVOLVING THE DISTAL EPIPHYSIS OF THE TIBIA

The ossific nucleus of the distal tibial epiphysis appears during the second year of life. The medial malleolus ossifies as a downward prolongation from the main nucleus, appearing at the age of seven years in girls and eight years in boys (Fig. 8–120). Occasionally the medial malleolus develops from a separate center of ossification; this should not be mistaken for a fracture. By 14 or 15 years of age, the entire lower end of the tibia (including the medial malleolus) is completely ossified; it unites with the diaphysis at about the eighteenth year. The lower epiphysis contributes to 45 per cent of the growth of the tibia.

Classification and Mechanism of Injury

Fractures involving the lower tibial epiphyseal plate constitute 11 per cent of all physeal injuries. Poland believed it is difficult to classify these injuries on a mechanistic basis; however, Bishop, Carothers, and Crenshaw grouped them according to the general outline of Ashhurst and Bromer as follows: (1) abduction injuries; (2) external rotation injuries; (3) adduction injuries; (4) plantar flexion injuries; and (5) axial compression injuries and injuries caused by direct violence.[643-646]

The ankle is a true mortise joint that moves in only one plane into plantar flexion and dorsiflexion but is stable and distinctly limited in all other planes. This shape of the ankle joint renders the distal tibial epiphysis particularly vulnerable to crushing injuries.

The injury is commonly caused by indirect violence; the fixed foot is forced into either eversion, inversion, plantar flexion, external rotation, or dorsiflexion. The fracture may also be sustained by direct violence. The usual history given is that the child was in an automobile accident, fell from a height, or was engaged in contact sports. The fracture may be open in direct crush injuries.

This fracture is more frequent in boys (about 80 per cent of cases), and the common age of incidence is from 11 to 15 years (with a median age of 14 years in males and 12 years in females).

Abduction Injuries. These are the most frequent type and occur in 41 per cent of cases (in the series of 48 patients reported by Crenshaw).[646] There is lateral displacement of the entire distal tibial epiphysis, often accompanied by a lateral metaphyseal fragment of the tibia (Type II fracture, according to the classification of Salter and Harris). Frequently there is a fracture of the distal diaphysis of the fibula (Fig. 8–121 A). In this type of injury, the fracture usually does not involve the distal fibular epiphyseal plate. The degree of lateral displacement varies from one tenth to six tenths of the width of the distal tibial metaphysis. Displacement is never extreme, since it is checked by the fibula, which extends farther distally than does the tibia. The prognosis for future growth is excellent, as the germinal layer of the physis is not damaged.

External Rotation Injuries. The second most common form, this type occurs in about 23 per cent of cases.[646] It is characterized by posterior displacement of the entire distal tibial epiphysis and is always accompanied by a posterior metaphyseal fragment of the tibia. Posterior displacement of the inferior tibial epiphysis varies from 10 to 90

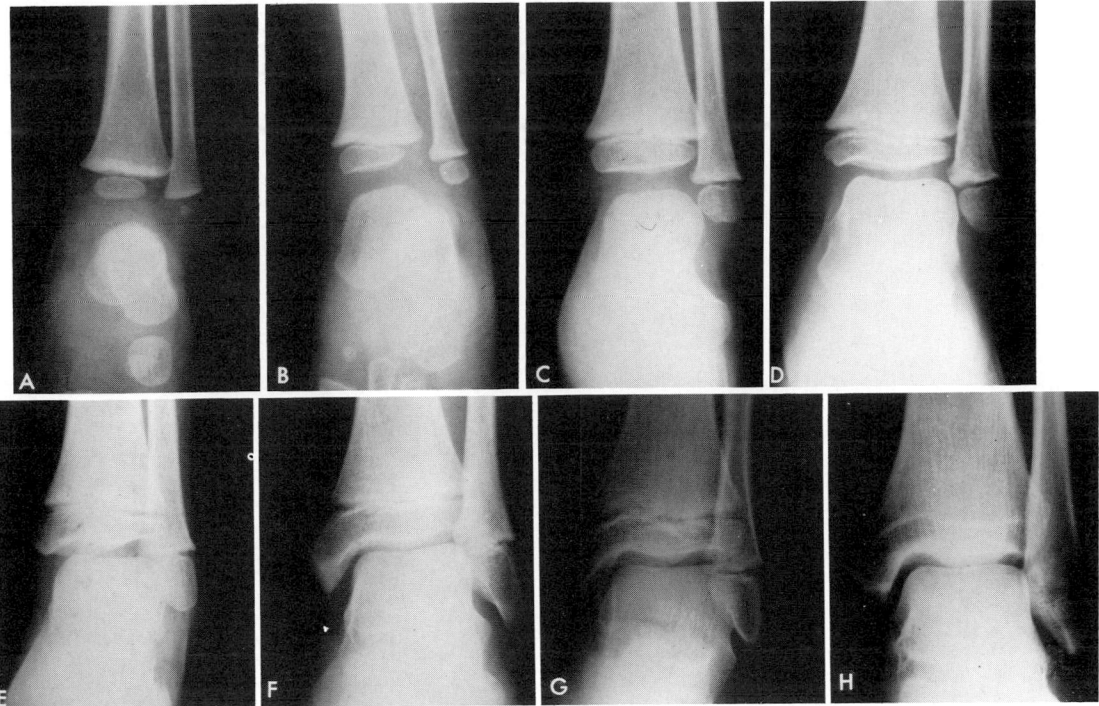

FIGURE 8–120. *Ossification of distal epiphyses of tibia and fibula.*

A. One year of age. **B.** Two years. **C.** Four years. **D.** Six years. **E.** Seven years. **F.** Ten years. **G.** Twelve years. **H.** Adult.

per cent of the metaphyseal width and is associated with an oblique fracture of the distal fibular shaft (Figs. 8–121 B and 8–122).

Adduction Injuries. Adduction injuries occur in approximately 14.5 per cent of cases and are characterized by medial displacement of either a part of or the entire distal tibial epiphysis. In this group, the affected children are usually younger; in the series of seven patients reported by Crenshaw, the median age was nine and one half years, the youngest being three and one half and the oldest, 15 years old.

In adduction injuries, the talus is forcibly adducted; after separation of the lower fibular epiphysis or fracture of the distal fibular shaft, the medial displacement of the talus is blocked by the medial malleolus. The medial border of the upper surface of the talus impinges on the medial half of the lower end of the tibia and exerts a crushing force at this point. The intra-articular shearing force causes a fracture that extends from the joint surface to the zone of the hypertrophic cartilage cells of the physis

and then along the plate to its medial border (Type III physeal injury of Salter and Harris). Displacement of the medial malleolus and the adjacent medial epiphyseal fragment may be slight or moderate (Figs. 8–121 C and 8–123). The germinal layer of the physis may be crushed by the compressive force. Occasionally an adduction injury will displace the distal tibial epiphysis medially with a medial metaphyseal tibial fragment attached to it (Type II physeal injury) (Fig. 8–124). Rarely, the intra-articular shearing force may completely split the epiphysis, physis, and a portion of the metaphysis, with upward and medial displacement of the medial fragment (Type IV physeal injury).

Plantar Flexion Injuries. This type occurs in 12.5 per cent of cases of those fractures that involve the distal tibial physis. It is distinguished by posterior displacement of the entire distal tibial epiphysis without fracture of the fibula. There is usually an associated posterior metaphyseal tibial fragment, and the degree of posterior

(Text continued on page 1730.)

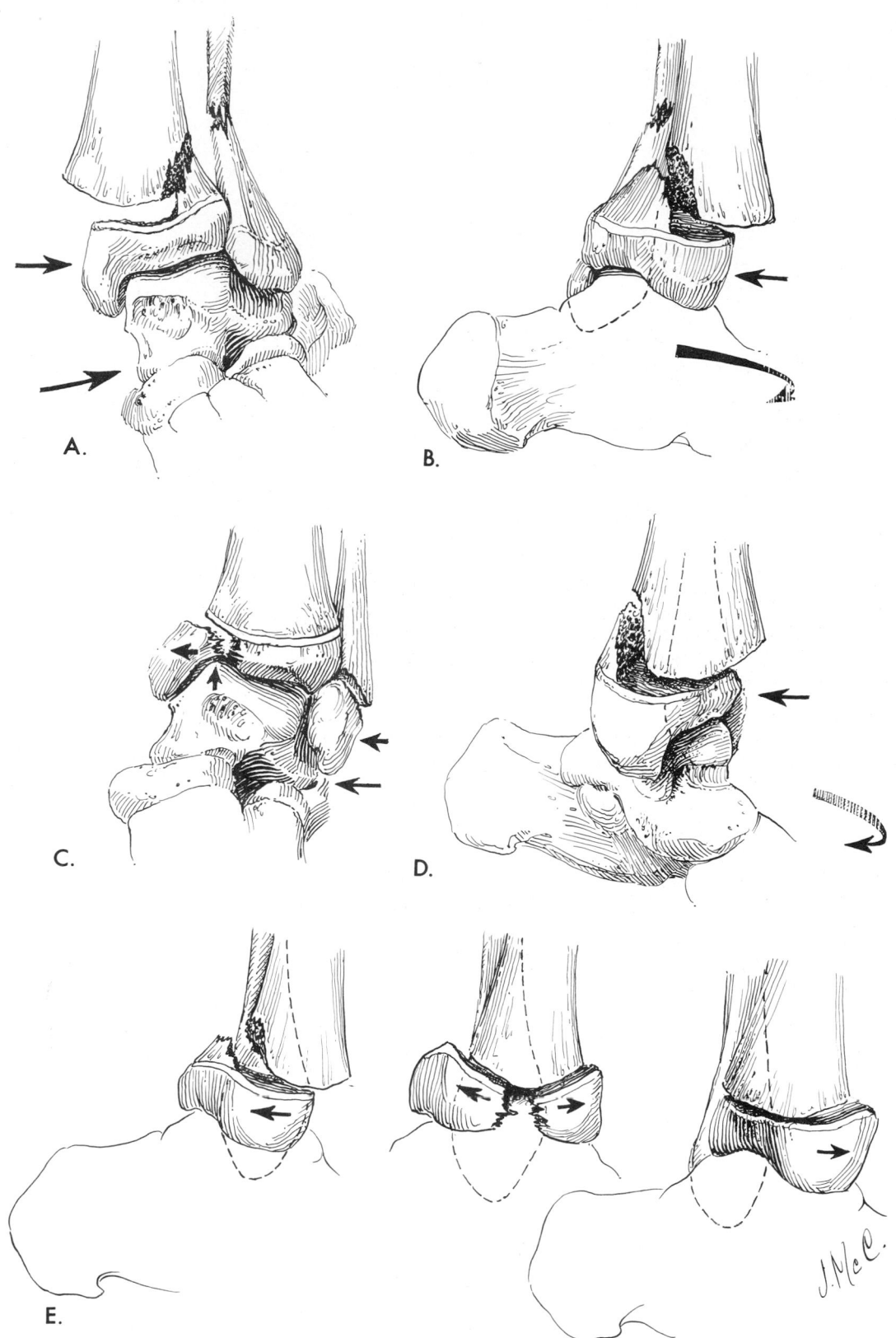

FIGURE 8–121. *Classification of fractures involving the distal physis of tibia.*

A. Abduction injury. **B.** External rotation injury. **C.** Adduction injury. **D.** Plantar flexion injury. **E.** Axial compression injury and injury caused by direct violence.

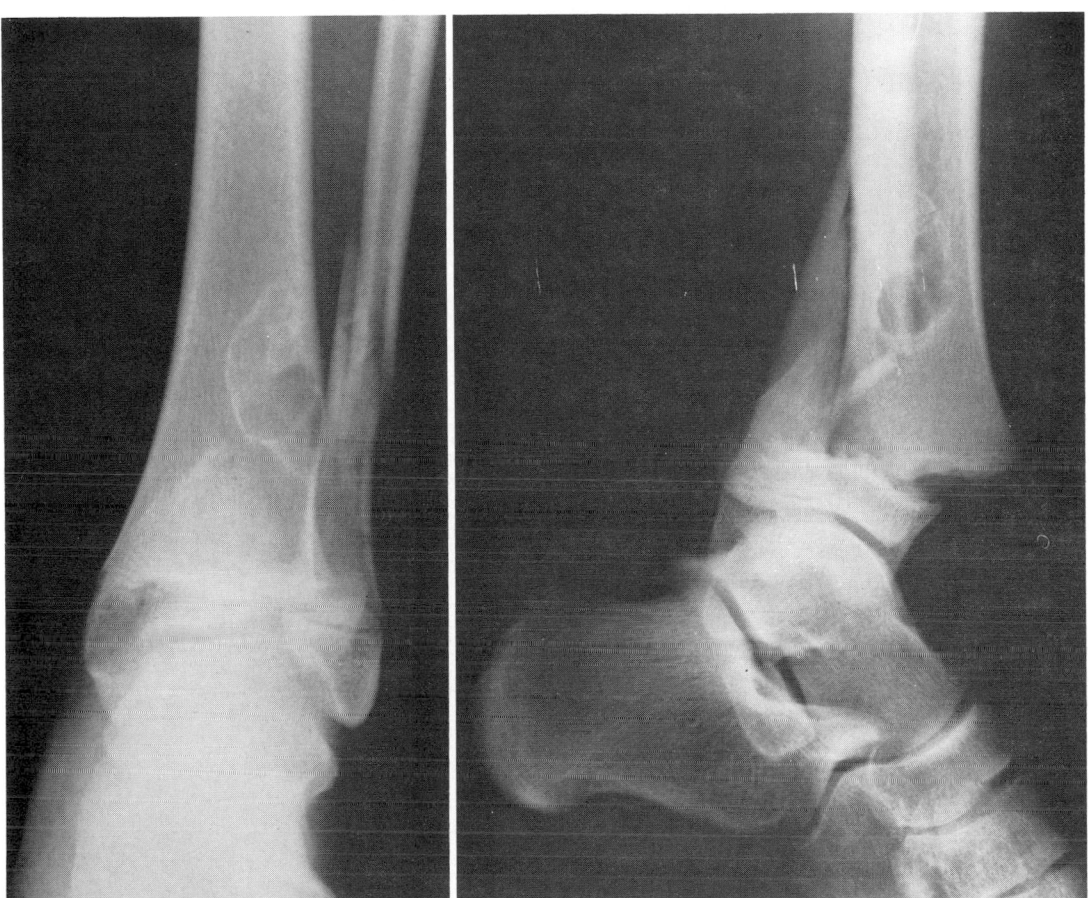

FIGURE 8-122. *External rotation injury causing Type II (Salter-Harris) fracture of distal tibial physis.*

Note posterior displacement of distal tibial epiphysis with posterior metaphyseal fragment and spiral fracture of fibular shaft. (There is also a fibrous cortical defect of the distal tibial diaphysis.)

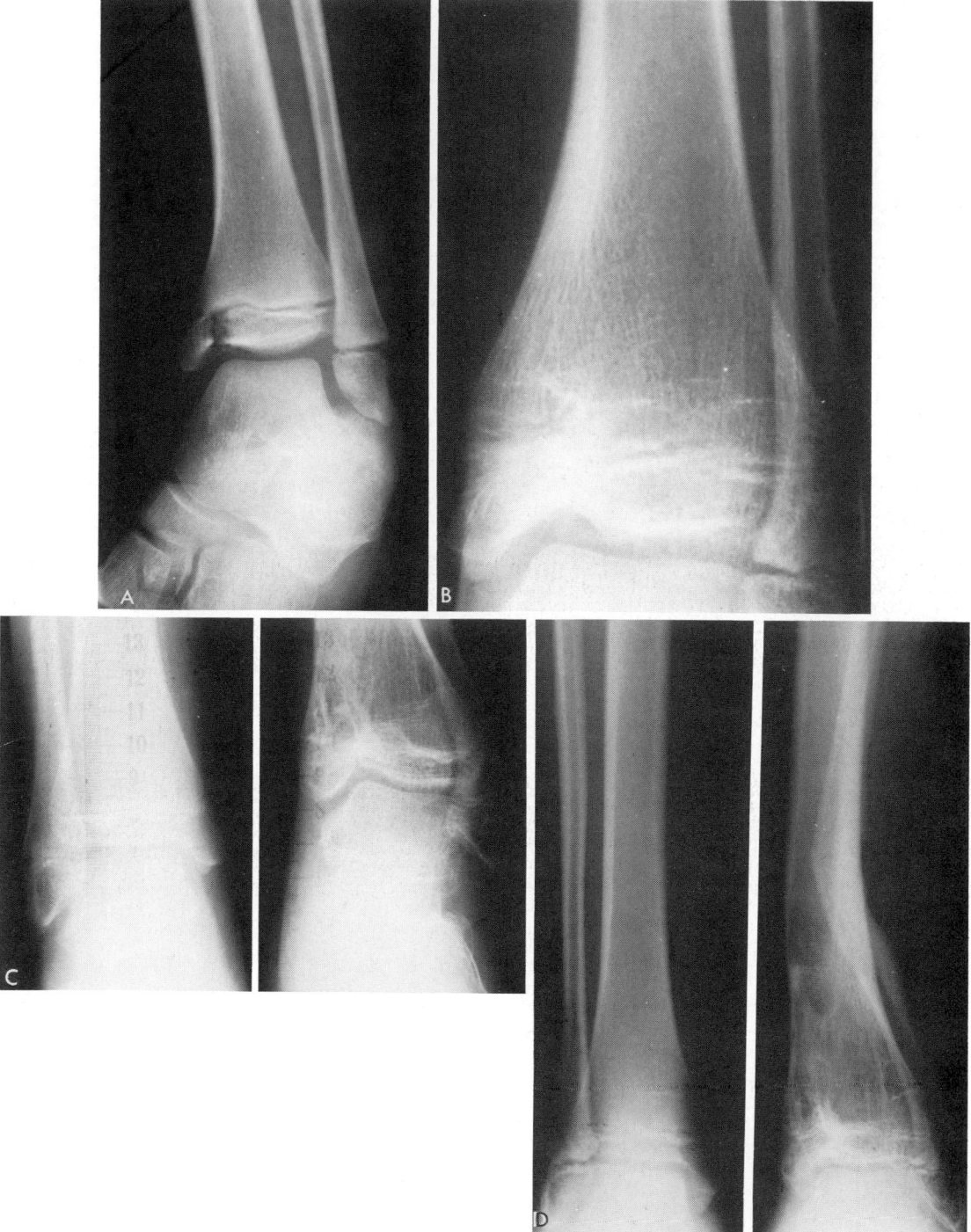

FIGURE 8–123.   *Adduction injury resulting in Type III (Salter-Harris) fracture involving the distal tibial physis.*

A. Initial roentgenogram. The fracture line extends from the joint surface to the zone of hypertrophic cartilage cells and then extends along the plate to its medial border. Note the moderate displacement of the medial epiphyseal fragment. **B.** Roentgenogram made one and one half years later, showing premature growth arrest of medial portion of the distal tibial physis. **C.** Two years later. Note the varus deformity of the ankle and overgrowth of the fibula. **D.** Note the correction of deformity following open-up supramalleolar osteotomy of the tibia.

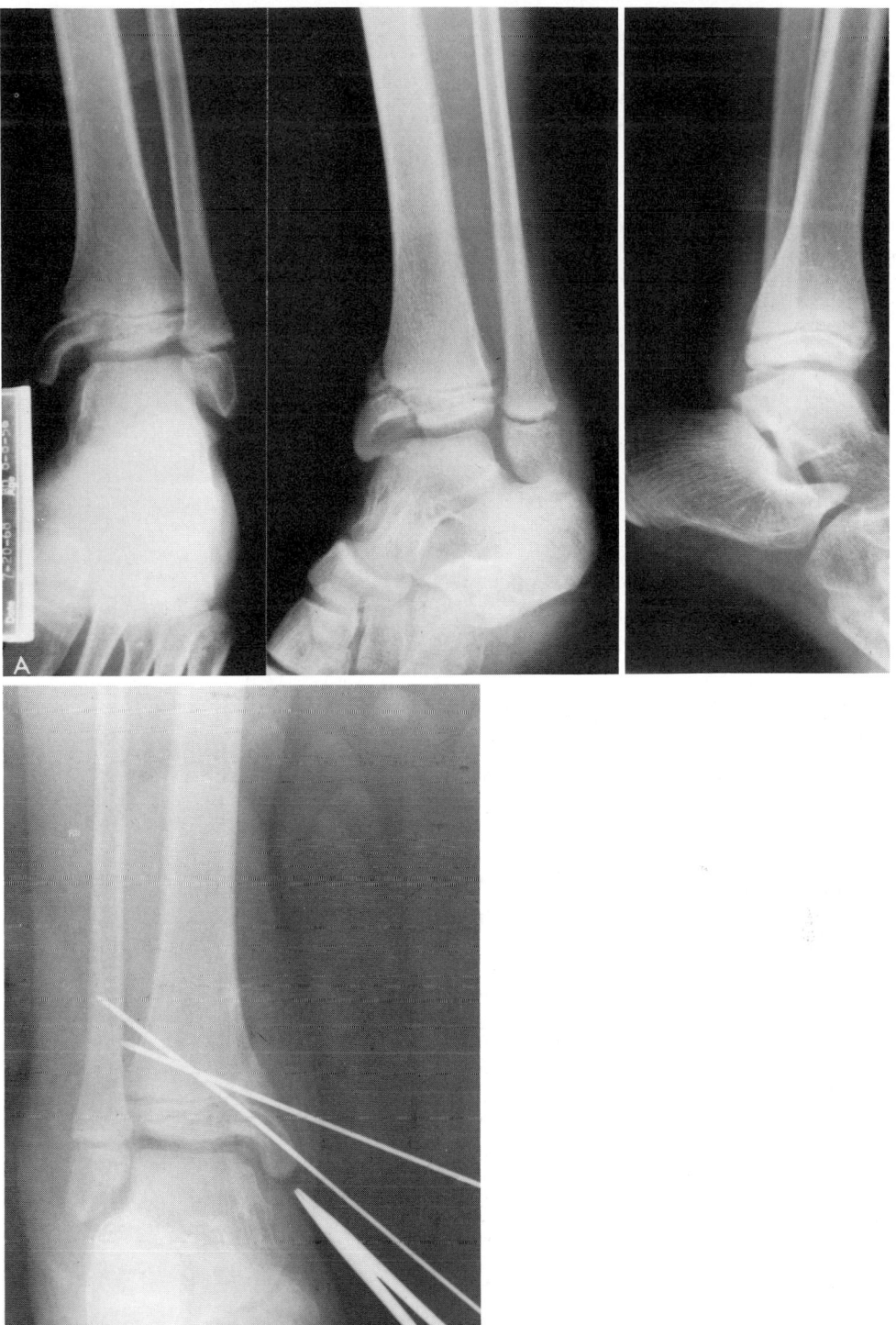

FIGURE 8–124. *Adduction injury resulting in Type II (Salter-Harris) fracture involving the distal tibial physis.*

A. Initial roentgenograms. Note the fracture line extending upward from the joint line, through the physis to include a portion of the medial metaphyseal fragment. **B.** Roentgenogram made in the operating room. Open reduction and internal fixation with two smooth Kirschner wires was carried out.

displacement varies up to 25 per cent of the width of the metaphysis (Fig. 8–121 D and Fig. 8–125).

Axial Compression Injuries and Those Caused by Direct Violence. In this group (9 per cent), the distal tibial epiphysis may be displaced anteriorly or posteriorly. In those caused by axial compression, there may be an intra-articular fracture through the central part of the epiphysis (Fig. 8–121 E and Fig. 8–126).

Treatment

Definitive treatment should be instituted immediately, whenever possible, since reactive swelling will develop soon after injury and make closed reduction much more difficult. In the emergency room, a well-padded compression dressing and a posterior splint should be applied before roentgenograms are made.

Gentle closed reduction is carried out under general anesthesia. Relaxation of muscles and absence of pain will make the manipulation easy and least traumatic. The knee is flexed 90 degrees and the foot is plantarflexed to relax the triceps surae muscle. An assistant applies countertraction by pulling up on the leg. With one hand, the surgeon grasps the foot by the heel, while steadying the anterior aspect of the lower one fourth of the tibia with the palm of his other hand. First, distal traction is applied in the line of deformity, i.e., in abduction injuries, distally and laterally; in external rotation and plantar flexion injuries, distally and posteriorly; and in adduction injuries, downward and medially. Then, while downward traction is maintained, the hindfoot and the distal fracture fragment are gently repositioned in normal anatomic alignment under the tibia. Overcorrection and forcible crushing of the physis should be avoided. In external rotation and plantar flexion injuries, the hindfoot is rotated to neutral position and dorsiflexed to 5 to 10 degrees beyond neutral to prevent recurrence of posterior displacement. In abduction and adduction injuries,

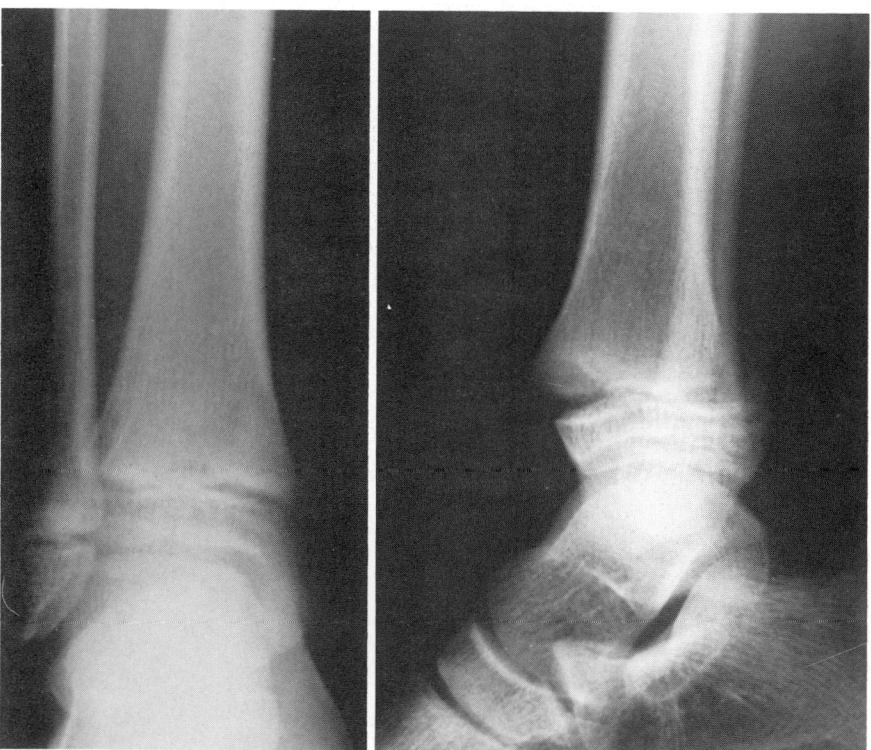

FIGURE 8–125. *Plantar flexion injury resulting in Type II (Salter-Harris) fracture involving distal tibial physis.*

The distal tibial epiphysis is displaced posteriorly. Note a small posterior metaphyseal fragment. The fibula is intact.

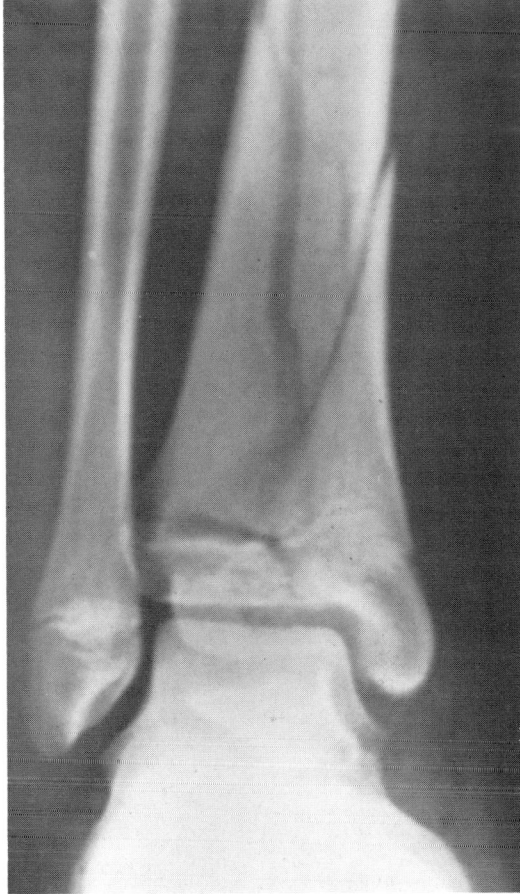

FIGURE 8–126. *Axial compression injury resulting in an intra-articular fracture with comminuted fracture of distal tibial diaphysis and metaphysis.*

the hindfoot is gently manipulated only into neutral position and not into inversion or eversion. Roentgenograms (anteroposterior and lateral views) are made to determine the accuracy of reduction. If there is still displacement, gentle manipulative reduction is repeated. If, however, after two attempts, accurate reduction cannot be achieved, it is wise to accept the deformed position.

After application of sheath wadding and pads of thin orthopedic felt over the malleoli, an above-knee cast is applied with the knee in 45 degrees of flexion. The plaster is carefully molded over the malleoli and the heel of the foot with the palms of the hands. The cast is extended above the flexed knee to relax the pull of the tendo Achillis and to prevent weight-bearing. Immobilization is continued for six weeks, and then gradual weight-bearing is allowed. Restraint from weight-bearing for longer periods is of no value in preventing deformity once the physis has been crushed.

Repeated forceful manipulation and open reduction in Type II fractures are contraindicated because moderate residual deformities tend to disappear spontaneously with subsequent growth and bone remodeling. Posterior or anterior displacements are corrected more readily, as they are in the plane of motion of the ankle joint. A valgus tilt of the ankle up to 15 degrees can be accepted. In the report of Crenshaw, roentgenograms made soon after the reduction showed a valgus tilt of the ankle in 6 of the 20 abduction fractures, and by the time of skeletal maturity, this tilt had disappeared spontaneously in every instance. The most severe tilt measured 12 degrees (in a 13½-year-old patient) and the least severe was 4 degrees (in a 10-year-old child). One case with external rotation fracture had a valgus tilt at the ankle of 10 degrees immediately following treatment, but the deformity disappeared completely during later growth.[646]

If a valgus tilt at the ankle of more than 15 degrees is present, a well-padded below-knee cast is applied, and after three or four days, gentle closed reduction is attempted again under general anesthesia; by then the reactive swelling will have subsided under the compression of cast immobilization and elevation of the leg. If reduction fails and lateral angulation of the ankle mortise greater than 15 degrees persists, open reduction is *not* carried out. The fracture is allowed to heal, and if, after two or three years, the deformity still persists, a supramalleolar osteotomy is performed to correct the valgus deformity at the ankle.

In Types III and IV fractures, accurate anatomic reduction is necessary; if this cannot be achieved by closed methods, open surgical reduction is performed and smooth Kirschner wires are used for internal fixation.

Prognosis and Complications

Growth arrest is likely to develop after adduction injury as a result of crushing of the germinal layer of the physis. The medial part of the tibial physis will fuse, whereas the lateral portion of the tibial physis and the distal fibular epiphysis will continue to grow with subsequent varus deformity at the ankle. The younger the patient, the worse will be the deformity.

Premature growth arrest of the entire distal tibial epiphysis will result in shortening of the tibia. In the older patient, this is of no clinical significance, whereas in the younger child, leg length discrepancy may be so marked that an epiphyseal arrest of the contralateral leg is indicated. An epiphyseodesis of the distal fibula on the affected side is performed to prevent its overgrowth.

The varus deformity at the ankle joint may be corrected by "close-up" or "open-up" supramalleolar osteotomy of the tibia. The age of the patient and the amount of shortening will determine the operative procedure chosen. In children and young adolescents (under 12 years of age for girls and under 14 years for boys), if surgery is to be postponed until complete ossification of the physis, structural changes in the ankle mortise may take place because of walking in inversion; also, resultant shortening of

the leg and overgrowth of the fibula may be of considerable magnitude. Thus, it is best to perform an open-up osteotomy without disturbing the lateral portion of the distal tibial physis. With growth, the varus deformity will recur, and a second osteotomy will be required for correction; this should be explained to the parents.

The technique of open-up supramalleolar wedge osteotomy is as follows: First, a 3-cm. linear incision is made over the lateral aspect of the distal diaphysis of the fibula. The peroneal tendons are retracted posteriorly, the periosteum is divided, and the fibula is osteotomized obliquely at a level 2 cm. proximal to its distal physis. Then a 5-cm. linear incision is made over the medial aspect of the tibia, beginning at the distal tibial physis and extending proximally. The subcutaneous tissue is divided, exposing the periosteum. The level of osteotomy is 1 cm. proximal to the distal tibial physis. A smooth Kirschner wire is drilled into the tibia and an anteroposterior roentgenogram is made to ascertain its site. Next, utilizing starters and a drill, holes are made through the medial four fifths of the tibia, which is divided transversely with sharp osteotomes, leaving the lateral cortex intact. The distal fragment of the tibia and the foot are angulated laterally, opening up the osteotomy site. Wedges of iliac bone of appropriate width are obtained and inserted into the gap on the medial side of the tibia (a laminectomy spreader may be used to keep the tibial bone fragments apart while inserting the iliac bone grafts). Roentgenograms are made to determine the degree of correction obtained. The wound is closed and an above-knee plaster cast is applied. The osteotomy will heal and the bone graft will be incorporated in about two months.

In the author's experience, supramalleolar open-up wedge osteotomy has been a very satisfactory procedure. The only pitfall, if significant varus inclination has already taken place, has been failure to correct overgrowth of the distal fibula. This can be accomplished either by wedge resection of the lower fibular diaphysis or by epiphyseodesis of the distal fibula.

In an older patient (girls over 12 years and boys over 14 years) epiphyseodesis of the distal fibula and of the lateral half of the distal tibial physis is performed to prevent the development of varus deformity of the ankle. If significant ankle varus deformity has already occurred, it is combined with an open-up wedge osteotomy of the medial aspect of the distal tibia.

If there is significant leg length discrepancy it is treated by epiphyseodesis of the opposite normal leg at the appropriate age.

The author does not recommend "close-up" supramalleolar osteotomy to correct varus deformity of the ankle joint because it will aggravate the leg length discrepancy.

Johnson and Fahl reported three additional complications, each of which occurred once following significant displacement of Salter Type II abduction fractures. In the first case, decreased circulation in the distal part of the foot was noted, but it quickly returned following reduction of the fracture. With the second (abduction injury), interposition of the anterior tibial tendon and periosteum occurred between the epiphysis and the tibia. Open reduction was necessary to remove the tendon and periosteum before accurate repositioning of the epiphysis could be carried out. In the third case, adhesions developed about the extensor hallucis longus tendon. Following operative lysis of these adhesions, full restoration of function was obtained.[648]

FRACTURES INVOLVING THE DISTAL PHYSIS OF THE FIBULA

The distal epiphysis of the fibula begins to ossify during the second year of life, usually between the ages of 18 and 20 months. Occasionally its ossification may be delayed until the end of the third year. Union with the diaphysis occurs around the twentieth year.

Fractures involving the distal fibular physis may occur alone or in association with those of the distal tibial physis. They usually take place in the age range of 8 to 15 years. Injury is usually by indirect trauma. Poland, in his experiments on autopsy specimens, found this to be one of the most readily separated epiphyses of the long bones, by either adduction or abduction injury; ordinarily the result is a Type II physeal injury

(Salter-Harris). The fracture may also result from direct violence on the outer aspect of the ankle, in which instance, it produces a Type IV injury (Salter-Harris).

Injury to the distal fibular physis usually goes undiagnosed because of the minimal displacement of the epiphysis. Following twisting of the ankle, the patient walks with an antalgic limp and complains of pain. There is local tenderness and swelling. In the routine anteroposterior and lateral roentgenograms of the ankle, the physeal injury is usually not visualized; oblique views are necessary to depict the minimal displacement (Fig. 8–127).

Treatment consists of a below-knee walking cast, which is worn for three weeks. When the fracture involving the distal fibular physis is associated with that of the distal tibial physis, treatment is the same as that described for fracture of the distal tibial physis.

FRACTURES OF THE FOOT*

The flexibility and resiliency of a child's foot make it relatively immune to injury. The forces of indirect violence are transmitted proximally, causing a fracture of the tibia or fibula.

Fractures of the foot in children are usually produced by the direct violence of a crushing injury, such as is caused by a heavy object being dropped on the child's foot, being run over by the wheels of an automobile, or falling from a height and landing on the heels. These squeezing and crushing forces may not break the skin, but may cause marked soft-tissue injury in the child's foot.

Fractures of the individual bones of the foot are not discussed here; for this, the reader is referred to general textbooks on fractures.

In treatment, the first step is to decrease the soft-tissue swelling by application of a Jones compression dressing, then reduce the fracture and immobilize it in a plaster of Paris cast. *Os calcis* fractures in children usually do not involve the subtalar joint. If displaced, *osteochondral fractures* of the articular surface of the trochlea of the *talus*

---

*See References 651 to 653 and 745 to 770.

(Text continued on page 1738.)

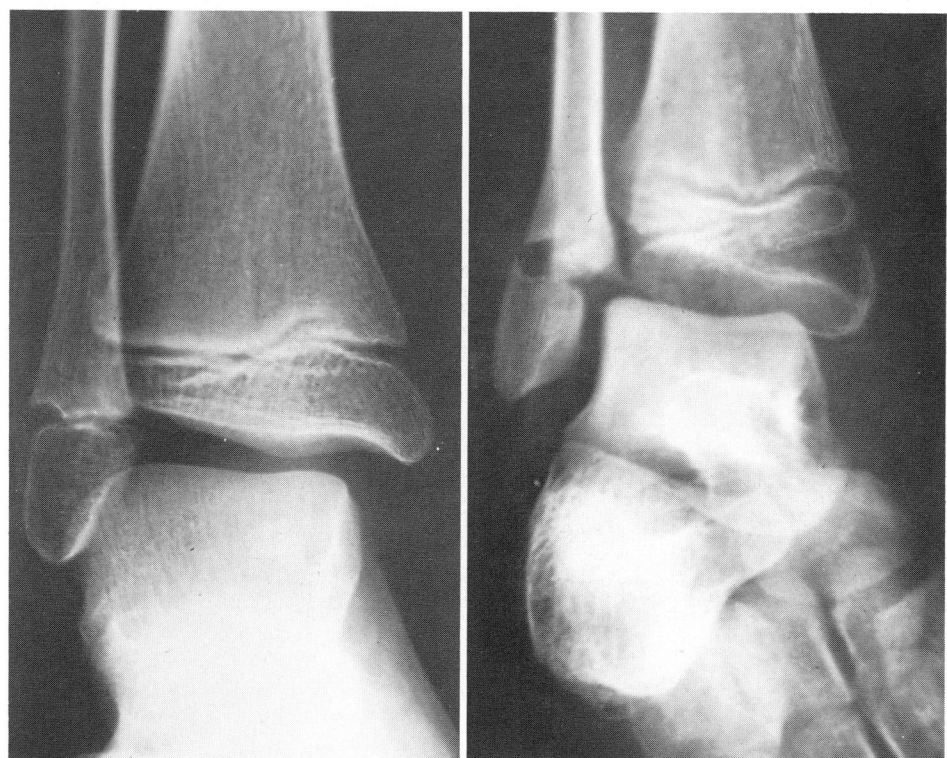

FIGURE 8–127.   Fracture involving distal fibular physis.

The importance of taking an oblique view is obvious.

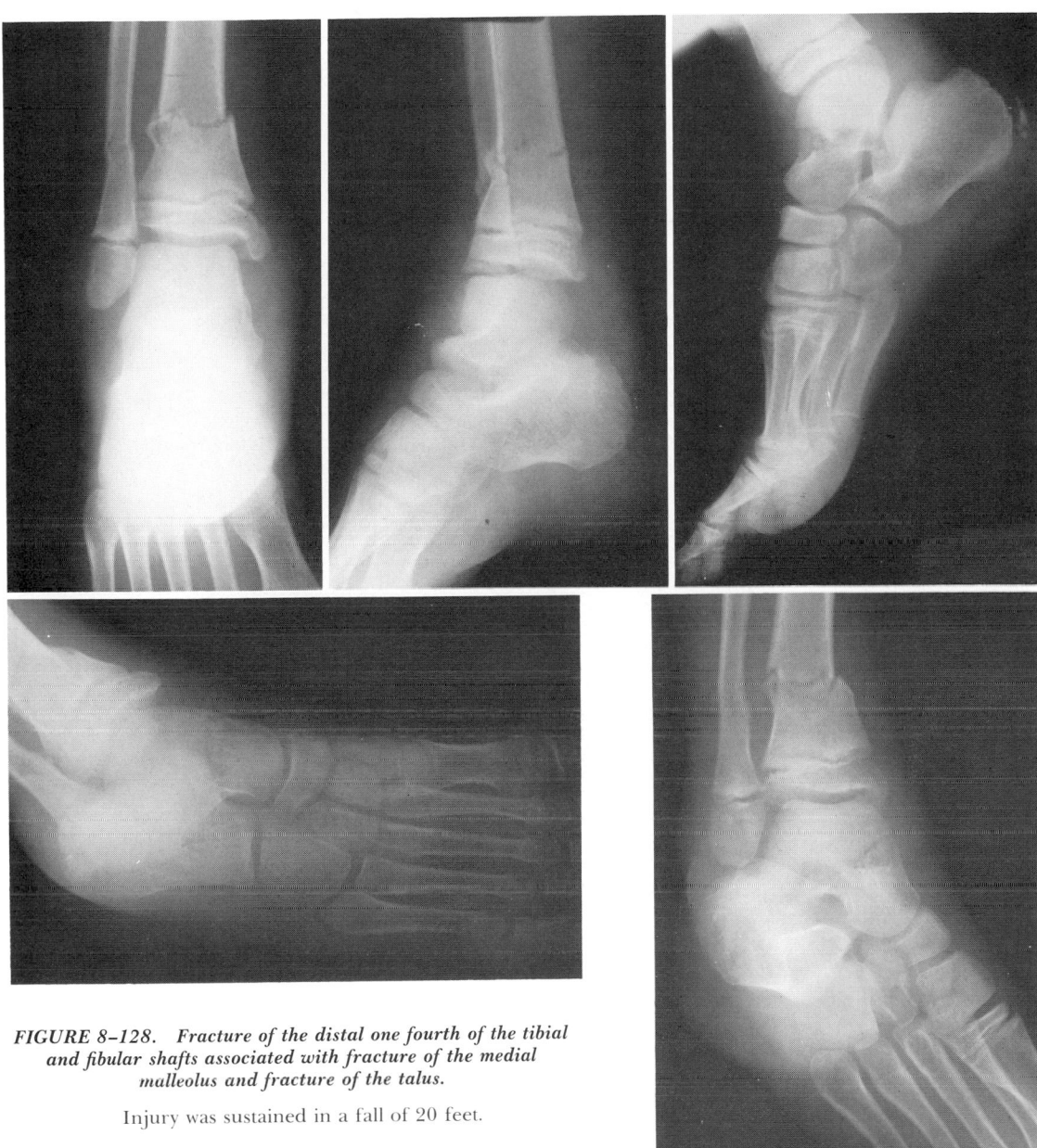

FIGURE 8–128. *Fracture of the distal one fourth of the tibial and fibular shafts associated with fracture of the medial malleolus and fracture of the talus.*

Injury was sustained in a fall of 20 feet.

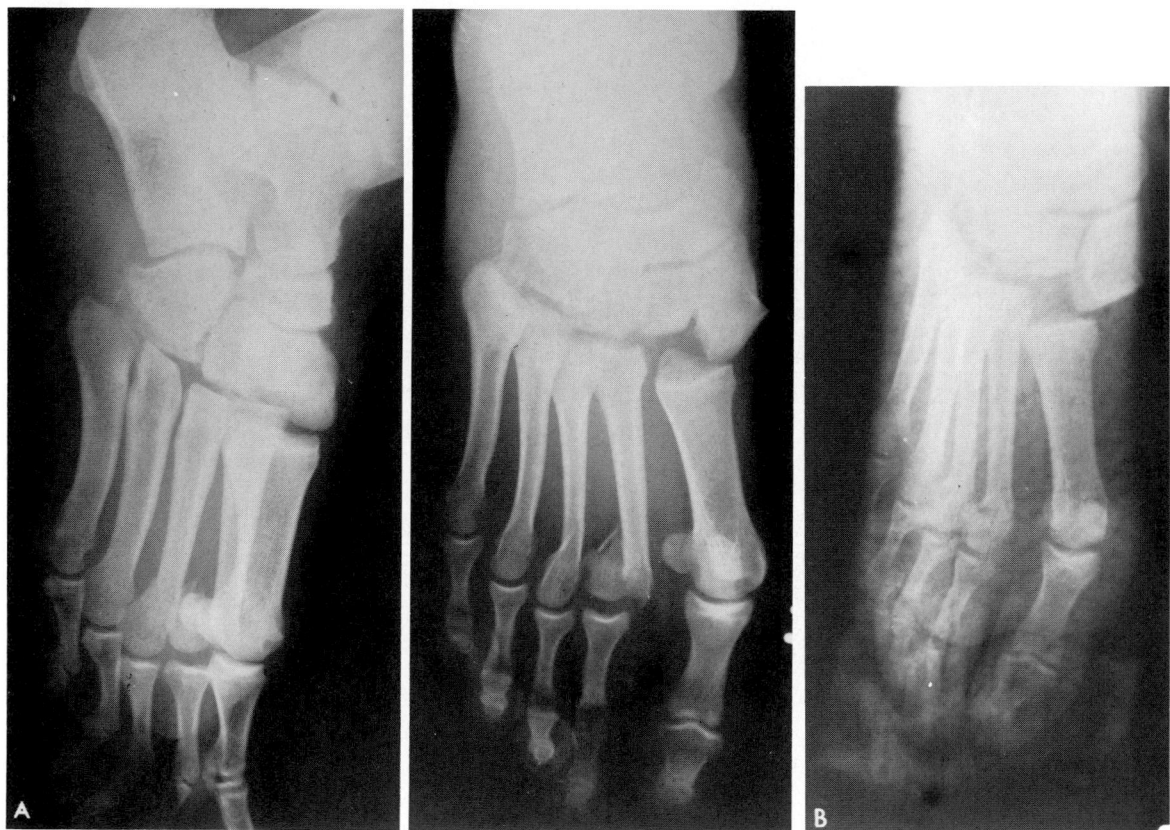

FIGURE 8–129. ***Lisfranc's tarsometatarsal dislocation with fracture of the second metatarsal neck.***

A and **B.** Initial roentgenograms.

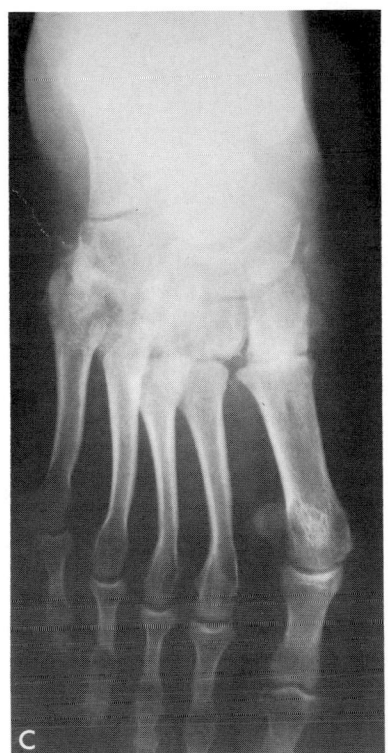

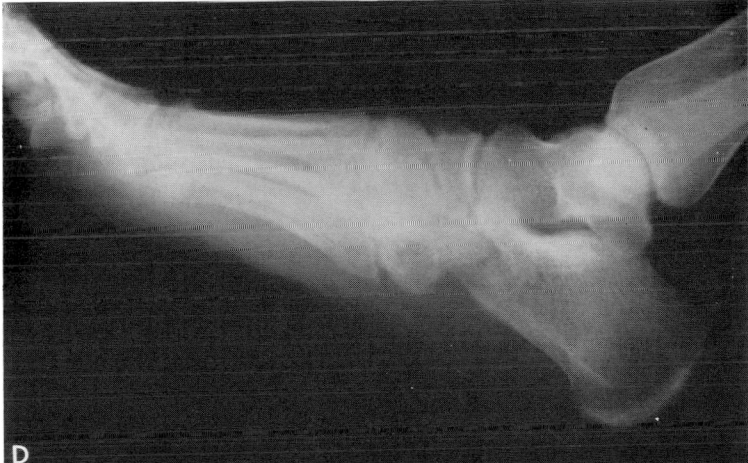

FIGURE 8–129 Continued. *Lisfranc's tarsometatarsal dislocation with fracture of the second metatarsal neck.*
C and **D.** Two years after closed reduction. Note the degenerative changes in the midtarsal joints.

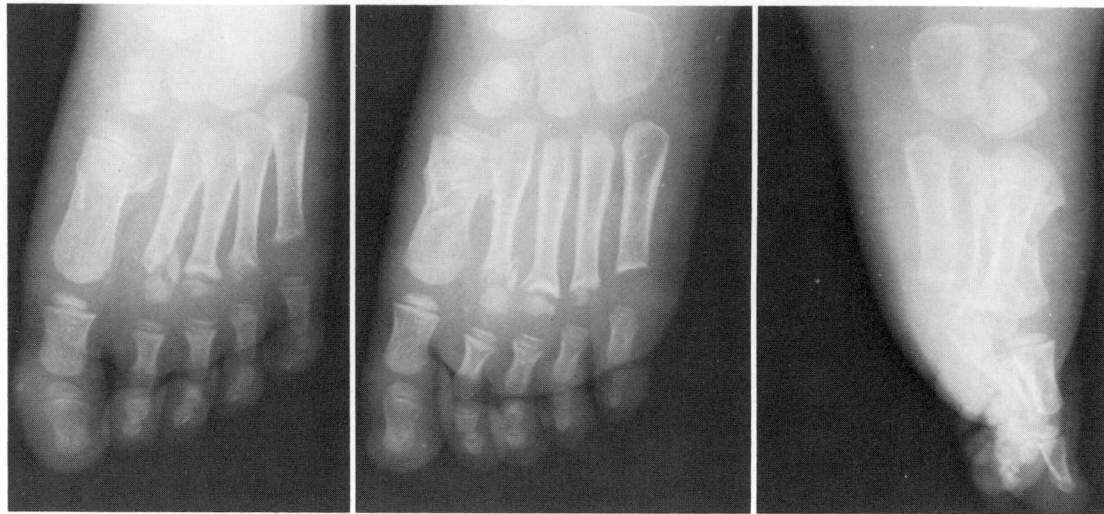

FIGURE 8–130. *Fracture of first metatarsal shaft and neck of second metatarsal caused by direct crushing injury.*

require arthrotomy of the ankle and removal of the loose fragment; if undisplaced, they are treated in a below-knee cast for four weeks. Fractures of the *body of the talus* usually result from severe violence (Fig. 8–128). If they are markedly displaced, open reduction may be necessary. Lisfranc's tarsometatarsal fracture-dislocation may be treated closed; if accurate reduction is not achieved, open surgery is indicated (Fig. 8–129).

Fractures of the tarsal navicular, cuboid, and cuneiform bones result from crushing injury; avulsion fracture of the base of the fifth metatarsal is caused by inversion force of sudden twisting of the foot. Fractures of the metatarsals are produced by a crushing force and usually more than one metatarsal is involved (Fig. 8–130). Treatment of all these fractures consists of simple immobilization in a below-knee walking cast for a period of four weeks.

Injuries to the Spine and Pelvis

INJURIES TO THE SPINE

Fracture-dislocations of the vertebral column are very rare in children; they usually are sustained by adolescents. For a detailed discussion of these injuries, the reader is referred to general textbooks on fractures.[745–770]

Rotatory Subluxation of Atlantoaxial Joint

This is a relatively common injury in a child, particularly if he has an upper respiratory infection; the associated hyperemia softens the ligaments that support the upper cervical spine and make the atlan-toaxial joint unstable. The subluxation is produced by suddenly twisting the neck, rotating it beyond its normal range.

The child is presented with painful torticollis accompanied by marked spasm of the sternocleidomastoid muscle. He may support his head with his hands or prefer to be recumbent. On palpation of the posterior aspect of the neck, there is local tenderness over the atlantoaxial joint. A neurologic examination is performed to rule out intraspinal lesions, such as tumors of the spinal cord (see pages 862 to 876 in Chapter 5).

Roentgenograms will disclose persistent asymmetry at the atlantoaxial joint in the open mouth view. Partial anterior subluxation of the second or third cervical vertebra is a normal variant in the appearance of lateral roentgenograms of the flexed cervical spine. Dunlop, Morris, and Thompson surveyed 47 *normal* children and found that 5 had marked subluxation of the second or the third cervical vertebra, and that 3 had borderline dislocations.[657] The width of the intraspinal canal should always be measured to detect the presence of slowly growing neoplasms of the cord.

Treatment consists of continuous traction with a head halter. The subluxation will be reduced within a few days and muscle spasm will subside. The neck is then supported in a soft cervical collar (stockinette filled with white orthopedic felt) for two or three weeks.

Fracture of Odontoid Process with Anterior Dislocation of Atlas

This is an extremely rare injury caused by a direct blow on the side or top of the head. It is incurred when a child is thrown out of an automobile and lands on his head, dives into shallow water, or is injured during body contact sports. Spinal cord injury is common in this fracture-dislocation. Treatment consists of reduction by continuous traction through skull tongs followed by immobilization in a halo fixation apparatus.[658] The fracture usually heals in three months. If it fails to unite, the joint should be stabilized by a posterior arthrodesis.

Compression Fractures of Vertebrae in Thoracic and Lumbar Spine

These are rare in childhood because of the flexibility of the spinal column. The injury is sustained when a child falls from a height and lands on his feet (Fig. 8–131). Rupture of the posterior longitudinal ligament and injury to the spinal cord or cauda equina usually do not occur. Treatment consists of immobilization of the spine in a body cast for two months. The prognosis is excellent for full recovery. Occasionally in fracture-dislocations of the lumbar spine, some residual instability may persist and spinal fusion will be required.

FRACTURES OF THE PELVIS

The pelvic ring is formed by the combination of the two innominate bones, which are united anteriorly at the symphysis and the sacrum, which closes the ring posteriorly by its articulations with the innominate bones at the sacroiliac joints. The pelvis supports the spine and transmits the body weight to the lower limbs; it also contains and protects the intrapelvic viscera.

In children, serious fractures of the pelvis usually do not occur, as its cartilaginous components—that at the symphysis pubis, the triradiate cartilage, and that of the sacroiliac joints—give a certain flexibility and elasticity to a child's pelvis.

Fractures of the pelvis may be divided into four groups: (1) unstable fractures with disruption of the pelvic ring; (2) intra-articular fractures of the acetabulum; (3) isolated fractures with continuity of the pelvic ring; (4) avulsion fractures resulting from muscular violence. The clinical picture and treatment vary according to the type of fracture. Fractures of the acetabulum are described in the section on central dislocation of the hip.

Unstable Fractures with Disruption of the Pelvic Ring

These are caused by direct crushing or compression violence, such as the wheels of an automobile running over the pelvis. Symptoms consist of severe local pain and inability to stand or walk. On examination, there is local swelling and tenderness. Frequently there is associated injury to the bladder or urethra. This possibility should be ruled out immediately by inserting a catheter into the bladder. If it cannot be introduced into the bladder, the urethra is crushed; if the catheter can be passed into the bladder and bloody urine is obtained, the bladder has been lacerated; if no fluid is obtained, most probably the bladder has been ruptured and the urine has extravasated into the peritoneal cavity. A definite diagnosis is established by a cystogram.

Severe shock due to massive intrapelvic hemorrhage is of common occurrence in fractures of the pelvis. The source of bleed-

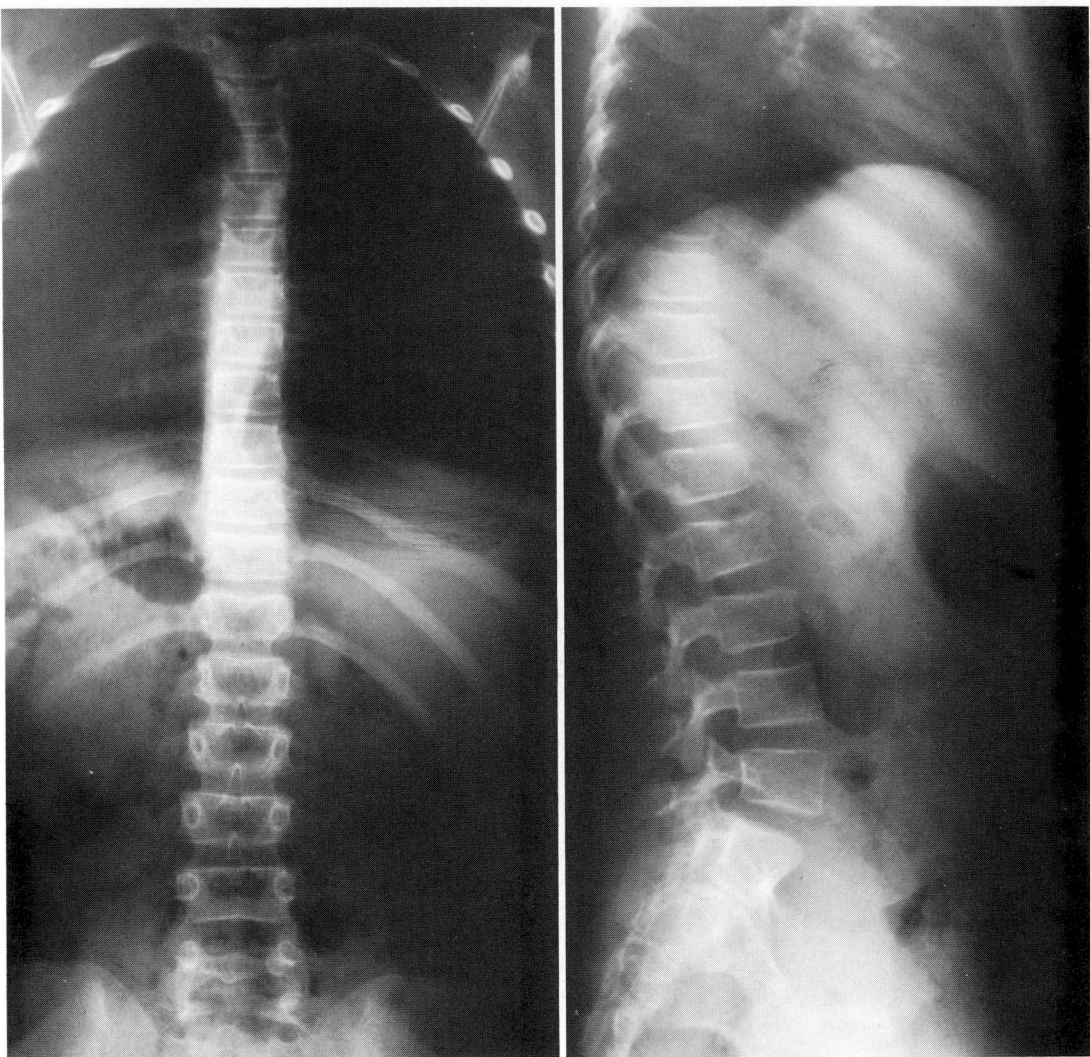

FIGURE 8–131. *Compression fracture of first, second, and third lumbar vertebrae.*

In children, collapse of cancellous bone will increase the height of intervertebral disc interspace.

ing may be the cancellous bone or a torn major vessel. These require immediate attention by transfusion. Over 50 per cent of the circulating blood volume may be lost by a child with a major fracture of the pelvis. The ensuing resultant hematoma will cause paralytic ileus. Sciatic nerve palsy may develop, but it is usually incomplete and transient. The intrapelvic visceral complications and the severe hemorrhagic shock require more immediate care than the fracture itself.

Adequate roentgenograms are essential to delineate the nature and extent of the fractures; these should include an anteroposterior projection, a tangential projection with the x-ray tube directed 50 degrees cephalad, and a pelvic inlet view with the x-ray tube directed inferiorly 60 degrees.

Treatment depends upon the type of the fracture. Anteroposterior compression of the pelvis will produce combined fractures of the pubic and iliac segments of the pelvic ring; this may result in either fractures of both pubic rami with luxation of the sacroiliac joint, a dislocation of the symphysis pubis with fracture of the ilium near the sacroiliac joint (Fig. 8–132), or a dislocation of the symphysis pubis with luxation of the sacroiliac joint. These fracture-dislocations are reduced in lateral recumbency (the patient lying on his normal side) according to the technique of Watson-Jones. The reduction is maintained in a well-molded bilateral hip spica cast with the hips in internal rotation. The pelvic bones have abundant blood supply and unite within four weeks. Any malunion will be remodeled with growth.

Lateral compression of the pelvis will result in either a bilateral fracture of both pubic rami or a unilateral fracture of the pubic ramus with separation of the symphysis pubis. Inequality of limb length or malalignment of weight-bearing joints does not occur in these fractures. Treatment consists of simple bed rest in supine posture—the child should not be allowed to lie on his side. These fractures consolidate in three to four weeks.

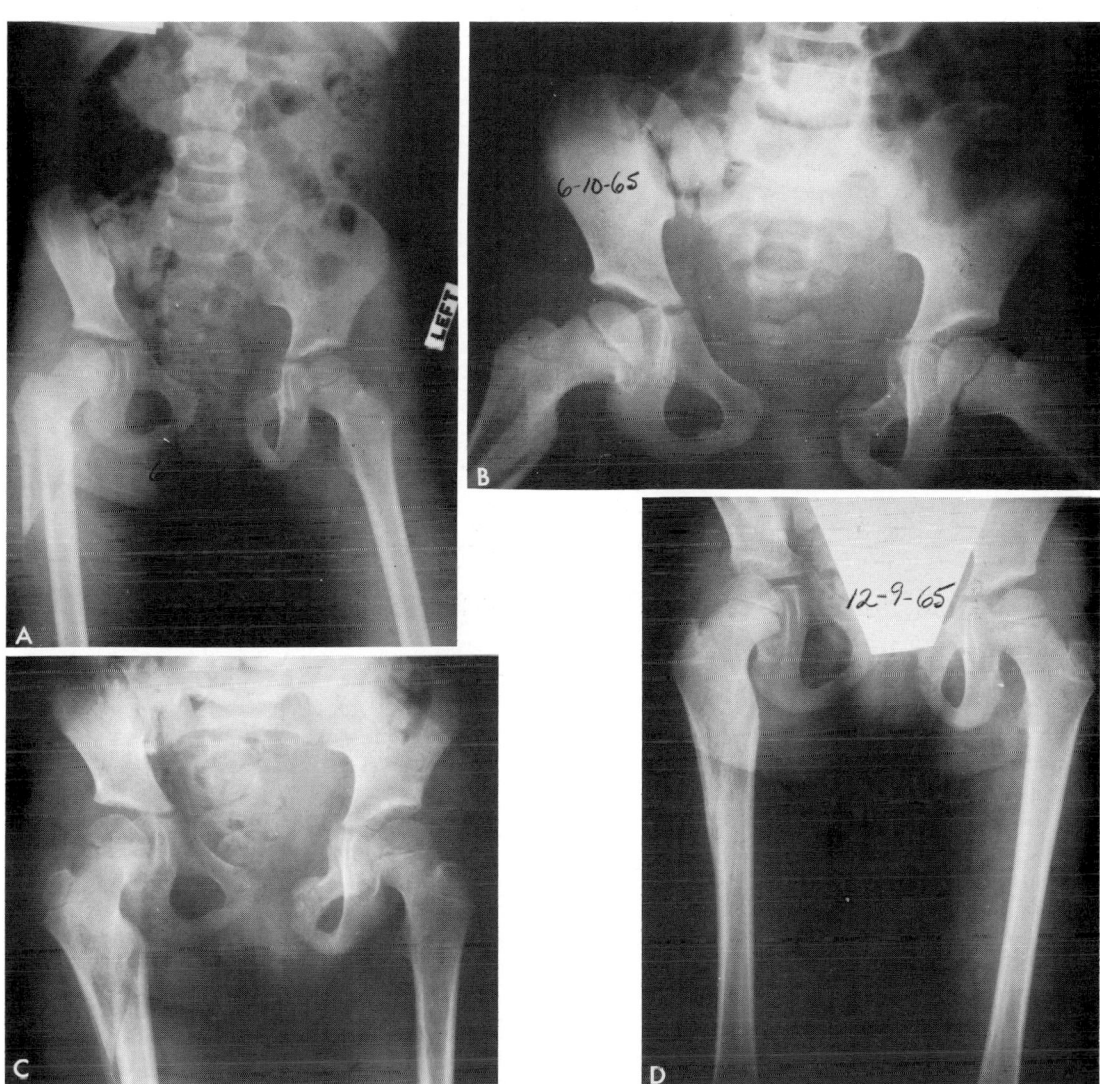

FIGURE 8–132. *Fracture of right ilium with separation of symphysis pubis associated with subtrochanteric fracture treated by skeletal traction through the distal femur.*

A and **B.** Initial roentgenograms. **C.** Six weeks later showing healing. **D.** Four months thereafter there is solid union of subtrochanteric fracture.

Isolated Fractures with Stable Pelvic Ring

These include a unilateral fracture of one or both pubic rami and fractures of the ilium, sacrum, or coccyx. Displacement of fragments is minimal, usually resulting from direct violence. Treatment consists of bed rest until the patient is comfortable; he is then allowed to begin walking with a three-point crutch gait, protecting the injured side. Within three to four weeks, full weight-bearing is permitted. The prognosis for complete recovery is excellent.

Avulsion Fractures of the Pelvis

These result from sudden and severe contraction of muscles attached to the pelvis. The ischial apophysis is avulsed by the action of the hamstrings; forceful contraction of the sartorius detaches the anterior superior iliac spine, and the anterior inferior iliac spine is avulsed by the action of the rectus femoris muscle (Fig. 8–133). Treatment is by simple bed rest until the patient is comfortable; he is then allowed to ambulate. *Os acetabuli* should not be misdiagnosed as a fracture.

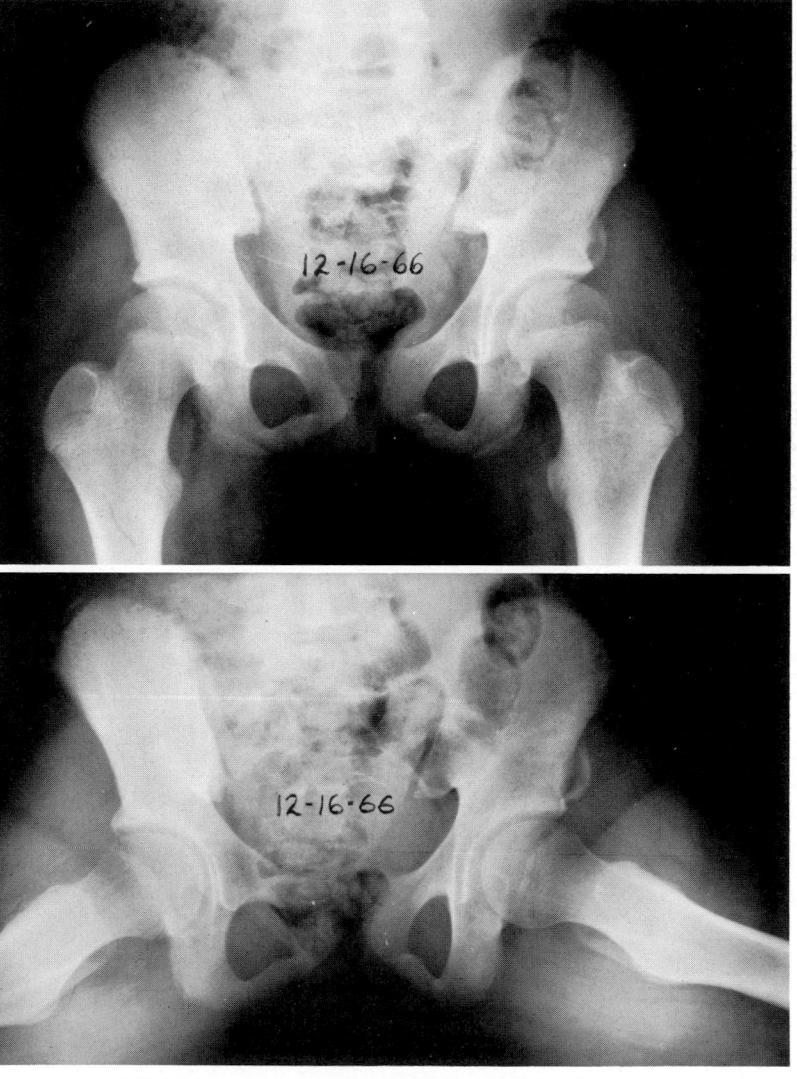

FIGURE 8–133. *Avulsion of anterior inferior iliac spine.*

Miscellaneous Fractures

OBSTETRICAL OR BIRTH INJURIES

Trauma to long bones in the newly born is sustained during a difficult delivery, particularly when the baby is especially large and the presentation is breech. Fetal anoxia and urgency of delivery often necessitate forceful extraction. These injuries are of special concern to the obstetrician, pediatrician, radiologist, and orthopedic surgeon. The skeletal injuries in order of decreasing frequency are: fractures of the clavicle, fractures of the humeral shaft, fractures of the femoral shaft, traumatic fracture-separation of the upper humeral and lower humeral epiphysis, and displacement of the upper and lower femoral epiphyses. Fractures distal to the elbow and knee are very rare. In fact, fracture of the tibia in a newborn is almost always pathologic, and congenital pseudarthrosis of the tibia should be ruled out. When multiple fractures are present, they are most probably pathologic, osteogenesis imperfecta being the commonest cause. Multiple birth fractures also occur in arthrogryposis multiplex congenita, particularly when the knees and elbows are rigidly fixed in extension. Traumatic dislocation of a previously normal joint rarely, if ever, occurs. Epiphyseal separations at birth were frequently misdiagnosed in the past as acute traumatic dislocation.

Birth Fractures of Shafts of Long Bones

Fracture of the diaphysis of the humerus usually occurs in its middle third; it is either transverse or oblique and angulated laterally by the pull of the deltoid muscle. Often it is associated with radial nerve palsy, which recovers completely within six to eight weeks. Diagnosis is readily made by the obstetrician, who feels and often hears the bone break. The infant's arm dangles by his side without active motion. Roentgenograms disclose the fracture. Treatment consists of immobilizing the arm, with the elbow acutely flexed across the chest, with an ace bandage. Soft pads are placed in the axilla to maintain the arm in abduction. The fracture will heal within two weeks, and angular deformities will be spontaneously corrected with growth.

Birth fractures of the shafts of the clavicle and femur are discussed in the treatment of fractures of the individual bones.

Birth Fractures Involving Physes of Long Bones

Epiphyseal fracture-displacement or traumatic separation of the *upper femoral epiphysis* is a rare injury and is often confused with congenital dislocation of the hip.[667, 668, 672, 674, 675, 677, 679, 681, 683] The term *pseudodislocation* of the hip has been used to describe it.[674, 675] Presentation in the birth canal is frequently abnormal, the baby being delivered by version and extraction. The mechanism of injury is one of hyperextension, abduction, and rotation by forceful traction in the leg as it is brought forward.

The line of separation is distal to the combined upper growth cartilage, extending in a crescentic line from the greater to the lesser trochanter. The "snap" is usually not felt by the obstetrician as the epiphysis slides off the metaphysis. On closer examination, however, there is obvious shortening of the involved lower limb, which is held in flexion, abduction, and external rotation at the hip. Acute injury is suggested by pseudoparalysis—the infant holds the leg still, avoiding active movements.

Since at birth, the femoral head, neck, and greater trochanter are entirely cartilaginous, roentgenographic diagnosis may be difficult. The upper end of the femoral diaphysis is displaced upward and laterally. Because the femoral head is in its normal position, the acetabula are symmetrically developed. As was stated earlier, this injury is often misdiagnosed as congenital dislocation of the hip; however, in traumatic separation of the upper femoral epiphysis, the hip appears reduced when held in abduction, medial rotation, and extension, but is grossly displaced when maintained in flexion, abduction, and external rotation (the so-called "frog-leg" position). Arthrography of the hip will establish the diagnosis. Commonly, the injury is not detected until fracture callus appears in the roentgenogram (cf. Fig. 8–84).

If the diagnosis is made at birth, treatment consists of immobilization of the hip in abduction, partial flexion, and medial rotation in a spica cast for two to three weeks. However, diagnosis is frequently delayed until the healing phase, when the coxa vara has become fixed and irreducible. Though there is a high potential for remodeling and spontaneous correction in infants, it should be pointed out that there are several case reports of coxa vara persisting until four years of age.[677, 683] Avascular necrosis is not a complication, as the entire cartilaginous proximal femur (head, neck, and greater trochanter) is displaced, and the blood supply is not disturbed. The ossification center of the femoral head appears first and is larger than on the normal side. Michael et al. reported a case in which the ossification center of the femoral head appeared at the exceptionally early age of 15 days.[681]

Traumatic Separation of Distal Femoral Epiphysis

This presents no problem in roentgenographic diagnosis, since the ossification center of the distal femoral epiphysis is present at birth.[666] However, the injury is not suspected until the knee becomes enlarged by ossification of the massive subperiosteal hematoma. The lower femoral epiphysis is almost always displaced posteriorly, with extensive stripping of the periosteum from the back of the lower femoral shaft. The fracture is a Type I physeal injury (Salter-Harris) with an excellent prognosis for subsequent growth. Care must be taken to avoid injury to the popliteal vessels by manipulative reduction of the posteriorly displaced epiphysis. If the degree of separation of the epiphysis is minimal or moderate, a single hip spica is applied for two weeks with the knee in partial flexion. Any residual angular deformity will spontaneously correct itself with growth. Markedly displaced lower femoral epi-

physes are treated by split Russell traction with a proximal sling behind the knee for two weeks. Bryant's traction should not be employed because of the possible danger of compressing the popliteal vessels and causing ischemia of the foot.

Traumatic Displacement of Distal Humeral Epiphysis

Displacement of the distal humeral epiphysis at birth is a very rare injury. Siffert reported three cases and described its characteristic diagnostic features.[687] The infants are the product of a difficult delivery, either total breech or vertex presentation with shoulder dystocia. The involved elbow is swollen, and on flexion-extension, definite crepitus can be palpated. The medial and lateral epicondyles and the tip of the olecranon are in a normal relationship to one another as the elbow is manipulated—a finding that distinguishes displacement of the distal humeral epiphysis from dislocation of the elbow. Roentgenographic diagnosis is difficult because the distal humeral epiphysis is entirely cartilaginous. In the lateral projection, the upper part of the radius and ulna are posteriorly displaced in relation to the long axis of the humerus; in the anteroposterior projection, the distance between the ossified lower end of the humeral diaphysis and the upper end of both bones of the forearm is foreshortened, as compared with the normal side. When the diagnosis is made at birth, treatment consists of gentle traction and forward manipulation of the olecranon. The elbow is immobilized in a posterior plaster splint for two to three weeks. Often the diagnosis is delayed until the appearance of callus of the healing fracture on the roentgenogram; in such an instance, immobilization of the elbow is not indicated (Fig. 8–134). Siffert points out that the condition is not altogether innocuous; in one child, there was residual limitation of flexion and cubitus varus at the end of two years, and in a second child, a follow-up examination after nine months disclosed persistent slight limitation of flexion and angulation of the distal end of the humerus.[687]

Birth fracture involving the *proximal humeral physis* may occur alone or in assocation with brachial plexus paralysis.[682, 686, 691] The

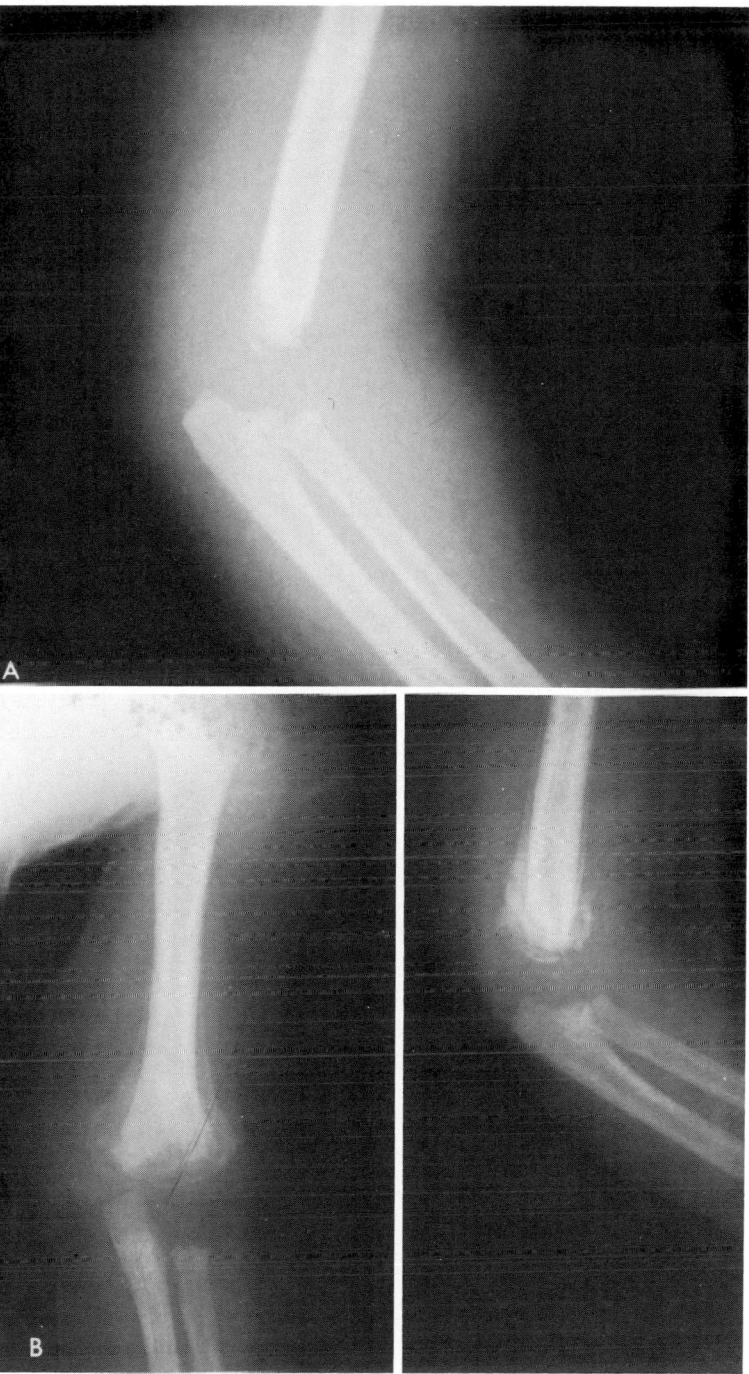

FIGURE 8–134.   Metaphyseal birth fracture of distal humerus.

A. Initial roentgenogram; note the distal metaphyseal fragment. **B.** Three weeks after, extensive subperiosteal new bone formation extends beyond the ossified lower end of the diaphysis.

shoulder will be markedly swollen. Often the condition is mistaken for suppurative arthritis of the shoulder with secondary dislocation. Diagnosis is again initially difficult because of the cartilaginous state of the humeral head. If doubt exists, aspiration of the joint and arthrography may be indicated. The diagnosis is established with the appearance of callus of the healing fracture (Fig. 8–135). Treatment consists of simply bandaging the arm across the chest. The prognosis is excellent.

Other Obstetrical Injuries

Nerve palsies are not rare at birth; obstetrical brachial plexus palsy and sciatic nerve palsy have been discussed in the chapter on the neuromuscular system. Trauma to the spinal cord may occur at birth with breech delivery.[665, 669, 670, 673] If the level of transection is above the fifth cervical segment, it results in sudden death due to respiratory paralysis; if it is distal to the fifth cervical segment, diaphragmatic function is preserved and respiration can be maintained by the infant with adequate assistance. Initially there is complete flaccid paralysis of the trunk and both upper and lower limbs. Anesthesia in all modalities is present distal to the level of injury. Sphincter control is lost. Within a few days, or a few weeks, with gradual recovery from spinal shock, muscle tone and reflex activity return, the degree of functional return being dependent on the extent of cord damage. Meticulous nursing care will keep these infants alive. Later orthopedic management will follow the principles outlined in the discussion of cerebral palsy.

Depressed fracture of the skull at birth is extremely rare because of the pliability of the skull with wide open sutures. The parietal bones are usually involved, injury arising either from forceps pressure or from compression by the walls of a contracted pelvis. Spontaneous recovery is the rule.

Intrauterine fractures of normal bones are of extremely rare occurrence.[666, 678, 688, 690] They may result from indirect violence to the fetus during pregnancy when the mother sustains a direct blow to her abdomen, as in an automobile accident. The diagnosis of intrauterine fracture is es-

tablished when roentgenograms obtained immediately after birth show evidence of fracture callus in normal bone. (A delay of one week would not rule out a birth fracture). Pathologic intrauterine fractures are common, particularly in osteogenesis imperfecta.

STRESS FRACTURES

A stress (or fatigue) fracture is a gradual localized dissolution of bone caused by repeated vigorous strain to which the limb is generally unaccustomed; it may or may not result in complete discontinuity of bone.

Stress fractures in children are rare, with the tibia and fibula most frequently affected. The fibula sustains stress fracture at a younger age than does the tibia. Other rare sites of stress fracture in children are the humerus, first rib, ischiopubic ramus of the pelvis, sesamoid bones, metatarsal bones, and femur (Fig. 8–136). Their clinical course and roentgenographic findings differ from those in the adult because bones in children have a richer blood supply and greater biologic plasticity.[701-704]

Pathogenesis

Resorption of cortical bone is a normal process that takes place in childhood, adolescence, and early adult life. Osteoclastic activity results in many microscopic channels through the cortex. Eventually these resorption cavities are filled by mature Haversian systems and the circumferential lamellar bone is gradually replaced by the structurally more sound osteomal bone of the adult.

Bone responds to excessive stress and strain by acceleration of the normal process of cortical resorption. The bony cortex is weakened by the formation of numerous resorption channels. In an attempt to splint the cortex, the endosteal and periosteal tissues respond by new bone formation adjacent to the areas of cortical resorption. If this buttressing process does not take place rapidly enough, and if continued excessive stress is applied to the bone, fracture will occur. If the buttressing process is adequate, the periosteal and endosteal new bone will

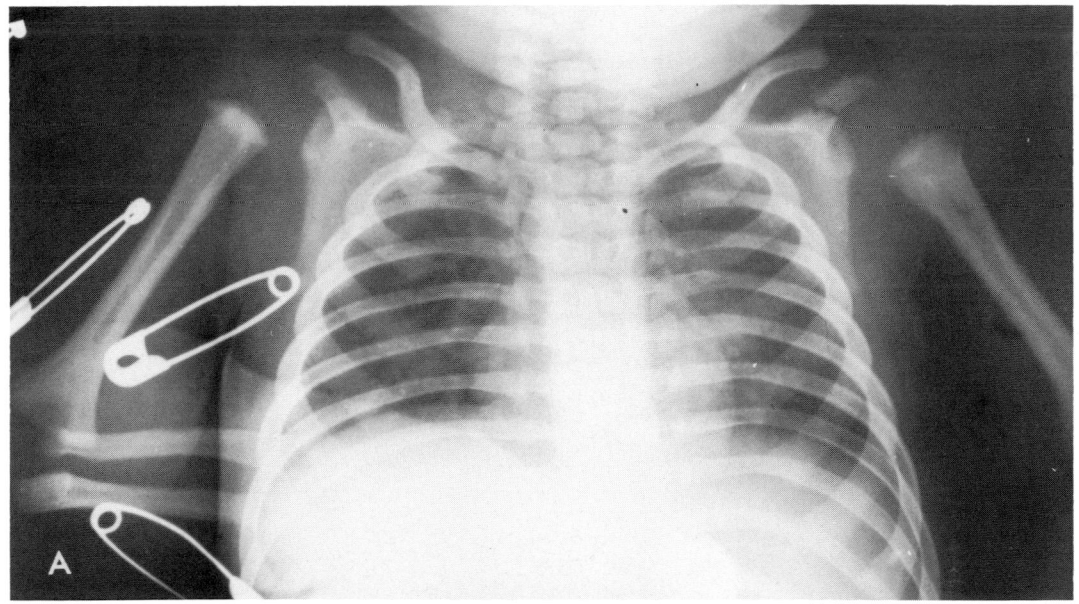

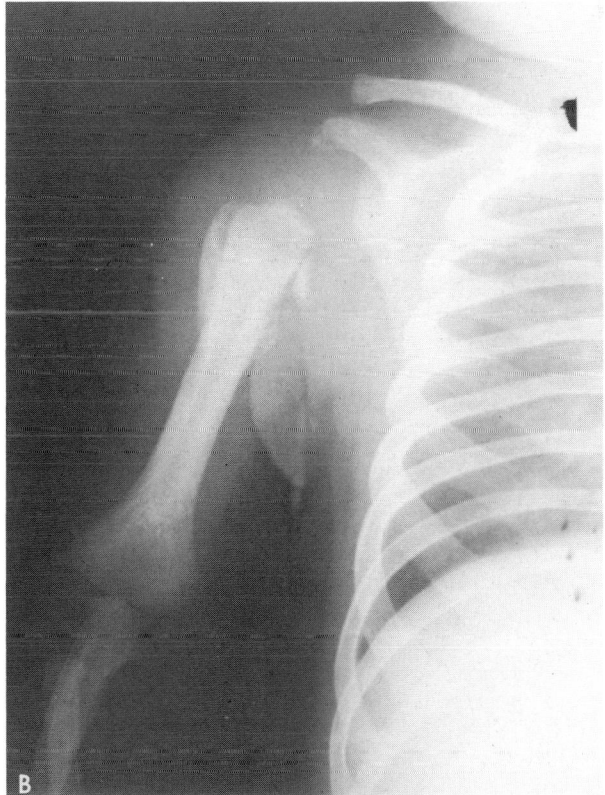

FIGURE 8–135. *Metaphyseal fracture of proximal left humerus.*

A. Initial roentgenograms. **B.** Three weeks later.

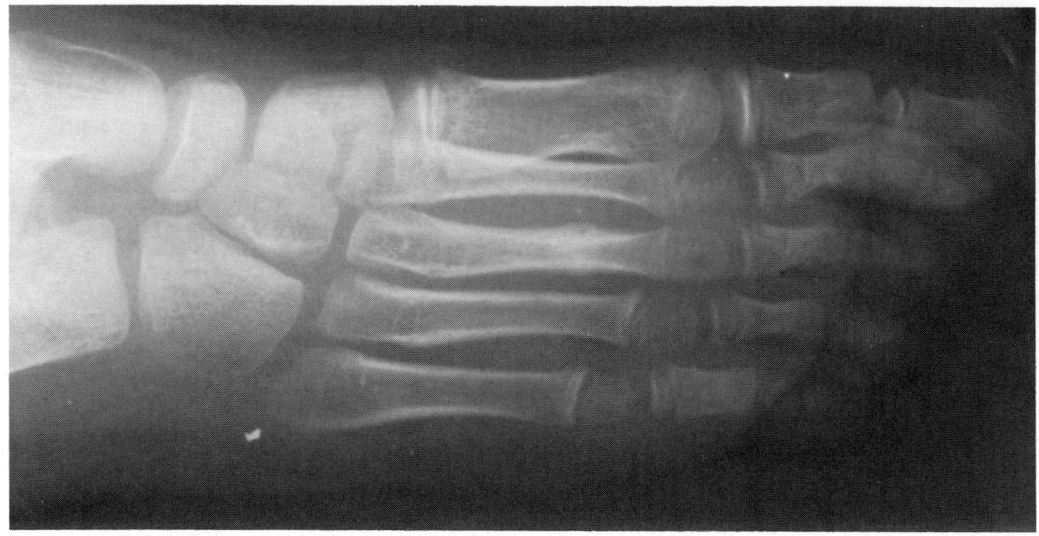

FIGURE 8–136.   *Stress fracture of the third metatarsal (March fracture).*

mature, and the cortical resorption cavities will fill in and eventually become osteomal bone. Thus, the histopathologic process in stress fracture is as follows: first, there is increased cortical resorption; this is followed by periosteal and endosteal new bone formation, which, in turn, is followed by filling in of the resorption cavities in the cortex and maturation of the periosteal and endosteal new bone.[705]

Clinical Findings

When the bones in the lower limb are affected, the child has an antalgic limp, usually of gradual, but occasionally of sudden onset. There is no history of acute trauma, although it may be ascertained that the child has recently taken part in some vigorous activity to which he has previously been unaccustomed.

Local pain is commonly present; it is aggravated by activity and relieved by rest. When the first rib or the humerus is involved, the pain is referred to the arm; when the ischiopubic ramus or the neck of the femur is the site of stress fracture, the pain radiates to the inner aspect of the thigh.

On palpation, there is a varying degree of local swelling and tenderness. The adjacent joints have full range of motion; but when the ischiopubic ramus or the femoral neck is involved, the hip joint is restricted in abduction and rotation (medial rotation with femoral neck fracture and lateral rotation with that of ischiopubic ramus).

Roentgenographic Findings

In the *tibia* the site of stress fracture is nearly always in its proximal third, involving the posteromedial or posterolateral cortex; it does not occur on the anterior aspect of the tibia (Fig. 8–137). There is a haze of internal callus across the diaphysis, subperiosteal new bone formation, and slight disruption of the cortex. An actual linear fracture across the shaft is not seen.

In the *fibula* the earliest roentgenographic sign is the presence of thin layers of "egg shell" callus along the diaphysis. The fracture itself cannot be visualized because it is obscured by the exuberant callus that extends up and down the shaft.

In the differential diagnosis, one should rule out Ewing's sarcoma, osteogenic sarcoma, infantile cortical hyperostosis, and osteomyelitis. In stress fractures, the obvious rapidity of formation and consolidation of subperiosteal callus will make the diagnosis clear in a few days. Oblique roentgenographic views and laminagraphy will assist in delineating osseus detail. Biopsy and pathologic examination of tissues are occasionally necessary to establish the diagnosis.

Treatment consists of rest of the affected part. In stress fractures of the tibia, an above-knee walking plaster of Paris cast is applied for three to four weeks; when the fibula is involved, adhesive elastic strapping and abstinence from strenuous physical activity are all that is necessary.

PATHOLOGIC FRACTURES

Pathologic fractures are those that are caused by minimal trauma in bones that have been weakened by some generalized abnormality or local disease. Pathologic fractures may be classified as follows:

Those due to generalized abnormalities of the skeleton

    Developmental affections

        Osteogenesis imperfecta

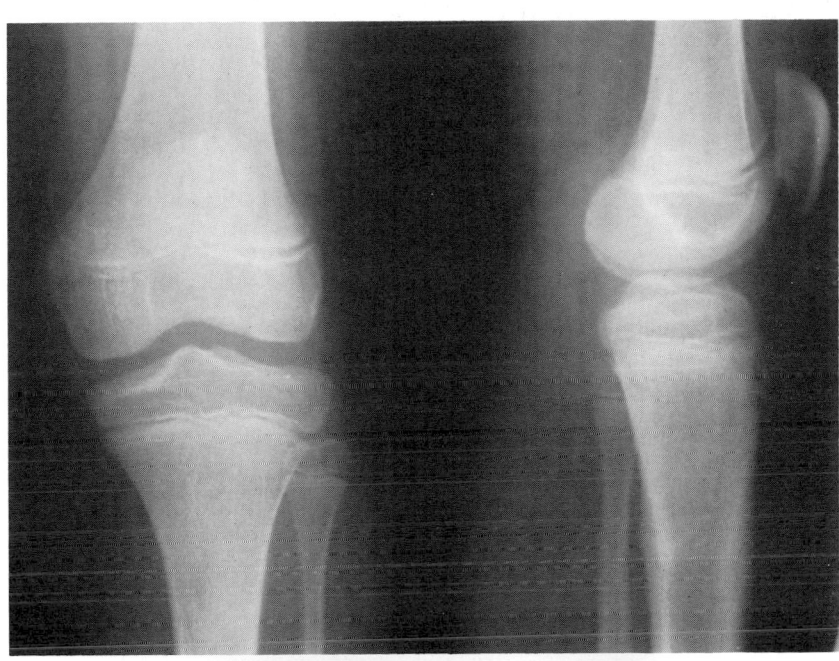

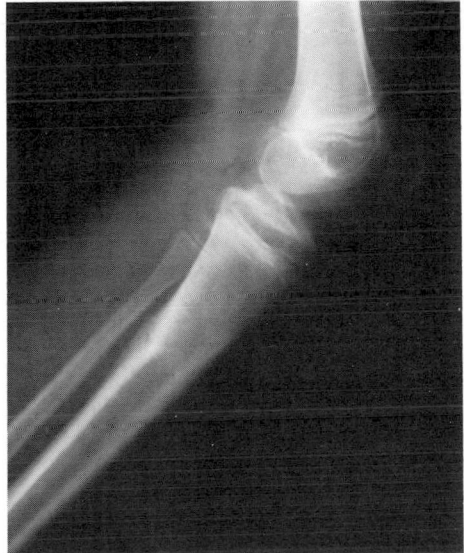

FIGURE 8–137. Stress fracture of proximal tibial diaphysis.

Osteopetrosis or marble bone disease
Arachnodactyly
Vitamin deficiency and endocrine disorders
  Scurvy
  Rickets
  Hyperparathyroidism—primary and secondary
  Hyperpituitarism or Cushing's syndrome.
  From cortisone treatment
Disuse atrophy
  Due to immobilization
  Paralytic diseases of neuromuscular system—myelomeningocele, poliomyelitis, cerebral palsy, arthrogryposis multiplex congenita
Those due to local causes
Inflammatory conditions
  Osteomyelitis
  Rheumatoid arthritis

Postirradiation local osteoporosis
Benign tumors or tumorous lesions
  Nonossifying fibroma (Fig. 8–138)
  Fibrous dysplasia
  Unicameral bone cyst (Fig. 8–139)
  Enchondroma
  Aneurysmal bone cyst
  Neurofibromatosis
Malignant bone tumors
  Primary—such as osteogenic sarcoma
  Metastatic—such as Wilms' tumor (Fig. 8–140) or neuroblastoma

The possibility that a fracture is pathologic should be suspected whenever it is produced by trivial injury. The roentgenograms should be carefully studied to rule out the presence of local or generalized bone disease. The diagnosis and treatment of the foregoing entities have been described under the individual lesions elsewhere in the textbook.

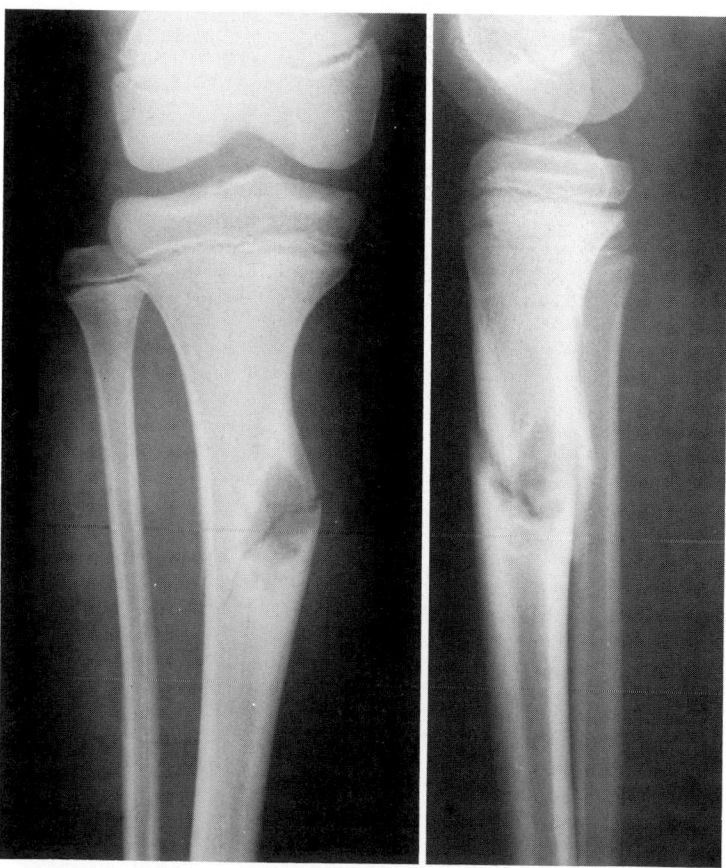

FIGURE 8–138. *Pathologic fracture through a nonossifying fibroma.*

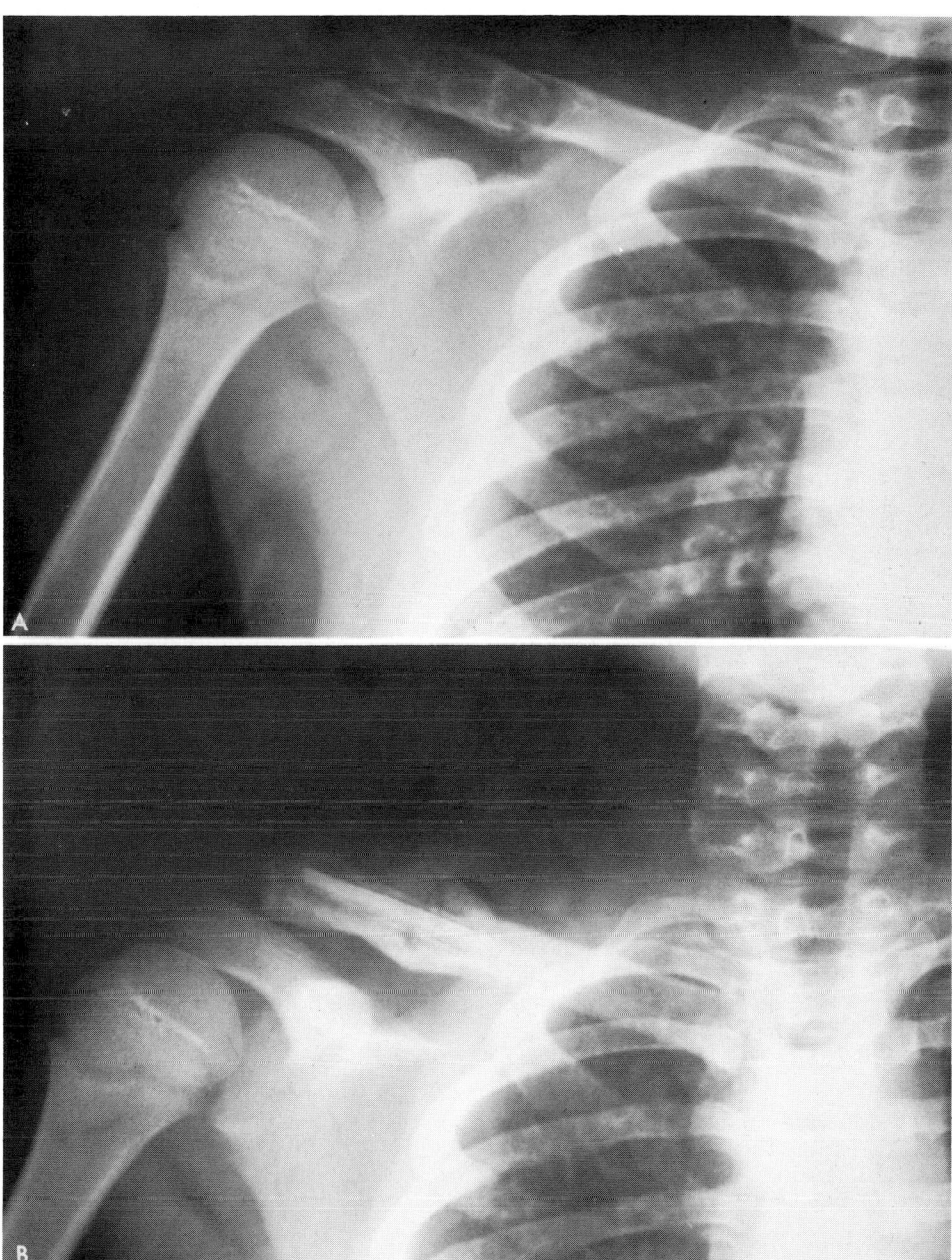

FIGURE 8–139. *Pathologic fracture through unicameral bone cyst of right clavicle.*

Fracture was treated by curettage and bone grafting. **A.** Preoperative roentgenograms. **B.** Postoperative roentgenograms.

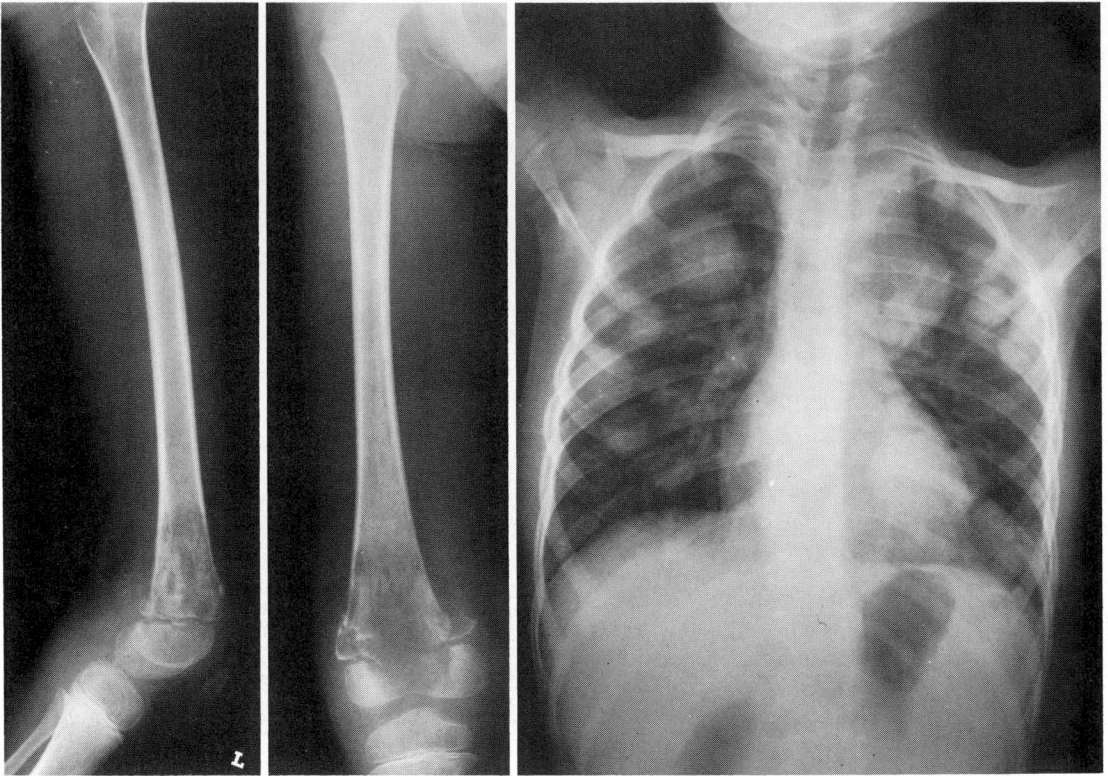

FIGURE 8–140. *Pathologic fracture of distal femur with pulmonary metastasis; original lesion was Wilms' tumor.*

THE BATTERED CHILD

A battered child is one who is a victim of deliberate nonaccidental physical trauma that has been inflicted by a person or persons responsible for his care.

Although reports of physical abuse of children antedate the discovery of roentgen rays, the syndrome of the battered child was not recognized until the signs of bone injury and repair were depicted in the roentgenograms. Caffey, in 1946, first drew attention to the association of multiple fractures of long bones with a significant number of cases of subdural hematoma.[726] Initially, these fractures were thought to be pathologic, occurring spontaneously in bones with some structural abnormality. In 1953, Silverman presented a report on multiple long bone fractures without subdural hematoma in three children, and established their traumatic basis.[741] The condition is sometimes referred to as Silverman's syndrome. Woolley emphasized that the roentgenographic manifestations of injury and its repair were identical, whether a history of injury was or was not obtained and regardless of the presence or absence of subdural hematoma. He also reviewed the undesirable environmental factors and family circumstances that led to physical attack on these children.[744] Since then, numerous reports have appeared in the literature, which lucidly delineate the syndrome of the battered child. The problem is complex, with many psychopathologic, social, and legal aspects; for a discussion of these, the reader is referred to the monograph on the subject by Helfer and Kempe.[733]

Battered children tend to be very young, about two thirds of them being under three years and one third under six months of age. Boys are slightly more subject to parent-induced trauma than girls. The abused child is usually in poor general health, underweight, malnourished, and retarded in development.

Suspicion is usually aroused when, on

presentation of the child at the emergency room, the history of injury as given by the parents is obviously unsatisfactory or too facile. The parents of these children are usually in their midtwenties and are emotionally maladjusted. Multiple fractures, evidence of repeated trauma, and bruises and lacerations should make the condition further suspect. The deformity of gross fractures is obvious.

The characteristic features of skeletal lesions in the battered child syndrome are well described by Silverman; there is predilection for the metaphysis, exaggerated periosteal reaction, and multiplicity of lesions in various stages of healing and repair.[741]

Trauma is inflicted by vigorous pulling on the limbs, direct blows, or throwing the child around. Since the victim is usually an infant or a young child, physeal injuries with gross or minimal displacement of the epiphysis are common. Recent injury may show only soft-tissue swelling in the roentgenogram; the older injury will be evident by abundant subperiosteal new bone formation and later by the relatively thick, dense cortex. The repetitive nature of the injury is hallmarked by the presence of various stages of bone repair. In the diagnostic work-up of a battered child, a roentgenographic skeletal survey is essential. The possibility of subdural hematoma must always be considered. Injuries to visceral organs can occur; rupture of the small intestine, laceration of the liver, perforation of the stomach, laceration of the lung, and subpleural hemorrhage have been reported.[736]

In the differential diagnosis, one should rule out osteogenesis imperfecta, congenital insensitivity to pain, scurvy, congenital lues, and infantile cortical hyperostosis.

Management of various skeletal injuries is described in the sections on treatment of fractures of the specific bones.

It is the duty of physicians to report their suspicions to appropriate authorities, with the understanding that the reporter is granted immunity from legal liability that might follow from making such a report.

In the United States, protective child legislation requires that a welfare department investigate and offer social services to families in cases of alleged child abuse. If this is refused, the case is brought to the attention of the juvenile court.

The battered child should be placed in a foster home and should not be returned to his original environment. The probability of abuse of other children in the same family should be investigated, as well as the possibility of a neighbor or sibling being the person who inflicted the trauma.

References

THE NORMAL PHYSIS AND ITS RESPONSE TO TRAUMA

1. Aitken, A. P.: The end results of the fractured distal radial epiphysis. J. Bone Joint Surg., *17:*302, 1935.
2. Aitken, A. P.: The end results of the fractured distal tibial epiphysis. J. Bone Joint Surg., *18:*685, 1936.
3. Aitken, A. P.: End results of fractures of the proximal humeral epiphysis. J. Bone Joint Surg., *18:*1036, 1936.
4. Aitken, A. P.: Fractures of the epiphyses. Clin. Orthop., *41:*19, 1965.
5. Banks, S. W., and Compere, E. L.: Regeneration of epiphyseal cartilage. An experimental study. Ann. Surg., *114:*1076, 1941.
6. Bergenfeldt, E.: Beiträge zur Kenntnis der traumatischen Epiphysenlösungen an den langen Röhrenenden der Extremitäten. Acta Chir. Scand., *73:*Suppl. 28, 1933.
7. Brashear, H. R., Jr.: Epiphyseal fractures. A microscopic study of the healing process in rats. J. Bone Joint Surg., *41 A:*1055, 1959.
8. Brodin, H.: Longitudinal bone growth. The nutrition of the epiphyseal cartilages and the local blood supply. Acta Orthop. Scand., Suppl. 20, 1955.
9. Campbell, C. J., Grisolia, A., and Zanconato, G.: The effects produced in the cartilaginous epiphyseal plate of immature dogs by experimental surgical traumata. J. Bone Joint Surg., *41-A:*1221, 1959.
10. Dale, G. G., and Harris, W. R.: Prognosis of epiphyseal separation. J. Bone Joint Surg., *40-B:*116, 1958.
11. Ford, L. T., and Key, J. A.: A study of experimental trauma to the distal femoral epiphysis in rabbits. J. Bone Joint Surg., *38-A:*84, 1956.
12. Foucher: Annales du Congrés Medical de Rouen, 1863. Quoted in Poland, J.: Traumatic Separation of the Epiphyses. London, Smith, Elder, & Co., 1898, p.72.
13. Friedenberg, Z. B.: Reaction of the epiphysis to partial surgical resection. J. Bone Joint Surg., *39-A:*332, 1957.
14. Green, W. T., and Cohen, J.: Personal communication to Campbell, C., et al. J. Bone Joint Surg., *41-A:*1239, 1959.
15. Haas, S. L.: The localization of the growing point in the epiphyseal cartilage plate of bones. Amer. J. Orthop. Surg., *15:*563, 1917.
16. Haas, S. L.: The relation of the blood supply to the longitudinal growth of bone. Amer. J. Orthop. Surg., *15:*157, 305, 1917.
17. Haas, S. L.: Restriction of bone growth by pins through the epiphyseal cartilage plate. J. Bone Joint Surg., *32-A:*338, 1950.
18. Harris, W. R.: The endocrine basis for slipping of the upper femoral epiphysis. J. Bone Joint Surg., *32-B:*5, 1950.
19. Harris, W. R., and Hobson, K. W.: Histological changes in experimentally displaced upper femoral epiphysis in rabbits. J. Bone Joint Surg., *38-B:*914, 1956.
20. Imbert, R.: Pathologie expérimentale de l'appareil de croissance des os longs. Marseille Chir., *3:*581, 1951.
21. Morgan, J. D.: Blood supply of growing rabbits' tibia. J. Bone Joint Surg., *41-B:*185, 1959.

22. Ollier, L.: Traité Expérimental et Clinique de la Régénération des Os et de la Production Artificielle du Tissu Osseux. Paris, Masson et Fils, 1867, Vol. I, pp. 236, 386.
23. Phemister, D. B.: Operative arrestment of longitudinal growth of bones in the treatment of deformities. J. Bone Joint Surg., *15:*1, 1933.
24. Poland, J.: Traumatic separation of the epiphyses in general. Historical. Clin. Orthop., *41:*7, 1965 (reprinted from Pediatrics, *4:*49, 1897.).
25. Reynolds, F. C.: Discussion of paper of Campbell, C. J., Grisolia, A., and Zanconato, G. J. Bone Joint Surg., *41-A:*1240, 1959.
26. Ross, D.: Disturbance of longitudinal growth associated with prolonged disability of the lower extremity. J. Bone Joint Surg., *30-A:*103, 1948.
27. Salter, R. B., and Harris, W. R.: Injuries involving the epiphyseal plate. J. Bone Joint Surg., *45-A:*587, 1963.
28. Siffert, R. S.: The effect of staples and longitudinal wires on epiphyseal growth. J. Bone Joint Surg., *38-A:*1077, 1956.
29. Sissons, H. A.: Osteoporosis and epiphyseal arrest in joint tuberculosis. J. Bone Joint Surg., *34-B:*275, 1952.
30. Trueta, J.: Studies of the Development and Decay of the Human Frame. Philadelphia, W. B. Saunders Co., 1968.
31. Trueta, J., and Amato, V. P.: The vascular contribution of osteogenesis. III. Changes in the growth cartilage caused by experimentally induced ischaemia. J. Bone Joint Surg., *42-B:*571, 1960.
32. Trueta, J., and Morgan, J. O.: The vascular contribution to osteogenesis. I. Studies by the injection method. J. Bone Joint Surg., *42-B:*97, 1960.
33. Trueta, J., and Trias, A.: The vascular contribution to osteogenesis. IV. The effect of pressure upon the epiphyseal cartilage of the rabbit. J. Bone Joint Surg., *43-B:*800, 1961.
34. Vogt, P.: Die traumatische Epiphysenntreimung und deren Einfluss auf des Längenwachsthum der Röhrenknochen. Arch. Klin. Chir., *22:*343, 1878.

FRACTURES OF THE CLAVICLE

35. Aikalaj, I.: Internal fixation of a severe clavicular fracture in a child. Israel Med. J., *19:*306, 1960.
36. Billington, R. W.: A new plaster yoke for fracture of the clavicle. Southern Med. J., *24:*667, 1931.
37. Calandi, C., and Bartolozzi, G.: On 110 cases of fracture of the clavicle in the newborn. Riv. Clin. Pediat., *64:*541, 1959.
38. Cappelo, N., and Longhi, G.: Fractures of the clavicle in children and adults. Minerva Med., *54:*408, 1963.
39. Conwell, H. E.: Fractures of the clavicle. Simple fixation dressing with summary of treatment and results attained in 92 cases. J.A.M.A., *90:*838, 1928.
40. DeBlasio, A., and Iafusco, F.: Fracture of the clavicle in newborn infants. Pediatria (Napoli), *68:*815, 1960.
41. Dickson, J. W.: Death following fractured clavicle. Lancet, *2:*666, 1952.
42. Eliason, E. L.: Fractures of clavicle. J.A.M.A., *91:*1974, 1928.
43. Farkas, R., and Levine, S.: X-ray incidence of fractured clavicle in vertex presentation. Amer. J. Obstet. Gynec., *59:*204, 1950.
44. Fawcett, J.: The development and ossification in the human clavicle. J. Anat. Physiol., *47:*225, 1913.
45. Fetisenko, I.: On the treatment of clavicular fracture in children. Khirugiia (Moska), *39:*36, 1963.
46. Greenwood, H. H.: Treatment of fractures of the clavicle. Brit. Med. J., *1:*1021, 1928.
47. Lehmacher, K., and Lehmann, C.: Clavicular fracture in newborn infants after spontaneous delivery in the occipital position. Z. Geburtsh. Gynaek., *158:*134, 1962.
48. Lester, C. W.: Treatment of fractures of the clavicle. Ann. Surg., *89:*600, 1929.

49. McCally, W. C., and Kelly, D. A.: Treatment of fractures of the clavicle, ribs, and scapulae. Amer. J. Surg., *50:*558, 1940.
50. Marinoni, R., and Blini, V.: Contribution to the knowledge and treatment of fractures of the clavicle in the newborn. Osped. Maggiore, *49:*506, 1961.
51. Mourigan, H.: Fractures de la clavicula en el recien nacido. Arch. Pediat. Uruguay, *25:*539, 1954.
52. Nasso, S., and Verga, A.: La frattura della clavicola nel neonato. Minerva Pediat., *6:*593, 1954.
53. Picchio, A. A.: Fractures of the clavicle in infants. Minerva Ortop., *3:*124, 1952.
54. Rolandi, L.: Fracture of the clavicle in the newborn. Osped. Maggiore, *48:*651, 1960.
55. Spina, G. M.: Clinical aspects and therapy of obstetric fractures of the clavicle. Minerva Ortop., *12:*160, 1961.
56. Stubbins, S. G., and McGaw, W. H.: Suspension case for acromioclavicular separations and clavicular fractures. J.A.M.A., *169:*672, 1959.
57. Swolinzky, K., and Borell, H.: Clavicular fracture in newborn infants. Geburtsch. Frauenheilk., *21:*749, 1961.
58. Wong, P. C.: Fractures of the clavicle in the children of Singapore. J. Singapore Paediat. Soc., *8:*55, 1966.
59. Zardini, V.: On the semeiology of clavicle fracture in the newborn. Minerva Ortop., *13:*491, 1962.

EPIPHYSEAL SEPARATION OF MEDIAL END OF CLAVICLE

60. Denham, R. H., Jr., and Dingley, A. F., Jr.: Epiphyseal separation of the medial end of the clavicle. J. Bone & Joint Surg., *49-A:*1179, 1967.
61. Karlèn, M. A.: Traitamiento quirurgico de la epifiseolosis clavicular. Bol. Soc. Cir. Uruguay, *14:*94, 1943.

ACROMIOCLAVICULAR DISLOCATION

62. Horn, J. S.: The traumatic anatomy and treatment of acute acromioclavicular dislocation. J. Bone Joint Surg., *36-B:*194, 1954.
63. Kennedy, J. G., and Cameron, H.: Complete dislocation of the acromioclavicular joint. J. Bone Joint Surg., *36-B:*202, 1954.
64. Lazcano, M. A., Anzel, S. H., and Kelly, P. J.: Complete dislocation and subluxation of the acromioclavicular joint. End results in 73 cases. J. Bone Joint Surg., *43-A:*379, 1961.
65. Urist, M. A.: Complete dislocation of the acromioclavicular joint. J. Bone Joint Surg., *28:*813, 1946.
66. Urist, M. A.: Treatment of dislocations of the acromioclavicular joint, a survey of the past decade. Amer. J. Surg., *98:*423, 1959.

FRACTURES INVOLVING THE PROXIMAL HUMERAL PHYSIS

67. Aitken, A. P.: End results of fractures of the proximal humeral epiphysis. J. Bone Joint Surg., *18:*1036, 1936.
68. Aitken, A. P.: Fractures of the proximal humeral epiphysis. Surg. Clin. N. Amer., *43:*1573, 1963.
69. Astedt, B.: A method for the treatment of humerus fractures in the newborn using the S. Von Rosch splint. Acta Orthop. Scand., *40:*234, 1969.
70. Austin, L. J.: Fractures of the morphological neck of the humerus in children. Canad. Med. Ass. J., *40:*546, 1939.
71. Bourdillon, J. F.: Fracture separation of the proximal epiphysis of the humerus. J. Bone Joint Surg., *32-B:*35, 1950.
72. Conwell, H. B.: Fractures of the surgical neck and epiphyseal separations of the upper end of the humerus. J. Bone Joint Surg., *8:*508, 1926.
73. Dameron, T. B., and Reibel, D. S.: Fractures involving the proximal humeral epiphyseal plate. J. Bone Joint Surg., *51-A:*289, 1969.
74. Divis, G.: Epiphyseolysis humeri unter beträchlicher

Dislokation des Gelenkskopfes. Arch. Orthop. Un-fallchir., *25*:342, 1927.

75. Jeffery, C. C.: Fracture separation of the upper humeral epiphysis. Surg. Gynec. Obstet., *96*:205, 1953.

76. Lee, H. G.: Operative reduction of an unusual fracture of the upper epiphyseal plate of the humerus. J. Bone Joint Surg., *26*:401, 1944.

77. Neer, C. S. II, and Horwitz, B. S.: Fractures of the proximal humeral epiphyseal plate. Clin. Orthop., *41*:24, 1965.

78. Nilsson, S., and Svartholm, F.: Fracture of the upper end of the humerus in children. Acta. Chir. Scand., *130*:433, 1965.

79. Robin, G. C., and Kedar, S. S.: Separation of the upper humeral epiphysis in pituitary gigantism. J. Bone Joint Surg., *44-A*:189, 1962.

80. Roche, A. E.: The ultimate result of a case of separated upper epiphysis of the humerus. Clinical Journal, *55*:478, 1926.

81. Scaglietti, O.: The obstetrical shoulder trauma. Surg. Gynec. Obstet., *66*:868, 1938.

82. Smith, F.: Fracture separation of the proximal humeral epiphysis. Amer. J. Surg., *91*:627, 1956.

83. Vivian, D. N., and Janes, J. M.: Fractures involving the proximal humeral epiphysis. Amer. J. Surg., *87*:211, 1954.

84. Zanolli, R.: Fratture dell'epifisi superiore dell'omero. Chir. Organi Mov., *12*:445, 1928.

FRACTURES OF THE SHAFT OF THE HUMERUS

85. Griswold, R. A., Goldberg, H., and Robertson, J.: Fractures of the humerus. Amer. J. Surg., *43*:31, 1939.

THE ELBOW

GENERAL

86. Ashhurst, A. P. C.: Fractures of the Elbow. An Anatomical and Surgical Study of Fractures of the Lower End of the Humerus. Philadelphia, Lea and Febiger, 1910.

87. Douglas, G. J.: Injuries to the elbow in children. Med. J. Aust., *2*:353, 1961.

88. Fahey, J. J.: Fractures of the elbow in children. A.A.O.S. Instructional Course Lectures. Vol. 17. St. Louis, C. V. Mosby Co., 1960, p. 13.

89. Keon-Cohen, B. T.: Fractures at the elbow. J. Bone Joint Surg., *48-A*:1623, 1966.

90. Smith, F. M.: Surgery of the Elbow. 2nd Ed. Philadelphia, W. B. Saunders Co., 1972.

SUPRACONDYLAR FRACTURE

91. Aebi, H.: Der Ellbogenwinkel, seine Beziehungen zu Geschlect, Körperbay und Hüftbreite. Acta Anat., *3*:228, 1947.

92. Aitken, A. P., Smith, L., and Blackett, C. W.: Supracondylar fractures in children. Amer. J. Surg., *59*:161, 1943.

93. Allen, P. D., and Gramse, A. E.: Transcondylar fractures of the humerus treated by Dunlop traction. Amer. J. Surg., *67*:217, 1945.

94. Attenborough, C. G.: Remodelling of the humerus of the supracondylar fractures in childhood. J. Bone Joint Surg., *35-B*:386, 1953.

95. Basom, W. C.: Supracondylar and transcondylar fractures in children. Clin. Orthop., *1*:43, 1953.

96. Beck, A.: Therapy of supracondylar fracture in children. Zbl. Chir., *60*:2242, 1933.

97. Bertola, L.: On supracondylar fractures of the humerus in childhood. Minerva Ortop., *10*:543, 1959.

98. Blount, W. P.: Fractures in Children. Baltimore, Williams & Wilkins Co., 1955, p. 26.

99. Brandberg, R.: Treatment of supracondylar fractures by reduction followed by fixation in plaster splint. Acta Chir. Scand., *82*:400, 1939.

100. Brewster, A. H., and Karp, M.: Fractures in the region of the elbow in children. Surg. Gynec. Obstet., *71*:643, 1940.

101. Carli, C.: Wire traction for supracondylar fracture of the elbow in children. Chir. Organi Movi., *18*:311, 1933.

102. Celoria, F.: Rupture of humeral artery in supracondylar fracture of elbow. Rev. Soc. Pediat. Litoral, *11*:133, 1946.

103. Christensen, L. O.: Method for bandaging of supracondylar extension fracture in children. Ugeskr, Laeg., *97*:1216, 1935.

104. Cooper, A., Sr.: A Treatise on Dislocations and Fractures of Joints. Philadelphia, Carey and Lea, 1825.

105. Corkery, P. H.: The management of supracondylar fractures of the humerus in children. Brit. J. Clin. Pract., *18*:583, 1964.

106. Coventry, M. B., and Henderson, C. C.: Supracondylar fractures of the humerus. Rocky Mountain Med. J., *53*:458, 1956.

107. Denis, R., and Guilleret, F.: Supracondyloid fractures of elbow irreducible by external maneuvers. Lyon Chir., *36*:620, 1940.

108. Deutschländer, K.: Therapy of supracondylar fractures. Chirurg, *6*:733, 1934.

109. Donchess, J. C.: Treatment of supracondylar fracture of the humerus. J. Indiana Med. Ass., *42*:717, 1949.

110. Dunlop, J.: Transcondylar fractures of the humerus in childhood. J. Bone Joint Surg., *21*:59, 1939.

111. Edman, P., and Lohr, G.: Supracondylar fractures of the humerus treated with olecranon traction. Acta Chir. Scand., *126*:505, 1963.

112. Ekesparre, W. V.: Treatment of supracondylar fractures of the humerus in child. Ann. Chir. Infant., *11*:213, 1970.

113. El-Sharkawi, A. H., and Fattah, H. A.: Treatment of displaced supracondylar fractures of the humerus in children in full extension and supination. J. Bone Joint Surg., *47 B*:111, 1965.

114. Eliason, E. L.: Dressing for supracondylar fractures of the humerus. J.A.M.A., *82*:1934, 1924.

115. Felsenreich, F.: Supracondylar fractures and post-traumatic deformities of elbow joint in children. Arch. Orthop. Unfallchir., *29*:555, 1931.

116. Finochietto, R., and Liambias, A.: Supracondylar fractures of elbow in children. Semana Med., *2*:1837, 1933.

117. French, P. R.: Varus deformity of the elbow following supracondylar fractures of the humerus in children. Lancet, *2*:439, 1959.

118. Garnier, C.: Surgical reduction of supracondylar fractures in children. Sem. Hôp. Paris, *23*:455, 1947.

119. Gartland, J. J.: Management of supracondylar fractures of the humerus in children. Surg. Gynec. Obstet., *109*:145, 1959.

120. Giannestras, N. J.: Displaced supracondylar fractures in children. Amer. J. Orthop., *7*:92, 1965.

121. Godfrey, J.: Trauma in Children. J. Bone Joint Surg., *46-A*:422, 1964.

122. Gruber, M. A., and Hudson, O. C.: Supracondylar fracture of the humerus in childhood—end result study of open reduction. J. Bone Joint Surg., *46-A*:1245, 1964.

123. Hagen, R.: Skin-traction-treatment of supracondylar fractures of the humerus in children. Acta Orthop. Scand., *35*:138, 1964.

124. Hammond, G.: Supracondylar fractures of the humerus in children treated by skeletal suspension traction. Guthrie Clin. Bull., *19*:5, 1949.

125. Hammond, G.: The management of supracondylar fractures of the humerus in children. Surg. Clin. N. Amer., *32*:747, 1952.

126. Hart, V. L.: Reduction of supracondylar fracture in children. Surgery, *11*:33, 1942.

127. Hey-Groves, E. W.: Direct skeletal traction in the treatment of fractures. Brit. J. Surg., *16*:149, 1928.

128. Hill, S. A.: Practical points in elbow fractures. Southern Med. J., *47*:26, 1954.

129. Hofmann, V.: On the management of supracondylar humeral fracture in childhood. Zbl. Chir., *93:*1678, 1968.

130. Holmberg, L.: Fractures of distal end of humerus in children. Acta Chir. Scand., *92:*1, 1945.

131. Hoyer, A.: Treatment of supracondylar fracture of the humerus by skeletal traction in an abduction splint. J. Bone Joint Surg., *34-A:*623, 1952.

132. Hudson, O. C., Lawrence, A. W., Sweet, R. T., and Murphy, H. K. S.: Injuries about the elbow with emphasis on supracondylar and Monteggia fractures. J. Int. Coll. Surg., *28:*332, 1957.

133. Jewett, E. L.: New closed method of treating supracondylar fractures. Amer. J. Surg., *44:*572, 1939.

134. Jonasch, E.: V-Osteotomie bei cubitus varus nach supracondylären Oberarmbrüchen bei Kindern. Arch. Orthop. Unfallchir., *48:*659, 1957.

135. Judet, H.: Exact immediate nonsurgical reduction of transverse supracondylar fracture in children. Bull. Soc. Chir. Paris, *28:*542, 1936.

136. Keller, E.: Supracondylar fractures in children and their treatment with special consideration of muscular mechanism. Arch. Klin. Chir., *192:*702, 1938.

137. King, D., and Secor, C.: Bow elbow (cubitus varus). J. Bone Joint Surg., *33-A:*572; 1951.

138. Klages, F.: Supracondyloid fractures in child. Deutsch. Med. Wschr., *58:*810, 1932.

139. Klinefelter, E. W.: Influence of position on measurement of projected bone angle. Amer. J. Roentgen., *55:*722, 1946.

140. Lagrange, J., and Rigault, P.: Fractures supracondyliennes. Rev. Chir. Orthop., *48:*337, 1962.

141. Lavik, K.: Supracondylar fracture of the humerus in children treated with traction using Semb's abduction splint. Nord. Med., *63:*422, 1960.

142. Lawrence, W.: Supracondylar fractures of the humerus in children. Brit. J. Surg., *44:*143, 1956.

143. Leveuf, J.: Treatment of supracondylar fractures in children. Rev. Orthop., *32:*263, 1946.

144. Leveuf, J., and Godard, H.: Open reduction of supracondyloid fractures in children. Fixation by transplanted bone. J. Chir., *45:*358, 1935.

145. Lusk, W. C.: Reduction of supracondylar fractures of humerus. Ann. Surg., *37:*433, 1908.

146. Madsen, E.: Supracondylar fractures of the humerus in children. J. Bone Joint Surg., *37-B:*241, 1955.

147. Malgaigne, J. F.: Treatise on fractures. Philadelphia, J. B. Lippincott Co., 1859.

148. Mann, T. S.: Prognosis in supracondylar fractures. J. Bone Joint Surg., *45-B:*516, 1963.

149. Maylahn, D. J., and Fahey, J. J.: Fractures of the elbow in children. J.A.M.A., *166:*220, 1958.

150. Miller, E. M., Fell, E. H., Brock, C., Todd, M. C., and Requarth, W. H.: Progress in the management of severe supracondylar fractures of the elbow. Ann. Surg., *113:*1098, 1941.

151. Minne, J.: Late results of orthopaedic and surgical therapy of transverse supracondylar fractures in children. Echo Med. Nord., *1:*129, 1936.

152. Mitchell, W. J., and Adams, J. P.: Supracondylar fractures of the humerus in children. A 10 year review. J.A.M.A., *175:*119, 1961.

153. Morwood, J. B.: Supracondylar fracture with absent radial pube: 2 cases. Brit. Med. J., *1:*163, 1939.

154. Ritchkin, J.: Treatment of supracondylar fractures. S. Afr. Med. J., *12:*742, 1938.

155. Rocher, H. L.: Surgical reduction of supracondylar transverse fracture of elbow in children. Bordeaux Chir., *3:*431, 1932.

156. Sandegard, E.: Fractures of the lower end of the humerus in children. Treatment and end results. Acta Chir. Scand., *89:*1, 1943.

157. Seghini, G.: Outcome of therapy of supracondylar fractures. Arch. Chir. Ortop., *20:*33, 1955.

158. Sgrosso, J. A.: Skeletal traction in therapy of supracondylar fractures in childhood. Rev. Ortop. Traumatol., *5:*381, 1936.

159. Siris, I. E.: Supracondylar fractures of the humerus. Surg. Gynec. Obstet., *68:*201, 1939.

160. Smith, F. M.: Kirschner wire traction in elbow and upper arm injuries. Amer. J. Surg., *74:*770, 1947.

161. Smith, L.: Deformity following supracondylar fractures of the humerus. J. Bone Joint Surg., *42-A:*235, 1960.

162. Sorrel, E.: Supracondylar fractures in children. Rev. Orthop., *32:*383, 1946.

163. Staples, O. S.: Supracondylar fractures of the humerus in children. Complications and problems associated with traction. J.A.M.A., *168:*730, 1958.

164. Swenson, A. L.: Treatment of supracondylar fractures of humerus by Kirschner wire transfixation. J. Bone Joint Surg., *30-A:*993, 1948.

165. Thorgersen, E.: Supracondylar fractures treated by Böhler method in children. Norsk. Mag. Laegevidensk., *96:*121, 1935.

166. Van der Hoff, H. L. M.: One hundred uncomplicated supracondylar fractures in children. Acta Chir. Scand., *88:*99, 1943.

167. Van Gorder, G. W.: Surgical approach in supracondylar "T" fractures requiring open reduction. J. Bone Joint Surg., *22:*278, 1940.

168. Verde, D.: Osteosynthesis in supracondylar fractures in child. Arch. Putti *1:*22, 1951.

169. Wade, F. V., and Batdorf, J.: Supracondylar fractures of the humerus. A 12 year review with follow-up J. Trauma, *1:*269, 1961.

170. Watson-Jones, R.: Fractures and Joint Injuries. 4th Ed. Edinburgh and London, E. & S. Livingstone, Ltd., 4th Ed. Vol. 2, p. 501. 1955.

171. Wiedhopf, O.: Therapy of supracondylar fractures in children by wire extension at elbow. Chirurg, *8:*395, 1936.

172. Wilson, J. C., and McDonnell, D. P.: Fractures of the lower end of the humerus in children. J. Bone Joint Surg., *30-A:*347, 1948.

VOLKMANN'S ISCHEMIA AND NEURAL COMPLICATIONS
FOLLOWING SUPRACONDYLAR FRACTURES OF THE HUMERUS

173. Bailey, G. G.: Nerve injuries in supracondylar fractures of the humerus in children. New Eng. J. Med., *221:*261, 1939.

174. Blount, W. P.: Volkmann's ischemic contracture. Surg. Gynec. Obstet., *90:*244, 1950.

175. Bristow, W. R.: Myositis ossificans and Volkmann's paralysis. Brit. J. Surg., *10:*475, 1923.

176. Brooks, B.: Pathologic changes in muscle as a result of disturbance of circulation. Arch. Surg., *5:*188, 1922.

177. Brower, T. D.: Volkmann's ischemic paralysis. Surg. Clin. N. Amer., *40:*491, 1960.

178. Bruce, J.: Localized Volkmann's contracture. J. Bone Joint Surg., *22:*738, 1940.

179. Bunnell, S.: Ischemic contracture, local, in the hand. J. Bone Joint Surg., *35-A:*101, 1953.

180. Bunnell, S., Coherty, E. W., and Curtis, R. M.: Ischemic contracture, local, in the hand. Plast. Reconstr. Surg., *3:*424, 1948.

181. Cohen, H. H.: Adjustable volar flexion splint for Volkmann's contracture. J. Bone Joint Surg., *24:*189, 1942.

182. Eaton, R. G., and Green, W. T.: Epimysiotomy and fasciotomy in the treatment of Volkmann's ischemic contracture. Orthop. Clin. N. Amer., *3:*175, 1972.

183. Eaton, R. G., Green, W. T., and Stark, H. A.: Volkmann's ischemic contracture. J. Bone Joint Surg., *47-A:*1289, 1965.

184. Eichler, G. R., and Lipscomb, P. R.: The changing treatment of Volkmann's ischemic contractures from 1955 to 1965 at the Mayo Clin. Clin. Orthop., *50:*215, 1967.

185. Flemming, C. W.: A case of impending Volkmann's ischaemic contracture treated by incision of the deep fascia. Lancet, *2:*293, 1931.

186. Foisie, P. S.: Volkmann's ischemic contracture. New Eng. J. Med., *226:*671, 1942.
187. Garber, J. N.: Volkmann's contracture as a complication of fractures of the forearm and elbow. J. Bone Joint Surg., *21:*154, 1939.
188. Griffiths, D. L.: Volkmann's ischaemic contracture. Brit. J. Surg., *28:*239, 1940.
189. Griffiths, D. L.: Volkmann's ischaemic contracture. J. Bone Joint Surg., *33-B:*299, 1951.
190. Harmon, J. W.: The significance of local vascular phenomena in the production of ischemic necrosis in skeletal muscles. Amer. J. Path., *24:*625, 1948.
191. Hill, R. L.: Volkmann's ischemic contracture in hemophilia. Trans. Hawaii Territor. Med. Ass., 26, 1929.
192. Hill, R. L., and Brooks, B.: Volkmann's ischemic contracture in hemophilia. Ann. Surg., *103:*444, 1936.
193. Hodgson, N.: Volkmann's ischaemic contracture treated by transplantation of internal epicondyle. Brit. J. Surg., *17:*317, 1929.
194. Holmes, W., Highet, W. B., and Seddon, H. J.: Ischaemic nerve lesions occurring in Volkmann's contracture. Brit. J. Surg., *32:*259, 1944.
195. Hordegen, K. M.: Neurologic complications of supracondylar humeral fractures in children. Arch. Orthop. Unfallchir., *68:*294, 1970.
196. Horwitz, T.: Significance of venous circulation about the elbow in pathomechanics of Volkmann's contracture. Surg. Gynec. Obstet., *74:*871, 1942.
197. Jepson, P. N.: Ischaemic contracture: Experimental study. Ann. Surg., *84:*785, 1926.
198. Jones, E. B.: Volkmann's ischaemia: Observations at open operation. Brit. Med. J., *1:*1053, 1940.
199. Jones, S.: Volkmann's contracture. J. Bone Joint Surg., *17:*669, 1935.
200. Kinmonth, J. B.: The physiology and relief of traumatic arterial spasm. Brit. Med. J., *1:*59, 1952.
201. Kulowski, J.: Tendon lengthening for Volkmann's ischemic clawhand. Southern Med. J., *53:*1241, 1960.
202. Laigle, L.: Evolution of ideas concerning Volkmann's syndrome. Medecine, *19:*893, 1938.
203. Leriche, R.: A propos du mecanisme et de la therapeutique de la maladie de Volkmann. J. Internat. Chir., *3:*81, 1938.
204. Lipscomb, P. R.: The etiology and prevention of Volkmann's ischaemic contracture. Surg. Gynec. Obstet., *103:*353, 1956.
205. Lipscomb, P. R., and Burleson, R. J.: Vascular and neural complications in supracondylar fractures of the humerus in children. J. Bone Joint Surg., *37-A:*487, 1955.
206. Malan, E., and Tattoni, G.: Physio-anatomo-pathology of acute ischemia of the extremities. J. Cardiovasc. Surg., *1:*212, 1963.
207. Massart, R.: La maladie de Volkmann. Rev. Orthop., *22:*385, 1935.
208. Meyerding, H. W.: Volkmann's ischemic contracture. J.A.M.A., *94:*394, 1930.
209. Meyerding, H. W.: Volkmann's ischemic contracture. Surg. Clin. N. Amer., *10:*49, 1930.
210. Meyerding, H. W.: Volkmann's ischemic contracture associated with supracondylar fractures of the humerus. J.A.M.A., *106:*1139, 1936.
211. Meyerding, H. W., and Krusen, F. H.: Treatment of Volkmann's ischemic contracture. Ann. Surg., *110:*417, 1939.
212. Middleton, D. S.: Discussion of Volkmann's ischemic contracture. Lancet, *2:*299, 1928.
213. Nario, C. V.: La enfermedad de Volkmann experimental. J. Internat. Chir., *3:*87, 1938.
214. Nisbet, N. W.: Volkmann's ischaemic contracture benefited by muscle slide operation. J. Bone Joint Surg., *34-B:*245, 1952.
215. Page, C. M.: Operation for relief of flexion contracture in forearm. J. Bone Joint Surg., *5:*233, 1923.
216. Parkes, W.: The treatment of established Volkmann's contracture by tendon transplantation. J. Bone Joint Surg., *33-B:*359, 1951.

217. Plewes, L. W.: Occlusion of brachial artery and Volkmann's ischemic contracture. Brit. Med. J., *1:*1054, 1945.
218. Pollock, G. A.: Early operation for Volkmann's ischaemic contracture. Brit. Med. J., *1:*783, 1944.
219. Seddon, H. J.: Volkmann's contracture. Treatment by excision of the infarct. J. Bone Joint Surg., *38-B:*152, 1956.
220. Seddon, H. J.: L'ischemie de Volkmann. Rev. Chir. Orthop., *46:*149, 1960.
221. Seddon, H. J.: Volkmann's ischaemia. Brit. Med. J., *1:*1587, 1964.
222. Spear, H. C., and James, J. M.: Rupture of the brachial artery accompanying dislocation of the elbow or supracondylar fracture. J. Bone Joint Surg., *33-A:*889, 1951.
223. Spinner, M.: Injuries to the Major Branches of Peripheral Nerves of the Forearm. Philadelphia, W. B. Saunders Co., 1972.
224. Spinner, M., and Schreiber, S. N.: Anterior interosseous-nerve paralysis of a complication of supracondylar fractures of the humerus in children. J. Bone Joint Surg., *51-A:*1584, 1969.
225. Staples, O. C.: Dislocation of the brachial artery—a complication of supracondylar fracture of the humerus in childhood. J. Bone Joint Surg., *47-A:*1525, 1965.
226. Stanford, S.: Traumatic ischaemia in forearm and leg. Lancet, *1:*462, 1944.
227. Steindler, A.: Ischemic contracture. Surg. Gynec. Obstet., *62:*358, 1936.
228. Tavernier, L., Dechaume, J., and Pouzet, E.: Infarctus musculaires et lésions nerveuses dans le syndrome de Volkmann. J. Med. Lyon, *17:*815, 1936.
229. Volkmann, R.: Die ischaemischen Mustellahmungen und Kontrakturer. Zbl. Chir., *8:*801, 1881.
230. White, J. W., and Stubbins, S. G.: Carpectomy for intractable flexion deformities of the wrist. J. Bone Joint Surg., *26:*131, 1966.
231. Zancolli, E.: Tendon transfers after ischaemic contracture of the forearm. Amer. J. Surg., *109:*356, 1965.

FRACTURE-SEPARATION OF THE DISTAL HUMERAL EPIPHYSIS

232. Kaplan, S. S., and Reckling, F. W.: Fracture separation of the lower humeral epiphysis with medial displacement. J. Bone Joint Surg., *53-A:*1105, 1971.
233. Marmor, L., and Bechtol, C. O.: Fracture separation of the lower humeral epiphysis. Report of a case. J. Bone Joint Surg., *42-A:*333, 1960.
234. Smith, R. W.: Observations on disjunction of the lower epiphysis of the humerus. Dublin Quart. J. Med. Sci., *9:*63, 1850.

FRACTURES OF THE LATERAL CONDYLE OF THE HUMERUS

235. Brenken, M., and Kuttner, H.: Die Ulnarisspatlahmung in folge Frakhn des Condyles lateralis Humeri. Arch. Orthop. Unfallchir., *28:*182, 1930.
236. Broca: Décollements épiphysaires et fractures de la région condylienne externe. J. Practiciens, *97:*117, 1914.
237. Conner, A. N., and Smith, M. G. H.: Displaced fractures of the lateral humeral condyle in children. J. Bone Joint Surg., *52-B:*460, 1970.
238. Crabbee, W. A.: The treatment of fracture-separation of the capitular epiphysis. J. Bone Joint Surg., *45-B:*722, 1963.
239. Fabian, E.: Zur Behandlung der Fractura Condyli externi Humeri mittcb. Exstirpation des freien Fragmente. Deutsch. Z. Chir., *128:*409, 1914.
240. Flynn, J. C., and Richards, J. F.: Non-union of minimally displaced fractures of the lateral condyle of the humerus in children. J. Bone Joint Surg., *53-A:*1096, 1971.
241. Freeman, R. H.: Fractures of the lateral humeral condyle. J. Bone Joint Surg., *41-B:*631, 1959.
242. Hardacre, J. A., Nahigian, S. H., Froimson, I., and

Brown, J. E.: Fractures of the lateral condyle of the humerus in children. J. Bone Joint Surg., *53-A:*1083, 1971.

243. Heyl, J. H.: Fracture of external condyle of humerus in children. Ann. Surg., *51:*1069, 1935.

244. Jones, K. G.: Percutaneous pin fixation of fractures of the lower end of the humerus. Clin. Orthop., *50:*53, 1967.

245. Kini, M. G.: Fractures of the lateral condyle of the lower end of the humerus with complications. J. Bone Joint Surg., *24:*270, 1942.

246. McDonnell, D. P., and Wilson, J. C.: Fractures of the lower end of the humerus in children. J. Bone Joint Surg., *30-A:*347, 1948.

247. McLearie, M., and Merson, R. D.: Injuries to the lateral condyle epiphysis of the humerus in children. J. Bone Joint Surg., *36-B:*84, 1954.

248. Massart, C.: Les fractures du condyle externe chez l'enfant—étude clinique et radiographique de ces fractures et de leurs resultats éloignes. Rev. Orthop., *15:*475, 1928.

249. Miller, E. M.: Late ulnar nerve paralysis. Surg. Gynec' Obstet., *38:*37, 1924.

250. Moorhead, E. L.: Old untreated fracture of the external condyle of humerus—factors in influencing choice of treatment. Surg. Clin., *3:*987, 1919.

251. Pelle, A.: Décollement du condyle externe de l'humerus passé inaperçu au cours d'un traumatisme du coude. Rev. Orthop., *19:*48, 1932.

252. Riess, J.: Fractures of the lateral humeral condyle in children. Zr. Orthop., *80:*427, 1951.

253. Rocher, H. L., and Guerin, R.: Luxation ouverte du coude avec fracture du condyle externe. Arch. Franco-Belg. Chir., *32:*627, 1930.

254. Smith, F. M., and Joyce, J. J.: Fractures of the lateral condyle of the humerus in children. Amer. J. Surg., *87:*324, 1954.

255. Smith, M. K.: Fractures of the external condyle of the humerus with rotation. Ann. Surg., *86:*304, 1927.

256. Speed, J. S., and Macey, H. B.: Fractures of the humeral condyles in children. J. Bone Joint Surg., *15:*903, 1933.

257. Stone, J. S.: Fractures of the external condyle of the humerus in childhood with rotation of the condylar fragment. Boston Med. Surg. J., *176:*151, 1917.

258. Wilson, J. N.: Fractures of the external condyle of the humerus in children. Brit. J. Surg., *43:*88, 1955.

259. Wilson, P. D.: Fractures and dislocations in the region of the elbow. Surg. Gynec. Obstet., *56:*335, 1933.

260. Wilson, P. D.: Fracture of the lateral condyle of the humerus in childhood. J. Bone Joint Surg., *18:*301, 1936.

FRACTURES OF THE MEDIAL EPICONDYLE OF THE HUMERUS

261. Fairbank, H. A. T., and Buxton, St. J. D.: Displacement of the internal epicondyle into the elbow joint. Lancet, *2:*218, 1934.

262. Granger, B.: On a particular fracture of the inner condyle of the humerus. Edinburgh Med. Surg. J., *14:*196, 1818.

263. Roberts, N. W.: Displacement of the internal epicondyle into the elbow joint. Four cases successfully treated by manipulation. Lancet, *2:*78, 1934.

264. Walker, H. B.: Displacement of the epicondyle into the elbow joint. Brit. J. Surg., *15:*677, 1928.

265. Watson-Jones, R.: Nerve lesions in injuries of the elbow. J. Bone Joint Surg., *12:*121, 1930.

DISLOCATION OF THE ELBOW

266. Albert, E.: Lehrbuch der Chirurgie und Operationslehre. Zweite Auflage. Band 2, 377. Wein, Urban & Schwarzenberg., 1881.

267. Cohn, I.: Forward dislocation of both bones of the forearm at the elbow. Surg. Gynec. Obstet., *35:*776, 1922.

268. Cotton, F. J.: Elbow dislocation and ulnar nerve injury. J. Bone Joint Surg., *11:*348, 1929.

269. Crosby, E. H.: Elbow dislocations reduced by traction in four different directions. J. Bone Joint Surg., *18:*1077, 1936.

270. Eliason, E. L., and Brown, R. B.: Posterior dislocation at the elbow with rupture of the radial and ulnar arteries. Ann. Surg., *106:*1111, 1937.

271. Gayton, W.: Recurrent dislocation of the elbow. J. Bone Joint Surg., *42–B:*406, 1960.

272. Gossman, J. A.: Recurrent dislocation of the ulna at the elbow. J. Bone Joint Surg., *25:*448, 1943.

273. Kapel, O.: Operation for habitual dislocation of the elbow. J. Bone Joint Surg., *33–A:*707, 1951.

274. King, T.: Recurrent dislocation of the elbow. J. Bone Joint Surg., *35–B:*50, 1953.

275. Kini, M. G.: Dislocation of the elbow and its complications. J. Bone Joint Surg., *22:*107, 1940.

276. Knoflach, J. G.: Zur Operation der habituellen Ellogenluxation. Zbl. Chir., *62:*2897, 1935.

277. Lavine, L. S.: A simple method of reducing dislocations of the elbow joint. J. Bone Joint Surg., *35–A:*785, 1953.

278. Linscheid, R. L., and Wheeler, D. K.: Elbow dislocation. J.A.M.A., *194:*1171, 1965.

279. Loomis, L. K.: Reduction and after treatment of posterior dislocation of the elbow. Amer. J. Surg., *63:*56, 1944.

280. Milch, H.: Bilateral recurrent dislocation of the ulna at the elbow. J. Bone Joint Surg., *18:*777, 1936.

281. Osborne, G., and Cotterill, P.: Recurrent dislocation of the elbow. J. Bone Joint Surg., *48–B:*340, 1966.

282. Prior: Severe compound dislocation of the elbow joint successfully treated. Lancet, *2:*366, 1844.

283. Reichenheim, P. P.: Transplantation of the biceps tendon as a treatment for recurrent dislocation of the elbow. Brit. J. Surg., *35:*201, 1947.

284. Richet: Observation de luxation en avant de l'extremité superieure des os de l'avant bras, compliqué de fracture du cubitus suivie de réflexions sur ces luxations. Arch. Gen., *6:*472, 1839.

285. Robertson, D. E.: Fractures and dislocation involving the elbow joint in children. Amer. J. Surg., *39:*327, 1938.

286. Silva, J. F.: Old dislocation of elbow. Ann. Roy. Coll. Surg., *22:*363, 1958.

287. Siris, P. E.: Elbow fractures and dislocations. Surg. Gynec. Obstet., *40:*665, 1925.

288. Sorrel, E.: Luxation récidivante du coude. Bull. et Mém. Soc. Nat. Chir., *61:*790, 1935.

289. Spear, H. C., Jancs, J. M.: Rupture of the brachial artery accompanying dislocation of the elbow or supracondylar fracture. J. Bone Joint Surg., *33–A:*889, 1951.

290. Speed, J. S.: An operation for unreduced posterior dislocation of the elbow. Southern Med. J., *18:*193, 1925.

291. Spring, W. E.: Report of a case of recurrent dislocation of the elbow. J. Bone Joint Surg., *35–B:*55, 1953.

292. Staunton, F. W.: Dislocation forward of the forearm without fracture of the olecranon. Brit. Med. J., *2:*1570, 1905.

293. Steiger, R. N., Larrick, R. B., and Meyer, T. L.: Median-nerve entrapment following elbow dislocation. J. Bone Joint Surg., *51–A:*381, 1969.

294. Wainwright, D.: Recurrent dislocation of the elbow joint. Proc. Roy. Soc. Med., *40:*885, 1947.

295. Wainwright, D.: Fractures involving the elbow joint. *In* Clark, J. P. (ed.): Modern Trends in Orthopedics. Vol. 2. London, Butterworth Co., 1962.

296. Wheeler, D. K., and Linscheid, R. L.: Fracture dislocations of the elbow. Clin. Orthop., *50:*95, 1967.

297. Wilson, P. D.: Fractures and dislocations in the region of the elbow. Surg. Gynec. Obstet., *56:*335, 1933.

298. Woods, R. S.: Backward dislocation of the elbow. Brit. Med. J., *1:*15, 1935.

FRACTURES INVOLVING THE PROXIMAL RADIAL PHYSIS AND RADIAL NECK

299. Dougall, A. J.: Severe fractures of the neck of the radius in children. J. Roy. Coll. Surg. Edin., *14:*220, 1969.

300. Fielding, J. W.: Radio-ulnar crossed union following dis-

placement of the proximal radial epiphysis. J. Bone Joint Surg., *46–A:*1277, 1964.

301. Henrikson, B.: Isolated fractures of the proximal end of the radius in children. Acta Orthop. Scand., *40:*246, 1969.
302. Jeffrey, C. C.: Fractures of the head of the radius in children. J. Bone Joint Surg., *32–B:*314, 1950.
303. Jones, E. R. W., and Esah, M.: Displaced fractures of the neck of the radius in children. J. Bone Joint Surg., *53–B:*429, 1971.
304. Key, J. A.: Treatment of fractures of the head and neck of the radius. J.A.M.A., *96:*101, 1939.
305. Lewis, R. W., and Thibodeau, A. A.: Deformity of the wrist following resection of the radial head. Surg. Gynec. Obstet., *64:*1079, 1937.
306. Mouchet, A.: Fractures of the neck of the radius. Rev. Chir., *22:*596, 1900.
307. Murray, R. C.: Fractures of the head and neck of the radius. Brit. J. Surg., *28:*109, 1940.
308. O'Brien, P. I.: Injuries involving the proximal radial epiphysis. Clin. Orthop., *41:*51, 1965.
309. Patterson, R. F.: Treatment of displaced fracture of the neck of the radius in children. J. Bone Joint Surg., *16:*695, 1934.
310. Reidy, J. A., and Van Gorder, G. W.: Treatment of displacement of the proximal radial epiphysis. J. Bone Joint Surg., *45–A:*1355, 1963.
311. Schwartz, R. P., and Young, F.: Treatment of fractures of the head and neck of the radius and slipped radial epiphysis in children. Surg. Gynec. Obstet., *57:*528, 1933.
312. Speed, K.: Fractures of the head of the radius. Amer. J. Surg., *38:*157, 1924.
313. Speed, K.: Traumatic lesions of the head of the radius. Surg. Clin. N. Amer., *4:*651, 1924.
314. Wood, S. K.: Reversal of the radial head during reduction of fracture of the neck of the radius in children. J. Bone Joint Surg., *51–B:*707, 1969.

PULLED ELBOW

315. Anderson, S. A.: Subluxation of the head of the radius, a pediatric condition. Southern Med. J., *35:*286, 1942.
316. Beegel, P. M.: "Slipped Elbow" in Children. J. Maine Med. Ass., *45:*293, 1954.
317. Blodgett, W. E.: Congenital luxation of the head of the radius. Amer. J. Orthop. Surg., *3:*253, 1906.
318. Bourquet: Mémoire sur les luxations dites incomplètes de l'extrémité. Rev. Med. Chir., *15:*287, 1854.
319. Boyette, B. P., Ahoskie, N. C., and London, A. H., Jr.: Subluxation of the head of the radius, "nursemaid's elbow." J. Pediat., *32:*278, 1948.
320. Broadhurst, R. W., Buhr, A. J.: The pulled elbow. Brit. Med. J., *1:*1018, 1959.
321. Caldwell, C. E.: Subluxation of the radial head by elongation. Cincinnati Lancet Clinic, *66:*496, 1891.
322. Chaissaignac: Paralysie douloureuse des jeunes enfants. Arch. Gen. Med., *1:*653, 1856.
323. Corrigan, A. B.: The pulled elbow. Med. J. Aust., *2:*187, 1965.
324. Costigan, P. G.: Subluxation of the annular ligament at the proximal radioulnar joint. Alberta Med. Bull., *17:*7, 1952.
325. Cushing, H. W.: Subluxation of the radial head in children. Boston Med. Surg. J., *114:*77, 1886.
326. Davis, J. H.: Subluxation of the radial head in children (nursemaid's elbow). Med. Times, *13:*1379, 1965.
327. Duverney, J. G.: Traité des Maladies des Os. Paris, De Bure l'aine, 1751.
328. Fournier, D.: L'Oeconomic Chirurgical, 250, Paris, Francoise Clouzier & Cie, 1671.
329. Gardner, J.: On an undescribed displacement of the bones of the forearm in children. London Med. Gaz., *20:*878, 1837.

330. Green, J. T., and Gay, F. H.: Traumatic subluxation of the radial head in young children. J. Bone Joint Surg., *36–A:*655, 1954.
331. Griffin, M. E.: Subluxation of the head of the radius in young children. Pediatrics, *15:*103, 1955.
332. Hart, G. M.: Subluxation of the head of the radius in young children. J.A.M.A., *169:*1734, 1959.
333. Hutchinson, J., Jr.: On certain obscure sprains of the elbow occurring in young children. Ann. Surg., *2:*91, 1885.
334. Kanter, A. J., and Bruton, O. C.: Subluxation of the head of the radius. Amer. Practit., *31:*39, 1952.
335. Lindeman, S. H.: Partial dislocation of the radial head peculiar to children. Brit. Med. J., *2:*1058, 1885.
336. McRae, R., and Freeman, P. A.: The lesion in pulled elbow. J. Bone Joint Surg., *47–A:*808, 1965.
337. McVeagh, T. C.: The slipped elbow in young children. Calif. Med., *74:*260, 1951.
338. Magill, H. K., and Aitken, A. P.: Pulled elbow. Surg. Gynec. Obstet., *98:*753, 1954.
339. Matles, A. L., and Eliopoulous, K.: Internal derangement of the elbow in children. Int. Surg., *48:*259, 1967.
340. Moore, E. M.: Subluxation of the radius from extension in young children. Trans. N.Y. Med. Ass., *3:*18, 1886.
341. Poinsot, G.: Dislocations of the head of the radius downward (by elongation). New York Med. J., *41:*8, 1885.
342. Ryan, J. R.: The relationship of the radial head to the radial neck diameters in fetuses and adults with reference to radial head subluxation in children. J. Bone Joint Surg., *51–A:*781, 1969.
343. Salter, R. B., and Zaltz, C.: Anatomic investigations of the mechanism of injury and pathologic anatomy of "pulled elbow" in children. Clin. Orthop., *77:*134, 1971.
344. Silquini, P. L.: La pronazione dolorosa. Minerva Ortop., *14:*481, 1963.
345. Silver, C. M., and Simon, S. D.: Subluxation of head of the radius in children. Rhode Island Med. J., *43:*722, 1960.
346. Smith, E. E.: Subluxation of the head of the radius in children. Ohio Med. J., *45:*1080, 1949.
347. Snellman, O.: Subluxation of the radial head in children. Acta Orthop. Scand., *28:*311, 1959.
348. Stone, C. A.: Subluxation of the head of the radius—report of a case and anatomical experiments. J.A.M.A., *1:*28, 1916.
349. Sweetman, R.: Pulled elbow. Practitioner, *182:*487, 1959.
350. Van Arsdale, W. H.: On subluxation of the head of the radius in children with a resume of one hundred consecutive cases. Ann. Surg., *9:*401, 1889.
351. Van Santvoordt, R.: Dislocation of the radial head downward. New York Med. J., *45:*63, 1887.

MONTEGGIA FRACTURE DISLOCATION

352. Bado, J. L.: The Monteggia lesion. Springfield, Ill., Charles C Thomas, 1962.
353. Bado, J. L.: The Monteggia lesion. Clin. Orthop., *50:*71, 1967.
354. Boyd, H. B.: Treatment of fractures of the ulna with dislocation of the radius. J.A.M.A., *115:*1699, 1940.
355. Boyd, H. B.: Surgical exposure of the ulna and proximal third of the radius through one incision. Surg. Gynec. Obstet., *71:*87, 1940.
356. Creer, W. S.: Some points about the Monteggia fracture. Proc. Roy. Soc. Med., *40:*241, 1947.
357. Cunningham, S. R.: Fracture of the ulna with dislocation of the head of the radius. J. Bone Joint Surg., *16:*351, 1934.
358. Curry, G. J.: Monteggia fracture. Amer. J. Surg., *73:*613, 1947.
359. Evans, E. M.: Rotational deformity in the treatment of fractures of both bones of the forearm. J. Bone Joint Surg., *27:*373, 1945.
360. Evans, E. M.: Pronation injuries of the forearm, with

special reference to the anterior Monteggia fracture. J. Bone Joint Surg., *31–B:*578, 1949.

361. Hunt, G. H.: Fracture of the shaft of the ulna with dislocation of the head of the radius. J.A.M.A., *112:*1241, 1939.

362. Kini, M. G.: Dislocation of the head of the radius associated with fracture of the upper third of the ulna. Antiseptic, *37:*1059, 1940.

363. Monteggia, G. B.: Istituzione Chirurgiche. 2a. Ed. G. Maspero, Milan, 1813–1815.

364. Naylor, A.: Monteggia fractures. Brit. J. Surg., *29:*323, 1942.

365. Penrose, J. H.: The Monteggia fracture with posterior dislocation of the radial head. J. Bone Joint Surg., *33–B:*65, 1951.

366. Perrin, J.: Les fractures du cubitus accompagnées de luxation de l'extremité superieur du radius. Paris, Thése de Paris, G. Steinheil, 1909.

367. Ray, R., Johnson, K. J., and Jameson, K. M.: Rotation of the forearm. J. Bone Joint Surg., *33–A:*993, 1951.

368. Smith, F. M.: Monteggia fractures; analysis of 25 consecutive fresh injuries. Surg. Gynec. Obstet., *85:*630, 1947.

369. Solcard, R.: Fracture de Monteggia vicieusement consolidée avec synostose radiocubitale. Rev. Orthop. Chirurgie de l'Appareil Moteur, *19:*37, 1932.

370. Speed, J. S., and Boyd, H. B.: Treatment of fractures of the ulna with dislocations of the radius. J.A.M.A., *115:*1699, 1940.

371. Thompson, H. A., and Hamilton, A. T.: Monteggia fracture; internal fixation of fractured ulna with intramedullary pin. Amer. J. Surg., *73:*579, 1950.

372. Tompkins, D. G.: The Monteggia fracture. J. Bone Joint Surg., *53–A:*1109, 1971.

373. Wise, R. A.: Lateral dislocation of the head of the radius with fracture of the ulna. J. Bone Joint Surg., *23:*379, 1941.

FRACTURES OF THE SHAFT OF THE RADIUS AND ULNA

374. Ashhurst, A. C., and John, R. L.: The treatment of fractures of the forearm with notes of the end results. Episcopal Hosp. Rep., *1:*224, 1913.

375. Bagley, C. H.: Fractures of both bones of the forearm. Surg. Gynec. Obstet., *42:*95, 1926.

376. Blount, W. P.: Fractures of the forearm in children. Indust. Med. Surg., *32:*9, 1963.

377. Blount, W. P.: Forearm fractures in children. Clin. Orthop., *51:*93, 1967.

378. Blount, W. P.: Schaeffer, A. A., and Johnson, J. H.: Fractures of the forearm in children. J.A.M.A., *120:*111, 1942.

379. Destot, E.: De la perte des mouvements de pronation et de supination dans les fractures de l'avant bras. Lyon Med., *112:*61, 1909.

380. Destot, E.: Pronation and supination of the forearm in traumatic lesions. Presse Méd., *21:*41, 1913.

381. Giberson, R. G., and Ivins, J. C.: Fractures of the distal part of the forearm in children. Minn. Med., *35·*744, 1952.

382. Levinthal, D. H.: Fractures of the lower one third of both bones of the forearm in children. Surg. Gynec. Obstet., *57:*790, 1933.

383. Onne, L., and Sandblom, P.: Late results in fractures of the forearm in children. Acta Chir. Scand., *98:*549, 1949.

384. Thorndike, A., Jr., and Dimmler, C. L., Jr.: Fractures of the forearm and elbow in children. New Eng. J. Med., *225:*475, 1941.

385. Wilson, J.: Fractures of the forearm. Pediat. Clin. N. Amer., *14:*664, 1967.

FRACTURES INVOLVING THE DISTAL RADIAL PHYSIS

386. Aitken, A. P.: The end results of the fractured distal radial epiphysis. J. Bone Joint Surg., *17:*302, 1935.

387. Aitken, A. P.: Further observations on fractured distal radial epiphysis. J. Bone Joint Surg., *17:*922, 1935.

388. Bragdon, R. A.: Fractures of the distal radial epiphysis. Clin. Orthop., *41:*59, 1965.

FRACTURES OF THE PHALANGES AND METACARPALS IN THE HAND

389. Flatt, A. E.: The Care of Minor Hand Injuries. 2nd Ed. St. Louis, C. V. Mosby Co., 1963.

390. Griffiths, J. C.: Bennett's fracture in childhood. Brit. J. Clin. Pract., *20:*582, 1966.

391. Lee, M. L. H.: Intra-articular and peri-articular fractures of the phalanges. J. Bone Joint Surg., *45–B:*103, 1963.

392. Leonard, M. H., and Dubravcik, P.: Management of fractured fingers in the child. Clin. Orthop., *73:*160, 1970.

393. Mansoor, I. A.: Fractures of the proximal phalanx of the fingers J. Bone Joint Surg., *51–A:*196, 1969.

394. Pulvertaft, R. G.: Injuries of the phalanges and metacrpal bones and joints. *In* The Hand. Clinical Surgery. Washington and London, Butterworths, Inc., 1966.

395. Seymour, N.: Juxta-epiphyseal fracture of the terminal phalanx of the finger. J. Bone Joint Surg., *48–B:*347, 1966.

WRINGER INJURY

396. Adams, J. B., and Fowler, P. D.: Wringer injuries of the upper extremity. Southern Med. J., *52:*798, 1959.

397. Allen, H. S.: Wringer injuries of the upper extremity. Ann. Surg., *113:*1101, 1941.

398. Bell, J. L., Mason, M. L., and Allen, H. S.: Management of acute crushing injuries of the hand and forearm over a five year period. Amer. J. Surg., *87:*370, 1954.

399. Entin, M. A.: Roller and wringer injuries; clinical and experimental studies. Plast. Reconstr. Surg., *15:*290, 1955.

400. Hardin, C. A., and Robinson, D. W.: Coverage problems in the treatment of wringer injuries. J. Bone Joint Surg., *36–A:*292, 1954.

401. Iritani, R. I., and Siler, V. E.: Wringer injuries of the upper extremity. Surg. Gynec. Obstet., *113:*677, 1961.

402. Luck, J. V., and Maddux, R.: Washing machine wringer injuries in children. G. P., *12:*87, 1955.

403. Lynn, R. B., and Reed, R. C.: Wringer injuries. J.A.M.A., *174:*500, 1960.

404. MacCollum, D. W.: Wringer arm. New Eng. J. Med., *218:*549, 1938.

405. MacCollum, D. W., Bernhard, W. F., and Banner, R. L.: The treatment of wringer arm injuries. New Eng. J. Med., *247:*750, 1952.

406. Posch, J. L., and Weller, C. N.: Mangle and severe wringer injuries of the hand in children. J. Bone Joint Surg., *36–A:*57, 1954.

407. Poulos, E.: The open treatment of wringer injuries in children. Amer. Surg., *24:*458, 1958.

408. Schulz, I.: Wringer injury. Surgery, *20:*301, 1946.

TRAUMATIC DISLOCATION OF THE HIP

409. Allis, O. A.: An Inquiry into the Difficulties Encountered in the Reduction of Dislocations of the Hip. Philadelphia, 1896.

410. Armstrong, J. R.: Traumatic dislocation of the hip joint. J. Bone Joint Surg., *30–B:*430, 1948.

411. Aufranc, O. E., Jones, W. N., and Harris, W. H.: Recurrent traumatic dislocation of the hip in a child. J.A.M.A., *90:*291, 1964.

412. Badgley, C. E.: Orthopedic correspondence club letter. Jan., 1952, as cited in personal communication, Liebenberg and Downmisse, 1968.

413. Banks, S. W.: Aseptic necrosis of the femoral head following traumatic dislocation of the hip. J. Bone Joint Surg., *23:*753, 1941.

414. Bigelow, H. J.: The Mechanism of Dislocation and Fracture of the Hip with the Reduction of the Dislocations by the Flexion Method. Philadelphia, Henry C. Lea & Co., 1869.

415. Bigelow, H. J.: The Mechanism of Dislocations and Fracture of the Hip. Boston, Little, Brown and Co., 1900.

416. Böhler, J.: Die sogenannten Schenkelkopfnekrosen nach traumatischen Hüftverrenkungen. Wiederherstellungschir. Traum., *4*:75, 1957.

417. Brav, E. A.: Traumatic dislocation of the hip joint. J. Bone Joint Surg., *44–A*:1115, 1962.

418. Caamaño, A.: Luxaciones traumáticas de la carderna en el niño. Semana Méd., *1*:450, 1941.

419. Charry, V.: Luxation traumatique invétérée de la hanche chez un enfant de sept ans et demi réduite par voie sanglante deux mois après l'accident. Rev. Orthop., *23*:147, 1936.

420. Charry, V.: Résultat éloigné d'une luxation traumatique de la hanche datant de deux mois et réduite par voie sanglante chez un enfant. Bull. Soc. Chir. Paris, *29*:160, 1937.

421. Choyce, C. C.: Traumatic dislocation of the hip in childhood and relation of trauma to pseudocoxalgia. Brit. J. Surg., *12*:52, 1924.

422. Clarke, H. O.: Traumatic dislocation of the hip joint in a child. Brit. J. Surg., *16*:690, 1929.

423. Cros, J. A.: Osteochondrosis of the upper femoral epiphysis following traumatic dislocation of the hip joint. J. Bone Joint Surg., *41–A*:1335, 1959.

424. Dehne, E., and Immerman, E. W.: Dislocation of the hip combined with fracture of the shaft of the femur on the same side. J. Bone Joint Surg., *33–A*:731, 1951.

425. Duytjes, F.: Recurrent dislocation of the hip joint in a boy. J. Bone Joint Surg., *45–B*:432, 1963.

426. Elmslie, R. C.: Pseudocoxalgia following traumatic dislocation of the hip in a boy aged four years. J. Orthop. Surg., *1*:109, 1919.

427. Elmslie, R. C.: Traumatic dislocation of the hip in a child aged seven, with subsequent development of coxa plana. Proc. Roy. Soc. Med. (Section of Orthopedics), *25*:1100, 1932.

428. Fairbank, H. A. T.: Case of pseudo-coxalgia following traumatic dislocation in a boy. Proc. Roy. Soc. Med. (Section of Orthopedics), *17*:40, 1924.

429. Fineschi, G.: Die traumatische Hüftverrenkung bei Kindern, Literaturübersicht und statistischer Beitrag von 7 Fällen. Arch. Orthop., *48*:225, 1956.

430. Freeman, G. E., Jr.: Traumatic dislocation of the hip in children. J. Bone Joint Surg., *43–A*:401, 1961.

431. Funk, F. J., Jr.: Traumatic dislocation of the hip in children. Factors influencing prognosis and treatment. J. Bone Joint Surg., *44–A*:1135, 1962.

432. Giraud, D. E. A.: Contribution à l'étude de la luxation traumatique de la hanche chez l'enfant. Thèses de Bordeaux, Geof-Josp., 1927.

433. Glass, A., and Powell, H. D. W.: Traumatic dislocation of the hip in children. An analysis of 47 patients. J. Bone Joint Surg., *43–B*:29, 1961.

434. Glynn, P.: Two cases of traumatic dislocation of the hip in children. Lancet, *1*:1093, 1932.

435. Goldenberg, R. R.: Traumatic dislocation of the hip followed by Perthes' disease. J. Bone Joint Surg., *20*:770, 1938.

436. Haines, C.: Traumatic dislocation of the head of the femur in a child. J. Bone Joint Surg., *19*:1126, 1937.

437. Haliburton, R. A., Brockenshire, F. A., and Barber, J. R.: Avascular necrosis of the femoral capital epiphysis after traumatic dislocation of the hip in children. J. Bone Joint Surg., *13–B*:43, 1961.

438. Hamada, G.: Unreduced anterior dislocation of the hip. J. Bone Joint Surg., *39–B*:471, 1957.

439. Hammond, G.: Posterior dislocations of the hip associated with fracture. Proc. Roy. Soc. Med., *37*:281, 1944.

440. Helal, B., and Skevis, X.: Unrecognized dislocations of the hip in fractures of the femoral shaft. J. Bone Joint Surg., *49–B*:293, 1967.

441. Henderson, R. S.: Traumatic anterior dislocation of the hip. J. Bone Joint Surg., *33–B*:602, 1951.

442. Henry, A. K., and Bayumi, M.: Fracture of the femur with luxation of the ipsilateral hip. Brit. J. Surg., *22*:204, 1934.

443. Hensley, C. D., and Schofield, G. W.: Recurrent dislocation of the hip. A case report. J. Bone Joint Surg., *51–A*:573, 1969.

444. Hohmann, D.: Rezidivierende traumatische Hüftluxation beim Kind nach fehlerhafter Gipsfixation. Mschr. Unfallheilk., *67*:352, 1964.

445. Hunter, G. A.: Posterior dislocation of fracture dislocation of the hip. J. Bone Joint Surg., *51–B*:38, 1969.

446. Ingram, A. J., and Turner, T. C.: Bilateral traumatic posterior dislocation of the hip complicated by bilateral fracture of the femoral shaft. J. Bone Joint Surg., *36–A*:1249, 1954.

447. King, D., and Richards, V.: Fracture-dislocation of the hip joint. J. Bone Joint Surg., *23*:533, 1941.

448. Kleiman, S. G., Stevens, J., Kolb, L., and Pankovich, A.: Late sciatic nerve palsy following posterior fracture-dislocation of the hip. J. Bone Joint Surg., *53–A*:781, 1971.

449. Kleinberg, S.: Aseptic necrosis of the femoral head following traumatic dislocation. Report of two cases. Arch. Surg., *39*:637, 1939.

450. Liebenberg, F., and Dommisse, G. F.: Recurrent posttraumatic dislocation of the hip. J. Bone Joint Surg., *51–B*:632, 1969.

451. Litton, L. O., and Workman, C.: Traumatic anterior dislocation of the hip in children. J. Bone Surg., *40–A*:1419, 1958.

452. Lyddon, D. W., and Hartman, J. T.: Traumatic dislocation of the hip with ipsilateral femoral fracture. J. Bone Joint Surg., *53–A*:1012, 1971.

453. McFarland, J. A.: Anterior dislocation of the hip. Brit. J. Surg., *23*:607, 1935.

454. Maffei, F.: Contributo allo studio della lussazione traumatica dell'anca nell'infanzia. Chir. Organi Mov., *6*,604, 1922.

455. Marsh, H. O.: Intertrochanteric and femoral neck fractures in children. Proc. A.A.O.S. J. Bone Joint Surg., *49–A*:1024, 1967.

456. Mason, M. L.: Traumatic dislocation of the hip in childhood. J. Bone Joint Surg., *36–B*:630, 1954.

457. Meng, C. I.: Traumatic dislocation of the hip in childhood. Chinese Med. J., *48*:736, 1934.

458. Merle D'Aubigné, R., and Cormier: Nécrose traumatique de la tête du fémur en dehors des pseudarthroses. Rev. Chir. Orthop., *12*:246, 1956.

459. Morton, K. S.: Traumatic dislocation of the hip in children. J.A.M.A., *47*:223, 1959.

460. Murphy, D. P.: Traumatic luxation of the hip in childhood. J.A.M.A., *80*:549, 1923.

461. Mutschler, H. M.: Sekundäre Oberschenkelkopf-necrose nach traumatischer Ausrenkung des Hüftgelenkes bei einem 14 Jahrigen. München. Med. Wschr., *86*:258, 1939.

462. Nelson, C. L.: Traumatic recurrent dislocation of the hip. Report of a case. J. Bone Joint Surg., *52–A*:128, 1970.

463. Nicoll, E. A.: Traumatic dislocation of the hip joint. J. Bone Joint Surg., *34–B*:503, 1952.

464. Niloff, R., and Petrie, J. G.: Traumatic anterior dislocation of the hip. Canad. Med. Ass. J., *62*:574, 1950.

465. Paus, B.: Traumatic dislocations of the hip. Acta Orthop. Scand., *21*:99, 1951.

466. Pennsylvania Orthopedic Society. Traumatic Dislocations of the hip joint in children. A report by the scientific research committee. J. Bone Joint Surg., *42–A*:705, 1960.

467. Pennsylvania Orthopedic Society. Traumatic dislocation of the hip joint in children. Final report by the Scientific Research Society. J. Bone Joint Surg., *50–A*:79, 1968.

468. Piggot, J.: Traumatic dislocation of the hip in childhood. J. Bone Joint Surg., *41–B*:209, 1959.

469. Piggot, J.: Traumatic dislocation of the hip in childhood. J. Bone Joint Surg., *43–B*:38, 1961.

470. Platt, H.: Traumatic dislocation of the hip joint in a child. Lancet, *1*:80, 1916.

471. Quist-Hanssen, S.: Caput necrosis after traumatic dislo-

cation of the hip in a 4-year-old boy. Acta Chir. Scand., 95:344, 1945.

472. Rocher, H. L., Rocher, C., and Cuzard, M.: Luxation traumatique de la hanche chez l'enfant. Bordeaux Chir., 8:255, 1937.

473. Stewart, M. J., and Milford, L. W.: Fracture-dislocation of the hip. An end-result study. J. Bone Joint Surg., 36–A:315, 1954.

474. Sullivan, C. R., Bickel, W. H., and Lipscomb, P. R.: Recurrent dislocation of the hip. J. Bone Joint Surg., 37–A:1266, 1955.

475. Thompson, V. P., and Epstein, H. C.: Traumatic dislocation of the hip. J. Bone Joint Surg., 33–A:746, 1951.

476. Townsend, R. G., Edwards, G. E., and Bazant, F. J.: Post-traumatic recurrent dislocation of the hip without fracture. J. Bone Joint Surg., 51–B:194, 1969.

477. Tronzo, R. G.: Traumatic dislocation of the hip in children. A problem in anesthetic management. J.A.M.A., 176:526, 1961.

478. Urist, M. R.: Fracture-dislocation of the hip joint. J. Bone Joint Surg., 30–A:1699, 1948.

479. Wadsworth, T. G.: Traumatic dislocation of the hip with fracture of the shaft of the ipsilateral femur. J. Bone Joint Surg., 43–B:47, 1961.

480. Wiltberger, B. R., Mitchell, C. L., and Hedrick, D. W.: Fracture of the femoral shaft complicated by hip dislocation. J. Bone Joint Surg., 30–A:225, 1948.

481. Wilson, D. W.: Traumatic dislocation of the hip in children. A report of four cases. J. Trauma, 6:739, 1966.

FRACTURE OF THE NECK OF THE FEMUR

482. Allende, G., and Lezama, L. G.: Fractures of the neck of the femur in children. A clinical study. J. Bone Joint Surg., 33–A:387, 1951.

483. Barber, E. T.: Fracture of the neck of the femur in a child seven years of age. Suit for Malpractice etc. Pacific Med. Surg. J., N.S. 5:61, 1871.

484. Bhansali, R. M.: Preliminary report on the use of defunctioning osteotomy for fracture of the femoral neck in children. In Proceedings of the Orthopaedic Section of the Association of Surgeons of India, Vol. 2. 1:7, 1965.

485. Bland-Sutton, J.: Spolia Opima—Presidential address to the Surgical Section, Royal Society of Medicine. Brit. Med. J., 2:595, 1918.

486. Böhler, L.: The treatment of fractures. 4th English Ed. (Trans. from 4th German edition by E. W. Hey Groves.) Baltimore, William Wood & Co., 1935.

487. Carrell, B., and Carrell, W. B.: Fractures in the neck of the femur in children, with particular reference to aseptic necrosis. J. Bone Joint Surg., 23:225, 1941.

488. Chigot, P. L., and Vialas, M.: Fracture du col du femur chez l'enfant. Ann. Chir. Infant., 4:209, 1963.

489. Colonna, P. C.: Fracture of the neck of the femur in childhood. Ann. Surg., 88:902, 1928.

490. Colonna, P. C.: Fracture of the neck of the femur in children. Amer. J. Surg., 6:793, 1929.

491. Cromwell, B. M.: A case of intra-capsular fracture of the neck of the femur in a young subject. North Carolina Med. J., 15:309, 1885.

492. Delbet, P.: Quoted by Colonna, P. C.: (Fractures of the neck of the femur in children.) Amer. J. Surg., 6:793, 1929.

493. Durbin, F. C.: Avascular necrosis complicating undisplaced fractures of the neck of the femur in children. J. Bone Joint Surg., 41–B:658, 1959.

494. Green, W. T.: Discussion on fractures of the hip in children. J. Bone Joint Surg., 35–A:886, 1953.

495. Greig, D. M.: Fracture of the cervix femoris in children. Edinburgh Med. J., 22:75, 1919.

496. Ingram, A. J., and Bachynski, B.: Fractures of the hip in children. Treatment and results. J. Bone Joint Surg., 35–A:867, 1953.

497. Johansson, S.: Über Epiphysennekrose bei geheilten Collumfrakturen. Zbl. Chir., 54:2214, 1927.

498. Jungbluth, K. H., Daum, R., and Metzger, E.: Schenkel-

halsfrakturen im Kindesalter. Z. Kinderchir., 6:392, 1968.

499. Khattab, A. S.: Fractures of the neck of the femur in children. Egyptian Orthop., 3:68, 1968.

500. Lam, S. F.: Fractures of the neck of the femur in children. J. Bone Joint Surg., 53–A:1165, 1971.

501. McDougall, A.: Fracture of the neck of the femur in childhood. J. Bone Joint Surg., 43–B:16, 1961.

502. Meershoek, P. E. M.: Fractures of the femoral neck in children. Arch. Chir. Neerl., 20:65, 1968.

503. Mitchell, J. I.: Fracture of the neck of the femur in children. J.A.M.A., 107:1603, 1936.

504. Naeraa, A.: On secondary epiphyseal necrosis after collum femoris fracture in young persons. Report of two cases. Acta Chir. Scand., 80:238, 1937.

505. Nielsen, B.: Om Calve-Perthes Sygdom after Fractura coli femoris hos unge og dens betydning for Forstaaelsen af de aseptiiske Epifysenekrosers Patogenese. Hospitalstidende, 81:773, 1938.

506. Ratliff, A. H. C.: Fractures of the neck of the femur in children. J. Bone Joint Surg., 44–B:528, 1962.

507. Ratliff, A. H. C.: Fractures of the femoral neck in children (A clinical study of 120 cases). Excerpta Medica, Internatl. Congr. Series, No. 116, p. E13, 25, 1966.

508. Russell, R. H.: A clinical lecture on fracture of the neck of the femur in childhood. Lancet, 2:125, 1898.

509. Schmorl, G.: Die pathologische Anatomie der Schenkelhals Frakturen. Munchen. Med. Wschr., 71:1381, 1924.

510. Seddon, H. J.: Necrosis of the head of the femur following fracture of the neck in a child. Proc. Roy. Soc. Med. (Section of Orthopaedics), 30:210, 1936.

511. Sullivan, R. H.: Discussion on fractures of the hip in children. J. Bone Joint Surg., 35–A:887, 1953.

512. Taylor, H. L.: Fractures of the neck of the femur in children. New York J. Med., 17:508, 1917.

513. Trueta, J.: The normal vascular anatomy of the human femoral head during growth. J. Bone Joint Surg., 39-B:358, 1957.

514. Trueta, J., and Harrison, M. H. M.: The normal vascular anatomy of the femoral head in adult man. J. Bone Joint Surg., 35-B:442, 1953.

515. Tucker, F. R.: Arterial supply to the femoral head and its clinical importance. J. Bone Joint Surg., 31-B:82, 1949.

516. Wedlikowski, A., and Dymala, L.: Fractures of the femoral neck in children. Chir. Narzad. Ruchu., Artop. Pol., 30:459, 1965.

517. Weiner, D. S., and O'Dell, H. W.: Fractures of the hip in children. J. Trauma, 9:62, 1969.

518. Whitman, R.: Fracture of neck of the femur in a child. Med. Rec., 39:165, 1891.

519. Whitman, R.: Observations on fracture of the neck of the femur in childhood with especial reference to treatment and differential diagnosis from separation of the epiphysis. Med. Rec., 43:227, 1893.

520. Whitman, R.: Further observations on fracture of the neck of the femur in childhood, with especial reference to its diagnosis and to its more remote results. Ann. Surg., 25:673, 1897.

521. Whitman, R.: Further observations on depression of the neck of the femur in early life; including fracture of the neck of the femur, separation of the epiphysis and simple coxa vara. Ann. Surg., 31:145, 1900.

522. Whitman, R.: Further observations on injuries of the neck of the femur in early life; with reference to the distinction between fracture of the neck and epiphyseal disjunction as influencing positive treatment. Med. Rec., 75:1, 1909.

523. Wilson, J. C.: Fracture of the neck of the femur in childhood. J. Bone Joint Surg., 22:531, 1940.

524. Wolcott, W. E.: The evolution of the circulation in the developing femoral head and neck. Surg. Gynec. Obstet., 77:61, 1943.

525. Zur Verth, M.: Sekundare Nekrose des Schenkelkopfes nach Schenkelhalsbruchen Jungendlicher. Zbl. Chir., 62:2549, 1935.

FRACTURES OF THE FEMORAL SHAFT

526. Abbott, L. C.: Fractures of the femur: with special reference to the treatment of ununited and malunited cases by manipulation and caliper extension. Arch. Surg., 9:413, 1924.

527. Aitken, A. P.: Overgrowth of the femoral shaft following fracture in children. Amer. J. Surg., 49:147, 1940.

528. Aitken, A. P., Blackett, C. W., and Cincotti, J. J.: Overgrowth of the femoral shaft following fractures in children. J. Bone Joint Surg., 21:334, 1939.

529. Anderson, M., Griffin, P. P., and Green, W. T.: Femoral shaft fractures in childhood. A report of later changes in growth and in angulation of the injured bone. Personal communication.

530. Anderson, R. L.: Conservative treatment of fractures of the femur. J. Bone Joint Surg., 49-A:1371, 1967.

531. Ashhurst, A. C., and Newell, W. A.: Conservative treatment of fractures of the femur. Ann. Surg., 48:749, 1908.

532. Barford, B., and Christiansen, J.: Fractures of the femoral shaft in children with special reference to subsequent overgrowth. Acta Chir. Scand., 116:235, 1958–1959.

533. Bisgard, J. B.: Longitudinal overgrowth of long bones with special reference to fractures. Surg. Gynec. Obstet., 62:823, 1936.

534. Bloch, R.: Les fractures de cuisse chez l'enfant. Rev. Orthop., 9:447, 1922.

535. Blount, W. P., Schaefer, A. A., and Fox, G. W.: Fractures of the femur in children. Southern Med. J., 37:481, 1944.

536. Bombelli, R.: Risultati anatomo-funzionali della fratture dia fisaria del femore nei bambini. Minerva Ortop., 6:125, 1955.

537. Broca, A.: Fractures du femur chez les enfants. Bull. Soc. Chir. Paris., 47:973, 1921.

538. Bryant, T.: The Practice of Surgery. London, J. & A. Churchill, 1876, Vol. 2, p. 405.

539. Burdick, C. G., and Siris, I. E.: Fractures of the femur in children. Treatment and end result in 286 cases. Ann. Surg., 77:736, 1923.

540. Clark, W. A.: Fractures of the femur in children. J. Bone Joint Surg., 8:273, 1926.

541. Cole, W. H.: Results of treatment of fractured femurs in children, with especial reference to Bryant's overhead traction. Arch. Surg., 5:702, 1922.

542. Cole, W. H.: Compensatory lengthening of the femur in children after fracture. Ann. Surg., 32:609, 1925.

543. Conwell, H. E.: Acute fractures of the shaft of the femur in children. J. Bone Joint Surg., 11:593, 1929.

544. Dameron, T. B., Jr., and Thompson, H. A.: Femoral shaft fractures in children. Treatment by closed reduction and double spica cast immobilization. J. Bone Joint Surg., 41-A:1201, 1959.

545. David, V. C.: Shortening and compensatory overgrowth following fractures of the femur in children. Arch. Surg., 9:438, 1924.

546. Ehalt, W.: Extension und Lagerung bie kindlichen Unterschenkel–und Oberschenkelbruchen. Chirurg, 21:386, 1950.

547. Eikenbary, C. F., and LeCoo, J. F.: Fractures of the femur in children. J. Bone Joint Surg., 14:801, 1932.

548. Eliason, E. L.: Results of treatment of 115 cases of fracture of the shaft of the femur at the University of Pennsylvania Hospital. Ann. Surg., 74:206, 1921.

549. Estes, W. L.: Fractures of the femur. Ann. Surg., 64:74, 1916.

550. Ferry, A. M., and Edgar, M. S.: Modified Bryant's traction. J. Bone Joint Surg., 48-A:533, 1966.

551. Firor, W. M.: The use of plaster in the treatment of fractured femurs. Bull. Johns Hopk. Hosp., 35:412, 1924.

552. Gallant, A. E.: Van Arsdale's triangular splint in thirty three cases of fracture of the femur in infants and children under six years. J.A.M.A., 29:1239, 1897.

553. Gatti, G.: Le fratture del femore nell' Infanzia. Arch. Atti. Soc. Ital. Chir., 27:359, 1921.

554. Greville, N. R., and Ivins, J. C.: Fractures of the femur in children; an analysis of their effect on the subsequent length of both bones in the lower limb. Amer. J. Surg., 93:376, 1957.

555. Griffin, P. P., Anderson, M., and Green, W. T.: Fractures of the shaft of the femur. Orthep. Clin. N. Amer., 3:213, 1972.

556. Hinz, R.: X-ray studies of fractures healed with deformity. Arch. Klin. Chir., 161:49, 1930.

557. Horst, J. M.: The prognosis of defective callus in fractures of the lower extremity in the child. Acta Chir. Belg., 60:27, 1961.

558. Humberger, F. W., and Eyring, E. J.: Proximal tibial 90–90 traction in treatment of children with femoral shaft fractures. J. Bone Joint Surg., 51-A:499, 1969.

559. Johnston, L. B.: The treatment of fractures of the shaft of the femur in children. Arch. Surg., 10:730, 1925.

560. Jones, J. P.: The treatment of fractures of the femur from an orthopaedic point of view. J. Orthop. Surg., 2:13, 1920.

561. Jones, S. G., and Cotton, F. J.: Ischaemic paralysis of leg simulating Volkmann's contracture. J. Bone Joint Surg., 17:659, 1935.

562. Judet, J., and Judet, R.: Traitement des fractures de cuisse chez l'enfant. Rev. Chir. Orthop. Paris, 39:658, 1953.

563. Kidner, F. C., and Laxoff, C. B.: Muscle interposition: A cause of delayed union in fracture of the femur. J.A.M.A., 79:200, 1922.

564. Kirmisson, E.: Des fractures du femur au cours des ankyloses du genou chez l'enfant. Bull. Méd., 24:767, 1910.

565. Lansche, W. E., Mishkin, M. R., and Stamp, W. G.: The management of complications of femoral shaft fractures in children. Southern Med. J., 56:1001, 1963.

566. LeMesurier, A. B.: The treatment of fractures of the shaft of the femur in children. Amer. J. Surg., 49:140, 1940.

567. Levander, G.: Increased growth of long bones of the lower extremities after they have been fractured. Acta Chir. Scand., 65:5, 1929.

568. Lidge, R. T.: Complications following Bryant's traction. J. Bone Joint Surg., 41-A:1540, 1959.

569. McMurray, T. P.: Thomas and his splint. Brit. Med. J., 1:872, 1946.

570. Miller, D. S., Markin, L., and Grossman, E.: Ischemic fibrosis of the lower extremity in children. Amer. J. Surg., 84:317, 1952.

571. Moore, R. A., and Schafer, E. W.: Treatment of simple fracture of the shaft of the femur by a fixed traction spica. A preliminary report. North Carolina Med. J., 9:514, 1948.

572. Moorhead, E. L.: Fracture of the femur in a boy five years of age; open treatment following failure of non-operative methods. Surg. Clin. Chicago, 3:1215, 1919.

573. Moorhead, J. J.: Transfixation method of treatment of fractured femur in children. Med. Rec., 85:1098, 1918.

574. Mustard, W. T., and Simmons, E. H.: Experimental arterial spasm in the lower extremities produced by traction. J. Bone Joint Surg., 35-B:437, 1953.

575. Neer, C. S., II, and Cadman, E. F.: Treatment of fractures of the femoral shaft in children. J.A.M.A., 163:634, 1957.

576. Nicholson, J. T., Foster, R. M., and Heath, R. D.: Bryant's traction: A provocative cause of circulation complications. J.A.M.A., 157:415, 1955.

577. Obletz, B. E.: Vertical traction in the early managment of certain compound fractures of the femur. J. Bone Joint Surg., 28:113, 1946.

578. Oeconomas, N.: Follow-up results of fractures of the femoral shaft in children. Rev. Orthop., 34:375, 1948.

579. Orr, T. G.: Conservative treatment of fractures of the femur in children. J. Kansas Med. Soc., 26:55, 1926.

580. Pavlik, A.: Treatment of obstetrical fractures of the femur. J. Bone Joint Surg., 21:939, 1939.

581. Pease, C. N.: Fractures of the femur in children. Surg. Clin. N. Amer., 37:213, 1957.

582. Pick, J. W., Stack, J. K., and Anson, B. J.: Measurements on the human femur: I. Lengths, diameters and angles. Quart. Bull. Northwest. Univ. Med. School, *15:*281, 1941; *17:*121, 1943.

583. Rice, J. D.: A new method of treating femoral fractures in the infant. Lancet, *2:*1130, 1900.

584. Russell, R. H.: Fractures of the femur. Brit. J. Surg., *11:*491, 1924.

585. Schenk, K. M.: Der Femurschaftbruch beim Kind: Spätergebnisse. Arch. Klin. Chir., *286:*144, 1957.

586. Scudder, C. L.: The Treatment of Fractures. 10th Ed. Philadelphia, W. B. Saunders Co., 1926, pp. 591–600.

587. Silver, D.: A modification of the Bradford frame for the treatment by suspension of fracture of the femur in young children. Ann. Surg., *49:*105, 1909.

588. Speed, K.: Analysis of the results of treatment of fractures of the femoral diaphysis in children under twelve years of age. Surg. Gynec. Obstet., *32:*57, 1921.

589. Staheli, L. T.: Femoral and tibial growth following femoral shaft fractures in childhood. Clin. Orthop., *55:*159, 1967.

590. Stern, W. O.: Successful method of treating fracture of the femur in infancy. New York Med. J., *81:*992, 1905.

591. Stryker, H. H.: Safe traction in children with fractured femurs. J.A.M.A., *160:*388, 1956.

592. Thompson, S. A., and Mahoney, L. J.: Volkmann's ischemic contracture: relationship to fracture of the femur. J. Bone Joint Surg., *33-B:*336, 1951.

593. Truesdell, E. D.: Inequality of lower extremity following fracture of the shaft of the femur in children. Ann. Surg., *74:*498, 1921.

594. Van Eden, P. H.: Results in the treatment of fractures of the shaft of the femur. Acta Chir. Scand., *67:*320, 1930.

595. Winant, E. M.: The use of skeletal traction in the treatment of fractures of the femur. J. Bone Joint Surg., *31-A:*87, 1949.

FRACTURE INVOLVING THE DISTAL FEMORAL EPIPHYSIS

596. Abbott, L., and Gill, G.: Valgus deformity of the knee resulting from injury to the lower femoral epiphysis. J. Bone Joint Surg., *24:*97, 1942.

597. Aitken, A. P., and Magill, H. K.: Fractures involving the distal femoral epiphyseal cartilage. J. Bone Joint Surg., *34-A:*96, 1952.

598. Bassett, F. H., III, and Goldner, L.: Fractures involving the distal femoral epiphyseal growth line. Southern Med. J., *55:*545, 1962.

599. Bellin, H.: Traumatic separation of epiphysis of lower end of femur. Amer. J. Surg., *37:*306, 1937.

600. Brashear, H. R., Jr.: Epiphyseal fractures of the lower extremities. Southern Med. J., *51:*845, 1958.

601. Brashear, H. R., Jr.: Discussion of paper by Bassett, F., III, and Goldner, J. L.: Fractures involving the distal femoral epiphyseal growth line. Southern Med. J., *55:*545, 1962.

602. Burman, M. S., and Langsam, M. J.: Posterior dislocation of the lower femoral epiphysis in breech delivery. Arch. Surg., *38:*250, 1939.

603. Cassebaum, W. H., and Patterson, A. H.: Fractures of the distal femoral epiphysis. Clin. Orthop., *41:*79, 1965.

604. Caffey, J., Madell, S. H., Royer, C., and Morales, P.: Ossification of the distal femoral epiphysis. J. Bone Joint Surg., *40-A:*647, 1958.

605. Griswold, A. S.: Early motion in the treatment of separation of the lower femoral epiphysis. J. Bone Joint Surg., *10:*75, 1928.

606. Heller, E. P.: Fracture separation ("slipping") of the lower femoral epiphysis. J. Bone Joint Surg., *15:*474, 1933.

607. Hutchinson, J., Jr.: Lectures on injuries to the epiphysis and their results. Brit. Med. J., *1:*669, 1894.

608. Kurlander, J. J.: Slipping of the lower femoral epiphysis. J.A.M.A., *96:*513, 1931.

609. Leavitt, P. H.: Traumatic separation of the lower femoral epiphysis. New Eng. J. Med., *245:*565, 1951.

610. Levinthal, D. H.: Old traumatic displacement of the distal femoral epiphysis. J. Bone Joint Surg., *18:*199, 1936.

611. Neer, C. S.: Separation of the lower femoral epiphysis. Amer. J. Surg., *99:*756, 1960.

612. Nicholson, J. T.: Epiphyseal fractures about the knee. A.A.O.S. Instructional Course Lectures. Vol. 18. St. Louis, C. V. Mosby Co., 1961, p. 74.

613. Patterson, W. J.: Separation of the lower femoral epiphysis. Canad. Med. Ass. J., *21:*301, 1929.

614. Sideman, S.: Traumatic separation of the lower femoral epiphysis. J. Bone Joint Surg., *25:*913, 1943.

TRAUMATIC DISLOCATION OF THE PATELLA AND OSTEOCHONDRAL FRACTURES OF THE KNEE

615. Ahstrom, J. P.: Osteochondral fracture in the knee joint associated with hypermobility and dislocation of the patella. J. Bone Joint Surg., *47-A:*1491, 1965.

616. Chaklin, V. D.: Injuries to the cartilage of the patella and femoral condyles. J. Bone Joint Surg., *21:*133, 1939.

617. Coleman, H. M.: Recurrent osteochondral fracture of the patella. J. Bone Joint Surg., *30-B:*153, 1948.

618. Harmon, P. H.: Intra-articular osteochondral fracture as a cause for internal derangement of the knee in adolescents. J. Bone Joint Surg., *27:*703, 1945.

619. Kleinberg, S.: Vertical fracture of the articular surface of the patella. J.A.M.A., *81:*1205, 1923.

620. Krida, A.: Osteochondral fractures of the knee joint. Surg. Gynec. Obstet., *39:*791, 1924.

621. Makin, M.: Osteochondral fracture of the lateral femoral condyle. J. Bone Joint Surg., *33-A:*262, 1951.

622. Milgram, J. E.: Tangential osteochondral fracture of the patella. J. Bone Joint Surg., *25:*271, 1943.

623. Millard, D. G., and Lee, T. H.: "The twist" fracture dislocation of the patella. New Eng. J. Med., *267:*246, 1962.

624. Rosenberg, N. J.: Osteochondral fracture of the lateral femoral condyle. J. Bone Joint Surg., *46-A:*1013, 1964.

625. Stewart, S. F.: Frontal fractures of the patella. Ann. Surg., *81:*536, 1925.

FRACTURES OF THE PATELLA

626. Oetteking, B.: Anomalous patellae. Anat. Rec., *23:*269, 1922.

627. George, R.: Bilateral bipartite patellae. Brit. J. Surg., *22:*555, 1935.

FRACTURES OF THE INTERCONDYLAR EMINENCE OF THE TIBIA

628. Meyers, M. H., and McKeever, F. M.: Fracture of the intercondylar eminence of the tibia. J. Bone Joint Surg., *41-A:*209, 1959.

FRACTURES INVOLVING THE PROXIMAL TIBIAL PHYSIS AND APOPHYSIS OF THE TIBIAL TUBERCLE

629. Aitken, A. P.: Fractures of the proximal tibial epiphyseal cartilage. Clin. Orthop., *41:*92, 1965.

630. Aitken, A. P., and Ingersoll, R. E.: Fractures of the proximal tibial epiphyseal cartilage plate. J. Bone Joint Surg., *33-A:*787, 1956.

631. Borch-Madsen, P.: On symmetrical bilateral fractures of the tuberosities tibiae and eminentia intercondyloidea. Acta Orthop. Scand., *24:*44, 1954.

632. Hand, W. H., Hand, C. R., and Dunn, A. W.: Avulsion fractures of the tibial tubercle. J. Bone Joint Surg., *53-A:*1579, 1971.

633. Smillie, I. S.: Injuries to the Knee Joint. 4th Ed. Baltimore, Williams & Wilkins Co., 1970.

634. Watson-Jones, R.: Fractures and Joint Injuries. 4th Ed. Vol. 2. Baltimore, Williams & Wilkins Co., 1955.

635. Welch, P. H., and Wynne, G. H.: Proximal tibial epiphy-

seal fracture separation. J. Bone Joint Surg., *45–A:*782, 1963.

FRACTURES OF THE SHAFT OF THE TIBIA AND FIBULA

636. Beekman, F., and Sullivan, J. E.: Some observations on fractures of the long bones in children. Amer. J. Surg., *51:*736, 1941.
637. Cozen, L.: Fracture of the proximal portion of the tibia in children, followed by valgus deformity. Surg., Gynec. Obstet., *97:*183, 1953.
638. Cozen, L.: Knock knee deformity after fracture of the proximal tibia in children. Orthopedics, *1:*230, 1959.
639. Holderman, W. D.: Results following conservative treatment of fractures of the tibial shaft. Amer. J. Surg., *98:*593, 1959.
640. Stanford, J. C., Rodriguez, R. P., and Hayes, J. T.: Tibial shaft fractures in adults and children. J.A.M.A., *195:*1111, 1966.
641. Taylor, S. L.: Tibial overgrowth: A cause of genu valgum. J. Bone Joint Surg., *45–A:*659, 1963.

FRACTURES INVOLVING THE DISTAL EPIPHYSIS OF THE TIBIA

642. Aitken, A. P.: The end results of the fractured distal tibial epiphysis. J. Bone Joint Surg., *18:*685, 1936.
643. Ashhurst, A. P. C., and Bromer, R. S.: Classification and mechanism of fractures of the leg bones involving the ankle. Arch. Surg., *4:*51, 1922.
644. Bishop, P. A.: Fractures and epiphyseal separation fractures of the ankle. A classification of 332 cases according to the mechanism of their production. Amer. J. Roentgen., *28:*49, 1932.
645. Carothers, C. O., and Crenshaw, A. H.: Clinical significance of a classification of epiphyseal injuries of the ankle. Amer. J. Surg., *89:*879, 1953.
646. Crenshaw, A. H.: Injuries to the distal tibial epiphysis. Clin. Orthop., *41:*98, 1965.
647. Gill, G., and Abbot, L.: Varus deformity of ankle following injury to the distal epiphyseal cartilage of the tibia in growing children. Surg. Gynec. Obstet., *72:*659, 1941.
648. Johnson, E. W., and Fahl, J. C.: Fractures involving the distal tibial epiphysis of the tibia and fibula in children. Amer. J. Surg., *93:*778, 1957.
649. Kleiger, B., and Mankin, H. J.: Fracture of the lateral portion of the distal tibial epiphysis. J. Bone Joint Surg., *46–A:*25, 1964.
650. McFarland, B.: Traumatic arrest of epiphyseal growth at the lower end of the tibia. Brit. J. Surg., *19:*1931–1932.

FRACTURES OF THE FOOT

651. Spak, I.: Fractures of the talus in children. Acta Chir. Scand., *107:*553, 1966.
652. Stephens, N. A.: Fracture dislocation of the talus in childhood: A report of two cases. Brit. J. Surg., *43:*600, 1956.
653. Thomas, H. M.: Calcaneal fracture in childhood. Brit. J. Surg., *56:*664, 1969.

INJURIES TO THE SPINE AND PELVIS

654. Bailey, D. K.: The normal cervical spine in infants and children. Radiology, *59:*712, 1952.
655. Berkheiser, E. J., and Seidler, F.: Nontraumatic dislocations of the atlanto-axial joint. J.A.M.A., *96:*517, 1931.
656. Donaldson, J. S.: Acquired torticollis in children and young adults. J.A.M.A., *160:*458, 1956.
657. Dunlop, J. P., Morris, M., and Thompson, R. G.: Cervical spine injuries in children. J. Bone Joint Surg., *40–A:*681, 1958.
658. Ewald, F. C.: Fracture of the odontoid process in a 17-month-old infant treated with a halo. J. Bone Joint Surg., *53–A:*1636, 1971.

659. Fielding, J. W.: Disappearance of the central portion of the odontoid process. A case report. J. Bone Joint Surg., *47–A:*1228, 1965.
660. Hamilton, A. R.: Injuries of the atlanto-axial joint. J. Bone Joint Surg., *33–B:*434, 1951.
661. Lipscomb, P. R.: Cervico-occipital fusion for congenital and post-traumatic anomalies of the atlas and axis. J. Bone Joint Surg., *39–A:*1289, 1957.
662. Sherk, H. H., and Nicholson, J. T.: Fractures of the atlas. J. Bone Joint Surg., *52–A::*1017, 1970.

Fractures of the Pelvis

663. Dunn, A. W., and Morris, H. D.: Fractures and dislocations of the pelvis. J. Bone Joint Surg., *50–A:*1639, 1968.
664. Peltier, L. F.: Complications associated with fractures of the pelvis. J. Bone Joint Surg., *47–A:*1060, 1965.

OBSTETRICAL INJURIES

665. Byers, R. K.: Transection of the spinal cord in the newborn. Arch. Neurol. Psychiat., *27:*585, 1923.
666. Burman, M. S., and Langsam, M. J.: Posterior dislocation of the lower femoral epiphysis in breech delivery. Arch. Surg., *38:*250, 1939.
667. Camera, R.: Il distacco epifisario ostetrico dell'estremita prossimale del femore. Chir. Organi Mov., *33:*331, 1949.
668. Caritat, R. J., and Peluffo, E.: El decolamiento de la epifisis superior del humero por traumatismo obstetrico. Arch. Pediat. Uruguay, *12:*785, 1941.
669. Crothers, B.: Injury of the spinal cord in breech extractions as an important cause of fetal death and paraplegia in childhood. Amer. J. Med. Sci., *165:*94, 1923.
670. Crothers, B., and Putnam, M. C.: Obstetrical injuries of the spinal cord. Medicine, *6:*41, 1927.
671. Dawson, G. R.: Intrauterine fractures of the tibia and fibula. J. Bone Joint Surg., *31–A:*406, 1949.
672. Elizalde, E. A.: Obstetrical dislocation of the hip associated with fracture of the femur. J. Bone Joint Surg., *28–A:*838, 1946.
673. Ford, F. R.: Breech delivery with special reference to infantile paraplegia. Arch. Neurol. Psychiat., *14:*742, 1925.
674. Halliburton, R. A., Barber, J. R., and Fraser, R. L.: Pseudo-dislocation—an unusual birth injury. J. Bone Joint Surg., *50–B:*437, 1968.
675. Harrenstein, R. J.: Pseudoluxatio coxae durch Abreissen der Femur Epiphyse bei der Geburt. Bruns' Beitr. Klin. Chir., *146:*592, 1929.
676. Jones, R.: Treatment of fractures of the femur in the newly born. Brit. Med. J., *1:*1358, 1908.
677. Kennedy, P. C.: Traumatic separation of the upper femoral epiphysis. A birth injury. Amer. J. Roentgen., *51:*707, 1944.
678. Koch, K.: Ein Beitrag zur Pathogenese der intrauterinen Frakkurer. Mschr. Geburtsch. Gynak, *101:*11, 1935.
679. Lindseth, R. E., and Rosene, H. A.: Traumatic separation of the upper femoral epiphysis in a newborn infant. J. Bone Joint Surg., *53–A:*1641, 1971.
680. Madsen, E. T.: Fractures of the extremities in the newborn. Acta Obstet. Gynec. Scand., *34:*41, 1955.
681. Michael, J. P., Theodorou, S., Houliaras, K., and Siatis, N.: Two cases of obstetrical separation (epiphyseolysis) of the upper femoral epiphysis. Appearance of ossification center of the femoral head in a 15 day old child. J. Bone Joint Surg., *40–B:*477, 1958.
682. Michel, L.: Obstetrical dislocation of the upper humeral epiphysis. Rev. Orthop., *24:*201, 1937.
683. Mortens, J., and Christianson, P.: Traumatic separation of the upper femoral epiphysis as an obstetrical lesion. Acta Orthop. Scand., *34:*239, 1964.
684. Robinson, W. H.: Treatment of birth fractures of the femur. J. Bone Joint Surg., *20:*778, 1938.

685. Ruiz Moreno, M.: Obstetrical fractures of the humerus and femur. Prensa Med. Argent., *25:*321, 1938.
686. Scaglietti, O.: The obstetrical shoulder trauma. Surg. Gynec. Obstet., *66:*868, 1938.
687. Siffert, R. S.: Displacement of distal humeral epiphysis in the newborn infant. J. Bone Joint Surg., *45–A:*105, 1963.
688. Smith, R. R.: Intra-uterine fracture. Report of a case and a review of the literature. Surg. Gynec. Obstet., *17:*346, 1913.
689. Snedecor, S. T., and Wilson, H. B.: Some obstetrical injuries in the long bones. J. Bone Joint Surg., *31–A:*378, 1949.
690. Snure, H.: Intrauterine fracture: Case report and review of roentgenologic findings. Radiology, *13:*362, 1929.
691. Tavernier: Sequelle d'un décollement épiphysaire obstetrical de l'extrémité superieure de l'humerus. Lyon Chir., *32:*465, 1935.
692. Weston, W. J.: Metaphyseal fractures in infancy. J. Bone Joint Surg., *39–B:*694, 1957.

STRESS FRACTURES

693. Beck, A.: Obstetrician's stress fracture. Brit. Med. J., *5423:*1509, 1964.
694. Blickenstaff, L. D., and Morris, J. M.: Fatigue fractures of the femoral neck. J. Bone Joint Surg., *48–A:*1031, 1966.
695. Branch, H. E.: March fractures of the femur. J. Bone Joint Surg., *26:*387, 1944.
696. Burrows, H. J.: Spontaneous fracture of the apparently normal fibula in its lowest third. Brit. J. Surg., *28:*82, 1940.
697. Burrows, H. J.: Fatigue fractures of the fibula. J. Bone Joint Surg., *30–B:*266, 1948.
698. Burrows, H. J.: Fatigue infraction of the middle of the tibia in ballet dancers. J. Bone Joint Surg., *38–B:*83, 1956.
699. Childress, H. M.: March foot in a seven year old child. J. Bone Joint Surg., *28:*877, 1946.
700. Darby, R. E.: Stress fractures of the os calcis. J.A.M.A., *200:*1183, 1967.
701. Devas, M. B.: Stress fractures of the patella. J. Bone Joint Surg., *42–B:*71, 1960.
702. Devas, M. B.: Compression stress fractures in man and the greyhound. J. Bone Joint Surg., *43–B:*540, 1961.
703. Devas, M. B.: Stress fractures in children. J. Bone Joint Surg., *45–B:*528, 1963.
704. Devas, M. B., and Sweetnam, B.: Stress fractures of the fibula. J. Bone Joint Surg., *38–B:*818, 1956.
705. Engh, C. A., Robinson, R. A., and Milgram, J.: Stress fractures in children. J. Trauma, *10:*532, 1970.
706. Ernst, J.: Stress fractures of the femoral neck. J. Trauma, *4:*71, 1964.
707. Evans, D. L.: Fatigue fracture of the ulna. J. Bone Joint Surg., *37–B:*618, 1955.
708. Griffiths, A. L.: Fatigue fracture of the fibula in childhood. Arch. Dis. Child., *27:*552, 1952.
709. Ingersoll, C. F.: Ice skater's fracture. Amer. J. Roentgen., *50:*469, 1943.
710. Kelly, R. P., and Murphy, F. E.: Fatigue fractures of the tibia. Southern Med. J., *44:*290, 1951.
711. Kitchin, I. D.: Fatigue fracture of the ulna. J. Bone Joint Surg., *30–B:*622, 1948.
712. Kroenig, P. M., and Shelton, M. L.: Stress fractures. Amer. J. Roentgen., *89:*1281, 1963.
713. Levine, D. C., Blazina, M. E., and Levine, E.: Fatigue fractures of the shaft of the femur. Simulation of malignant tumor. Radiology, *89:*883, 1967.
714. Miller, J. E.: Javelin thrower's elbow. J. Bone Joint Surg., *42–B:*788, 1960.
715. Morris, J. M., and Blickenstaff, L. D.: Fatigue Fractures. Clinical Study. Springfield, Ill., Charles C Thomas, 1967.
716. North, K. A.: Multiple stress fractures simulating osteomalacia. Amer. J. Roentgen., *97:*672, 1966.
717. Roberts, S. M., and Vogt, E. C.: Pseudofracture of the tibia. J. Bone Joint Surg., *21:*891, 1939.
718. Samuel, E.: Fatigue (insufficiency) fracture of the tibia. S. Afr. Med. J., *29:*89, 1955.
719. Weaver, J. B., and Francisco, C. B.: Pseudofractures. J. Bone Joint Surg., *22:*610, 1940.
720. Wolfe, H. R. I., and Robertson, J. M.: Fatigue fracture of femur and tibia. Lancet, *2:*11, 1945.

THE BATTERED CHILD

721. Adelson, L.: Murder of children. New Eng. J. Med., *264:*1345, 1961.
722. Altman, D. H., and Smith, R. L.: Unrecognized trauma in infants and children. J. Bone Joint Surg., *42–A:*407, 1960.
723. Astley, R.: Multiple metaphyseal fractures in small children. Brit. J. Radiol., *26:*577, 1953.
724. Bakwin, H.: Multiple skeletal lesions in young children due to trauma. J. Pediat., *49:*7, 1956.
725. Brailsford, J. F.: Ossifying hematoma and other simple lesions mistaken for sarcomata. Brit. J. Radiol., *21:*157, 1948.
726. Caffey, J.: Multiple fractures in the long bones of infants suffering from chronic subdural hematoma. Amer. J. Roentgen., *56:*163, 1946.
727. Caffey, J.: Significance of the history in the diagnosis of traumatic injury to children. J. Pediat., *67:*1008, 1965.
728. Fisher, S. H.: Skeletal manifestations of parent-induced trauma in infants and children. Southern Med. J., *51:*956, 1958.
729. Friedman, M. S.: Traumatic periostitis in infants and children. J.A.M.A., *166:*1840, 1958.
730. Godrey, J. D.: Trauma in children. J. Bone Joint Surg., *46–A:*422, 1964.
731. Griffiths, D. L., and Moynihan, F. J.: Multiple epiphyseal injuries in babies ("battered baby syndrome"). Brit. Med. J., *2:*1, 558, 1963.
732. Gwinn, J. L., Lewin, K. W., and Peterson, H. G., Jr.: Roentgenographic manifestations of unsuspected trauma in infancy. J.A.M.A., *176:*926, 1961.
733. Helfer, R. E., and Kempe, C. H.: The Battered Child. Chicago, London, University of Chicago Press, 1968.
734. Kempe, C. H., Silverman, F. N., Steele, B. F., Droegemueller, W., and Silver, H. K.: The battered child syndrome. J.A.M.A., *181:*17, 1962.
735. Lis, E. F., and Frauenberger, G. S.: Multiple fractures associated with subdural hematoma in infancy. Pediatrics, *6:*890, 1950.
736. McCort, J., and Vandagua, J.: Visceral injuries in battered children. Radiology, *82:*424, 1964.
737. McHenry, T., Girdany, B. R., and Elmer, E.: Unsuspected trauma with multiple skeletal injuries during infancy and childhood. Pediatrics, *31:*903, 1963.
738. Milowe, I., and Lourie, R.: The child's role in the battered child syndrome. J. Pediat., *65:*1079, 1964.
739. Rose, C. B.: Unusual periostitis in children. Radiology, *27:*131, 1936.
740. Shaw, A.: The surgeon and the battered child. Surg. Gynec. Obstet., *119:*355, 1964.
741. Silverman, F. N.: The roentgen manifestations of unrecognized skeletal trauma in infants. Amer. J. Roentgen., *69:*413, 1953.
742. Skinner, A. E., and Castle, R. L.: 78 Battered Children. London, National Society for the Prevention of Cruelty to Children, 1969.
743. Smith, M. J.: Subdural hematoma with multiple fractures. Am. J. Roentgen., *63:*342, 1950.
744. Woolley, P. V., Jr.: The pediatrician and the young child subjected to repeated physical abuse. J. Pediat., *62:*628, 1963.

GENERAL – FRACTURES

745. Böhler, L.: The Treatment of Fractures. 5th English Ed. (Translated from German 13th Ed. by Hans Tretter et al.) New York, Grune & Stratton, Inc., 1956–1958.

746. Blount, W. P.: Fractures in Children. Baltimore, Williams & Wilkins Co., 1955.

747. Bonnin, J. G.: A Complete Outline of Fractures. 2nd Ed. London, William Heinemann Ltd., 1946.

748. Cave, E. F. (ed.): Fractures and Other Injuries. Chicago, Year Book Medical Publishers, Inc., 1958.

749. Charnley, J.: The Closed Treatment of Common Fractures. Edinburgh, E. S. Livingstone, Ltd., 1950.

750. Compere, E. L., Banks, S. W., and Compere, C. L.: Pictorial Handbook of Fracture Treatment. 5th Ed. Chicago, Year Book Medical Publishers, Inc., 1963.

751. Cooper, A.: A Treatise on Dislocations and on Fractures of Joints. 2nd Ed. London, the author, 1823; Boston, T. R. Marvin, 1844.

752. Conwell, H. E., and Reynolds, F. C.: Key and Conwell's Management of Fractures, Dislocations, and Sprains. 7th Ed. St. Louis, C. V. Mosby Co., 1961.

753. Cotton, F. J.: Dislocations and Joints Fractures. Philadelphia, W. B. Saunders Co., 1924.

754. De Palma, A. F.: The Management of Fractures and Dislocations. An Atlas. 2nd Ed. Philadelphia, W. B. Saunders Co., 1970.

755. Furlong, R. (ed.): Fractures and Dislocations. Washington, Butterworth, Inc., 1966.

756. Groves, E. W. H.: On Modern Methods of Treating Fractures. Bristol, England, John Wright & Sons, Ltd., 1916.

757. Hamilton, F. H.: A Practical Treatise on Fractures and Dislocations. 5th Ed. Philadelphia, Henry C. Lea, 1875.

758. Judet, R., Judet, J., and LaGrange, J.: Les Fractures des Membres chez l'Enfant. Paris, Librairie Maloine, 1958.

759. McLaughlin, H. L.: Trauma. Philadelphia, W. B. Saunders Co., 1960.

760. Malgaigne, J. F.: Traité des Fractures et des Luxations. Paris, J. B. Bailliére, 1847.

761. O'Donoghue, D. H.: Treatment of Injuries to Athletes. 2nd Ed. Philadelphia, W. B. Saunders Co., 1970.

762. Poland, J.: Traumatic Separation of the Epiphyses. London, Smith, Elder & Co., 1898.

763. Salter, R. B.: Textbook of Disorders and Injuries of the Musculoskeletal System. Baltimore, Williams & Wilkins Co., 1970.

764. Scudder, C. L.: The Treatment of Fractures. 7th Ed. Philadelphia, W. B. Saunders Co., 1938.

765. Speed, K.: A Textbook of Fractures and Dislocations. Covering Their Pathology, Diagnosis and Treatment. Philadelphia, Lea and Febiger, 1942.

766. Stimpson, L. A.: Fractures and Dislocations. Philadelphia, Lea and Febiger, 1910.

767. Stimpson, L. A.: A Manual of Fractures and Dislocations. 2nd Ed. Philadelphia, Lea and Febiger, 1947.

768. Truesdell, E. D.: Birth Fractures and Epiphyseal Dislocations. New York, Paul B. Hoeber, Inc., 1917.

769. Watson-Jones, R., Sr.: Fractures and Joint Injuries. 4th Ed. Baltimore, Williams & Wilkins Co., 1962.

770. Wiles, P.: Fractures, Dislocations and Sprains. 2nd Ed. Baltimore, Williams & Wilkins Co., 1969.

Index

Index

In this index page numbers in *italic* type refer to illustrations; in **bold** type, to plates. Those followed by (t) indicate tables; the abbreviation *vs.* indicates differential diagnosis.

Phelps classification of cerebral palsy, 772, 772(t)

Phemister classification of bone tumors, 492(t)

Phemister epiphyseodesis (Green modification of), of distal femur, 1489, **1490–1493,** *1495–1497*

Phenobarbital, minimal brain dysfunction and, 859

Phenylbutazone, in rheumatoid arthritis, 708

Philippson's reflex, *27, 30, 32*

Phocomelia, classification of, 108, 109(t), *110, 113*

Phosphate depletion, in renal rickets, 437–443, *439, 442*

Phosphate therapy, in vitamin D-refractory rickets, 440

Photosensitivity, in dermatomyositis, 1104

Physical therapy, after tendon transfer, 955 in poliomyelitis, 950

Physiologic bowleg, vs. tibia vara, 349

Physis, 1470
  birth fractures of, 1743–1744
  blood supply to, epiphyseal side, 1536, *1538, 1539*
    metaphyseal side, 1539, *1539*
  fractures of, 1544
    distal fibular, 1733, *1734*
    distal radial, 1643
    proximal humeral, 1555–1560
    proximal radial, 1613–1619, *1614–1617*
    proximal tibial, 1716–1719, *1717*
  in slipped capital femoral epiphysis, 464
  pathogenesis of osteochondroma and, 493
  trauma and, 1533–1545
    circulation loss in, 1536, *1538, 1539*
    compression in, 1540
    direct, 1534, 1537(t)
    surgical, 1536, 1537(t)
  zones of, 1533, *1534*

"Pigeon-breast" deformity, in vitamin D deficiency rickets, 435

Pigeon toe, 1448. See also *Femur, torsional deformity of.*

Pigmented villonodular synovitis, 747–752
  of foot, 1437, *1438*
  synovial fluid in, 663, 664–665(t)
  vs. popliteal cyst, 744

Pin fixation, in femoral neck fracture, dangers of, 1671, 1681
  in slipped capital femoral epiphysis, 468, *468*

Pin tract infection, in femoral lengthening, 1505

Pinealoma, incidence of, *861*

Pisiform bone, ossification center of, *41*

Pituitary dwarfism, 459–460, *459*

Placing reaction, *27, 28, 30, 31*

Plagiocephaly, idiopathic scoliosis and, 1195, *1195*

Planovalgus deformity, of foot, 1397, 1399

Plantar fasciotomy, in pes cavus, 1381, **1388–1389**

Plantar flexion injury, of distal tibial epiphysis, 1725, *1726, 1730*

Plantar grasp reflex, 25, *27, 28*

Plantar soft-tissue release, in talipes equinovarus, 1314, *1315, 1316,* **1388–1389**

Plantar wart, 1441

Platybasia, 124

Poland's classification of fractures, 1541, *1541*

Poliomyelitis, 944–1036
  deformity and loss of function in, 949, *949*
  elbow in, 1013, *1016,* **1018–1027,** *1029, 1030, 1032–1035*
  electromyographic response in, 46
  exercise in, active, 949
    passive, 948
  fatigue in, 949
  foot and ankle in, 975, 978–979(t), *980, 981,* **982–985,** *986,* **988–991,** *992,* **994–995,** 996(t), **998–1002,** *1002–1004,* **1006–1009**
  forearm in, 1031
  hip in, 956, *957, 962, 960, 964, 966*
  idiopathic scoliosis and, 1194
  knee in, 967, *968, 969, 971–973, 975*
  moist heat in, 947
  motor activity patterns in, 948
  muscle examination in, 946
  muscle spasm in, 947
  orthoses and apparatus in, 951, *952*
  pathology of, 944
  phases of, 945
    acute, 946
    chronic, 950, *952*
    convalescent, 948, *949*
  physical therapy in, 950
  shoulder in, 1010, 1011(t), *1012–1016*
  tendon transfer in, principles of, 953
  treatment of, 945
    surgical, in, 953
  trunk in, 1010
  vs. myasthenia gravis, 1112

Pollock hamstring transfer, in hip abduction deformity, 818

Pollock-Eggers hamstring lengthening, 824

Polyarthritis, rheumatoid, 699
  systemic disease with, 701

Polydactylism, in Ellis-van Creveld syndrome, 256, *260, 261*
  of toes, 1422, *1423*

Polymyositis, 1104–1107
  differential diagnosis of, 881(t)
    Duchenne type muscular dystrophy, 1097(t)

Polyneuropathy, vs. myasthenia gravis, 1112

Polyradiculoneuritis, acute, 1070–1071

Ponseti Y coordinate, 139, *140*

Popliteal cyst, 735–747
  clinical features of, 742, *746*
  excision of, **748–749**
  pathology of, 735, *745*
  roentgenographic findings in, 744, *746*
  treatment of, 747